OSTERGARD'S Textbook of

Urogynecology

Female Pelvic Medicine and Reconstructive Surgery

Seventh Edition

Ali Azadi, MD, MSc, MBA, FACOG, FPMRS
Clinical Associate Professor
University of Arizona College of
  Medicine
Department of Obstetrics and
  Gynecology
Associate Professor
Creighton University School of
  Medicine
Department of Obstetrics and
  Gynecology
Phoenix Regional Campus
Phoenix, Arizona

Jeffrey L. Cornella, MD, FACS
Professor Emeritus
Department of Obstetrics and
  Gynecology
Mayo Clinic College of Medicine
Phoenix, Arizona

Peter L. Dwyer, OAM, FRACOG, FRCOG, CU
Professor
Department of Obstetrics and
  Gynecology
The University of Melbourne
Melbourne, Victoria, Australia
Head
Department of Urogynecology
Mercy Hospital for Women
Heidelberg, Victoria, Australia

Felicia L. Lane, MS, MD, FACOG, FPMRS
Professor and Vice Chair
Division and Program Director
Female Pelvic Medicine and
  Reconstructive Surgery
Department of Obstetrics and
  Gynecology
University of California, Irvine
Orange, California

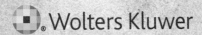 Wolters Kluwer

Philadelphia · Baltimore · New York · London
Buenos Aires · Hong Kong · Sydney · Tokyo

Acquisitions Editor: Chris Teja
Senior Development Editor: Stacey Sebring
Editorial Coordinator: Lesley Drewitt
Marketing Manager: Kirsten Watrud
Production Project Manager: Frances M. Gunning
Manager, Graphic Arts & Design: Stephen Druding
Manufacturing Coordinator: Beth Welsh
Prepress Vendor: Absolute Service Inc.

7th edition

9 8 7 6 5 4 3 2 1

Printed in Mexico

Library of Congress Cataloging-in-Publication Data
ISBN: 978-1-975162-33-7
Library of Congress Control Number: 2022906932

shop.lww.com

QUADM0922

My contributions to this textbook are dedicated to my loving wife, Charlene,
and our children, Derolyn, Derek, Brett, Kristen, and Kyle,
and their children, Cheyne, Chelsea, Christion, Cecilia, Kellen, Asher,
and our great granddaughter Remi.
-Donald R. Ostergard

To my wife, Tara for her love and support
and to my beautiful daughters, Lillian and Melody.
-Ali Azadi

To my loving wife, Kathryn
and our children, Johnathan, Krystiana, Julia, Joseph, and Kiara.
-Jeffrey L. Cornella

To my beautiful wife Pam
and my family who have given me a lifetime of love and support.
-Peter L. Dwyer

Gratitude to my family for their unconditional love and support;
to my peers and mentors for sharing their knowledge within these pages,
may their wisdom help those suffering from pelvic floor disorders.
-Felicia L. Lane

Contents

Contributing Authors

Jonia Alshiek, MD, MSc
Clinical Assistant Professor
Department of Obstetrics and Gynecology
Technion Israel Institute of Technology Ruth and
    Bruce Rappaport Faculty of Medicine
Hadera, Israel

Jennifer T. Anger, MD, MPH
Professor and Vice Chair of Research
Department of Urology
UC San Diego
Gender Affirming Surgery, Urologic Reconstruction,
    and Female Pelvic Medicine
Department of Urology
UC San Diego Health
La Jolla, California

Breffini Anglim, MB, BCh, BAO, MSc, MRCPI, MRCOG
Assistant Professor
Department of Urogynecology
University College Dublin
Consultant Obstetrician and Gynecologist
Department of Urogynecology
Coombe Women and Infants University Hospital
Dublin, Ireland

Steven D. Arrowsmith, MD
Medical Advisor for Fistula Direct Relief
Fistula Foundation
San Jose, California
Medical Advisor for Fistula
Direct Relief
Santa Barbara, California

Afiba Arthur, MD
Clinical Instructor
Department of Obstetrics and Gynecology
University of California, Irvine
University of California, Irvine Medical Center
Orange, California

Ali Azadi, MD, MSc, MBA, FACOG, FPMRS
Clinical Associate Professor
University of Arizona College of Medicine
Department of Obstetrics and Gynecology
Associate Professor
Creighton University School of Medicine
Department of Obstetrics and Gynecology
Phoenix Regional Campus
Phoenix, Arizona

Mary Van Meter Baker, MD, MBA
Clinical Fellow
Department of Obstetrics and Gynecology
Vanderbilt University Medical Center
Nashville, Tennessee

Kari Bø, PhD
Full Professor
Department of Sports Medicine
Norwegian School of Sport Sciences
Oslo, Norway
Project Leader
Department of Obstetrics and Gynecology
Akershus University Hospital
Lørenskog, Norway

Brittni A. J. Boyd, MD
Clinical Instructor
Department of Obstetrics and Gynecology
University of California, Irvine
Orange, California

Douglas Brown, PhD
Surgical Ethics Specialist
Department of Surgery
Washington University in St. Louis School of Medicine
St. Louis, Missouri

Taylor John Brueseke, MD
Assistant Professor of Clinical Health Sciences
Department of Obstetrics and Gynecology
University of California, Irvine
Orange, California

Linda Burkett, MD, MSc
Assistant Professor
Department of Obstetrics and Gynecology
Virginia Commonwealth University School of Medicine
Faculty
Department of Obstetrics and Gynecology
Virginia Commonwealth University Health
Richmond, Virginia

Kristina A. Butler, MD, MS
Gynecologic Surgeon, Urogynecologist, and
   Gynecologic Oncologist
Department of Obstetrics and Gynecology
Mayo Clinic Arizona
Phoenix, Arizona

Olivia O. Cardenas-Trowers, MD
Assistant Professor
Senior Associate Consultant
Department of Medical and Surgical Gynecology
Mayo Clinic
Jacksonville, Florida

Frida Carswell, BMed, FRANZCOG, CU
Urogynecologist
Department of Urogynecology
Mercy Hospital for Women
Melbourne, Victoria, Australia

Megan Cesta, MD
Clinical Assistant Professor of Obstetrics and Gynecology
Department of Obstetrics and Gynecology
Northeast Ohio Medical University
Rootstown, Ohio
Pelvic Health and Gynecology Surgery
Department of Obstetrics and Gynecology
Summa Health
Akron, Ohio

Anita H. Chen, MD
Assistant Professor
Department of Obstetrics and Gynecology
Mayo Clinic Alix College of Medicine
Consultant
Division of Female Pelvic Medicine and Reconstructive
   Pelvic Surgery
Program Director
Minimally Invasive Gynecologic Surgery Fellowship
Department of Medical and Surgical Gynecology
Mayo Clinic
Jacksonville, Florida

Zhuoran Chen, MBBS, PhD
Senior Lecturer
Department of Medicine
University of New South Wales
Urogynecologist
Women's and Children's Health
St. George Hospital
Sydney, New South Wales, Australia

Christopher John Chermansky, MD
Assistant Professor
Department of Urology
University of Pittsburgh School of Medicine
Chief
Department of Urology
UPMC Magee-Womens Hospital
Pittsburgh, Pennsylvania

Ralph Raymond Chesson, Jr., MD
Professor Emeritus of Obstetrics and Gynecology
Department of Obstetrics and Gynecology
Section of Female Pelvic Medicine and Reconstructive
   Surgery
Louisiana State University Health Sciences Center
New Orleans, Louisiana

Jeffrey L. Cornella, MD, FACS
Professor Emeritus
Department of Obstetrics and Gynecology
Mayo Clinic College of Medicine
Phoenix, Arizona

Marlene M. Corton, MD, MSCS
Professor
Department of Obstetrics and Gynecology
UT Southwestern Medical Center
Dallas, Texas

Carly Crowder, MD
Fellow Physician
Division of Female Pelvic Medicine and Reconstructive
   Surgery
Department of Obstetrics and Gynecology
University of California, Irvine
Irvine, California

Michael D. Crowell, PhD
Professor of Medicine
Department of Gastroenterology and Hepatology
Mayo Clinic
Phoenix, Arizona

Patrick Culligan, MD
Co-Director
Department of Urogynecology
Valley Hospital Medical Center
Ridgewood, New Jersey

Kristina Cvach, MBBS, FRANZCOG, MPHTM
Urogynecologist
Department of Urogynecology
Mercy Hospital for Women
Melbourne, Victoria, Australia

John O. L. DeLancey, MD
Norman F. Miller Professor of Gynecology
Department of Obstetrics and Gynecology
University of Michigan Medical School
Attending Physician
Department of Obstetrics and Gynecology
University of Michigan, Michigan Medicine
Ann Arbor, Michigan

Hans Peter Dietz, MD, PhD, FRANZCOG, DDU, CU
Obstetrician, Gynecologist, and Urogynecologist
Partner, Sydney Urodynamic Centres
Springwood, New South Wales, Australia

Alexandra Dubinskaya, MD
Female Pelvic Medicine and Reconstructive Surgery
  Fellow
Department of Urology
Cedars-Sinai Medical Center
Los Angeles, California

Peter L. Dwyer, OAM, FRACOG, FRCOG, CU
Professor
Department of Obstetrics and Gynecology
The University of Melbourne
Melbourne, Victoria, Australia
Head
Department of Urogynecology
Mercy Hospital for Women
Heidelberg, Victoria, Australia

Nicola Dykes, MBChB, FRANZCOG, CU
Urogynecologist
Department of Women's Health
North Shore Hospital, Waitematā District Health Board
Auckland, New Zealand

Sarah E. Eckhardt, MD
Fellow Physician
Female Pelvic Medicine and Reconstructive Surgery
Department of Obstetrics and Gynecology
Harbor-UCLA Medical Center
Torrance, California

Brendan Thomas Frainey, MD
Urology Resident
Glickman Urological and Kidney Institute
Cleveland Clinic
Cleveland, Ohio

Sean L. Francis, MD, MBA
Chairman
Department of Female Pelvic Medicine and
  Reconstructive Surgery
University of Louisville School of Medicine
Urogynecologist
University of Louisville Health
Louisville, Kentucky

Emily Helena Frisch, MD
Resident Physician
Women's Health Institute
Cleveland Clinic
Cleveland, Ohio

Bobby Garcia, MD
Assistant Program Director, OB-GYN Residency
Female Pelvic Medicine and Reconstructive Surgeon
Department of Obstetrics and Gynecology
NYC Health and Hospitals—Lincoln
Bronx, New York

John B. Gebhart, MD, MS
Professor of Obstetrics and Gynecology, Urology, and
  Surgery
Chair, Division of Urogynecology
Department of Obstetrics and Gynecology
Mayo Clinic
Rochester, Minnesota

Howard B. Goldman, MD, FACS
Professor and Vice Chairman
Center for Female Pelvic Medicine and Reconstructive
  Surgery
Glickman Urologic and Kidney Institute
Lerner College of Medicine, Cleveland Clinic
Department of Urology
Cleveland Clinic
Cleveland, Ohio

Meghan L. Good, MD
Fellow
Department of Colon and Rectal Surgery
Mayo Clinic Hospital
Phoenix, Arizona

Cara Grimes, MD, MAS
Associate Professor of Obstetrics and Gynecology
  and Urology
Associate Chair of Research in Obstetrics and Gynecology
Departments of Obstetrics and Gynecology and Urology
New York Medical College
Chief of Urogynecology and Female Pelvic Medicine
  and Reconstructive Surgery
Department of Obstetrics and Gynecology
Westchester Medical Center
Valhalla, New York

Ankita Gupta, MD, MPH
Associate Fellowship Director
Female Pelvic Medicine and Reconstructive Surgery
University of Louisville School of Medicine
Urogynecologist
Department of Obstetrics and Gynecology
University of Louisville Health
Louisville, Kentucky

Robert E. Gutman, MD
Professor
Departments of Obstetrics and Gynecology and Urology
Georgetown University
Program Director, Female Pelvic Medicine and
  Reconstructive Surgery Fellowship
Department of Obstetrics and Gynecology
MedStar Washington Hospital Center
Washington, District of Columbia

Victoria L. Handa, MD, MHS
Professor
Department of Gynecology and Obstetrics
Johns Hopkins University School of Medicine
Chair
Department of Gynecology and Obstetrics
Johns Hopkins Bayview Medical Center
Baltimore, Maryland

Bernard T. Haylen, MB, BS, MD, FRCOG, FRANZCOG, CU
Professor
Department of Gynecology
University of New South Wales
Sydney, New South Wales, Australia
Professor
Department of Gynecology
St. Vincent's Clinic
Darlinghurst, New South Wales, Australia

Bhumy Dave Heliker, MD
Assistant Professor
Department of Obstetrics and Gynecology
University of California, Irvine
Orange, California

J. Eric Jelovsek, MD, MMEd, MSDS
Professor
Director, Data Science for Women's Health
Department of Obstetrics and Gynecology
Duke University
Durham, North Carolina

Sarah E.S. Jeney, MD
Assistant Professor
Department of Obstetrics and Gynecology
University of New Mexico
University of New Mexico Hospital
Albuquerque, New Mexico

Debjyoti Karmakar, MBBS, MD, MRCOG, FRANZCOG
Consultant Gynecologist
Department of Obstetrics and Gynecology
Joan Kirner Hospital, Western Health
University Hospital Geelong, Barwon Health
Melbourne, Victoria, Australia

James Oliver Keck, MBBS, FRACS
Lecturer
Department of Surgery
University of Melbourne
Director
Department of Colorectal Surgery
St. Vincent's Hospital
Melbourne, Australia

Aqsa Azam Khan, MD
Assistant Professor
Urologist
Department of Urology
Mayo Clinic
Phoenix, Arizona

Gaurav Khatri, MD
Associate Professor
Chief, Division of Body Magnetic Resonance Imaging
Interim Chief, Division of Abdominal Imaging
Department of Radiology
University of Texas Southwestern Medical Center
Dallas, Texas

Rosanne M. Kho, MD
Professor
Department of Obstetrics, Gynecology and
  Reproductive Biology
Cleveland Clinic Lerner College of Medicine and Case
  Western Reserve University
Head, Section of Medical Gynecology & MIGS
Ob/Gyn &Women's Health Institute, Cleveland Clinic
Cleveland, Ohio

Cassandra K. Kisby, MD, MS
Assistant Professor
Department of Obstetrics and Gynecology
Division of Urogynecology
Duke University
Duke University Medical Center
Durham, North Carolina

Niels Klarskov, MD, DMSc
Professor
Department of Clinical Medicine
University of Copenhagen
Copenhagen, Denmark
Consultant
Department of Obstetrics and Gynecology
Herlev and Gentofte University Hospital
Herlev, Denmark

Yuko M. Komesu, MD
Howard Friedman Endowed Professor
Department of Obstetrics and Gynecology
Division of Female Pelvic Medicine and Reconstructive
  Surgery
University of New Mexico
Albuquerque, New Mexico
Professor
Department of Obstetrics and Gynecology
University of New Mexico
University of New Mexico Health Sciences Center
Albuquerque, New Mexico

Felicia L. Lane, MS, MD, FACOG, FPMRS
Professor and Vice Chair
Division and Program Director
Female Pelvic Medicine and Reconstructive Surgery
Department of Obstetrics and Gynecology
University of California, Irvine
Orange, California

Nathan Lawrentschuk, MBBS, PhD, FRACS Urol
Professor
Department of Surgery
The University of Melbourne
Director
Department of Urology
The Royal Melbourne Hospital
Melbourne, Victoria, Australia

Joseph Kim-sang Lee, BhB, MbChB, FRANZCOG, CU
Associate Professor
University of New South Wales
Sydney, New South Wales, Australia
Urogynecologist
St. Vincent's Clinic
Darlinghurst, New South Wales, Australia

Brian J. Linder, MD, MS
Associate Professor of Urology and Obstetrics and
  Gynecology
Consultant
Department of Urology
Mayo Clinic
Rochester, Minnesota

Lioudmila Lipetskaia, MD, Msc
Assistant Professor
Department of Obstetrics and Gynecology
Cooper Medical School of Rowan University
Fellowship Director for Female Pelvic Medicine and
  Reconstructive Surgery
Department of Obstetrics and Gynecology
Cooper Health University
Camden, New Jersey

Gunnar Lose, MD, DMSc
Overlæge, dr. med.
Professor emeritus Københavns Universitet
Afdeling for Kvindesygdomme, Graviditet og Fødsler
Herlev Universitetshospital

Tisha N. Lunsford, MD
Associate Professor of Gastroenterology
Director of Motility
Division of Gastroenterology and Hepatology
Mayo Clinic
Scottsdale, Arizona

Javier F. Magrina, MD
Professor Emeritus
Department of Obstetrics and Gynecology
Mayo Clinic
Phoenix, Arizona

Christopher Maher, FRANZCOG, CU, PhD
Professor
Department of Urogynecology
University of Queensland
Royal Brisbane and Women's Hospital
Wesley Hospital
Brisbane, Australia

Bahar Mansoori, MD
Assistant Professor of Abdominal Imaging
Department of Radiology
University of Washington
Seattle, Washington

Donna Mazloomdoost, MD
Medical Officer and Project Scientist for the Pelvic
    Floor Disorders Network
Gynecologic Health and Disease Branch
Eunice Kennedy Shriver National Institute of Child
    Health and Human Development/National Institutes
    of Health
Bethesda, Maryland
Associate Professor
University of Virginia School of Medicine
MidAtlantic Urogynecology and Pelvic Surgery/INOVA
    Fairfax Hospital
Annandale, Virginia

Aoife McVey, MBBS
Urology Research Fellow
Division of Cancer Surgery
Urology Registrar
Department of Urology
Peter MacCallum Cancer Centre
Melbourne, Victoria, Australia

Daniel Jacob Meller, MD, MS
Resident Physician
Department of Obstetrics and Gynecology and
    Women's Health
Montefiore Medical Center
Albert Einstein College of Medicine
Bronx, New York

Kate V. Meriwether, MD
Assistant Professor
Department of Obstetrics and Gynecology
University of New Mexico
Albuquerque, New Mexico

Isuzu Meyer, MD, MSPH
Associate Professor
Department of Obstetrics and Gynecology
University of Alabama at Birmingham
Birmingham, Alabama

John R. Miklos, MD, FPMRS
Director
Urogynecology/Reconstructive and Vaginal Surgery
Miklos and Moore Urogynecology
Atlanta, Georgia/Beverly Hills, California/Dubai,
    United Arab Emirates

Nitin Mishra, MBBS, MS, MPH
Associate Professor
Department of Surgery
Mayo Clinic Alix School of Medicine
Program Director
Department of Surgery
Mayo Clinic Hospital
Phoenix, Arizona

Robert D. Moore, DO, FPMRS, FACS
Co-director
Urogynecology/Reconstructive and Vaginal Surgery
Miklos and Moore Urogynecology
Atlanta, Georgia/Beverly Hills, California/Dubai,
    United Arab Emirates

Daniel M. Morgan, MD
Professor
Department of Obstetrics and Gynecology
University of Michigan
Ann Arbor, Michigan

Ceana Nezhat, MD
Fellowship Director, Nezhat Medical Center
Medical Director of Training & Education and
    Director of Minimally Invasive Surgery and Robotics
Northside Hospital
Atlanta, Georgia

Victor W. Nitti, MD
Professor
Departments of Urology and Obstetrics and Gynecology
David Geffen School of Medicine at UCLA
Chief, Division of Female Pelvic Medicine and
    Reconstructive Surgery
Departments of Urology and Obstetrics and Gynecology
UCLA Medical Center
Los Angeles, California

Karen L. Noblett, MD, MBA
Professor
Division of Female Pelvic Medicine and Reconstructive
    Surgery
Department of Obstetrics and Gynecology
University of California, Irvine
Orange, California

John A. Occhino, MD, MS
Associate Professor
Director, Female Pelvic Medicine and Reconstructive
    Surgery Fellowship
Division of Urogynecology
Department of Obstetrics and Gynecology
Mayo Clinic
Rochester, Minnesota

Ellen O'Connor, MBBS
Urology Research Fellow
Division of Cancer Surgery
Peter MacCallum Cancer Centre
Melbourne, Victoria, Australia
Urology Registrar
Department of Urology
Barwon Health
Geelong, Victoria, Australia

Barry A. O'Reilly, MB, BCh, BAO, MD, FRCOG, FRANZCOG, FRCPI
Clinical Professor
Department of Obstetrics and Gynecology
University College Cork
Head of Urogynecology
Department of Obstetrics and Gynecology
Cork University Maternity Hospital
Cork, Ireland

Suzanne L. Palmer, MD, FACP, FACR
Professor of Clinical Radiological Sciences
University of California, Irvine
Chief of Imaging HCG
Veterans Administration Medical Center
Long Beach, California

Resad Pasic, MD, PhD
Professor
Director, Minimally Invasive Gynecologic Surgery
    Fellowship
Department of Obstetrics and Gynecology and
    Women's Health
University of Louisville
University of Louisville Hospital
Louisville, Kentucky

Danielle Patterson, MD, SM
Assistant Professor
Department of Gynecology and Obstetrics
Johns Hopkins University School of Medicine
Director, Female Pelvic Medicine and Reconstructive
    Surgery Fellowship
Department of Gynecology and Obstetrics
Johns Hopkins Bayview Medical Center
Baltimore, Maryland

Kenneth M. Peters, MD
Professor and Chair
Department of Urology
Oakland University William Beaumont School of
    Medicine
Rochester, Michigan
Chief
Department of Urology
Beaumont Health
Royal Oak, Michigan

Joseph B. Pincus, MD
Urogynecology Fellow
Department of Urogynecology
NorthShore University HealthSystem
Skokie, Illinois

Marc Possover, Prof, Prof (DA), Prof he (Ch), Dr, Med
Director, Head of Department
Departments of Obstetrics and Gynecology and
    Neuropelveology
Possover International Medical Center
Zürich, Switzerland

Rubin Raju, MBBS
Assistant Professor
Department of Obstetrics and Gynecology
Mayo Clinic Alix School of Medicine
Female Pelvic Medicine and Reconstructive Surgery
    Fellow
Department of Obstetrics and Gynecology
Mayo Clinic
Rochester, Minnesota

Alanna Rebecca, MD, MBA
Plastic Surgeon
Department of Surgery
Mayo Clinic
Phoenix, Arizona

Anna Rosamilia, MB, BS, FRANZCOG, CU, PhD
Adjunct Associate Professor
Department of Obstetrics and Gynecology
Monash University
Head, Pelvic Floor Unit
Women's and Children's Program
Monash Medical Centre
Clayton Road Clayton, Victoria, Australia

Anne G. Sammarco, MD, MPH
Assistant Professor
Female Pelvic Medicine and Reconstructive Surgery
Department of Obstetrics and Gynecology
University Hospitals Cleveland Medical Center
Case Western Reserve University
Cleveland, Ohio

Peter K. Sand, MD
Clinical Professor
Department of Urogynecology
NorthShore University HealthSystem
Skokie, Illinois

Polina Sawyer, MD
Fellow
Department of Obstetrics and Gynecology
UT Southwestern Medical Center
Dallas, Texas

Payton Schmidt, MD
Assistant Professor
Department of Obstetrics and Gynecology
University of Michigan
University of Michigan, Michigan Medicine
Ann Arbor, Michigan

Shefali Sharma, MD
Clinical Assistant Professor
Gynecologic Surgical Subspecialties
Spectrum Health Medical Group
Grand Rapids, Michigan

S. Abbās Shobeiri, MD, MBA, FACS, FACOG, CMPE
INOVA Health System Division Chief of Benign
    Gynecology
INOVA Health System Director of Pelvic Floor Program
Professor of Medical Education, The University of
    Virginia, Affiliate Faculty, Bioengineering, George
    Mason University, INOVA Fairfax Hospital
Department of Obstetrics & Gynecology
Falls Church, Virginia

Bob L. Shull, MD
Retired
Department of Obstetrics and Gynecology
Baylor Scott and White Health
Temple, Texas

Larry T. Sirls, MD, FACS
Professor
Oakland University William Beaumont School of
    Medicine
Program Director, Female Pelvic Medicine and
    Reconstructive Surgery
Department of Urology
Beaumont Hospital
Royal Oak, Michigan

Meagan Slate, MD
Attending
Department of Obstetrics and Gynecology
Sibley Memorial Hospital
Washington, District of Columbia

S. L. Stanton, FRCS, FRCOG, FRANZCOG (Hon)
Former Professor of Gynecology
St. George's Hospital Medical School
London, United Kingdom

Assia Stepanian, MD
Medical Director
Academia of Women's Health and Endoscopic Surgery
Gynecology Surgeon
Department of Obstetrics and Gynecology
Northside Hospital
Atlanta, Georgia

Surabhi Tewari, BS
Medical Student
Cleveland Clinic Lerner College of Medicine
Case Western Reserve University School of Medicine
Cleveland, Ohio

Nia Thompson Jenkins, MD, MPH
Assistant Professor
Department of Obstetrics and Gynecology
Female Pelvic Medicine and Reconstructive Surgery
University Health, Truman Medical Center
Kansas City, Missouri

Emanuel C. Trabuco, MD
Associate Professor
Department of Obstetrics and Gynecology
Mayo Clinic Alix School of Medicine
Consultant
Department of Obstetrics and Gynecology
Mayo Clinic
Rochester, Minnesota

Annah Vollstedt, MD
Assistant Clinical Professor
Department of Urology
University of Iowa
Iowa City, Iowa

L. Lewis Wall, MD, DPhil
Selina Okin Kim Conner Professor Emeritus for
    Medical Anthropology in Arts and Sciences
Emeritus Professor of Anthropology, College of Arts
    and Sciences
Emeritus Professor of Obstetrics and Gynecology,
    School of Medicine
Washington University in St. Louis
St. Louis, Missouri

Emily L. Whitcomb, MD, MAS
Assistant Clinical Professor
Department of Obstetrics and Gynecology
University of California, Irvine
Orange, California
Partner Physician
Department of Obstetrics and Gynecology
Southern California Permanente Medical Group
Irvine, California

Christopher E. Wolter, MD
Assistant Professor
Department of Urology
Mayo Clinic Arizona
Consultant and Assistant Professor
Department of Urology
Mayo Clinic Hospital
Phoenix, Arizona

Katherine L. Woodburn, MD
Clinical Instructor
Department of Obstetrics and Gynecology
Georgetown University
Fellow
Department of Obstetrics and Gynecology
MedStar Washington Hospital Center
Washington, District of Columbia

Tajnoos Yazdany, MD, FACOG
Associate Professor
Department of Obstetrics and Gynecology
UCLA David Geffen School of Medicine
Los Angeles, California
Program Director and Division Chief
Female Pelvic Medicine and Reconstructive Surgery
Harbor-UCLA Medical Center
Torrance, California

Johnny Yi, MD
Assistant Professor
Department of Obstetrics and Gynecology
Department of Medical and Surgical Gynecology
Mayo Clinic Arizona
Phoenix, Arizona

Ariel Zilberlicht, MD
Department of Obstetrics and Gynecology
Technion Institute of Technology
Consultant
Department of Obstetrics and Gynecology
Carmel Medical Center
Haifa, Israel

Foreword

The first edition of this textbook was published in 1980 with 10 authors and 30 chapters. The goal of that first edition was "the education of the physician in the establishment of specific therapies based upon an appropriate diagnosis." The fifth edition was published in 2003 with Dr. Alfred E. Bent as the lead editor with Drs. Geoffrey W. Cundiff and Steven E. Swift as the associate editors. It was translated into Korean, Spanish, and Chinese. Dr. Bent stated in the preface, "A brief look at the contents should point the reader to a specific section that will assist in the management of patients with a wide number of problems including the pelvic floor, urinary incontinence, colorectal dysfunction, and pelvic organ prolapse." The scope of the textbook was widened considerably with the notable interaction with another medical specialty. New up-to-date chapters on ethics, neuropelveology, functional aspects and biomechanics of pelvic floor and viscera, innovation and evolution of medical devices, cosmetic gynecology, laparoscopic and robotic surgery, principles of electrosurgery, and sacral neuromodulation are included in this seventh edition.

The physician education and research aspects were further increased by the establishment of the International Urogynecologic Association (IUGA) in 1976 at the International Federation of Gynecology & Obstetrics (FIGO) meeting in Mexico City. Professor Axel Ingelman-Sundberg of Sweden, who was a long-standing editor of *Acta Obstetricia et Gynecologica Scandinavica*, felt the need for a society devoted to the study of urinary incontinence in the female along with related lower urinary tract issues. Dr. Ingelman-Sundberg convened a group of about 50 like-minded physicians at that meeting where this society was established. He was elected president, and Ulf Ulmsten became secretary-treasurer. IUGA currently has 38 affiliate societies worldwide and has sponsored international symposia for all levels of training in urogynecology with registrants representing 55 countries. The last joint in person meeting with AUGS had 2,250 registrants.

These physician education and research efforts were also facilitated by the establishment of the American Urogynecology Society (AUGS, initially called the Gynecologic Urology Society). The organizing event was in an Orange County, California, living room in 1979 with four prominent urogynecologists in attendance. Jack Robertson became its first president.

The inaugural meeting occurred in 1980 with about 60 physicians attending compared to the recent meetings with more than 1,000 attendees. AUGS continues the educational process by sponsoring many in-depth clinical webinars including special meetings for fellows.

Physician education as well as dissemination of current research in urogynecology was greatly enhanced by the establishment of the *International Urogynecology Journal* by Professor Oscar Contreras Ortiz of Buenos Aires University, Buenos Aires, Argentina, in 1990. He became the editor-in-chief, and I became the managing editor. Volume 33 is current in 2022.

Physician training in urogynecology reached a new level in 1979 at Harbor UCLA Medical Center in Torrance, California, with the establishment of the first fellowship program in urogynecology. That fellowship program continues to date under the direction of Dr. Taji Yazdani, and many other such fellowships have been established, many by the graduates of this program. In 2016, Astellas Pharma researched the graduates of this program and their subsequent graduates which at that time numbered about 202 physician specialists. The American Board of Obstetrics and Gynecology has recognized this field as a subspeciality known as female pelvic medicine and reconstructive surgery with its own scientific journal affiliated with AUGS. AUGS has sponsored many local conferences as well as virtual educational events.

The importance of the educational process for physicians and other health care providers in urogynecology certainly results in better patient care. We have seen the establishment of urogynecology specialist societies worldwide each with their own outreach efforts to educate health care providers in this new field of medicine. The International Continence Society and the Society of Gynecologic Surgeons also contribute to this educational effort.

The pioneers in urogynecology set the stage for ongoing enhanced patient care for women with urogynecologic disorders by establishing the means to provide specific diagnoses with subsequent application of specific therapies for these diagnoses. The goal of this 61-chapter textbook with contributions by more than 100 national and international leaders in the field of urogynecology is to collate and organize the current scope of knowledge in urogynecology, to continue to educate physicians in this field, and, most importantly, to further enhance patient care.

Donald R. Ostergard, MD, FACOG

Preface to the First Edition

The first edition of this book was in 1980 when I wrote the following preface for its publication by the Williams & Wilkins Co. This older preface is included to provide a comparison with the current preface to emphasize how far we have come in the understanding of the urogynecologic aspects of the lower urinary tract.

The multiplicity of different procedures, operations, concepts and evaluations relating to female urinary incontinence bespeaks the complexity of this problem. In spite of the "80%" surgical cure rate reported by various writers, all too often the gynecologist must care for the patient who is still incontinent after more than one operative procedure. There is genuine uneasiness by all who are confronted by the patient's question: Will *this* operation cure my incontinence?

The custom of performing a vaginal reparative operation on the basis of history alone continues to be the norm. When the vaginal operation fails, a retropubic procedure follows. The physician refers those patients who are still incontinent after the second operation with an air of resignation that little hope is in prospect.

From time-to-time questions arise about the scope of responsibility of the obstetrician-gynecologist regarding urinary tract symptoms in the female and the nature of the preoperative evaluation. All too often failures of operative treatment are due to the lack of proper assessment of the lower urinary tract before surgery.

The goal of this text is to promote a more active role of the obstetrician-gynecologist in the evaluation of the lower urinary tract regardless of how obvious the patient's symptoms of stress incontinence may seem. Office procedures are now available to adequately screen the lower urinary tract. More sophisticated techniques are now available to accurately diagnose alterations of vesicourethral physiology. The physician rapidly learns the skills necessary to perform or interpret the results of these evaluations.

The medical literature of the past few years contains information concerning the neurophysiology, maturation of micturition, new techniques for evaluation of the lower urinary tract and the fascinating new field of urodynamics. Unfortunately, most of this material is in publications which the practicing obstetrician-gynecologist does not regularly review. This text collates the relevant medical literature in a readily comprehensive format. The contributors to this text are experts in such areas of medicine as neurology, urology, gynecology and psychiatry. The foundation of their collective clinical experience with a sound basis in the medical literature leads to the formulation of a logical, orderly, practical evaluation of the patient's lower urinary tract. The thoroughness of this evaluation ensures the likeliness of clinical success. The clinical evaluation and triage plans provide a clinical diagnosis and treatment programs which are unique for each individual patient.

This text brings together the known facets of lower urinary tract physiology and pathophysiology which are needed for an in-depth understanding of the basis of urinary complaints of the individual patient. The "anatomy of failure" in the past has largely been a failure to apply the correct treatment to the specific urinary malfunction and to a preoccupation with incontinence as the only symptom of the female urinary tract. The availability of modern urodynamic evaluation equipment now allows us to alter this myopic view of the lower urinary tract. A comprehensive urodynamic evaluation of the patient in a step-by-step fashion allows the establishment of a specific diagnosis. The physician then treats specific problems either medically or surgically. Surgical procedures are applied only when indicated for that patient with true anatomic stress incontinence. The education of the physician in the establishment of specific therapies based on appropriate diagnosis is the goal of this text.

The material in this text is based upon presentations by the authors to *Postgraduate Courses in Gynecologic Urology Theory and Practice*, in Los Angeles, California, June 22–23, 1978; Anaheim, California, March 14–16, 1979; and North Hollywood, California, December 5–9, 1979.

Donald R. Ostergard, MD, FACOG

Preface to the Seventh Edition

We are honored to introduce the seventh edition of *Ostergard's Textbook of Urogynecology*. Since the first edition's release in 1980, the specialty of urogynecology and pelvic reconstructive surgery has experienced advancements that have been reflected in each edition of the book. We acknowledge the outstanding work of prior authors and editors.

In this edition of the book, many new chapters have been introduced to reflect the countless updates of science and literature added to the field of urogynecology. The new format, illustrations, and surgical videos provide a comprehensive education for an audience interested in the field of pelvic medicine and reconstructive surgery. We are grateful for the contributions of our authors who deliver cutting-edge, state-of-the-art content in each chapter. Our outstanding international authors are the strength of this book.

Ultimately, we are most thankful to our patients. Despite the complexity of practicing medicine in a modern world influenced by technology, industry, and increasingly complicated health systems, our patients are always the valued focus of our profession. We strive not only to provide them with the highest quality of care but also to ensure that their rights as human beings are preserved. The ethical considerations of practicing medicine are essential aspects of health care, as the rights of every individual person needs to be reconciled with the demands of scientific enterprise.

Ali Azadi, MD, MSC, MBA
Jeffrey L. Cornella, MD
Peter L. Dwyer, OAM, FRANZCOG, FRCOG, CU
Felicia L. Lane, MD

SECTION 1

Female Pelvis and Epidemiology of Pelvic Floor Disorders

CHAPTER 1

Brief History of Female Pelvic Reconstructive Surgery

Peter L. Dwyer • Bob L. Shull • S. L. Stanton

Introduction

Over the 20th century, advances in medicine have improved the quality and length of people's lives everywhere. This ballooning of medical knowledge has occurred through diligent research into the causation of disease with a better understanding of pathophysiology and careful and better assessment, leading to accurate diagnosis and appropriate treatment. There has been increasing specialization in medicine with the development of divisions initially into medicine and surgery, then specialist, Colleges of Obstetrics and Gynaecology and subspeciality interest groups such as urogynecology. It is appropriate that the first chapter in this book is devoted to the development of urogynecology as a subspecialty—what were the important contributions that led to advancing our knowledge in the assessment and treatment of disorders of the pelvic floor and lower urinary tract in the female. Our increasing knowledge was not solely by gynecologists but also from scientists, other specialist areas such as urologists and colorectal surgeons, physiotherapists, and nursing colleagues for there should be no barriers to knowledge, just as there are no borders within the pelvis to effective treatment of pelvic floor disorders.

We discuss the people and the events that moved the specialty of urogynecology forward, although this road has not always been smooth and without controversy. The advancement of medical knowledge occurred through the diligence of inquisitive people asking simple questions such as why is that so, or how can I do this better? Chance also played a part, as when Florey found the penicillin mold growing on the petri dish on the windowsill or Sims using the knee-chest position to distend the vagina with air and examine the vesicovaginal fistula with his speculum or Kelly dropping and breaking the glass partition of his primitive cystoscope seeing the inside of the air-filled bladder for the first time. The accumulation of knowledge is slow and is based on improvements in many areas, including technology such as Edison electric light in endoscopy, so his quote "if I see further it is because I sit on the shoulders of giants" is so true.

The evolution of our understanding of urogynecologic conditions and their treatment with improved outcomes has occurred slowly and, at times, erratically. Rather than look at a timeline of milestones and people, we explore the key areas in urogynecology and discuss what events and people in our opinion made a real difference.

The areas to be explored are the following:

- Urinary stress incontinence
- Endoscopy with cystourethroscopy and laparoscopy and their contribution to the assessment and management of pelvic floor disorders
- Painful bladder conditions
- Lower urinary tract and anorectal fistulas
- Uterovaginal prolapse

STRESS URINARY INCONTINENCE

Anterior Colporrhaphy with Bladder Neck Buttress

The anterior colporrhaphy was being performed in the 1870s. Leon Le Fort, a French surgeon, describes his procedure for partial colpocleisis for prolapse in 1877, and Archibald Donald (1908) and Fothergill (1915), both English surgeons, describe the Manchester repair with vaginal repair, cervical amputation, and reattachment of the uterosacral ligaments. Kelly[1] published his classic description in 1913, describing "the torn or relaxed tissues of the vesical neck should be sutured together using two or three vertical mattress sutures of fine silk linen passed from side to side" (Fig. 1.1). Victor Bonney in 1923 stated that "incontinence depends in some way upon a sudden and abnormal displacement of the urethra and urethrovesical junction immediately behind the symphysis." Aldridge et al.[2] in 1952 thought that lack of support of the bladder base and neck and proximal urethra, and prolapse of the urethrovesical junction outside the environment of the intra-abdominal pressure, was associated with incontinence. The vaginal repair was a simple, low-risk vaginal

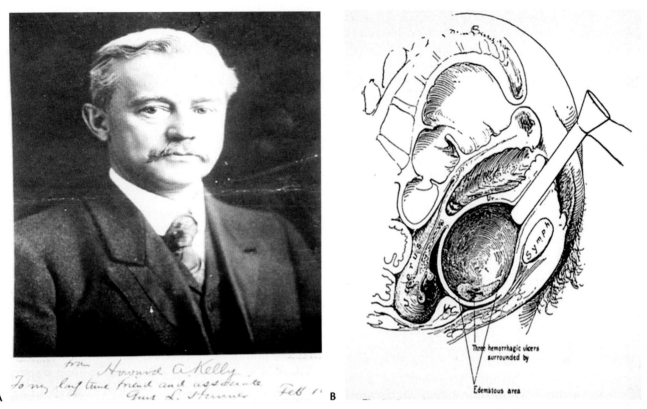

FIGURE 1.1 Howard Kelly circa 1910 (**A**) and his air cystoscope with a woman with interstitial cystitis in the knee-chest position to insufflate the bladder (**B**). (Reprinted from Hunner GL. A rare type of bladder ulcer in women; report of cases. *Boston Med Surg J* 1915;172:660–664.)

operation which became the primary surgery used by gynecologists to treat urinary stress incontinence for a century until thinking started to change in the 1970s with the introduction of the Burch colposuspension.

The first reported elective hysterectomy was performed by Conrad Langenbeck in 1813 and was through a vaginal approach. Interestingly, after 200 years, despite the vaginal approach having the lowest morbidity and cost, it remains less popular today than the alternatives of abdominal, laparoscopic, and robotic hysterectomy. Trends in medicine are not always driven solely by science.

Urethral Suspensions

The first retropubic operation for the treatment of stress urinary incontinence (SUI), the Marshall-Marchetti-Krantz procedure, was said to be described in a 1949 paper entitled "The Correction of Stress Incontinence by Simple Vesicourethral Suspension."[3] Marshall, a urologist, believed that elevation of the junction to its normal position restores continence. He developed an operation for treating voiding dysfunction that developed after rectal resection in men as a result of pronounced urethral hypermobility. He, with two gynecologists, Marchetti and Krantz, employed a

suprapubic approach to suspend the bladder neck by placement of interrupted chromic catgut sutures to the periosteum of the symphysis and posterior rectus sheath for the treatment of SUI in women. However, 30 years earlier in 1920, Thomas Hepburn, a urologist from Hartford, Connecticut, described a retropubic urethral suspension for females with urethral prolapse. Initially performed in children, he reported a further two cases in adult women. "When the neck of the bladder has been freed enough, so that traction on the bladder reduces the prolapse, it is sutured with 20 day catgut" to the periosteum.[4] There is no record of him using this operation to treat women with stress incontinence. Hepburn had a large family of six children, including a son who became a urologist and a daughter, Katharine, who became a Hollywood actress.

John Christopher Burch, a professor at Vanderbilt, described his retropubic colposuspension technique in 1961[5] after noting that when performing a Marshall-Marchetti-Krantz procedure, the sutures in the periosteum of the pubic symphysis often pulled out, and there was the added risk of osteitis pubis.

Robert Zacharin described in 1963[6] the anatomical supports of the urethra and their importance in the continence mechanism and prevention of urinary stress incontinence. Based on his findings, he developed his own urethral suspension operation for SUI. Eventually, it was these ideas that lead to the placement of the midurethral slings (MUS) at the midurethral rather than the bladder neck. The midurethral placement of slings without tension decreased the incidence of postoperative voiding difficulty without adversely affecting the continence success rate.

In 1959, Pereyra,[7] an American gynecologist, performed the first needle endoscopic bladder neck suspensions, and subsequently, modifications were made by Raz, Stamey, and Gittes. Although initially popular, particularly with urologists in the 1970s and 1980s as it was a simple procedure with low morbidity, the continence outcomes were not as good as the retropubic procedures. Peattie and Stanton[8] reported a cure rate in women over 65 years as only 41% at 3 months.

Sling procedures

Allographic slings

The first suburethral sling procedure was described in 1907 by von Giordano who suggested the use of the gracilis muscle by wrapping it around the urethra. In 1910, Goebel[9] described detaching the pyramidalis muscle and suturing it beneath the urethra, and Frangenheim[10] modified the technique in 1914 by attaching a vertical strip of rectus fascia to the pyramidalis muscle. Price[11] described the first sling constructed from fascia lata in 1933, and Aldridge[12] in 1942 described a rectus fascia sling with two strips of rectus fascia sutured in the midline below the urethra via a separate vaginal incision. Other autographic material, including fascia lata and round ligament (Hodgkinson), have been used. The Aldridge sling has two bilateral fascial strips, which are left attached medially to the rectus sheath, passed behind the symphysis pubis, and sutured together beneath the bladder neck. These slings were used mainly for recurrent severe SUI by gynecologists. A simple modification named the pubovaginal sling, using a strip of detached rectus fascia fashioned as a free graft through a Pfannenstiel incision and passed under the urethra with a vaginal incision, was popularized by urologists McGuire and Blaivas in the 1970s and 1980s to treat women with severe or recurrent incontinence and/or intrinsic sphincter deficiency.[13] Although very successful, fascial slings were associated with an increased rate of voiding dysfunction and morbidity when compared to urethral suspension operations. In the 1990s, the incidence of voiding dysfunction decreased with the MUS placement under minimal tension.

Synthetic slings

The use of synthetic slings was introduced in the 1960s with the Moir's gauze hammock operation[14] and the Morgan sling[15] using Mersilene and polypropylene mesh, which they placed under the bladder neck through an abdominal and vaginal incision. Stanton et al.[16] used a silastic sling in the 1980s again, which was introduced through abdominal and vaginal incisions. Although all had good results in small trials, they were not widely used. In the 1970s and 1980s, the Burch colposuspension was popularized by Hilton and Stanton[17] and performed globally in over 80% of SUI operations with fascial slings less than 10%.[18]

Midurethral sling procedures

In the 1990s, urinary stress incontinence surgery was revolutionized by the advent of minimally invasive MUS procedures. The tension-free vaginal tape (TVT) was developed by Petros and Ulmsten.[19] Petros first met Ulf Ulmsten at a conference in Melbourne in 1989 organized by one of the chapter's authors. Based on Zacharin's anatomical studies, Petros was experimenting in animals attempting to recreate pubourethral ligaments initially by the temporary placement of Mersilene tapes placed at the insertion of pubourethral ligaments at the midurethra. This led to a collaboration with Ulmsten and the development of the TVT, a loosely woven suburethral polypropylene sling attached to trocars passed through vaginal and abdominal stab incisions and performed under local anesthesia as same day surgery.[20] This proved to be as safe and effective procedure as the Burch colposuspension but required less dissection and had less postoperative complications, pain, and hospital stay. There was a rapid uptake of MUS from 1998 and a corresponding decline in colposuspensions.[18] MUS are currently the most commonly performed operations for SUI.

In view of the success of the MUS, it is not surprising there have been further modifications.

The transobturator sling was developed in 2001 by Delorme[21] using the obturator foramina approach to place the midurethral tape, and DeLeval[22] described an inside-out approach in 2003. These two transobturator approaches could reduce potential injury to the bladder, bowel, and other major vessels compared to the retropubic approach but have a higher incidence of postoperative pain. The third generation of slings was the single-incision mini-slings, also placed at the midurethra, and attached to the obturator fascia and muscle without exit incisions. Potentially, this may cause less postoperative pain, but the longer term effectiveness remains to be proven.

Urethral Injections with Bulking Agents

The first reported use of urethral injections was by Murless in 1938 using sodium morrhuate.

In 1974, Politano injected polytetrafluoroethylene or Teflon first to treat postprostatectomy incontinence in men and then used it in women with urinary stress incontinence in the early 1980s. This was followed by periurethral and transurethral of bovine dermal collagen. In the 1990s, silicone microparticles and cross-linked polysaccharides and hyaluronic acid in the 2000s. More recently, in the 2010s, autologous fat, skeletal cells, and stem cells have all been studied but not used widely.

The urethral injections can also be performed under local anesthesia as day surgery and have low morbidity which makes them particularly suited to the elderly. With the adverse media attention of synthetic products, there has been a considerable increase in their usage. However, continence success is low on follow-up and the injections frequently need repeating.

ENDOSCOPY

Cystourethroscopy

In 1804, Bozzini, a German physician, investigated possible options to examining "deeply seated organs" including the bladder and urethra. He advocated the inspection of all "interior cavities" by looking through natural openings or at least small wounds.[23] He designed a number of long thin funnels, which he called a "lichtleiter" (light conductor), with illumination provided by a light reflected from a box containing a wax candle (Fig. 1.2). He presented his instrument to the Faculty of Medicine of Vienna, but they were reportedly alarmed at his invention. They ridiculed Bozzini's lichtleiter, which effectively stopped any further development for many decades, and there is no evidence that it was used in a human. However, his ideas lived on, and he foresaw the future of diagnostic and operative endoscopy of the urinary tract (cystourethroscopy) and abdominal cavity (laparoscopy) and vaginal surgery (natural

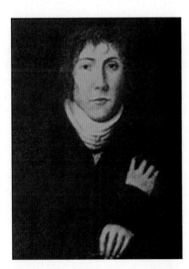

FIGURE 1.2 Philippe Bozzini, a German physician, circa 1804. (Reprinted from Alkatout I, Mechler U, Mettler L, et al. The development of laparoscopy—A historical overview. *Front Surg* 2021;8:799442.)

opening). He wrote, "Surgery will not only develop new and previously impossible procedures, but all uncertain operations which rely on luck and approximation will become safe under the influence of direct vision, since the surgeon's hands will now be guided by his eyes."

In 1826, Pierre Ségalas had more success using a simplified version of Bozzini's instrument. It was a funnel with a polished interior to reflect light. It was used to illuminate the bladder and ureteral orifices with illumination from candles and a concave mirror which focused the light which allowed 3 mm of aperture for viewing and heralded the advent of cystoscopy for the diagnosis and treatment of lower urinary tract conditions.[24]

In 1853, Antonin Jean Desormeaux, a French surgeon, used a modified *lichtleiter* to examine his patients with urinary problems. A system of mirrors, lenses, and larger angulated tubes was used to improve visualization and a much brighter lamp flame burning a mixture of alcohol and turpentine instead of a wax candle improved visualization but caused burns both to himself and his patients.

Max Nitze, a German physician, is generally credited as the "father of the modern cystoscope." He, with Josef Leiter in 1869, devised a combination of lenses, which enlarged the field of vision, and electricity to illuminate the inside of the bladder as never before. He filled the bladder with ice water to prevent thermal injury and used the glow of a platinum wire as the light source.[25] Later, Thomas Edison's incandescent lamp dramatically improved illumination in cystoscopy, although the heat of the bulb still required a water medium to prevent overheating.[26]

Josef Grünfeld, born in Gyor, Hungary, was the first to successfully catheterize the ureters under vision, using malleable catheters introduced into the bladder alongside his glass-ended endoscope in 1876. He also was the first surgeon to remove a bladder tumor by cystoscope in 1881 after developing an endoscopic loop threader, scissors, forceps, and knives.

Howard A. Kelly, professor of obstetrics and gynecology at Johns Hopkins Hospital in Baltimore, United States, and a pioneer in female urology, developed operations for stress incontinence and vaginal prolapse. In 1893, he constructed a cystoscope from a handled, hollow tube with a glass partition (see Fig. 1.1). He accidentally broke the glass partition and then wondered, like Sims before him, with his vaginal speculum if the bladder could be distended with air. He inserted the broken cystoscope into the bladder in the knee-chest position; the bladder ballooned with air with the removal of the obturator giving excellent vision and performing the first air cystoscopy. He was able to see the bladder mucosa and ureters and was able to insert a ureteral catheter under direct vision and was said by some to be the first, a gynecologist, to do so.[27] However, Hunner, a protégé of Kelly, latter concluded that "Grunfeld of Vienna" was the first to pass a metal catheter into the ureter under direct vision.

In the early 20th century, cystoscopy was rarely used as the instrumentation was imperfect and dangerous often resulting in injuries from the use of large tubes. Air cystoscopy was a simple and inexpensive method of examining the female bladder but had disadvantages of external illumination and lack of a lens system, and it is necessary to position the patient in the knee-chest position.

The invention of the rod lens system and flexible fiber-optic endoscopes led to rapid improvements in diagnosis and treatment of lower urinary conditions. The development of the Hopkins fiber-optic telescope in 1954 using glass fibers in place of an air chamber dramatically improved light transmission and resolution and provided a wider viewing area with various angled scopes to improve the extent of visualization of the bladder epithelium. However, the angled telescope did not allow good urethral distension and visualization of the urethral epithelium because the irrigation fluid escaped through the urethral meatus. Jack Robertson addressed these issues by inventing a shorter straight-on fiber-optic telescope which he called a urethroscope. In 1968, he together with a German instrument maker, Karl Storz, of Tuttlingen produced a female urethroscope, 8 inches long with a straight forward view, the Robertson carbon dioxide endoscopy telescope. The scope fits into an airtight handle, through which the carbon dioxide is insufflated. Urethral and bladder pressure measurements were made during endoscopy and charted on an X-Y recorder with bladder sensations during bladder filling documented.[28]

The modern rigid cystoscopes use fluid irrigation with water, saline, or glycine with three digital chip cameras attached to provide excellent vision and photography. Flexible cystoscopes use a fiber-optic lens system to provide a scope that is smaller and pliable, increasing patient comfort and the range of vision and allowing outpatient cystoscopy with local anesthetic ointment.

Endoscopy of the urinary tract is a developing science with new endoscopes to visualize the upper urinary tracts and new instruments to perform procedures that previously required open surgery, such as the removal of calculi, tumors, or foreign bodies.

Laparoscopy

Gynecologists were one of the first specialists to understand the importance and benefits of the laparoscope. However, early laparoscopic surgery in the 1960s and 1970s was hindered by limited optical and instrumental technology. Important milestones in laparoscopic surgery technology include the first tube camera in 1981 and the solid-state medical video camera in 1981 by William Chang. The first three digital chip cameras introduced in 1989 significantly improved clarity of vision and digital enhancement and zoom technology again improved our capabilities in 1999. Improved instrumentation and better understanding of energy sources have made laparoscopy safer and suitable for a wider range of pelvic surgeries including diagnosing and treating women with pelvic disorders.

Laparoscopy provided excellent vision and exposure so that open procedures could be performed through the retropubic space and pelvis. John C. Burch described the Burch colposuspension for the surgical management of SUI in 1961, and Vancaille and Schuessler[29] first reported the laparoscopic colposuspension in 1991. Prospective randomized control trials, where similar operating procedures are performed in both arms by suitably trained surgeons, have demonstrated that the laparoscopic colposuspension is as effective as the open procedure laparoscopic colposuspensions take longer time to perform but are associated with less blood loss, less pain, and quicker return to normal activities. The laparoscopic colposuspension in well conducted studies has been shown to be effective as the TVT in primary[4] and repeat continence surgery.[5]

The sacral colpopexy was first described by Lane in 1982 where he suspended the posthysterectomy upper vagina from the sacral promontory using permanent synthetic mesh. Laparoscopic sacral colopexy became popular in the 1990s pioneered by Tony Smith from the United Kingdom[30] and others.

PAINFUL BLADDER CONDITIONS

Skene[31] in 1887 was the first to describe and name interstitial cystitis "when the disease has destroyed the mucous membrane partly or wholly and extended to the muscular parietes, we have what is known as interstitial cystitis." He also described the anatomy of the female urethra and Skene glands which still bear his name.

Max Nize[32] with his improved cystoscope was able to get better visualization of the bladder pathologies including interstitial cystitis. However, it was Guy Hunner, a protégé of Howard Kelly and a gynecologist from Johns Hopkins Hospital in Baltimore, United States, who was the first to clearly describe the condition of interstitial cystitis. In two classical manuscripts published in 1915 and 1918,[33] he discussed the clinical presentation, diagnosis, etiology, pathology, and treatment. He also gave very clear descriptions of interstitial cystitis using an early air distension cystoscope pioneered by Kelly in the knee-chest position. There were many who criticized Hunner's description. In 1977, Walsh[34] stated that "the ulcers Hunner originally described were secondary to optic deficiency of early cystoscopes." However, Hunner's original descriptions of his cystoscopic findings have stood the test of time even using modern endoscopic equipment.

"The crucial test in cystoscopy is the finding of a small abrasion on the mucosa surface which, if not bleeding on discovery, will easily bleed on being touched." "The ulcer is usually found in the vertex or free portion of the bladder." "Occasionally the distention of the bladder by air as the patient assumes the knee-breast posture causes this area to split and a tiny stream of blood flows to the vertex." "One may see a dead white scar area with a small congested area in the immediate neighborhood and while one is examining this area the congestion becomes marked and may even begin to ooze blood."[33]

Progress in the treatment of painful bladder syndrome has been slow. Consensus on diagnostic criteria has been attempted by groups of interested clinicians[35] who stated that for a positive diagnosis of interstitial cystitis, either widespread glomerulations or a classic Hunner ulcer were required in the presence of bladder pain or urgency.

LOWER URINARY TRACT FISTULAE

The basic surgical principles for the vaginal approach to vesicovaginal fistula repair were described in 1663 by Hedrik Van Roonhuyse, a Dutch surgeon. He published his clinical treatise entitled *Medico-Chirurgical Observations* in 1672. The technique for vesicovaginal fistula repair included essential steps including the use of the lithotomy position, exposure of the fistula with a speculum, sharp paring of the fistula edge prior to attempted closure, careful approximation of the denuded edges of the fistula using Swan quills, dressing of the wound with absorbent vaginal packing, and immobilization of the patient in bed until the repair has healed.[36]

Johann Fatio, who may be considered the true father of pediatric surgery, reported a successful closure of a vesicovaginal fistula also using Swan quills in 1675.[37]

A French surgeon, Antoine Jobert de Lamballe was the first physician to use a labial skin flap for repair of a vesicovaginal fistula. Among Jobert's works, stand his masterpiece *Traité de chirurgie plastique* on plastic surgery (1849), where he had described his innovative technique to cure vesicovaginal fistulas.[38]

The first use of metallic sutures to close a wound was reported in 1833 by John Peter Mettauer, a Virginia surgeon, in the *American Journal of the Medical Science*. In 1838, he reported his first successful closure of a vesicovaginal fistula using metal sutures with the patient in the knee-chest position.[39]

Mackenrodt was first to perform a layered repair of a vesicovaginal fistula in 1894. Latzko[40] described his technique for vesicovaginal fistula repair in 1942 with excision of the vaginal epithelium around the fistula site, leaving the bladder mucosa and wall intact minimizing the risk of ureteric injury. Although classified by some as an upper vaginal colpocleisis, removal of minimal amounts of vaginal skin only is necessary once adequate mobilization of the bladder has occurred which allows a tension-free suture closure of the fistula in multiple layers.

Another major innovation in vesicovaginal fistula repair was the use of grafts particularly the use of labial fat pad harvesting described by Martius[41] in 1932, providing a well-vascularized fat graft to provide additional support to the tension-free closure and improve healing. Martius initially used the graft to improve postrepair incontinence which also contained parts of the bulbocavernosus muscle, but he found that continence was not improved but it did improve his primary closure success. Garlock in 1928 described the use of a pedicled gracilis muscle graft, and Axel Ingleman-Sundberg[42] from the Karolinska Institute in Stockholm performed transplantation of levator muscles for repairing rectovaginal fistula. Axel was a doyen of urogynecology in the Scandinavian countries and is well known to older members of the International Urogynecological Association which he cofounded with Jack Robertson, attending annual scientific meetings into his 90s.

Abdominal Repairs

The abdominal route using the transvesical or transperitoneal approach is indicated when vaginal access is very limited or the fistulas are high and fixed in the vault. Trendelenburg pioneered the transvesical approach in 1890.[43] Other reasons for the abdominal approach would be the presence of complex fistulas including vesicoureteric vaginal fistula where ureteric reimplantation is necessary and the vesicovaginal fistula was inaccessible per vaginam. Transvesical repair has the advantage of being entirely extraperitoneal.

PELVIC ORGAN PROLAPSE

In the 19th and early 20th century, there were no objective descriptions of pelvic organ prolapse on physical findings (Table 1.1).[44] Dr. Wayne Baden and his colleagues[45] described the halfway system of prolapse grading in the 1968. In 1996, Dr. Richard Bump and his colleagues[46] published the Pelvic Organ Prolapse Quantification (POP-Q) system, which has become the most universally used method to describe the vaginal physical examination. Now, 21st century authors report not only anatomic but also functional results including bowel, bladder, and sexual function as well as acquired pain complaints and quality-of-life measurements. Earlier authors did not routinely report data on the durability of prolapse surgery or on quality-of-life measurements. In the 21st century, anatomic durability is considered a critical factor in assessing and comparing operative outcomes.

TABLE 1.1

Milestones in the History of Pelvic Reconstructive Surgery

1846	Introduction of general anesthesia
1867	Antisepsis—Joseph Lister
1878–1884	Asepsis in surgery—Gustav Adolf Neuber
1881	Steam autoclave—Charles Chamberland
1889	Surgical education evolution began in 1889 at Johns Hopkins School of Medicine with institution of residency programs
1890	Rubber gloves commercially available—William Halstead
1900	A, B, O blood groups—Karl Landsteiner
1907	First transfusion of cross-matched blood
1928	Penicillin—Alexander Fleming
1930	Commercial antibiotic era—Sulfonamide
1945	Penicillin commercially available
1968	Objective description of pelvic organ prolapse
	Baden-Walker halfway system
1970s	Laparoscopy in gynecology
1990s	Synthetic mesh products in transvaginal surgery
1996	Standardization of terminology for pelvic organ prolapse and POP-Q[a]
2000s	Robotic surgery in gynecology
2020	Joint Report on Terminology for Surgical Procedures to Treat Pelvic Organ Prolapse

[a]From Bump RC, Mattiasson A, Bø K, et al. The standardization of terminology of female pelvic organ prolapse and pelvic floor dysfunction. *Am J Obstet Gynecol* 1996;175(1):10–17.

LESSONS FROM OUR COLLEAGUES

We have learned from general surgeons that anatomic success following hernia surgery is a function of the preoperative size of the original hernia as well as the duration of postsurgical follow-up.[47,48] It is reasonable to conclude that anatomic outcomes in pelvic organ prolapse surgery also depend on the duration of follow-up as well as the size of the original support defects. In addition, the reconstructive surgeon is required to establish the proper preoperative diagnosis and skillfully execute the appropriate surgical procedure.

Oncologists have proven that earlier stage disease is more likely to have longer disease-free intervals or cure, provided the proper diagnosis is established and effective therapy is instituted. Conversely, late-stage disease uniformly has a worse prognosis. The accurate preoperative diagnosis and expert execution of a proven surgical treatment for pelvic organ prolapse should lead to improved anatomic and functional outcomes in prolapse surgery. Surgeons who use an objective descriptive technique such as the POP-Q to report anatomic findings before and after surgery include data on symptom relief, quality-of-life measurements, and complications which help us make data-driven decisions regarding procedures. The most recent effort to add standardization to our literature is the 2020 Joint Report on Terminology for Surgical Procedures to Treat Pelvic Organ Prolapse developed by the Joint Writing Group of the American Urogynecologic Society and the International Urogynecological Association.[49] In 2021, the primary surgical anatomic challenge continues to be successful treatment of anterior compartment prolapse.[50]

For the first 100 years of gynecologic surgery, all procedures were performed with an open abdominal incision or through a vaginal approach. Because of innovations in lighting and instrumentation during the last 30 years of the 20th century, minimally invasive surgery has become practical and popular and offers advantages in perioperative morbidity, recovery times, reduced hospitalization times, as well as earlier return to normal activities as compared to open abdominal techniques. By the beginning of the 21st century, robotic surgery was beginning to find a place in reconstructive pelvic surgery. Because of the greater costs for purchase and maintenance of equipment, robotic surgery is currently more frequently used in a few developed countries than in many developing countries. When the cost differences between laparoscopic and robotic surgery disappear, robotic surgery may be used more widely around the world. Presently, the most cost-effective and universally available minimally invasive surgery is vaginal hysterectomy with or without reconstructive procedures and transvaginal repair of posthysterectomy vaginal prolapse.

Because reports in our literature have documented anatomic and functional failure rates associated with reconstructive pelvic surgery,[51–54] innovative surgeons and industry partners in the later part of the 20th century began working on surgical techniques which incorporate biologic or synthetic graft materials in both abdominal and vaginal repairs. To date in 2021, the abdominal use of synthetic grafts in abdominal sacral colpopexy procedures is universally accepted as an effective, durable procedure with well-described risk/benefit profiles.

On the other hand, transvaginal use of synthetic mesh graft in reconstructive surgery has been more controversial. The initial enthusiasm for transvaginal mesh implantation has subsided following numerous reports of acquired postoperative complaints leading to medicolegal cases, government restrictions on its use, and finally to products being withdrawn from production. In 2021, there is a more measured approach to the use of synthetic products placed transvaginally. It is not clear which products will prove to be safe and effective and which patients are suitable candidates for such procedures.

Another significant change over the past 50 years is the greatly increased role of women surgeons and scientists in the fields of pelvic organ prolapse education, research, leadership, and patient care. Some of our more senior women surgeons and researchers such as Professors Linda Cardozo, Linda Brubaker, Peggy Norton, and Renee Thacker have mentored and educated an entire generation of leading pelvic floor specialists around the world, both men and women.

One of the continuing unsolved problems which has defied solution to date is the accurate identification of women at greatest risk for disorders of the pelvic floor and subsequent interventions to prevent, rather than treat, those disorders. Once that happens, the need for surgical intervention may be significantly reduced.

CONCLUSION

Future change has the possibility to be driven by corporations rather than individuals. Change must be driven by science, and changes in our practices guided by proven benefit confirmed by prospective randomized trials where possible. Too often, new surgical treatments are introduced in haste before fully evaluated under the banner of being minimally invasive and new but in reality are more expensive, take longer to do, and have a higher morbidity.

We should take pride in what medicine has achieved and how it has dramatically improved the quality and longevity of life in women and men. The history of medicine like humanity has not always been just and inspirational but needs to be documented accurately rather than erased and rewritten as many authoritative governments are doing worldwide. We need to learn from it and not repeat past mistakes. We need to strive personally for a better world. One example of this from our urogynecologic recent past is the work of Catherine and Reginald Hamlin who toward the end of their medical careers in Australia and New Zealand went to Ethiopia and opened a fistula hospital to treat obstetric fistulas and improve the life of African women.[55] It is a self-evident truth that all people should be treated equally regardless of race, gender, age, geography, or economic or social circumstances. Perhaps it was best said in that less fashionable publication the Bible that we should treat all as we would like to be treated ourselves.

References

1. Kelly HA. Incontinence of urine in women. *Urol Cutaneous Rev* 1913;17:291–293.
2. Aldridge A, Jeffcoate TNA, Roberts H. Stress incontinence of urine. *J Obstet Gynaecol Br Emp* 1952;59(5):681–720.
3. Marshall VF, Marchetti AA, Krantz KE. The correction of stress incontinence by simple vesicourethral suspension. *Surg Gynecol Obstet* 1949;88(4):509–518.
4. Hepburn TN. Prolapse of the urethra in female children. *Surg Gynecol Obstet* 1920:40–41.
5. Burch JC. Cooper's ligament urethrovesical suspension for stress incontinence. Nine years' experience—Results, complications, technique. *Am J Obstet Gynecol* 1968;100(6):764–774.
6. Zacharin RF. The suspensory mechanism of the female urethra. *J Anat (London)* 1963;97:423–427.
7. Pereyra AJ. A simplified procedure for the correction of stress incontinence in women. *West J Surg Obstet Gynecol* 1959;67(4):223–226.
8. Peattie AB, Stanton SL. The Stamey operation for the correction of genuine stress incontinence. *Br J Obst Gynecol* 1989;96(8):983–986.
9. Goebel R. Zur operitaven beseitigung der angebornen incontinentia vesicae. *Zeitscher Gynakol* 1910;2:187–191.
10. Frangenheim P. Zu operativen behandlung der inkontinenz der mannlichen harnohre. *Ver Dtsch Ges Chir* 1914;43:149–154.
11. Price PB. Plastic operations for incontinence of urine and feces. *Arch Surg* 1933;26:1043–1053.
12. Aldridge AH. Transplantation of fascia for relief of urinary stress incontinence. *Am J Obstet Gynecol* 1942;44:398–411.
13. McGuire EJ, Lytton B. Pubovaginal sling procedure for stress incontinence. *J Urol* 1978;119(1):82–84.
14. Moir JC. The gauze/hammock operation (a modified Aldridge sling procedure). *J Obstet Gynaecol Br Commonw* 1968;75(1):1–9.
15. Morgan JE. A sling using Marlex polypropylene mesh for treatment of recurrent stress incontinence. *Am J Obstet Gynec* 1970;106(3):369–377.
16. Stanton SL, Brindley GS, Holmes DM. Silastic sling for urethral sphincter incompetence in women. *Br J Obstet Gynaecol* 1985;92(7):747–750.
17. Hilton P, Stanton SL. A clinical and urodynamic assessment of the Burch colposuspension for genuine stress incontinence. *Br J Obstet Gynaecol* 1983;90(10):934–939.
18. Lee JK, Dwyer PL. Surgery for stress urinary incontinence in Australia: Current trends from Medicare data. *Med J Aust* 2010;192(7):422.
19. Petros PE, Ulmsten UI. An integral theory of female urinary incontinence. Experimental and clinical considerations. *Acta Obstet Gynecol Scand Suppl* 1990;153:7–31.
20. Ulmsten U, Henriksson L, Johnson P, et al. An ambulatory surgical procedure under local anesthesia for treatment of female urinary incontinence. *Int Urogynecol J Pelvic Floor Dysfunct* 1996;7(2):81–85.
21. Delorme E. Transobturator urethral suspension: Mini-invasive procedure in the treatment of stress urinary incontinence in women. *Prog Urol* 2001;11(5):1306–1313.
22. DeLeval J. Novel surgical technique for the treatment of female stress urinary incontinence: Transobturator vaginal tape inside-out. *Eur Urol* 2003;44(6):724–730.
23. Bozzini P. Lichtleiter, eine Erfindung zur Anschauung innerer Theile und Krankheiten nebst der Abbildung. *Journal der practischen Arzneykunde und Wundarzneykunst* 1806;24:107–124.
24. Pousson A, Besnos E, eds. *Encyclopedie Francaise d'Urologie.* Paris: Doin et Fils, 1914.
25. Macalpine JB. *Cystoscopy and urography*, 2nd ed. Baltimore: William Wood, 1936.
26. Encyclopedia Britannica, Thomas Edison *Encyclopedia Britannica*, Thomas Edison.
27. Kelly HA. *Medical gynecology*. New York: Appleton, 1908.

28. Robertson JR. Robertson method. In: *Genitourinary problems in women*. Springfield: Charles C. Thomas, 1978:42–64.

29. Vancaille T, Schuessler W. Laparoscopic bladder-neck suspension. *J Laparoenosc Surg* 1991;1(3):169–173.

30. Higgs PJ, Chua HL, Smith ARB. Long term review of laparoscopic sacrocolpopexy. *BJOG* 2005;112(8):1134–1138.

31. Skene A. The anatomy and pathology of two important glands of the female urethra. *Am J Obstet Dis Women Child* 1880;13(2):265–270.

32. Nize M. *Lehbuch der Kystoskopie: Ihre Technik und Klinische Bedeuting*. Berlin: J. Bergman, 1907.

33. Hunner GL. A rare type of bladder ulcer in women; report of cases. *Boston Med Surg J* 1915;172:660–664.

34. Walsh A. Interstitial cystitis. Observations on diagnosis and on treatment with anti-inflammatory drugs, particularly benzydamine. *Eur Urol* 1977;3:216–217.

35. Gillenwater JY, Wein AJ. Summary of the National Institute of Arthritis, Diabetes, Digestive and Kidney Diseases workshop on interstitial cystitis, National Institutes of Health, Bethesda, Maryland, August 28–29, 1987. *J Urol* 1988;140(1): 203–206.

36. Wall LL. Henry van Roonhuyse and the first repair of vesico-vaginal fistula (~1676). *Int Urogynecol J* 2020;31(2):237–241.

37. Stanford E, Romanzi L. Vesicovaginal fistula: What is the preferred closure technique? *Int Urogynecol J* 2012;23(4): 383–385.

38. Tsoucalas G, Laios K, Sgantzos M, et al. The ingenious Antoine Jobert de Lambelle (1799-1867) and his innovative autoplastic cure of vesicovaginal fistulas. *Surg Innov* 2014;21(6):649–650.

39. Bickers W. John Peter Mettauer of Virginia. *JAMA* 1963;184(11): 870–871.

40. Latzko W. Postoperative vesicovaginal fistulas: Genesis and therapy. *Am J Surg* 1942;58:211–228.

41. Martius H. Uber die Behandlung von Blasenscheidenfisteln, insbesondere met Hilfe einer Lappenplastik. *Geburtshilfe Gynakol* 1932;103:22–34.

42. Ingleman-Sundberg A. Transplantation of levator muscles in repair of complete tear and rectovaginal fistula. *Acta Chir Scand* 1948;96:313–316.

43. Trendelenburg F. Uber Blasenscheidenfisteloperationen und uber Beckenhochlagerung bei Operationen in der Bauchhohle. *Samml Klin Vortr* 1890;355:3373–3392.

44. Randall CL, Nichols DH. Surgical treatment of vaginal inversion. *Obstet Gynecol* 1971;38(3):327–332.

45. Baden WF, Walker TA, Lindsey JH. The vaginal profile. *Tex Med* 1968;64(5):56–58.

46. Bump RC, Mattiasson A, Bø K, et al. The standardization of terminology of female pelvic organ prolapse and pelvic floor dysfunction. *Am J Obstet Gynecol* 1996;175(1):10–17.

47. Anthony T, Bergen PC, Lawrence TK, et al. Factors affecting recurrence following incisional herniorrhaphy. *World J Surg* 2000;24(1):95–101.

48. Wantz GE, Chevrel JP, Flament JB, et al. Incisional hernias symposium. *J Am Coll Surg* 1999;188(4):429–447.

49. Joint report on terminology for surgical procedures to treat pelvic organ prolapse. Developed by the Joint Writing Group of the American Urogynecologic Society and the International Urogynecological Association. *Int Urogynecol J* 2020;31(3): 429–463.

50. Sheyn D, El-Nashar S, Mahajan ST, et al. Apical suspension utilization at the time of vaginal hysterectomy for pelvic organ prolapse varies with surgeon specialty. *Female Pelvic Med Reconstr Surg* 2020;26(6):370–375.

51. Shull BL, Capen CV, Riggs MW, et al. Preoperative and postoperative analysis of site-specific pelvic support defects in 81 women treated with sacrospinous ligament suspension and pelvic reconstruction. *Am J Obstet Gynecol* 1992;166(6 Pt 1):1764–1771.

52. Shull BL, Benn SJ, Kuehl TJ. Surgical management of prolapse of the anterior vaginal segment: An analysis of support defects, operative morbidity, and anatomic outcome. *Am J Obstet Gynecol* 1994;171(6):1429–1436.

53. Shull BL. Pelvic organ prolapse: Anterior, superior, and posterior vaginal segment defects. *Am J Obstet Gynecol* 1999;181(1):6–11.

54. Shull B. Reasonable people disagree: Lessons learned from the sling and mesh story. *Int Urogynecol J* 2016;27:1289–1291.

55. Zacharin RF. *Obstetric fistula*. Vienna: Springer-Verlag, 1988.

CHAPTER 2

PELVIC AND SUPPORT ANATOMY

Polina Sawyer • Marlene M. Corton

Introduction

Support of the pelvic organs is provided by the complex interactions between pelvic viscera, musculature, and connective tissues and their attachments to the inner surface of the bony pelvis. The bony pelvis serves as a unique scaffolding that enables the pelvic viscera to expand, store and expel contents, all while maintaining the dynamic positions of the organs in three-dimensional space.

BONY PELVIS

The paired hip or coxal bones are formed by the fusion of three bones: *ilium, ischium,* and *pubic bones* (Fig. 2.1). These bones fuse at the *acetabulum,* the cup-shaped structure which articulates with the head of the femur. Anteriorly, the pubic bones articulate with each other at the *pubic symphysis,* and posteriorly, the ilium articulates with the sacrum at the *sacroiliac joint.*

The *pelvic inlet* separates the pelvic cavity into a *true pelvis* (below the inlet) and a *false pelvis* (above the inlet) (Fig. 2.2). The pelvic brim is the edge of the pelvic inlet. The brim is circumscribed by the sacral promontory, the arcuate and pectineal lines, pubic crest, and the upper margin of the pubic symphysis. The *false* pelvis is bounded laterally by the *alae of the ilium,* which serve as attachment sites for the large muscles of locomotion. The pelvic outlet is bordered by the pubic arch anteriorly, the ischial tuberosities laterally, and the coccyx posteriorly (Fig. 2.3).

In the anatomic or standing position, the pelvic cavity tilts anteriorly. This adaption, which evolved to allow humans bipedal locomotion, brings the internal surface of the sacrum forward and downward and tilts the pelvic outlet so that it lies in a plane 60° to 65° from the horizontal. In this position, the anterior superior iliac spines and anterior surface of the pubic symphysis are in the same vertical plane and the ischiopubic rami and genital hiatus are parallel to the ground. This orientation directs the pressure of the intra-abdominal and pelvic contents toward the bones of the pelvis rather than toward the muscles and connective tissue of the pelvic floor.[1]

Deviations from stated configuration may predispose to pelvic organ prolapse.[2,3] For example, a loss of lumbar lordosis, which can occur following spinal fusion, shifts the orientation of the pelvic outlet into a more horizontal plane, and this has been more commonly noted in women with prolapse.[4,5]

LIGAMENTS AND OPENINGS OF THE PELVIS

The *sacrospinous, sacrotuberous, sacroiliac,* and *anterior longitudinal ligaments* of the sacrum are dense connective tissue condensations which join bony structures and contribute significantly to the stability of the bony pelvis.

Sacrospinous and Sacrotuberous Ligaments

Both sacrospinous and sacrotuberous ligaments attach to the lateral and anterior aspect of the lower sacrum and coccyx medially and are fused in this region (see Fig. 2.2). Laterally, the sacrospinous ligament attaches to the ischial spine and the sacrotuberous ligament to the ischial tuberosity.

Greater and Lesser Sciatic Foramen

The *sacrospinous* and *sacrotuberous ligaments* divide the greater and lesser sciatic notches of the ischium into the *greater sciatic foramen* and *lesser sciatic foramen.*

Structures that pass through the greater sciatic foramen include the piriformis muscle, sciatic nerve, internal pudendal vessels and pudendal nerve, superior and inferior gluteal vessels and nerves, and other branches of the lumbosacral nerve plexus. These structures pass through the foramen dorsal to the sacrospinous ligament and near the ischial spine. Understanding these anatomic relationships is critical to avoiding neurovascular injury during sacrospinous ligament fixation and pudendal nerve blocks.

Structures which pass through the lesser sciatic foramen include the internal pudendal vessels and pudendal nerve and the obturator internus tendon.

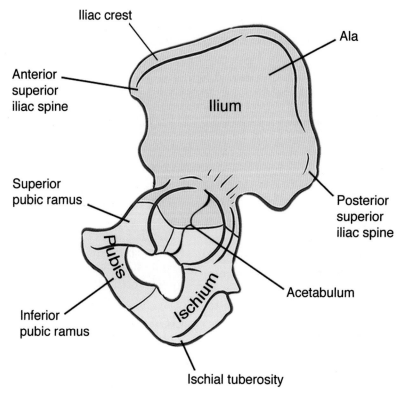

FIGURE 2.1 Left hip bone.

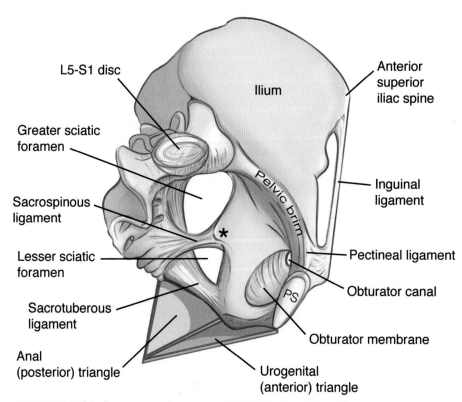

FIGURE 2.2 Pelvic ligaments and openings. *, ischial spine; PS, pubic symphysis.

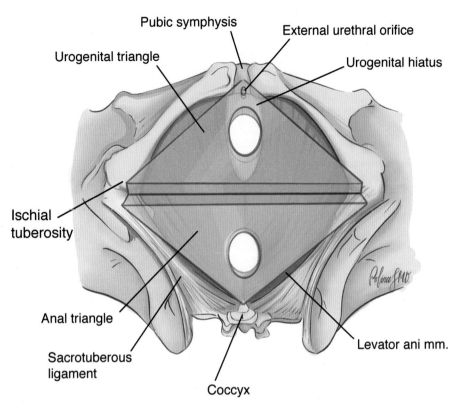

FIGURE 2.3 Perineal triangles. mm., muscle.

Anterior Longitudinal Ligament

The anterior longitudinal ligament consists of a broad and strong band of connective tissue fibers that extends along the anterior surfaces of the vertebral bodies and intervertebral discs, from the base of the skull to the sacrum. This ligament is composed of several layers of fibers of varying length and thickness that are closely interlaced with each other. These fibers limit extension of the vertebral column and reinforce the intervertebral disc, to which it is densely adherent. On the anterior surface of the first sacral vertebra, the average ligament thickness is 1.2 to 2.5 mm.[6] It is in this region that the ligament serves as the optimal site for mesh fixation during sacrocolpopexy.[7,8]

Obturator Membrane and Obturator Canal

The obturator membrane is a dense fibrous structure that almost completely covers the *obturator foramen* between the ischium and pubis. Within the superior portion of this membrane is a small aperture, the *obturator canal*, through which the obturator neurovascular bundle exits the pelvis to reach the medial compartment of the thigh. This canal is found 5 to 6 cm from the midline of the upper pubic symphysis and 1.5 to 2 cm below the upper margin of the pectineal ligament.[9,10]

The *pectineal (Cooper)* ligament is a thickening in the pubic bone periosteum formed by the deep and medial fibers of the inguinal ligament; it serves as the anchoring site for retropubic colposuspension procedures.

PELVIC WALL MUSCLES

The lateral, inferior, and posterior walls of the pelvis are partially covered by striated muscles and their investing layers of fascia. These muscles include the *piriformis*, *obturator internus*, and the muscles of the *pelvic diaphragm*.

Piriformis Muscle

The *piriformis muscle* lines the posterolateral walls of the pelvis and is found directly posterior to the sacral nerves (Fig. 2.4). It arises from the anterior and lateral surface of the sacrum and exits the pelvis through the greater sciatic foramen to attach to the greater trochanter of the femur, where it functions as an external hip rotator. This muscle has a precise and intimate relationship with the sciatic nerve and has been implicated as a cause of nondiscogenic sciatica in cases where the muscle impinges on the nerve.[11,12]

Beaton and Anson[13] described the existence of six different anatomic variations between the sciatic nerve and the piriformis muscle. In this cadaveric study, an undivided sciatic nerve emerging inferior to the piriformis

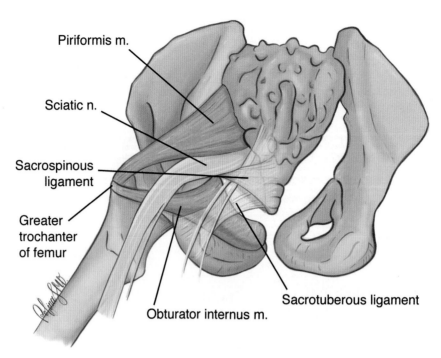

FIGURE 2.4 Posterior view of pelvis. m., muscle; n., nerve.

muscle was the most common and accounted for 90% of specimens examined. However, a recent magnetic resonance imaging study showed 20% aberrant anatomic relationships between the piriformis muscle and sciatic nerve.[14] Although the clinical significance of these findings is uncertain, it has been suggested that these anatomic aberrations may have a role in pelvic floor dysfunction.[15]

Obturator Internus Muscle

The *obturator internus muscle* arises from the pelvic surfaces of the ischium and ilium and from the obturator membrane and fills the lateral sidewalls of the pelvis (Fig. 2.5). The muscle tendon exits the pelvis through the lesser sciatic foramen and attaches to the greater trochanter of the hip. Like the piriformis muscle, it serves as an external hip rotator.

Along its medial pelvic surface, the obturator internus fascia condenses into two structures that are critical to pelvic organ support: the arcus tendineus fascia pelvis (ATFP) and the arcus tendineus levator ani (ATLA). The ATLA serves as origin for part of the levator ani muscles, and the ATFP serves as the attachment site for the mid anterior vaginal wall. In the perineum, a splitting of the obturator internus fascia forms the pudendal (Alcock) canal, through which the pudendal nerve and internal pudendal vessels pass before separating into the three terminal branches that innervate structures in the perineum.[9,16]

Pelvic Diaphragm

The muscles that span the pelvic floor are collectively known as the *pelvic diaphragm* (Fig. 2.6). The diaphragm

consists of the *levator ani* and *coccygeus muscles* as well as their investing layers of fascia.

The levator ani muscle represents the "active" support of the pelvis and is functionally composed of three distinct parts: the *iliococcygeus*, *pubococcygeus*, and *puborectalis*. The connective tissue covering both the superior and inferior surfaces of these muscles is called the *superior and inferior fascia of the levator ani*. Below the pelvic diaphragm, the perineal membrane and perineal body also provide contributions to pelvic floor support.

Coccygeus muscle

The *coccygeus muscle* lies on the superior (pelvic) surface of the sacrospinous ligament and together with the levator ani muscles form the pelvic diaphragm. This muscle has the same bony attachments and runs an identical course to the sacrospinous ligament; thus, these two structures are commonly referred to as the *coccygeus-sacrospinous ligament complex (C-SSL)*. Nerves which supply the coccygeus and levator ani muscles course over the midportion of the C-SSL complex, making these nerves particularly vulnerable during sacrospinous ligament fixation procedures (see Fig. 2.6).[17,18] Postoperative dyspareunia and pelvic pain may potentially result from nerve or muscle disruption; thus, examination of the pelvic floor muscles is warranted when these symptoms present.

Pubococcygeus muscle

The *pubococcygeus* part of the levator ani muscle arises from the inner surface of the pubic bone and the ATLA

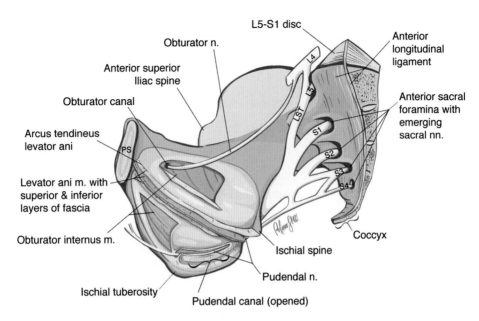

FIGURE 2.5 Pelvic sidewall and pudendal canal. n., nerve; nn., nerves; LST, lumbosacral trunk; PS, pubic symphysis; m., muscle.

and attaches medially to the distal walls of the vagina, rectum, and perineal body (Fig. 2.7). Accordingly, this muscle consists of three subdivisions: The *puboperinealis* attaches to the perineal body, the *pubovaginalis* to the vaginal wall, and the *puboanalis* to the anus at the intersphincteric groove between the internal and external anal sphincters. Some fibers of the pubococcygeus also attach to the coccyx. However, given the significant attachments

of muscle fibers to the pelvic viscera, the pubococcygeus is also known as the pubovisceralis muscle.[19]

Although the levator ani muscles have no direct attachments to the urethra in women, the fibers of the pubococcygeus muscle that attach to the vagina are responsible for elevating the anterior vaginal wall and indirectly the urethra and hence may contribute to urinary continence, as discussed later.[20,21]

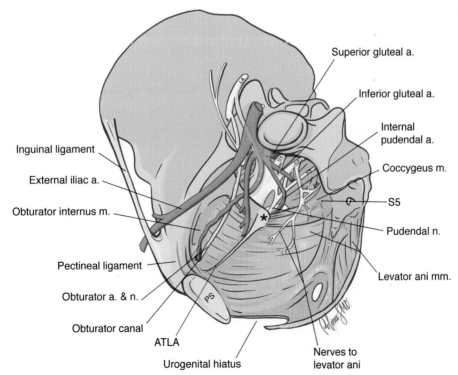

FIGURE 2.6 Levator ani muscles and innervation. *, ischial spine; a., artery; m., muscle; n., nerve; PS, pubic symphysis.

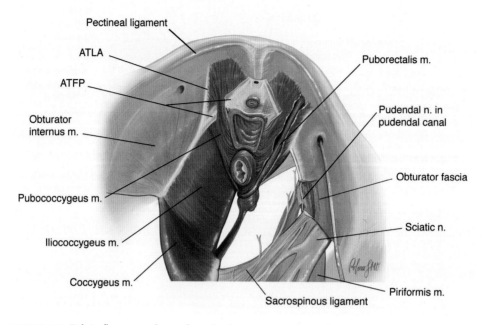

FIGURE 2.7 Pelvic floor muscles and urethral support. m., muscle; n., nerve.

Iliococcygeus muscle

The *iliococcygeus*, the most posterior part of the levator ani muscles, arises from the ATLA and the ischial spines. Muscle fibers from one side join those from the opposite side in the midline between the anus and coccyx. This meeting line is termed the *iliococcygeal raphe*, which contributes to the *anococcygeal body*. This portion forms a relatively flat, horizontal shelf, which spans the potential gap from one pelvic sidewall to the other. In addition to the iliococcygeus, some fibers of the pubococcygeus muscle pass behind the rectum and attach to the coccyx. These fibers course cephalad to the iliococcygeus muscle, and along with attachments of the superficial part of the external anal sphincter, also contribute to the anococcygeal body. The *levator plate* is a clinical term used to describe the anococcygeal body (Fig. 2.8); it forms a supportive shelf on which the rectum, upper vagina, and uterus rest.[22]

Puborectalis muscle

The *puborectalis* represents the medial and most inferior fibers of the levator ani muscle that arise on either side from the pubic bone and form a U-shaped sling behind the anorectal junction. Fibers of this muscle blend with the deep part of the external anal sphincter muscle. The puborectalis muscle fibers are oriented such that muscular contraction draws the anorectal junction toward the pubic bones and contributes to the *anorectal angle*.[20] The importance of the puborectalis and anorectal angle in anal continence is best appreciated in women with chronic fourth-degree lacerations who maintain fecal continence.

Urogenital hiatus and levator hiatus

Within the pelvic diaphragm is a U-shaped opening in the pelvic floor muscles, called the levator hiatus, through which the urethra, vagina, and rectum pass. This is also the opening through which pelvic organ prolapse occurs. The opening through which the urethra and vagina pass is the *urogenital hiatus* (see Fig. 2.6). This latter hiatus is separated from the anus by the perineal body (see Fig. 2.8).

Innervation of the pelvic diaphragm

The pelvic diaphragm muscles are primarily innervated by direct somatic efferents from the third through the fifth sacral nerve roots (S3–S5). These are appropriately called the nerve to the coccygeus and nerve to the levator ani muscles (see Fig. 2.6). However, a dual innervation to the levator muscle has traditionally been described, where the perineal (or inferior) surface of the muscle is supplied by branches of the pudendal nerve.[23,24] Recent data, however, suggests the pudendal does not contribute significantly to levator muscle innervation.[16,25]

CONNECTIVE TISSUE ELEMENTS OF SUPPORT

The pelvic connective tissue represents the "passive" support of the pelvis. It consists of parietal fascia, which lines the walls of the abdominopelvic cavity and

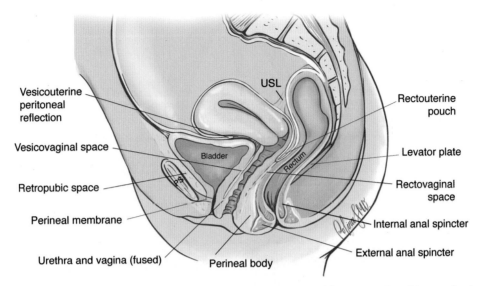

FIGURE 2.8 Pelvic organs and surgical spaces. USL, uterosacral ligament; PS, pubic symphysis.

covers the pelvic sidewall and pelvic floor muscles; the visceral fascia, which surrounds the pelvic viscera and allows for independent organ function; and the extra-serosal fascia, which surrounds blood vessels, nerves, and lymph channels in their path from the pelvic side-wall to the pelvic organs. The most obvious example of extraserosal fascia in the pelvis is the cardinal ligament of the uterus.

Pelvic Fascia

All connective tissue within the pelvis is interconnected and is collectively known as the endopelvic fascia. However, the composition of this tissue varies depending on function.

The fascia that invests the striated muscles that lines the walls of the abdomen and pelvis is known as *parietal fascia*. This fascia consists of a mechanically dense matrix of predominantly collagen fibers which weave together to form a tough three-dimensional sheet. A common example of parietal fascia in the ab-domen is the rectus fascia, which can be easily dissected away from the rectus muscles and reapproximated with sutures during closure of an abdominal incision. In the pelvis, condensations of the obturator fascia, such as the ATFP and ATLA, serve important functions, as dis-cussed earlier.

In contrast to parietal fascia, *visceral pelvic fascia* surrounds the pelvic viscera, and it allows for indepen-dent and proper function of each organ. It consists of a loose mesh-like matrix of collagen, elastin, and smooth muscle, and it lacks the dense collagen composition associated with conventional fascia, such as the rec-tus fascia.[26] Nonetheless, it contributes to pelvic organ support.

Lastly, *extraserosal fascia* is a term used to de-scribe condensations of connective tissue that join

pelvic viscera to pelvic side wall structures. It is a generic term of exclusion used to describe any other fascia lying inside the parietal fascia and outside the visceral fascia. Examples of this tissue include the car-dinal and uterosacral ligaments. Extraserosal fascia provides a flexible conduit for pelvic nerves, vessels, and lymphatics, and thus, it resembles a mesentery-like structure.[27] A critical role of the cardinal and utero-sacral ligaments is to mechanically suspend the pelvic viscera over the pelvic floor.

Levels of Support

Although the connective tissue support of the pelvis is a seamless, interdependent web, pelvic organ support can be better understood when separated into three levels described by DeLancey (Fig. 2.9).[21]

Level 1 (apical support)

Level 1 refers to support of the cervix and upper one-third of the vagina and is provided by the parametrium (cardinal and uterosacral ligaments) and its distal exten-sions, the paracolpium. This tissue attaches the upper vagina and cervix to the pelvic wall, suspending it over the pelvic floor. Thus, level 1 support is also known as the suspensory axis, and it provides connective tissue support to the vaginal apex after hysterectomy.[28] In the standing or anatomic position, level 1 support fibers are both vertically oriented (cardinal ligaments) and hori-zontally oriented (uterosacral ligaments).[29]

Uterosacral ligament

The uterosacral ligaments attach broadly at the pre-sacral and coccygeus fascia proximally and to the pos-terolateral walls of the cervix and upper vagina distally. They define the lateral boundaries of the rectouterine

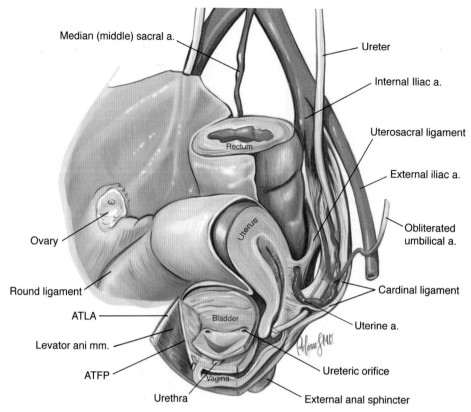

FIGURE 2.9 Pelvic organ support structures. a., artery; mm., muscles.

pouch (posterior cul-de-sac) and are positioned lateral to the rectum and medial to the ureters. The ureters are thus susceptible to injury during surgical procedures that involve the uterosacral ligaments.

The ureter courses lateral to the uterosacral ligament and lies closest to the ligament at the level of the cervix. In one cadaveric study, the mean distance from the ureter to the uterosacral ligament was 4.1, 2.3, and 0.9 cm at the levels of the sacrum, ischial spine, and cervix, respectively.[17,30,31]

The sacral nerves lie close to the ligament at the level of the ischial spine, where suspension sutures are typically placed. Cadaveric studies have shown that sacral nerves S1, S2, and S3 are in proximity to the ligament, but S3 seems most susceptible to entrapment during uterosacral ligament suspensions.[17,32,33]

The uterosacral ligament is divided into a superficial and a deep component. Although the superficial portion of the ligament is largely composed of smooth muscle and connective tissue, higher content of autonomic nerve fibers is found in the deep part.[27]

Cardinal ligament

In contrast to the uterosacral ligaments, the attachment points of the cardinal ligament are less well defined. They extend from the pelvic sidewalls, near the origin of the internal iliac artery to the lateral walls of the pelvic organs. The cardinal ligaments consist of a "mesentery-like" connective tissue network that convey blood vessels and nerves to target organs.[34]

The cranial part of the ligament consists of a perivascular sheath of connective tissue that conveys internal iliac branches to the pelvic viscera. The caudal or deeper portion of the ligament is relatively less vascular and has higher density of nerve fibers from the inferior hypogastric plexus.

The ureter passes within a parametrial "tunnel" before entering the bladder wall at the ureterovesical junction. This tunnel roughly separates the anterior fibers of the cardinal ligament from the posterior fibers of the uterosacral ligament. A higher density of nerve tissue is found posterior to the ureter.[31]

Level 2 (midvaginal support)

Level 2 refers to support of the midvagina and is provided by the attachments of paracolpium to the ATFP and to the fascia of the levator ani muscles (see Figs. 2.7 and 2.9). This level of support is also known as the attachment axis.

The paracolpium represents the distal extension of the parametrium along the lateral walls of the vagina. It transmits blood vessels and nerves and is continuous with the visceral fascia that surrounds the vagina and the vaginal adventitia.[26] These lateral attachments of the vaginal walls create the anterior and posterior vaginal sulci which give the vagina an "H" shape when viewed in cross section. This continuity of connective tissue from one pelvic sidewall to the other provides support to the bladder and urethra.[35]

Attachment of the anterior vaginal wall to the levator ani muscles can aid bladder neck elevation and may have significance for stress urinary continence and vaginal wall prolapse.

Similar to the anterior vaginal wall, the posterior vaginal wall also attaches to the pelvic sidewall fascia.

Level 3 (distal vaginal support)

Level 3 refers to support for the distal vagina and is provided by the fusion of the distal vaginal walls with its surrounding structures (Fig. 2.10). Level 3 supports is also known as the fusion axis. Anteriorly, the vagina is fused with the urethra.[36,37] Laterally, it attaches to the perineal membrane and pubovaginalis muscle and posteriorly to the perineal body.

Perineal membrane

The perineal membrane, previously known as the urogenital diaphragm, is a complex three-dimensional mass of connective tissue with attachments to the urethra, distal vagina, ATFP, ischiopubic rami, and the perineal body (see Fig. 2.10). Although it has been traditionally described as a trilaminar musculofascial structure pierced by the vagina and urethra, this simplistic view of the perineal membrane fails to recognize its interconnectivity with the rest of the endopelvic fascial components of the pelvic floor. Rather, it has been described as consisting of a dorsal and a ventral as well as a pelvic (proximal) and a perineal (distal) portion.[38,39]

The perineal membrane separates the superficial pouch from the deep pouch of the urogenital (anterior) perineal triangle. The dorsal portion of the membrane consists of bilateral transverse fibrous bands of connective tissue that attach the perineal body and lateral walls of the vagina to the ischiopubic rami. This portion is associated with the ischioanal fossa fat cranially and with the vestibular bulbs, clitoral crura, and perineal muscles caudally. The ventral part of the membrane is part of a solid, three-dimensional mass of tissue within which the external urethral sphincter, compressor urethrae, and sphincter urethrovaginalis are embedded.[40] The pelvic margin of the ventral part blends with the ATFP as this structure inserts into the pubic bone. Here, the perineal membrane complex is also continuous with the levator ani muscle fascia. Medially, the perineal membrane fuses with the walls of the urethra and distal vagina and with itself at the midline, where it contributes to the perineal body.

Perineal body

The perineal body is a three-dimensional mass of fibromuscular tissue found between the distal vagina and vestibule anteriorly and the anus posteriorly (see Fig. 2.10). It is formed by contributions from several structures. The bulbospongiosus, transverse perineal, and anal sphincter muscles contribute at superficial level; the perineal

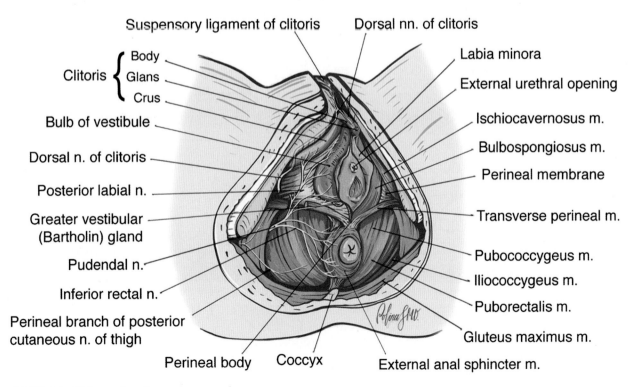

FIGURE 2.10 Vulva and perineum. m., muscle; n., nerve.

membrane, which attaches to the vaginal wall at the level of the hymen, contributes at a deeper level; lastly, the puboperinealis portion of the pubococcygeus muscle adds to the perineal body at a deeper level.[38] In the midsagittal plane, the perineal body has a triangular shape with a distal base (see Fig. 2.8). The perineal body is thickest and densest distally, below the hymen level, and then becomes progressively thinner at its cranial end, by the anorectal junction. Both the length (from hymen to midanus) and the height (from skin to apex) of the perineal body in this plane are 3 to 4 cm. The perineal body typically extends 2 to 3 cm above the level of the hymen.[41]

Mechanical studies of the perineal body have shown that when the distal rectum is subjected to increased force directed caudally, the fibers of the perineal membrane become tight and resist further displacement. These fibers derive their lateral support from their attachment to the pelvic bones at the ischiopubic rami.[42,43] With disruptions in these fibers (as would be observed during an obstetric laceration), the distal posterior vagina wall loses its normal support and rectocele may develop.

LOWER URINARY TRACT

Within the pelvis, the urinary tract includes the pelvic ureters, bladder, vesical neck, and urethra.

Ureters

The ureters are flexible muscular tubes that transmit urine from the kidneys to the bladder. They are approximately 22 to 30 cm long with approximately half their length in the pelvis. The lumen of the ureters is lined by transitional epithelium, which lies on a substratum of smooth muscle arranged in a circular orientation. The muscular wall is surrounded by an adventitial connective tissue layer that is closely adherent to the peritoneum and carries the ureter's blood supply.[31] In the abdomen, the ureter receives its blood supply from medially derived vessels such as the renal, ovarian, and common iliac arteries (Fig. 2.11).

The ureters exit the medial aspect of the renal pelvis and course inferiorly and medially over the psoas

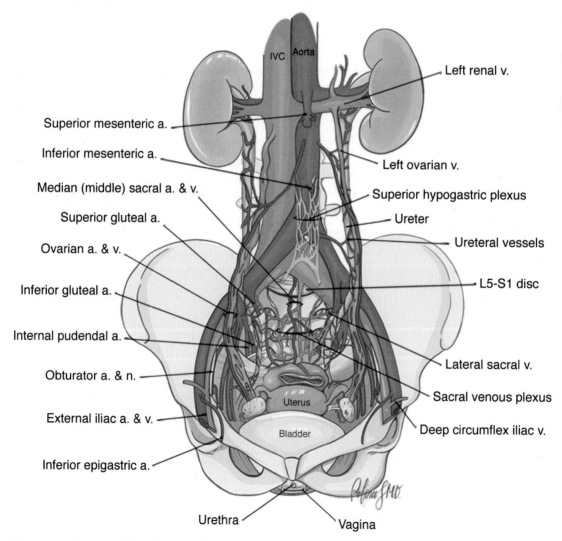

FIGURE 2.11 Ureter and blood vessels. IVC, inferior vena cava; v., vein; a., artery; n., nerve.

muscles in the retroperitoneal space. They enter the pelvis by passing over the bifurcation of the common iliac artery or the proximal part of the external iliac artery, just medial to the ovarian vessels. The ureter then descends on the pelvic sidewall retroperitoneal space where its adventitial layer remains attached to the peritoneum. This explains why the ureter remains adhered to the peritoneum, in the "medial leaf" of the broad ligament, when the retroperitoneal space is entered. Along this course, the ureter lies lateral and ventral to the uterosacral ligaments and medial to the internal iliac artery branches (internal iliac, uterine, superior vesicals, and vaginal arteries). Thus, the plane of dissection for ureterolysis should be kept medial to the ureter to avoid devascularization injuries.[31]

The ureter then passes under the uterine artery near the level of the uterine isthmus, and here, it lies approximately 1 to 2 cm lateral to the cervix. It then enters the parametrium and courses within a "ureteral tunnel" surrounded by loose areolar tissue that allows for its peristalsis. Within this tunnel, the ureter roughly separates the anterior fibers of the cardinal ligament from the posterior fibers of the uterosacral ligament. The ureter then travels anteromedially toward the bladder base and in this path, it runs close to the proximal third of the anterior vaginal wall. Lastly, the ureter courses obliquely within the bladder wall for approximately 1.5 cm to terminate at the ureteric orifices.[30,31]

Bladder

The bladder is a hollow viscus, the wall of which is composed of course bundles of smooth muscle fibers, known as the *detrusor muscle*, which extends to the upper part of the urethra. The mucosal lining of the bladder consists of transitional epithelium and lamina propria, which rests on a loose submucosal layer.

Anteriorly, the bladder lies against the inner surface of the pubic bones, and when it fills, it also lies against the anterior abdominal wall. Here, the bladder is in contact with the loose areolar tissue that fills the retropubic space and lacks a peritoneal covering. This extraperitoneal portion is preferred for intentional cystotomy to prevent fistula formation with abdominopelvic organs. Posteriorly, the bladder rests against the vagina and cervix and also lacks a peritoneal covering. In the midline, the apex of the bladder is continuous with the *median umbilical* ligament, which is a remnant of the embryologic urachus.

The bladder is divided into a body (dome) and fundus (base) approximately at the level of the ureteric orifices. The dome of the bladder is thin walled and distensible and is covered by peritoneum. The bladder base is thicker and undergoes less distension with filling than the bladder dome.[21] It consists of the trigone and the detrusor loops. The detrusor loops are two bands of muscle fibers found at the *vesical neck*, which is the

part of the urinary bladder immediately surrounding the internal orifice of the urethra.

The blood supply to the bladder arises from the superior vesical arteries and variably from the middle and inferior vesical arteries. In women, the latter two vessels are often replaced by the vaginal and internal pudendal arteries.[44] The bladder muscle is innervated by the vesical plexus, a component of the inferior hypogastric plexus, which also supplies the smooth muscle of the urethra.[45]

Urethra

The female urethra is 3.5 to 4 cm long, and its distal two-thirds are fused with the anterior vaginal wall. The proximal urethral lumen begins within the bladder at the *internal urethral orifice* (meatus). It then courses within the wall of the bladder in the region called the *bladder neck*. The external urethral orifice is found at the vestibule, between the clitoral body and vaginal orifice.

The lumen of the urethra is lined by hormonally sensitive stratified squamous epithelium. Pseudostratified columnar and transitional epithelium are also found. A spongy submucosal layer that contains a prominent vascular plexus is thought to contribute to continence by forming a watertight seal via "coaptation" of the mucosal surface. Within the submucosal layer, on the dorsal (vaginal) surface of the urethra, is a group of glands known as the paraurethral glands, which open into the urethral lumen. Infection and obstruction of these glands can lead to urethral diverticula.[46] The duct openings of the two most prominent glands, called the Skene glands, are seen on the surface of the external urethral orifice at the vestibule, at approximately the 5 and 7 o'clock positions. Surrounding the submucosa are two layers of smooth muscle: an inner longitudinal and an outer circular layer, which are in turn surrounded by a circular layer of skeletal muscle known as the external urethral sphincter. Approximately at the junction between the middle and lower third of the urethra, and just proximal (deep) to the perineal membrane, two small skeletal muscles, called the compressor urethrae and sphincter urethrovaginalis, are found. These two muscles were previously known as the deep transverse perineal muscles in females.[47] Together with the external urethral sphincter, they form the striated urogenital sphincter complex (Fig. 2.12). These three skeletal muscles function as a unit and have an incompletely understood innervation. Direct branches of S2–S4 that reach the muscles from their pelvic surface as well as the perineal branch of the pudendal nerve are thought to contribute.[25]

This complex primarily consists of type 1 (slow twitch) fibers and thus contributes to urinary continence by providing constant tone; it also provides emergency reflex activity, mainly in the distal half of the urethra, when continence is threatened.[37]

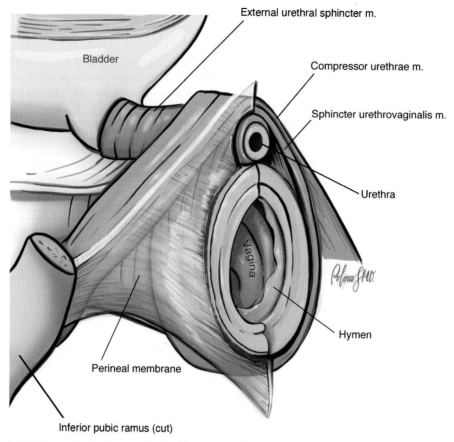

FIGURE 2.12 Striated urogenital sphincter muscles. m., muscle.

The walls of the urethra in its distal third, below the perineal membrane, primarily consist of fibrous tissue and serves as the nozzle that directs the urine stream.

Anatomy of Urinary Continence

In order for urinary continence to be maintained, the pressure within the urethra must be higher than that within the bladder. Given the dynamic nature of the bladder and the pelvic floor, this is a complex process that is not fully understood. Current theories suggest that urethral closing pressure is maintained by a combination of urethral constriction and urethral support.

The constrictive forces of the urethra are maintained by the urethral submucosal vasculature, smooth muscle, and striated musculature. Each of these elements is believed to contribute equally to urinary continence.

In addition to the constrictive forces, the endopelvic fascia associated with the anterior vaginal wall is also important in maintenance of urinary continence, especially during times of increased intra-abdominal pressure. Because the distal two-thirds of the urethra are fused with the anterior vaginal wall, urethral support functionally hinges on the presence of intact vaginal wall support. The fascia that invests the striated urethral muscles blends with the connective tissue within the paracolpium, which in turns attaches to the distal part of the ATFP,

levator muscle, and the ventral part of the perineal membrane. Thus, increases in intra-abdominal pressure—as may take place during a cough or a sneeze—accompanied by contraction of the pelvic floor results in vaginal and urethral elevation. Functionally, the anterior vaginal wall and its endopelvic fascial attachments to the pelvic sidewall create a backstop against which the urethra compresses, effectively preventing the leakage of urine by increasing the pressure within the lumen of the urethra relative to the bladder.[21] Thus, constriction of the urethral lumen via its intrinsic structures maintains urine in the bladder at rest but during sudden increases in abdominal pressure, continence is additionally maintained through a passive reliance on the endopelvic fascia.

PELVIC INNERVATION

Components of the autonomic nervous system in the pelvis include the *superior and inferior hypogastric plexuses* and hypogastric nerves (Fig. 2.13). The pelvic viscera (bladder, urethra, vagina, uterus, and rectum) and erectile structures in the perineum (clitoris and vestibular bulbs) are innervated by fiber extensions from the inferior hypogastric plexus.

The *superior hypogastric plexus*, often called the *presacral nerve*, is an extension of the aortic and inferior mesenteric plexuses, found anterior and below the aortic bifurcation. This plexus primarily contains sympathetic

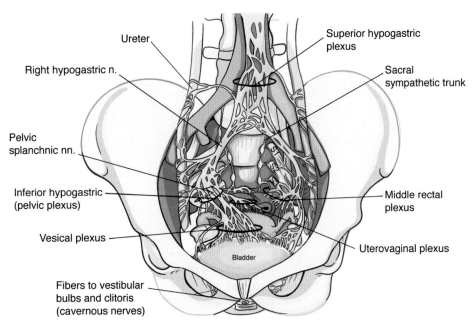

FIGURE 2.13 Pelvis autonomic innervation. n., nerve; nn., nerves.

fibers and sensory afferent fibers from the uterus and terminates by dividing into the right and left hypogastric nerves. These nerves join parasympathetic efferents from the second through the fourth sacral nerve roots (pelvic splanchnic nerves) to form the *inferior hypogastric plexus*, also known as the *pelvic plexus*. In addition, the inferior hypogastric plexus generally receives contributions from the *sacral sympathetic trunk*.[45]

The inferior hypogastric plexus is a mixed plexus containing sympathetic and parasympathetic fibers that variably accompany the distal branches of the internal iliac artery to the pelvic viscera. Accordingly, this plexus is divided into three portions: the *vesical, uterovaginal* (Frankenhäuser ganglion), and *middle rectal plexuses*. Extensions of the inferior hypogastric plexus reach the perineum by passing through the paracolpium and innervate the clitoris and vestibular bulbs via the cavernous nerve.

Injury to the inferior hypogastric plexus during cancer debulking, lymphadenectomy, or other extensive pelvic surgeries can lead to varying degrees of voiding, defecatory, and sexual dysfunction. For example, radical hysterectomy is associated with 70% to 85% rates of bladder dysfunction, 17% to 91% bowel dysfunction, and 33% to 65% sexual dysfunction.[48,49] Although less documented, similar dysfunction is also possible during incontinence or prolapse procedures where sutures or trocars are passed through the paravaginal and paraurethral tissue.[50,51]

Pudendal Nerve

The pudendal nerve provides both motor and sensory innervation to the perineal region. The cell bodies of the motor neurons of the pudendal nerve are located in the anterior horn of the sacral spinal cord, in a region called Onuf's nucleus. Its fibers are primary derived from S3 with variable contributions from S2 and S4. The pudendal nerve forms within the pelvis, close to the superior surface of the sacrospinous ligament and inferior to the piriformis muscle. It exits the pelvis through the greater sciatic foramen by passing behind the sacrospinous ligament, just medial to the ischial spine. It then enters the perineum through the lesser sciatic foramen. On the lateral walls of the ischioanal fossa, the pudendal nerve enters a fascial tunnel known as the pudendal canal (Alcock canal). This canal is formed from a splitting of the fascia covering the medial surface of the obturator internus muscle and is approximately 4 cm long (Figs. 2.5 and 2.14).[9,18] The nerve then separates into three terminal branches. Of these, the largest is the perineal nerve, which supplies the labia via the posterior labial nerves and the muscles in the superficial perineal pouch (bulbospongiosus, ischiocavernosus, and transverse perineal). A branch of this nerve contributes to the innervation of the striated urogenital sphincter muscles within the deep perineal pouch. The dorsal nerve of the clitoris innervates the glans and prepuce of the clitoris. The inferior rectal nerve innervates the external anal sphincter and the skin in the perianal region. Thus, the pudendal nerve is important for urinary and anal continence and also for sexual function.

PELVIC BLOOD SUPPLY

The pelvic organs are supplied by the visceral branches of the internal iliac artery and by direct branches of the abdominal aorta. The internal iliac artery generally divides in the area of the greater sciatic foramen into two clinically recognized divisions (see Fig. 2.6). The *iliolumbar*, *lateral sacral*, and *superior gluteal arteries*

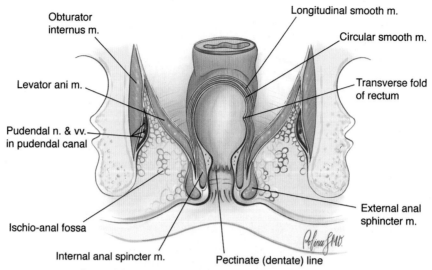

FIGURE 2.14 Ischioanal fossa and anal sphincter complex. m., muscle; n., nerve; vv., veins.

are branches of the posterior division that supply non-visceral structures. These branches generally arise from the posterolateral wall of the internal iliac artery, approximately 3 to 4 cm from its origin.[52] The *internal pudendal, obturator,* and *inferior gluteal arteries* are parietal (nonvisceral) branches that arise from the anterior division. The remaining branches of the anterior division supply pelvic viscera (uterus, vagina, rectum, and bladder). These include the *uterine, vaginal, middle rectal,* and the *superior vesical arteries.* The superior vesical arteries commonly arise from the patent part of the umbilical arteries. Branches that supply the inferior part of the bladder and proximal urethra are present in women, but typically stem from the vaginal arteries and internal pudendal, respectively. The middle rectal arteries are generally small-caliber vessels and may be absent.

The two most important direct branches of the aorta that contribute to pelvic organ blood supply are the superior rectal and ovarian arteries. The *superior rectal artery* is the terminal branch of the inferior mesenteric artery; it anastomoses with the middle rectal arteries on the dorsal surface of the rectum and thus contributes to its blood supply. The *ovarian arteries* anastomose with the ascending branch of the uterine artery within the mesosalpinx and contribute to the blood supply of the uterus and adnexa. Other important anastomoses between the aorta and internal iliac arteries include those between the median (middle) sacral and lateral sacral arteries and between the lumbar and iliolumbar arteries.

EXTRAPERITONEAL SURGICAL SPACES

Retropubic Space

The *retropubic space,* also called the *prevesical space,* is a potential extraperitoneal surgical space that lies between the bladder and the pubic bones. This space is filled with loose connective and adipose tissue and contains important neurovascular structures. The space is bounded by the pubic bones and pelvic sidewall muscles (obturator internus and levator ani) anterolaterally. The bladder and proximal urethra, as well as their endopelvic fascial attachments to the pelvic sidewall and to the cardinal ligament, represent the posterior boundary. When the bladder fills, the retropubic space extends into the abdominal cavity, and consequently, the anterior abdominal wall also contributes to its anterior boundary. The adipose tissue within this space is continuous with that of the extraperitoneal layer of the anterior abdominal wall (preperitoneal fat), which is found between the transversalis fascia and the peritoneum.

Vessels and nerves that pass through this space include the dorsal vein of the clitoris, which passes below the inferior border of the pubic symphysis before draining into the vesical venous plexus. This plexus consists of several rows of veins which are embedded in the paravaginal connective tissue and eventually drain into the internal iliac vein (Fig. 2.15).

Fibers of the inferior hypogastric plexus that innervate the bladder, urethra, and erectile structures in the vulva are also embedded within the paravaginal tissue and course on the inferolateral walls of the bladder and urethra.[53] Disruption of these fibers during incontinence or prolapse procedures may lead to voiding and sexual dysfunction.[50]

The obturator neurovascular bundle courses along the lateral pelvic sidewall and passes through the obturator canal to supply the muscles and skin of the medial thigh compartment. In most women, accessory obturator vessels, which arise from or drain into the inferior epigastric or external iliac vessels, cross the superior pubic rami and connect with the main obturator vessels near the obturator canal. Bleeding in this area may be difficult to control as veins retract into the pelvic bones.

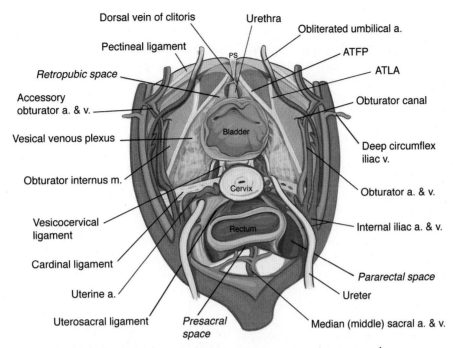

FIGURE 2.15 Extraperitoneal surgical spaces. a., artery; v., vein; m., muscle.

The *paravesical space* is a surgical term used to describe that portion of the retropubic space found lateral to the obliterated umbilical or the superior vesical arteries. The external iliac vessels represent the superolateral boundary and the cardinal ligament the posterior boundary. The main and accessory obturator vessels are found in this part of the retropubic space.

Presacral Space

Surgical entry into the presacral space is required for sacrocolpopexy and other procedures such as presacral neurectomies, lymphadenectomy, and tumor resection.

This extraretroperitoneal space lies between the rectosigmoid and posterior abdominal wall peritoneum anteriorly and the sacrum posteriorly. The presacral space begins below the aortic bifurcation and extends inferiorly to the pelvic diaphragm muscles. The lateral boundaries are the common and internal iliac vessels and the fascia covering the piriformis muscle and lumbosacral nerve plexus.

Between the peritoneum and the sacrum lies a substantial adipose tissue layer which contains the superior hypogastric plexus and hypogastric nerves. The right hypogastric nerve is often encountered during sacrocolpopexy dissection. As discussed earlier, the hypogastric nerves course toward the lateral pelvic walls to join the pelvic splanchnic nerves in forming the inferior hypogastric plexus. In addition, the sacral sympathetic trunk, a continuation of the lumbar trunk, is found on the anteromedial aspect of sacral foramina.

The presacral space contains an extensive venous plexus called the *sacral venous plexus*. This plexus is primarily formed by connections between the median (middle) and lateral sacral veins and is adherent to the ventral surface of the sacrum. The plexus also receives contributions from the lumbar veins of the posterior abdominal wall and from the basivertebral veins that pass through the anterior sacral foramina. Thus, bleeding in this region may be difficult to control as veins retract into the sacral foramina. The *middle sacral vein* generally drains into the left common iliac vein, but in some cases, it drains directly into the inferior vena cava or into the right common iliac vein. The *lateral sacral veins* drains into the internal iliac vein and ultimately into the caval system. The *middle sacral artery* courses in proximity to the vein and arises from the posterior and distal part of the abdominal aorta. It passes posterior to the left common iliac vein to reach the presacral space (see Fig. 2.15).

Cadaveric studies of the presacral space suggest that the anterior surface of the first sacral vertebra (S1) is the optimal location for mesh fixation during sacrocolpopexy.[6,54,55] Several critical structures are found within 3 cm from the midpoint of the sacral promontory, which represents the most superior aspect of the first sacral vertebra. These include the ureter, iliac vessels, and the first sacral nerve.

In the supine, surgical position, the most prominent nonvascular presacral space structure is the L5–S1 disc, which extends approximately 1.5 cm cephalad to the "true" sacral promontory.[55] Thus, surgeons often use this area for graft fixation. However, septic discitis and osteomyelitis are reported complications of sacrocolpopexy. In addition, the left common iliac vein is the closest major vessel identified both cephalad and lateral to the midsacral promontory. The average distance of this vein from the midsacral promontory is 2.7 cm (range 0.9 to 5.2 cm).[6,54] Thus, precise identification of the ligament and the left common iliac vein is critical if sutures or metal tacks are placed above the sacral promontory. Awareness of the average 60° drop between the anterior surfaces of L5 and S1 vertebrae helps with intraoperative localization of the anatomic or "true" promontory and avoidance of the L5–S1 disc.

Vesicocervical and Vesicovaginal Space

The *vesicocervical space* begins below the vesicouterine peritoneal fold, which represents the loose attachments of the peritoneum in the vesicouterine pouch (anterior cul-de-sac) (see Fig. 2.8). This potential surgical space continues inferiorly as the *vesicovaginal space*, which extends to the junction of the proximal and middle thirds of the urethra. Below this point, the urethra and vagina fuse.[36] These spaces are filled with loose connective tissue or visceral fascia, which allows for ease of dissection when separating the bladder from the cervix and anterior vaginal walls during abdominal hysterectomy and sacrocolpopexy.

The vaginal walls consist of three layers. A nonkeratinized squamous epithelium with underlying lamina propria line the vaginal lumen. This is surrounded by a muscular layer and then an outer adventitial layer. These latter two form the fibromuscular component of the vagina. The visceral fascia is intimately associated with the vaginal adventitia, and together, this connective tissue is continuous with the paracolpium (paravaginal connective tissue), which attaches the vaginal wall to the pelvic sidewall at the ATFP.

When dissected in the operating room, this fibromuscular combination of muscularis and adventitia represents the surgeon's "fascia."[26,46]

Rectovaginal Space

The rectovaginal space is a potential surgical space that lies immediately adjacent to the posterior surface of the midvagina. It extends from the rectouterine pouch (posterior cul-de-sac) superiorly to the superior border (apex) of the perineal body inferiorly. As discussed earlier, the perineal body extends 2 to 3 cm cephalad to the hymen (see Fig. 2.8).[41] The posterior cul-de-sac peritoneum extends down the posterior vaginal wall 2 to 3 cm inferior to the cervicovaginal junction.[41] The inferior extensions of the uterosacral ligament fibers, also known as rectal pillars, are fibers of the posterior parametrium that extend down from the cervix and attach to the upper portion of the posterior vaginal wall. These fibers connect the vagina to the lateral walls of the rectum and to the sacrum. They also separate the midline rectovaginal space from the more lateral pararectal space. Similar to the vesicovaginal space, the rectovaginal space contains loose areolar tissue and is easily

opened with finger dissection during sacrocolpopexy or rectopexy procedures.[56]

A topic that remains controversial in this region is the existence of a separate layer of fascia, the so-called rectovaginal fascia (rectovaginal septum) between the walls of the vagina and rectum in females. Although some studies have found evidence of this fascia, many histologic studies have failed to show a separate layer of surgically useful fascia between the walls of the vagina and the rectum.[57,58] Thus, similar to the anterior vaginal wall, the fibromuscular combination of muscularis and adventitia in the posterior vaginal wall represents the surgeon's "fascia."

The visceral fascia in the rectovaginal space is also intimately associated with the vaginal adventitia and together, this connective tissue is continuous with the paracolpium, which attaches the posterior vaginal wall to the obturator and levator fascia.

PUDENDUM (VULVA) AND UROGENITAL TRIANGLE

The female external genitalia consists of the pudendum, or vulva, which lie within the urogenital (anterior) triangle of the perineum (see Fig. 2.10). The vulva consists of the *mons pubis, labia majora, labia minora, clitoris, bulbs of vestibule,* and the *vestibule* with its associated vestibular and paraurethral glands and urethral and vaginal orifice.

Urogenital (Anterior) Triangle

An arbitrary line between the ischial tuberosities separates the perineum into an anterior or *urogenital triangle* and a posterior or *anal triangle* (see Fig. 2.3). Vulvar structures are found within the *urogenital triangle.* This triangle is further divided into a subcutaneous, superficial, and deep pouches (also called spaces or compartments).

Subcutaneous pouch

This is a potential space between the deep membranous layer of the subcutaneous tissue (previously called Colles fascia) and the fascia that invests the perineal muscles. The membranous layer of subcutaneous tissue attaches to the ischiopubic rami laterally and to each other posteriorly. Medially, this layer of tissue attaches to the vestibule and to the perineal body. These medial, lateral, and posterior attachments prevent the spread of fluid, blood, or infection from the subcutaneous perineal pouch to the thighs, posterior perineal triangle, or contralateral side. However, as the deep membranous layer of the subcutaneous tissue in the abdominal wall (previously called Scarpa fascia) is continuous with that of the perineum, extravasations or collections in this compartment may extend into the anterior abdominal wall or into the labia majora.

Superficial pouch

This space of the anterior triangle is a fully enclosed compartment that lies between the fascia that invests the perineal muscles and the perineal membrane. The perineal muscles include the *ischiocavernosus*, *bulbospongiosus*, and *transverse perineal*. Also included within this compartment are the vestibular bulbs, clitoral crus, clitoral body, greater vestibular (Bartholin) glands, and branches of the internal pudendal vessels and pudendal nerve. The urethra and vagina traverse this space.

The perineal membrane attaches firmly to the ischiopubic rami laterally and to each other posteriorly. Medially, the membrane firmly attaches to the urethra, distal vagina, and perineal body. These medial, lateral, and posterior attachments prevent the spread of fluid, blood, or infection from the superficial perineal pouch to the thighs, posterior perineal triangle, or contralateral side.[38]

Deep pouch

This space is found between the perineal membrane and the inferior fascia of the pelvic diaphragm. In contains the anterior recess of the ischioanal fossa fat, parts of the urethra and striated urogenital sphincter complex, and branches of the pudendal nerve and internal pudendal vessels. This space is continuous with the posterior perineal triangle and thus with the contralateral side (see Fig. 2.10).

Vulvar Structures

The *mons pubis* lies over the pubic bones and consists of fatty tissue covered in hair-bearing skin. The *labia majora* are the posterior continuation of the mons pubis and are similarly composed of adipose tissue covered by hair-bearing skin. The subcutaneous tissues of the labia majora and the mons pubis are a continuation of the subcutaneous tissues of the anterior abdominal wall. They consist of a fatty superficial layer and a deeper membranous layer which are known as the *fatty layer of subcutaneous tissue* (formerly Camper fascia), and the *membranous layer of subcutaneous tissue* (formerly Colles fascia). The round ligament of the uterus, a remnant of the embryonic *gubernaculum* and the obliterated *processus vaginalis* (canal of Nuck), an embryonic developmental outpouching of peritoneum, pass through the inguinal ligament and terminate in the subcutaneous tissue of the labia majora. Incomplete obliteration of the processus vaginalis may lead to indirect inguinal hernias or hydrocele of the canal of Nuck.

The mons pubis and labia majora are innervated by the genital branch of the genitofemoral nerve and by the anterior labial nerves, which are branches of the ilioinguinal nerve. The labia majora also receives innervation from the posterior labial nerves, which are derived from the perineal branch of the pudendal nerve.

Seen between the two labia majora within the *pudendal cleft* are the *labia minora, vestibule,* and *glans of the clitoris*. Unlike the labia majora, the labia minora are hairless and do not contain adipose. Rather, these cutaneous folds lie on a loosely organized connective-tissue stratum which permits mobility of the labial skin during intercourse. Posteriorly, the labia join in the midline to form the *frenulum of the labia minora* (also known as *fourchette*). Anteriorly, each labium minus bifurcates to form two folds that surround the glans of the clitoris. The more anterior folds unite to form the distal end of the prepuce, which partially or completely covers the glans of clitoris and is often referred to as the hood of the clitoris. The more posterior folds insert into the underside of the glans as the frenulum of clitoris. Although devoid of erectile tissue, the labia minora are adjacent to the vestibular bulbs and in contact with the glans of the clitoris. Thus, stimulation of these highly innervated structures may contribute to sexual arousal.

The vaginal vestibule lies between the clitoris anteriorly and the fourchette posteriorly and is bordered laterally by the line of Hart (where labial epithelial pigmentation ends) and by the hymen medially. The vestibule contains the urethral and vaginal orifices and the openings of the greater vestibular (Bartholin) and paraurethral (Skene) glands. The greater vestibular glands open into the vaginal vestibule via two small duct openings at the 5 and 7 o'clock positions.

Clitoris and Associated Structures

The clitoris and bulbs of the vestibule are two prominent erectile structures found in the superficial pouch of the urogenital perineal triangle.

The vestibular bulbs are 3 to 5 cm oblong erectile structures which lay lateral to the vaginal vestibule and are firmly adherent to the perineal membrane. Their posterior ends are wider and are in contact with the greater vestibular glands. Their anterior ends are tapered and connect to one another at the commissure of the bulbs, found between the undersurface of the clitoral body and the ventral surface of the distal urethra. The vestibular bulbs are composed of erectile tissue that is less dense than that found in the body and crura of the clitoris, with wider lacunae lined by finer trabeculae. The bulbs are innervated by distal extensions of the inferior hypogastric plexus.

The clitoris consists of the body, crura, and the glans. The *body of the clitoris* is lined by the *prepuce*. The glans is partially covered by the distal part of the prepuce, colloquially called the hood of the clitoris. This part is continuous with the anterior fold of the labia minora.

The glans is approximately 8 mm long and is the only part of the clitoris that is directly visualized during examination. It consists of dense fibroconnective tissue with interspersed blood vessels and prominent nerve bundles. The glans is innervated by the *dorsal nerves of the clitoris, which also innervates the skin of the prepuce.*

The body and the crura of the clitoris consist of erectile tissue that is surrounded by a dense fibroconnective tissue layer known as the tunica albuginea. The paired crura are attached to the medial surface of the inferior pubic rami and are partially covered by the ischiocavernosus muscle. Each crus courses anteriorly and medially and joins at the lower part of the anterior pubic symphysis to form the *body of clitoris.* The body of the clitoris consists of paired corpora cavernosa which are separated in the midline by a fibrous septum, the septum of corpora cavernosa. The clitoral body consists of a proximal part, which is firmly attached to the pubic symphysis, and a distal part that is covered anteriorly and laterally by the prepuce of the clitoris. The distal body is oriented inferoposteriorly at an approximately 90° angle from the proximal body. The body is approximately 2 to 3 cm in length and is partially external.[59] The body is capped distally by the glans of the clitoris. The body and crura of the clitoris are innervated by the cavernous nerves, which are distal extensions of the inferior hypogastric plexus. These nerves course at the 2 and 10 o'clock positions of the anterior vaginal wall and then 5 and 7 o'clock positions along the urethra; they enter the perineum by passing under the pubic arch (Fig. 2.16). On the dorsal surface of the body of the clitoris, the cavernous nerves course alongside the dorsal nerves of the clitoris.[60]

The clitoris is supported by deep and superficial suspensory structures known as the *fundiform ligament* and the *suspensory ligament of the clitoris,* respectively. The fundiform ligament is a condensation of fibroconnective tissue that descends from the linea alba above the pubic symphysis and then splits and surrounds the body of the clitoris before fusing with the clitoral fascia. The suspensory ligament of the clitoris is a superficial condensation of the membranous layer of the subcutaneous tissue which helps to support and position the clitoral body.

The *dorsal nerves of the clitoris* are the terminal branches of the pudendal nerve that innervate the glans and prepuce of the clitoris (see Figs. 2.10 and 2.16). These nerves perforate the dorsal part of the perineal membrane and course within a connective tissue sheath between the crus of the clitoris and the medial surface of the ischiopubic ramus. They then emerge from the lateral surface of the crus and pass deep to the dense connective tissue layers that blend with the suspensory ligament and the clitoral fascia. On the surface of the clitoral body that is covered by the prepuce, the nerves pass between the tunica albuginea and the clitoral fascia, approximately at the 11 and 1 o'clock positions, before penetrating the substance of the glans, which it innervates. Along this latter course, the dorsal nerves give multiple cutaneous branches to the skin of the prepuce.[25,53,61] Removal of the prepuce and vulvar skin lateral to the midline of the clitoral body might lead to injury during dissection or suture placement that extends deep to the subcutaneous tissue and clitoral fascia. As this nerve provides sensation to the glans, injury may result in decreased sensation, pain syndromes, and sexual dysfunction.

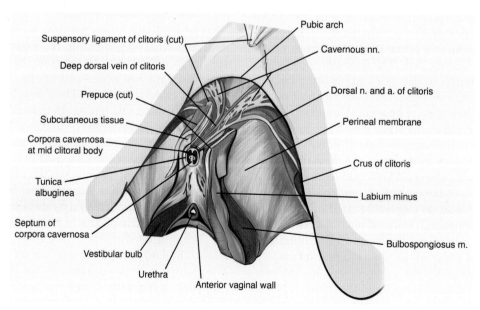

FIGURE 2.16 Clitoral body cross section and clitoris innervation. NOTE: Suspensory ligament cut and clitoral body displaced from pubic symphysis to expose autonomic nerves. nn., nerves; n., nerve; a., artery; m., muscle.

CONCLUSION

In order to reduce risk of surgical complications and improve patient safety, the gynecologic surgeon should have a thorough understanding of female pelvic anatomy. Although there are guiding principles and relationships that are seen in most cases, pelvic anatomy is not a static set of structures and should be understood in terms of function as well as structure. As pelvic surgeons, we should recognize that our current understanding is a dynamic process which will continue to grow and change as the literature evolves.

References

1. Barber MD. Contemporary views on female pelvic anatomy. *Cleve Clin J Med* 2005;72(Suppl 4):S3–S11.
2. Mattox TF, Lucente V, McIntyre P, et al. Abnormal spinal curvature and its relationship to pelvic organ prolapse. *Am J Obstet Gynecol* 2000;183(6):1381–1384.
3. Nguyen JK, Lind LR, Choe JY, et al. Lumbosacral spine and pelvic inlet changes associated with pelvic organ prolapse. *Obstet Gynecol* 2000;95(3):332–336.
4. Sze EH, Kohli N, Miklos JR, et al. Computed tomography comparison of bony pelvis dimensions between women with and without genital prolapse. *Obstet Gynecol* 1999;93(2):229–232.
5. Handa VL, Pannu HK, Siddique S, et al. Architectural differences in the bony pelvis of women with and without pelvic floor disorders. *Obstet Gynecol* 2003;102(6):1283–1290.
6. Florian-Rodriguez ME, Hamner JJ, Corton MM. First sacral nerve and anterior longitudinal ligament anatomy: Clinical applications during sacrocolpopexy. *Am J Obstet Gynecol* 2017;217(5):607.e1–607.e4.
7. Balgobin S, Good MM, Dillon SJ, et al. Lowest colpopexy sacral fixation point alters vaginal axis and cul-de-sac depth. *Am J Obstet Gynecol* 2013;208(6):488.e1–488.e6.
8. White AB, Carrick KS, Corton MM, et al. Optimal location and orientation of suture placement in abdominal sacrocolpopexy. *Obstet Gynecol* 2009;113(5):1098–1103.
9. Montoya TI, Calver L, Carrick KS, et al. Anatomic relationships of the pudendal nerve branches. *Am J Obstet Gynecol* 2011;205:504.e1–504.e5.
10. Drewes PG, Marinis SI, Schaffer JI, et al. Vascular anatomy over the superior pubic rami in female cadavers. *Am J Obstet Gynecol* 2005;193(6):2165–2168.
11. Varenika V, Lutz AM, Beaulieu CF, et al. Detection and prevalence of variant sciatic nerve anatomy in relation to the piriformis muscle on MRI. *Skeletal Radiol* 2017;46(6):751–757.
12. Wan-Ae-Loh P, Huanmanop T, Agthong S, et al. Evaluation of the sciatic nerve location regarding its relationship to the piriformis muscle. *Folia Morphol (Warsz)* 2020;79(4):681–689.
13. Beaton LE, Anson B. The sciatic nerve and the piriformis muscle: Their interrelation a possible cause of coccygodynia. *J Bone Joint Surg* 1938;20(3):686–688.
14. Bartret AL, Beaulieu CF, Lutz AM. Is it painful to be different? Sciatic nerve anatomical variants on MRI and their relationship to piriformis syndrome. *Eur Radiol* 2018;28(11):4681–4686.
15. Natsis K, Totlis T, Konstantinidis GA, et al. Anatomical variations between the sciatic nerve and the piriformis muscle: A contribution to surgical anatomy in piriformis syndrome. *Surg Radiol Anat* 2014;36(3):273–280.
16. Barber MD, Bremer RE, Thor KB, et al. Innervation of the female levator ani muscles. *Am J Obstet Gynecol* 2002;187(1):64–71.
17. Wieslander CK, Roshanravan SM, Wai CY, et al. Uterosacral ligament suspension sutures: Anatomic relationships in unembalmed female cadavers. *Am J Obstet Gynecol* 2007;197(6):672.e1–672.6.
18. Maldonado PA, Stuparich MA, McIntire DD, et al. Proximity of uterosacral ligament suspension sutures and S3 sacral nerve to pelvic landmarks. *Int Urogynecol J* 2017;28(1):77–84.
19. Kim J, Betschart C, Ramanah R, et al. Anatomy of the pubovisceral muscle origin: Macroscopic and microscopic findings within the injury zone. *Neurourol Urodyn* 2015;34(8):774–780.
20. Betschart C, Kim J, Miller JM, et al. Comparison of muscle fiber directions between different levator ani muscle subdivisions: In vivo MRI measurements in women. *Int Urogynecol J* 2014;25(9):1263–1268.
21. Ashton-Miller JA, Howard D, DeLancey JO. The functional anatomy of the female pelvic floor and stress continence control system. *Scand J Urol Nephrol Suppl* 2001;(207):1–7; discussion 106–125.
22. Nandikanti L, Sammarco AG, Kobernik EK, et al. Levator ani defect severity and its association with enlarged hiatus size, levator bowl depth, and prolapse size. *Am J Obstet Gynecol* 2018;218:537–539.
23. Enck P, Hinninghofen H, Wietek B, et al. Functional asymmetry of pelvic floor innervation and its role in the pathogenesis of fecal incontinence. *Digestion* 2004;69(2):102–111.
24. Wallner C, Maas CP, Dabhoiwala NF, et al. Innervation of the pelvic floor muscles: A reappraisal for the levator ani nerve. *Obstet Gynecol* 2006;108(3 Pt 1):529–534.
25. Yucel S, De Souza A Jr, Baskin LS. Neuroanatomy of the human female lower urogenital tract. *J Urol* 2004;172(1):191–195.
26. Otcenasek M, Baca V, Krofta L, et al. Endopelvic fascia in women: Shape and relation to parietal pelvic structures. *Obstet Gynecol* 2008;111(3):622–630.
27. Ramanah R, Berger MB, Parratte BM, et al. Anatomy and histology of apical support: A literature review concerning cardinal and uterosacral ligaments. *Int Urogynecol J* 2012;23(11):1483–1494.
28. Balgobin S, Jeppson PC, Wheeler T II, et al. Standardized terminology of apical structures in the female pelvis based on a structured medical literature review. *Am J Obstet Gynecol* 2020;222(3):204–218.
29. Chen L, Ramanah R, Hsu Y, et al. Cardinal and deep uterosacral ligament lines of action: MRI based 3D technique development and preliminary findings in normal women. *Int Urogynecol J* 2013;24(1):37–45.
30. Rahn DD, Bleich AT, Wai CY, et al. Anatomic relationships of the distal third of the pelvic ureter, trigone, and urethra in unembalmed female cadavers. *Am J Obstet Gynecol* 2007;197(6):668.e1–668.e4.
31. Jackson LA, Ramirez DMO, Carrick KS, et al. Gross and histologic anatomy of the pelvic ureter: Clinical applications to pelvic surgery. *Obstet Gynecol* 2019;133(5):896–904.
32. Montoya TI, Dillon SJ, Balgobin S, et al. Functional and anatomic comparison of 2 versus 3 suture placement for uterosacral ligament suspension: A cadaver study. *Am J Obstet Gynecol* 2013;209:486.e1–486.e5.
33. Siddiqui NY, Mitchell TRT, Bentley RC, et al. Neural entrapment during uterosacral ligament suspension: An anatomic study of female cadavers. *Obstet Gynecol* 2010;116(3):708–713.

34. Luo J, Smith TM, Ashton-Miller JA, et al. In vivo properties of uterine suspensory tissue in pelvic organ prolapse. *J Biomech Eng* 2014;136(2):021016–0210166.

35. Yavagal S, de Farias TF, Medina CA, et al. Normal vulvovaginal, perineal, and pelvic anatomy with reconstructive considerations. *Semin Plast Surg* 2011;25(2):121–129.

36. Hamner JJ, Carrick KS, Ramirez DMO, et al. Gross and histologic relationships of the retropubic urethra to lateral pelvic sidewall and anterior vaginal wall in female cadavers: Clinical applications to retropubic surgery. *Am J Obstet Gynecol* 2018;219(6):597.e1–597.e8.

37. Li J-R, Lei L, Luo N, et al. Architecture of female urethral supporting structures based on undeformed high-resolution sectional anatomical images. *Anat Sci Int* 2021;96(1):30–41.

38. Stein TA, DeLancey JO. Structure of the perineal membrane in females: Gross and microscopic anatomy. *Obstet Gynecol* 2008;111(3):686–693.

39. Kato M, Matsubara A, Murakami G, et al. Female perineal membrane: A study using pelvic floor semiserial sections from elderly nulliparous and multiparous women. *Int Urogynecol J Pelvic Floor Dysfunct* 2008;19(12):1663–1670.

40. Hinata N, Murakami G. The urethral rhabdosphincter, levator ani muscle, and perineal membrane: A review. *Biomed Res Int* 2014;2014:906921.

41. Maldonado PA, Carrick KS, Montoya TI, et al. Posterior vaginal compartment anatomy: Implications for surgical repair. *Female Pelvic Med Reconstr Surg* 2020;26(12):751–757.

42. Clark NA, Brincat CA, Yousuf AA, et al. Levator defects affect perineal position independently of prolapse status. *Am J Obstet Gynecol* 2010;203(6):595.e17–595.e22.

43. Lewicky-Gaupp C, Yousuf A, Larson KA, et al. Structural position of the posterior vagina and pelvic floor in women with and without posterior vaginal prolapse. *Am J Obstet Gynecol* 2010;202(5):497.e1–497.e6.

44. de Treigny OM, Roumiguie M, Deudon R, et al. Anatomical study of the inferior vesical artery: Is it specific to the male sex? *Surg Radiol Anat* 2017;39(9):961–965.

45. Ripperda CM, Jackson LA, Phelan JN, et al. Anatomic relationships of the pelvic autonomic nervous system in female cadavers: Clinical applications to pelvic surgery. *Am J Obstet Gynecol* 2017;216(4):388.e1–388.e7.

46. Mazloomdoost D, Westermann LB, Mutema G, et al. Histologic anatomy of the anterior vagina and urethra. *Female Pelvic Med Reconstr Surg* 2017;23(5):329–335.

47. Oelrich TM. The striated urogenital sphincter muscle in the female. *Anat Rec* 1983;205(2):223–232.

48. Unger CA, Tunitsky-Bitton E, Muffly T, et al. Neuroanatomy, neurophysiology, and dysfunction of the female lower urinary tract: A review. *Female Pelvic Med Reconstr Surg* 2014;20(2):65–75.

49. Derks M, van der Velden J, Frijstein MM, et al. Long-term pelvic floor function and quality of life after radical surgery for cervical cancer: A multicenter comparison between different techniques for radical hysterectomy with pelvic lymphadenectomy. *Int J Gynecol Cancer* 2016;26(8):1538–1543.

50. Bekker MD, Hogewoning CR, Wallner C, et al. The somatic and autonomic innervation of the clitoris; preliminary evidence of sexual dysfunction after minimally invasive slings. *J Sex Med* 2012;9(6):1566–1578.

51. Pace G, Vicentini C. Female sexual function evaluation of the tension-free vaginal tape (TVT) and transobturator suburethral tape (TOT) incontinence surgery: Results of a prospective study. *J Sex Med* 2008;5(2):387–393.

52. Bleich AT, Rahn DD, Wieslander CK, et al. Posterior division of the internal iliac artery: Anatomic variations and clinical applications. *Am J Obstet Gynecol* 2007;197(6):658.e1–658.e5.

53. Jackson LA, Hare AM, Carrick KS, et al. Anatomy, histology, and nerve density of clitoris and associated structures: Clinical applications to vulvar surgery. *Am J Obstet Gynecol* 2019;221(5):519.e1–519.e9.

54. Wieslander CK, Rahn DD, McIntire DD, et al. Vascular anatomy of the presacral space in unembalmed female cadavers. *Am J Obstet Gynecol* 2006;195(6):1736–1741.

55. Good MM, Abele TA, Balgobin S, et al. Preventing L5-S1 discitis associated with sacrocolpopexy. *Obstet Gynecol* 2013;121(2 Pt 1):285–290.

56. Baessler K, Schuessler B. Abdominal sacrocolpopexy and anatomy and function of the posterior compartment. *Obstet Gynecol* 2001;97(5 Pt 1):678–684.

57. Zhu X-M, Yu G-Y, Zheng N-X, et al. Review of Denonvilliers' fascia: The controversies and consensuses. *Gastroenterol Rep (Oxf)* 2020;8(5):343–348.

58. Dariane C, Moszkowicz D, Peschaud F. Concepts of the rectovaginal septum: Implications for function and surgery. *Int Urogynecol J* 2016;27(6):839–848.

59. O'Connell HE, Sanjeevan KV, Hutson JM. Anatomy of the clitoris. *J Urol* 2005;174(4 Pt 1):1189–1195.

60. Oakley SH, Mutema GK, Crisp CC, et al. Innervation and histology of the clitoral-urethal complex: A cross-sectional cadaver study. *J Sex Med* 2013;10(9):2211–2118.

61. Puppo V. Anatomy and physiology of the clitoris, vestibular bulbs, and labia minora with a review of the female orgasm and the prevention of female sexual dysfunction. *Clin Anat* 2013;26(1):134–152.

CHAPTER 3

BIOMECHANICS OF THE PELVIC FLOOR

John O. L. DeLancey • Anne G. Sammarco • Payton Schmidt

Introduction

Understanding pelvic floor disorders requires an understanding of biomechanics, which is the study of how structures of the body (e.g., muscles, ligaments, and connective tissues) respond to forces or displacements. This is just as important as, for example, knowing the principles of endocrinology is to understanding many reproductive gynecologic abnormalities. First, one must understand normal pelvic support—including what the critical components are and how they provide support individually and in combination. Then, pelvic floor disorders that occur due to failures in this biomechanical system can be understood. Furthermore, how operative approaches attempt to correct these failures can help us understand why treatments succeed and fail. This chapter describes the basic principles and experimental evidence in support of—normal pelvic support, failures that lead to pelvic organ prolapse, and how treatments aim to address these failures.

BASIC PRINCIPLES: HOW DO THE PELVIC FLOOR STRUCTURES WORK TOGETHER?

Structural Factors that Prevent Prolapse

As is true throughout the body, both muscles and connective tissues work together and are essential for structural support. Normal pelvic organ support is provided by the interaction between the levator ani muscles (LAMs) and the connective tissues that attach the uterus and vagina to the pelvic sidewalls (cardinal and uterosacral ligaments).

There are three basic structural strategies involved in normal pelvic support (Fig. 3.1). First, connective tissues attach the uterus and vaginal walls to the inside of the pelvis and provide stability by absorbing load and limiting movement. Second, the pelvic floor muscles provide closure of the vaginal opening, which prevents prolapse from occurring. Vaginal closure within the high-pressure zone acts in the same way that, for

example, the anal sphincters work. Stool does not fall out of the rectum because of the occlusive effect of the high-pressure anal canal. And third, as seen in a lateral view, these two individual biomechanical systems interact with and complement one another, thereby maintaining support even if an imbalance in one of these systems occurs.

Biomechanical Principles

The way in which these factors interact to provide pelvic organ support can be seen in Figure 3.2[1] and a glossary of selected biomechanical terms needed to understand pelvic organ support is provided in Table 3.1.

The LAMs hold the pelvic floor closed and provide closing forces to prevent pelvic floor descent by creating a high-pressure zone in the lower vagina.[2] In this situation, the closing forces in the anterior and posterior compartments are equal and opposing, creating **balanced pressures** (pressure is the measure of how much force is acting on an area). The LAMs maintain a balanced system and therefore remain closed—in response to increased forces (e.g., rise in abdominal pressure during Valsalva), thereby preventing prolapse. The cardinal and uterosacral ligaments provide lifting forces that resist persistent downward descent of the pelvic organs by temporarily lengthening in response to increased force (due to their elastic properties) and absorbing any increases in force (due to their stiffness). This illustrates the principle of **alignment** within the biomechanical system of the pelvis, which depends on the muscles being strong enough to keep the hiatus closed and the connective tissues strong enough to resist deformation in order to hold the organs in place in response to increased load (e.g., during a cough).

When the muscles, nerves, and fascial structures involved in creating the vaginal high-pressure zone that holds the hiatus closed are damaged or weakened, the hiatus in the LAM complex can easily be pushed open. This is the principle of **deformation under load**. If the muscles, under the control of complex neural reflexes, fail to hold the hiatus closed, the vaginal walls descend so that one or both vaginal walls protrude below and through the levator hiatus. When the vaginal walls

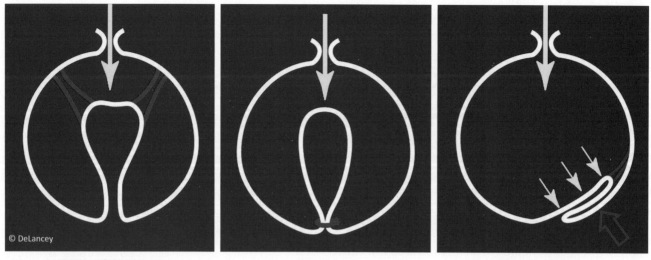

**Attachment:
Suspension**

**Hiatus:
Closure**

**Alignment:
Interactions**

FIGURE 3.1 Concepts of pelvic organ support. The basic principles of support are shown. Attachment of the vagina to the pelvic walls, closure of the vagina by muscle action at the hiatus, and the role of alignment allowing interactions between vaginal walls and surrounding structures. The *yellow arrow* indicates increased pressure, and the *red arrow*, support provided by the pelvic muscles. NOTE: **Right panel** is a lateral view. (© John O. L. DeLancey.)

descend below the hymen to the level where the levators no longer maintain proper alignment of the system, **unbalanced pressures** occur, creating a **pressure differential** between abdominal and atmospheric pressure. The **force** created by this pressure differential is like the one that moves a sailboat. The difference in pressure between two sides of a sail, for example, creates a force that propels the boat in a certain direction. In an anterior vaginal wall prolapse, abdominal pressure acts on the vaginal wall to create a downward force due to its **misalignment**. This force then places abnormal tension on the tissues that attach the uterus and vagina to the pelvic walls.

The size of the surface that is exposed to this pressure differential of exposed vagina matters. **Pressure can**

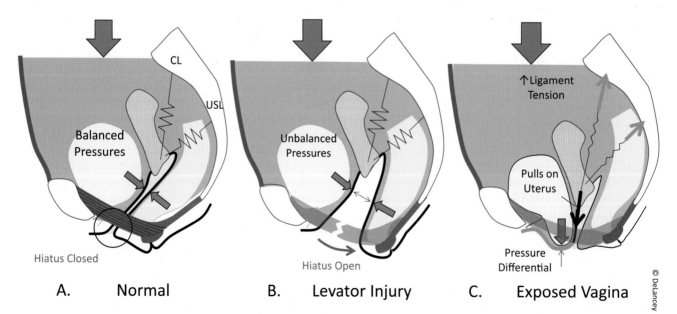

FIGURE 3.2 Diagrammatic representation of interactions between LAM, anterior vaginal wall prolapse, and cardinal ligament (CL)/uterosacral ligament (USL) suspension. With normal levator function (**A**), the vaginal walls are in apposition, and anterior and posterior pressures are balanced. Levator damage (**B**) results in hiatal opening, and the vagina becomes exposed to a pressure differential between abdominal and atmospheric pressures. This pressure differential (**C**) creates a traction force on the CL and USL. (© John O. L. DeLancey.)

TABLE 3.1	
Glossary of Terms	
TERM	**DEFINITION**
Pressure	The amount of force exerted over an area. This parameter has no direction.
Alignment	Correct positioning of the muscles, ligaments, and tendons within a biomechanical system that allows the system to effect optimal functioning
Deformation	Change in shape, length, or location in response to increased load
Deformation under load	The ability of a material, tissue, or complex structure to withstand permanent deformation in response to applied forces
Force	Any interaction (e.g., push or pull) on an object that affects the object's position or movement
Structural interaction	Interaction between two or more subsystems allowing them to withstand and respond to forces on the system as a whole
Elasticity	The ability of a material to return to its original size and shape after deformation
Hyperelastic property	Nonlinear elastic response to large deformation loads

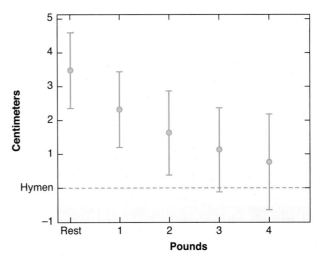

FIGURE 3.3 Location of the cervix relative to the hymeneal ring with varying amounts of traction force in 73 patients without clinical evidence of prolapse. Decreasing location of the cervix with varying amounts of traction. Positive numbers are cephalic to the hymen and measurements are made to the lateral border of the cervix.

be expressed as force per unit area. That means that if there is 1 sq in of vagina exposed and the pressure differential is 1 lb/sq in, then there would be 1 lb of force on the ligaments and fascia resisting this downward force. The same 1 lb/sq in of pressure applied to 2 sq in results in 2 lb of force, etc. In more familiar units, 100 cm H_2O applied during Valsalva to 1 sq in results in 1.42 lb. Now, the larger the exposed area, the greater the force. As a cystocele enlarges, the force produced by the same pressure increases in a **positive feedback loop**. This explains why a woman can push hard with only a small descent of the anterior wall, but as the prolapse becomes a little more exposed, a greater change is seen.

The cardinal and uterosacral ligaments that attach the uterus and vagina to the pelvic walls are important to support of the pelvic organs by providing lifting forces. Their ability to maintain alignment in the pelvis is dictated by their material properties of stiffness, which is the ability to resist deformation (change in shape or length) in response to increased load, and elasticity, which is the ability to stretch (or lengthen) in response to increased force and then return to the original state when that force is removed. The cardinal and uterosacral ligaments have a normal range of lengthening, and in response, the pelvic organs have a normal range of movement. When you pull on the cervix as you would during a dilation and curettage (D&C), it

lengthens the cardinal ligament somewhat like a spring. However, unlike an elastic spring, where doubling the force doubles the descent, the ligament gets stiffer the more it is elongated (Fig. 3.3). This is called a **hyperelastic property**. With increasing load, there is less and less elongation until an elastic limit is reached. At this point, additional load does not increase descent, as the cardinal ligament cannot stretch anymore. Any further descent would involve tearing in the short term or tissue changes in the long term.

Because the ligaments are elastic, this lengthening phenomenon is reversible and the pull on the cervix during D&C does not cause prolapse. However, Davis law states that connective tissue responds to *chronic* and *excessive* force with **tissue adaptation**. A skin expander is a good example of this, where it is possible to double the amount of skin present in 6 to 8 weeks by subjecting it to constant increased force. If the cardinal ligament is subjected to excessive downward force over time because the hiatus is not closed and the vaginal wall is subjected to a pressure differential, it can remodel to become longer.

The degree to which the vaginal wall moves downward in this situation has to do with the properties of the ligaments and fascial structures connecting it to the pelvic walls. Both the **stiffness and length** of the ligaments are involved. If the connective tissues are too lax or too long to hold the organs in alignment, the vaginal walls and uterus descend below the normal LAMs and the same imbalance in pressure can occur. Because these tissues are "stretchy," some movement is normal, such as that seen during D&C, where the cervix can easily be drawn down to the introitus.

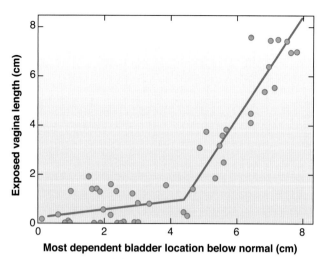

FIGURE 3.4 Illustration of bilinear relationship, or threshold effect. The threshold effect is illustrated here in the relationship between bladder descent and the size of a cystocele, measured as the length of the vagina exposed at the introitus to atmospheric pressure on magnetic resonance imaging (MRI). Note that at about 4 cm, the relationship changes.

Another important concept concerns the principle of **structural interactions**. All the different anatomical elements in the pelvic floor interact with one another. The muscles that close the pelvic floor may be strong enough to support the organs under light loads. Under these conditions, increases in abdominal pressure may not cause any displacement. However, once the threshold that overcomes the ability of the muscles to resist the downward force is reached, the pelvic floor opens. This is a **threshold effect**.[3] In some systems, if you double

the load, you double the displacement. In other systems, a certain load must be reached before any change happens. The pelvic floor remains closed until enough force develops to open it. Once the hiatus is opened, the vaginal wall descends and is exposed to a pressure differential. With less than that opening force, it does not matter how much pressure there is—no opening occurs and no exposed vagina is subjected to the pressure differential. But once this threshold is exceeded, the pelvic floor opens, the structures become misaligned, and the pressure differential comes into play (Fig. 3.4). Failure of the hiatus to remain closed affects connective tissue loading.

Failure analysis is a foundational aspect of engineering. If a plane crashes or a bridge falls, the exact cause of the failure is rigorously sought and lessons learned. This type of failure analysis has now been applied to the pelvic floor to determine the causes of prolapse and, as a powerful tool, to understand why certain women have recurrence after surgery. The next section describes the evidence to support how these support systems fail. 3D stress magnetic resonance imaging (MRI) has facilitated this type of analysis, allowing the many competing hypotheses to be tested scientifically.

Levels of Support

A brief overview of the regional differences or levels of support will help in our further consideration of how these principles affect normal and abnormal pelvic organ support (Fig. 3.5). We briefly describe the levels of

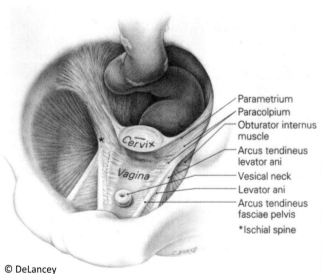

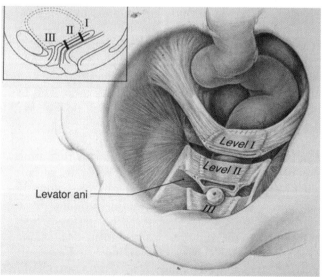

FIGURE 3.5 Lateral attachments of the vagina and cervix to the lateral sidewalls. The **left panel** shows a view of the pelvic organs from above looking over the pubic symphysis showing structures of the pelvic sidewall in relationship to the vagina (outlined by *dotted line*) after removal of the bladder and uterine corpus. The **right panel** shows different levels of support in a posthysterectomy cadaver. The parametrium and paracolpium are two portions of the cardinal ligament. Arcus tendineus fasciae pelvis and arcus tendineus levator ani refer to the fascial and levator arches respectively. (Reprinted from DeLancey JO. Anatomic aspects of vaginal eversion after hysterectomy. *Am J Obstet Gynecol* 1992;166[6 Pt 1]:1717–1728. Copyright © 1992, with permission from Elsevier.)

support and then provide more detail on how the attachment factors and the hiatal closure factors are each known to fail in prolapse.

In level 1, the cervix and upper third of the vagina are attached to the pelvic walls by mesenteric structures that suspend these organs (cardinal and uterosacral ligaments). In level 2, the middle third of the vagina is attached laterally to the arcus tendineus fascia pelvis (ATFP), which we refer to as the fascial arch for simplicity's sake. This fascial arch can also be seen from the posterior compartment.[4] It is important to remember that the cardinal and uterosacral "ligaments" have the structure of a mesentery, carrying neurovascular tissue to the organs. They do have a structural function of attachment but should never be confused with the dense regular connective tissue that comprises skeletal ligaments.

HIATUS FUNCTION AND FAILURE

The word *hiatus* derives from the Latin *hiare* meaning to gape or yawn. The ability of various structures to keep the hiatus from gaping is one of the most fundamental aspects of pelvic organ support. The connective tissue and neuromuscular structures surrounding the lower third of the vagina create a high-pressure zone[2] that holds the vagina closed (Fig. 3.6). If the hiatus is closed, it protects the connective tissues from being subjected to forces that would injure them. The advent of clinical assessment and modern imaging—both ultrasound and MRI—has proven the central role that hiatal closure failure plays in the cause of prolapse and prolapse recurrence after surgery.[5-8] The structures that lie in this high-pressure zone that affect hiatal closure include the medial portion of the levator ani, the perineal membrane, and the perineal body.

Perineal Membrane

The perineal membrane (formerly known as the urogenital diaphragm) is a dense triangular membrane with a central opening through which the vagina and urethra pass.[9,10] In its ventral aspect, the urethra, anterior vaginal wall, and perineal membrane are fused together as a single solid mass that is attached to the pubic bone laterally. This is quite different than the dorsal aspect, which is like a sheet of tissue. The LAMs attach to the cranial surface of the perineal membrane and to the perineal body, forming the perineal complex responsible for hiatal closure. Failures in the perineal membrane and perineal body are poorly understood at this time. Their structure clearly indicates their importance; yet, the exact role these structures play in maintaining hiatal closure is unclear.

Levator Ani Anatomy

Activity and integrity of the LAMs are primary factors in hiatal closure. This unusual muscle demonstrates constant tonic activity that is adjusted to offset changes in loading that occur during activities.[11] The LAM consists of three primary subdivisions: pubovisceral (i.e., pubococcygeal), iliococcygeal, and puborectal (Fig. 3.7). The pubovisceral muscle originates from the inner surface of the pubis and has three components: the pubovaginal, which attaches to the vagina; the puboperineal, which attaches in the perineal body; and the puboanal, which inserts between the internal and external anal sphincters.[12] We have chosen to use the term *pubovisceral muscle* rather than *pubococcygeal* because it more accurately describes the origin and insertion.[13] The iliococcygeal muscle (ICM) is a thin sheet of muscle that spans the pelvic canal between its bilateral

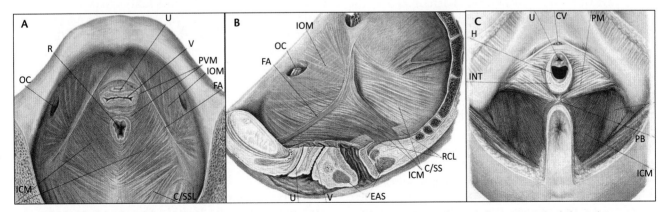

FIGURE 3.6 Three views of the hiatus, levator ani, and perineal membrane. Views shown after removal of the pelvic organs, from above (**A**), in sagittal view (**B**), and from below (**C**), including the perineal membrane. OC, obturator canal; R, rectum; U, urethra; V, vagina; PVM, pubovisceral muscle; IOM, internal obturator muscle; FA, fascial arch; ICM, iliococcygeal muscle; C/SSL, coccygeus/sacrospinous; EAS, external anal sphincter; RCL, recto-coccygeal ligament; H, hymen; CV, clitoral vessels; PM, perineal membrane; INT, introitus; PB, perineal body. (From Halban J, Tandler J. *Anatomie und Atiologie der Genital prolapse biem Weibe.* Vienna and Leipzig: Wilhelm Braumüller, 1907.)

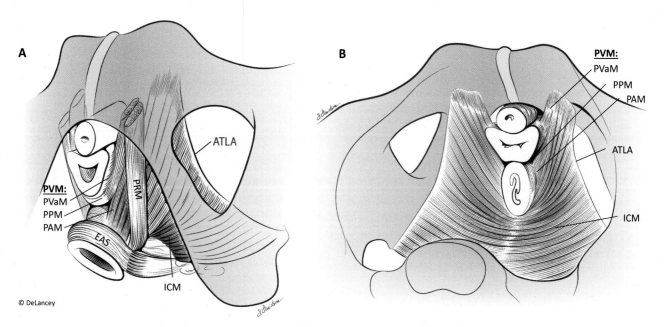

FIGURE 3.7 Levator ani anatomy. **A:** LAMs from below after the vulvar structures and perineal membrane have been removed. ATLA, arcus tendineus levator ani ("levator arch"); PRM, puborectal muscle; PVM, pubovisceral muscle; PVaM, pubovaginal muscle; PPM, puboperineal muscle; PAM, puboanal muscle; EAS, external anal sphincter; ICM, iliococcygeal muscle. (© DeLancey; modified from Kearney R, Sawhney R, DeLancey JO. Levator ani muscle anatomy evaluated by origin-insertion pairs. *Obstet Gynecol* 2004;104[1]:168–173.)

origin at the arcus tendineus levator ani, we refer to as the "levator arch" for simplicity's sake. The puborectal muscle originates on the inside of the pubic bones, near the perineal membrane, and courses laterally to the other parts of the LAMs. It forms a sling behind the rectum and is distinct from the pubovisceral muscle.

Levator Ani and Anal Sphincter Lines of Action

The action of pelvic floor muscles is determined by the muscle fiber direction, the muscle shape, and the points of attachment. Each muscle of the LAM complex provides action in a different vector, but they all activate at roughly the same time so that their combined actions result in one coordinated motion. If one component (muscle) of the LAM complex is lost, only that specific vector is affected. Understanding each muscle's direction of action provides insight into how injury to a specific muscle contributes to overall failure of the system. This is particularly important given that the pubovisceral muscle is involved in obstetrical injury while others remain intact.[14] Figure 3.8 shows the mean fiber directions for the pubovisceral and puborectal components[15] measured in MRI images of normal women. The pubovisceral muscle fibers course 41° above the horizontal in the standing posture. By contrast, the puborectal muscles act 19° below the horizontal. Therefore, with loss of the pubovisceral muscle, both

hiatal elevation and muscle constriction are affected, whereas if the puborectal were to be injured or weakened, only constriction would be affected.

Conceptual Model for Changes that Happen in the Pelvic Floor

There are several ways in which changes in the pelvic floor are discussed and measured. Figure 3.9 shows a conceptual model. The most familiar changes are those in the urogenital and levator hiatus that enlarge with childbirth and prolapse. In addition, the more dorsal component of the pelvic floor, in the region of the ICM, expands with age—even in the absence of childbirth.[16] It is possible to see how these changes affect both the levator plate angle that is often discussed as well as the levator bowl volume—that is, the volume held within the shape of the pelvic floor.

Evidence that Hiatal Closure Is Important

There is strong evidence that hiatal failure is associated with prolapse.[7] Hiatal enlargement precedes the occurrence of prolapse, indicating a causal relationship.[8] During the first 20 years after giving birth, a quarter of women with an enlarged hiatus who were followed prospectively developed prolapse at least 1 cm below the hymenal ring.[17] For a woman with

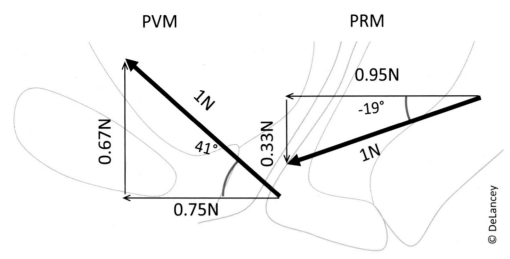

FIGURE 3.8 Horizontal and vertical components of the pubovisceral muscle (PVM) and puborectal muscles (PRM) in the standing posture. The *thick arrows* show the average direction of the lines of action of the pubovisceral and puborectal muscles relative to the horizontal with a theoretical 1-N force. *Thin arrows* indicate the portion of each horizontal force related to a closing function and vertical force related to a lifting function. NOTE: Vectors are shown larger than the background anatomy to avoid an overlap in the display. (Modified from Betschart C, Kim J, Miller JM, et al. Comparison of muscle fiber directions between different levator ani muscle subdivisions: In vivo MRI measurements in women. *Int Urogynecol J* 2014;25[9]:1263–1268.)

a 3-cm hiatus (distance from urethra to perineal body) on physical exam, the estimated median time to develop prolapse would be 33 years, whereas for a woman with a hiatus of 4.5 cm, it would be 6 years.[17] Prolapse is also more common with reduced muscle strength (odds ratio, 0.87 per 5 cm H_2O). Prolapse was associated with levator avulsion (odds ratio, 4.2) and hiatus area and strength mediated 61% of the association is between avulsion and prolapse. This proves the first hypothesis in our model (see Fig. 3.2) indicating the essential role of hiatal closure in the development of prolapse.

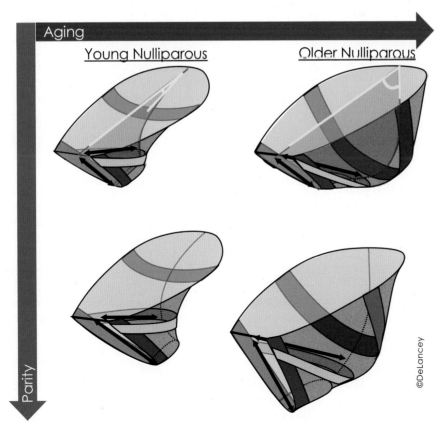

FIGURE 3.9 Conceptual model for pelvic floor changes. Pelvic floor changes resulting from aging and vaginal parity, where parity primarily affects urogenital and levator hiatus size *(black arrows)* and age affects the midsagittal area *(light blue shading)*. Levator plate angle *(yellow lines)* is also shown. Muscle bands: *red,* pubovisceral; *gold,* puborectal; *blue,* iliococcygeal. (© DeLancey; modified from Swenson CW, Masteling M, DeLancey JO, et al. Aging effects on pelvic floor support: A pilot study comparing young versus older nulliparous women. *Int Urogynecol J* 2020;31[3]:535–543.)

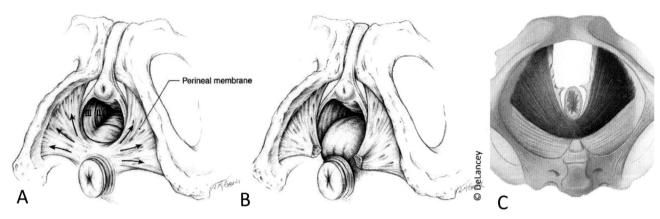

FIGURE 3.10 Perineal anatomy. Peripheral attachments of perineal membrane to ischiopubic rami (**A**) and direction of tension on fibers uniting through perineal body *(arrows)*. The U-shaped contour of the posterior vaginal wall in level 3 and W-shaped contour in level 2 are demonstrated. Loss of connection (**B**) shown as it would occur due to obstetrical trauma that could lead to distal rectocele. The effect of midline separation causing a widened hiatus and diastasis of the LAMs (**C**) is shown. (**A,B**, © DeLancey; from DeLancey JO. Structural anatomy of the posterior pelvic compartment as it relates to rectocele. *Am J Obstet Gynecol* 1999;180[4]:815–823; C, from DeLee JB. *The principles and practice of obstetrics*. Philadelphia: W.B. Saunders, 1933.)

Muscle Tearing and Hiatal Enlargement

Muscle tearing, often referred to as avulsion, occurs during at least 15% of vaginal deliveries[18] and is strongly associated with prolapse. In women with prolapse, 55% have levator tears, whereas these injuries are seen in only 16% of women of similar age and parity who do not have prolapse, an odds ratio of greater than 7.[19] The women with prolapse generated 37% less vaginal closure force during pelvic muscle contraction than controls (2.0 vs. 3.2 N), whereas those with major levator defects generated 35% less force than women without defects. In addition, the genital hiatus was 50% longer in cases than controls. Similar findings of muscle weakness with injury have been seen using a pressure-based device to compare women with and without prolapse, where pelvic floor muscle strength was associated with prolapse (odds ratio, 7.5) and endurance (odds ratio, 11.5).[20]

As one might expect with a muscle injury, the severity of the injury matters. Analysis of 503 patients from case-control studies of prolapse reveals that only cases in which 50% or more of the muscle is missing are associated with prolapse.[21] This cutoff has been independently confirmed using ultrasounds.[22]

Other Factors Involved in Hiatal Enlargement

It is important to recognize that visible levator muscle damage is not the only factor leading to an enlarged hiatus. Several other independent factors have been identified, such as muscle strength, perineal elevation with muscle contraction, descent during Valsalva, and visible muscle on MRI.[23] The degree of muscle damage only explains less than a quarter of the variation in hiatus size.[24]

Correlations between these factors reveal that no one factor explains more than 20% of the variation in others. The only significant association was between levator defect status and both resting urogenital hiatus and change in urogenital hiatus size with straining, but these were weak associations, only explaining 13% of variation in hiatus size.

Throughout the body, connective tissue and muscle work together to achieve physiologically important mechanical effects; this is also true of the connective tissues that make up the perineum. Figure 3.10 shows several structural hypotheses. Because the LAMs are connected to the perineal body, disruption of this structure can be associated with hiatal enlargement separate from injury to the muscle itself. In addition, the activity of the levator muscle can affect the configuration of the perineal membrane and size of the hiatus as shown in Figure 3.11.

FASCIAL FAILURES

Anatomy Anterior and Apical Supports

Anterior and apical support are intimately connected and are discussed together. When hiatal closure fails, or even sometimes when it does not, the connective tissues no longer hold the organs in place. The connective tissues of the pelvis attach the vagina and uterus laterally to the pelvic walls as outlined in Figure 3.5[25] and discussed earlier based on the "Levels of Support" section.

Anterior Compartment Failure Conceptual Model

Our conceptual model for anterior vaginal descent, based on intraoperative findings during transabdominal paravaginal defect repairs[26] and subsequently evaluated

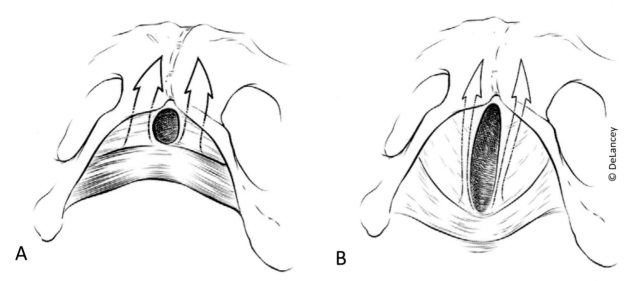

FIGURE 3.11 Effects of perineal elevation and depression mediated by the levator ani *(arrows)* involved hiatal enlargement. **A,B:** The effect of the levator ani on the hiatus and perineal structures is shown. Loss of levator tone results in an enlarged hiatus. (© DeLancey.)

in 3D stress MRI as described later in this chapter, is shown in Figure 3.12. Apical descent explains 60% of cystocele size and anterior vaginal wall factors contribute 30%, so together these are the two key factors affecting anterior vaginal wall prolapse.[27]

The lines of action for ligaments connecting two points are determined by the angle at which they act, their length, and their stiffness (Fig. 3.13) in the same way that the tension on two cables suspending a weight determine their relative tension. In the standing posture, the **cardinal ligaments** are in a relatively upright orientation 18° from the vertical—a logical direction for them to resist downward forces (see Fig. 3.13).[28] They are on average 5.7 cm long. The uterosacral

ligaments are more dorsally directed toward the sacrum. They are oriented at 92° from vertical on average in an orientation where they can prevent the uterus and upper vagina from sliding down the inclined plane of the levator plate toward the opening in the levator muscles through which prolapse occurs. They are normally 2.7 cm long. Using the lines of action for the cardinal and uterosacral ligaments and the inclination of the levator plate (the portion of the LAMs in the midline behind the rectum), it is possible to make a theoretical calculation of the tensions on the two ligaments for a given 1-N unit load. Analysis shows a cardinal ligament load that is 52% larger than the load on the uterosacral ligament.

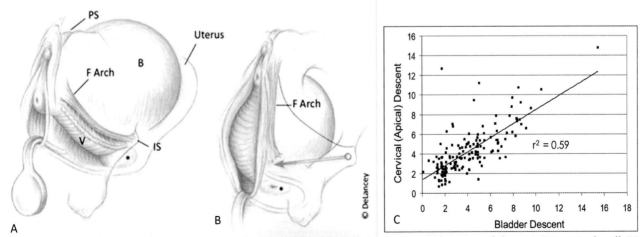

FIGURE 3.12 Anterior vaginal wall conceptual illustration. Diagrams show the normal location of the anterior vaginal wall (V) and descent and appearance through the vaginal opening (**A**) and the location in anterior vaginal prolapse or cystocele with weighted speculum in place (**B**). PS, pubic symphysis; B, bladder; IS, ischial spine; *asterisk,* cervix. The mechanical effect of apical descent *(arrow)* and concomitant downward movement of the fascial arch (F Arch; normal position is indicated with a *dashed line*) are shown. **C:** Association of apical and anterior wall descent. (© DeLancey; from Delancey JO. Fascial and muscular abnormalities in women with urethral hypermobility and anterior vaginal wall prolapse. *Am J Obstet Gynecol* 2002;187[1]:93–98.)

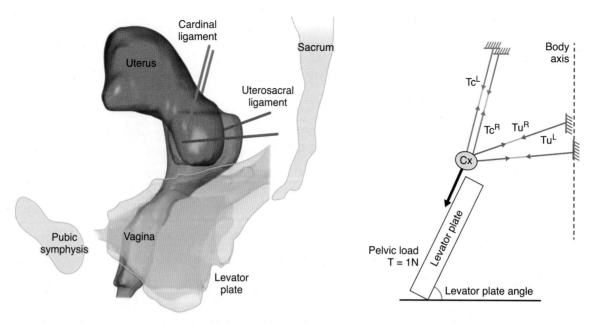

FIGURE 3.13 Cardinal and uterosacral loading. **Left panel** shows the magnetic resonance–based 3D model of the uterus and vagina and transparent LAM *(blue)*. **Right panel** shows four-cable suspension biomechanical model showing lines of action for the cardinal and uterosacral ligaments.

Clinically, sacral colpopexy tends to mimic the support of the cardinal ligaments, whereas sacrospinous and uterosacral ligament suspension mimics the support of the uterosacral ligaments. The vertical orientation is most effective in anterior compartment support, whereas the more dorsal support favors posterior compartment correction.

Cardinal and Uterosacral Biomechanics

Apical mechanics affect how treatment for patients is selected and must therefore be based on a sound scientific foundation rather than opinion. The cardinal and uterosacral ligaments allow a normal range of movement for the cervix; for example, its lower extent can be seen during D&C, where downward traction is placed upon it. Data from 73 normal women show that the normal range of cervical descent under anesthesia extends to the hymeneal ring, as shown in Figure 3.3 earlier in this chapter.[29] This data refers to the lateral margin of the cervix (at the 3 o'clock position) to avoid anterior lip stretching from the tenaculum. Any movement of the cervix to this point is therefore within the normal range of cardinal/uterosacral extension.

As previously discussed, if the LAMs hold the pelvic floor closed as they do in nulliparas or normal parous women, then no matter how high abdominal pressure becomes, there is little if any tension on the ligaments. When the pelvic floor is pushed open and the anterior wall descends, the pressure differential acting on the anterior vaginal wall creates a downward force on the cervix that, in turn, puts tension on the apical ligaments (Fig. 3.14). In this way, it acts the same as a tenaculum. This explains why women who underwent anterior colporrhaphy may postoperatively on pelvic examination have a cervix that is higher than it was preoperatively[30] and why apical prolapse is so rarely encountered if the uterus is within this normal range of movement.[31] Understanding ligament properties and behavior will aid in understanding whether women with prolapse do or do not have normal ligaments, which is key to rational surgical correction.

Clinical Evaluation of Apical Support

The way in which clinical evaluation of the status of apical support matters. The difference between evaluating ligament properties on pelvic examination and in the operating room (OR) is illustrated in Figure 3.15. When normal women perform a maximal Valsalva, the uterus moves on average 2 cm as measured during MRI. When one measures the amount of force that causes this amount of descent with traction on a tenaculum, it shows that almost no force is needed—just 3 oz, or the weight of a chicken egg. This 2 cm is much less movement than the ligaments would allow, indicating that while the muscles are active, very little ligament tension is needed to hold the uterus in place. This shows clearly that the properties of the ligaments alone do not determine uterine position. During surgery, we place much more force on the ligaments—an average of 8 lb, or 40 times more than the 3 oz of force generated from Valsalva that occurs during a Pelvic Organ Prolapse Quantification (POP-Q) exam.[32] On average, the cervix

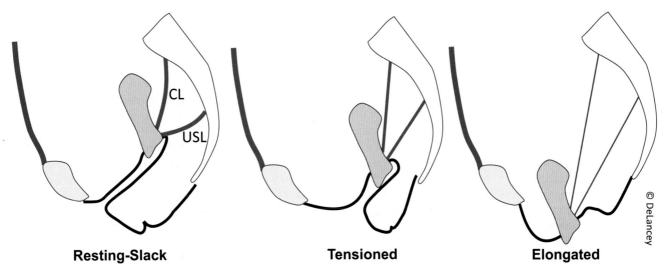

Resting-Slack　　**Tensioned**　　**Elongated**

© DeLancey

FIGURE 3.14 Ligament behavior. At rest, the ligaments are loose and not under any tension. With descent of the uterus, they straighten, become tensioned, and elongate within the normal range. In some women with prolapse, they remodel to become elongated, allowing the uterus to descend below the normal range. CL, cardinal ligament; USL, uterosacral ligament. (Reprinted by permission from Springer: Luo J, Betschart C, Chen L, et al. Using stress MRI to analyze the 3D changes in apical ligament geometry from rest to maximal Valsalva: A pilot study. *Int Urogynecol J* 2014;25[2]:197–203.)

is 3.5 cm lower in the OR under traction versus POP-Q exam in clinic during maximal Valsalva.[33]

Clinical decisions are made for each woman based on her specific situation. The information obtained in the clinic can differ from what is seen in the OR. To illustrate this, consider data comparing three groups of women.[34] One group is normal asymptomatic volunteers who have normal anterior and apical support (N/N); one group has

normal apical support on POP-Q but anterior or posterior wall prolapse with Ba or Bp >0 (N/P); and one group has both uterine (C > −5 cm) and anterior or posterior wall prolapse (P/P). By definition, clinical POP-Q apical support was in the normal range for the first two groups. When assessed in the OR with standardized traction at 1 N (0.25 lb) or 18 N (4 lb) of traction, 40% to 50% of the women judged to have normal support in clinic

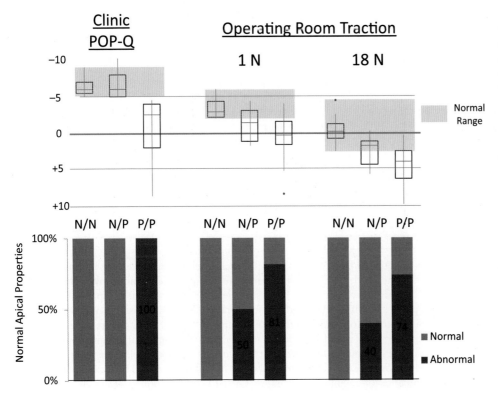

FIGURE 3.15 Cervix location. The **top graph** shows cervix location measured on Pelvic Organ Prolapse Quantification (POP-Q) and with 1-N (0.25 lb) and 18-N (4 lb) traction in the OR in the same women. The percentage of women outside the normal range *(red)* is shown in the **bottom graph**.

had abnormal support in the OR, and 20% to 25% of women whose uterus was below the normal location in clinic had normal ligament properties. This means that a substantial number of women who might have had a hysterectomy or an apical suspension have normal ligaments, whereas some would not have had these interventions might actually need them. This occurs because the cystocele pulls the uterus down, within the normal range of its elongation.

Biomechanical modeling demonstrates the relationship between unbalanced pressures on the anterior vaginal wall that create tension on the apical supports as shown in Figures 3.2, 3.14, and 3.16.[35] If muscle function is normal, the anterior wall remains in contact with the posterior wall and no downward tension on the ligaments is seen. With progressive failure of the hiatus to remain closed, the vagina becomes exposed and the ligaments lengthen. The threshold effect has been discussed and illustrated earlier in Figure 3.4.

Further evidence of this threshold effect comes from investigating exposed vagina and bladder descent (see Fig. 3.4). There is a very strong relationship between the exposed vaginal wall length and how far the bladder descends ($R^2 = 0.91$).[3] Initial descent while the vaginal wall is still in contact with the posterior vaginal wall does not increase the amount exposed to a pressure differential, but when the bladder descends 4 cm below its normal position, exposed vaginal wall length increases linearly and is highly correlated with hiatus diameter ($R^2 = 0.85$)—consistent with the relationship between hiatus status and prolapse.

Apical Ligament Defects and Prolapse

There are two ways in which abnormal ligaments may contribute to prolapse—one is that they are not stiff enough to resist downward force and the other is that they have become too long. Biomechanical testing of

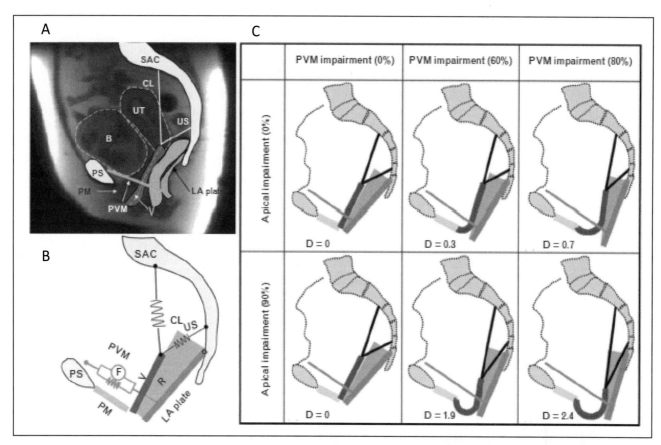

FIGURE 3.16 Two-dimensional biomechanical model created from MRI scan. **A:** Model development, including midsagittal MRI and modeled element traced or projected on midsagittal MRI. **B:** The lumped parameter biomechanical model, with the pubovisceral muscle modeled as a spring in parallel with an active force generator. SAC, sacrum; CL, cardinal ligament spring; UT, uterus; US, uterosacral ligament spring; B, bladder; PS, pubic symphysis; PM, perineal membrane; PVM, pubovisceral muscle; LA plate, levator plate; F, force; V, vagina; R, rectum. **C:** Simulated deformation of the model anterior vaginal wall, and its support system, under maximal Valsalva with various degrees of pubovisceral muscle and cardinal and uterosacral ligament impairment (indicated in percentage). The value for D, which presents the size of prolapse measured as the decent of the most dependent point of the vaginal wall from the end of the perineal membrane, is provided. (Modified from Chen L, Ashton-Miller JA, Hsu Y, et al. Interaction among apical support, levator ani impairment, and anterior vaginal wall prolapse. *Obstet Gynecol* 2006;108[2]:324–332.)

ligaments in vivo in women with and without prolapse reveals that 46% of the degree of uterine prolapse is explained by ligament length and 19% is explained by ligament stiffness.[36] It is important to consider in vivo data because standard biomechanical testing of these tissues creates a situation far outside of the physiologic range by "preconditioning" the ligaments. Classical in vitro experiments on small, excised ligament pieces suggest that it would take 26 N (or 5.8 lb) to stretch the uterosacral ligament by 1 mm.[37] In vivo studies of the ligaments in living women, by contrast, reveal that 1 lb of force moves the uterus 12 mm—a 650-fold difference.[29,38] The fact that it is length rather than stiffness that is the predominant factor involved in apical descent has clinical importance. It explains why reattaching the vagina to shortened ligaments or attaching them to a higher point (uterosacral suspension) is effective in correcting prolapse.[39,40] If it was the stiffness that was primarily at fault, then shortening or reattaching would fail.

The length and angle of action for the cardinal and uterosacral ligaments behave differently in the development of prolapse (Fig. 3.17).[41] The primary change in the cardinal ligament is lengthening, whereas the deep uterosacral ligament primarily rotates. The cardinal ligament is 20% longer at rest in women with prolapse compared to women with normal support (71 vs. 59 mm, $P < .05$). By contrast, the deep uterosacral ligament at rest has a similar length in women with prolapse and those with normal support. During maximal Valsalva, the cardinal ligament lengthens by 30 mm in prolapse versus 15 mm in normal women, whereas the deep uterosacral ligament lengthens by 15 versus 7.4 mm ($P = .09$). In contrast, the cardinal ligaments

remain at roughly the same angle relative to the body axis from rest to strain, whereas the deep uterosacral ligament angle is significantly different. This rotation contributes to misalignment, thereby inhibiting the lifting forces provided by the uterosacral ligaments.

Repetitive Loading

These considerations all focus on ligament behavior at a specific time. Examining what happens over decades is also an important consideration. As discussed in the "Biomechanical Principles" section, tissue remodels in response to forces placed on it (Davis law). If pelvic floor closure is inadequate, then the ligaments are called on to carry more of the load. If they are weak and subjected to repetitive loads, they can elongate. In many women, damage to the hiatal closure mechanism that results from vaginal birth occurs decades before prolapse becomes evident. This property, in which repetitive loading can result in material property changes and elongation under a constant load is resisted less over time, indicates that the types of repetitive loading over time can result in increasing descent of the pelvic organs. These are difficult to study because of the long time course of the forces applied but can be inferred from the observation that birth-related injury occurs to young women, whereas uterine descent often occurs many years later.

Posterior Compartment Biomechanics

The posterior wall shares support from the cardinal/uterosacral complex, but the uterosacral ligaments—especially the deep portion that suspends the upper

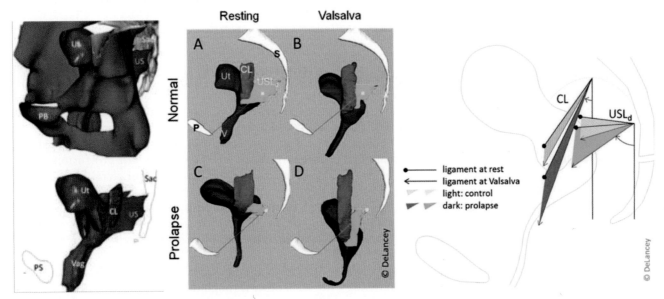

FIGURE 3.17 Cardinal and uterosacral ligament dynamics. The **left panels** show model construction, with the cardinal ligament in *blue* and the uterosacral ligaments in *pink*. The **middle panels A** to **D** reveal ligament orientations for women with normal support and prolapse at rest and during maximal Valsalva. The **right panel** shows the summary indicating the aggregate data. Ut, uterus; Sac, sacrum; US, uterosacral; PB, perineal body; CL, cardinal ligament; Vag, vagina; PS, pubic symphysis; S, sacrum; USL, uterosacral ligament.

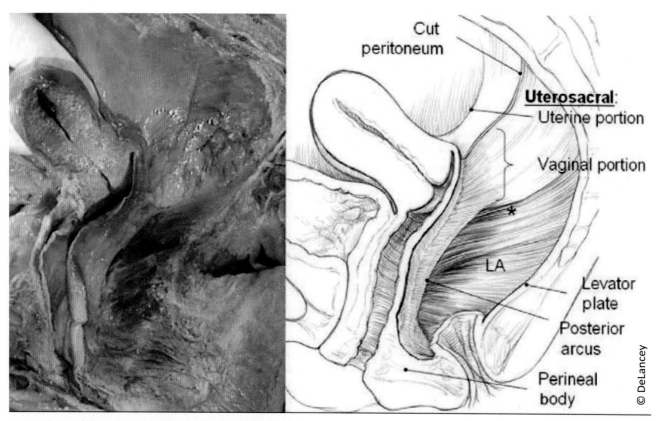

FIGURE 3.18 Posterior compartment anatomy. Cadaver dissection (**left**) and illustration (**right**) of posterior compartment after the rectum has been removed. *Asterisk* (*), sacrospinous ligament; LA, levator ani. (© DeLancey; from Hsu Y, Lewicky-Gaupp C, DeLancey JO. Posterior compartment anatomy as seen in magnetic resonance imaging and 3-dimensional reconstruction from asymptomatic nulliparas. *Am J Obstet Gynecol* 2008;198[6]:651.e1–651.e7.)

posterior wall—play a more important role in posterior vaginal wall support. This portion of the suspensory system holds the upper posterior vaginal wall dorsally over the levator plate—a vector that cannot be achieved by the more vertically oriented cardinal ligament (Fig. 3.18).[42]

The midportion of the posterior vaginal wall (level 2) is connected laterally to the posterior fascial arch[4] in a way that is analogous to the anterior vaginal wall's attachment. The posterior fascial arch is stretched between an attachment near the ischial spine and the perineal body. The distal attachment of the ATFP/fascial arch to the moveable perineal body differs from the anterior fascial arch, whose distal end has an immovable attachment to the pubic bone (see Fig. 3.5).

There are conflicting views on the presence and importance of rectovaginal fascia (i.e., Denonvilliers fascia). Whether or not one believes that there is a structurally important rectovaginal fascia that is separate from the vaginal wall is not important. Understanding the connections between the posterior vaginal wall and its connective tissue, whatever you call it, and the deep uterosacral ligament, perineal body, and posterior ATFP/fascial arch is critical to normal upper vaginal support.

In level 3, the lower third of the vagina is fused laterally with the perineal membrane and medial aspect of the LAMs and distally to the perineal body (see Fig. 3.18).

Differences between Posterior Vaginal Wall Shape in Women with and without Rectocele

There has been a century of conjecture about the structural defects that are involved in rectocele formation, and many competing hypotheses have been put forward.

The 3D stress MRI reconstructions demonstrate that a rectocele involves a forward protrusion of the posterior vaginal wall and anterior rectal wall through the urogenital hiatus in the LAM (Fig. 3.19).[43] In addition, there is overall descent of the posterior vaginal wall and perineal body that is easily seen on MRI, although not appreciated on physical examination. It can be presumed that this is associated with descent of the LAMs.

The perineal membranes on either side are connected to each other through the perineal body (see Fig. 3.5 earlier in chapter). This connection helps limit the degree to which the perineal body can descend. If the fibers that connect one side with the other rupture, the bowel may protrude downward, resulting in a posterior vaginal wall

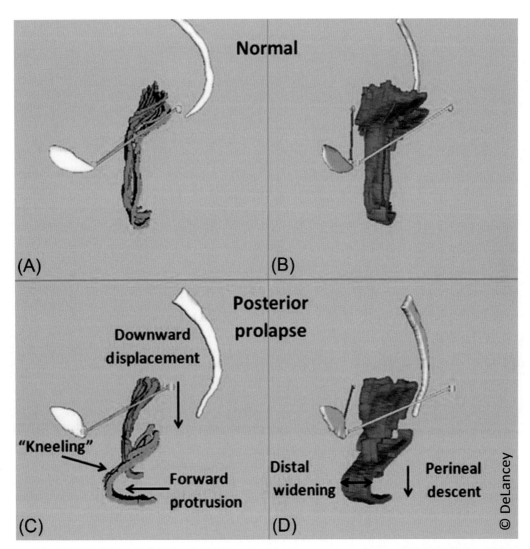

FIGURE 3.19 Posterior vaginal prolapse shape and position changes. Comparison of control (**A,B**) and case (**C,D**) in lateral view (**A,C**) and oblique view (**B,D**) showing five characteristic features (**C,D**) during rest *(blue)* and Valsalva *(pink)*: (1) increased folding (kneeling), (2) downward displacement in the upper two-thirds of the vagina, (3) forward protrusion, (4) perineal descent, and (5) distal widening in the lower third of the vagina. Pubis and sacrum are shown in *white*. The *line* from the inferior pubis to ischial spine (P-IS line) is shown in *turquoise*. (© 2011 DeLancey; posterior vaginal prolapse shape and position changes at maximal Valsalva seen in 3D MRI-based models from Luo J, Larson KA, Fenner DE, et al. Posterior vaginal prolapse shape and position changes at maximal Valsalva seen in 3-D MRI-based models. *Int Urogynecol J* 2012;23[9]:1301–1306.)

prolapse. In addition, because the LAMs are fused with the other tissues in this area, distention of the vaginal opening is also associated with enlargement of the levator hiatus through which prolapse occurs.

STRUCTURAL FAILURE ANALYSIS

The traditional approach to discussing prolapse has been to focus on which organ fell: uterus, anterior wall and bladder, posterior wall, or rectum. This is like saying that a bridge fell or a plane crashed. Engineering failure analysis focuses on understanding **why** the structure fell or where the mechanism broke down. There have been many conflicting theories about what failures

were responsible for prolapse; therefore, studies were needed to discern which theories were supported by evidence. Because many practitioners base their treatment on these theories, identifying which women had which failure and having data that are supported by evidence is important.

The 3D stress MRI has provided a technique capable of identifying structural failure sites by comparing measurements of supports between women with and without prolapse. This allows hypotheses to be tested—for example, regarding the relative contribution of apical descent, paravaginal defect size, and changes in vaginal width and length that would be associated with the connective tissue fascia of the pelvis (Figs. 3.20 and 3.21).[44,45]

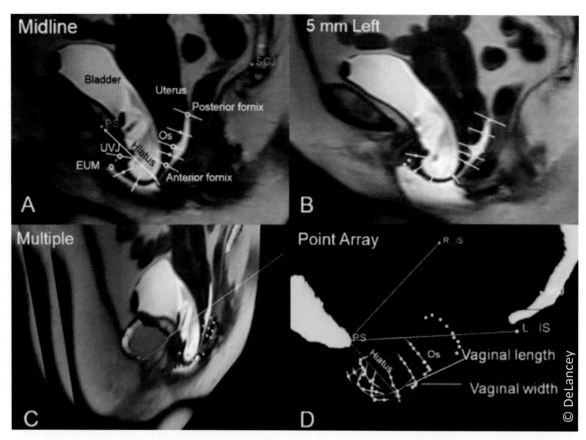

FIGURE 3.20 System for measuring vaginal wall location and dimensions. **A:** Midsagittal MRI with prolapse. **B:** Parasagittal scan showing point placement. **C:** Multi-slice illustration (three shown). **D:** Resulting point array. PS, pubic symphysis; UVJ, urethrovesical junction; EUM, external urethral meatus; SCJ, sacrum coccyx junction; R_IS, right ischial spine; L_IS, left ischial spine. (© DeLancey; from Chen L, Lisse S, Larson K, et al. Structural failure sites in anterior vaginal wall prolapse: Identification of a collinear triad. *Obstet Gynecol* 2016;128[4]:853–862.)

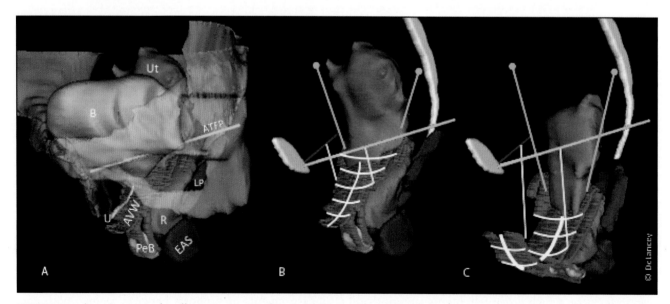

FIGURE 3.21 Anterior vaginal wall measurement scheme. **A:** 3D reconstruction of the pelvic organs and bones (semitransparent) from MRI at rest, with the line of the arcus tendineus fascia pelvis (ATFP) indicated. Ut, uterus; B, bladder; LP, levator plate; U, urethra; AVW, anterior vaginal wall; R, rectum; PeB, perneal body; EAS, external anal sphincter. **B:** The organs at rest with the measuring lines indicated. Vaginal wall parameters are shown with *white lines*; vaginal width is measured at five locations and length in the midline. *Green lines* indicate apical support as the distance from the uterus to the top of the greater sciatic foramen where the cardinal ligament is fixed to the pelvic wall. Paravaginal distance is indicated by a *yellow line* (shown for one of five sampling locations). **C:** The same distances at maximal Valsalva.

3D Stress MRI Technique

The technique of 3D stress MRI is shown in Figure 3.20.[44] A woman performs and holds a maximal Valsalva maneuver for about 15 seconds, during which serial sagittal slices are made from one side of the pelvis to another and the location of various structures is systematically plotted. Figure 3.20A shows the system with reference points at the pubis symphysis and sacrococcygeal junction and points placed along the length of the vagina at regular intervals in the midsagittal plane. These include the posterior fornix, external cervical os, anterior fornix, urethrovesical junction, and distal end of the vagina, which are marked with blue dots, and other equally spaced sampling locations, which are marked with yellow dots. Figure 3.20C is an example of anterior vaginal wall points in multiple sagittal MRIs. Figure 3.20D illustrates the resulting point array for the anterior vaginal wall at maximum Valsalva in three dimensions, which allows for both the measurement of the length and width of various vaginal wall segments and the location relative to the body axis ("high" or "low").

The scheme for making measurements is shown in Figure 3.21. In the first panel, a 3D reconstruction of the pelvic organs and bones (semitransparent) is shown from MRI at rest with organs in situ and a reference line representing the normal location of the ATFP indicated. The measurement system in women with normal support and pelvic organ prolapse are also shown as described in the figure caption.

Anterior Wall Failure Analysis

The results of comparing measurements of normal women with prolapse to women with prolapse who were of similar age, race, and parity are shown in Figure 3.22.[44] The measures are grouped by the different structural subsystem that they relate to. Vaginal wall factors have to do with the "pubocervical fascia" that represents the fibromuscular tissues of the anterior vaginal wall and are represented by its length and width. Attachments of the anterior vaginal wall and uterus are grouped as "attachment factors" and concern how high or low these points are. Although in the previous figure, this is illustrated conceptually as the distance to the ATFP, because this structure is not visible in these scans, the measurement is made to a horizontal line at the level of the inferior pubic point corrected for differences in pelvic inclination.[46]

Figure 3.22 shows that the largest differences between women with and without anterior prolapse exist in the attachment factors (apical and paravaginal) and hiatus. The next largest differences are each of the five paravaginal distances between cases and controls, with effect sizes between 2.2 and 2.8, as well as in apical support (effect size, 1.7). Effect size is a statistic that describes how different measurements are between groups. An effect size of 1 means that the mean values in the two groups differ by 1 standard deviation unit. The relationship between these different factors is shown in Figure 3.23. There is also a strong correlation between apical descent and paravaginal gap size ($r = 0.77$ to 0.93) that is greatest in the segments closest to the apex, indicating that apical descent and paravaginal gap are essentially two components of the same phenomenon. This is consistent with clinical observations showing a strong relationship between apical descent and cystocele size.[47]

The next largest effect size (1.9) was in the size of the urogenital hiatus, which was 55% larger in the women with prolapse during maximal Valsalva. Major levator tears are also much more common, occurring in 50% of women with prolapse as opposed to 20% in controls. Of the vaginal wall factors, vaginal length differed the most between the groups, being 24% longer in women with prolapse—an effect size of 1.1.[27] The only statistically significant difference in vaginal width occurred in the upper vagina near the anterior fornix, which was actually 15% narrower in the women with prolapse. This is probably because with prolapse, the normally wider upper portion of the vagina descends to the narrower opening in the LAMs, where it is limited in its lateral extent and made narrower itself.

Why does clinical intuition suggest that the vagina is wider in cystocele? This is somewhat of an optical illusion. Normally, the vagina is narrowest in its lower third and widest in its upper third.[48] When this wider upper portion becomes visible, it is clearly wider than one is used to seeing in this location. So why does anterior colporrhaphy work if its side-to-side plicating sutures do not address a widened vagina? This is because the anterior repair also returns the vaginal wall to a more normal length.[49] When coupled with elevating the apex, these steps correct two of the major factors causing cystocele. Paravaginal separation is the result of apical descent as indicated by the strong correlation between these factors. Correction of the apical support, when indicated, restores the location of paravaginal points.

Correlations among vaginal wall factors

The correlations among the various factors show that many are strongly related to one another. The correlation between apical descent and paravaginal location supports the earlier hypothesis that they are largely two different measurements of the same phenomenon. This is not universally the case, as there are women with cervical elongation who have normal anterior wall support, but in general, these factors go together. The correlation between hiatal diameter and both apical and paravaginal descent confirms the observation that hiatal failure exposes the vaginal wall and is associated with apical descent.

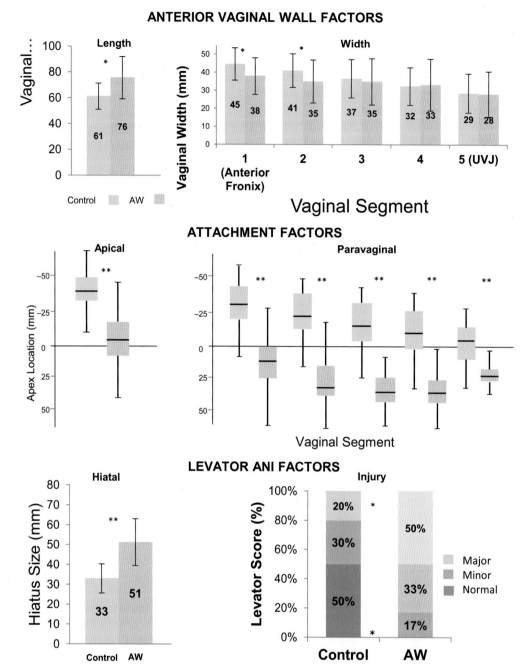

FIGURE 3.22 Anterior vaginal wall measurements at maximal Valsalva. Comparison of anterior vaginal wall factors (**first row**), attachment factors (**second row**), and levator ani factors (**third row**) by group between women with and without anterior vaginal wall prolapse; error bars show the standard deviation. *Denotes statistical significance, $P < .05$. **Denotes statistical significance, $P < .001$.

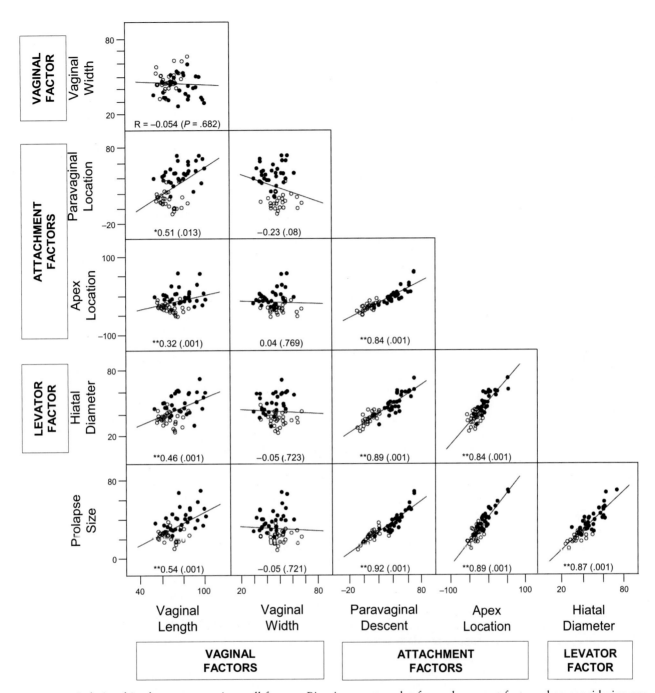

FIGURE 3.23 Relationships between anterior wall factors. Bivariate scatter plot for each support factor when considering prolapse size. Note the highly correlated nature of paravaginal descent, apex location, and hiatal diameter. Cases shown as *filled circles* and controls as *open circles*.

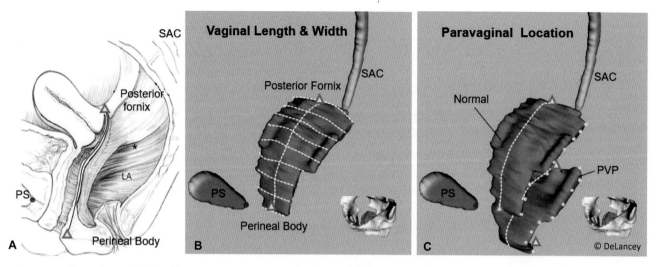

FIGURE 3.24 Posterior vaginal wall measurement strategy. Conceptual framework of posterior wall support showing normal posterior wall support anatomy (**A**): vaginal wall, posterior fornix support, distal support for the perineal body, and the LAM. The *blue line* indicates the portion that was modeled. **B:** Length and width of a normally supported posterior vaginal wall. **C:** The paravaginal and perineal location in normal women changes in women with posterior vaginal prolapse. SAC, sacrum; *Asterisk* (*), sacrospinous ligament; LA, levator ani; PS, pubic symphysis; PVP, posterior vaginal prolapse. (© 2020 DeLancey.)

Posterior Wall Failure Analysis

As in the analysis of the anterior wall, 3D stress MRI has also allowed quantitative assessment of structural failure sites in the posterior compartment (Fig. 3.24).[45] Many of the concepts discussed previously about the support of the apex and genital hiatus apply as posterior wall support is discussed. In patients with average support with a normal genital hiatus, these structures balance against the anterior vaginal wall. Once posterior wall descent happens, the posterior vaginal wall becomes exposed to a pressure differential, which the suspensory tissues must resist.

Comparison of vaginal wall, attachment, and levator ani factors (hiatus) are shown in Figure 3.25. The posterior vagina is almost 19% longer and 50% wider at the level of the perineal body in prolapse than in women with normal support. Loss of apical support at the level of the uterosacral ligaments allows for descent of the posterior vaginal wall in much the same way it can for the anterior wall. However, as the data will show, this factor is not as prominent as it is in the anterior compartment. Logically, with loss of apical support comes a lower location of the paravaginal attachments of the posterior wall to the ATFP in patients with posterior vaginal prolapse. Paravaginal descent in posterior wall prolapse has an effect size around 2. Failure of the posterior vaginal wall's upper suspension is associated with enterocele and prolapse of the vaginal vault (see Fig. 3.25). This loss of attachment to the sacrum allows forward protrusion of the posterior vaginal wall. This often occurs with the downward tipping (or more vertical orientation) of the levator plate that is associated with pelvic organ prolapse

in general. This is an area currently under active investigation so that the mechanics can be as well understood as those of the anterior compartment.

In the distal portion of the vagina, failure of perineal membrane fusion in the midline at the level of the perineal body can result in a widened genital hiatus (see Fig. 3.10). Failure of the LAMs, whether related to muscle avulsion or age-related change, can also account for part of this hiatal widening. This opened hiatus can allow for protrusion of the posterior vaginal wall; the hiatus is found to be widened in 74% of patients with posterior wall prolapse and has an effect size of greater than 2. By contrast, the levator hiatus plays less of a role in posterior wall prolapse and is widened in only 4% of cases with posterior predominant prolapse. In addition to hiatal widening, the position of the perineal body is also lower in patients with posterior vaginal prolapse. The effect size of the height of the perineal body is 2.1 (see Fig. 3.25).

As with the factors that affect anterior wall prolapse, there is a correlation between different factors. For the posterior wall, paravaginal descent, perineal body descent, and urogenital hiatus size are highly correlated with one another (Fig. 3.26). However, as can be seen in the overlap between individuals with normal and abnormal values, not all of these factors are found to be abnormal in every patient with posterior wall prolapse. In contrast to the anterior wall, where apical support seems to play a large role, the perineal body location is a stronger factor in posterior wall prolapse. This highlights the complex and individualized nature of support in this compartment.

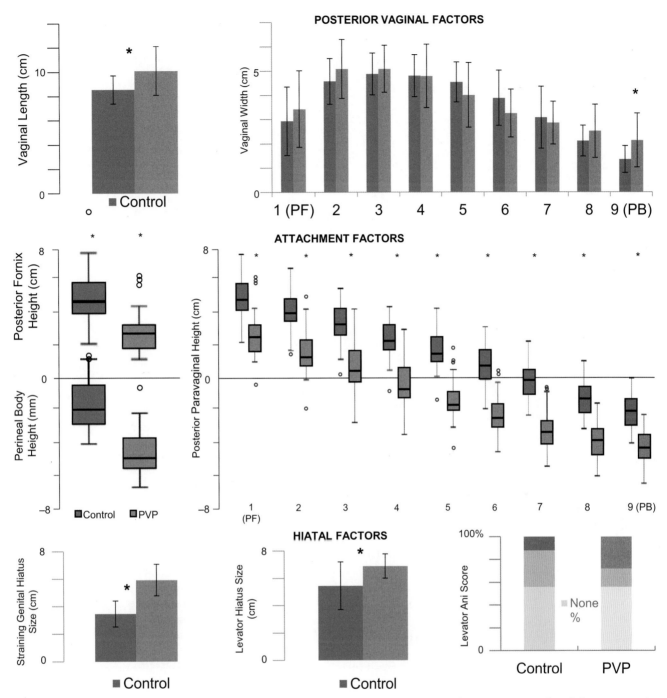

FIGURE 3.25 Posterior vaginal wall measurements at maximal Valsalva. Comparison of posterior vaginal wall factors, attachment factors, and levator ani factors by group. Error bars show standard deviations. *Denotes statistical significance, $P < .05$. PF, posterior fornix; PB, perineal body; PVP, posterior vaginal prolapse group.

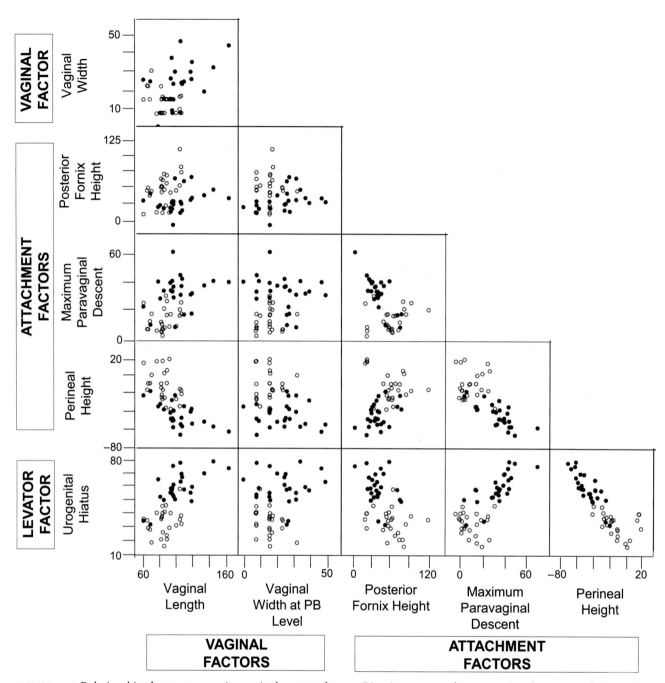

FIGURE 3.26 Relationships between posterior vaginal support factors. Bivariate scatter plot comparing the support factors. Cases shown as *filled circles* and controls as *open circles*.

CONCLUSION

The pelvic floor is an elegantly structured system that provides for normal pelvic organ support, excretory continence, and reproduction. The biomechanical principles that explain normal pelvic floor function and the location and nature of structural failures are now well understood. These principles and evidence-based system failure sites form the foundation for understanding pelvic floor disorders. Understanding these facts will help in understanding how operations and treatments work and why they fail.

References

1. DeLancey JO. Surgery for cystocele III: Do all cystoceles involve apical descent? Observations on cause and effect. *Int Urogynecol J* 2012;23(6):665–667.
2. Raizada V, Bhargava V, Jung SA, et al. Dynamic assessment of the vaginal high-pressure zone using high-definition manometry, 3-dimensional ultrasound, and magnetic resonance imaging of the pelvic floor muscles. *Am J Obstet Gynecol* 2010;203(2): 172.e1–172.e8.
3. Yousuf A, Chen L, Larson K, et al. The length of anterior vaginal wall exposed to external pressure on maximal straining

MRI: Relationship to urogenital hiatus diameter, and apical and bladder location. *Int Urogynecol J* 2014;25(10):1349–1356.

4. Leffler KS, Thompson JR, Cundiff GW, et al. Attachment of the rectovaginal septum to the pelvic sidewall. *Am J Obstet Gynecol* 2001;185(1):41–43.

5. Vaughan MH, Siddiqui NY, Newcomb LK, et al. Surgical alteration of genital hiatus size and anatomic failure after vaginal vault suspension. *Obstet Gynecol* 2018;131(6):1137–1144.

6. Andrew BP, Shek KL, Chantarasorn V, et al. Enlargement of the levator hiatus in female pelvic organ prolapse: Cause or effect? *Aust N Z J Obstet Gynaecol* 2013;53(1):74–78.

7. DeLancey JO, Hurd WW. Size of the urogenital hiatus in the levator ani muscles in normal women and women with pelvic organ prolapse. *Obstet Gynecol* 1998;91(3):364–368.

8. Handa VL, Blomquist JL, Carroll M, et al. Longitudinal changes in the genital hiatus preceding the development of pelvic organ prolapse. *Am J Epidemiol* 2019;188(12):2196–2201.

9. Stein TA, DeLancey JO. Structure of the perineal membrane in females: Gross and microscopic anatomy. *Obstet Gynecol* 2008;111(3):686–693.

10. Brandon CJ, Lewicky-Gaupp C, Larson KA, et al. Anatomy of the perineal membrane as seen in magnetic resonance images of nulliparous women. *Am J Obstet Gynecol* 2009;200(5):583.e1–583.e6.

11. Taverner D, Smiddy FG. An electromyographic study of the normal function of the external anal sphincter and pelvic diaphragm. *Dis Colon Rectum* 1959;2(2):153–160.

12. Kearney R, Sawhney R, DeLancey JO. Levator ani muscle anatomy evaluated by origin-insertion pairs. *Obstet Gynecol* 2004;104(1):168–173.

13. Lawson JO. Pelvic anatomy. I. Pelvic floor muscles. *Ann R Coll Surg Engl* 1974;54(5):244–252.

14. DeLancey JO, Sørensen HC, Lewicky-Gaupp C, et al. Comparison of the puborectal muscle on MRI in women with POP and levator ani defects with those with normal support and no defect. *Int Urogynecol J* 2012;23(1):73–77.

15. Betschart C, Kim J, Miller JM, et al. Comparison of muscle fiber directions between different levator ani muscle subdivisions: In vivo MRI measurements in women. *Int Urogynecol J* 2014;25(9):1263–1268.

16. Swenson CW, Masteling M, DeLancey JO, et al. Aging effects on pelvic floor support: A pilot study comparing young versus older nulliparous women. *Int Urogynecol J* 2020;31(3):535–543.

17. Handa VL, Blomquist JL, Carroll MK, et al. Genital hiatus size and the development of prolapse among parous women. *Female Pelvic Med Reconstr Surg* 2021;27(2):e448–e452.

18. Dietz HP, Lanzarone V. Levator trauma after vaginal delivery. *Obstet Gynecol* 2005;106(4):707–712.

19. DeLancey JO, Morgan DM, Fenner DE, et al. Comparison of levator ani muscle defects and function in women with and without pelvic organ prolapse. *Obstet Gynecol* 2007;109(2 Pt 1):295–302.

20. Braekken IH, Majida M, Ellström Engh M, et al. Pelvic floor function is independently associated with pelvic organ prolapse. *BJOG* 2009;116(13):1706–1714.

21. Berger MB, Morgan DM, DeLancey JO. Levator ani defect scores and pelvic organ prolapse: Is there a threshold effect? *Int Urogynecol J* 2014;25(10):1375–1379.

22. Dietz HP, Simpson JM. Levator trauma is associated with pelvic organ prolapse. *BJOG* 2008;115(8):979–984.

23. English EM, Chen L, Sammarco AG, et al. Mechanisms of hiatus failure in prolapse: A multifaceted evaluation. *Int Urogynecol J* 2021;32(6):1545–1553.

24. Nandikanti L, Sammarco AG, Kobernik EK, et al. Levator ani defect severity and its association with enlarged hiatus size, levator bowl depth, and prolapse size. *Am J Obstet Gynecol* 2018;218(5):537–539.

25. DeLancey JO. Anatomic aspects of vaginal eversion after hysterectomy. *Am J Obstet Gynecol* 1992;166(6 Pt 1):1717–1728.

26. DeLancey JO. Fascial and muscular abnormalities in women with urethral hypermobility and anterior vaginal wall prolapse. *Am J Obstet Gynecol* 2002;187(1):93–98.

27. Hsu Y, Chen L, Summers A, et al. Anterior vaginal wall length and degree of anterior compartment prolapse seen on dynamic MRI. *Int Urogynecol J Pelvic Floor Dysfunct* 2008;19(1):137–142.

28. Chen L, Ramanah R, Hsu Y, et al. Cardinal and deep uterosacral ligament lines of action: MRI based 3D technique development and preliminary findings in normal women. *Int Urogynecol J* 2013;24(1):37–45.

29. Bartscht KD, DeLancey JO. A technique to study the passive supports of the uterus. *Obstet Gynecol* 1988;72(6):940–943.

30. Swenson CW, Morgan DM, George J, et al. Effect of cystocele repair on cervix location in women with uterus in situ. *Female Pelvic Med Reconstr Surg* 2018;24(1):56–59.

31. Madhu C, Foon R, Agur W, et al. Does traction on the cervix under anaesthesia tell us when to perform a concomitant hysterectomy? A 2-year follow-up of a prospective cohort study. *Int Urogynecol J* 2014;25(9):1213–1217.

32. Foon R, Agur W, Kingsly A, et al. Traction on the cervix in theatre before anterior repair: Does it tell us when to perform a concomitant hysterectomy? *Eur J Obstet Gynecol Reprod Biol* 2012;160(2):205–209.

33. Crosby EC, Sharp KM, Gasperut A, et al. Apical descent in the office and the operating room: The effect of prolapse size. *Female Pelvic Med Reconstr Surg* 2013;19(5):278–281.

34. Swenson CW, Smith TM, Luo J, et al. Intraoperative cervix location and apical support stiffness in women with and without pelvic organ prolapse. *Am J Obstet Gynecol* 2017;216(2):155.e1–155.e8.

35. Chen L, Ashton-Miller JA, Hsu Y, et al. Interaction among apical support, levator ani impairment, and anterior vaginal wall prolapse. *Obstet Gynecol* 2006;108(2):324–332.

36. Smith TM, Luo J, Hsu Y, et al. A novel technique to measure in vivo uterine suspensory ligament stiffness. *Am J Obstet Gynecol* 2013;209(5):484.e1–484.e7.

37. Rivaux G, Rubod C, Dedet B, et al. Comparative analysis of pelvic ligaments: A biomechanics study. *Int Urogynecol J* 2013;24(1):135–139.

38. Swenson CW, Luo J, Chen L, et al. Traction force needed to reproduce physiologically observed uterine movement: Technique development, feasibility assessment, and preliminary findings. *Int Urogynecol J* 2016;27(8):1227–1234.

39. Fairchild PS, Kamdar NS, Rosen ER, et al. Ligament shortening compared to vaginal colpopexy at the time of hysterectomy for pelvic organ prolapse. *Int Urogynecol J* 2017;28(6):899–905.

40. Jelovsek JE, Barber MD, Brubaker L, et al. Effect of uterosacral ligament suspension vs sacrospinous ligament fixation with or without perioperative behavioral therapy for pelvic organ vaginal prolapse on surgical outcomes and prolapse symptoms at 5 years in the OPTIMAL randomized clinical trial. *JAMA* 2018;319(15):1554–1565.

41. Luo J, Betschart C, Chen L, et al. Using stress MRI to analyze the 3D changes in apical ligament geometry from rest to maximal Valsalva: A pilot study. *Int Urogynecol J* 2014;25(2):197–203.

42. Hsu Y, Lewicky-Gaupp C, DeLancey JO. Posterior compartment anatomy as seen in magnetic resonance imaging and 3-dimensional reconstruction from asymptomatic nulliparas. *Am J Obstet Gynecol* 2008;198(6):651.e1–651.e7.

43. Luo J, Larson KA, Fenner DE, et al. Posterior vaginal prolapse shape and position changes at maximal Valsalva seen in 3-D MRI-based models. *Int Urogynecol J* 2012;23(9):1301–1306.

44. Chen L, Lisse S, Larson K, et al. Structural failure sites in anterior vaginal wall prolapse: Identification of a collinear triad. *Obstet Gynecol* 2016;128(4):853–862.

45. Chen L, Xie B, Fenner DE, et al. Structural failure sites in posterior vaginal wall prolapse: Stress 3D MRI-based analysis. *Int Urogynecol J* 2021;32(6):1399–1407.

46. Betschart C, Chen L, Ashton-Miller JA, et al. On pelvic reference lines and the MR evaluation of genital prolapse: A proposal for standardization using the Pelvic Inclination Correction System. *Int Urogynecol J* 2013;24(9):1421–1428.

47. Summers A, Winkel LA, Hussain HK, et al. The relationship between anterior and apical compartment support. *Am J Obstet Gynecol* 2006;194(5):1438–1443.

48. Luo J, Betschart C, Ashton-Miller JA, et al. Quantitative analyses of variability in normal vaginal shape and dimension on MR images. *Int Urogynecol J* 2016;27(7):1087–1095.

49. Swenson CW, Simmen AM, Berger MB, et al. The long and short of it: Anterior vaginal wall length before and after anterior repair. *Int Urogynecol J* 2015;26(7):1035–1039.

CHAPTER 4

ANATOMIC NEUROUROLOGY

Annah Vollstedt • Larry T. Sirls • Kenneth M. Peters

Introduction: Neuro-anatomy of the Female Lower Urinary Tract

The lower urinary tract (LUT) has two discrete modes: bladder storage and bladder emptying. These two processes are dependent on the coordination of peripheral, spinal and central neuropathways. Continence, or bladder storage, is maintained by inhibition of detrusor muscle contraction and activation of the external urethral sphincter (EUS). After sensation of a full bladder, voiding, or bladder emptying, is initiated by a neural reflex that causes the EUS to relax and the detrusor muscle to contract. In general, storage of urine is a sympathetic nervous system response and voiding is a parasympathetic response. This can be considered in the context of the flight-or-fight response, with the large sympathetic burst when running from a predator one would not want to leave a trail of urine.

The brain and the spinal cord make up the central nervous system (CNS). The peripheral nervous system (PNS) consists of afferent (sensory) and efferent (motor) neurons that communicate with the CNS. The parasympathetic, sympathetic, and the pudendal nerves are the nerves with afferent and efferent fibers that are involved in the coordination of storage and emptying. Figure 4.1 shows an overview of these neural pathways. Lesions along any of these neural pathways may result in LUT dysfunction. The clinical symptoms that are observed are dependent on the area affected. Application of the knowledge of these complex systems can be used to treat neurologic causes of LUT dysfunction, such as with neuromodulation or nerve rerouting. In this chapter, we discuss these neural pathways as well as some of the pertinent clinical applications.

EFFERENT INNERVATION TO THE LOWER URINARY TRACT

Efferent nerve fibers send impulses from the CNS to the limbs and organs. The efferent innervation of the female LUT includes the parasympathetic, sympathetic, and pudendal nerves.

The **parasympathetic** nerves originate in the intermediolateral gray matter of the sacral spinal cord at the level of S2–S4. The axons then travel a long distance within the **pelvic nerve** to the ganglia (pelvic plexus), which is located immediately adjacent to the end organ (bladder).[1,2] **The preganglionic and postganglionic parasympathetic fibers release acetylcholine (ACh), which is an excitatory neurotransmitter.** ACh acts on the muscarinic receptors on the detrusor muscle, which then results in bladder contractions. There are five subtypes of the muscarinic cholinergic receptor (M1 to M5). The bladder contains M2 and M3 receptors. M2 is the more abundant subtype, but **M3 is the primary receptor that mediates detrusor contraction.** Activation of M3 receptors triggers intracellular calcium release, whereas activation of M2 receptors inhibits adenylate cyclase. The latter may contribute to bladder contractions by suppressing adrenergic inhibitory mechanisms which are mediated by β-adrenergic receptors and stimulation of adenylate cyclase.[3]

> **CLINICAL CORRELATION**
>
> Anticholinergic medications, such as **oxybutynin**, **tolterodine**, and **solifenacin**, are used to treat overactive bladder (OAB) because they decrease bladder contractions. Inhibition of muscarinic receptors outside the bladder can cause side effects.
>
> - Inhibition of M3 in the eye can cause pupil dilation and blurry vision.
> - Inhibition of M3 in the salivary glands can cause decreased saliva secretion and dry mouth.
> - Inhibition of M3 in the intestine causes decreased motility and constipation.
> - Inhibition of M2 in the sinus node of the heart can cause tachycardia.
> - Inhibition of M1 in the brain impairs cognition and memory.

Because the parasympathetic postganglionic neurons are located in the both the detrusor wall and the pelvic plexus, patients with cauda equina syndrome or pelvic plexus injury may not be completely denervated.[4]

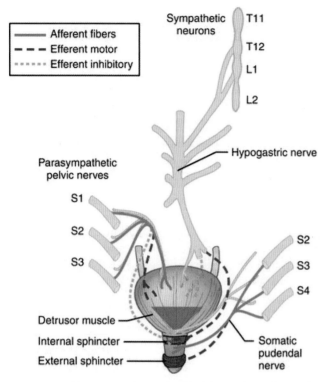

FIGURE 4.1 Nerve supply to the bladder and urethra. The bladder is innervated by the sympathetic, parasympathetic, and somatic nervous systems. The pudendal nerve maintains external sphincter and pelvic muscle tone. The pelvic nerve (parasympathetic) stimulates bladder contraction. The hypogastric nerve (sympathetic) stimulates internal sphincter closure and detrusor relaxation. (Reprinted from Norris TL. *Porth's pathology: Concepts of altered health states*, 10th ed. Philadelphia: Wolters Kluwer, 2018.)

The **preganglionic sympathetic** nerves arise from the thoracolumbar spinal cord at the level of **T10–L2**. The sympathetic efferent nerves to the LUT are located in the bilateral **hypogastric nerves.**[2] These noradrenergic nerves originate in the sympathetic chain ganglia and travel to the inferior mesenteric ganglia and then through the hypogastric nerves to the pelvic ganglia. They provide inhibitory input during bladder filling via β-3 receptors and excitatory input to the urethra and the bladder neck via α-1 receptors during filling/storage, which results in detrusor relaxation and EUS contraction. **The primary neurotransmitter for postganglionic sympathetic fibers is norepinephrine, but the primary neurotransmitter for preganglionic sympathetic fibers is ACh.**

Figure 4.2 shows the distribution of the sympathetic and parasympathetic contributions to the autonomic pelvic plexus.

surgery can lead to a decrease in bladder capacity and relaxation of the bladder neck, causing a decrease in outflow resistance. Clinically, patients may present with increased voiding frequency, "bladder spasms," and urge incontinence.

The **pudendal nerve is a somatic nerve** whose efferents innervate the striated muscle of the EUS and the pelvic floor muscles. **The nerve bodies originate in Onuf nucleus,** along the lateral border of the ventral gray matter at the S2–S4 region of the spinal cord (Fig. 4.3).[5]

The efferent nerve fibers travel within the pudendal nerve to the EUS.[2] Its **nerve terminals release ACh, which acts on nicotinic cholinergic receptors within the EUS, causing contraction of the EUS during storage/filling.**

During voiding/emptying, activation of the parasympathetic pathway leads to the release of nitric oxide (NO), which causes removal of the adrenergic and somatic cholinergic excitation and relaxation of the urethral smooth muscle.[6]

AFFERENT INNERVATION TO THE LOWER URINARY TRACT

Afferent nerves receive information from the sensory organs and transmit the input to the CNS. Afferent nerves have been identified both in the detrusor muscle and the suburothelium.[2] The suburothelial afferent nerve fibers form a plexus, with some nerve terminals extending into the urothelium itself. This plexus is more prominent in the trigone and bladder neck compared to the bladder dome.[2] **The pelvic, hypogastric, and pudendal nerves carry afferent input from the LUT to the lumbosacral spinal cord.**[7] These peripheral nerves carry both afferent and efferent information between the end organs and the spinal cord.[2] **The majority of afferent input from the bladder and urethra is transmitted via the pelvic nerve, with a smaller amount carried by the hypogastric nerve. The pudendal nerve carries input from the striated muscle of the EUS and the pelvic floor.** The afferent nerves release several different neurotransmitters, including vasoactive intestinal polypeptide, substance P, neurokinins, and calcitonin gene–related polypeptide.[2]

The **primary afferent neurons of the pelvic and pudendal nerves** are contained in the **sacral dorsal root**

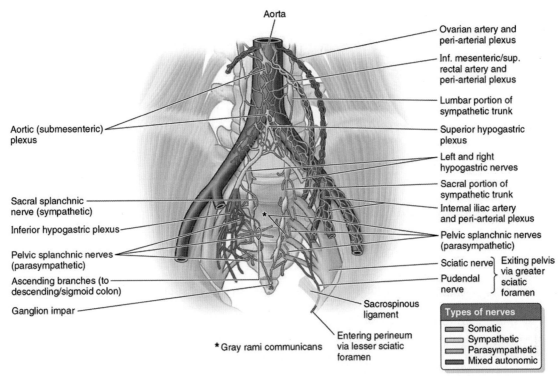

Aorta

Ovarian artery and peri-arterial plexus

Inf. mesenteric/sup. rectal artery and peri-arterial plexus

Lumbar portion of sympathetic trunk

Superior hypogastric plexus

Left and right hypogastric nerves

Sacral portion of sympathetic trunk

Internal iliac artery and peri-arterial plexus

Pelvic splanchnic nerves (parasympathetic)

Sciatic nerve ⎫ Exiting pelvis
Pudendal ⎬ via greater
nerve ⎭ sciatic foramen

Aortic (submesenteric) plexus

Sacral splanchnic nerve (sympathetic)

Inferior hypogastric plexus

Pelvic splanchnic nerves (parasympathetic)

Ascending branches (to descending/sigmoid colon)

Ganglion impar

Sacrospinous ligament

Entering perineum via lesser sciatic foramen

* Gray rami communicans

Types of nerves
- Somatic
- Sympathetic
- Parasympathetic
- Mixed autonomic

Anterior view

FIGURE 4.2 Sympathetic and parasympathetic contributions to the pelvic autonomic nervous plexus. The **superior hypogastric plexus** is formed by sympathetic fibers from the celiac plexus and the first four lumbar splanchnic nerves. Anterior to the bifurcation of the aorta, it divides into two **hypogastric nerves** that enter the pelvis medial to the internal iliac vessels, anterior to the sacrum, and deep to the endopelvic fascia. The pelvic continuations of the sympathetic trunks pass deep to the common iliac vessels and medial to the sacral foramina and fuse in front of the coccyx at the **ganglion impar**. Each chain comprises four to five ganglia that send branches anterolaterally to participate in the formation of the **inferior hypogastric plexus**. Presynaptic parasympathetic innervation arises from the intermediolateral cell column of the sacral cord. Fibers emerge from the second, third, and fourth sacral spinal nerves as the parasympathetic pelvic splanchnic nerves (nervi erigentes) to join the hypogastric nerves and branches from the sacral sympathetic ganglia to form the **inferior hypogastric plexus**. Note that in older texts, the superior hypogastric plexus is called the hypogastric plexus or presacral plexus and the that inferior hypogastric plexus is called the pelvic plexus. (Reprinted from Dalley AF, Agur AM. *Moore's clinically oriented anatomy*, 9th ed. Philadelphia: Wolters Kluwer, 2022.)

Serotonin & Norepinephrine Effects at Onuf's Nucleus

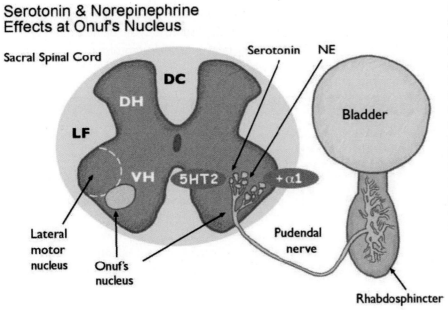

Sacral Spinal Cord

Serotonin   NE

DC

DH

LF

Bladder

VH   5HT2   +α1

Lateral motor nucleus

Onuf's nucleus

Pudendal nerve

Rhabdosphincter

FIGURE 4.3 Onuf nucleus. In the sacral spinal cord, Onuf nucleus is the origin of the pudendal nerve. Serotonin and norepinephrine (NE) stimulate the receptors 5-hydroxytryptamine-2 receptor (5HT2) and α1-adrenergic receptors (α1) to increase activity of the pudendal nerve and cause contraction of the skeletal component of the EUS. DC, dorsal column; DH, dorsal horn; LF, lateral funiculus; VH, ventral horn. (Reprinted by permission from Springer: Jost W, Marsalek P. Duloxetine: Mechanism of action at the lower urinary tract and Onuf's nucleus. *Clin Auton Res* 2004;14[4]:220–227.)

FIGURE 4.4 Location of afferent sensory information and efferent motor information within the spinal cord.

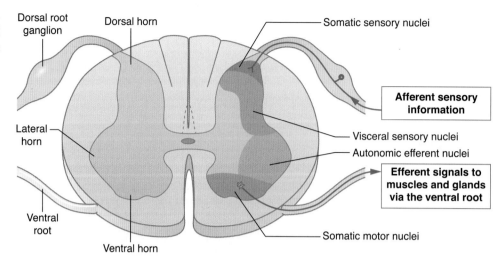

ganglia (DRG) (Fig. 4.4).[7] The **afferent neurons of the hypogastric nerve** arise in the **lumbar DRG**.[7] Afferent fibers enter the spinal cord through the dorsal horn and then diverge and project either locally to interneurons or to second-order neurons and then ascend to supraspinal centers in the micturition centers in the brain.[8]

The pelvic nerve afferent fibers monitor bladder volume and amplitude of bladder contractions. **These afferent fibers are made up of myelinated (A-delta) and unmyelinated (C) fibers** (Table 4.1). The A-delta fibers are located with the detrusor smooth muscle and communicate a sense of fullness, responding to detrusor stretching during bladder filling and are quiescent when the bladder is empty.[9] Compared to the unmyelinated C fibers, the A-delta fibers are more sensitive to increases in volumes and gradually increase in discharge frequency at intravesical pressures less than 25 mm Hg.[10,11] The unmyelinated C fibers are located within both the detrusor muscle and the lamina propria, adjacent to urothelial cells.[12] Those located in the muscle function as nociceptors, responding to overdistention by discharging at a higher range of physiologic bladder volumes.[10] In animal studies, C fibers have been described as mechanoinsensitive and have

been termed "silent C fibers" because of the lack of response to normal bladder stretching.[7] Instead, they respond to other stimuli, such as cold, chemical, or noxious stimulation like high potassium, low pH, high osmolality, or irritants like capsaicin.[13–15] In spinal cord injury (SCI) patients, the C fibers can become sensitized leading to a new type of spinal cord reflex that results in aberrant bladder contractions.[16] In patients with pelvic pain, there is evidence that neuropathy/inflammation/injury of the bladder/pelvic floor can lead to recruitment of C fibers to form a new functional afferent pathway, which may lead to bladder pain and urgency incontinence.[7,17] Thus, C fibers may be important targets for clinical interventions.

CLINICAL CORRELATION

Chronic inflammation, like that seen in interstitial cystitis/bladder pain syndrome, can lead to an increase in sensitizing agents such as cytokines and chemokines, which in turn leads to hyperexcitability of C fiber afferents. This may lead to a "cycle" of increasing pain and/or worsening urination symptoms.[10]

TABLE 4.1			
Bladder Afferent Properties			
FIBER TYPE	**LOCATION**	**NORMAL FUNCTION**	**INFLAMMATION EFFECT**
A-delta (finely myelinated)	Smooth muscle	Sense bladder fullness (wall tension)	Increase discharge at lower pressure threshold
C fiber (unmyelinated)	Mucosa	Respond to stretch (bladder volume sensors)	Increase discharge at lower threshold
C fiber (unmyelinated)	Mucosa Muscle	Nociception to overdistention Silent afferent	Sensitive to irritant Becomes mechanosensitive and unmasks new afferent pathway during inflammation

Reprinted from Yoshimura N C, MB. Pathophysiology and pharmacology of the bladder and urethra. In: McDougal WS, Wein AJ, Kavoussi LR, et al, eds. *Campbell-Walsh urology*, 10th ed. Philadelphia: Elsevier, 2012:329–334, with permission from Elsevier.

SUMMARY

Parasympathetic Pathway: Emptying

S2–S4 spinal cord → pelvic nerve → inferior pelvic plexus → nerves to the bladder → release ACh → stimulates <u>M3</u>/M2 receptors in the bladder → bladder contraction

Sympathetic Pathway: Storage

T10–L2 spinal cord → hypogastric nerve → inferior pelvic plexus →

> Nerves to bladder → release norepinephrine → stimulates β-3 receptors in bladder → detrusor relaxation
>
> Nerves to sphincter smooth muscle → release of norepinephrine → stimulates α-1 receptors → sphincter contraction

Somatic Pathway: Voluntary sphincter

S2–S4 spinal cord in Onuf nucleus → pudendal nerve → nerves to striated sphincter → release ACh → stimulates nicotinic cholinergic receptors in the voluntary EUS → contraction

Figure 4.5 summarizes the innervation of the female LUT and the neural pathways.

A WORD ON THE PUDENDAL NERVE

The pudendal nerve originates from spinal roots S2–S4 and is the major nerve to the perineum. Although we are focusing on the motor function of the pudendal nerve (i.e., innervation to the EUS), it should be noted that the pudendal nerve also supplies motor function to the anal sphincter and the

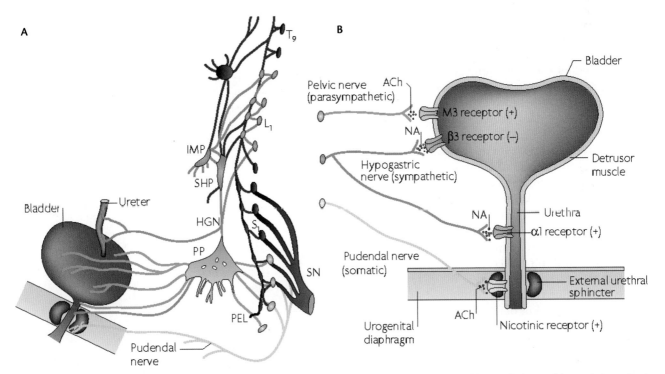

FIGURE 4.5 Efferent pathways of the LUT. **A:** Innervation of the female LUT. **Sympathetic fibers** (shown in *blue*) originate in the **T11–L2** segments in the spinal cord and run through the inferior mesenteric plexus (IMP) and the **hypogastric nerve** (HGN) or through the paravertebral chain to enter the pelvic nerves at the base of the bladder and urethra. **Parasympathetic** preganglionic fibers (*green*) arise from the **S2–S4** spinal segments and travel in sacral roots and pelvic nerves (PEL) to ganglia in the **pelvic plexus** (PP) (also called the **inferior hypogastric plexus**) and in the bladder wall. This is where the postganglionic nerves that supply parasympathetic innervation to the bladder arise. **Somatic motor nerves** (*yellow*) that supply the striated muscles of the external EUS arise from S2–S4 motor neurons and pass through the **pudendal nerves. B:** Efferent pathways and neurotransmitter mechanisms that regulate the LUT. **Parasympathetic postganglionic** axons in the **pelvic nerve** release ACh, which produces a bladder contraction by stimulating **M3** muscarinic receptors in the bladder smooth muscle. **Sympathetic postganglionic neurons** release noradrenaline (NA) (also known as **norepinephrine**), which activates **β3-adrenergic receptors** to relax bladder smooth muscle and activates **α1-adrenergic receptors** to contract urethral smooth muscle. Somatic axons in the **pudendal nerve also release ACh,** which produces a contraction of the external sphincter striated muscle by **activating nicotinic cholinergic receptors.** T₉, ninth thoracic root; L₁, first lumbar root; S₁, first sacral root; SHP, superior hypogastric plexus; SN, sciatic nerve. (From de Groat WC, Griffiths D, Yoshimura N. Neural control of the lower urinary tract. *Compr Physiol* 2015;5[1]:327–396.)

levator ani as well as sensory function to the skin of perineum, including the labia, vagina, and clitoris.

Because of the relationship to the palpable ischial spine, a pudendal block can be administered for local anesthesia for chronic pain syndromes. The injection can be given transvaginally, just medial to the ischial spine.

CLINICAL APPLICATION OF EFFERENT AND AFFERENT SPINAL CORD ANATOMY

An example of how the afferent/sensory nerve input entering the spinal cord through the dorsal nerve root and the efferent/motor neurons leaving the spinal cord through the ventral nerve root can be used clinically is with the "nerve rerouting" surgery of Xiao et al.[18] (Fig. 4.6).

This procedure was developed for children with myelomeningocele in an attempt to recover spontaneous voiding. In myelomeningocele patients, the sacral nerve sheaths are lacking axons due to the spinal lesion, and the bowel and bladder are poorly innervated resulting in urinary and fecal dysfunction. The concept of nerve rerouting to improve bladder and bowel function is based on a simple reflex such as a knee jerk. When one taps the knee, an afferent sensory signal is sent through the dorsal root to the cord and immediately transmitted to a motor nerve through the ventral root, resulting in a knee jerk at the site of stimulation. This surgery involves a laminectomy and isolation of the L5 dorsal and ventral root. The ventral root (efferent) is cut and anastomosed to S3 distal to the lesion. The dorsal root is left intact to preserve thigh skin sensation and so the cutaneous reflex can be stimulated. In theory, over 6 to 9 months, the ventral root axons extend down the axonal sheath to innervate the bladder. When innervation is complete, a voiding reflex can be initiated by scratching the L5 dermatome (skin of the thigh) sending an afferent signal through the dorsal root, to the reanastomosed ventral root and leading to reflex bladder contraction.

Although illustrative of the principles of neuroanatomy, nerve rerouting procedures have not shown long-term success.

SUPRASPINAL MICTURITION REFLEX CENTERS

The neural circuitry of the LUT behaves as a switch between filling/storage and voiding, which is under control of a network of interconnected brain regions. **The pontine micturition center (PMC), or Barrington nucleus, mediates the normal micturition reflex by coordinating the activity of the detrusor and EUS muscles.**[2] Therefore, **lesions in the spinal cord below this level can**

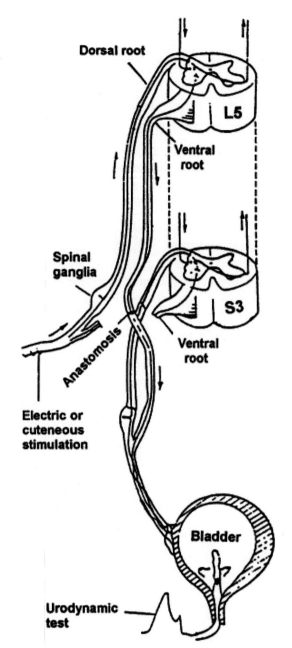

FIGURE 4.6 CNS-skin-bladder reflex pathway. (From Xiao C-G, Du M-X, Dai C, et al. An artificial somatic-central nervous system-autonomic reflex pathway for controllable micturition after spinal cord injury: Preliminary results in 15 patients. *J Urol* 2003;170[4 Pt 1]:1237–1241.)

result in detrusor external sphincter dyssynergia (DESD), which is a discoordination between the bladder and EUS where the detrusor muscle contracts and the external sphincter contracts instead of relaxing, causing a functional obstruction. The neurons of the PMC provide direct synaptic input to the sacral preganglionic neurons and carry excitatory outflow to the bladder. They also provide input to GABAergic (gamma-aminobutyric acid) neurons in the sacral dorsal commissure, providing an inhibitory influence on the EUS.[7]

The periaqueductal gray (PAG) is the gray matter that is located around the cerebral aqueduct within the tegmentum of the midbrain. The **PAG functions as a relay center between the PMC and the spinal cord neurons** that are needed for excitatory and inhibitory control of the micturition reflex.[7] During filling/urine storage, afferents from the bladder increase in strength until they exceed a threshold set in the brainstem, specifically, the PAG in the midbrain. Once the threshold is met, the PMC is activated, and voiding is initiated by relaxation of the EUS and bladder contraction.[19]

Brain imaging in the rat has confirmed that during filling/storage, the PAG is activated and the PMC is quiet.[20] However, studies regarding the importance of the PAG in micturition are conflicting. Although some animal studies have shown the PAG to be essential in micturition,[21] other cat models have found that when the connections between the PMC and PAG are interrupted, reflex bladder contractions persist. This indicates that the PAG does not have a critical role in reflex micturition, but rather transmits sensory information about bladder filling to higher brain centers.[22]

Figure 4.7 illustrates a conceptual model by Griffiths et al. of the current understanding of the control system, broken down into neural circuits that plat different roles.[19] *Circuit 1* describes the perception of fullness and consists of the lateral prefrontal cortex and the insula. Whereas the prefrontal cortex involves cognition and working memory, the insula receives "homeostatic" information via the afferent input relayed in the thalamus. Thus, insular activation has been reported in studies of urine storage. In healthy individuals, activation increases with bladder filling and the desire to void.[19] Interestingly, in women with impaired bladder sensation (i.e., Fowler syndrome), activation of the insula is absent.[23]

Circuit 2 describes the perception of urgency and involves the anterior cingulate cortex (ACC) and the supplementary motor area. The ACC is responsible for motivation and modulation of bodily arousal states.[3] Studies have demonstrated that ACC activation helps to suppress voiding by activating the sympathetic nervous system that inhibits bladder contraction and contracts urethral smooth muscle. Furthermore, the ACC can be activated along with the adjacent supplementary motor cortex, which in turn activates the pelvic floor muscles. Thus, when an individual senses urgency, the ACC and the supplementary motor cortex act together to

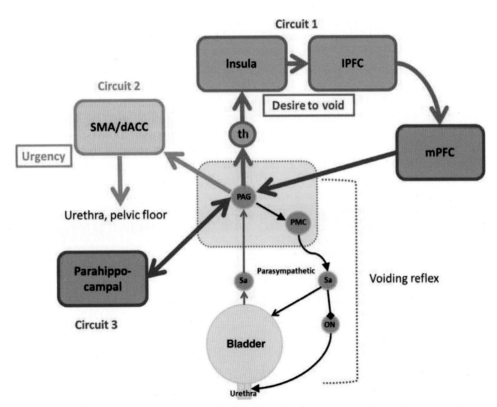

FIGURE 4.7 A simple working model of the LUT control system, showing the voiding reflex with its rostral terminus in the brainstem (*green*) and circuits 1, 2, and 3 of the control network (in *red, orange,* and *blue,* respectively). The return path of circuit 1 is in *blue* to signify that medial prefrontal cortex (mPFC) deactivation plays an important role in continence control. lPFC, lateral prefrontal cortex; SMA, supplementary motor area; dACC, dorsal anterior cingulate cortex; th, thalamus; PAG, periaqueductal gray; PMC, pontine micturition center; Sa, sacral parasympathetic area; ON, Onuf nucleus. (Reprinted from de Groat WC, Griffiths D, Yoshimura N. Neural control of the lower urinary tract. *Compr Physiol* 2015;5[1]:327–396.)

generate a sensation of urgency and a contraction of the EUS, thus "hastening a toilet visit while reinforcing the ability to postpone voiding until the toilet is reached."[3]

Circuit 3 involves subcortical structures, including the PAG and parahippocampal cortex, and can be thought of as the unconscious monitoring of bladder fullness by the brain when the bladder volume is small and there is little sensation.[3]

The PAG is the location of the switch from storage to voiding and back. The PAG has connections to and from the forebrain, amygdala, hypothalamus, thalamus, and the stria terminalis. The PAG also receives ascending afferents from the bladder and sends descending signals back to the bladder and the urethra via the PMC. Unlike the complex connections to and from the PAG, the PMC receives input almost exclusively from the PAG.[19] When activated by the PAG, the PMC passes on a signal to the sacral cord, where inhibitory neurons in Onuf nucleus relaxes the EUS while the bladder contracts. Thus, bladder sphincter synergy is coordinated by the PMC.[19]

BRAIN IMAGING STUDIES

Although the clinical role of brain imaging studies has yet to be defined, functional brain imaging has emerged as a powerful tool for studying the relationship between activities in certain areas of the brain and specific bodily functions. Initially, single photon computerized tomography[24] was used, followed by positron emission tomography (PET). Both involve injection of a radioactive substance that concentrates in the metabolically active areas of the brain.[19] With the advantage of being noninvasive and free of radioactivity, functional magnetic resonance imaging (fMRI) started to be used.[19] Both PET and fMRI provide indirect measures of regional blood flow, an indirect measure of local neural activity. The temporal relationship for

PET is several minutes versus a few seconds for fMRI. For this reason, PET is used to measure long-lasting states, whereas fMRI can follow relatively fast events.[25]

Researchers have used PET to study brain activity during bladder emptying and filling in normal males and females. Initial studies by Blok et al.[26] demonstrated activation in the medial prefrontal cortex and the dorsal pons, the presumptive location of the PMC, during the voiding phase (Fig. 4.8).[26]

fMRI has been the functional neuroimaging technique most widely used for the last 10 years because of its relatively high spatial resolution compared to other functional neuroimaging techniques, as well as lack of radiation and radioactivity.[27] Due to technical challenges related to voiding in the magnetic resonance imaging machine, research has focused on the storage phase and initiation of micturition. However, recently, researchers have been able to study the voiding phase and even pair fMRI findings with simultaneous urodynamic tracings.[28] fMRI in healthy females has confirmed what was previously seen in PET studies. Bladder filling shows a complex activation pattern involving areas of the prefrontal cortex, orbitofrontal/frontopolar cortex, ACC, left and right insulae, hypothalamus, and left basal ganglia.[29] The end of bladder storage and the strong desire to void shows activation of the prefrontal cortex, anterior cingulate gyrus, hypothalamus, temporal lobes, and the left caudate nucleus.[30] The voiding phase involves activation of the PAG, pons, insula, thalamus, prefrontal cortex, the parietal operculum, and the cingulate cortex.[31]

Although functional brain imaging has advanced our understanding of these complex higher-order connections, one potential issue with interpretation of the data is that neuronal activations may represent either excitatory or inhibitory activity.[19]

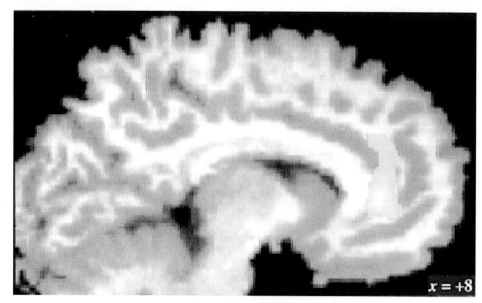

FIGURE 4.8 The medial frontal region and presumptive PMC are activated during voiding, as shown in *yellow* on a sagittal cross-section of the brain. (Reprinted from Blok BF, Willemsen AT, Holstege G. A PET study on brain control of micturition in humans. *Brain* 1997;120[Pt 1]:111–121, by permission of Oxford University Press.)

SENSORY ROLE OF THE UROTHELIUM

Traditionally, the urothelium has been regarded as a passive "barrier" that prevents toxins in the urine from entering the underlying bladder interstitium. More recently, it has been shown that the **urothelial cells display properties similar to sensory neurons and play an active role in communication with the bladder nerves, smooth muscle, interstitial cells, and blood vessels.**[2,3] Researchers have shown that the urothelium expresses various receptors for "sensory molecules," including receptor for bradykinin, neurotrophins (TrkA and p75), purines (P2X and P2Y), norepinephrine (alpha and beta), ACh (muscarinic and nicotinic), protease activated receptors, amiloride/mechanosensitive sodium channels, prostaglandin E2 receptors, and transient receptor potential channels.[3]

In response to these receptors, the urothelium releases chemical mediators such as NO, adenosine triphosphate (ATP), ACh, prostaglandins, and substance P peptide.[32] These chemical mediators have excitatory or inhibitory effects on the close-by afferent nerves, which, in turn, is relayed to the CNS. For instance, NO is released by urothelial cells in response to inflammation, and it has been shown that NO levels in the bladder of interstitial cystitis/bladder pain syndrome patients is increased, especially in those with Hunner lesions.[33] During bladder stretching, the urothelium releases ATP which activates bladder afferents expressing P2X and P2X3 receptors, relaying the sensation of fullness and pain.[3]

Additionally, researchers have shown that the muscarinic receptors in the bladder are not limited to detrusor contractility. Muscarinic receptors are found on the urothelium in high density, and ACh is released at a basal rate from urothelium that increases with age and bladder stretching. This activation of the muscarinic receptors in the urothelium then causes release of substances that modulate the afferent nerve and smooth muscle activity.[7]

NEUROMODULATION

The most contemporary application of our bladder neuroanatomy is neuromodulation that acts directly on the sacral, pudendal, tibial, and other nerves by delivering electrical impulses directly to a target area. Neuromodulation has many applications to the field of urology and urogynecology, including treatment of OAB, urinary and fecal incontinence, urinary retention, and chronic pelvic pain. Devices may be percutaneous, such as that with percutaneous tibial nerve stimulation, or implantable, like the Medtronic or Axonics sacral neuromodulation devices.

Sacral Neuromodulation Foramen

Currently, **the S3 sacral nerve is the only U.S. Food and Drug Administration (FDA)-approved site for treatment of bladder and bowel dysfunction using an** implantable device. Sacral neuromodulation devices can be used to treat various pathologies, including OAB, urinary urgency incontinence, nonobstructive urinary retention, and fecal incontinence. The exact mechanism of action is unclear; however, it is hypothesized that electrical stimulation of the afferent nerves in the spinal roots leads to modulation of voiding and continence reflex pathways in the CNS by inhibiting sensory processing in the spinal cord.[7] Specifically for the treatment of OAB, sacral neuromodulation is thought to work by either blocking transmission of information from the bladder to the PMC by inhibition of the ascending limb of the micturition reflex or by direct inhibition to the bladder preganglionic neurons.[7] For the treatment of idiopathic urinary retention, animal studies have found that stimulation of the somatic afferent fibers within the pudendal nerve from the perineum lead to activation of the bladder efferents and inhibition of excitatory pathways to the bladder outlet, leading to voiding.[34]

Tibial Neuromodulation

The tibial nerve is a sensory-motor nerve that arises from the L4, L5, S1, S2, and S3 spinal roots. Currently, percutaneous tibial nerve stimulation is used as a third-line treatment of OAB. Like sacral neuromodulation, the mechanism of action of tibial neuromodulation is not completely understood.[35] However, the burden of weekly tibial nerve treatments limits compliance, and work is ongoing to develop an implantable device at this location. Although, there is not yet an FDA-approved implantable device for neuromodulation of the tibial nerve, there is ongoing research that takes advantage of wireless technologies that are office based and less invasive. These new devices allow for neurostimulation without the burden of an office visit as well the potential for improving outcomes with daily stimulation.[36]

Pudendal Neuromodulation

Modulation of the pudendal nerve allows stimulation to all three sacral nerve roots: S2, S3, and S4. This allows the pudendal nerve to have a wider range of effects because it innervates the bladder, external urethral and anal sphincters, the pelvic organs, and the pelvic floor musculature.[37] Compared to sacral stimulation, studies have shown that pudendal stimulation has greater impact on improvement in urinary urgency, frequency, and bowel function.[38] The pudendal nerve can be considered an alternative approach for the treatment of OAB if refractory to sacral neuromodulation. In addition, pudendal neuromodulation has been used for the treatment of neuralgia, pelvic pain, and other complex voiding disorders.[37]

CLINICAL CORRELATION

Some evidence suggests that the stimulation of nerves that have several afferent nerve roots provides better clinical response than stimulation of a single nerve root. For example, in one study, patients had simultaneous placement of both a sacral nerve stimulation lead (S3) and a pudendal nerve stimulation lead (S2, S3, and S4). Patients reported that pudendal nerve stimulation provided greater improvement in their pelvic pain than S3.[38] The tibial nerve, with five afferent nerve roots (L4, L5, S1, S2, and S3), is an exciting new target for chronic stimulation.

CONCLUSION

The two functions of the bladder, storage and emptying, are regulated by a complex of communication between nervous systems in the brain and the spinal cord, bladder and urethra muscles, as well as the urothelium. Insult to any of these components can disrupt the functions of storage and emptying, leading to bladder dysfunction with symptoms of OAB and incontinence. Understanding the physiology of the neuroanatomy of LUT is essential for the management of urinary tract dysfunction.

References

1. Fowler CJ, Griffiths D, de Groat WC. The neural control of micturition. *Nat Rev Neurosci* 2008;9(6):453–466.
2. Clemens JQ. Basic bladder neurophysiology. *Urol Clin North Am* 2010;37(4):487–494.
3. de Groat WC, Griffiths D, Yoshimura N. Neural control of the lower urinary tract. *Compr Physiol* 2015;5(1):327–396.
4. de Grout WC, Booth AM. Synaptic transmission in pelvic ganglia. In: Maggi CA, ed. *The autonomic nervous system*. London: Harwood Academic Publishers, 1993:291–347.
5. Jost W, Marsalek P. Duloxetine: Mechanism of action at the lower urinary tract and Onuf's nucleus. *Clin Auton Res* 2004;14(4):220–227.
6. Benson JT, Griffis K. Pudendal neuralgia, a severe pain syndrome. *Am J Obstet Gynecol* 2005;192(5):1663–1668.
7. Yoshimura N, Chancellor MR. Pathophysiology and pharmacology of the bladder and urethra. In: McDougal WS, Wein AJ, Kavoussi LR, et al, eds. *Campbell-Walsh urology*, 10th ed. Philadelphia: Elsevier, 2012:329–334.
8. Tennyson L, Chermansky CJ. Basic neuroanatomy and neurophysiology of the lower urinary tract. In: Gilleran J, Alpert S, eds. *Adult and pediatric neuromodulation*. Switzerland: Springer International Publishing, 2018:3–11.
9. Sengupta JN, Gebhart GF. Mechanosensitive properties of pelvic nerve afferent fibers innervating the urinary bladder of the rat. *J Neurophysiol* 1994;72(5):2420–2430.
10. Birder LA, de Groat W, Mills I, et al. Neural control of the lower urinary tract: Peripheral and spinal mechanisms. *Neurourol Urodyn* 2010;29(1):128–139.
11. Bruns TM, Gaunt RA, Weber DJ. Multielectrode array recordings of bladder and perineal primary afferent activity from the sacral dorsal root ganglia. *J Neural Eng* 2011;8(5):056010.
12. Wakabayashi Y, Tomoyoshi T, Fujimiya M, et al. Substance P-containing axon terminals in the mucosa of the human urinary bladder: Pre-embedding immunohistochemistry using cryostat sections for electron microscopy. *Histochemistry* 1993;100(6):401–407.
13. Chancellor MB, de Groat WC. Intravesical capsaicin and resiniferatoxin therapy: Spicing up the ways to treat the overactive bladder. *J Urol* 1999;162(1):3–11.
14. McMahon SB, Abel C. A model for the study of visceral pain states: Chronic inflammation of the chronic decerebrate rat urinary bladder by irritant chemicals. *Pain* 1987;28(1):109–127.
15. Fall M, Lindström S, Mazieres L. A bladder-to-bladder cooling reflex in the cat. *J Physiol* 1990;427:281–300.
16. de Groat WC, Yoshimura N. Mechanisms underlying the recovery of lower urinary tract function following spinal cord injury. *Prog Brain Res* 2006;152:59–84.
17. Yoshimura N, Oguchi T, Yokoyama H, et al. Bladder afferent hyperexcitability in bladder pain syndrome/interstitial cystitis. *Int J Urol* 2014;21(Suppl 1):18–25.
18. Xiao C-G, Du M-X, Dai C, et al. An artificial somatic-central nervous system-autonomic reflex pathway for controllable micturition after spinal cord injury: Preliminary results in 15 patients. *J Urol* 2003;170(4 Pt 1):1237–1241.
19. Griffiths D. Functional imaging of structures involved in neural control of the lower urinary tract. *Handb Clin Neurol* 2015;130:121–133.
20. Tai C, Wang J, Jin T, et al. Brain switch for reflex micturition control detected by FMRI in rats. *J Neurophysiol* 2009;102(5):2719–2730.
21. Stone E, Coote JH, Allard J, et al. GABAergic control of micturition within the periaqueductal grey matter of the male rat. *J Physiol* 2011;589(Pt 8):2065–2078.
22. Takasaki A, Hui M, Sasaki M. Is the periaqueductal gray an essential relay center for the micturition reflex pathway in the cat? *Brain Res* 2010;1317:108–115.
23. Kavia R, Dasgupta R, Critchley H, et al. A functional magnetic resonance imaging study of the effect of sacral neuromodulation on brain responses in women with Fowler's syndrome. *BJU Int* 2010;105(3):366–372.
24. Fukuyama H, Matsuzaki S, Ouchi Y, et al. Neural control of micturition in man examined with single photon emission computed tomography using 99mTc-HMPAO. *Neuroreport* 1996;7(18):3009–3012.
25. Drake MJ, Fowler CJ, Griffiths D, et al. Neural control of the lower urinary and gastrointestinal tracts: Supraspinal CNS mechanisms. *Neurourol Urodyn* 2010;29(1):119–127.
26. Blok BF, Willemsen AT, Holstege G. A PET study on brain control of micturition in humans. *Brain* 1997;120(Pt 1):111–121.
27. Coolen RL, Groenendijk IM, Blok BFM. Recent advances in neuroimaging of bladder, bowel and sexual function. *Curr Opin Urol* 2020;30(4):480–485.
28. Shy M, Fung S, Boone TB, et al. Functional magnetic resonance imaging during urodynamic testing identifies brain structures initiating micturition. *J Urol* 2014;192(4):1149–1154.
29. Walter M, Leitner L, Michels L, et al. Reliability of supraspinal correlates to lower urinary tract stimulation in healthy participants—A fMRI study. *Neuroimage* 2019;191:481–492.
30. Gao Y, Liao L, Blok BFM. A resting-state functional MRI study on central control of storage: Brain response provoked by strong desire to void. *Int Urol Nephrol* 2015;47(6):927–935.

31. Michels L, Blok BFM, Gregorini F, et al. Supraspinal control of urine storage and micturition in men—An fMRI study. *Cereb Cortex* 2015;25(10):3369–3380.

32. Birder LA, de Groat WC. Mechanisms of disease: Involvement of the urothelium in bladder dysfunction. *Nat Clin Pract Urol* 2007;4(1):46–54.

33. Hosseini A, Ehrén I, Wiklund NP. Nitric oxide as an objective marker for evaluation of treatment response in patients with classic interstitial cystitis. *J Urol* 2004;172(6 Pt 1):2261–2265.

34. de Groat WC, Booth AM, Yoshimura N. Neurophysiology of micturition and its modification in animal models of human disease. In: Maggi CA, ed. *The autonomic nervous system*. London: Harwood Academic Publishers, 1993:227–290.

35. Wolff GF, Krlin RM. Posterior tibial nerve stimulation. In: Gilleran JP, Alpert SA, eds. *Adult and pediatric neuromodulation*. Switzerland: Springer International Publishing, 2018:131–141.

36. Vollstedt A, Gilleran J. Update on implantable PTNS devices. *Curr Urol Rep* 2020;21(7):28.

37. Gilleran JP, Gaines N. Pudendal neuromodulation. In: Gilleran JP, Alpert SA, eds. *Adult and pediatric neuromodulation*. Switzerland: Springer International Publishing, 2018:89–104.

38. Peters KM, Feber KM, Bennett RC. Sacral versus pudendal nerve stimulation for voiding dysfunction: A prospective, single-blinded, randomized, crossover trial. *Neurourol Urodyn* 2005;24(7):643–647.

CHAPTER 5

CONGENITAL ANOMALIES AND CREATION OF THE NEOVAGINA

Cassandra K. Kisby • Assia Stepanian • John B. Gebhart

Introduction

Female genital malformations are common. They are seen in 5.5% to 6.7% of the general population, 7.3% of the females with infertility, and 16.7% of patients with recurrent miscarriages.[1,2] This chapter briefly explores the embryology of the female genital system and reviews the diagnosis and management of congenital anomalies, with a focus on vaginal agenesis and creation of the neovagina.

EMBRYOLOGY OF THE FEMALE REPRODUCTIVE TRACT

At birth, the urologic and genital system are functionally separate; however, embryologically, they are interconnected due to their common mesodermal origin. The urogenital system differentiates through complex epithelial–mesenchymal interactions in the presence of promoting or inhibiting factors. Anomalies arise when these processes fail to occur normally. Anomalies of the urogenital system are common and knowledge of the embryologic origins is imperative to understanding the causes and treatments of these conditions.

The cloacal membrane is located on the ventral embryo and becomes partitioned into the urogenital sinus and anorectal canal by the urorectal septum, the eventual perineal body (Fig. 5.1A). The mesonephric ducts attach to the urogenital sinus around the fourth to seventh week of development as the urinary bladder is expanding. A pair of each of the mesonephric (wolffian) and paramesonephric ducts (müllerian) is present in male and female embryos. The paired paramesonephric ducts form the bilateral fallopian tubes and broad ligaments cephalad and fuse to form the uterus, cervix, and upper vagina caudally. In the absence of müllerian inhibiting substance, the mesonephric ducts regress in the female (Fig. 5.1B). The distal vagina forms from the urogenital sinus, from which the sinovaginal bulbs emanate and form the vaginal plate. The vaginal plate canalizes by the fifth month of development to form the

vaginal lumen. Given the interconnectedness of the embryologic pathways, error in formation, fusion, or resorption pathways often results in combined congenital anomalies.

CONGENITAL ANOMALIES OF THE FEMALE REPRODUCTIVE TRACT

Müllerian anomalies and malformation of the genitalia can impart significant consequences for sexual function and reproductive potential. The prevalence of female congenital anomalies is estimated to be as high as 5.5% in an unselected population and 24.5% in women who have experienced miscarriage and/or infertility.[2] Patients often seek care for primary amenorrhea or for workup of pregnancy loss or infertility; however, many congenital anomalies may go undiagnosed if the patient is asymptomatic.

No one classification system exists for female reproductive tract anomalies given the number of variations and combinations of variations that exist. The American Society of Reproductive Medicine has a naming convention specific to uterine anomalies (Fig. 5.2).[3] Dr. Leila Adamyan authored a morphologic-functional classification of müllerian anomalies targeted at creating protocols for treatment and rehabilitation of each class of malformation; the 2014 version contains 10 classes and 25 groups of malformations (Table 5.1).[4,5] Common anomalies and syndromes of the female reproductive tract are presented in Table 5.2. The remainder of this chapter focuses on diagnosis and management of vaginal agenesis.

DIAGNOSIS AND WORKUP OF SUSPECTED VAGINAL AGENESIS

Although vaginal agenesis can arise from sex-steroid pathway defects, a majority of cases are of unknown etiology and suspected to result from multifactorial inheritance. The most common clinical presentation of vaginal agenesis is with Mayer-Rokitansky-Küster-Hauser

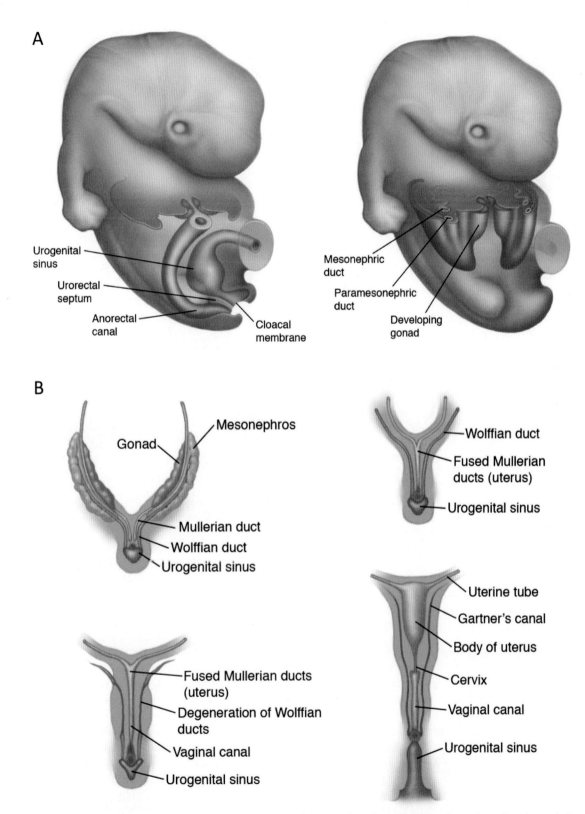

FIGURE 5.1 Female reproductive system embryogenesis. **A:** By the seventh to eighth weeks, the embryo has formed the essential structures of the urogenital system. The urorectal septum is shown dividing the cloaca into the anorectal canal and urogenital sinus. The mesonephric and paramesonephric ducts are present in male and female embryos and will later fuse or regress to form the genitals, a process guided by the presence or absence of the Y chromosome and estrogen. **B:** The paramesonephric (müllerian) ducts and mesonephric (wolffian) ducts are paired structures. During embryogenesis of the female embryo, the müllerian ducts fuse to form the uterus, fallopian tubes, and upper vagina. The wolffian ducts regress due to the absence of testosterone. The urogenital sinus is present distally and fuses with the distal müllerian ducts. The vaginal plate is eventually formed, and this canalizes to form the vagina. (Images used with permission of Mayo Foundation for Medical Education and Research, all rights reserved.)

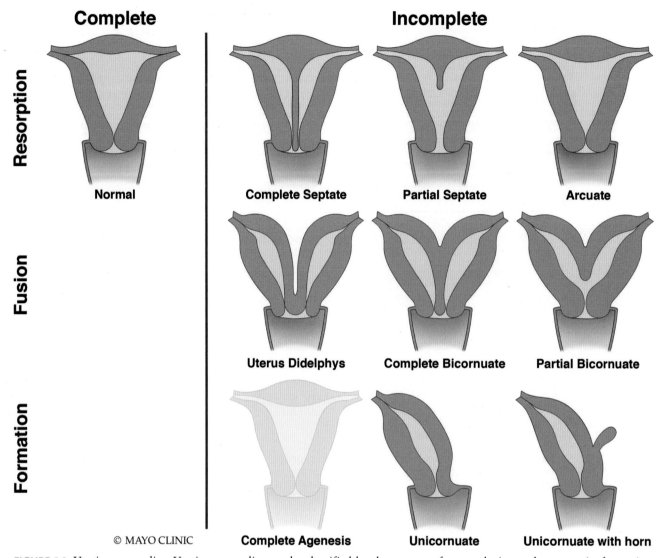

FIGURE 5.2 Uterine anomalies. Uterine anomalies can be classified by three types of errors during embryogenesis: formation, fusion, and resorption. These processes may be complete or incomplete. (Images used with permission of Mayo Foundation for Medical Education and Research, all rights reserved.)

syndrome (MRKH). The incidence of MRKH is estimated to be 1 per 4,500 to 5,000 female births.[6] So as not to make assumptions regarding concomitant anomalies or etiologies, the following sections on workup and management focus generically on absence of the vagina and refer to it as vaginal agenesis.

Patients with vaginal agenesis typically present at the time of puberty for primary amenorrhea or at coitarche due to their inability to have penetrative intercourse. Depending on the presence or absence of the rudimentary uterine horns and functional endometrium, presenting symptoms may also include cyclic abdominal pain due to hematometra of the uterine remnants, which are present in 90% of patients. Concomitant anomalies of the urinary and gastrointestinal tracts are present in 53% of patients and skeletal anomalies in 12%.

The patient presenting with vaginal agenesis is reliant on the physician to guide her, determine the extent of the pathology, offer support and reassurance, and provide guidance on options to achieve penetrative sexual function and, possibly, reproductive potential. It is imperative to have a kind and open discussion with the patient regarding her goals and expectations because these will direct counseling and management. A thorough history should be collected to evaluate the degree of psychological and sexual development, identify prior interventions and additional pathology, guide further investigation, and select the best approach to address the needs of the patient. Surgical histories may reveal neonatal intervention, which may suggest history of more extensive anomalies such as bladder or cloacal exstrophy. Depending on the patient's comfort, the exam may be performed in the clinic or deferred to the operating room to be conducted under anesthesia. The latter option allows for more complete assessment with cystoscopy, vaginoscopy, and diagnostic

TABLE 5.1
Adamyan Morphologic-Functional Classification of Müllerian Anomalies

1. Uterovaginal aplasia (MRKH)
   - With nonfunctional uterine rudiments or functional rudiments

2. Vaginal aplasia
   - Atresia of hymen
   - Partial vaginal aplasia (1/3 or 2/3 part of vagina)

3. Cervicovaginal aplasia
   - Complete vaginal and cervical aplasia with functional uterus
   - Cervical canal aplasia with functional uterus

4. Unicornuate uterus
   - With functional uterine horn
   - Nonfunctional uterine horn
   - Without rudimental horn

5. Uterus duplex
   - Symmetric form with duplication of (1/3, 2/3, full) vagina
   - Asymmetric form—with aplasia of the hemivagina

6. Bicornuate uterus
   - Complete form, incomplete form
   - Arcuate uterus

7. Septate uterus
   - Incomplete septum
   - Complete septum (with vaginal duplication or with normal vagina)

8. Fallopian tube anomalies: congenital absence of tubes or adnexa

9. Gonadal dysgenesis: fibrous streak, ovarian dysgenesis

10. Complex urinary and anorectal anomalies

laparoscopy, as appropriate. An exam should include evaluation of the perineum for the presence of a vaginal dimple or pouch. If a pouch is present, the apex may contain a palpable longitudinal band, which represents the rudimentary uterosacral ligament. The uterine remnants and adnexa are often not palpable unless hematometra is present. It is important to distinguish vaginal agenesis from obstructive anomalies such as a distal transverse septum or imperforate hymen, where the patient may present with pain and hematocolpos. To do this, imaging is beneficial. Transperineal and transabdominal imaging may be performed to delineate pelvic anatomy. Alternatively, magnetic resonance imaging may be preferred due to the ability to concurrently assess for uterovaginal, urologic, and spinal anomalies. Figure 5.3 demonstrates common concomitant anomalies found on imaging in patients with vaginal agenesis.

SURGICAL PROCEDURES FOR CREATION OF A NEOVAGINA

After defining the patient's anatomy, the clinician should, through shared decision-making, decide if penetrative intercourse is a goal and if creation of a neovagina is an appropriate next step. Diagnosis of vaginal agenesis is often distressing and can significantly impact a patient's self-esteem and future intimacy. Psychological support should be provided and interventions only undertaken when the patient is psychologically ready and willing to participate in the care and maintenance of her neovagina. Finally, management of the uterine remnants should be discussed. Although the majority are rudimentary and nonfunctional, a small number may require menstrual suppression or surgical excision if active endometrium or pain is present.

Nonsurgical Management

The primary and least invasive means to create a neovagina is by use of vaginal dilators. In 1938, Frank[7] first described a nonoperative means of creating a neovagina by applying pressure to the vaginal dimple with progressively longer and wider dilators to elongate the vagina. Ingram[8] subsequently described a technique of passive dilation by instructing patients to sit on a dilator that had been affixed to a bicycle seat. Dilation should be performed by applying firm pressure (with a slight posterior angle) on the vaginal dimple three times daily for at least 20 minutes. With consistent dilation, anatomic and functional success can be achieved. In a multicenter study of 131 patients, a mean vaginal depth of 9.6 cm was achieved with the dilator method, compared to 11 cm with surgical intervention.[9]

McIndoe Neovagina

If, following counseling, the patient desires surgical intervention or if she has failed nonsurgical management, she should be presented with options for neovagina creation. The most widely used operation for neovagina creation is the Abbe-Wharton-McIndoe operation, commonly known as the McIndoe operation.[10] This method was first described by Wharton, in 1938, as a combination of simple dissection of the vaginal space and maintenance with a form. It was not until later that Sir Archibald McIndoe incorporated a split-thickness graft and achieved excellent success in clinical trials. The McIndoe technique has three main principles:

1. Dissection of the space between the rectum and bladder
2. Inlay of a graft and temporary mold
3. Dilation with dilators and/or intercourse to maintain patency

TABLE 5.2

Congenital Anomalies of the Female Reproductive Tract

PROCEDURE	ETIOLOGY	PRESENTATION	MANAGEMENT	EXAMPLES
Vaginal septum	Longitudinal septum: Lateral fusion defect of the paramesonephric ducts or urogenital sinus. Transverse septum: Failure of fusion or canalization of the urogenital sinus and paramesonephric ducts	• Difficulty inserting tampons or persistent bleeding despite inserting a tampon • Dyspareunia or inability to have penetrative intercourse • If obstructing, a vaginal mass may be present	Simple surgical excision and suture reapproximation, with temporary postoperative dilator use is often sufficient. If excision leaves a large defect, a graft may be required.	Longitudinal vaginal septum. Transverse vaginal septum. (Illustrations used with permission of Mayo Foundation for Medical Education and Research, all rights reserved.)

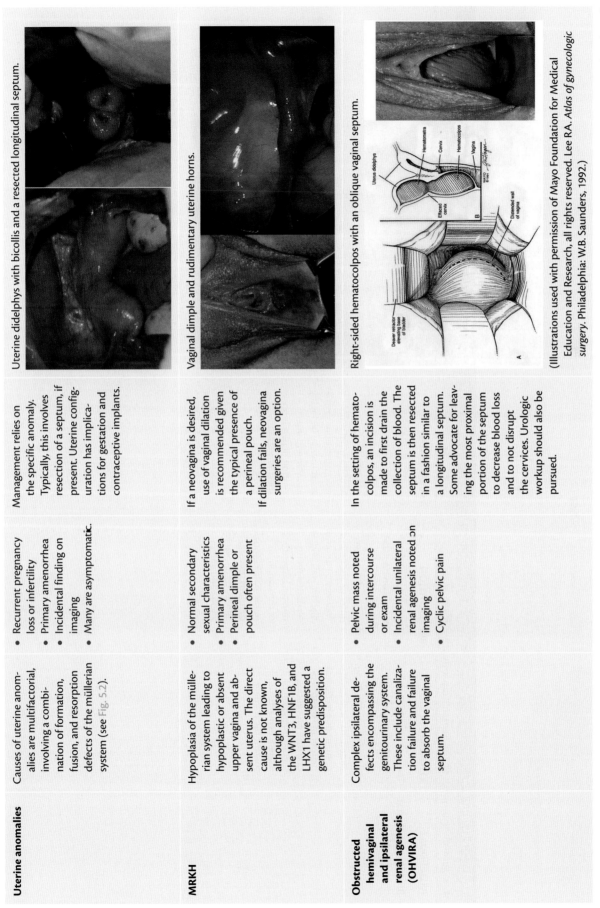

Uterine anomalies	Causes of uterine anomalies are multifactorial, involving a combination of formation, fusion, and resorption defects of the müllerian system (see Fig. 5.2).	• Recurrent pregnancy loss or infertility • Primary amenorrhea • Incidental finding on imaging • Many are asymptomatic.	Management relies on the specific anomaly. Typically, this involves resection of a septum, if present. Uterine configuration has implications for gestation and contraceptive implants.	Uterine didelphys with bicollis and a resected longitudinal septum.
MRKH	Hypoplasia of the müllerian system leading to hypoplastic or absent upper vagina and absent uterus. The direct cause is not known, although analyses of the WNT3, HNF1B, and LHX1 have suggested a genetic predisposition.	• Normal secondary sexual characteristics • Primary amenorrhea • Perineal dimple or pouch often present	If a neovagina is desired, use of vaginal dilation is recommended given the typical presence of a perineal pouch. If dilation fails, neovagina surgeries are an option.	Vaginal dimple and rudimentary uterine horns.
Obstructed hemivaginal and ipsilateral renal agenesis (OHVIRA)	Complex ipsilateral defects encompassing the genitourinary system. These include canalization failure and failure to absorb the vaginal septum.	• Pelvic mass noted during intercourse or exam • Incidental unilateral renal agenesis noted on imaging • Cyclic pelvic pain	In the setting of hematocolpos, an incision is made to first drain the collection of blood. The septum is then resected in a fashion similar to a longitudinal septum. Some advocate for leaving the most proximal portion of the septum to decrease blood loss and to not disrupt the cervices. Urologic workup should also be pursued.	Right-sided hematocolpos with an oblique vaginal septum.

(continued)

TABLE 5.2 (Continued)

Congenital Anomalies of the Female Reproductive Tract

PROCEDURE	ETIOLOGY	PRESENTATION	MANAGEMENT	EXAMPLES
Bladder and cloacal exstrophy	The exact mechanism is not known, although theorized to involve disruption of the lower abdominal wall development due to cloacal membrane overdevelopment, preventing medial migration of mesenchymal tissue toward the midline.	• Anomalies are often detected on prenatal ultrasound: Absence of the lower anterior abdominal wall, absent anterior bladder wall, widely separated rectus muscles, absence of the symphysis pubis, bifid clitoris, patulous urethra, anteriorly displaced vagina and anus	Management after birth may include urinary and/or gastrointestinal diversion as well as abdominal wall reconstruction. Vaginal anatomy can be highly variable and intervention depends on specific anatomy.	Patient with cloacal exstrophy status post end ileostomy, bladder neck closure with Monti catheterizable urinary diversion, and failed prior neovagina surgery.

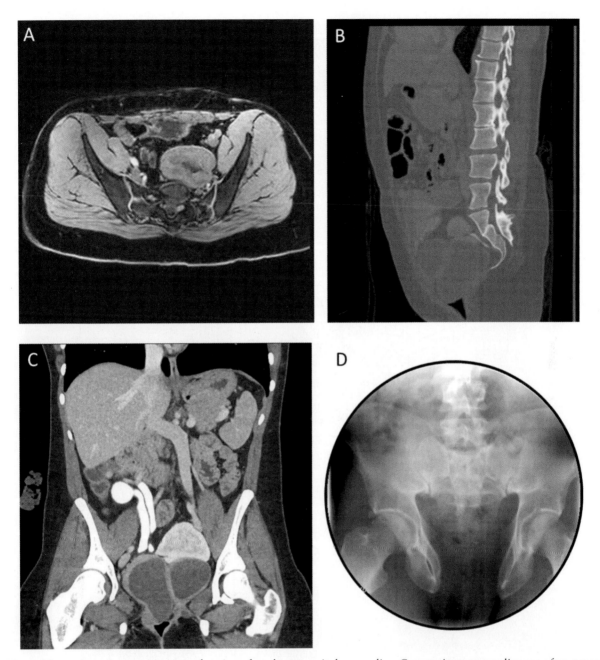

FIGURE 5.3 Magnetic resonance imaging of various female congenital anomalies. Concomitant anomalies are often present in patients with congenital genital anomalies. **A:** Magnetic resonance imaging depicting a left pelvic kidney. **B:** Magnetic resonance imaging demonstrating coccygeal agenesis and sacral fusion. **C:** Computed tomography scan with contrast showing a duplicated right renal collecting system and rudimentary uterine horns with hematocolpos. **D:** A kidney ureter and bladder x-ray depicting agenesis of the symphysis pubis and separation of the pubic rami.

Technique of the McIndoe operation (Video 5.1)

With the patient in lithotomy position, a 3- to 4-cm transverse incision is made in the apex of the vaginal pouch, if present. In the absence of a pouch, the transverse incision is made just beneath the urethral meatus. The neovaginal space is then sharply and bluntly dissected cephalad, with the guidance of a finger in the rectum, to the level of the peritoneal reflection (Fig. 5.4).

The dissection space should easily accommodate two fingerbreadths. If necessary, the levator muscles can be divided laterally to provide sufficient space. Meticulous hemostasis is then achieved. Next, the foam rubber vaginal form is shaped with scissors (Fig. 5.5A). The form is placed into a sterile condom and compressed. The compressed form is then inserted into the vagina and allowed to expand for 1 to 2 minutes. The distal end of the condom is tied, the form removed, and a second condom is placed over the form and the end tied.

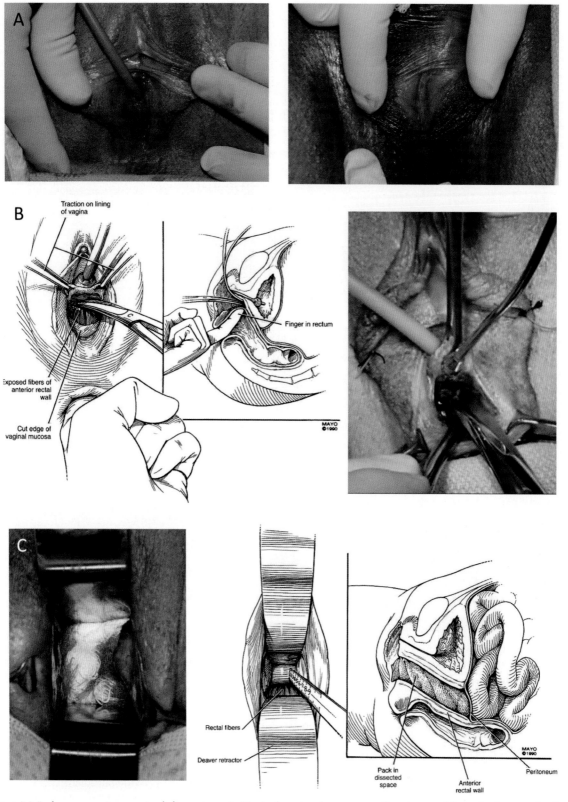

FIGURE 5.4 McIndoe neovagina: vaginal dissection. **A:** Typical perineal anatomy of patients with vaginal agenesis. A vaginal pouch is absent, and the labia minora terminate at approximately the urethral meatus. **B:** McIndoe dissection is carried out bluntly and sharply following an initial transverse incision in the perineum. A finger in the rectum is used to guide dissection. **C:** Dissection is carried out until the peritoneal reflection is encountered. An adequate dissection is approximately 10 to 12 cm in depth and loosely accommodates two fingerbreadths. Hemostasis is essential and achieved by a combination of cautery, suture ligation, and pressure from a vaginal pack. (Illustrations used with permission of Mayo Foundation for Medical Education and Research, all rights reserved. Lee RA. *Atlas of gynecologic surgery*. Philadelphia: Saunders, 1992.)

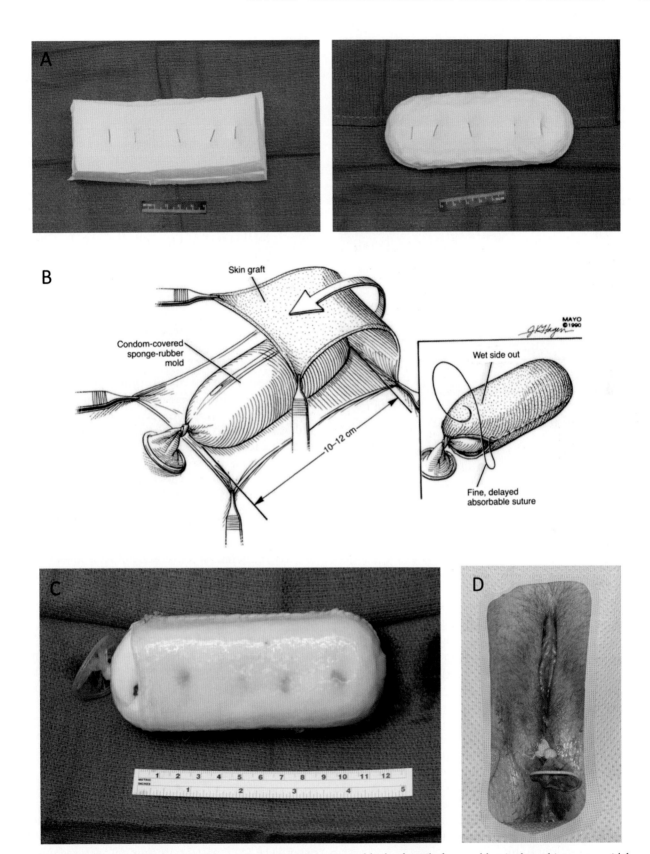

FIGURE 5.5 McIndoe neovagina: vaginal form. **A:** A 10 × 10 × 20 cm block of sterile foam rubber is shaped into an ovoid form using scissors. **B:** The form is placed within a condom, and the split-thickness skin graft is placed over it, with the skin side facing the condom. **C:** The edges of the graft are approximated over the form with interrupted 4-0 absorbable sutures, followed by a running suture of the same. **D:** The form covered with the graft is gently placed into the neovaginal space and the labia sutured overtop. (Illustrations used with permission of Mayo Foundation for Medical Education and Research, all rights reserved. Lee RA. *Atlas of gynecologic surgery*. Philadelphia: Saunders, 1992.)

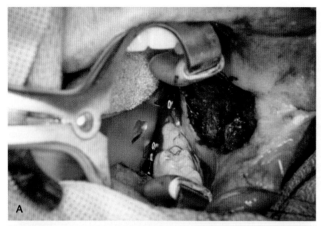

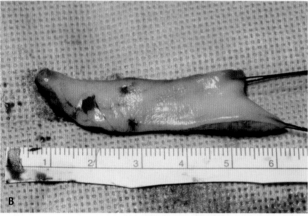

FIGURE 5.6 McIndoe neovagina: buccal graft harvest. **A:** To harvest a buccal graft, retractors are placed in the mouth and a full-thickness graft is taken sharply, bilaterally. **B:** The grafts are defatted and meshed to increase the size as indicated. The graft site may be closed with 4-0 absorbable suture or allowed to reepithelialize naturally. (Photos courtesy of Katherine Theissen, MD and Bridget Findlay, MD.)

Next, the graft is harvested. The authors favor a split-thickness skin graft due to the adequacy of the size of the graft; however, buccal grafts are also acceptable (Fig. 5.6).[11,12] To obtain a split-thickness skin graft, the patient is repositioned and the donor site (commonly the buttock or lateral thigh) is prepared with an antiseptic solution. The skin is then lubricated with sterile mineral oil. A 10-cm Padgett electrodermatome blade is set to 0.45 mm (0.017″). With uniform pressure across the dermatome, a 20-cm graft is obtained (Fig. 5.7B). The graft should be without breaks in continuity and of uniform thickness. The donor site is dressed with gauze soaked with a dilute solution of epinephrine to achieve hemostasis. The patient is then repositioned in lithotomy.

Interrupted 4-0 absorbable sutures are used to affix the graft over the condom-covered vaginal mold, ensuring the skin is facing the condom (Fig. 5.5B,C). Running 4-0 absorbable suture is then used to reinforce and approximate the edges of the skin, avoiding

the underlying condom. The graft and form are then placed in the neovaginal space (Fig. 5.5D). Sutures are applied to the bilateral labia to aid in retention of the form. The graft donor site is then re-dressed with a petrolatum-based gauze infused with bismuth and covered with a waterproof sterile dressing (Fig. 5.8D).

Ten days later, the patient is brought back to the operating room. The form is gently removed, and the neovagina irrigated and the graft assessed for viability. Small nonviable areas may be excised and allowed to heal spontaneously; however, repeat grafting should be performed if large areas of necrosis are present or if there is total failure of the graft. If the graft is successful, the edges are trimmed and sutured to the introitus circumferentially with 2-0 absorbable suture (Fig. 5.8A). A permanent vaginal mold is then placed into the vagina, lubricated with an antibiotic-containing cream (Fig. 5.8B,C). This mold should be worn continuously for 3 to 6 months and removed twice daily for cleansing. The patient may choose to then wear the mold nightly or maintain patency with intercourse or a dilator.

Complications of the procedure include rectal or bladder injury during dissection, postoperative fistula (4.2%), infection, new-onset stress urinary incontinence, and graft failure. Overall, the rate of serious complications has declined with the use of a compressible form, perioperative antibiotics, and nonreactive suture.[13] It is imperative that the patient consistently uses the permanent mold because the risk of stenosis and contracture is highest during the first 3 months after surgery.

Long-term functional outcomes of the McIndoe operation are excellent, with a success rate of 80% (Fig. 5.9). In a long-term retrospective study of 86 women who had undergone a McIndoe operation (mean time from surgery 23 years), Klingele et al.[14] found that 79% reported improved quality of life, 91% remained sexually active, and 75% were able to achieve orgasm. Moreover, 55% of women reported an improved self-image.[14] These findings are consistent with several earlier and smaller case series.[15–19] Regarding cosmetic outcomes, although skin grafting has cosmetic consequences, the donor site will continue to fade in appearance with time (Figs. 5.7C,D and 5.9). Some have proposed use of regenerative medicine techniques to allow for a scarless McIndoe operation[20]; this topic is discussed further in Chapter 22.

Vecchietti Procedure

The Vecchietti procedure was first described by Giuseppe Vecchietti in 1965, and he later reported his initial 14-year experience (522 patients) using an open technique.[21] Minimally invasive modifications to the original technique were first described by Dr. L. Fedele and colleagues, and this approach is now the preferred method due to comparable outcomes and a faster recovery.[22–25] The Vecchietti procedure is a surgical technique to create a

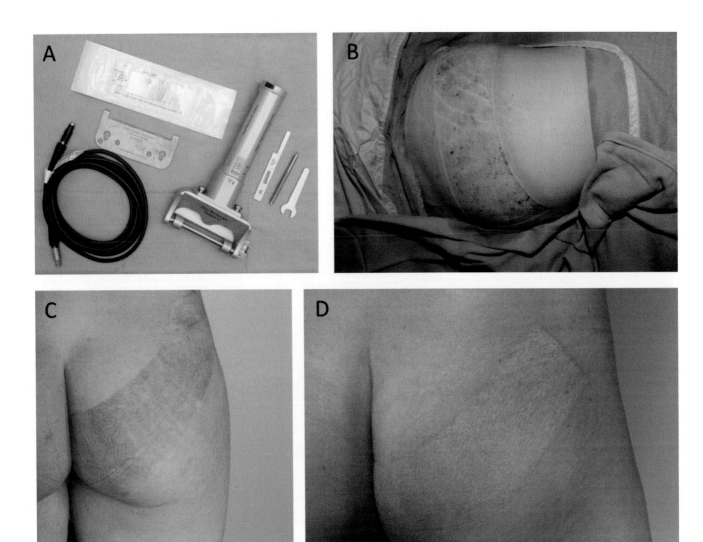

FIGURE 5.7 McIndoe neovagina: graft harvest and insertion. **A:** After preparation with an antiseptic solution and mineral oil, a split-thickness graft is obtained by use of a Padgett electrodermatome. A 10-cm wide blade is used on a setting of 0.45 mm. **B:** Appearance of the graft donor site immediately after harvest. This site should be dressed with a dilute epinephrine-soaked gauze to aid in hemostasis. **C:** Appearance of the graft donor site 6 weeks postoperatively. **D:** Appearance of the graft donor site 1 year postoperatively.

neovagina in 7 to 10 days by traction on sutures attached to an acrylic olive which are affixed to an external tension device on the abdomen (Fig. 5.10). Like vaginal dilation, this technique avoids the use of a graft. This procedure requires frequent follow-up in the early stage, and, like the McIndoe, continued dilation is essential to success.

Technique of the Vecchietti procedure (Video 5.2)

Due to wide adoption of the minimally invasive approach, the laparoscopic technique is described here. Laparoscopic access is typically obtained with two ports: one for the laparoscope and one for a blunt grasper. A single or connected chain of 3-cm synthetic olives is affixed to the end of a no. 2 polyglycolic acid suture. Under laparoscopic guidance, the

sharp ligature carrier holding the olive's suture tails is inserted between the bladder and rectum into the peritoneal cavity. Cystoscopy should then be performed to evaluate for bladder perforation. The blunt ligature carrier is then passed through the lateral, lower abdominal cavity to the preperitoneal space. It is burrowed in this space toward the peritoneal fold just superior to the bladder. At this point, the blunt ligature is pierced intraperitoneally and one suture tail is threaded into the eye of the ligature carrier and carried cephalad through the created tunnel. This is performed bilaterally, such that sutures are passed from the perineum, briefly intraperitoneally, preperitoneally along the anterior abdominal wall, and exit through the skin. The laparoscope and ports are removed and the bilateral suture tails are attached to the external Vecchietti spring traction device (Fig. 5.11).

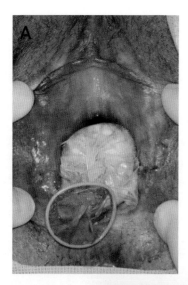
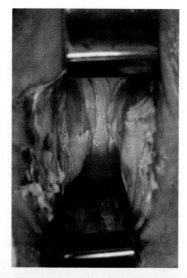
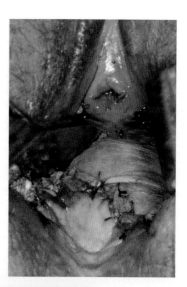

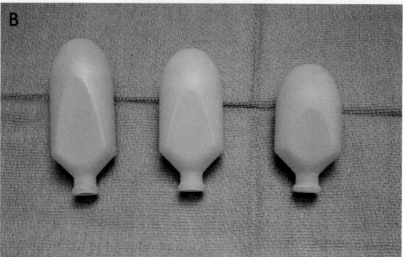

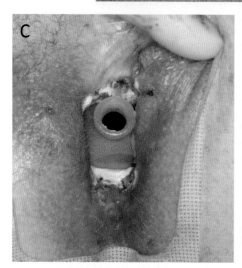
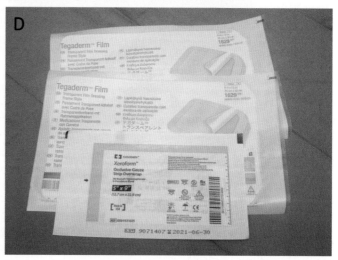

FIGURE 5.8 McIndoe neovagina: stage 2 and postoperative cares. **A:** Seven to 14 days after the stage 1 procedure, the patient returns to the operating room and the form is removed. The neovaginal space is irrigated and the graft edges sutured to the introitus with 2-0 absorbable interrupted sutures. **B:** Permanent vaginal molds of various sizes may be 3D printed. The authors favor molds with a deep and distal drainage hole to allow for egress of vaginal discharge. Furthermore, the distal anterior and posterior edges of the mold are tapered to prevent compression of the urethra and anus. **C:** Permanent vaginal mold in place, lubricated with silver-impregnated cream. **D:** The authors prefer dressing the graft donor site with a petrolatum-based gauze infused with bismuth and a waterproof sterile dressing on top.

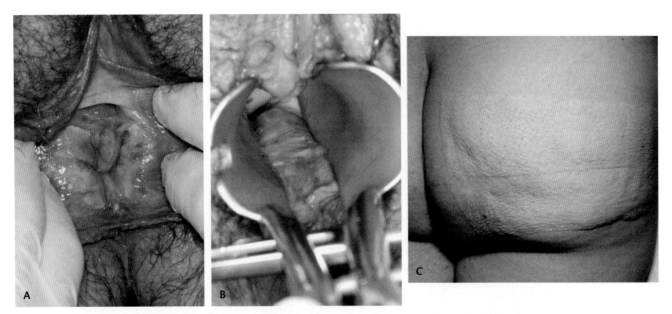

FIGURE 5.9 McIndoe neovagina: outcomes. **A:** Outcomes status post McIndoe neovagina 32 years prior. **B:** The neovagina is patent, with adequate depth and caliber, and the graft donor site has faded remarkably (**C**).

Postoperatively, constant traction is applied to the perineal olive(s) by adjusting tension on the suture tails attached to the traction device. Tension is increased daily, resulting in an approximate neovaginal lengthening of 1 cm per day. Within 7 to 10 days, a 10- to 12-cm neovagina is created. Synthetic olives are then removed under sedation and a vaginal mold placed. After surgery, the patient should maintain patency and depth by use of regular sexual activity or routine use of dilators.

Complications of this technique include bowel and bladder perforation with the ligature carrier, infection, and vaginal vault hemorrhage. Some experts advocate

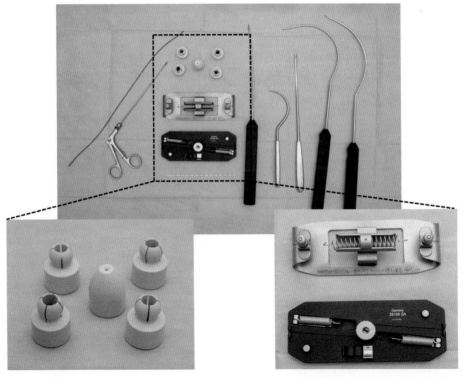

FIGURE 5.10 Vecchietti instruments. Instrument tray with equipment necessary to perform the Vecchietti procedure. Centrally are the acrylic olives and spring-loaded traction device. To the left is the sharp ligature passer. And, to the right, are the blunt ligature passers of various configurations.

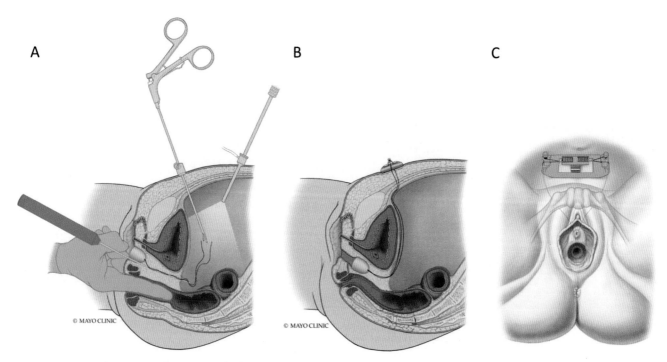

A   B   C

FIGURE 5.11 Vecchietti procedure. **A:** Under laparoscopic guidance, the sharp ligature device is passed from the perineal dimple to the abdominal cavity, passing the suture strings containing the acrylic olive. The blunt ligature carrier is tunneled from the bilateral lower quadrants of the abdomen, preperitoneally, and is then passed intraperitoneally above the bladder-peritoneal reflection (not pictured). The bilateral suture ends are threaded onto the ligature carrier and brought out to the skin. **B,C:** The strings attached to the olive are attached to the Vecchietti spring-loaded device to allow tensioning of the olive. (Illustrations used with permission of Mayo Foundation for Medical Education and Research, all rights reserved.)

for dissection of the vesicorectal space to reduce the risk of perforation, although this step increases the risk of bleeding and hematoma formation.

Anatomic outcomes are well-described for the Vecchietti procedure; however, sexual satisfaction is poorly documented. In Vecchietti's report of outcomes on 522 cases, he reported a 100% success rate in the 2 years following surgery and only nine complications.[21] Kaloo and Cooper[26] reported outcomes in a five-case series; all women maintained a functional vagina at 3 years postoperatively and reported improvements in self-esteem, self-confidence, and general well-being. Using a laparoscopic approach, Borruto et al.[22] reported 100% anatomic success in 86 cases, with a 98.1% functional success rate.

Peritoneal (Davydov) Colpopoiesis

Introduced by D.O Ott in 1898, the method of neovagina creation using peritoneum underwent five modifications until S.N. Davydov performed the one-stage abdominovaginal colpopoiesis in 1974. This approach to abdominovaginal peritoneal colpopoiesis thus acquired the name Davydov colpopoiesis or Davydov surgery or procedure.[27-29] Although Davydov described an abdominovaginal technique, Dr. L.V. Adamyan, in

1991, performed the first laparovaginal peritoneal colpopoiesis, in which three of the 6 main steps of the procedure were carried out laparoscopically.[30-32] The author subsequently reported two additional techniques: total laparoscopic and laparovaginal suture-down technique.[33,34] These techniques are used interchangeably depending on the elasticity of the peritoneum and of the vaginal dimple. This experience is the largest in the world and currently includes over 570 patients with MRKH form of vaginal agenesis alone.[35] Predicated on the success of Drs. Adamyan and Davydov, others have made modifications to their technique with varied success.[36-39]

Technique of the Adamyan laparovaginal peritoneal colpopoiesis (Videos 5.3 and 5.4)

Following evaluation under anesthesia, Foley catheter placement, and diagnostic laparoscopy take place in order to plan the course of vesicorectal canal dissection, assess the elasticity of the pelvic peritoneum, establish topographic relationships in the pelvis (including the appearance of the fibrous streaks or rudimentary uterine horns), and identify any pathology requiring treatment prior to undertaking colpopoiesis.

A transverse 3- to 3.5-cm incision is then made between the posterior aspects of the labia minora. With a preference for blunt/digital dissection, the canal is formed in the vesicorectal space; this dissection is conducted via the vaginal route under laparoscopic guidance. The canal formed needs to allow for easy passage of two slightly separated fingers.

In an effort to facilitate tensionless tissue approximation and to prevent labial pulling into the neovaginal canal, the most mobile aspect of the pelvic peritoneum is identified laparoscopically and gently introduced into the newly formed vesicorectal canal using the laparoscopic pusher. The peritoneum is then grasped with hemostats vaginally and incised.

The next step is approximation of the peritoneum with the mucosa of the vaginal dimple using interrupted stitches of 3-0 absorbable suture. This can be done vaginally or laparoscopically, depending on the elasticity of the peritoneum and the perineum, as well as the position of their incisional edges. Should the peritoneum be prematurely entered, the suture-down technique can be used. After the peritoperineal approximation is concluded, the 4-inch tampon or inflatable vaginal dilator, lubricated with estrogen vaginal cream or a combination of Vaseline and antibiotic cream, is placed into the neovaginal canal.

The apex of the vagina is formed by laparoscopic placement of one or two purse-string stitches of 0 or #1 permanent suture at a distance of about 11 to 13 cm from the opening of the neovagina, depending on the natural pelvic dimensions. This stitch involves the peritoneum overlying the bladder, the fibromuscular streaks, the peritoneum overlying the pelvic sidewall, and serosa of the sigmoid colon or perirectal gutter. A neovagina is thus created (Figs. 5.12 and 5.13).

Postoperatively, patients stay one night in the hospital and are given instructions to follow a regular diet and

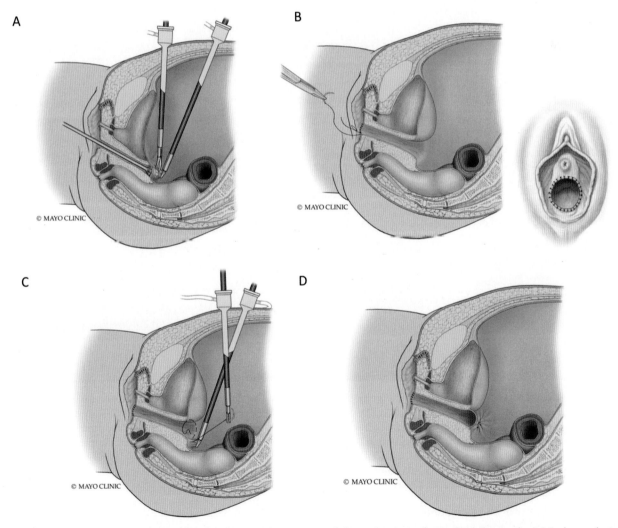

FIGURE 5.12 Minimally invasive peritoneal colpopoiesis. **A:** Vaginal dissection is performed similar to the McIndoe technique, until the peritoneum is reached. A dilator is placed in the neovaginal space. Laparoscopically, an incision is made over the cephalad tip of the dilator. **B:** The peritoneum is dissected free and pulled toward the introitus. The peritoneal edges are affixed to the introital skin with interrupted sutures. **C,D:** The upper vaginal apex is created by placing one-two purse-string sutures laparoscopically. (Illustrations used with permission of Mayo Foundation for Medical Education and Research, all rights reserved.)

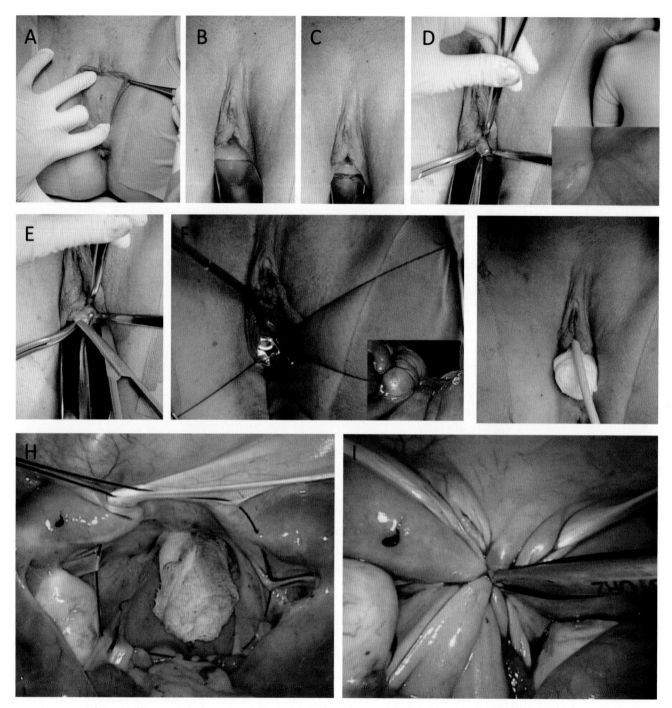

FIGURE 5.13 Adamyan laparovaginal peritoneal colpopoiesis. After the mobile aspects of the peritoneum are laparoscopically identified and mobilized the following steps are performed. **A–C:** Examination under anesthesia and perineal incision. **D:** Introduction of the peritoneum and attached tissue into the perineal incision. **E:** Clearing of the introduced peritoneum from attached tissue, peritoneal incision. **F:** Approximation of the peritoneum and the mucosa of the vaginal dimple. **G:** Placement of the neovaginal tampon. **H,I:** Purse-string suture placement for formation of the apex of the neovagina. (Photographs provided by Dr. Assia Stepanian on behalf of Dr. Leila Adamyan.)

to return for removal of the Kling and Foley after 48 to 72 hours. Oral antibiotics are used while the vaginal Kling and Foley catheter remain in place. At 1-week, patients are reexamined with attention to the tissue reaction, vaginal width and length, the condition of the vaginal apex, and the state of the suture line. Sexual intercourse may occur not

earlier than 4 weeks after the procedure or earlier, if the examiner's glove or maintenance dilator no longer shows evidence of bloodstaining. No maintenance dilation is needed after initiation of regular (at least twice a week) intercourse. When not sexually active, the patients are instructed to use a maintenance dilator.

TABLE 5.3		
Advantages and Disadvantages of Neovagina Techniques		
	ADVANTAGES	**DISADVANTAGES**
McIndoe	Well-described technique with high-level evidence Graft use increases the likelihood of achieving adequate vaginal depth.	Cosmesis at the donor graft site Risk of graft failure Need for second-stage procedure/anesthesia Delayed use of neovagina during convalescence
Vecchietti	Graftless technique Ability to achieve a functional vagina in 7–10 d	Special equipment is required. Initial intensive care during spring traction device use Requires laparotomy or laparoscopic incisions Need for second-stage procedure/anesthesia Need to dilate to increase vaginal diameter
Davydov	No special equipment is required. Short operative time No need for a second stage Local graft harvest (peritoneum)	Requires laparotomy or laparoscopic incisions Short-term delayed use of neovagina during convalescence

The presented technique has excellent functional and anatomic outcomes.

In 269 patients with MRKH who were operated on between 1995 and 2013, scores for the Female Sexual Function Index (FSFI) were obtained for a 10- to 15-year follow-up in 57 patients, 5- to 10-year follow-up in 90 patients, and 1- to 5-year follow-up in 111 patients.[40] The average *functional* length of the neovagina equaled 12.46 ± 1.16 cm, whereas *anatomic* vaginal length was found to be 10.87 ± 1.0 cm. Two hundred twenty-four (87.8%) of 255 sexually involved patients were satisfied with the sexual results of their surgeries, as compared with 38 (76.0%) of 50 women in the control group. The questions related to libido, excitability, lubrication, orgasm, and satisfaction identified no significant statistical differences between the patients and the control group based on FSFI scores.

Complications are a rare occurrence using this technique. Out of 570 patients operated on between 1991 and November of 2020, rectovaginal fistula formation was seen in 1 patient (0.18%), rectal injury in 1 patient (0.18%), bladder injury in 2 patients (0.36%), short (<6 cm) vaginal length in 2 patients (0.36%), vaginal stricture in 6 patients (1.05%), and dyspareunia in 12 patients (2.1%). Both vaginal stricture and failure to achieve the appropriate vaginal length occurred in patients who did not perform maintenance dilation and did not engage in regular intercourse. No pelvic prolapse, abscesses, hematoma, apical dehiscence, or urethral damage seen in earlier smaller abdominal studies were reported in this group.

In Davydov's account of his 12-year experience performing the procedure, he noted that all but 1 of 30 patients was able to achieve penetrative intercourse within several weeks following surgery. Mean vaginal length achieved by his technique was 8 to 11 cm.[27] In a case series of 28 women, sexual function, as measured by the FSFI, was equivalent between women having undergone the Davydov and a control group of women with normal genital development.[38] In this series, there was 1 vesicovaginal fistula, 1 apical dehiscence, and vaginal length was greater than 6 cm in 26 out of 28 patients.

Peritoneal colpopoiesis presents multiple advantages: It results immediately in the creation of a neovagina of normal size and elasticity, spares skin and the sigmoid colon utilization for grafting, reduces dependency on tractional devices, and allows for early commencement of satisfying sexual activity.

Advantages and Disadvantages of Neovagina Techniques

This chapter presented three techniques for creation of a neovagina, each with its individual complication profile and success rates. These points are summarized in Table 5.3. Although not described here, alternative options for neovagina creation include a bowel vaginoplasty, biologic grafting, and use of myocutaneous and fasciocutaneous flaps. The ultimate choice of technique is determined by the patient, using her goals and counseling by her surgeon to guide her decision.

References

1. Acien P, Acien M. The presentation and management of complex female genital malformations. *Hum Reprod Update* 2016;22(1):48–69.
2. Chan YY, Jayaprakasan K, Zamora J, et al. The prevalence of congenital uterine anomalies in unselected and high-risk populations: A systematic review. *Hum Reprod Update* 2011;17(6):761–771.
3. The American Fertility Society classifications of adnexal adhesions, distal tubal occlusion, tubal occlusion secondary to tubal ligation, tubal pregnancies, mullerian anomalies and intrauterine adhesions. *Fertil Steril* 1988;49(6):944–955.

4. Makiyan Z, Adamyan L. Systematization of female genital anomalies. *Geburtshilfe Frauenheilkd* 2011;71(10):A14.

5. Adamyan LV, Kurilo LF, Okulov AB, et al. Classification of female genital malformations (part II). *Prob Reprod* 2011.

6. Committee on Adolescent Health Care. ACOG Committee Opinion No. 728: Müllerian agenesis: Diagnosis, management, and treatment. *Obstet Gynecol* 2018;131(1):e35–e42.

7. Frank R. The formation of an artificial vagina without operation. *Am J Obstet Gynecol* 1938;35(6):1053–1055.

8. Ingram JM. The bicycle seat stool in the treatment of vaginal agenesis and stenosis: A preliminary report. *Am J Obstet Gynecol* 1981;140(8):867–873.

9. Cheikhelard A, Bidet M, Baptiste A, et al. Surgery is not superior to dilation for the management of vaginal agenesis in Mayer-Rokitansky-Kuster-Hauser syndrome: A multicenter comparative observational study in 131 patients. *Am J Obstet Gynecol* 2018;219(3):281.e1–281.e9.

10. McIndoe A. An operation for the cure of congenital absence of the vagina. *J Obs Gyn Brit Emp* 1938;45:490–494.

11. Grimsby GM, Bradshaw K, Baker LA. Autologous buccal mucosa graft augmentation for foreshortened vagina. *Obstet Gynecol* 2014;123(5):947–950.

12. van Leeuwen K, Baker L, Grimsby G. Autologous buccal mucosa graft for primary and secondary reconstruction of vaginal anomalies. *Semin Pediatr Surg* 2019;28(5):150843.

13. McQuillan SK, Grover SR. Dilation and surgical management in vaginal agenesis: A systematic review. *Int Urogynecol J* 2014;25(3):299–311.

14. Klingele CJ, Gebhart JB, Croak AJ, et al. McIndoe procedure for vaginal agenesis: Long-term outcome and effect on quality of life. *Am J Obstet Gynecol* 2003;189(6):1569–1573.

15. Keser A, Bozkurt N, Taner OF, et al. Treatment of vaginal agenesis with modified Abbe-McIndoe technique: Long-term follow-up in 22 patients. *Eur J Obstet Gynecol Reprod Biol* 2005;121(1):110–116.

16. Thompson JD, Wharton LR Sr, Te Linde RW. Congenital absence of the vagina; an analysis of thirty-two cases corrected by the McIndoe operation. *Am J Obstet Gynecol* 1957;74(2):397–404.

17. Khanna S, Khanna NN. Congenital absence of vagina: An analysis of 18 cases corrected by the McIndoe operation using a condom mould. *Int Surg* 1982;67(4):345–346.

18. Højsgaard A, Villadsen I. McIndoe procedure for congenital vaginal agenesis: Complications and results. *Br J Plastic Surg* 1995;48(2):97–102.

19. Buss JG, Lee RA. McIndoe procedure for vaginal agenesis: Results and complications. *Mayo Clin Proc* 1989;64(7):758–761.

20. Panici PB, Ruscito I, Gasparri ML, et al. Vaginal reconstruction with the Abbe-McIndoe technique: From dermal grafts to autologous in vitro cultured vaginal tissue transplant. *Semin Reprod Med* 2011;29(1):45–54.

21. Borruto F. Mayer–Rokitansky–Kuster syndrome: Vecchietti's personal series. *Clin Exp Obstet Gynecol* 1992;19(4):273–274.

22. Borruto F, Camoglio FS, Zampieri N, et al. The laparoscopic Vecchietti technique for vaginal agenesis. *Int J Gynaecol Obstet* 2007;98(1):15–19.

23. Borruto F, Chasen ST, Chervenak FA, et al. The Vecchietti procedure for surgical treatment of vaginal agenesis: Comparison of laparoscopy and laparotomy. *Int J Gynaecol Obstet* 1999;64(2):153–158.

24. Nahas S, Yi J, Magrina J. Mayo Clinic experience with modified Vecchietti procedure for vaginal agenesis: It is easy, safe, and effective. *J Minim Invasive Gynecol* 2013;20(5):553.

25. Wang Y-Y, Duan H, Zhang X-N, et al. Neovagina creation: A novel improved laparoscopic Vecchietti procedure in patients with Mayer–Rokitansky–Küster–Hauster syndrome. *J Minim Invasive Gynecol* 2021;28(1):82–92.

26. Kaloo P, Cooper M. Laparoscopic-assisted Vecchietti procedure for creation of a neovagina: An analysis of five cases. *Aust N Z J Obstet Gynaecol* 2002;42(3):307–310.

27. Davydov SN. 12-Year experience with colpopoiesis using the peritoneum. *Gynakologe* 1980;13(3):120–121.

28. Davydov SN. Colpopoeisis from the peritoneum of the uterorectal space. *Akush Ginekol (Mosk)* 1969;45(12):55–57.

29. Davydov SN, Zhvitiashvili OD. Formation of vagina (colpopoiesis) from peritoneum of Douglas pouch. *Acta Chir Plast* 1974;16(1):35–41.

30. Adamyan L, inventor. Laparoscopic peritoneal colpopoiesis. RU2,015,126,640.

31. Davis G, Redwine DB, Perez JJ, et al. Gynecology. In: Arregui ME, Fitzgibbons RJ, Katkhouda N, et al, eds. *Principles of laparoscopic surgery: Basic and advanced techniques.* New York: Springer, 1995:537–679.

32. Adamyan L. Additional international perspectives: Colpopoiesis in vaginal and uterine aplasias. In: Nichols D, eds. *Gynecologic and obstetric surgery.* Maryland Heights: Mosby, 1993:1167–1182.

33. Adamyan L, inventor. Total laparoscopic colpopoiesis. RU2,015,199,396.

34. Adamyan L, inventor. Total laparoscopic colpopoiesis with 2 provisionary sutures. RU2,585,739.

35. Adamyan LV, Stepanian AA. Neovagina creation with the use of the pelvic peritoneum. In: Grimbizis GF, Campo R, Tarlatzis BC, et al, eds. *Female genital tract congenital malformations: Classification, diagnosis and management.* London: Springer, 2015:201–210.

36. Moriarty CR, Miklos JR, Moore RD. Surgically shortened vagina lengthened by laparoscopic Davydov procedure. *Female Pelvic Med Reconstr Surg* 2013;19(5):303–305.

37. Langebrekke A, Istre O, Busund B, et al. Laparoscopic assisted colpoiesis according to Davydov. *Acta Obstet Gynecol Scand* 1998;77(10):1027–1028.

38. Giannesi A, Marchiole P, Benchaib M, et al. Sexuality after laparoscopic Davydov in patients affected by congenital complete vaginal agenesis associated with uterine agenesis or hypoplasia. *Hum Reprod* 2005;20(10):2954–2957.

39. Acar O, Sofer L, Dobbs RW, et al. Single port and multiport approaches for robotic vaginoplasty with the Davydov technique. *Urology* 2020;138:166–173.

40. Adamyan LV, Stenyayeva NN, Makiyan ZN. Sexual function of women after surgical correction of the vaginal and uterine aplasia. *Proceedings of the XXVII Congress of New Technologies for Diagnosis and Treatment of Gynecologic Disease.* National Medical Research Center for Obstetrics, Gynecology and Perinatology. 2014.

CHAPTER 6

ETIOLOGY OF PELVIC ORGAN PROLAPSE AND URINARY INCONTINENCE

Daniel M. Morgan

Introduction

Pelvic organ prolapse (POP) and urinary incontinence (UI) are distinct conditions but often treated and studied concurrently, as they are in this chapter. The role of pelvic relaxation in treating both of these conditions may account for how they have become linked in our thinking. Nonetheless, it is worthwhile to remember that the association between prolapse and UI is weak at best. Many women with prolapse are not affected by UI and vice versa.[1]

The lifetime risk of surgical intervention for POP and UI increases with age[2] and ranges from 11% to 20%[3–6] by age 80 to 85 years. Women are increasingly more likely to seek care for prolapse and UI as they age.[7] With an aging population in the United States, it is estimated that by 2050, the number of women with POP will increase from 3.3 to 4.9 million and the number with UI will increase from 18.3 million to 28.4 million. Surgical management is projected to increase annually for POP from 166,000 to 245,970 and for stress urinary incontinence (SUI) from 210,700 to 310,050.[8] An analysis of a large managed care organization has raised concerns that there may be a shortage of health care personnel to meet this need.[9]

DEFINITIONS

Consensus is developing around definitions for POP. To consider it a clinical problem, there should be a combination of symptoms and findings consistent with the condition.

The American College of Obstetricians and Gynecologists (ACOG) and the American Urogynecologic Society (AUGS) define POP as descent of the vagina or uterus that allows the bladder or bowel to herniate into the vaginal space. They advise that prolapse be considered a problem when it causes symptoms of bulging or pressure or when it alters bladder or bowel function. Mild relaxation is common and should not be considered pathologic.[10] The International Continence Society (ICS) and the International Urogynecological Association (IUGA) define prolapse as the "descent of one or more of the anterior vaginal wall, posterior vaginal wall, uterus (cervix), or apex of the vagina (vaginal vault or cuff scar after hysterectomy)" and advise that "the presence of any such sign should be correlated with relevant POP symptoms." These symptoms of POP are described by ICS/IUGA as the "departure from normal sensation, structure or function, experienced by the woman in reference to the position of her pelvic organs." ICS/IUGA further recognize how symptoms may be "generally worse . . . when gravity makes prolapse worse (e.g. long periods of standing or exercise) . . . better when . . . lying supine," and "more prominent at times of abdominal straining, e.g. defecation."

Both societies also recognize that there is a threshold in prolapse at which symptoms are more common. ACOG/AUGS have noted that protrusion of the vagina 0.5 cm beyond the hymen is associated with symptoms of prolapse,[11] whereas ICS/IUGA have commented that the "correlation" of signs and symptoms would most often "occur at the level of the hymen or beyond."[12]

PROLAPSE STAGING AND PREVALENCE

The Pelvic Organ Prolapse Quantification (POP-Q) staging system is used most often to describe pelvic organ support. Prolapse is assessed with respect to the hymen, with negative numbers indicating support above it, positive numbers beyond it, and zero at the hymen. In Figure 6.1, support of the vagina and uterus are shown with respect to common reference points of vaginal and vulvar anatomy.[13] The proportion of women who have support in these different stages—also analyzed by centimeters in relationship to the hymen—is illustrated in Figure 6.2.[14] Due to the definition of stage 2 prolapse being within 1 cm of the hymen, it is important to recognize that two-thirds of women have vaginal support that is categorized as having some prolapse.

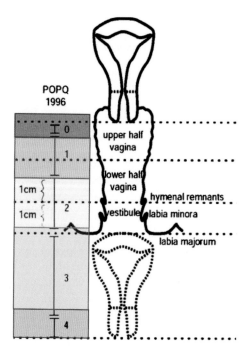

FIGURE 6.1 Prolapse staging. (Reprinted by permission from Springer: Haylen BT, de Ridder D, Freeman RM, et al. An International Urogynecological Association [IUGA]/ International Continence Society [ICS] joint report on the terminology for female pelvic floor dysfunction. *Int Urogynecol J* 2010;21[1]:5–26.)

Symptom questionnaires and exam findings are useful in establishing the prevalence of vaginal prolapse considered a clinical issue. Vaginal prolapse that is bothersome enough for treatment is reported by 6% of women[15] and prolapse beyond the hymen is also present in 5% to 5.7%.[14,16] These findings make it appear that there is a nearly perfect correlation between subjective and objective findings of POP. Although symptoms are important in establishing a diagnosis of POP, there are limitations—especially when support is at or just above the hymen. When the criterion for prolapse on pelvic exam is vaginal support 0.5 cm proximal to the hymen, only 72% were correctly identified with the question "Can you feel with your hand or see something bulging out of your vagina?"

ETIOLOGY

Disease models are helpful in conceptualizing the development of prolapse and UI. In 1998, Bump and Norton[17] described how risk factors can be sorted into those that predispose, incite, promote, or decompensate structure or function and how medication or surgery can intervene and return structure or function to normal. In 2008, DeLancey et al.[18] described a lifespan model (Fig. 6.3) to emphasize the temporal relationship between these factors and development of symptoms. Phase 1 consists of the interaction of genetics,

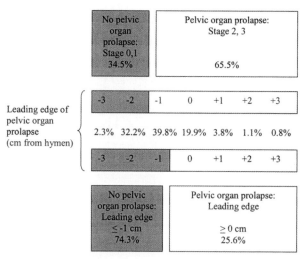

FIGURE 6.2 The proportion of women with leading edge of prolapse at centimeter intervals from the hymen. Two methods of defining prolapse are presented (discussed in text), along with the prevalence of prolapse depending on definition. (Reprinted from Nygaard I, Bradley C, Brandt D; for the Women's Health Initiative. Pelvic organ prolapse in older women: Prevalence and risk factors. *Obstet Gynecol* 2004;104[3]:489–497.)

environment, and social training that lead to variation in health status. Phase 2 is characterized by inciting factors such as childbirth. In Phase 3, there are intervening factors (considered promoting and decompensating in the Bump and Norton model) that can hasten the onset of symptoms. Aging and conditions such as constipation that leads to excessive straining, obesity that increases abdominal pressure, or any number of medical conditions that require chronic corticosteroids can hasten deterioration in tissue health and function and cause a patient to cross the symptom threshold.

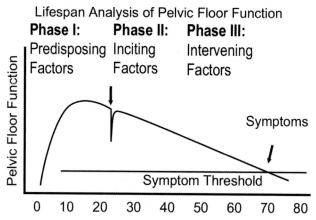

FIGURE 6.3 Lifespan analysis of pelvic floor function. (Reprinted from Delancey JO, Kane Low L, Miller JM, et al. Graphic integration of causal factors of pelvic floor disorders: An integrated life span model. *Am J Obstet Gynecol* 2008;199[6]:610.e1–610.e5. Copyright © 2008, with permission from Elsevier.)

PREDISPOSING FACTORS

There is a complex interplay of genetics and environment with evidence that heritability is a factor in the development of prolapse. A twin study identified a higher concordance rate for surgically treated POP and SUI among monozygotic than dizygotic twins,[19] and the sisters of women presenting for treatment with stage 3 or 4 prolapse were fivefold more likely to develop prolapse than the general population.[20] Many investigators have focused on genes that are associated with connective tissue and extracellular matrix. A meta-analysis of the genetic epidemiology of prolapse identified 4.79 increased odds (95% confidence interval [CI], 1.91 to 11.98) for developing prolapse when a gene that affects type 3 collagen fibers (COL3A1 rs1900255 genotype AA) is present. This type of collagen is found predominantly in the loose areolar tissue surrounding the vagina and pelvic organs.[21]

Patients with spina bifida, characterized by an incomplete closure of the spinal column, are also at higher risk of symptomatic prolapse than women in the general population. The underdeveloped sacral nerves, which supply innervation to the levator ani and other pelvic floor muscles, lead to a flaccid pelvic floor and high rates of POP. In two cohorts of patients with spina bifida, the rates of prolapse approached 50%. Among the 24 nulliparous women, 50% had at least stage 2 POP.[22] Bladder management is associated with their risk for prolapse. The rate of de novo vaginal prolapse or rectal intussusception for patients with acontractile neurogenic bladder who empty the bladder by Valsalva was 32.1% compared to 3.7% in those using clean intermittent catheterization with 5-year follow-up.[23]

Social determinants of health are important to consider when comparing the prevalence of prolapse between populations. Differences observed among women analyzed by race are likely related to socioeconomic factors. For instance, women who have physically demanding occupations and fewer financial resources may be at higher risk of developing prolapse.[24] These findings are beginning to demonstrate how race is "more accurately described as a social construct and not a biological one."[25]

INCITING FACTORS

Vaginal childbirth influences the risk of developing prolapse. The cumulative incidence rates for developing prolapse at 5 and 15 years are 1.6% and 30% for spontaneous vaginal birth and 4% and 45% for operative vaginal delivery, compared to 0.2% and 9.4% for cesarean delivery.[26]

Many events of labor are potentially associated with the development of POP. These include length of the second stage of labor, use of episiotomy, mode of delivery (spontaneous vs. instrumented vs. cesarean), anal sphincter injury, and occult injuries (levator ani avulsion and connective tissue injuries). Memon et al. (Fig. 6.4) illustrated the clustering of childbirth events in 418 primiparous women to show how individual women may have one or multiple exposures.[27]

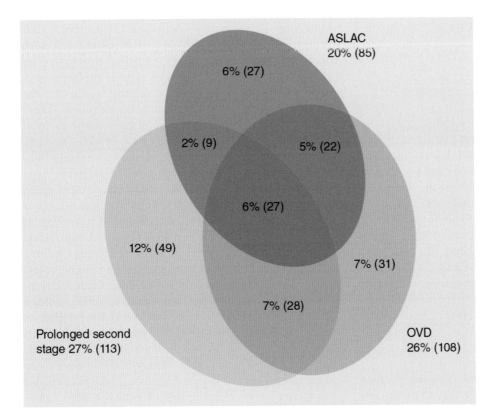

FIGURE 6.4 Clustering of obstetrical exposures in a population of 418 primiparous women who delivered vaginally. ASLAC, anal sphincter laceration; OVD, operative vaginal delivery. (From Memon HU, Handa VL. Vaginal childbirth and pelvic floor disorders. *Womens Health [Lond]* 2013;9[3]:265–277. Reprinted by permission of SAGE Publications.)

Levator avulsion injury is associated with a significant increase in risk for POP. The prevalence of levator ani injury with first birth ranges from 15% to 36%.[28-32] Several studies have confirmed the importance of this injury in the development of prolapse.[33,34] In age- and parity-matched groups of women with prolapse and normal support, DeLancey et al.[34] found that 55% of women with prolapse had magnetic resonance imaging consistent with a levator ani injury compared to 16% of controls—a sevenfold increased odds of prolapse. With a median of 11 years follow-up after first vaginal birth, Handa et al.[32] found that 55% of women with levator avulsion injury diagnosed by ultrasound had developed prolapse compared to 21% of those without levator avulsion—a fourfold increased risk.

Levator ani injury is associated with functional and physiologic change in the pelvic floor, but it is not clear how this injury mediates prolapse. It has been argued that levator ani injury leads to an increase in levator hiatus size and decreased contraction strength.[35] However, there is also evidence that a levator ani defect accounts for only a proportion of the changes in the size of the levator hiatus and prolapse.[36] Among patients recruited 5 to 10 years after delivery, Handa et al.[37] found that a larger genital hiatus led to a significantly increased risk of prolapse and that the effect of parity was attenuated with adjustment for genital hiatus.

There are several risk factors for levator ani injuries. Forceps-assisted vaginal birth is associated with injury.[38] Compared to noninstrumented vaginal delivery, operative delivery by forceps or vacuum significantly increases the odds for all pelvic floor disorders, with the highest increase for POP (odds ratio 7.5, 95% CI 2.7 to 20.9).

PHASE 3 FACTORS

Aging is frequently cited as a factor in prolapse.[16,39,40] It seems likely that there is an interaction between aging and parity and other risk factors. In matched cohorts recruited from the Swedish Medical Birth Register, the rate of prolapse for those with one vaginal delivery increased from 3.8% at age 40 years to 13.8% by age 64 years. In contrast, the rate of symptomatic prolapse did not exceed 5% among nulliparous women and those who had one cesarean delivery.[41] There was no difference in pelvic organ support assessed by POP-Q among nulliparous women stratified by deciles between ages 20 and 70 years.[42] In a large epidemiologic study, the odds of prolapse did not increase for women up to age 84 years compared to those 25 to 39 years when adjustments were made for birth experience, menopausal status, hysterectomy, and obesity.[15]

Hysterectomy

Although posthysterectomy prolapse rates are less than 1%, epidemiologic analyses indicate that hysterectomy is associated with an increased risk of vaginal prolapse.

This complication was most common among those who had a vaginal hysterectomy for prolapse, followed by those who had a vaginal hysterectomy for nonprolapse indications, and then by those who underwent a total abdominal hysterectomy for nonprolapse indications. The lowest rates of prolapse were identified among women who did not undergo hysterectomy.[43] It is not possible to disentangle the relative impact of the underlying reasons for an increased rate of prolapse—it could be the hysterectomy itself, the pelvic anatomy allowing for vaginal hysterectomy, or the indication of uterovaginal prolapse.

Surgical technique is believed to reduce the risk of posthysterectomy prolapse. Shortening and plication of the uterosacral and cardinal ligaments have long been used to restore apical vaginal support. In 1927, Miller described reattachment of these ligaments to the vaginal cuff using chromic catgut as "lifting sutures passed through the peritoneum and underlying fascial and muscular structures at the base of the sacro-uterine ligament."[44] The technique of posterior culdoplasty to treat enterocele at the time of hysterectomy was published by McCall[45] in 1957. The principles of this approach underlie the treatment of posthysterectomy vaginal vault prolapse.[46]

Obesity is a risk factor for POP. Studies with larger sample sizes are more likely to report an increased risk of prolapse.[47] In a meta-analysis of 22 studies providing estimates for overweight (body mass index [BMI] 25 to <30) and obese (BMI ≥30), there was a 36% (risk ratio [RR] 1.36, 95% CI 1.20 to 1.53) and 47% (RR 1.47, 95% CI 1.35 to 1.59) higher risk of prolapse, respectively, compared to women of normal (<25) BMI.[48]

Chronic straining also plays a role in prolapse. Obstructed defecation syndrome, dyssynergic defecation, and constipation are often associated with prolapse—especially posterior vaginal prolapse. The anatomic defects leading to this type of prolapse were first described according to the relative location in the posterior vagina—low, middle, and upper vagina. These forms of prolapse correlate with injuries to the perineal membrane, failure of the levator ani muscles to close the genital hiatus, and failure of the uterosacral ligaments to provide upward suspension, respectively.

Physical stressors and socioeconomic status (SES) are risk factors about which little is known. In a cross-sectional analysis, women found to have POP at least 1 cm beyond the hymen were sevenfold more likely to work as laborers/factory workers and to have income <$10,000. It is not clear to what extent nutrition, access to care, and health status might confound this relationship.[24] In the only other study evaluating SES, women living in Massachusetts were surveyed about whether or not a health care provider had advised them if they had uterine prolapse or vaginal prolapse involving the bladder or rectum. Those with income >$70,000 were more likely to be aware of such a diagnosis. These patients did not have a pelvic exam to describe the severity of prolapse and were not asked about symptoms.[49]

URINARY INCONTINENCE

Prevalence and Impact

In population-based studies, UI symptoms affect 25% to 60% of women,[39,50–56] with several clustering around a 30% prevalence for any incontinence. Managing UI symptoms is a burden for patients, caregivers, and the community. Women who are incontinent are more likely to experience anxiety and depression,[57] in addition to being more likely to have unmet care needs and to be dependent on others.[55] The average annual cost per woman to manage UI was $873 in community-dwelling settings and $5,325 for those older than age 65 years in an institutionalized setting. The total costs of UI for women in the United States was $11.2 billion in 2000.[58]

Definitions

The ICS describes UI symptoms and signs separately. The symptom of UI is any complaint of involuntary loss of urine. The sign of UI is the observation of involuntary loss of urine on examination, which "may be urethral or extra-urethral" and is specified as

- Stress incontinence that occurs from the urethra synchronous with effort or physical exertion
- Urgency UI that occurs from the urethra synchronous with the sensation of a sudden, compelling desire to void that is difficult to defer
- Extraurethral incontinence that occurs through channels other than the urethral meatus[13]

Natural History

Minassian et al.[59] (Fig. 6.5) proposed a model to conceptualize risk factors as a series of exposures leading from mild, subclinical symptoms to more severe, clinically recognized symptoms. Environmental or genetic factors do not usually lead to sequelae but may predispose a woman to symptoms. Childbirth and weight gain are a potentially biologically effective dose exposure and can lead to episodic UI symptoms. Comorbidities such as diabetes or neurologic disease can further modify risk, leading to persistent or chronic UI, altered structure and function, and clinically recognizable disease.

An important aspect of this model is the effort to identify opportunities for secondary prevention. This is in contrast to a now-retired UI definition by ICS, which required the involuntary loss of urine to be objectively demonstrable and a social or hygienic problem.[60] Because this definition placed such emphasis on the exam finding of UI, women who did have not demonstrable incontinence too often received little attention or treatment. The goal of management today is to identify and modify potential risk when possible.

The subtypes of UI change across the age span. A pooled estimate of several epidemiologic trials is shown (Fig. 6.6).[59] The prevalence of SUI without urgency peaks in the fifth decade. Mixed UI symptoms—a combination of stress and urgency UI—become increasingly common, surpassing SUI as the most common symptom

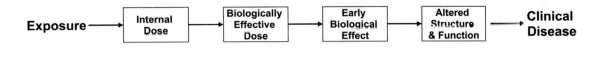

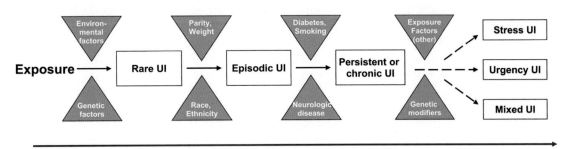

FIGURE 6.5 Natural history of UI. Exposure represents the interaction of the individual with a risk factor, internal dose is the amount of injury sustained with few to no sequelae; a biologically effective dose of an exposure represents the threshold needed to be crossed to produce an effect (i.e., UI); early biologic effect is the untoward expression of symptoms of UI as a result of prolonged or sustained exposure but which may still be reversible; the altered structure and function represent advanced disease (stress, urgency, or mixed UI) that is not spontaneously reversible without an intervention. (Reprinted by permission from Springer: Minassian VA, Bazi T, Stewart WF. Clinical epidemiological insights into urinary incontinence. *Int Urogynecol J* 2017;28[5]:687–696.)

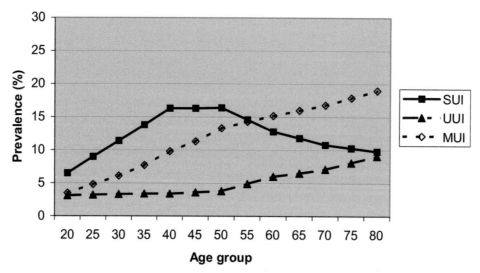

FIGURE 6.6 Prevalence of stress, urgency, and mixed UI by age group. Prevalence estimates of stress, urgency, and mixed incontinence represent pooled estimates of several population-based studies, including Hannestad et al., Hunskaar et al., Melville et al., and Minassian et al. (Reprinted by permission from Springer: Minassian VA, Bazi T, Stewart WF. Clinical epidemiological insights into urinary incontinence. *Int Urogynecol J* 2017;28[5]:687–696.)

subtype in the sixth decade. The prevalence of urgency UI without SUI is 2% to 3% until the sixth decade, after which it increases steadily.

Severity of Urinary Incontinence

The severity of incontinence is highly associated with bother.[61] Questionnaire studies have established population-based estimates for the range of UI symptoms. Several have used the 2-item Sandvik severity index,[56,62] which is estimated by multiplying patient-reported leakage by the frequency of leakage. Melville et al.[52] identified an essentially linear dose response between aging and the likelihood of UI symptoms. The prevalence of severe UI was 8% among women ages 30 to 39, nearly tripled among women ages 50 to 59, and increased to 33% among those ages 80 to 89. Furthermore, moderate UI symptoms were present in another approximately 15% of women in each age decile. In summary, the burden of moderate and severe UI symptoms is striking, reported by one in five women ages 30 to 39 to almost one in two women age 70 and older.

There are limitations to recognize with questionnaire-based studies. Studies examining the differences between self-report and exam findings of continence versus incontinence reveal agreement in only 83% of cases. There are women who report continence but are found to be incontinent on exam and vice versa—a contradiction in classification that occurs in roughly equal proportions.[63] It is also apparent that UI symptoms go into remission and the course is not always a progressive, unyielding condition. With 5-year follow-up for any degree of UI, the mean annual incidence rate was 2.9% and the mean annual remission rate was 5.9%. With 12-year follow-up of a Norwegian county, the remission rate was 34.1%.[56] Women who experienced remission were on average younger, had less severe symptoms, and had a lower BMI.[53,56] There are much lower remission rates reported as well, such as those of the Nurses' Health Studies, which ranged from 3% to 13.9%.

Pregnancy, Role of Delivery, Forceps versus Vacuum

Pregnancy and mode of delivery are associated with UI symptoms. Pregnancy itself is associated with an increased risk of incontinence compared to age-matched nulliparous controls.[64] The first pregnancy is associated with the largest increase in risk, which continues to increase slightly with each subsequent pregnancy.[39,54,65] In a population of women in Washington state, each parous event was estimated to increase the risk of UI by 17%.[52] An increase in symptom risk is observed for term pregnancy compared to nulliparous women,[66] cesarean compared to spontaneous vaginal birth,[54] and assisted vaginal delivery compared to spontaneous vaginal birth.[54] Additional risk factors for UI 1 year after delivery among primiparous women include prepregnancy BMI ≥30 and UI symptoms during pregnancy.[67]

The effect of delivery on rates of UI is modified by age (Fig. 6.7). The increased odds of incontinence are greatest among younger women. The prevalence of incontinence increases each decade for women who delivered vaginally or by cesarean. At age 30 years, there is two- to threefold increased odds of SUI attributable

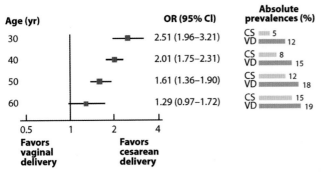

FIGURE 6.7 Relative and absolute risk of SUI between vaginal delivery (VD) and cesarean section (CS) by age group. OR, odds ratio; CI, confidence interval. (Reprinted from Tähtinen RM, Cartwright R, Tsui JF, et al. Long-term impact of mode of delivery on stress urinary incontinence and urgency urinary incontinence: A systematic review and meta-analysis. *Eur Urol* 2016;70[1]:148–158.)

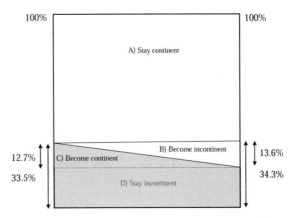

FIGURE 6.8 Continence status 4 to 12 years after first delivery. Group A: women who were continent at baseline and follow-up; group B: women continent at baseline who became incontinent at follow-up; group C: women incontinent at baseline who became continent at follow-up; and group D: women incontinent at baseline and follow-up. (Reprinted from Pizzoferrato AC, Fauconnier A, Quiboeuf E, et al. Urinary incontinence 4 and 12 years after first delivery: Risk factors associated with prevalence, incidence, remission, and persistence in a cohort of 236 women. *Neurourol Urodyn* 2014;33[8]:1229–1234.)

to vaginal delivery. By age 60 years, however, the odds of SUI are no longer statistically attributable to vaginal delivery.[68] There are similar distinctions with respect to assisted vaginal delivery and UI symptoms. For women aged younger than 50 years, forceps vaginal delivery confers an increased risk of SUI compared to spontaneous vaginal delivery. Vacuum-assisted vaginal delivery, however, is not associated with an increased risk compared to spontaneous vaginal delivery, and among women aged 50 years and older, there was no association between stress or urgency incontinence and mode of delivery.[69]

These observations are consistent with findings that cesarean delivery is unlikely to be an effective strategy to prevent pelvic floor morbidity. Simple math—taking into account that most women in the United States deliver vaginally and that only 11% to 20% undergo surgery for a pelvic floor disorder—illustrates that cesarean delivery to prevent pelvic floor disorders would expose many women to unnecessary surgery.[3,4,70] A cost-effectiveness analysis of elective cesarean delivery versus a trial of labor at term for nulliparous women planning only one child also failed to reveal a preferable method of delivery.[71]

Remission of symptoms after pregnancy is common, but symptoms often recur. SUI most often resolves after pregnancy. Viktrup et al.[72] reported that SUI resolved in 99% of primiparous women within 1 year after delivery. However, the prevalence of SUI increases remarkably during longer term follow-up, with a 5-year incidence of 19% and a 12-year incidence of 30%.[73,74] There is a significant amount of crossover from continence to incontinence and vice versa during this time. This phenomenon is illustrated in a longitudinal retrospective cohort study (Fig. 6.8). Incontinence was reported by 33.5% of patients at 4 years and by

34.3% at 12 years after first delivery, but during that time, 12.7% who were incontinent became continent and 13.6% became incontinent.[75]

HYSTERECTOMY: TOTAL VERSUS SUBTOTAL

In a national registry for hysterectomy performed in Sweden, 29.4% of women had incontinence at least one to three times per week. Among those with incontinence, 45% experienced remission of UI symptoms and 55% had residual symptoms. In this same registry, de novo UI symptoms after hysterectomy were reported by 8.5%.[76] In trials of subtotal versus total hysterectomy, authors have universally reported that the proportion of women with UI decreased with each technique.[77,78] In a meta-analysis of hysterectomy surgical technique for benign disease, women who had a total hysterectomy were less likely to have postoperative UI symptoms.[79]

Race

Many authors have reported an association between race and UI symptoms. In the Kaiser Permanente Medical Care Program of Northern California, age-adjusted rates of incontinence were highest among Hispanic women, followed by white, black, and Asian American women (36%, 30%, 25%, and 19%, respectively, $P < .001$). Risk-adjusted rates of stress incontinence were significantly lower in black and Asian American women compared to white women, but the racial groups did not differ for urge UI symptoms.[80] Authors have differed in findings regarding health-seeking behaviors. Among a population-based cohort of black and white women in Southeastern Michigan who reported bothersome incontinence, there were no significant differences in reasons for not seeking care among doctor not asking, embarrassment, nothing to be done, unable to afford doctor/no health insurance, or fear of doctors. The same group also reported that black women were more likely to restrict fluids and to practice Kegel exercise than white women in their attempts at self-care.[81] In contrast, another group reported that women of color were significantly less likely to have knowledge of preventive and curative treatment for pelvic floor disorders.[82] At nursing home admission among continent women, black women received fewer provider orders regarding timed voiding and bladder retraining designed to prevent incontinence than white women.[83]

Menopause and Estrogen Replacement Therapy

It has been difficult to discern the relationship between menopause and UI. Among women aged 45 to 59 years, the range of incidence rates for UI are 4% to 8%, whereas those for remission are 4% to 7%. Cohort studies have not revealed an association between menopause and UI, but they have noted that aging and weight gain are associated with UI. Symptomatology changes during menopause, with urge UI increasing after menopause and SUI decreasing. The effects of estrogen replacement during menopause vary with the route of administration. Vaginal estrogen replacement, in the presence of postmenopausal vaginal atrophy and lower urinary tract symptoms, increases bladder capacity and decreases urge incontinence symptoms and nocturia. Systemic estrogen therapy, however, increased rates of UI in two large randomized controlled trials—the Women's Health Initiative and the Heart and Estrogen/Progestin Replacement Study.[84]

Obesity and Role of Weight Loss

Population-based studies demonstrate that excessive BMI is associated with any incontinence and severe incontinence.[52] Women with a BMI >30 are at the highest risk.[52,85] The predicted probability of progressing from stress incontinence only to mixed incontinence was 30% higher for those with a BMI >25 and 36% for those with a BMI >30.[86] Several studies have identified that increased intravesical pressure is associated with SUI in obese women,[87] but there are also biologic changes such as the production of ghrelin, a

28–amino-acid peptide gut hormone that might adversely affect urinary tract function.[88]

Weight loss is effective in reducing the severity of UI. Weekly incontinence episodes were reduced more effectively with an intensive 6-month program of diet, exercise, and behavior modification compared to a structured education program (47% vs. 27%, $P = .01$).[89] Weight loss achieved with bariatric surgery is also effective in inducing remission of UI symptoms regardless of incontinence subtype and severity of symptoms.[90,91]

Chronic Illnesses

Women older than age 65 years with chronic illnesses such as Parkinson disease, dementia, cerebral vascular disease, depression, congestive heart failure, and osteoarthritis are at increased risk for developing UI. They also have greater health care needs, with a 30% to 40% higher odds of hospitalization and 2.5-fold higher odds of admission to a skilled nursing facility compared to continent patients during 9 years of follow-up.[92] In a meta-analysis of 38 observational studies, the risk of death increased with severity of incontinence in a dose-dependent fashion among nonstroke patients versus continent controls.[93]

Cognitive factors and mobility are associated with incontinence.[94,95] Community-dwelling women older than age 65 years who had cognitive or physical decline were more likely to report UI that interfered with activities.[96] However, continent and incontinent women were not found to be more likely to need formal home care or home nursing care with 11 years of follow-up in a well-characterized epidemiologic study in Norway.[97]

Parkinson disease is an extrapyramidal neurologic syndrome presenting with motor symptoms such as tremor, hypokinesia, and postural instability. Nonmotor symptoms affect more than half of patients with Parkinson disease,[98] with UI experienced by 71%.[99] In a study of aging and cognition among recruited individuals without known dementia, the frequency of UI was associated with impairment of activities of daily living, incident Parkinsonism, and more severe neurologic disease but not with mild cognitive impairment.[100]

Studies evaluating an association between diabetes mellitus (DM) and UI are nuanced, with some confirming higher rates of incontinence for women with both type 2 and type 1 DM.[101] However, there are many studies in which obesity confounds the relationship between UI and DM. For instance, among women in Washington state, UI was not associated with diabetes with adjustment for BMI, but severe UI was associated with DM, even with adjustment for obesity (BMI ≥30).[52] The complexity of this relationship is further underscored by the findings that UI severity is not associated with diabetic management including duration of diagnosis, treatment or control, or diabetic complications including retinopathy and microalbuminuria.[102]

Smoking is associated with UI. One study reported that current and former smoking was associated with both stress and urge UI symptoms.[103] A more recent study found a higher prevalence of storage symptoms including urgency UI symptoms, nocturnal enuresis, coital incontinence, and urodynamic detrusor overactivity among smokers compared to nonsmokers. This same study reported similar rates of SUI symptoms and unexpectedly lower rates of urodynamic stress incontinence among smokers and nonsmokers.[104] An increased prevalence of urgency UI among current and former smokers has been reported among Japanese women.[105]

Chronic lung disease is associated with UI.[106,107] Women with cystic fibrosis and chronic obstructive pulmonary disease are more likely to develop incontinence and those with chronic obstructive pulmonary disease report more bother related to UI.[108]

The relationship between UI and depression is challenging to untangle. Although numerous studies have identified depression as a risk factor for UI, the analyses could not identify if depression causes pathophysiologic changes leading to UI symptoms or whether the potential chronic embarrassment and social isolation due to incontinence leads to depression. A longitudinal cohort of female Health and Retirement Study participants provides some insight into this question. Among community-dwelling women who were followed for 6 years, those who had major depression at baseline measurement were more likely to develop incontinence than those who did not, and the women who had incontinence at baseline were no more likely to develop major depression.[62] Use of psychotropic drugs did not influence the association between UI and depression.[109] A trial of solifenacin for overactive bladder symptoms found that women with concomitant depressive symptoms experienced significant improvement in both urinary and depression symptoms.[110] The coping strategies that patients develop to manage their symptoms are complex and interrelated, pointing to how multimodal interventions will be needed in future trials.[111]

Microbiome

The microbiome of the vagina and urinary tract and its role in the pathophysiology of UI is a relatively new area of research. Studies using 16S rRNA gene sequencing provide evidence that numerous bacteria reside in the urine, the most common of which are *Lactobacillus*, with a high degree of correlation between specimens found in the vagina and urine. Also commonly found in both the vagina and urine are *Gardnerella*, *Prevotella*, and *Ureaplasma*.[112] A group of proteomics investigators has identified a large number of proteins found among stress incontinent patients and a smaller group

of proteins not found in stress incontinent patients compared to controls.[113,114]

Genetics

Evidence from studies regarding the heritability of UI is mixed. In a survey of 765 identical and 117 nonidentical twin sisters, shared and unique environmental factors were statistically associated with SUI, but genetics were not.[115] However, a genome-wide association analysis recently identified six loci on chromosomes 5, 10, 11, 12, and 18 and three genetic variants in genes.[116] There are studies regarding gene products encoding matrix metalloproteinases, which have a role in collagen breakdown and smooth muscle signaling. These cellular mechanisms may have a role in the development of SUI.

UI is a common condition with many recognized risk factors. Disease models for UI now seek to account for how these risk factors interact and where there are opportunities to prevent symptom progression and to induce remission when possible. Although demographics such as aging and genetics predispose individuals to a higher risk, there may be opportunities to modify risk. Successful management of life events such as pregnancy, delivery, genitourinary syndrome in menopause, and comorbid conditions such as smoking, constipation, and weight gain have the potential to mitigate the risk for UI among other medical comorbidities.

References

1. Ellerkmann RM, Cundiff GW, Melick CF, et al. Correlation of symptoms with location and severity of pelvic organ prolapse. *Am J Obstet Gynecol* 2001;185(6):1332–1338.
2. Mant J, Painter R, Vessey M. Epidemiology of genital prolapse: Observations from the Oxford Family Planning Association Study. *Br J Obstet Gynaecol* 1997;104(5):579–585.
3. Wu JM, Matthews CA, Conover MM, et al. Lifetime risk of stress urinary incontinence or pelvic organ prolapse surgery. *Obstet Gynecol* 2014;123(6):1201–1206.
4. Olsen AL, Smith VJ, Bergstrom JO, et al. Epidemiology of surgically managed pelvic organ prolapse and urinary incontinence. *Obstet Gynecol* 1997;89(4):501–506.
5. Smith FJ, Holman CD, Moorin RE, et al. Lifetime risk of undergoing surgery for pelvic organ prolapse. *Obstet Gynecol* 2010;116(5):1096–1100.
6. Fialkow MF, Newton KM, Lentz GM, et al. Lifetime risk of surgical management for pelvic organ prolapse or urinary incontinence. *Int Urogynecol J Pelvic Floor Dysfunct* 2008;19(3):437–440.
7. Morrill M, Lukacz ES, Lawrence JM, et al. Seeking healthcare for pelvic floor disorders: A population-based study. *Am J Obstet Gynecol* 2007;197(1):86.e1–86.e6.
8. Wu JM, Hundley AF, Fulton RG, et al. Forecasting the prevalence of pelvic floor disorders in U.S. women: 2010 to 2050. *Obstet Gynecol* 2009;114(6):1278–1283.
9. Kirby AC, Luber KM, Menefee SA. An update on the current and future demand for care of pelvic floor disorders in the United States. *Am J Obstet Gynecol* 2013;209(6):584.e1–584.e5.

10. American College of Obstetricians and Gynecologists. Pelvic organ prolapse: ACOG Practice Bulletin, Number 214. *Obstet Gynecol* 2019;134(5):e126–e142.

11. Gutman RE, Ford DE, Quiroz LH, et al. Is there a pelvic organ prolapse threshold that predicts pelvic floor symptoms? *Am J Obstet Gynecol* 2008;199(6):683.e1–683.e7.

12. Haylen BT, Maher CF, Barber MD, et al. An International Urogynecological Association (IUGA)/International Continence Society (ICS) joint report on the terminology for female pelvic organ prolapse (POP). *Int Urogynecol J* 2016;27(4):655–684.

13. Haylen BT, de Ridder D, Freeman RM, et al. An International Urogynecological Association (IUGA)/International Continence Society (ICS) joint report on the terminology for female pelvic floor dysfunction. *Int Urogynecol J* 2010;21(1):5–26.

14. Nygaard I, Bradley C, Brandt D; for the Women's Health Initiative. Pelvic organ prolapse in older women: Prevalence and risk factors. *Obstet Gynecol* 2004;104(3):489–497.

15. Lawrence JM, Lukacz ES, Nager CW, et al. Prevalence and co-occurrence of pelvic floor disorders in community-dwelling women. *Obstet Gynecol* 2008;111(3):678–685.

16. Swift S, Woodman P, O'Boyle A, et al. Pelvic Organ Support Study (POSST): The distribution, clinical definition, and epidemiologic condition of pelvic organ support defects. *Am J Obstet Gynecol* 2005;192(3):795–806.

17. Bump RC, Norton PA. Epidemiology and natural history of pelvic floor dysfunction. *Obstet Gynecol Clin North Am* 1998;25(4):723–746.

18. DeLancey JO, Kane Low L, Miller JM, et al. Graphic integration of causal factors of pelvic floor disorders: An integrated life span model. *Am J Obstet Gynecol* 2008;199(6):610.e1–610.e5.

19. Altman D, Forsman M, Falconer C, et al. Genetic influence on stress urinary incontinence and pelvic organ prolapse. *Eur Urol* 2008;54(4):918–922.

20. Jack GS, Nikolova G, Vilain E, et al. Familial transmission of genitovaginal prolapse. *Int Urogynecol J Pelvic Floor Dysfunct* 2006;17(5):498–501.

21. Ward RM, Velez Edwards DR, Edwards T, et al. Genetic epidemiology of pelvic organ prolapse: A systematic review. *Am J Obstet Gynecol* 2014;211(4):326–335.

22. Liu JS, Vo AX, Doolittle J, et al. Characterizing pelvic organ prolapse in adult spina bifida patients. *Urology* 2016;97:273–276.

23. El Akri M, Brochard C, Hascoet J, et al. Risk of prolapse and urinary complications in adult spina bifida patients with neurogenic acontractile detrusor using clean intermittent catheterization versus Valsalva voiding. *Neurourol Urodyn* 2019;38(1):269–277.

24. Woodman PJ, Swift SE, O'Boyle AL, et al. Prevalence of severe pelvic organ prolapse in relation to job description and socioeconomic status: A multicenter cross-sectional study. *Int Urogynecol J Pelvic Floor Dysfunct* 2006;17(4):340–345.

25. National Human Genome Research Institute. Race. Accessed May 31, 2021. https://www.genome.gov/genetics-glossary/Race.

26. Blomquist JL, Munoz A, Carroll M, et al. Association of delivery mode with pelvic floor disorders after childbirth. *JAMA* 2018;320(23):2438–2447.

27. Memon HU, Blomquist JL, Dietz HP, et al. Comparison of levator ani muscle avulsion injury after forceps-assisted and vacuum-assisted vaginal childbirth. *Obstet Gynecol* 2015;125(5):1080–1087.

28. Chan SS, Cheung RY, Yiu KW, et al. Effect of levator ani muscle injury on primiparous women during the first year after childbirth. *Int Urogynecol J* 2014;25(10):1381–1388.

29. Dietz HP, Lanzarone V. Levator trauma after vaginal delivery. *Obstet Gynecol* 2005;106(4):707–712.

30. DeLancey JO, Kearney R, Chou Q, et al. The appearance of levator ani muscle abnormalities in magnetic resonance images after vaginal delivery. *Obstet Gynecol* 2003;101(1):46–53.

31. Caudwell-Hall J, Kamisan Atan I, Martin A, et al. Intrapartum predictors of maternal levator ani injury. *Acta Obstet Gynecol Scand* 2017;96(4):426–431.

32. Handa VL, Blomquist JL, Roem J, et al. Pelvic floor disorders after obstetric avulsion of the levator ani muscle. *Female Pelvic Med Reconstr Surg* 2019;25(1):3–7.

33. Dietz HP, Simpson JM. Levator trauma is associated with pelvic organ prolapse. *BJOG* 2008;115(8):979–984.

34. DeLancey JO, Morgan DM, Fenner DE, et al. Comparison of levator ani muscle defects and function in women with and without pelvic organ prolapse. *Obstet Gynecol* 2007;109(2 Pt 1):295–302.

35. Handa VL, Roem J, Blomquist JL, et al. Pelvic organ prolapse as a function of levator ani avulsion, hiatus size, and strength. *Am J Obstet Gynecol* 2019;221(1):41.e1–41.e7.

36. Nandikanti L, Sammarco AG, Kobernik EK, et al. Levator ani defect severity and its association with enlarged hiatus size, levator bowl depth, and prolapse size. *Am J Obstet Gynecol* 2018;218(5):537–539.

37. Handa VL, Blomquist JL, Roem J, et al. Longitudinal study of quantitative changes in pelvic organ support among parous women. *Am J Obstet Gynecol* 2018;218(3):320.e1–320.e7.

38. Kearney R, Miller JM, Ashton-Miller JA, et al. Obstetric factors associated with levator ani muscle injury after vaginal birth. *Obstet Gynecol* 2006;107(1):144–149.

39. MacLennan AH, Taylor AW, Wilson DH, et al. The prevalence of pelvic floor disorders and their relationship to gender, age, parity and mode of delivery. *BJOG* 2000;107(12):1460–1470.

40. Samuelsson EC, Victor FT, Tibblin G, et al. Signs of genital prolapse in a Swedish population of women 20 to 59 years of age and possible related factors. *Am J Obstet Gynecol* 1999;180(2 Pt 1):299–305.

41. Akervall S, Al-Mukhtar Othman J, Molin M, et al. Symptomatic pelvic organ prolapse in middle-aged women: A national matched cohort study on the influence of childbirth. *Am J Obstet Gynecol* 2020;222(4):356.e1–356.e14.

42. Trowbridge ER, Wei JT, Fenner DE, et al. Effects of aging on lower urinary tract and pelvic floor function in nulliparous women. *Obstet Gynecol* 2007;109(3):715–720.

43. Forsgren C, Lundholm C, Johansson AL, et al. Vaginal hysterectomy and risk of pelvic organ prolapse and stress urinary incontinence surgery. *Int Urogynecol J* 2012;23(1):43–48.

44. Miller NF. A new method of correcting complete inversion of the vagina. *Surg Gynecol Obstet* 1927;44:550–554.

45. McCall ML. Posterior culdeplasty; surgical correction of enterocele during vaginal hysterectomy; a preliminary report. *Obstet Gynecol* 1957;10(6):595–602.

46. Symmonds RE, Williams TJ, Lee RA, et al. Posthysterectomy enterocele and vaginal vault prolapse. *Am J Obstet Gynecol* 1981;140(8):852–859.

47. Vergeldt TF, Weemhoff M, IntHout J, et al. Risk factors for pelvic organ prolapse and its recurrence: A systematic review. *Int Urogynecol J* 2015;26(11):1559–1573.

48. Giri A, Hartmann KE, Hellwege JN, et al. Obesity and pelvic organ prolapse: A systematic review and meta-analysis of observational studies. *Am J Obstet Gynecol* 2017;217(1):11–26.e13.

49. Brazell HD, O'Sullivan DM, Tulikangas PK. Socioeconomic status and race as predictors of treatment-seeking behavior for pelvic organ prolapse. *Am J Obstet Gynecol* 2013;209(5): 476.e1–476.e5.

50. Hannestad YS, Rortveit G, Sandvik H, et al. A community-based epidemiological survey of female urinary incontinence: The Norwegian EPINCONT study. Epidemiology of Incontinence in the County of Nord-Trøndelag. *J Clin Epidemiol* 2000;53(11):1150–1157.

51. Minassian VA, Drutz HP, Al-Badr A. Urinary incontinence as a worldwide problem. *Int J Gynaecol Obstet* 2003;82(3):327–338.

52. Melville JL, Katon W, Delaney K, et al. Urinary incontinence in US women: A population-based study. *Arch Intern Med* 2005;165(5):537–542.

53. Herzog AR, Diokno AC, Brown MB, et al. Two-year incidence, remission, and change patterns of urinary incontinence in noninstitutionalized older adults. *J Gerontol* 1990;45(2):M67–M74.

54. Rortveit G, Daltveit AK, Hannestad YS, et al; for the Norwegian EPINCONT Study. Urinary incontinence after vaginal delivery or cesarean section. *N Engl J Med* 2003;348:900–907.

55. Yang E, Lisha NE, Walter L, et al. Urinary incontinence in a national cohort of older women: Implications for caregiving and care dependence. *J Womens Health (Larchmt)* 2018;27(9): 1097–1103.

56. Ebbesen MH, Hunskaar S, Rortveit G, et al. Prevalence, incidence and remission of urinary incontinence in women: Longitudinal data from the Norwegian HUNT study (EPINCONT). *BMC Urol* 2013;13:27.

57. Nygaard I, Turvey C, Burns TL, et al. Urinary incontinence and depression in middle-aged United States women. *Obstet Gynecol* 2003;101(1):149–156.

58. Hu T-W, Wagner TH, Bentkover JD, et al. Costs of urinary incontinence and overactive bladder in the United States: A comparative study. *Urology* 2004;63(3):461–465.

59. Minassian VA, Bazi T, Stewart WF. Clinical epidemiological insights into urinary incontinence. *Int Urogynecol J* 2017;28(5):687–696.

60. Bates P, Bradley WE, Glen E, et al. The standardization of terminology of lower urinary tract function. *J Urol* 1979;121(5):551–554.

61. Samuelsson E, Victor A, Tibblin G. A population study of urinary incontinence and nocturia among women aged 20–59 years. Prevalence, well-being and wish for treatment. *Acta Obstet Gynecol Scand* 1997;76(1):74–80.

62. Melville JL, Fan M-Y, Rau H, et al. Major depression and urinary incontinence in women: Temporal associations in an epidemiologic sample. *Am J Obstet Gynecol* 2009;201(5): 490.e1–490.e7.

63. Herzog AR, Fultz NH. Prevalence and incidence of urinary incontinence in community-dwelling populations. *J Am Geriatr Soc* 1990;38(3):273–281.

64. Hansen BB, Svare J, Viktrup L, et al. Urinary incontinence during pregnancy and 1 year after delivery in primiparous women compared with a control group of nulliparous women. *Neurourol Urodyn* 2012;31(4):475–480.

65. Rortveit G, Hannestad YS, Daltveit AK, et al. Age- and type-dependent effects of parity on urinary incontinence: The Norwegian EPINCONT study. *Obstet Gynecol* 2001;98(6):1004–1010.

66. McKinnie V, Swift SE, Wang W, et al. The effect of pregnancy and mode of delivery on the prevalence of urinary and fecal incontinence. *Am J Obstet Gynecol* 2005;193(2):512–518.

67. Svare JA, Hansen BB, Lose G. Risk factors for urinary incontinence 1 year after the first vaginal delivery in a cohort of primiparous Danish women. *Int Urogynecol J* 2014;25:47–51.

68. Tahtinen RM, Cartwright R, Tsui JF, et al. Long-term impact of mode of delivery on stress urinary incontinence and urgency urinary incontinence: A systematic review and meta-analysis. *Eur Urol* 2016;70(5):148–158.

69. Tahtinen RM, Cartwright R, Vernooij RWM, et al. Long-term risks of stress and urgency urinary incontinence after different vaginal delivery modes. *Am J Obstet Gynecol* 2019;220(2): 181.e1–181.e8.

70. Patel DA, Xu X, Thomason AD, et al. Childbirth and pelvic floor dysfunction: An epidemiologic approach to the assessment of prevention opportunities at delivery. *Am J Obstet Gynecol* 2006;195(1):23–28.

71. Xu X, Ivy JS, Patel DA, et al. Pelvic floor consequences of cesarean delivery on maternal request in women with a single birth: A cost-effectiveness analysis. *J Womens Health (Larchmt)* 2010;19:147–160.

72. Viktrup L, Lose G, Rolff M, et al. The symptom of stress incontinence caused by pregnancy or delivery in primiparas. *Obstet Gynecol* 1992;79(6):945–949.

73. Viktrup L, Lose G. The risk of stress incontinence 5 years after first delivery. *Am J Obstet Gynecol* 2001;185(1):82–87.

74. Viktrup L, Rortveit G, Lose G. Risk of stress urinary incontinence twelve years after the first pregnancy and delivery. *Obstet Gynecol* 2006;108:248–254.

75. Pizzoferrato AC, Fauconnier A, Quiboeuf E, et al. Urinary incontinence 4 and 12 years after first delivery: Risk factors associated with prevalence, incidence, remission, and persistence in a cohort of 236 women. *Neurourol Urodyn* 2014;33(8):1229–1234.

76. Bohlin KS, Ankardal M, Lindkvist H, et al. Factors influencing the incidence and remission of urinary incontinence after hysterectomy. *Am J Obstet Gynecol* 2017;216(1):53.e1–53.e9.

77. Learman LA, Summitt RL Jr, Varner RE, et al. A randomized comparison of total or supracervical hysterectomy: Surgical complications and clinical outcomes. *Obstet Gynecol* 2003;102:453–462.

78. Thakar R, Ayers S, Clarkson P, et al. Outcomes after total versus subtotal abdominal hysterectomy. *N Engl J Med* 2002;347:1318–1325.

79. Gimbel H. Total or subtotal hysterectomy for benign uterine diseases? A meta-analysis. *Acta Obstet Gynecol Scand* 2007;86:133–144.

80. Thom DH, van den Eeden SK, Ragins AI, et al. Differences in prevalence of urinary incontinence by race/ethnicity. *J Urol* 2006;175:259–264.

81. Berger MB, Patel DA, Miller JM, et al. Racial differences in self-reported healthcare seeking and treatment for urinary incontinence in community-dwelling women from the EPI Study. *Neurourol Urodyn* 2011;30(8):1442–1447.

82. Mandimika CL, Murk W, McPencow AM, et al. Racial disparities in knowledge of pelvic floor disorders among community-dwelling women. *Female Pelvic Med Reconstr Surg* 2015;21(5):287–292.

83. Bliss DZ, Gurvich OV, Eberly LE, et al. Racial disparities in primary prevention of incontinence among older adults at nursing home admission. *Neurourol Urodyn* 2017;36(4):1124–1130.

84. Legendre G, Ringa V, Fauconnier A, et al. Menopause, hormone treatment and urinary incontinence at midlife. *Maturitas* 2013;74:26–30.

85. Linde JM, Nijman RJM, Trzpis M, et al. Urinary incontinence in the Netherlands: Prevalence and associated risk factors in adults. *Neurourol Urodyn* 2017;36(6):1519–1528.

86. Minassian VA, Hagan KA, Erekson E, et al. The natural history of urinary incontinence subtypes in the Nurses' Health Studies. *Am J Obstet Gynecol* 2020;222:163.e1–163.e8.

87. Swenson CW, Kolenic GE, Trowbridge ER, et al. Obesity and stress urinary incontinence in women: Compromised continence mechanism or excess bladder pressure during cough? *Int Urogynecol J* 2017;28(9):1377–1385.

88. Agur W, Rizk DE. Obesity and urinary incontinence in women: Is the black box becoming grayer? *Int Urogynecol J* 2011;22(3):257–258.

89. Subak LL, Wing R, West DS, et al. Weight loss to treat urinary incontinence in overweight and obese women. *N Engl J Med* 2009;360:481–490.

90. Subak LL, King WC, Belle SH, et al. Urinary incontinence before and after bariatric surgery. *JAMA Intern Med* 2015;175(8):1378–1387.

91. Nygaard CC, Schreiner L, Morsch TP, et al. Urinary incontinence and quality of life in female patients with obesity. *Rev Bras Ginecol Obstet* 2018;40(9):534–539.

92. Thom DH, Haan MN, Van Den Eeden SK. Medically recognized urinary incontinence and risks of hospitalization, nursing home admission and mortality. *Age Ageing* 1997;26(5):367–374.

93. John G, Bardini C, Combescure C, et al. Urinary incontinence as a predictor of death: A systematic review and meta-analysis. *PloS One* 2016;11(7):e0158992.

94. Hsu A, Conell-Price J, Stijacic Cenzer I, et al. Predictors of urinary incontinence in community-dwelling frail older adults with diabetes mellitus in a cross-sectional study. *BMC Geriatr* 2014;14:137.

95. Suskind AM, Quanstrom K, Zhao S, et al. Overactive bladder is strongly associated with frailty in older individuals. *Urology* 2017;106:26–31.

96. Huang AJ, Brown JS, Thom DH, et al; for the Study of Osteoporotic Fractures Research Group. Urinary incontinence in older community-dwelling women: The role of cognitive and physical function decline. *Obstet Gynecol* 2007;109(4):909–916.

97. Omli R, Hunskaar S, Mykletun A, et al. Urinary incontinence and risk of functional decline in older women: Data from the Norwegian HUNT-study. *BMC Geriatr* 2013;13:47.

98. Yeo L, Singh R, Gundeti M, et al. Urinary tract dysfunction in Parkinson's disease: A review. *Int Urol Nephrol* 2012;44(2):415–424.

99. Hely MA, Reid WG, Adena MA, et al. The Sydney multicenter study of Parkinson's disease: The inevitability of dementia at 20 years. *Mov Disord* 2008;23:837–844.

100. Buchman NM, Leurgans SE, Shah RJ, et al. Urinary incontinence, incident parkinsonism, and Parkinson's disease pathology in older adults. *J Gerontol A Biol Sci Med Sci* 2017;72(9):1295–1301.

101. Phelan S, Grodstein F, Brown JS. Clinical research in diabetes and urinary incontinence: What we know and need to know. *J Urol* 2009;182:S14–S17.

102. Phelan S, Kanaya AM, Subak LL, et al. Prevalence and risk factors for urinary incontinence in overweight and obese diabetic women: Action for health in diabetes (look ahead) study. *Diabetes Care* 2009;32:1391–1397.

103. Bump RC, McClish DK. Cigarette smoking and urinary incontinence in women. *Am J Obstet Gynecol* 1992;167(5):1213–1218.

104. Madhu C, Enki D, Drake MJ, et al. The functional effects of cigarette smoking in women on the lower urinary tract. *Urol Int* 2015;95(5):478–482.

105. Kawahara T, Ito H, Yao M, et al. Impact of smoking habit on overactive bladder symptoms and incontinence in women. *Int J Urol* 2020;27(12):1078–1086.

106. Schreiber Pedersen L, Lose G, Høybye MT, et al. Prevalence of urinary incontinence among women and analysis of potential risk factors in Germany and Denmark. *Acta Obstet Gynecol Scand* 2017;96(8):939–948.

107. Jackson RA, Vittinghoff E, Kanaya AM, et al. Urinary incontinence in elderly women: Findings from the Health, Aging, and Body Composition Study. *Obstet Gynecol* 2004;104(2):301–307.

108. Button BM, Holland AE, Sherburn MS, et al. Prevalence, impact and specialised treatment of urinary incontinence in women with chronic lung disease. *Physiotherapy* 2019;105(5):114–119.

109. Felde G, Engeland A, Hunskaar S. Urinary incontinence associated with anxiety and depression: The impact of psychotropic drugs in a cross-sectional study from the Norwegian HUNT study. *BMC Psychiatry* 2020;20(1):521.

110. Kim KS, Moon HS. Antimuscarinic agent treatment affecting patient-reported outcomes in overactive bladder syndrome with depressive symptoms. *Int Neurourol J* 2016;20:349–355.

111. Molinuevo B, Batista-Miranda JE. Under the tip of the iceberg: Psychological factors in incontinence. *Neurourol Urodyn* 2012;31:669–671.

112. Komesu YM, Dinwiddie DL, Richter HE, et al. Defining the relationship between vaginal and urinary microbiomes. *Am J Obstet Gynecol* 2020;222(2):154.e1–154.e10.

113. Koch M, Mitulovic G, Hanzal E, et al. Urinary proteomic pattern in female stress urinary incontinence: A pilot study. *Int Urogynecol J* 2016;27(11):1729–1734.

114. Koch M, Umek W, Hanzal E, et al. Serum proteomic pattern in female stress urinary incontinence. *Electrophoresis* 2018;39(8):1071–1078.

115. Nguyen A, Aschkenazi SO, Sand PK, et al. Nongenetic factors associated with stress urinary incontinence. *Obstet Gynecol* 2011;117(2 Pt 1):251–255.

116. Richter HE, Whitehead N, Arya L, et al. Genetic contributions to urgency urinary incontinence in women. *J Urol* 2015;193(6):2020–2027.

CHAPTER 7

CLINICAL RESEARCH METHODOLOGY AND STATISTICS

Donna Mazloomdoost

Introduction

Clinicians often express discomfort with statistical methods, even those actively engaged in research.[1] While they believe research is important, few practitioners agree that more emphasis should be placed on research education during residency training.[2] Not surprisingly, skills learned by clinicians diminish as the years lapse,[3] feasibly as a result of time constraints and workload pressures.[4] Nonetheless, an understanding of research methodologies can improve critical appraisal and interpretation of research and ultimately aid in determining if the results should be implemented into clinical practice.

ETHICS AND INTEGRITY IN CLINICAL RESEARCH

Human subjects research is critical to advancing the understanding of human pathologies and enhancing medical care, yet subjects involved are asked to incur potential risk from which society may ultimately benefit.[5] Ethical principles are, therefore, imperative to protect the rights of research participants.

Codes and Regulations

Prior to formalized research, medical treatments were mostly experimental as large data rarely existed.[5] Much of medical ethics at this point relied on the Hippocratic oath,[6] and although most investigators likely had good intentions, concerns over deception, self-interests, or exploitation eventually led to a need for regulations. Some regulations were in response to specific situations, whereas others were developed as new information was obtained.[5] Among the first of these regulations was the Food and Drugs Act, also known as the Wiley Act, signed by President Roosevelt in 1906. This act paved the way for the regulatory and first consumer protection agency, the U.S. Food and Drug Administration, and prohibited transport or sale of altered or mislabeled food or drug products between states and required food and drugs to have labels of active ingredients.[7] Despite the attempted protections laid forth in the act, in 1937, a Tennessee drug company marketed an untested new sulfa drug geared toward children. The drug was found to contain a toxic analogue of antifreeze and resulted in over 100 deaths, many of whom were children. This prompted Congress to pass the Food, Drug, and Cosmetic Act in 1938, which mandated premarket approval of all new drugs.[8]

World War II ushered in a new era of ethical concerns as research saw tremendous growth. The Nuremberg trials set the foundation for modern-day ethical protection of human subjects.[9,10] The trials held in Nuremberg, Germany, accused Nazi physicians of conducting torturous and fatal experiments in concentration camp prisoners and led to the Nuremberg Code of 1947. The first principle of the Nuremberg Code asserts that the informed consent of the competent human subject is essential.[9] While the Nuremberg Code was widely accepted and resulted in guidelines from government agencies and the National Institutes of Health (NIH) Clinical Center regarding informed consent, some scientists continued to ignore these principles.[11]

In 1966, Henry Beecher, a respected Harvard anesthesiologist and researcher, published a groundbreaking article in *The New England Journal of Medicine* (*NEJM*), highlighting ethical problems in a preliminary sample of 17 studies, which ultimately expanded to 50 manuscripts.[12] Beecher called out reputable institutions such as Harvard and the NIH Clinical Center as well as journals such as *NEJM* and the *Journal of the American Medical Association* for their roles or complacency in these ethical violations. He described 22 examples of breaches including withholding of accepted disease treatments, active administration of viral infections to cause disease, and dispensing of medications with known serious adverse events. Of particular concern was the inclusion of vulnerable populations such as institutionalized mentally "defective" individuals, infants, and inmates. Beecher argued subjects in some cases had received harm without any clear benefit, whereas others may not have been appropriately counseled on the risks.

In 1972, the nation was shocked by the revelation of the U.S. Public Health Service Tuskegee syphilis study.[13,14] The study initiated in 1932 by the Public Health Service with the intent to study the natural history of syphilis, enrolling 399 black men from Macon County, Alabama, at the Tuskegee Institute with syphilis along with 201 men who were disease free. The men were promised medical examinations, meals, and burial insurance free of charge as an incentive to participate. The study was scheduled to last 6 months but continued for 40 years, while hundreds of black men had intervention deliberately withheld even once penicillin became the accepted treatment. An advisory panel was convened from the public outcry and found that the men had been misled and were not properly provided with informed consent. Publicization of Tuskegee along with Beecher's advocacy ultimately led to enough public scrutiny for Congress to pass the 1974 National Research Act.[5,14]

Belmont Report

The 1974 Act convened the National Commission for the Protection of Human Subjects of Biomedical and Behavioral Research, charged to identify basic ethical principles and develop guidelines for the conduct of research involving human subjects.[15] The Belmont Report described the following basic ethical principles necessary in research: (1) respect for persons, (2) beneficence, and (3) justice. These principles described the need to (1) respect the autonomous decision making of the participant, (2) protect them from intentional or unnecessary harm, and (3) select research subjects in a representative and just manner. The Commission then recommended that the application of these general principles to the conduct of research would require (1) informed consent, (2) risk/benefit assessment, and (3) the selection of subjects of research.[15] Influenced by the Belmont Report, in 1991, the "Common Rule" was published and required research funded by 17 federal agencies to comply with this Federal Policy for the Protection of Human Subjects which outlines provisions for human subjects protections, institutional review boards (IRBs), informed consent, and assurances of compliance.[16] Further protection developed to include traditionally neglected populations. The NIH now requires those receiving funding to include underrepresented populations such as women, minorities, and children when eligible or provide justification for their exclusion.[17,18] Although the Common Rule is enforced with regard to research involving federal funding through the U.S. Department of Health and Human Services (HHS), most research is impacted because the Common Rule applies to *any* research involving human

subjects conducted at institutions receiving direct or indirect federal funding.[19] Therefore, investigators are often bound to the Common Rule because their institution might receive applicable funding, and everyone at that institution must comply.

Informed Consent

Research is ever-evolving, and as new technologies and applications are introduced, a universal framework is necessary to guide investigators, IRBs, sponsors, and other involved personnel to determine whether a research protocol is ethically compliant.[20] Seven requirements have been suggested to provide this systematic framework: social or scientific value, scientific validity, fair selection of subjects, favorable risk-to-benefit ratio, independent review, informed consent, and respect for eligible/enrolled participants.[5,20] Of these seven principles, informed consent has potentially received the most attention, as it ensures that competent subjects or their decision makers voluntarily agree without coercion to participate only after being fully informed of the purpose, methods, risks, benefits, and alternatives of the research.[20] Unfortunately, the importance of the informed consent process was observed and verified through the historical scandals that led to the ethical discussions.

Informed consent should involve appropriate disclosure of the risks and benefits, allow for adequate comprehension of what the trial entails, and permit uncoerced enrollment.[21] The informed consent should also provide explanation of the randomization and potential assignment to placebo groups, though subjects show lower comprehension of this.[21,22] A particular challenge is verifying the subject's understanding, particularly when the participant is a minor or incapacitated. The most effective way to educate a participant appears to be a direct conversation explaining the study by a member of the research team.[23] Despite the burden, especially in an ever-increasing era of time demand and complex research methods, when possible, it is imperative that this be executed.[22] To decrease the burden, addition of a video explaining the study protocol appears to enhance patient understanding,[24] although alternative methods to the traditional consent process remain controversial.[22,23] Incentives or payments have always been debated to undermine the voluntary nature of consent due to concerns that payments unnecessarily coerce subjects into participation. However, most ethicists agree that because incentives do not involve threats, a method considered to coerce, payments unlikely coerce subjects into participation and can be used when appropriate for recruitment or retention of participants.[25] Consent is traditionally obtained by a written signature documenting the subject's willingness to participate.[5]

Institutional Review Boards

IRBs were established to assure that the well-being and rights of human subjects are considered in clinical trials.[26] While nonhuman research is exempt from IRB review, the use of animals in federally funded research is subject to the Animal Welfare Act (AWA), and NIH-funded research is subject to the U.S. Public Health Service's *Policy on Humane Care and Use of Laboratory Animals*.[27,28] The AWA seeks to ensure the humane treatment of animals in the research setting, recommending the establishment of an oversight committee, the Institutional Animal Care and Use Committee.[28] The AWA describes "the 3Rs," reduction, refinement, and replacement, which encourages reducing the number of animals used, minimizing suffering, and replacing them with technologies or other models when appropriate.[29]

As previously discussed, the Common Rule dictates that, with some exception, federally funded clinical trials involving human subjects must receive IRB approval.[30] Specifically, six categories were designated exempt from IRB approval as they were not deemed to expose subjects to physical, social, or psychological harm beyond what exists in daily life (Table 7.1).[26] Researchers, however, should consult with their institutions regarding institution-specific guidelines, particularly when not funded by applicable federal agencies.[31]

TABLE 7.1	
Research Exempt from Institutional Review Board Approval[a]	
RESEARCH TYPE	**DESCRIPTIONS**
1. Educational settings	Research conducted in typical educational settings, involving established or accepted practices that are unlikely to impact the students' opportunities to learn; may include the effectiveness of various instructional techniques, curricula, or management methods
2. Surveys, interviews, public observations, or educational tests	Requires the data to be collected in a de-identified manner and the disclosure of the data would not result in criminal/civil liability or damage the subjects' financial status or opportunities
3. Benign behavioral interventions	Requires an adult subject with data collected so that the individual cannot be identified. Interventions must be brief in duration, harmless, painless, not physically invasive, not be embarrassing or offensive, and should not have a lasting adverse impact.
4. Secondary analyses or research	If research involves identifiable data or biospecimens, they must either be a. Publicly available b. De-identified or compliant with *45 CFR parts 160 and 164*[b] c. Collected on behalf of the federal government for nonresearch purposes
5. Federal research	Performed by a federal department or agency, intended to evaluate public benefit or service programs. The research plan must be publicized and accessible.
6. Taste and food quality evaluation and consumer acceptance programs	Apply if wholesome foods without additives are involved and are consumed at levels at or below established safety concentrations

[a]Adapted from Part 46—Protection of human subjects. Code of Federal Regulations. Accessed September 1, 2021. https://www.ecfr.gov/cgi-bin/retrieveECFR?gp=&SID=83cd09e1c0f5c6937cd9d7513160fc3f&pitd=20180719&n=pt45.1.46&r=PART&ty=HTML#se45.1.46_1104, with permission.
[b]From The HIPPA Privacy Rule. U.S. Department of Health and Human Services. Accessed September 1, 2021. https://www.hhs.gov/hipaa/for-professionals/privacy/index.html, with permission.

Research involving minimal risk to subjects may be eligible for expedited review. Institutions who offer this option allow the IRB chair or a designee to approve the study on behalf of the entire group, allowing for a more prompt response than a fully convened IRB.[32]

Federal regulations require that an IRB have at least five members, with at least one individual whose expertise is in the scientific area of interest, someone with expertise in nonscientific areas, and one individual not affiliated with the institution. Obtaining IRB approval has become standard practice, and investigators can employ for-profit organizations, known as independent or commercial IRBs, if an institutionally provided IRB is not available.[19]

Multicenter trials have long struggled with the inefficiency of multiple IRB submissions and approvals, delaying research and potentially increasing costs, without any evidence that the duplicative approvals enhance human subject protection.[33,34] Therefore, beginning in January 2020, the Common Rule required relative federally funded multisite trials use a single IRB for approval, which hopes to improve the efficiency of trials and human subject protection.[34]

Data and Safety Monitoring

In addition to informed consent, randomized controlled trials (RCTs) raise further ethical considerations compared with alternative trials. A hallmark to the design of clinical trials is *equipoise*, or the uncertainty behind the intervention being examined.[35] Equipoise requires that, in the design of a clinical trial, the investigators should be certain that there is no evidence that either treatment provided to the subjects is more valuable such that a known beneficial therapeutic would be withheld. Subjects must not knowingly receive an inferior treatment or the study becomes invalid.[20] Equipoise influences another ethical dilemma in RCTs: the selection of controls. Choosing an appropriate control is paramount to the validity and generalizability of the study (to be discussed later); however, electing to compare a treatment to a placebo requires justification to withhold a potentially beneficial treatment, or equipoise.[5]

Because researchers are invested in their studies, an unobjective and independent safety review is necessary.[36] In the United States, data and safety monitoring boards (DSMBs) or safety monitors are often used and first surfaced in the 1950s under different titles.[36,37] Early experiences with safety monitoring occurred during the first chronic disease trials in the 1960s–1970s.[36,38] Though all clinical trials need safety oversight, not all need an independent DSMB, which can be confusing and frustrating to investigators. The World Health Organization has suggested a DSMB be used in eight areas of study involving: (1) mortality, (2) severe morbidity, (3) high-risk interventions, (4) novel interventions with limited safety, (5) complex design or data accrual, (6) potential early termination after an interim analysis, (7) emergency situations, and (8) vulnerable populations.[39] NIH now requires all its institutes and centers to designate a system to oversee and monitor funded clinical trials to ensure the safety of the participants, and multicenter trials require an independent DSMB composed of varying expertise to evaluate the safety of ongoing clinical trials.[40] The DSMB should evaluate the protocol prior to implementation and also review data while the trial is ongoing.[38] Importantly, the DSMB has the authority to stop a trial if there are safety concerns, clear efficacy with regard to a treatment, or futility.[37] Perhaps one of the best-known examples of this was from the Women's Health Initiative (WHI).

The WHI trial was an NIH-funded study designed in 1991–1992 to assess benefits and risks of postmenopausal hormone replacement therapy on multiple outcomes, a complicated approach which more closely resembled real-world scenarios where such outcomes can occur concurrently.[41] Women were randomized to one of two treatment groups and compared to controls receiving placebo. In the treatment groups, participants with a uterus received a combination estrogen/progesterone pill, whereas posthysterectomy subjects received oral estrogen alone. Over 164,500 women were projected to be enrolled in over 40 clinical sites, perhaps the most considerable and challenging trial to ever be undertaken.[42] Due to the preventive nature of the study design, the investigators placed more emphasis on global health, and therefore, traditional methods to determine needs to cease the study could not apply. They held discussions *a priori* with the DSMB to determine scenarios under which members would vote to continue versus stop the trial, and from this, they published that a mixed approach to finding statistical guidelines and would likely best represent appropriate monitoring of the trial.[43] One of the unanimous determinations from the DSMB members was the occurrence of breast cancer, and on May 31, 2002, the DSMB recommended early cessation of the combined treatment arm trial after only a mean 5.2 years of follow-up because a predesignated boundary regarding breast cancer was exceeded in the treatment group.[44] The estrogen-alone arm was continued. In February 2004, the NIH decided to halt the trial on the determination that the estrogen-alone arm after 7 years of follow-up had failed to demonstrate cardioprotection, but that stroke risk was elevated similarly to the combination group of the alternative arm. Of note, the breast cancer risk remained similar between the estrogen-alone and placebo groups.[45] A statement was issued by the National Heart, Lung, and Blood Institute director of NIH determining that enough data had been collected for analysis, and interim assessments deemed enough risks to halt subjecting healthy women to a preventative medication that was not showing prevention benefits.[46] The trial challenged traditional epidemiologic study and uncovered approaches that have and will continue to benefit future studies.[41]

STUDY DESIGNS AND CONDUCT

A fundamental and perhaps difficult step in research development can be the selection of a question and the subsequent appropriate study design. A proper understanding of the state of the science is imperative to pursuing a relevant study question. Often, the first step involves a literature search to evaluate what has already been discovered and understand the gaps about the topic of interest. Once the investigator has determined the question to be answered, the study design can be developed.

Study Designs

Clinical research is divided into two categories: observational versus experimental.[47] The determination relates to whether exposure was assigned. Observational studies are analytical or descriptive, whereas experimental studies may be randomized or nonrandomized (Fig. 7.1). Understanding study designs is critical to developing an appropriate protocol. The strength of a study is

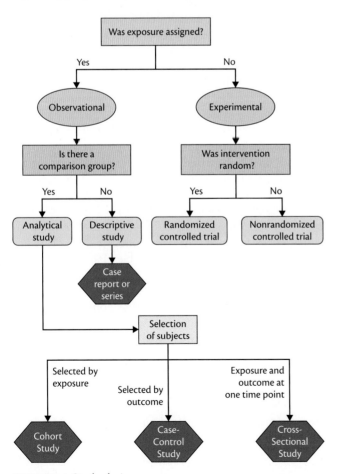

FIGURE 7.1 Study design.

TABLE 7.2	
Hierarchy of Study Designs	
QUALITY OF EVIDENCE	**DESCRIPTION**
I	Evidence obtained from at least one properly randomized controlled trial
II-1	Evidence obtained from well-designed controlled trials without randomization
II-2	Evidence obtained from well-designed cohort or case-control analytic studies, preferably from more than one center or research group
II-3	Evidence obtained from multiple time series with or without the intervention. Results from uncontrolled experiments (e.g., the introduction of penicillin treatment in the 1940s) could also be regarded as this type of evidence.
III	Opinions of respected authorities, based on clinical experience, descriptive studies and case reports, or reports of expert committees

Adapted from Harris RP, Helfand M, Woolf SH, et al; Methods Work Group, Third US Preventive Services Task Force. Current methods of the US Preventive Services Task Force: A review of the process. *Am J Prev Med* 2001;20(3 Suppl):21–35, with permission from Elsevier.

determined by its design, and guidelines impacting clinical practice are often based on the strength of the evidence obtained from studies. The U.S. Preventive Services Task Force (USPSTF) is an example of an agency which considers an evidence-based approach to clinical practice guidelines.[48] The USPSTF refers to an accepted hierarchy of study quality (Table 7.2), and practice recommendation are also graded with regard to strength (Table 7.3).[47]

TABLE 7.3	
Strength of Recommendations	
RECOMMENDATION	**EXPLANATION**
A	Good evidence to recommend the treatment or service
B	Fair evidence to recommend the treatment or service
C	Insufficient evidence to recommend for or against the treatment or service
D	Fair evidence against the treatment or service
E	Good evidence against treatment or service

Adapted from Schulz KF, Grimes DA. *The Lancet handbook of essential concepts in clinical research.* New York: Elsevier, 2006, with permission from Elsevier.

Observational Trials

Descriptive

While an RCT is considered the gold standard, it is not always feasible or even appropriate. Observational studies are acceptable when an intervention or exposure cannot be assigned, whether this is secondary to safety or practicality. Observational studies are further divided into descriptive or analytical (see Fig. 7.1). *Descriptive studies* do not include a comparison group and are commonly known as case reports, case series, or case studies. They can be used to describe the frequency, natural history, or possible factors of a condition.[47] Despite occupying the lowest tier of the study quality hierarchy, descriptive studies can be critical in announcing or understanding emerging medical issues.[49,50] Nonetheless, these studies may be minimized and even discouraged, but with quality review, publication can be invaluable to medical advancement.[51] The discovery of the HIV/AIDS is a well-known example[52] followed most recently by the 2020 pandemic caused by the novel coronavirus.[53] Although case reports or series can alert the medical community to new conditions, one must use caution changing clinical practice because of these discoveries.

Analytical

Analytical studies, alternatively, compare groups, which can allow for better understanding of associations. They are categorized as cohort studies, case-control studies, and cross-sectional studies (see Fig. 7.1). The classifications are based on how the groups are selected.

Cohort

A *cohort study* selects subjects on the basis of exposure and often follows them prospectively until the outcome is observed while comparing them to individuals not exposed.[47] A *retrospective cohort study* examines exposures and outcomes that have already occurred. It involves reviewing exposure information that was collected at a time in the past and examining for the outcome at the time of the study. For example, records documenting head injury from World War II veterans were reviewed to identify those with and without this exposure, and the sample was evaluated in the 1990s for dementia or Alzheimer disease.[54] The authors found that moderate and severe head injuries may be associated with the development of dementia or Alzheimer disease later in life. A common retrospective cohort within pelvic floor research is a review of charts from women who have undergone surgery and examining for risk factors potentially associated with a particular outcome.

General strengths of cohort studies include a better appreciation of exposure preceding the outcome, minimized recall bias (to be discussed later), and estimations of populations at risk.[55] Cohort studies allow for the calculation of incidence rates, relative risks (RRs), and attributable risks.[47] However, they cannot infer causality, may be lengthy and/or expensive, and are not appropriate for rare events.[47,55] Additionally, retrospective cohort studies may miss cases that were either of short duration or fatal.[56] Nonetheless, they provide invaluable information on potential disease development.

A prominent example of an effective cohort is the Nurses' Health study. This ambitious study with continued NIH funding launched in 1976, enrolling 121,700 married registered nurses aged 30 to 55 years, and remains one of the largest and longest running studies on women's health, boasting a continued 90% response rate of the original cohort after accounting for deaths.[57] The study's original focus was on contraceptive methods, smoking, cancer, and heart disease but has since expanded and contributed vital information about lifestyle factors, behaviors, personal characteristics, and more than 30 diseases.[58]

Case control

When a study begins with an outcome and looks back for an exposure, it is called a *case-control study*. These studies are often retrospective because the disease or condition of interest is identified first, and investigators evaluate for potential exposures prior to diagnosis that may have been associated with the development of the outcome. Case-control studies are advantageous when evaluating rare outcomes or those that have a prolonged period of development.[47] They are also typically shorter in duration and less expensive to conduct than cohort studies. However, one significant limitation is *recall bias*, a systematic error where participants do not recall memories accurately, with better recollection of exposures among cases compared to controls, potentially due to impaired memory, confusion, or even a desire to cooperate with an investigator.[47,59] Recall bias will be discussed further in the bias section.

Another limitation of case-control trials is the susceptibility to confounding and inability to determine incidence or prevalence. The data from case-control studies are often presented in a 2×2 table (Table 7.4). Due to the nature of the study, case-control studies cannot be used to obtain incidence rates, prevalence, relative risk, or attributable risks because the base population, which would be the denominator, is unknown.[56] The measure of association for a case-control study is the odds ratio (OR) (Table 7.5). Table 7.6 summarizes the advantages and disadvantages of cohort versus case-control studies.

Cross-sectional

Cross-sectional studies, *prevalence surveys*, and *incidence studies* examine the presence of the outcome and the exposure at the same time. A sample of the population is enrolled and their exposures and outcomes are simultaneously measured.[60] These studies can provide

TABLE 7.4			
Presentation of Case-Control Data			
EXPOSURE/RISK FACTOR	**OUTCOME/DISEASE**		**TOTAL**
	PRESENT	**ABSENT**	
Present	a	b	a + b
Absent	c	d	c + d
Total	a + c	b + d	

valuable information about the prevalence or incidence rates of the outcome in question and can be used to describe a population at a specific time point. One advantage of this design is that if a population-based sample is used, the bias conferred from a case series (cases who received medical attention might have been more severe or had improved access to care) can be avoided. Furthermore, cross-sectional studies are typically short, evaluate subjects specifically of interest, and can evaluate for multiple outcomes and exposures concurrently. However, such designs are costly for rare conditions as larger samples are needed and not appropriate for diseases of short duration because the window may have passed at the time of examination.[56] Another disadvantage is a high reliance on an adequate response rate or else selection bias can significantly impact results. Furthermore, cross-sectional studies cannot assess causality, as the temporal relationship between the exposure and outcome cannot be evaluated in a single time point. Such studies are appropriate to help generate further questions to be examined. Statistically, findings are often presented as prevalence estimates with a 95% confidence interval (CI) to help estimate the risk of error. Frequency or means can be used to compare data that is discovered (see Table 7.5).

A common example of a cross-sectional study is the decennial U.S. census. Another well-known cross-sectional study is the Centers for Disease Control and Prevention National Health and Nutrition Examination Survey.[61] The program began in the 1960s, combining interviews and physical examinations to obtain health and nutritional information about U.S. adults and children in the United States. It continues to provide important data, particularly on the increasing obesity rates in the United States.[62]

Challenges in observational studies

Selection of controls

Perhaps one of the major challenges in observational studies is the selection of appropriate controls because inappropriate controls can lead to incorrect conclusions

TABLE 7.5		
Observational Designs and Associated Statistical Findings		
DESIGN	**EXPLANATION**	**STATISTICAL DESCRIPTIONS**
Case reports	Description of an unusual or new clinical case	Typically, descriptions
Case series	Description of a series of unusual or new clinical cases and findings	Could involve simple statistics such as means, medians, ranges
Cross-sectional studies	Evaluates a single time point ("snapshot"), examines the presence or absence of an exposure and outcome at the same time; may also be referred to as a prevalence study	Means, SDs, percentages, Ors, risk ratios, risk differences, RRs
Case-control studies	Outcomes identified and then typically retrospectively examined for exposures; appropriate for rare diseases	Means, SDs, percentages, Ors
Cohort studies	Individuals with and without exposures are evaluated over time to observe for the outcome.	Means, SDs, percentages, Ors, risk ratios, attributable risk, incidence rates, RRs

Adapted from Johnson LL. Design of observational studies. In: Gallin JI, Ognibene FP, Johnson LL, eds. *Principles and practice of clinical research*, 4th ed. Boston: Academic Press, 2018:231–248, with permission from Elsevier.

	CASE CONTROL	COHORT
TABLE 7.6		
Comparison of Case-Control versus Cohort Studies		
Advantages	1. Appropriate for rare diseases or those with long latencies 2. Development and conduct of study are relatively quick. 3. Comparatively less expensive 4. Typically require less participants 5. Risk to subjects is minimized. 6. Can examine multiple associations of a condition	1. Examines the exposure prior to outcome development, allowing examination of the progression, staging, natural history 2. Can evaluate multiple possible effects of an exposure, examining both risks and benefits 3. Able to calculate rates of disease in the exposed and unexposed groups 4. Able to determine which variables to record 5. Able to have quality control in study variable measurements, better validating the data
Disadvantages	1. Requires subjects' recall or historical records for data 2. Often unable to validate data 3. Cannot always control for confounders 4. Difficult to select an appropriate control group 5. Cannot determine rates of diseased in the case versus control groups 6. Unable to study the disease process and mechanism of development	1. Not suitable for rare disease because a large number of subjects would be required 2. Often require a long follow-up period 3. Long duration may ultimately make findings irrelevant as practice or exposures may change over time. 4. Often expensive 5. Loss of subjects to follow-up is a concern. 6. Unable to always control for confounders 7. Cannot study the mechanism of disease development

Adapted from Schlesselman JJ. *Case-control studies: Design, conduct, analysis.* New York: Oxford University Press, 1982, with permission.

and even potential medical harm.[47] For example, if an investigator wanted to examine the impact of nonsteroidal anti-inflammatory medications (NSAIDs) on a particular condition in a hospital population, selecting controls from a rheumatology service that may have increased exposure to NSAIDs versus a gastroenterology service which may have decreased exposure to NSAIDs could alter the associations seen. A selected comparison group in observational studies should ideally be identical to the exposure/selected outcome group with the exception of the exposure or outcome.[63] Because identical is often not possible, controls should be selected such that they are comparable to the comparison group or population at risk, in other words, at equal risk of becoming exposed or having the outcome.[64] This is a particular challenge in observational studies where randomization cannot help to control for confounders or differences. Studies should always explain the rationale behind how and why the groups were selected.

Proposed strategies for selecting controls include drawing from (1) within the intervention area (such as a hospital), (2) a convenience sample or randomly chosen area, (3) matched areas, or (4) nationally.[65] Each approach has advantages and disadvantages. One relatively straightforward approach in a case-control study is a population control, where controls are randomly selected from the study base. This is an appropriate approach when a particular disease experience in a population during a specific time in a defined geographical area is being evaluated.[66] Advantages include having

the same study base which will allows for exclusions as well as easy extrapolation of the distribution of exposure in controls, allowing for the calculation of absolute or attributable risk. Disadvantages include possible inconvenience, more expense, and recall bias.[66] If a list of potential controls is not available, random digit dialing can be used to recruit population controls, with the obvious disadvantage that those without accessible numbers would be differentially excluded.[66] Neighborhoods may also be used to recruit controls, which involve selecting individuals from a geographical region attempted to reduce variables such as socioeconomic status or access to medical care.[66] Hospital or registries are also commonly used to select controls. They have the advantage of being convenient and may represent similar referral patterns to that institution, but there are inherent problems to selecting from this group of individuals.[67] Patients within teaching hospitals, for example, may unintentionally overrepresent individuals with poor access to care, have higher disease severity requiring hospitalization, or introduce confounders associated with the hospitalization and not represent the general population.[66,67] Controls may also be recruited from an investigator's medical practice or friends/relatives of cases.[66] Investigators should be cautious not to simply choose controls from other hospital populations or family/friends, as they may not truly represent populations at risk or have overlapping conditions that may also place these individuals at disproportional risks (such as the previous NSAIDs example).[64]

Controls can be matched for confounders, the ultimate form being selection of an identical twin.[68] Controls may also be matched based on age, gender, or risk factors thought to be related to the exposure that might not want to be investigated, with the intent to prevent confounding.[56] It is possible, however, to "overmatch" and cause bias or reduce efficiency.[68] Although detailed exploration of the advantages and disadvantages of control selection is beyond the scope of this chapter, it is imperative to evaluate the selection of controls to avoid introducing confounders or bias.

The number of controls needed is also important.[68] Most of the time, having an increased number of controls, however, will not greatly improve precision. Rather, widening the selection area geographically or extending the time frame might be more beneficial.[68]

Bias

Bias is another complication of observational trials.[69] Three common forms of bias exist in observational studies: selection bias, informational bias, and confounding.[70]

Selection bias. Selection bias describes a systematic error that causes intervention groups to differ with respect to what is being studied because of the way in which there were selected, which can then explain differences in the observed outcome between groups.[63,71] Joseph Berkson introduced a form of selection bias, *Berkson bias or paradox*, in the 1940s which described an inherent difference between admitted hospital patients and subjects from the community.[72] *Neyman bias* or prevalence–incidence bias is another form of selection bias where subjects that are more or less severely impacted are excluded due to a gap in time between the exposure and subject selection.[73] If prevalence over incidence (or "newer" cases) is used, individuals who have died or recovered may be excluded, skewing the findings. In general, selection bias may always be inherent to studies, as volunteers for a study are likely different from those who decline participation.[56] Although selection bias cannot always be eliminated, investigators need to be cognizant and acknowledge this in their result reporting.

Information bias. Information bias is a systematic measurement error resulting from how information may be collected.[70] Various types of this bias have been described and involve bias toward how information is obtained or strongly probed: diagnostic suspicion bias, interviewer bias, family information bias, and exposure suspicion.[56] *Recall bias* is perhaps one of the most well-known types of information bias which particularly impacts case-control studies. Recall bias occurs when cases are more likely to remember an exposure or perhaps even exaggerate or minimize potential risk factors because of their outcome.[69] With common knowledge of melanoma risk factors, subjects with the disease may be more likely to recall exposure to sun than those without a melanoma diagnosis.[74] Studies inflicted with recall bias can have consequences. Case-control studies in the late 20th century suggested a correlation with genital talc powder use and ovarian cancer.[75,76] Further prospective cohort studies lacked to show the association, and it became apparent that the significant media attention toward the topic might have influenced the recall in case-control studies.[77,78] Despite little prospective evidence of association, there remains concern among women regarding the use of talc.

Three methods can be employed to reduce bias in the design of case-control studies.[56] First, the selection of cases should be representative of those who could potentially develop the outcome. Secondly, controls should represent a healthy population who would not be anticipated to develop the disease. Lastly, information should be collected similarly for both cases and controls to reduce *interviewer bias* (another form of information bias), which can occur when the interviewer has knowledge of the study hypothesis and may unintentionally question cases differently from controls.[59]

Confounding. A *confounder* is a variable that is associated with both the exposure and outcome and can overestimate, underestimate, or change the direction of the relationship between an exposure and outcome.[71] In other words, a confounder differs between the groups being compared and predicts the result. Strategies implemented to reduce confounding may occur during the study design or after data collection through analytic methods. With regard to the study design, investigators may apply *restriction* (restrict inclusion to a certain category of a confounder or exclude those with the confounder) or *matching* (match a control to a case based on a particular criteria). To improve validity during the statistical analysis, one can apply *stratification* (groups are divided into subgroups based on the potential confounding variable) or *adjustment* (control/adjust for confounders; techniques include multivariate analysis, regression, propensity score, or instrumental variable).[69]

Experimental

Randomized clinical trials

When feasible, the gold standard design is the randomized controlled trial, which randomly assigns subjects to a treatment group, and the impacts are examined.[47(p8)] RCTs allow for controlling confounders and bias as subjects are randomly assigned to an intervention or exposure, creating "equal" groups in this sense. It allows for a direct correlation between a cause and effect of a treatment or exposure. Nonetheless, RCTs have their limitations. As described later in this chapter, RCTs often have internal validity but may be weaker on external validity, or generalizability. Volunteers for such trials, for example, may be inherently different than individuals who decline participation.[79] Furthermore, RCTs can introduce ethical dilemmas given that a potentially beneficial or harmful intervention may be involved, and therefore, equipoise is a necessity.[80] Additionally, RCTs can be costly and, therefore, not always possible.

In clinical trials, the RCT can aim to examine superiority, equivalence, or noninferiority.[81] *Superiority trials* are conducted to determine if one intervention is better than the other (e.g., whether drug A vs. drug B works better). A superiority trial might also be conducted on other parameters. For example, if drug A already improves a condition by 95%, one may not see significant improvement with drug B, but an investigator may be looking to see if drug B has less side effects (more "superior" adverse event profile).[82] *Equivalence trials* seek to evaluate whether one treatment may be therapeutically similar to another, often performed to see if a new intervention is equivalent to a traditional intervention ("active control").[83] In such a trial, drug A may be the active control (conventionally used treatment), and an investigator is curious to see if newly developed drug B is similar in efficacy. A *noninferiority trial* examines whether a treatment is not an "acceptable" amount worse than an existing treatment (within a chosen margin different from the conventional treatment). Noninferiority trials may be used to (1) compare a new treatment to an active control (e.g., when using a placebo is unethical), (2) evaluate a new treatment that may have desirable secondary endpoints (e.g., evaluating a minimally invasive approach over laparotomy), or (3) examine a new treatment that may be overall more efficient (e.g., more cost-effective or easier to implement).[82] A noninferiority trial has the potential to also demonstrate superiority using a prespecified test.[82]

Noninferiority trials have become more popular in recent years, but they may be more complicated to design and could even require a higher sample size than a superiority trial because the margin of difference being investigated might be smaller than a superiority trial. Furthermore, flaws in design are more likely to cause a type I error (to be discussed later) in a noninferiority design because this could make it *more difficult to find a difference*, which is the outcome of choice in this design, therefore increasing the chance of a false-positive result.[82] Nonetheless, both equivalence and noninferiority trials may be more clinically useful than superiority trials because they allow comparison to existing treatments (as opposed to placebo) and evaluation of secondary outcomes. In a clinical example, with regard to treatment of stress urinary incontinence, transobturator slings may have the benefit of less risk of bladder injury over retropubic slings, and, therefore, appropriately,

RCTs have examined and demonstrated transobturator slings to be both equivalent[84] as well as noninferior to retropubic slings.[84,85]

In addition to the aforementioned, clinical trials may be designed to test other assumptions. A *crossover design* involves participants receiving more than one treatment being evaluated, just at different times. The order in which the interventions are received is randomized. Such a design might be used because the subject serves as his or her own control, and the variability between subjects can be reduced.[86] A *factorial design* compares the impact multiple variables may have on one or more outcomes. In the Controlling Anal incontinence in women by Performing Anal Exercises with Biofeedback or Loperamide (CAPABLe) trial, a factorial design allowed comparison of two first-line treatments in a single population, which made studying these interventions more efficient and less costly.[87] Subjects in CAPABLe were randomized in what is called a 2 × 2 factorial design to receive: (1) usual care with placebo, (2) usual care with loperamide, (3) anal exercises with usual care plus placebo, or (4) combination loperamide with anal sphincter exercises with usual care. In *parallel group designs*, subjects are randomized to more than two interventions so that the effects of multiple treatments may be examined. Although clinically useful, parallel group designs are also expensive because large sample sizes are required.[86]

A *sequential trial with interim analysis* allows for parallel groups to be studied until a benefit is observed rather than for a fixed amount of time. The benefit of this trial is that they tend to be of shorter duration.[85] An *interim analysis* is, as can be inferred, that an analysis is performed at any time before formal trial completion and may be performed to assess safety, benefit, or futility.[71] Regarding clinical trials, investigators choose the design that will allow the most efficient route to the answer.

Design Selection, Validity, and Protocol Development

After determining a research question, a study design needs to be chosen. Critical factors to determining which design might be most appropriate are the internal and external validity.[71] *Internal validity* represents that the study measured what it was designed to, such that the results can be believed and trusted.[88] *External validity* involves the generalizability of the study to other individuals, settings, or time periods. Internal validity can be improved through development of and adherence to an appropriate study design, random assignment, and blinding. External validity can be improved by random selection when possible. To ensure appropriate reporting and transparency of studies, guidelines have been developed to help assess a study's validity. The Consolidated Standards of Reporting Trial (CONSORT) statement recommends a 25-item checklist and flow diagram to guide

TABLE 7.7
Sample Components of Protocols and Manual of Operations/Manual of Procedures (MOO/MOP)

	PROTOCOL	**MOO/MOP**

Included items	1. Background/rationale
	2. Specific aims
	3. Design description
	   a. Methods and statistical analysis
	   b. Population to be studied (inclusion/exclusion criteria)
	   c. Approach to recruiting subjects
	   d. Informed consent
	   e. Randomization, masking, blinding plan
	   f. Primary versus additional outcomes
	   g. Statistical analysis
	4. Data collection
	   a. Case report forms
	5. Safety assessment
	6. Funding source
	7. Timeline
	8. Data sharing plan
	   a. Presentations
	   b. Publications
	9. References
		1. Background/rationale
		2. Objectives and specific aims
		3. Study design
		   a. Design type
		   b. Outcome measures
		4. Participants
		   a. Inclusion/exclusion criteria
		   b. Screening
		   c. Recruitment
		   d. Retention
		5. Methods
		   a. Informed consent
		   b. Description of study interventions
		   c. Randomization, masking, blinding
		   d. Plan for follow-up visits
		   e. Data to be collected
		   f. Tools and questionnaires
		   g. Case report form
		6. Statistical analysis
		   a. Sample size
		   b. Power calculation
		7. Budget
		8. Project timeline and schedule
		9. References

Adapted from Stoney CM, Johnson LL. Development and conduct of studies. In: Gallin JI, Ognibene FP, Johnson LL, eds. *Principles and practice of clinical research*, 4th ed. Boston: Academic Press, 2018:203–218, with permission from Elsevier.

reporting of RCTs.[89] The Strengthening the Reporting of Observational Studies in Epidemiology (STROBE) initiative was similarly developed to improve the reporting of observational studies and involves 22-item checklist for all sections of a manuscript.[90] For systematic reviews and meta-analyses, the Preferred Reporting Items for Systematic Reviews and Meta-Analyses (PRISMA) statement contains a 27-item checklist.[91]

Once a design method has been determined, a protocol is drafted, and the details are documented in a manual of operations (MOO) or manual of procedures (MOP). The protocol describes the background knowledge and rationale for the study, study aims, methods, and statistical analysis plan.[92] The MOO/MOP provides the documentation that a coinvestigator would need to conduct the study step by step (Table 7.7).

STATISTICAL TERMINOLOGY AND METHODS

Understanding statistical methods is imperative to developing an appropriate protocol design. The design determines what may be extracted from the study.

For example, while either a cross-sectional or cohort study can allow for determination of *prevalence* (number of existing cases within the population at risk), *incidence* (new cases over a particular time period within the population at risk), may only be determined through a cohort study. The remainder of this chapter reviews common statistical methodologies used in research.

Sample Size, Error, and Power

RCTs require calculation of a *sample size* or the number of subjects needed in a trial to determine an effect.[71] If too few subjects are enrolled, the sample may be inadequate to determine a significant effect size, even though one might actually exist. Additionally, the sample size calculates the number of subjects ultimately available to be included in the analysis. Therefore, recruitment must account for possible withdrawals or "dropouts."

Sample sizes calculations require examining certain questions. First, the investigator must determine an effect size that is clinically relevant. Such assumptions may be made with available literature. Next, for the actual calculation, it is important to understand the null hypothesis, type I (α), and type II (β) errors.[47(pp107–117),81] The null hypothesis in a study is the proposition that no difference exists between the groups being examined, symbolized by H_0. Type I errors (α) measure the false-positive probability, for example, the chance that a study shows a difference between two groups when one does not exist. Conversely, type II (β) error measures the chance of a false negative, or when a study concludes there is no difference when one actually exists.

The α is typically (and arbitrarily) set between 0.01 and 0.10, with 0.05 being a commonly accepted value.[93] With an $\alpha = 0.05$, this means the investigator is willing to accept up to a 5% chance that an association found in the study is actually a false positive or due purely to chance or error. When α is set at 0.05, then the statistical analysis looks for a P value, or calculated probability, to be less than .05 in order to reject the null hypothesis (accept that a difference exists). In other words, if the P value is less than the predetermined .05, the authors can state there was a difference between the two groups. If the P value is greater than .05, it does not necessarily indicate that no difference existed but rather that the association observed is too small to ensure it was due to the intervention rather than to chance.

The α can be one or two sided.[94] A one-sided test looks for *one* direction of difference, for example, when an investigator is only interested if treatment A is better than treatment B (superiority trial) or if treatment A is noninferior to treatment B (noninferiority trial). A two-sided α test looks for *any* difference between groups and, thus, may be used for either a superiority trial or an equivalence trial. Another way to look at it is that a two-sided test is appropriate when there is no data to suggest that one intervention might be more efficacious than the other. The decision regarding which test to use must be made *a priori*.[94]

The β is conventionally set between 0.05 and 0.20. Traditionally, in many clinical trials, the β is chosen as 0.10 or 0.20, meaning the investigator is willing to accept a 10% or 20% chance, respectively, of missing a statistical difference in the study.[93]

The power of a study is drawn from the specified β.[47(p109)] Although the possibility of making a type II error is the β, *power* represents the probability of actually detecting a difference if a specified level of difference (the significance of which is represented by α) exists. Mathematically, power is represented as $(1 - \beta)$. Therefore, if an investigator chooses a β of 0.10, then the power is $1 - \beta = 0.90$. This translates to a 90% chance of detecting a true difference between groups.[93] If a study does not have enough power, it will be unable to precisely answer the scientific question or may result in insignificant results even when an important difference exists.[95] When reporting results of a trial, the authors must be diligent to report the sample size and power calculations.[89]

Confidence Intervals

A confidence interval (CI) is an important yet possibly overlooked value in research. The CI has great implications in the interpretation of study results. The CI represents a range and estimates the variability of the point estimate (such as proportion, RR, or OR) determined in a study. In other words, the CI represents the precision of a study.[47(p11)] CI is represented as $100 \times (1 - \alpha)$. When $\alpha = 0.05$, CI = $100 \times (1 - 0.05)$, or 95% CI. A 95% CI represents 95% probability that if the study were repeated, the CI would contain the mean value.[94] Although one may be tempted to use the CI as a marker for hypothesis testing, indicating a significance when it does not include the number 1, the importance of CI is in the range. The wider the CI, the less precise the results. Conversely, a narrow CI indicates less variability, or more precision, in the factor, increasing "confidence" in the results.[47] Therefore, a study with a narrow CI has findings that are more likely to be precise with less variability, and less likely to have different results if repeated.

Statistical Methods

Data distribution

Data comes as different forms: (1) nominal (categorical), (2) ordinal, or (3) interval (Table 7.8).[95] *Nominal* data do not have a quantitative value, such as gender (male/female) or presence/absence of a condition (prolapse vs. no prolapse). *Ordinal* data describe categories that have an *order* to them, for example, prolapse stage or mild/moderate/severe urinary incontinence. *Interval* data are measured along a scale and are *continuous*, such as age or body mass index. The type of data is relevant in order to determine how they should be analyzed.

Measures of central tendency

Measures of central tendency attempt to describe a measure of interest from a population by identifying the "center."[94] The *mean* is used to describe the average and can be used with interval (continuous) data. The *median* is the middle value, with half of values above and half of values below this value and is used with ordinal data or data that is continuous but does not have a normal distribution (bell-shaped curve, see below). The *mode* describes the most frequently occurring category and is used with nominal (categorical) data.

The concept of normal distribution being described as a bell-shaped curve refers to the appearance of the data when graphed out. The *standard deviation* (SD) refers to the variability of the data around the mean.[94] In normally distributed data, 95.4% of the values from the data collected fall within one SD of the mean, and

TABLE 7.8			
Choice of Statistical Test			
COMPARISON	**TYPE OF DATA**		
	INTERVAL/CONTINUOUS (PARAMETRIC)	**ORDINAL (NONPARAMETRIC)**	**NOMINAL (CATEGORICAL)**
One group	Mean	Median	Proportions
Two groups	Student's t test	Mann-Whitney U (Wilcoxon rank sum)	Chi-square (χ^2) Fisher exact
Three or more groups	One-way ANOVA	Kruskal Wallis	Chi-square (χ^2)
Predict dependent variable from an independent variable	Linear regression	Ordinal regression	Logistic regression
Two paired groups	Paired t test	Wilcoxon signed rank	McNemar
Association between two variables	Pearson correlation	Spearman correlation	Chi-square (χ^2)

ANOVA, analysis of variance.

99.74% fall within 2 SD of the mean, with an equal appearance on either side of the mean. As previously described, certain measures are appropriate for normally versus nonnormally distributed data.

Parametric methods rely on this distribution. *Parametric* methods are used when the data has a normal distribution, and *nonparametric* methods are for asymmetric distributions or data with an unusual number of extreme/outlier values.[94] Parametric methods are used for interval (continuous) data. Nonparametric procedures are often used for ordinal data. Importantly, nonparametric tests have lower power than parametric methods.[94]

An important concept related to statistics is *regression to the mean* (*RTM*). RTM describes the phenomenon that measured values, particularly those that are difficult to measure, will tend to be closer to the mean on repeated measures.[96] In other words, extreme measures become less extreme when repeatedly measured. This can falsely show an improvement in a study, when in reality, measures with greater variability will trend towards average as they are measured repetitively. One explanation for the "placebo effect" may actually be due to the RTM. If a subject enrolls in a study at the height of his or her symptoms, then even without an efficacious intervention, a repeated evaluation of symptoms may show an improvement because the measure will regress closer to the mean. This is particularly evident with conditions that are difficult to measure such as quality of life.[96]

Result Interpretation

Measures of risk

A rather confusing area of research results is the interpretation of risk measures. Most individuals are familiar with *probability*, which is the proportion or percentage of times an event would occur if repeated multiple times, such as the chance for rain today.[97] In contrast, *odds* refer to the probability of the event divided by the probably of the event not occurring, mathematically represented as (probability / 1 − probability). Most clinicians can understand *RR*, which is a ratio of probabilities: the probability of the outcome in those exposed divided by the probability of the outcome in those unexposed. RR is often used in cohort studies to describe the association between an exposure and outcome.[98] When the RR is greater than 1, it denotes a risk from the exposure, whereas RR less than 1 shows a protective association.[56] The *OR*, however, is the odds of an outcome in one group divided by the odds of the outcome in another group. The mathematical formula is a little more complicated than the RR. When the risk of an outcome is small or rare (probability less than 10% to 20%), the OR is similar to the RR and can be used interchangeably. However, with common outcomes, the OR will overexaggerate the RR, and it would, therefore, be incorrect to assume they are the same measure. Although the RR is a preferable measure, the OR is required in three situations. As mentioned previously, the OR is the risk measure in a case-control study because there is no denominator to calculate an RR. The OR is also used in meta-analyses and is the product in logistic regression, which was previously mentioned as a technique to control for confounders. When necessary, techniques are available to approximate RR from an OR.[97]

Once an effect is observed in a study, several terms may be used to describe the size of the effect: RR reduction, absolute risk reduction, and number needed to treat.[98] *RR reduction* refers to the estimated magnitude of the effect of an exposure on the outcome in relative terms, expressed as a *proportion*. The RR reduction can be thought of an estimation of the proportion of baseline outcome risk that is reduced because of the exposure. The *absolute risk reduction* describes the absolute difference in risk between the exposed and unexposed groups and can represent the amount of harm or benefit the exposure provides. This is mathematically described as the incidence in the exposed group minus the incidence in the unexposed group.[98] Finally, the *number needed to treat* describes how many individuals would need to undergo the treatment to prevent one event. For example, an investigator may be curious about the number of women who would need to undergo a cesarean delivery to prevent one case of pelvic organ prolapse.

Sensitivity, specificity, positive predictive value, and negative predictive value

When it comes to test interpretation, four measures (sensitivity, specificity, positive predictive value, and negative predictive value) are used to define test accuracy. Although these work on the assumption that disease and tests are dichotomous, which is not always the case, they are useful to help understand test results.[47] *Sensitivity* describes the ability of a test to detect those with the disease in question. *Specificity* represents a test's ability to identify those who do not have the disease. These are sometimes described with the mnemonics "SNOUT" (because a highly *Sensitive* test when *Negative* can rule *OUT* disease) and "SPIN" (because a highly *Specific* test when *Positive* rules *IN* disease).[99] These values can be placed in a 2 × 2 table format (Table 7.9).

Predictive values aid practitioners in clinically interpreting tests. *Positive predictive value* refers to the likelihood that someone with a positive test will have the disease, whereas *negative predictive value* denotes the probability that someone with a negative test does not have the disease.[47] A clinical example is the fetal fibronectin test for preterm labor. The negative predictive value has been shown to be 97% to 100%, which means that when negative, women can be reassured they will not deliver within 7 days.[100]

ANALYSES

Per-Protocol and Intent-to-Treat Analyses

Data may be analyzed in different forms based on the variables related to the study needs. A *planned analysis* is specified *a priori*. This is preferable to *exploratory*, *data-derived*, or *post hoc analyses*, which are unplanned and swayed by the data. When analysis is restricted to only those subjects who were enrolled, randomized, and completed the study fully adhering to the protocol, this is considered a *per-protocol* analysis.[71]

However, most studies do not go perfectly as planned, and to account for inconsistencies such as subjects who did not receive the randomized intervention or randomization of ineligible subjects, an *intent-to-treat* analysis may be conducted. In such an analysis, subjects are analyzed according to their original assignment randomization, regardless of whether they received that treatment. This analysis can prevent bias from loss of subjects.[71]

Survival Analysis

A *survival analysis* involves subjects either followed for different lengths of time or enrolled at different times. The focus of a survival analysis is the time it takes for an event to occur.[101] A *survival time* is the time from the initiation point to the event occurrence, often beginning at the time the subject enrolls in the study. In survival analyses, the follow-up time varies and is dependent on when the subject enrolls and when the outcome occurs. Subjects may enter the study at varying times and be followed for different time frames. Therefore, some subjects might be monitored for longer durations than others. Additionally, the outcome is often not observed in all subjects by the study completion. When the event does not occur by the study end point, the survival time is termed *censored*.

The statistical method used is the *Kaplan-Meier estimator* or *product–limit estimator*.[47,101] This estimates the risk of the event over time and can determine the probability of the event at any point in time because it uses all subjects in the study. The proportion surviving is then graphed against time, creating a *Kaplan-Meier curve*, an estimate of the true survival if censored cases are typical of the whole population being followed. Marks may be found on the curve where censoring has occurred. Interestingly, with longer follow-up time periods, because less and less subjects will be followed,

TABLE 7.9		
Test Validity		
	DISEASE	
	Positive	**Negative**
Positive	True positive **A**	False positive **B**
Negative	False negative **C**	True negative **D**

Sensitivity = a / a + c
Specificity = d / b + d

Positive predictive value = a / a + b
Negative predictive value = d / c + d

Adapted from Schulz KF, Grimes DA. *The Lancet handbook of essential concepts in clinical research.* New York: Elsevier, 2006, with permission from Elsevier.

the curve becomes less reliable. The *log-rank* statistical method is used to compare the overall survival between two groups. The log-rank test, however, denotes significance and does not describe the magnitude of difference between groups. For this task, the *Cox proportional-hazards model* can adjust for both categorial and continuous prognostic factors and is used to evaluate the effect of several variables on the time required for the outcome to occur.[101] Because it uses a regression method, it can control for covariates.[47] Survival analyses are useful in pelvic floor research to estimate the time to failure from a surgical repair.

Multiple Comparisons

Although it may appear convenient to test for many hypotheses in one study, statistically, this can result in type I errors.[71,94] If multiple analyses are performed on the same data, approximately $\alpha \times 100\%$ of the tests will be significant even when they are not in truth.[94] Using this calculation, with $\alpha = 0.05$, ultimately on average, 5% of the tests will be significant by chance. Therefore, adjustments need to be made to correct for this. One commonly used correction is the *Bonferroni* correction, which restates the type I error (α) as α / n, with n representing the number of tests being performed. Therefore, in any study with multiple comparisons in which an adjustment was not made, it is possible that any statistically significant findings may be due to chance.[94]

ALTERNATE FORMS OF RESEARCH

Meta-analyses and Systematic Reviews

When incomplete data exists in one given study, alternative methods can be used to describe effects. A *meta-analysis* pools data from multiple clinical studies to determine if similar effects of a treatment can be observed or to explain for differences in results.[102] To perform a meta-analysis, eligibility criteria for studies must be designated. Once this is performed, relevant studies are identified, reviewed, and data extracted. This data is then analyzed via methods developed for meta-analyses. Typically, OR or RR is used to describe treatment effects. One hallmark limitation of meta-analyses is that their quality is dependent on the quality of the original studies.[102] A *systematic review*, alternatively, systematically collects all relevant studies to review and analyze the results. Both forms of study can influence practice guidelines and are at the top of the hierarchy of study quality.[48]

"Big Data"

Finally, although original data is intriguing and exciting, often the work may have already been performed, and investigators can borrow from previously collected data to answer new questions. Historically, there was a concern that for financial reasons, medical information obtained through studies was not being shared.[103] Government regulation now mandates federally funded research to be registered and the data to ultimately be shared.[104] As a result of this resource sharing, investigators now have access to large data sets ("big data") that can be used to answer important clinical questions. New or underresourced investigators may take advantage of such opportunities through initiatives such as the National Institute of Child Health and Human Development (NICHD) Data and Specimen Hub (DASH), a cost-free centralized resource that allows access to de-identified data from NICHD-funded studies.[105]

CONCLUSION

Participation in research has become a mainstay in residency and fellowship training.[106] Although it may seem intimidating or even arduous to consider engaging in investigative study, it can be quite energizing to be involved in a new or improved discovery. Nonetheless, even if a practitioner opts not to participate in research in their practice, an understanding of research and research methods can aid critical appraisal of the literature. As practice guidelines are dependent on evidence-based medicine, understanding how to interpret data may be a useful tool.

References

1. Perneger TV, Ricou B, Boulvain M, et al. Medical researchers evaluate their methodological skills. *J Clin Epidemiol* 2004;57(12):1323–1329.
2. Leahy N, Sheps J, Tracy CS, et al. Family physicians' attitudes toward education in research skills during residency: Findings from a national mailed survey. *Can Fam Physician* 2008;54(3):413–414.
3. Ramsey PG, Carline JD, Inui TS, et al. Changes over time in the knowledge base of practicing internists. *JAMA* 1991;266(8):1103–1107.
4. Yew KS, Reid A. Teaching evidence-based medicine skills: An exploratory study of residency graduates' practice habits. *Fam Med* 2008;40(1):24–31.
5. Grady C. Ethical principles in clinical research. In: Gallin JI, Ognibene FP, Johnson LL, eds. *Principles and practice of clinical research*, 4th ed. Massachusetts: Academic Press, 2018:19–31.
6. Truog RD. Patients and doctors—The evolution of a relationship. *N Engl J Med* 2012;366(7):581–585.
7. U.S. Food and Drug Administration. Part I: The 1906 Food and Drugs Act and its enforcement. Updated April 24, 2019. Accessed September 1, 2021. https://www.fda.gov/about -fda/fdas-evolving-regulatory-powers/part-i-1906-food-and -drugs-act-and-its-enforcement
8. U.S. Food and Drug Administration. Part II: 1938, Food, Drug, Cosmetic Act. Updated November 28, 2018. Accessed September 1, 2021. https://www.fda.gov/about-fda/fdas -evolving-regulatory-powers/part-ii-1938-food-drug -cosmetic-act

9. Shuster E. Fifty years later: The significance of the Nuremberg Code. *N Engl J Med* 1997;337(20):1436–1440.

10. Shuster E. American doctors at the Nuremberg Medical Trial. *Am J Public Health* 2018;108(1):47–52.

11. Jones DS, Grady C, Lederer SE. "Ethics and clinical research"— The 50th anniversary of Beecher's Bombshell. *N Engl J Med* 2016;374(24):2393–2398.

12. Beecher HK. Ethics and clinical research. *N Engl J Med* 1966;274(24):1354–1360.

13. The Tuskegee timeline. Centers for Disease Control and Prevention. Accessed September 1, 2021. https://www.cdc.gov/tuskegee/timeline.htm

14. Adashi EY, Walters LB, Menikoff JA. The Belmont Report at 40: Reckoning with time. *Am J Public Health* 2018;108(10):1345–1348.

15. The Belmont Report. U.S. Department of Health and Human Services. Accessed September 1, 2021. https://www.hhs.gov/ohrp/regulations-and-policy/belmont-report/read-the-belmont-report/index.html

16. Federal policy for the protection of human subjects ('common rule'). U.S. Department of Health and Human Services. Accessed September 1, 2021. https://www.hhs.gov/ohrp/regulations-and-policy/regulations/common-rule/index.html

17. NIH policy and guidelines on the inclusion of children as participants in research involving human subjects. Accessed September 1, 2021. https://grants.nih.gov/grants/guide/notice-files/not98-024.html

18. NIH policy and guidelines on the inclusion of women and minorities as subjects in clinical research. National Institutes of Health. Accessed September 1, 2021. https://grants.nih.gov/policy/inclusion/women-and-minorities/guidelines.htm

19. Schwenzer KJ. Practical tips for working effectively with your institutional review board. *Respir Care* 2008;53(10):1354–1361.

20. Emanuel EJ, Wendler D, Grady C. What makes clinical research ethical? *JAMA* 2000;283(20):2701–2711.

21. Mandava A, Pace C, Campbell B, et al. The quality of informed consent: Mapping the landscape. A review of empirical data from developing and developed countries. *J Med Ethics* 2012;38(6):356–365.

22. Nishimura A, Carey J, Erwin PJ, et al. Improving understanding in the research informed consent process: A systematic review of 54 interventions tested in randomized control trials. *BMC Med Ethics* 14(1):28.

23. Flory J, Emanuel E. Interventions to improve research participants' understanding in informed consent for research: A systematic review. *JAMA* 2004;292(13):1593–1601.

24. Brubaker L, Jelovsek E, Lukacz ES, et al. Recruitment and retention: A randomized controlled trial of video-enhanced versus standard consent processes within the E-OPTIMAL study. *Clin Trials* 2019;16(5):481–489.

25. Millum J, Garnett M. How payment for research participation can be coercive. *Am J Bioeth* 2019;19(9):21–31.

26. Slutsman J, Nieman L. Institutional review boards. In: Gallin JI, Ognibene FP, Johnson LL, eds. *Principles and practice of clinical research*, 4th ed. Massachusetts: Academic Press, 2018:47–61.

27. U.S. Department of Health and Human Services, National Institutes of Health. Public Health Service policy on humane care and use of laboratory animals. Accessed September 1, 2021. https://olaw.nih.gov/sites/default/files/PHSPolicyLabAnimals.pdf

28. National Academy of Sciences, National Academy of Engineering, Institute of Medicine Committee on Science, Engineering, and Public Policy. Human participants and animal subjects in research. In: *On being a scientist: A guide to responsible conduct in research*, 3rd ed. Washington, DC: National Academies Press, 2009. https://www.ncbi.nlm.nih.gov/books/NBK214566/

29. 3Rs alternatives: Technologies and approaches. National Agricultural Library. Accessed September 1, 2021. https://www.nal.usda.gov/awic/3rs-alternatives-technologies-and-approaches

30. 45 CFR 46. U.S. Department of Health and Human Services. Accessed September 1, 2021. https://www.hhs.gov/ohrp/regulations-and-policy/regulations/45-cfr-46/index.html

31. Part 46—Protection of human subjects. Code of Federal Regulations. Accessed September 1, 2021. https://www.ecfr.gov/cgi-bin/retrieveECFR?gp=&SID=83cd09e1c0f5c-6937cd9d7513160fc3f&pitd=20180719&n=pt45.1.46&r=PART&ty=HTML#se45.1.46_1104

32. Expedited review: Categories of research that may be reviewed through an expedited review procedure (1998). U.S. Department of Health and Human Services. Accessed September 1, 2021. https://www.hhs.gov/ohrp/regulations-and-policy/guidance/categories-of-research-expedited-review-procedure-1998/index.html#:~:text=%5B1%5D%20An%20expedited%20review%20procedure

33. Hudson KL, Lauer MS, Collins FS. Toward a new era of trust and transparency in clinical trials. *JAMA* 2016;316(13):1353–1354.

34. Wolinetz CD, Collins FS. Single-minded research review: The common rule and single IRB policy. *Am J Bioeth* 2017;17(7):34–36.

35. Shamy M, Dewar B, Fedyk M. Different meanings of equipoise and the four quadrants of uncertainty. *J Clin Epidemiol* 2020;127:248–249.

36. Wakim PG, Shaw PA. Data and safety monitoring. In: Gallin JI, Ognibene FP, Johnson LL, eds. *Principles and practice of clinical research*, 4th ed. Massachusetts: Academic Press, 2018:127–140.

37. Harrington D, Drazen JM. Learning from a trial stopped by a data and safety monitoring board. *N Engl J Med* 2018;378(21):2031–2032.

38. Terrin ML. Evaluating and implementing data and safety monitoring plans. *J Investig Med* 2004;52(7):459–463.

39. Operational guidelines for the establishment and functioning of data and safety monitoring boards. World Health Organization. Accessed September 1, 2021. https://www.who.int/tdr/publications/documents/operational-guidelines.pdf?ua=1

40. NIH policy for data and safety monitoring. National Institutes of Health. Accessed September 1, 2021. https://grants.nih.gov/grants/guide/notice-files/not98-084.html

41. Lacey JV Jr. The WHI ten year's later: An epidemiologist's view. *J Steroid Biochem Mol Biol* 2014;142:12–15.

42. The Women's Health Initiative Study Group. Design of the Women's Health Initiative clinical trial and observational study. *Control Clin Trials* 1998;19(1):61–109.

43. Freedman L, Anderson G, Kipnis V, et al. Approaches to monitoring the results of long-term disease prevention trials: Examples from the Women's Health Initiative. *Control Clin Trials* 1996;17(6):509–525.

44. Rossouw JE, Anderson GL, Prentice RL, et al. Risks and benefits of estrogen plus progestin in healthy postmenopausal women: Principal results from the Women's Health Initiative randomized controlled trial. *JAMA* 2002;288(3):321–333.

45. Anderson GL, Limacher M, Assaf AR, et al. Effects of conjugated equine estrogen in postmenopausal women with

hysterectomy: The Women's Health Initiative randomized controlled trial. *JAMA* 2004;291(14):1701–1712.

46. Clinical alert: NIH asks participants in women's health initiative estrogen-alone study to stop study pills, begin follow-up phase. National Library of Medicine. Accessed September 1, 2021. https://www.nlm.nih.gov/databases/alerts/estrogen_alone.html

47. Schulz KF, Grimes DA. *The Lancet handbook of essential concepts in clinical research*. New York: Elsevier, 2006.

48. Harris RP, Helfand M, Woolf SH, et al. Current methods of the US Preventive Services Task Force: A review of the process. *Am J Prev Med* 2001;20(3 Suppl):21–35.

49. Morris BA. The importance of case reports. *CMAJ* 1989; 141(9):875–876.

50. Ortega-Loubon C, Culquichicón C, Correa R. The importance of writing and publishing case reports during medical training. *Cureus* 2017;9(12):e1964.

51. Ramulu VG, Levine RB, Hebert RS, et al. Development of a case report review instrument. *Int J Clin Pract* 2005;59(4):457–461.

52. Gottlieb MS, Schroff R, Schanker HM, et al. Pneumocystis carinii pneumonia and mucosal candidiasis in previously healthy homosexual men: Evidence of a new acquired cellular immunodeficiency. *N Engl J Med* 1981;305(24):1425–1431.

53. Zhu N, Zhang D, Wang W, et al. A novel coronavirus from patients with pneumonia in China, 2019. *N Engl J Med* 2020;382(8):727–733.

54. Plassman BL, Havlik RJ, Steffens DC, et al. Documented head injury in early adulthood and risk of Alzheimer's disease and other dementias. *Neurology* 2000;55(8):1158–1166.

55. Sedgwick P. Prospective cohort studies: Advantages and disadvantages. *BMJ* 2013;347:f6726.

56. Johnson LL. Design of observational studies. In: Gallin JI, Ognibene FP, Johnson LL, eds. *Principles and practice of clinical research*, 4th ed. Massachusetts: Academic Press, 2018:231–248.

57. Abbasi J. The Nurses' Health Study takes fresh aim at breast cancer as it heads into decade five. *JAMA* 2016;316(24):2583–2585.

58. History. Nurses' Health Study. Accessed September 1, 2021. https://www.nurseshealthstudy.org/about-nhs/history

59. Schlesselman JJ. *Case-control studies: Design, conduct, analysis*. New York: Oxford University Press, 1982.

60. U.S. Department of Health and Human Services. *Principles of epidemiology in public health practice: An introduction to applied epidemiology and biostatistics*, 3rd ed. Georgia: U.S. Department of Health and Human Services, 2006.

61. National Center for Health Statistics. About the National Health and Nutrition Examination Survey. Centers for Disease Control and Prevention. Accessed September 1, 2021. https://www.cdc.gov/nchs/nhanes/about_nhanes.htm

62. Hedley AA, Ogden CL, Johnson CL, et al. Prevalence of overweight and obesity among US children, adolescents, and adults, 1999-2002. *JAMA* 2004;291(23):2847–2850.

63. Rochon PA, Gurwitz JH, Sykora K, et al. Reader's guide to critical appraisal of cohort studies: 1. Role and design. *BMJ* 2005;330(7496):895–897.

64. Malay S, Chung KC. The choice of controls for providing validity and evidence in clinical research. *Plast Reconstr Surg* 2012;130(4):959–965.

65. Steventon A, Grieve R, Sekhon JS. A comparison of alternative strategies for choosing control populations in observational studies. *Health Serv Outcomes Res Methodol* 2015;15(3–4):157–181.

66. Wacholder S, Silverman DT, McLaughlin JK, et al. Selection of controls in case-control studies. II. Types of controls. *Am J Epidemiol* 1992;135(9):1029–1041.

67. Lasky T, Stolley PD. Selection of cases and controls. *Epidemiol Rev* 1994;16(1):6–17.

68. Wacholder S, Silverman DT, McLaughlin JK, et al. Selection of controls in case-control studies. III. Design options. *Am J Epidemiol* 1992;135(9):1042–1050.

69. Lu CY. Observational studies: A review of study designs, challenges and strategies to reduce confounding. *Int J Clin Pract* 2009;63(5):691–697.

70. Luijendijk HJ, Page MJ, Burger H, et al. Assessing risk of bias: A proposal for a unified framework for observational studies and randomized trials. *BMC Med Res Methodol* 2020;20(1):237.

71. Altman DG, Schulz KF, Moher D, et al. The revised CONSORT statement for reporting randomized trials: Explanation and elaboration. *Ann Intern Med* 2001;134(8):663–694.

72. Woodfine JD, Redelmeier DA. Berkson's paradox in medical care. *J Intern Med* 2015;278(4):424–426.

73. Swanson DM, Anderson CD, Betensky RA. Hypothesis tests for Neyman's bias in case-control studies. *J Appl Stat* 2018;45(11):1956–1977.

74. Parr CL, Hjartåker A, Laake P, et al. Recall bias in melanoma risk factors and measurement error effects: A nested case-control study within the Norwegian Women and Cancer Study. *Am J Epidemiol* 2009;169(3):257–266.

75. Cramer DW, Welch WR, Scully RE, et al. Ovarian cancer and talc: A case-control study. *Cancer* 1982;50(2):372–376.

76. Cramer DW, Liberman RF, Titus-Ernstoff L, et al. Genital talc exposure and risk of ovarian cancer. *Int J Cancer* 1999;81(3):351–356.

77. Trabert B. Body powder and ovarian cancer risk—What is the role of recall bias? *Cancer Epidemiol Biomarkers Prev* 2016;25(10):1369–1370.

78. O'Brien KM, Tworoger SS, Harris HR, et al. Association of powder use in the genital area with risk of ovarian cancer. *JAMA* 2020;323(1):49–59.

79. Ssali A, Nunn A, Mbonye M, et al. Reasons for participating in a randomised clinical trial: The volunteers' voices in the COSTOP trial in Uganda. *Contemp Clin Trials Commun* 2017;7:44–47.

80. Miller FG, Joffe S. Equipoise and the dilemma of randomized clinical trials. *N Engl J Med* 2011;364(5):476–480.

81. Sakpal TV. Sample size estimation in clinical trial. *Perspect Clin Res* 2010;1(2):67–69.

82. Vavken P. Rationale for and methods of superiority, noninferiority, or equivalence designs in orthopaedic, controlled trials. *Clin Orthop Relat Res* 2011;469(9):2645–2653.

83. Piaggio G, Elbourne DR, Pocock SJ, et al. Reporting of noninferiority and equivalence randomized trials: Extension of the CONSORT 2010 statement. *JAMA* 2012;308(24):2594–2604.

84. Richter HE, Albo ME, Zyczynski HM, et al. Retropubic versus transobturator midurethral slings for stress incontinence. *N Engl J Med* 2010;362(22):2066–2076.

85. Barber MD, Kleeman S, Karram MM, et al. Transobturator tape compared with tension-free vaginal tape for the treatment of stress urinary incontinence: A randomized controlled trial. *Obstet Gynecol* 2008;111(3):611–621.

86. Stoney CM, Johnson LL. Development and conduct of studies. In: Gallin JI, Ognibene FP, Johnson LL, eds. *Principles and practice of clinical research*, 4th ed. Massachusetts: Academic Press, 2018:203–218.

87. Jelovsek JE, Markland AD, Whitehead WE, et al. Controlling Anal incontinence in women by Performing Anal Exercises with Biofeedback or Loperamide (CAPABLe) trial: Design and methods. *Contemp Clin Trials* 2015;44:164–174.

88. Streiner DL. Statistics Commentary Series. Commentary No. 44: Internal and external validity. *J Clin Psychopharmacol* 2020;40(6):531–533.

89. Schulz KF, Altman DG, Moher D. CONSORT 2010 statement: Updated guidelines for reporting parallel group randomised trials. *BMJ* 2010;340:c332.

90. von Elm E, Altman DG, Egger M, et al. The Strengthening the Reporting of Observational Studies in Epidemiology (STROBE) statement: Guidelines for reporting observational studies. *J Clin Epidemiol* 2008;61(4):344–349.

91. Moher D, Liberati A, Tetzlaff J, et al. Preferred Reporting Items for Systematic Reviews and Meta-Analyses: The PRISMA statement. *J Clin Epidemiol* 2009;62(10):1006–1012.

92. Stoney CM, Johnson LL. Design of clinical trials and studies. In: Gallin JI, Ognibene FP, Johnson LL, eds. *Principles and practice of clinical research*, 4th ed. Massachusetts: Academic Press, 2018:249–268.

93. Banerjee A, Chitnis UB, Jadhav SL, et al. Hypothesis testing, type I and type II errors. *Ind Psychiatry J* 2009;18(2):127–131.

94. Johnson LL, Borkowf CR, Shaw PA. Hypothesis testing. In: Gallin JI, Ognibene FP, Johnson LL, eds. *Principles and practice of clinical research*, 4th ed. Massachusetts: Academic Press, 2018:341–357.

95. Borkowf CB, Johnson LL, Albert PS. Power and sample size calculations. In: Gallin JI, Ognibene FP, Johnson LL, eds. *Principles and practice of clinical research*, 4th ed. Massachusetts: Academic Press, 2018:359–372.

96. Shaw PA, Johnson LL, Proschan MA. Intermediate topics in biostatistics. In: Gallin JI, Ognibene FP, Johnson LL, eds. *Principles and practice of clinical research*, 4th ed. Massachusetts: Academic Press, 2018:383–409.

97. Grimes DA, Schulz KF. Making sense of odds and odds ratios. *Obstet Gynecol* 2008;111(2 Pt 1):423–426.

98. Replogle WH, Johnson WD. Interpretation of absolute measures of disease risk in comparative research. *Fam Med* 2007;39(6):432–435.

99. Baeyens J-P, Serrien B, Goossens M, et al. Questioning the "SPIN and SNOUT" rule in clinical testing. *Arch Physiother* 2019;9:4.

100. Cornelissen, van Oostrum, van der Woude DAA, et al. The diagnostic value of fetal fibronectin testing in clinical practice. *J Obstet Gynaecol Res* 2020;46(3):405–412.

101. Johnson LL. An introduction to survival analysis. In: Gallin JI, Ognibene FP, Johnson LL, eds. *Principles and practice of clinical research*, 4th ed. Massachusetts: Academic Press, 2018:373–381.

102. Sun J, Freeman BD, Natanson C. Meta-analysis of clinical trials. In: Gallin JI, Ognibene FP, Johnson LL, eds. *Principles and practice of clinical research*, 4th ed. Massachusetts: Academic Press, 2018:317–327.

103. Califf RM. Large clinical trials and registries—Clinical research institutes. In: Gallin JI, Ognibene FP, Johnson LL, eds. *Principles and practice of clinical research*, 4th ed. Massachusetts: Academic Press, 2018:411–444.

104. NIH Data Sharing Policy and Implementation Guidance. National Institutes of Health. Accessed September 1, 2021. https://grants.nih.gov/grants/policy/data_sharing/data_sharing_guidance.htm.

105. Eunice Kennedy Shriver National Institute of Child Health and Human Development Data and Specimen Hub. Welcome to the Data and Specimen Hub. Accessed February 4, 2022. https://dash.nichd.nih.gov/.

106. ACGME Program Requirements for Graduate Medical Education in Obstetrics and Gynecology. Accreditation Council for Graduate Medical Education. Accessed September 1, 2021. https://www.acgme.org/Portals/0/PFAssetsProgramRequirements/220_ObstetricsAndGynecology_2020pdf?ver=2020-06-29-162338-630.

CHAPTER 8

ETHICAL ISSUES IN UROGYNECOLOGY

L. Lewis Wall • Douglas Brown

WHAT IS "ETHICS"?

In its most basic form, medical ethics refers to the way we interact with each other as doctors, patients, and clinical colleagues and as members of health care teams, faculties, practice groups, and other institutions. Medical ethics lays out the priorities and responsibilities that should guide clinical performance and interpersonal behavior in the practice of medicine and surgery. Medical ethics helps us navigate difficult decisions by establishing a process by which to determine—and then to act on—what ought to be done, all things considered.

What priorities and responsibilities should guide us in clinical practice, be it in urogynecology or any other field of patient care? The anchoring admonition for the clinician is to put the best interests of the patient ahead of all other considerations. This observation may seem self-evident, but often, it is not. Many ethical dilemmas in clinical medicine today are fundamentally about whose interests are really being served by the way care is delivered or financed. Corporate and commercial interests have intruded into clinical care in ways that would have seemed incomprehensible to previous generations of clinicians.

Urogynecologists are fiduciaries for their patients.[1] The term *fiduciary* stems from a concept in ancient Roman law in which one person acted as a trustee for another, accepting the obligation to oversee the object placed in trust for the benefit of the person who entrusted it to the fiduciary. Patients expect their doctors to act in a similar way, to give them unbiased medical advice that serves their best interests as patients. What that "best interest" may be in any given clinical situation depends on the patient's free and full communication of her needs and desires to her doctor who respects her autonomy. However, this responsibility does not obligate the physician to "do whatever the patient wants." Clinicians are obliged to provide objective information and to give their best clinical advice, even when the patient resists such information and advice. Clinicians are certainly not obligated to provide treatment that is dangerous, harmful, or unwarranted. Clinicians should fully understand the patient's perspective and should tailor treatments (when possible) to patient preferences, but they are not obligated to override their own clinical judgment simply "because that's what the patient wanted."

SYSTEMATIC WAYS TO THINK ABOUT MEDICAL ETHICS

Ethicists have presented various systematic ways to help clinicians sort through ethical issues in clinical practice. One of the most commonly used systems, popularized by Tom Beauchamp and James Childress, is known as "principlism."[1] This approach—which is rooted in a highly legalistic background—proposes that the way to solve clinical ethical problems is to evaluate each situation using four landmark principles. These principles are (1) patient autonomy, or the right of patients to define the goals of their care, to have their wishes considered and respected (which is the basis for the practice of securing informed consent prior to undertaking operations or procedures); (2) nonmaleficence, or the obligation of clinicians not to inflict avoidable harm on their patients; (3) beneficence, or the responsibility to work to benefit the patients, striving always to act in the patients' best interest; and (4) fairness (sometimes also called the "principle of justice"), or the expectation that patients should be treated fairly, that like cases should be treated similarly.

Fairness has two components. Procedural fairness requires the health care system to treat patients equally within the system. Distributive fairness requires patients to have access to the same kinds of medical care. Distributive justice and procedural fairness are emerging as major areas of conflict and distress in the American health care system and are likely to be areas of conflict for some time. Many dilemmas arise in this domain. Fiduciary duty demands that urogynecologists be vigorous advocates for their patients within the health care system, just as lawyers have similar duties to their clients within the legal system.

The principlist approach evaluates ethically challenging clinical scenarios by first examining the various aspects of a case through the lens of each principle (i.e., autonomy, beneficence, nonmaleficence, and justice) and then, through a process of "balancing," deciding where the most important aspects of each case lie, leading the way to a proper decision.

Jonsen et al.'s[2] approach is similar, but their four categories of evaluation resonate more clearly with clinicians, largely because their clinical background is much stronger than that of Beauchamp and Childress. They segment the evaluation of clinical cases into (1) medical indications (beneficence and nonmaleficence); (2) patient preferences (respect for autonomy); (3) quality of life (beneficence, nonmaleficence, and respect for autonomy); and (4) contextual features (loyalty and fairness). They argue that clinicians who work through each quadrant will uncover the salient aspects of each case and will arrive at a reasonable ethical resolution (Table 8.1).[2]

Both frameworks are very useful for determining where the problem areas lie in any particular clinical dilemma, but they are somewhat limited in making real-time decisions. Another approach to medical ethics is known as virtue ethics.[3,4] This approach is less popular than principlism among professional academic ethicists who consult with hospital administrators, lawyers, and ethics committees during business hours but who also tend to have little experience on the wards or little interaction with working clinicians, particularly during the night or on weekends when pressing ethical dilemmas often arise. Virtue ethics, we believe, is as critical to the training of clinicians, medical students, residents, and fellows as is the more formal, legalistic approaches because virtue ethics focuses on the character and practice patterns of clinicians, their integrity,

TABLE 8.1

The "Four Topics Chart" for Analyzing Ethical Decisions in Medicine

MEDICAL INDICATIONS	PREFERENCES OF PATIENTS
The Principles of Beneficence and Nonmaleficence	The Principle of Respect for Autonomy
1. What is the patient's medical problem? Is the problem acute? Chronic? Critical? Reversible? Emergent? Terminal? 2. What are the goals of treatment? 3. In what circumstances are medical treatments not indicated? 4. What are the probabilities of success of the various treatment options? 5. In sum, how can this patient be benefitted by medical and nursing care, and how can harm be avoided?	1. Has the patient been informed of benefits and risks of diagnostic and treatment recommendations, understood this information, and given consent? 2. Is the patient mentally capable and legally competent, or is there evidence of incapacity? 3. If mentally capable, what preferences about treatment is the patient stating? 4. If incapacitated, has the patient expressed prior preferences? 5. Who is the appropriate surrogate to make decisions for an incapacitated patient? What standards should govern the surrogate's decision? 6. Is the patient unwilling or unable to cooperate with medical treatment? If so, why?
QUALITY OF LIFE	**CONTEXTUAL FEATURES**
The Principles of Beneficence and Nonmaleficence and Respect for Autonomy	The Principles of Justice and Fairness
1. What are the prospects, with or without treatment, for a return to normal life, and what physical, mental, and social deficits might the patient experience even if treatment succeeds? 2. On what grounds can anyone judge that some quality of life would be undesirable for a patient who cannot make or express such a judgment? 3. Are there biases that might prejudice the provider's evaluation of a patient's quality of life? 4. What ethical issues arise concerning improving or enhancing a patient's quality of life? 5. Do quality-of-life assessments raise any questions that might contribute to a change of treatment plan, such as forgoing life-sustaining treatment? 6. Are there plans to provide pain relief and provide comfort after a decision has been made to forgo life-sustaining treatment? 7. Is medically assisted dying ethically or legally permissible? 8. What is the legal and ethical status of suicide?	1. Are there professional, interprofessional, or business interests that might create conflicts of interest? 2. Are there parties other than clinician and patient, such as family members, who have a legitimate interest in clinical decisions? 3. What are the limits imposed on patient confidentiality by the legitimate interest of third parties? 4. Are there financial factors that create conflicts of interest in clinical decisions? 5. Are there problems of allocation of resources that affect clinical decisions? 6. Are there religious factors that might influence clinical decisions? 7. What are the legal issues that might affect clinical decisions? 8. Are there considerations of clinical research and medical education that might affect clinical decisions? 9. Are there considerations of public health and safety that might influences clinical decisions? 10. Does institutional affiliation create conflicts of interest that might influence clinical decisions?

and the characteristics on which trust is based—and trust is the ultimate foundation on which all clinical relationships rest.[5]

Several often unspoken but highly consequential questions are pivotal in clinical training: What kind of doctor do you want to be? What reputation do you want to have? How do you want to be regarded by colleagues and patients? When you appear on a call list with other doctors, what do you want their reaction to be to having to work with you? These questions are part of what has been called the "hidden curriculum," the unstated norms, values, beliefs, and behaviors that are enculturated informally by words and actions.[6] Through this professional socialization, physicians in training gravitate toward clinical role models after whom they pattern themselves. Every medical student, resident, and fellow can name those doctors whom they admire and "who they want to be like," either consciously or unconsciously. Selecting a role model is extraordinarily consequential. It is no surprise that a disproportionate percentage of doctors come from families where one or both parents are physicians themselves.

Virtue ethics concentrates on building the character of physicians and reinforcing the characteristics that make them active, reliable fiduciaries for their patients. This approach is ancient, going back to Aristotle.[7]

As an exercise, take out a piece of paper and make a list of the characteristics you would want in a doctor taking care of *you*. We expect that, at a minimum, the list will include compassion, professional competence, mindfulness (the ability to be fully present "in the moment" with patients, not distracted or "mentally elsewhere"), trustworthiness, courage, justice (fairness), integrity (having a strong set of ethical values and being willing to defend them), and also what Aristotle referred to as *phronesis*, "practical wisdom" (the ability to integrate these characteristics into a unified, coherent whole—the ability to "get your clinical act together").

Virtue ethics is not incompatible with principlism. In fact, we would argue that those with a strong commitment to virtue ethics will be much more concerned with and adept at using a four-part system of analysis than those who dismiss the virtue ethics approach.

INFORMED CONSENT

Although widely recognized, many clinicians have an incomplete grasp of informed consent and the concept's importance.[8,9] The justification for obtaining informed consent before treatment is rooted in the principle of autonomy (often also called "respect for persons"). Commitment to informed consent implicitly acknowledges that patients have a right to participate in their own care, to have their views considered, and to give their consent to undergo treatment based on their understanding of the reasons and indications for that treatment. The necessity for obtaining informed consent

was pushed to the forefront of ethical discussions in medicine by the discovery/disclosure of significant past abuses of patients as illustrated by the Nuremberg war crimes trials after World War II,[10,11] the Willowbrook State School hepatitis studies,[12,13] the Tuskegee syphilis study,[13,14] and the New Zealand cervical cancer scandal.[15] In each case, patients were subjected to involuntary treatment (or had proper treatment withheld) without their appropriate knowledge or consent. These studies were often poorly conceived from a scientific viewpoint, were carried out without proper oversight, and were abusive of the human subjects involved in them. Such instances led to the formation of institutional review boards (IRBs) for monitoring research and to the implementation of increasingly stringent requirements for obtaining and documenting patient consent before treatment.[16]

Informed consent is best understood as a process rather than as an event. Many clinicians regard obtaining informed consent as simply getting the patient to sign a document—a "permission slip"—before undergoing surgery. Once the form is signed, they think they have secured informed consent. In reality, all they have is a signed form. Truly informed consent is a process in which the patient and the clinician exchange information in dialogue in order to make sure the patient has the information she needs to consent to treatment.[17]

The urogynecologist's role in this process is to act as a fiduciary, to safeguard the patient's best interests. There are two standards in common use (varying by state) that clarify what should be communicated to the patient. One standard is the "reasonable patient standard," which means that the information conveyed about treatment options should be what a "reasonable patient" would want to know under similar circumstances.[17] The "prudent physician standard" proposes that the information conveyed to the patient should be what a "prudent physician" would be expected to communicate under similar circumstances. In reality, both of these standards have limited value. What should be communicated is what each individual patient needs to know about her specific circumstances and the proposed treatment. The volume and detail of information in the informed consent process should be tailored to the individual patient. Enough information has been imparted when the patient agrees that all of her questions have been answered and all of her concerns have been addressed.[1,8,9,17-19]

Meeting this standard of informed consent may require considerable time. Ideally, it should take place in advance of surgery as part of a thorough preoperative visit. The *least* appropriate time for this process is the morning of surgery in the preoperative holding area where the patient is handed a form to sign prior to the operation taking place. Responsibility for obtaining informed consent should never be delegated to a nurse because the surgeon "doesn't have the time"; it is the responsibility of the attending surgeon to make sure this process is completed. To reduce informed consent to a matter of routine paperwork is to court disaster. When an operation goes awry, if a reasonable and thorough informed consent process cannot be documented, the fact that a signed "permission slip" is present in the medical record will provide no protection to the surgeon at the center of the case, particularly if the patient has a shrewd and insightful lawyer.

Informed consent is also critical in human subjects research in which conflicting interests may arise between the research subject (who may also be a patient) and the researcher (who may also be a clinician). In a research setting—such as in a clinical trial for a new pharmacologic preparation in which the researcher is being paid to enroll study participants—a potential conflict exists between the research subject's best interests and the researcher's potential financial gain. Researchers are often paid a set amount per subject enrolled by the drug company sponsoring the trial. A related ethical concern in human subjects research is that the compensation offered to research participants should not be so great as to cause unreasonable pressure to participate. This is of special concern in situations where the subjects of the study are from easily exploited or vulnerable populations. Populations considered "vulnerable" are those who cannot protect their own interests, such as disadvantaged ethnic groups, pediatric populations, persons with certain mental or physical disabilities that diminish their capacity, individuals with medical needs that are not being met adequately by the health care system that is tasked with serving them, and so on. Numerous instances of human subjects research abuse (such as the Nuremberg medical crimes referred to previously) led to the creation of IRBs to oversee human subjects research and to the virtually universal requirement for research protocols involving human subjects to be reviewed in advance and formally approved by an ethics oversight committee before they begin enrolling subjects.

It is important to differentiate between therapeutic and nontherapeutic research. In therapeutic research, the study subject herself potentially stands to gain from the research—such as by having the opportunity to take a new drug that is not otherwise available for a particular condition. In nontherapeutic research, the potential for therapeutic benefit of this kind does not arise. In this case, the study subject agrees to participate without the prospect of personal benefit, except perhaps for feeling good about participating in research or in return for a particular payment. An example of nontherapeutic research would be a study of a new drug in which volunteers are participating in an attempt to understand the pharmacodynamics of the medication: How much of a dose is metabolized? What effect does the drug have on blood-clotting or liver function tests? How rapidly and by what mechanism is it excreted? Answering these questions is scientifically important but conveys no therapeutic benefit to the study participant—and in early-stage drug studies of this kind, there may be substantial risks that are not yet known.

Informed consent is ethically necessary (and legally required) before human subjects can participate in either therapeutic or nontherapeutic research. The exact requirements for the information that must be disclosed to research participants is specified in some detail by the particular IRB tasked with overseeing the project. Although researchers are legally obligated to follow the requirements of the appropriate IRB protocol, the ethical considerations parallel those previously discussed regarding surgical operations. The researcher must take as much time as necessary to answer the participant's questions about the study, just as a surgeon must take the time to answer all of the patient's inquiries about the proposed operation.

CORPORATISM AND THE DILEMMA OF BEING A "HEALTH CARE PROVIDER"

Modern urogynecologic care is provided in technically complex health care settings. The structure of the health care system frames the delivery of ethical care, which is the focus of organizational ethics; that is, the principles and standards by which health care systems operate.[20] Health care systems as well as clinicians are accountable to/for the principles of beneficence, nonmaleficence, autonomy, and fairness. Unfortunately, there is frequently a conflict between the standards by which health care systems operate and the standards which clinicians must uphold, particularly where issues of operational and distributional fairness are concerned. This conflict increases exponentially when a health care system is run as a profit-making enterprise.

An irreconcilable conflict exists between the profession of medicine which demands that the best interests of patients must come before all other considerations and for-profit businesses whose fundamental imperative is making money. The strategic plan by which many health care systems in the United States now operate reflects the maxim of Chicago economist Milton Friedman, who famously declared that "the social responsibility of business is to increase its profits."[21] Many health care systems are run by business executives with little or no training in medicine and almost no familiarity with the basic principles of medical ethics. This kind of leadership views the health care system as a capitalist "output" factory that delivers health care products to consumers or "clients."[22] This paradigm does not see clinicians as professionals with an ethical obligation to care for the sick and suffering by putting patients' best interests first.[23] In such systems, the special imperative to look after sick and suffering patients is eclipsed by pure economic transactionalism. In the corporate output paradigm of modern capitalist health care, clinicians have become health care providers, mere spigots of clinical output, rather than professionals.[23] They are only independent contractors who can be replaced at will. The consequences of such a system have been predictably and frequently dire for patients with limited economic means, lack of access to robust insurance plans, or the political connectivity to leverage the system to protect their interests. Conflicts between the fiduciary duty of clinicians to their patients and the corporate interests of health care systems will only increase unless meaningful health care reform takes place.

COMMERCIAL CONFLICTS OF INTEREST IN UROGYNECOLOGY

Overtly commercial interests have steadily intruded into medicine over the last century.[24] The pharmaceutical industry did not exist as a significant economic force until World War II, when there was a major government-funded push to develop penicillin as part of the war effort. "Big Pharma" emerged from these efforts after the war and has become increasingly powerful over the last seven decades.[25] Big Pharma and its younger sibling, the medical device industry, now exert enormous influence on the practice of medicine and the development of health policy.[26,27] Pharmaceutical companies routinely spend more money on advertising, marketing, and sales than they do on drug development.[28] There are 2.7 pharmaceutical company lobbyists for each member of congress,[29] and 70,000 pharmaceutical sales representatives serve 870,900 physicians, with roughly 1 sales representative for every 12 practicing physicians in the United States.[26,30] Why?

The market for medications and devices is different from the market for automobiles, soap, or Bermuda shorts. In transactions for such products, the consumer interfaces directly with the purveyor of the goods involved. Prescription drugs and medical devices are different. These regulated products have a gatekeeper between the "consumer" (patient) and the seller. That gatekeeper is the physician, who must write a prescription for a particular drug or authorize the use of a particular medical device. The physician or surgeon has a fiduciary ethic that puts the best interests of the patient before everything else, the mandate to do good and to avoid harm. Pharmaceutical sales representatives or medical device company representatives operate with different expectations. Their bottom line is to maximize shareholder value, to obtain the maximum profit possible for their companies and for themselves, often on the basis of incentive or bonus plans. At the most fundamental level, these two goals are both incompatible and irreconcilable.

Company sales representatives are trained to conceal this inherent conflict of interest.[31-35] They are uniformly affable, willing (and often able) to please their marks—their physician targets. Company representatives present themselves as the clinician's friend, providing heavily skewed information to their targets while they track and report each interaction with physicians to their companies. Many physicians do not know that the details of their prescriptions are available commercially to pharmaceutical sales representatives who track the prescribing habits of individual physicians through commercially available pharmacy databases. They use this information to target high-volume prescribers with special attention—which was one of the major tools employed by companies pushing opioid medications for profit that helped create the opioid pandemic. Purdue Pharma was an innovator and serial abuser of these techniques.[25,35,36]

Pharmaceutical representatives use gifting, free meals, and other enticements to develop an unconscious sense of obligation among the physicians with whom they interact.[31-35] They particularly target high-volume prescribers who can make enormous amounts of money through company speakers' bureaus and other entanglements. The pharmaceutical industry spends over $20 billion per year on marketing to medical professionals in the United States—and another $9.6 billion dollars in the United States on direct-to-consumer advertising (which is prohibited in every country in the world except in the United States and New Zealand).[26]

Many physicians protest—naively, in our judgment—that they "can't be bought by a free ham sandwich or a cup of coffee"—but the data show otherwise.[26,31,33] Pharmaceutical companies are not ignorant. They would not spend enormous sums of money per physician on advertising, gifting, and the like if they lost money using these tactics.[26,31,33-35] The companies bear this expense because it works—and because it works extremely well.

Big Pharma has been relentless in its efforts to manipulate physicians' prescribing habits in order to maximize profits, with scant regard for patient safety. For example, Parke-Davis relentlessly pushed doctors to use the antibiotic chloramphenicol even after the drug was shown to produce fatal aplastic anemia in large numbers of patients.[37] The opioid crisis in the United States that has led to over 400,000 deaths to date was fueled largely by ethically untethered marketing by sales representatives who persistently misinformed physicians about the risks of opioid addiction.[25,36] They were incentivized to maximize sales through high-volume prescribers who were complicit with the drug companies (sometimes criminally) for personal gain. They exploited ineffectively regulated distribution networks that allowed wholesale pharmaceutical suppliers to flood small towns with millions of doses of highly addictive opioid products for profits.

The medical device industry has a similar record. Medical devices have not been regulated as tightly in the past as pharmaceutical products have been.[38,39] This disparity has allowed device manufacturers to introduce products to the market with inadequate testing and inadequate attention to patient safety. In the field of urogynecology, this negligence has led to the two-decades-long controversy surrounding the use of vaginal mesh implants in the treatment of urinary stress incontinence and especially in the treatment of pelvic organ prolapse.[40–43] The vast majority (but still not all) of these products have now been withdrawn from the market by the U.S. Food and Drug Administration due to the serious complications resulting from their use.[40–45]

A crucial and urgent ethical problem exists with regard to the way medical devices have been introduced into the marketplace: The current approval process compromises the surgeon's ability to obtain truly informed consent from the patients in whom such products are to be used. Because medical devices are not regulated as tightly as are pharmaceuticals, urogynecologists who consider using these devices often have no data regarding either the immediate or the long-term complications that may arise. These data should be collected in clinical trials of the kind that are required for the introduction of new drugs. However, these data are not required for medical devices such as transvaginal mesh products. Because device companies can omit such trials, there are often no data on the seriousness of potential complications, on whether these complications are avoidable, on whether complications are reversible, and on what their long-term consequences might be. This is information that a reasonable patient will want to know and that a prudent physician will want to provide, but at present, the use of most new medical devices is governed only by the old economic adage, *caveat emptor*: "Let the buyer beware." Current industry practices undermine the ethical use of their products.

Physicians and surgeons also take on considerable medicolegal risk when using these devices. In addition to there being no good data on safety, efficacy, long-term outcomes, and the seriousness of potential complications, when adverse outcomes do arise (as they inevitably will), the device manufacturers consistently try to dump the responsibility onto physicians and surgeons by using a legal concept known as the "learned intermediary doctrine."[46] Because surgeons act as gatekeepers to the access of restricted products such as prescription drugs or medical devices, the companies argue that it is the *surgeon's* duty as a "learned intermediary" between the product and the patient to inform patients of possible complications. The companies maintain this responsibility is the surgeon's problem, not theirs. *Caveat emptor*. Thus, despite not having access to data on the occurrence, nature, severity, and prognosis of complications (because the necessary studies are never carried out by the companies), urogynecologists are left hanging in the wind as the device manufacturers walk to the bank.

Similar problems have been identified in the realm of organizational ethics, where the best interests of patients may conflict with the personal financial interests of practicing physicians and the organizations that represent them. This conflict has also played out with respect to the marketing and use of vaginal mesh products in urogynecology. In the absence of good data on complications and long-term outcomes, patients who undergo implantation of medical devices are actually participating in a large-scale medical experiment without appropriate review or controls. Because "experimental" operations often are not reimbursed by insurance companies, classifying the use of new medical devices as experimental procedures triggers alarm bells within industry and within some clinical practices. Professional organizations may therefore be tempted to minimize the ethical issues at stake in order to protect their members' financial interests. Such actions should be anticipated and resisted. Professional organizations have a fiduciary duty to look after the best interests of patients when the best interests of patients conflict with the financial interests of their members. Ethically grounded urogynecologists always stand in solidarity protecting the best interests of their patients.[47–50] Patients must not be forced to become mere consumers in a world of unfettered economic transactionalism. They are individuals whose interests should be protected by the physician's special fiduciary obligations. To be reduced to consumer status (which is the way they are viewed by pharmaceutical and medical device companies) only accelerates the loss of physicians' standing as professionals, reducing them to being little more than "providers" in a commercialized, profit-driven, industrialized health care machine.[23,51,52] Such changes also crack open the door to allowing the commercial exploitation of patients. Urogynecologists must continually be aware of these conflicts and the forces that promote them. These concerns involve not only individual physicians in practice but also the professional organizations that represent them.

INTERNATIONAL HUMANITARIAN MISSIONS

Interest in global medicine has been expanding for several years. The COVID-19 pandemic that struck the world in 2020 is demonstrating how interconnected the world has become. We ignore the health problems of less affluent parts of the world at our own peril. Medicine nurtures compassionate endeavors to help the sick, the injured, and those who suffer from preventable, treatable illnesses and maladies. This admirable desire to help comes with ethical obligations that must not be overlooked in the enthusiasm to put a service project together. This caution is particularly relevant for efforts to provide surgical services in less affluent parts of the world. Urogynecologists must be keenly attuned to the pitfalls inseparable from their participation in such initiatives.

Many years ago, Dr. Reginald Hamlin (who along with his wife, Dr. Catherine Hamlin, founded the Addis Ababa Fistula Hospital in Ethiopia) coined the term "fistula tourism" to characterize the phenomenon of well-intentioned surgeons coming to Africa to "try their hands" at fistula surgery, to do a "great case," and then to return home armed with the "trophy" of the stories of their adventures of encountering these exotic (to European or American eyes) injuries.[53] Dr. Hamlin saw this phenomenon as a particular problem in fistula surgery, where the pathologies were far more complex than anything many of these visitors had ever encountered in Europe or North America. Surgical visitors "hunting a fistula" in Africa sometimes led to bad outcomes of which the visitors never knew and for which they were never held responsible because they had already returned home without making adequate provision for the continuing care of the women on whom they had operated.

We have no problem with volunteer surgical missions when they are competently structured and properly overseen, provide continuing care for patients after the surgical team has returned home, and recruit surgeons extensively experienced with the conditions on which they are operating and who are using well-established surgical techniques. However, impoverished women in Africa and Asia should not be subjected to experimental procedures simply because they live in poverty, lack political and social power, and do not have regular access to standard medical or surgical services.[54,55] They are, by definition, "vulnerable populations."

Better than irregular, intermittent surgical visits by individual volunteers are the creation of long-lasting partnerships between in-country institutions such as established hospitals and accredited medical schools with partner institutions from overseas. The creation of ongoing institutional links and interchanges is far more likely to result in robust capacity building at the local level by promoting the elevation of surgical standards and clinical practices and also allowing for the development of training programs to improve the quality of in-country care. A recent example of the creation of a urogynecology fellowship training program in Ethiopia serves as a case in point.[56] In all such endeavors, careful attention to the organizational ethics of the institutions involved is of paramount importance.

CONCLUSION

How then does the ethical dimension of patient care matter to a busy surgeon? Ethics examines how well we respect those we encounter. To respect a person means to see that person again or afresh, to look back at that person expecting to "see more clearly." The same Latin root

verb (L., *re* + *specere*) has given us such related words as *speculate*, *inspect*, *spectacles*, and *speculum*. To respect someone is to be artistic, subjective, freeing, reciprocal, gentle, engaged, holistic, attentive, patient, modest, trusting, graceful, reconciling, and humanizing. But surgeons must also be scientific, objective, and detached. Therein exists the ethical complexity of the patient encounter. A surgeon's clinical mindset can deteriorate into being rough, indifferent, curt, suspicious, selfish, alienating, dehumanizing—in short, into being disrespectful.

To be reduced by a surgeon to "the fistula in Room 1" or "the uterine prolapse in Room 2" or "the acute abdomen in Room 3" is not necessarily damaging. Excellent surgical care is evidence based. The surgeon objectifies the patient with statistical associations and by concentrating on damaged or diseased body parts. Differential diagnoses reflect plausible explanations of cause and effect. The surgeon necessarily focuses on the patient's immediate problem more than on the patient's larger story. The surgeon must be sufficiently detached to achieve what Sir William Osler referred to as *aequanimitas* or balance.[57]

At some point, however, patient encounters that may be clinically competent may cease to be respectful. Only by being sufficiently disciplined to remember that patients are individuals worthy of respect, compassion, and fairness can a surgeon avoid succumbing to the indifference that turns patient encounters into interactions with mere "work objects"—encounters that may leave patients manipulated, exploited, and dehumanized.

For patient encounters to be truly respectful, another professional language is required—the language of respect, compassion, and fairness.[55] This language is clearly distinguishable from clinical/scientific language, from the language of risk management and the law, and from the language of billing offices and economics. Fluency in the professional language of respect, compassion, and fairness is *not* required to complete medical school, to pass postgraduate boards, to be rewarded economically, to secure hospital privileges, to pass recertification examinations, to be promoted, to be elected to national positions of leadership, or even to be on a hospital ethics committee. Fluency in the professional language of respect, compassion, and fairness is, however, essential for being a humane surgeon who cares deeply about patients—especially the most difficult patients—and who brings a resolute social conscience to the practice of surgery. This is the heart of medical ethics.

References

1. Beauchamp TL, Childress JF. *Principles of biomedical ethics*, 8th ed. New York: Oxford University Press, 2019.
2. Jonsen A, Siegler M, Winslade WJ. *Clinical ethics: A practical approach to ethical decision in clinical medicine*, 8th ed. New York: McGraw-Hill, 2015.

3. Pellegrino ED, Thomasma DC. *The virtues in medical practice*. New York: Oxford University Press, 1993.

4. Pellegrino ED, Thomasma DC. *The Christian virtues in medical practice*. Washington, DC: Georgetown University Press, 1996.

5. Hall MA. Law, medicine, and trust. *Stanford Law Rev* 2002;55(2):463–527.

6. Snyder BR. *The hidden curriculum*. New York: Alfred A. Knopf, 1971.

7. Aristotle. *Nichomachean ethics*. New York: Cambridge University Press, 2000.

8. Faden RR, Beauchamp TL. *A history and theory of informed consent*. New York: Oxford University Press, 1986.

9. Berg JW, Appelbaum PS, Lidz CW, et al. *Informed consent: Legal theory and clinical practice, 2nd ed*. New York: Oxford University Press, 2001.

10. Lifton RJ. *The Nazi doctors: Medical killing and the psychology of genocide*. New York: Macmillan, 1986.

11. Annas GJ, Grodin MA, eds. *The Nazi doctors and the Nuremberg codes: Human rights in human experimentation*. New York: Oxford University Press, 1992.

12. Krugman S. The Willowbrook hepatitis studies revisited: Ethical aspects. *Rev Infect Dis* 1986;8(1):157–162.

13. Rothman DJ. Were Tuskegee and Willowbrook 'studies in nature'? *Hastings Cent Rep* 1982;12(2):5–7.

14. Benedek TG, Erlen J. The scientific environment of the Tuskegee study of syphilis, 1920-1960. *Perspect Biol Med* 1999;43(1):1–30.

15. Committee of Inquiry into Allegations Concerning the Treatment of Cervical Cancer at National Women's Hospital and into Other Related Matters. *The report of the cervical cancer inquiry 1988*. New Zealand: Government Printing Office, 1988.

16. National Commission for the Protection of Human Subjects of Biomedical and Behavioral Research. *The Belmont report: Ethical principles and guidelines for the protection of human subjects in research*. Washington, DC: Department of Health, Education, and Welfare, 1979.

17. Peeters PG Jr. The reasonable physician standard: The new malpractice standard of care? *J Health Law* 2001;34(1):105–119.

18. Murray B. Informed consent: What must a physician disclose to a patient? *Virtual Mentor* 2012;14(7):563–566.

19. Spatz ES, Krumholz HM, Moulton BW. The new era of informed consent: Getting to a reasonable-patient standard through shared decision making. *JAMA* 2016;315(19):2063–2064.

20. Spencer EM, Mills AE, Rorty MV, et al. *Organization ethics in health care*. New York: Oxford University Press, 2000.

21. Friedman M. A Friedman doctrine—The social responsibility of business is to increase its profits. *The New York Times*. September 13, 1970:32–33, 122–124.

22. Weber LJ. *Profits before people? Ethical standards and the marketing of prescription drugs*. Indiana: Indiana University Press, 2006.

23. Wall LL. The nature of suffering, health care "providers," and the opioid crisis. *Obstet Gynecol* 2020;135(4):836–839.

24. Kassirer JP. *On the take: How medicine's complicity with big business can endanger your health*. New York: Oxford University Press, 2005.

25. Posner G. *Pharma: Greed, lies and the poisoning of America*. New York: Avid Reader Press, 2020.

26. Schwartz LM, Woloshin S. Medical marketing in the United States, 1997-2016. *JAMA* 2019;321(1):80–96.

27. Wouters OJ. Lobbying expenditures and campaign contributions by the pharmaceutical and health product industry in the United States, 1999-2018. *JAMA Intern Med* 2020;180(5):688–697.

28. Swanson A. Big pharmaceutical companies are spending far more on marketing than research. *The Washington Post*. February 11, 2015.

29. Politifact. Accessed February 17, 2021. https://www.politifact.com/factchecks/2019/jul/26/amy-klobuchar/21lobuchar-says-there-are-enough-drug-lobbyists-dc-/2

30. Michas F. U.S. physicians—Statistics & facts. Statista. Accessed February 17, 2021. https://www.statista.com/topics/1244/physicians/#dossierKeyfigures

31. Wall LL, Brown D. The high cost of free lunch. *Obstet Gynecol* 2007;110(1):169–173.

32. Wall LL, Brown D. Pharmaceutical sales representatives and the doctor/patient relationship. *Obstet Gynecol* 2002;100(3):594–599.

33. Oldani MJ. Thick prescriptions: Toward an interpretation of pharmaceutical sales practices. *Med Anthropol Q* 2004;18(3):325–356.

34. Sufrin CB, Ross JS. Pharmaceutical industry marketing: Understanding its impact on women's health. *Obstet Gynecol Surv* 2008;63(9):585–596.

35. Fugh-Berman A, Ahari S. Following the script: How drug reps make friends and influence doctors. *PloS Med* 2007;4(4):e150.

36. Meier B. *Pain killer: An empire of deceit and the origin of America's opioid epidemic*. New York: Random House, 2018.

37. Maeder T. *Adverse reactions*. New York: William Morrow, 1994.

38. Nygaard I. What does "FDA approved" mean for medical devices? *Obstet Gynecol* 2008;111(1):4–6.

39. Heneghan CJ, Goldacre B, Onakpoya I, et al. Trials of transvaginal mesh devices for pelvic organ prolapse: A systematic database review of the US FDA approval process. *BMJ Open* 2017;7(12):e017125.

40. Javadian P, Shobeiri SA. The disability impact and associated cost per disability in women who underwent surgical revision of transvaginal mesh kits for prolapse repair. *Female Pelvic Med Reconstr Surg* 2018;24(5):375–379.

41. Dunn GE, Hansen BL, Egger MJ, et al. Changed women: The long-term impact of vaginal mesh complications. *Female Pelvic Med Reconstr Surg* 2014;20(3):131–136.

42. Hansen BL, Dunn GE, Norton P, et al. Long-term follow-up of treatment for synthetic mesh complications. *Female Pelvic Med Reconstr Surg* 2014;20(3):126–130.

43. Unger CA, Abbott S, Evans JM, et al. Outcomes following treatment for pelvic floor mesh complications. *Int Urogynecol J* 2014;25(6):745–749.

44. U.S. Food and Drug Administration. FDA takes action to protect women's health, orders manufacturers of surgical mesh intended for transvaginal repair of pelvic organ prolapse to stop selling all devices. U.S. Food and Drug Administration. Published April 16, 2019. Accessed February 17, 2021. https://www.fda.gov/news-events/press-announcements/fda-takes-action-protect-womens-health-orders-manufacturers-surgical-mesh-intended-transvaginal

45. *Scottish independent review of the use, safety and efficacy of transvaginal mesh implants in the treatment of stress urinary incontinence and pelvic organ prolapse in women. Final report March 2017*. Scotland: The Scottish Government, 2017.

46. Kuhlmann-Capek MJ, Kilic GS, Shaw AB, et al. Enmeshed in controversy: Use of vaginal mesh in the current medicolegal environment. *Female Pelvic Med Reconstr Surg* 2015;21(5):241–243.

47. Wall LL, Brown D. Commercial pressures and professional ethics: Troubling revisions to the recent ACOG Practice Bulletins on surgery for pelvic organ prolapse. *Int Urogynecol J* 2009;20(7):765–767.

48. Wall LL, Brown D. The perils of commercially driven surgical innovation. *Am J Obstet Gynecol* 2010;202:30.e1–30.e4.

49. Lawrence HC III. Comments on Wall and Brown: "Commercial pressure and professional ethics: troubling revisions to the recent ACOG Practice Bulletins on surgery for pelvic organ prolapse." *Int Urogynecol J Pelvic Floor Dysfunct* 2009;20(12): 1519–1520.

50. Weber AM. Response to Wall and Brown: "Commercial pressures and professional ethics: Troubling revisions to the recent ACOG Practice Bulletins on surgery for pelvic organ prolapse." *Int Urogynecol J Pelvic Floor Dysfunct* 2009;20(12):1523.

51. Muffly TM, Giamberardino WL, Guido J, et al. Industry payments to obstetricians and gynecologists under the Sunshine Act. *Obstet Gynecol* 2018;132(1):9–17.

52. Wall LL. Obstetrician-gynecologists and industry: Let the sunshine in! *Obstet Gynecol* 2018;132(1):7–8.

53. Wall LL, Arrowsmith SD, Lassey AT, et al. Humanitarian ventures or 'fistula tourism'? The ethical perils of pelvic surgery in the developing world. *Int Urogynecol J Pelvic Floor Dysfunct* 2006;17(6):559–562.

54. Wall LL. Ethical concerns regarding surgical operations on vulnerable patient populations: The case of obstetric fistula. *HEC Forum* 2011;23(2):115–127.

55. Wall LL. *Tears for my sisters: The tragedy of obstetric fistula.* Maryland: Johns Hopkins University Press, 2018.

56. Nardos R, Ayenachew F, Roentgen R, et al. Capacity building in female pelvic medicine and reconstructive surgery: Global health partnership beyond fistula care in Ethiopia. *Int Urogynecol J* 2020;31:227–235.

57. Osler W. *Aequanimitas: With other addresses to medical students, nurses, and practitioners of medicine*, 2nd ed. Pennsylvania: Blakiston, 1928.

2

Evaluation and Treatment of Combined Pelvic Floor Disorders

CHAPTER 9

CLINICAL EVALUATION OF INCONTINENCE AND PROLAPSE

Lioudmila Lipetskaia • Cara Grimes • Shefali Sharma

Introduction

This chapter aims to provide a systematic and practical approach to the evaluation of pelvic organ prolapse (POP) and urinary incontinence (UI). There is significant overlap in these conditions with at least 34% women older than 40 years reporting one pelvic floor disorder and as many as 7% suffering from both POP and UI.[1] In the majority of cases, a diagnosis can be established through a carefully collected history and detailed physical examination; rarely invasive testing is required to confirm a diagnosis or guide management. In addition, assessing patient's goals prior to conducting an examination can save time and improve care. First-line treatments can be offered and started without establishing a definitive diagnosis.[2,3] In practice, the more complex the patient's history and the longer the list of bothersome symptoms, the higher likelihood that additional testing beyond a routine clinical evaluation will be needed.

A comprehensive approach to the evaluation of prolapse and UI is presented here in the following order: chief complaint, history of present illness, treatment goal assessment, detailed physical examination, and ancillary evaluation tools. Due to the significant overlap between prolapse and incontinence, the clinical evaluation is conducted as a single workflow rather than separate evaluation pathways for both conditions. This workflow should be tailored to the chief complaint and some steps described in the following text can be omitted if a diagnosis is established with the information already gathered.

CHIEF COMPLAINT

Urinary Incontinence

Patients with UI typically present with the very specific complaint of involuntary urinary loss. Occasionally, complaints of clear vaginal discharge or wetness are also reported.

Prolapse

Prolapse complaints tend to be more nuanced. The most specific chief complaint is feeling (or seeing) a bulge protruding past the vaginal opening. This complaint is associated with a confirmed diagnosis of prolapse 85% of the time.[4] Additional prolapse related complaints include a feeling of pressure in the pelvis, difficulty evacuating bladder or bowels, sensation of something falling out of the vagina, personal sexual complaints of "my vagina feels loose during sex," or partner-related complaints "my partner feels that he is hitting something during penetration." Those less specific complaints are not as predictive of prolapse and should be scrutinized more during careful history collection.

HISTORY OF PRESENT ILLNESS

Urinary Incontinence

In the assessment of UI, we find the following approach most practical: First, obtain a detailed description of the leakage episodes. Second, gather pertinent information on comorbidities, functional status, social situations, and environmental factors which can affect the management options and decisions.

Obtain a detailed description of leakage episodes

Eliciting a vignette of the patient's leakage episodes helps to clarify the timing, quality, frequency, quantity, and other factors of the incontinence. For example, leakage associated with exertion such as coughing, laughing, and sneezing (in the absence of urgency, frequency, or other pelvic symptoms) is highly predictive of stress UI (SUI); a diagnosis can easily be made with history and a physical examination alone.

It is more difficult to describe the gestalt of patients with urgency incontinence. The majority of patients describe a significant amount of urgency ("I've got to go and cannot make it on time to bathroom") prior to the leakage episode. A common misconception is that leaks due to urgency incontinence need to be preceded by urgency or some other irritative voiding complaints. In fact, it is possible for patients to have "leakage out of the blue while sitting on the couch and reading a book" without feeling any preceding urge; the absence of sensory urgency prior to leakage does not rule out urgency incontinence.

This picture can be frequently complicated by complaints of incomplete bladder emptying. A common chief complaint may be "It seems that I cannot empty my bladder and I leak all the time." This statement can falsely lead a physician toward the diagnosis of overflow incontinence, when in reality, their symptoms may be secondary to sensory urgency. Further questioning typically will uncover a scenario such as "I just finished urinating 15 minutes ago. Right after I left the bathroom, I suddenly felt the need to urinate again. When I'm on my way to the bathroom, I leak. I don't think I empty my bladder!"

Another important aspect in the description of urgency incontinence episodes is an assessment of triggers that provoke either urgency or leakage. Some of the most common triggers are hearing the sound of running water, doing dishes, inserting house keys into the lock, or pulling into the driveway at home. Identifying the triggers not only aids in diagnosis but also helps with the management of the condition.

The other types of incontinence (overflow incontinence and anatomic disruption of urinary tract) are encountered less frequently but should be considered. A complaint of continuous urinary leakage is highly suggestive of a fistula or abnormal ureteral implantation. If a patient states "I just leak all the time and feel like I am constantly wet," attention should be dedicated to the onset of the symptoms. Fistulas are very rarely spontaneous and in the vast majority of cases have an identifiable preceding event: typically surgery or radiation to the pelvic area in developed countries or complicated childbirth in underdeveloped countries. Abnormal ureteral implantation in the vagina is present at birth and is typically diagnosed in a patient's youth.

Overflow incontinence can frequently mimic stress incontinence as the majority of the most noticeable leaks will be similarly associated with external bladder compression (e.g., cough or sneeze). The key distinguishing characteristic is that patients typically report many more episodes of insensible urine loss and often suffer from conditions which make retention a more likely diagnosis. These conditions include advanced age, diabetes, and various neurologic conditions. The easiest way to distinguish overflow incontinence from SUI is to routinely incorporate a postvoid residual (PVR) check into clinical exams, as those with overflow typically present with elevated PVRs. PVRs more than 100 to 150 mL are concerning and should trigger further investigation.

The presence of nocturnal enuresis (leakage during nighttime while asleep) defines a specifically challenging subset of patients with urgency incontinence. The presence of sleep apnea is frequently associated with nocturia and subsequent nighttime leakage. An inquiry should be made into potential snoring or partner-observed short-term breathing cessation at night to see if sleep apnea testing is indicated.

The history of a patient's prior treatments and interventions for incontinence should be gathered at this stage and their efficacy noted. Prior surgical interventions for incontinence can prompt a subsequent, more complex evaluation with the possible need for invasive studies. Prior nonsurgical treatments should be assessed for quality: For example, pelvic floor therapy with a trained professional can yield very different results for incontinence control as compared to self-guided Kegel exercises.

The type of history gathering described earlier uses a "story-telling approach" wherein the majority of symptoms are provided by the patient. The specific details are elicited by the clinician with open-ended questions such as "What makes your symptoms worse?" or "Tell me more about your leakage episodes?" This approach allows for collection of a clinical vignette which serves as a "working theory" or theoretical framework for establishing the final diagnosis. Many physicians prefer to ask a standardized set of questions, in combination with the use of validated questionnaires. Table 9.1 lists some frequently used questions.

Assess incontinence comorbidities, functional status, social situations, and environmental factors

Comorbidities and modifiable factors can affect incontinence and choice of treatment. It is important to assess for medical conditions such as constipation, diabetes, hypertension, recurrent urinary tract infections (UTIs), and overall functional status.

Defecatory dysfunction can significantly worsen urgency incontinence. Persistent presence of hard stool in the rectum due to constipation or obstructed defecation can increase pressure exerted by the rectum onto the bladder, thereby decreasing functional bladder capacity. Poorly controlled diabetes worsens incontinence especially if it is accompanied by polyuria. Diabetes not only is predictive of less optimal treatment outcomes but also raises the probability of overflow incontinence given its association with neuropathy and retention. Diuretic treatments can worsen UI by leading to shifts in urine production throughout the day. UTIs can worsen or cause urinary leakage, especially in elderly

TABLE 9.1

Frequently Used Questions during Urinary Incontinence History Taking

QUESTION	TYPE OF INCONTINENCE
If you sneeze really hard, would you leak urine?	Stress
Do you leak urine when you exercise?	Stress
If you leak urine while running or jumping—do you leak the moment you bounce of the ground?	Stress
Does sound of running water make you leak?	Urgency
Do you feel an urge before you start leaking urine?	Urgency
Does urge to urinate wake you up at night?	Urgency
If you leak after changing position (e.g., from sitting to standing), do you feel urge before the urine leaks down your legs?	Urgency
Do you feel like you are constantly wet?	Fistula or insensible urine loss associated with urgency incontinence

patients whose initial presentation may be worsening incontinence rather than dysuria.

Assessment of patients' functional status is of great importance. Specifically, inquiring about their level of mobility, use of assisting walking devices, and dexterity helps in identifying functional incontinence. Access to bathrooms can be hindered for patients whose mobility status precludes them from moving quickly. Patients with altered dexterity might leak because they are unable to open bathroom doors easily or have trouble removing their undergarments. Functional status and ability to perform activities of daily living can be assessed formally or informally. Informal assessments include collecting data via simple conversation with questions such as "Did you have any trouble getting to our office? Do you like cooking? What did you cook for dinner last night?" Simple observations on how the patient moves in the room, gets up from the chair, climbs on the exam table, and/or moves into lithotomy position are revealing of patient functional status. Formal assessment can be performed by administering the Functional Status Questionnaire,[5] which takes about 15 minutes to complete and can be used for initial evaluation as well as monitoring of the patient's progress.

Cognitive impairment plays a major role in prognosis and management options. In some situations, cognitive impairment will be evident through basic patient interactions. Using a Mini-Mental State Examination is a quick and more formal way to assess mental status. Interviewing patients' caregivers and family members is a useful way to assess the level of mental decline, and it also provides insight into the level of social support your patient has.

Fluid intake measured as the amount and type of fluid consumed is important when considering the effectiveness of behavioral modifications for incontinence control. So-called "bladder irritants" such as alcohol, soda, artificial sweetener, carbonated, and caffeinated beverages can be modifiable factors in UI treatment. Fluid overconsumption (increases in fluid intake more than 80 to 90 oz/d) can significantly worsen urgency incontinence.

With a careful and detailed history collection, a differential diagnosis for UI can be established even prior to physical examination. The first aim should be to assess so called "transient (or modifiable) causes of UI" frequently described by mnemonic "DIAPPERS" described in Table 9.2.[8] When incontinence is established as a chronic nontransient condition, the physical examination will further assess the pelvic floor to guide the treatment plan.

Prolapse

We recommend gathering a history for prolapse in a similar fashion: Start with disease-specific symptoms and assess for comorbidities and social and environmental components. The key challenge in this aspect of history taking is not only to assess for all symptoms pertinent to prolapse but to also evaluate the symptoms in respect to their "cause-and-effect" relationship with prolapse. In contrast to the evaluation of incontinence, pelvic examination almost always provides the most definitive diagnosis of prolapse. It is important to realize that not all patient-reported symptoms will be related to prolapse, reiterating the importance of a thorough physical exam. The ultimate goal of history taking should be to assess whether the patient's most bothersome symptoms will be alleviated by prolapse treatment.

TABLE 9.2	
DIAPPERS: Transient/Modifiable Causes of Urinary Incontinence	
CAUSE	**DESCRIPTION**
Delirium	Incontinence as a symptom of delirium will abate when the cause of the patient's confusion is identified and treated.
Infection	Symptoms of UTI in elderly patients differ from those in younger patients as dysuria is often absent, and incontinence may be the patient's only symptom.
Atrophic vaginitis	Urogenital atrophy does not cause incontinence per se but exacerbates urgency and frequency and contributes to worsening of urgency incontinence.
Pharmacologic	Commonly prescribed medications may exacerbate incontinence as long as their mechanism of action alters the autonomic nervous system or urine production.[6] *α-Adrenergic agonists*: can precipitate urinary retention *α-Adrenergic antagonists*: can precipitate SUI and are linked to a threefold increase in the odds of having UI[7] *Angiotensin-converting* enzyme inhibitors: can cause a cough that can exacerbate SUI *Anticholinergics*: can cause impaired emptying, urinary retention, and constipation as well as cognitive impairment *Cholinesterase inhibitors*: increase in bladder contractility; can precipitate urgency UI *Diuretics*: cause increased diuresis and precipitate UI *Lithium*: polyuria via induced diabetes insipidus *Opioid analgesics*: urinary retention, constipation, confusion, and immobility *Psychotropic drugs, sedatives, hypnotics, antipsychotics, and histamine 1 receptor antagonists*: confusion and impaired mobility *Selective serotonin reuptake inhibitors*: increased cholinergic transmission can lead to urgency UI *Calcium channel blockers, gabapentin, glitazones and NSAIDs*: edema, which can lead to nocturnal polyuria causing nocturia and nocturnal enuresis
Psychological	Incontinence may occasionally be used to gain attention or to manipulate others. Patients may be so profoundly depressed that they do not care about continence.
Endocrine	Diabetes mellitus, diabetes insipidus, and hypercalcemia may induce an osmotic diuresis that exacerbates other causes of incontinence.
Restricted mobility	Inability to reach the bathroom on time due to gait instability, frailty, pain or deformity of the extremities is often referred to as functional incontinence. If mobility cannot be improved, a nearby commode may improve the incontinence.
Stool impaction	As the sigmoid and rectum enlarge, they act as a pelvic mass, compressing the bladder and exacerbating other forms of incontinence.

Obtain detailed description of the bulge

As stated earlier, feeling the sensation of a bulge and seeing a bulge protruding past the vaginal opening are the most predictive symptoms of prolapse. The more detailed description of a bulge that a patient is able to provide increases the likelihood that the diagnosis of prolapse will be confirmed. Specific references to bulge size (egg size, walnut size), complaints that the bulge worsens with prolonged standing, and descriptions of a bulge rubbing against clothing indicate that prolapse is likely to be discovered during examination.

Vague complaints include the sensation of pelvic pressure and pain and difficulty with voiding and defecation.[9,10] Pelvic pressure can result from pelvic floor muscle spasm which may or may not be related to prolapse. In cases where pelvic pressure and pain are the primary bothersome symptoms, it is worth assessing for alleviating factors. Pelvic pressure and pain worsening with standing and at the end of the day are more likely to

be associated with prolapse. When pressure is not time (or position) dependent, and if the pressure is quickly relieved by heat and nonsteroidal anti-inflammatory drugs (NSAIDs), the relationship becomes less obvious. Distinguishing muscle spasm as a primary compensatory response to worsening of prolapse versus muscle spasm caused by other conditions such as a prior episiotomy, high-impact exercise, surgery, endometriosis, or vulvodynia can be nebulous. Taking a thorough history is typically not enough in these more complicated situations, and these patients often require trials of different therapeutic approaches to establish the definitive relationship.

Voiding and defecatory dysfunction are other challenging presentations of prolapse.[11,12] Occasionally, the relationship to prolapse is obvious, such as in the case of feeling incomplete bladder emptying relieved by splinting. When patients report that their vaginal bulge needs to be reduced manually and replaced inside their body to help them urinate, it is likely that their voiding

TABLE 9.3

Differential Diagnosis of Prolapse-Associated Symptoms

SYMPTOM GROUP	SYMPTOM	OTHER ASPECTS OF DIFFERENTIAL DIAGNOSIS
Herniation symptoms	Pelvic pressure	Rectal prolapse
	Vaginal protrusion	
Voiding symptoms	Urinary hesitancy	Detrusor dysfunction
	Incomplete emptying	Detrusor sphincter dyssynergia
	Splinting to complete urination	Behavioral voiding disorders
Lower urinary tract symptoms	Urinary frequency	Overactive bladder
	Urinary urgency	Excessive fluid intake
	Dysuria	Interstitial cystitis
		Urinary tract infection
Urinary incontinence	Urinary incontinence	Stress incontinence
		Detrusor overactivity
Defecatory dysfunction	Dyschezia	Irritable bowel syndrome
	Incomplete defecation	Colonic inertia
	Splinting to complete defecation	Anismus
Fecal incontinence	Fecal urgency	Irritable bowel syndrome
	Fecal incontinence	Diarrhea
		External anal sphincter dysfunction
Sexual dysfunction	Dyspareunia	Levator ani syndrome
	Decreased sensation	Libido dysfunction

Reprinted from Cundiff GW. An 80-year-old woman with vaginal prolapse. *JAMA* 2005;293(16):2018–2027, with permission.

dysfunction is related to prolapse. Patients who report an ability to urinate freely in the morning followed by a complete blockage of their urinary stream in the evening when their prolapse worsens can help establish this "cause-and-effect relationship." Some voiding dysfunction symptoms, such as increased urgency and frequency, are less predictive of prolapse: Urinary frequency can be triggered by chronic displacement of the bladder out of its normal anatomic position or can be a sign of overactive bladder. Frequently, performing a trial of pessary placement can provide insight: Reduction of a patient's prolapse with a pessary that leads to subsequent improvement of frequency can help establish prolapse as a cause of irritative voiding symptoms.

Splinting with defecation is even less predictive of prolapse as a diagnosis. A thorough assessment of stool consistency using a tool such as the Bristol stool scale is needed if obstructive defecation symptoms such as splinting, straining, or manual evacuation is noted by the patient. When other symptoms consistent with constipation are present (e.g., lumpy and rare stools, straining with defecation), it is less likely that prolapse alone is responsible for splinting (Table 9.3). One helpful question that assists in determining whether splinting is due to prolapse or constipation is "Do you feel that your stool is stuck and gets out only when you press on the bulge?" Typically, a definitive relationship between defecatory dysfunction and a vaginal bulge can only be established after prolapse correction, a point that is important to explain when counseling your patients.

Assess prolapse comorbidities, functional status, social situations, and environmental factors

Gathering information on comorbidities and social and environmental factors should be based on potential therapeutic options. Surgical interventions for prolapse are typically more extensive compared to procedures to treat incontinence especially if apical correction of prolapse is required. Hence, comorbidities such as cardiac and pulmonary diseases and determination of physical status should be used to guide management: For high-risk patients, surgery is a less optimal management choice. Social support and cognitive status play a significant role in guidance of nonsurgical treatments. Patients with cognitive impairment and a lack of social support are at increased risk for inconsistent follow-up; hence, pessary trials and physical therapy might not be feasible.

History taking can be extensive and time-consuming but when done well constitutes a significant portion of the evaluation. Incorporating carefully considered validated questionnaires that patients complete prior to their appointments can be helpful and time-saving. There are a plethora of questionnaires designed to assess pelvic floor function, but we favor the Pelvic Floor Distress Inventory Questionnaire-20 as it covers urinary, prolapse, and defecatory domains using only 20 questions. For complete descriptions of questionnaire options, please refer to Chapter 11.

TREATMENT GOAL ASSESSMENT

We recommend assessing treatment goals prior to proceeding with pelvic examination. Very frequently, pelvic examinations can be tailored to the specific goals of the patient, thereby leading to a more efficient exam.

At this point, it is useful to assess your patient's understanding of the condition. We have found that this varies greatly and can provide useful insight for the provider. Some patients present with predetermined ideas regarding the cause and treatment options for their leakage or bulge. Some patients simply want reassurance that their bulge is not cancer or dangerous. This insight allows providers to focus their evaluation on pertinent factors, such as omitting the uncomfortable cotton swab hypermobility test or foregoing rectal examination.

This is also a good time to assess whether a patient desires future penetrative intercourse. Patients who are not currently sexually active, but desire the option for intercourse in their future, will not be candidates for obliterative procedures. This information is critical in surgical planning.

We include the patient's overall health goals assessment into this section of the evaluation. Weight management plans are important as obesity worsens pelvic floor dysfunction and as little as 10% loss in body weight can lead to improvement in incontinence and prolapse symptoms.[13] If an obese patient presents with incontinence but plans to undergo bariatric surgery in the near future, then the management of incontinence should be tied into her planned weight loss and surgical options should be delayed until after her weight loss surgery. No intervention may be needed as patients can have complete resolution of incontinence after weight loss.

Another important component of assessment is overall lifestyle. Patients who have physically demanding jobs which require heavy lifting or plan on being very physically active (traveling with a heavy backpack through the countryside) may require a different treatment approach. The likelihood of prolapse recurrence with chronic straining may be higher, and symptoms of minor incontinence can be more bothersome for more active patients compared to patients who live a more sedentary life.

Patient goals and expectations in regard to prolapse and incontinence treatments vary drastically and can affect treatment satisfaction. Assessing goals early in the evaluation process and linking them to the patients personal sexual, emotional, and health context helps in formulating a patient-centered care plan.[14,15]

PHYSICAL EXAMINATION

A thorough pelvic examination is crucial in the evaluation of UI and prolapse. Advancing therapies beyond the first line (behavioral modifications and physical therapy) without completing an in-depth pelvic exam is inadvisable. Performing a pelvic examination in both the standing/straining position and the lithotomy position with straining typically yields the most information. The pelvic exam should include a focused neurologic examination, an assessment of pelvic floor muscle function, and a bimanual and speculum examination as well as cough stress test. If pertinent symptoms are not elicited in lithotomy position, a patient can be evaluated in the standing position and during maximum straining. The assessment of PVR volume should be included in the pelvic examination.

It is best practice to start the pelvic exam with an evaluation of the neurologic integrity of sacral dermatomes, pelvic nerves, and muscle strength. Pain mapping should be performed prior to performing an internal exam for patients with pain to yield maximum precision in pain distribution and quality. The sensation component typically involves an assessment of light touch and pinprick sensation testing with a cotton swab. The softer end of the cotton swab is used to examine the sensation of touch and to elicit the bulbocavernosus reflex; the sharper end of the swab is used to assess pinprick sensation in all important sensory dermatomes (Table 9.4).

The same soft-ended cotton swab can be used for pain mapping. By sequentially touching the labia majora, labia minora, periurethral area, and posterior fourchette, a precise distribution of pain symptoms can be assessed along with the quality of the pain (sharp, burning, stabbing, etc). For detailed technique on pain mapping, see Chapter 18.

TABLE 9.4

Dermatomes in Relationship to Nerve and Nerve Root Structures

DERMATOME	NERVE	NERVE ROOT
Perineum and perianal skin	Pudendal nerve	S2–S4
Mons pubis and upper aspect of labia majora	Ilioinguinal and genitofemoral nerves	L1–L2
Front of the knees	Anterior femoral cutaneous nerve	L1–L2
Posterior sole of the foot	Tibial nerve	S1

The quality of vaginal and perineal tissue should be noted, particularly for atrophy and the presence or absence of vaginal rugae. This is not only necessary for the assessment of pain and dyspareunia but also allows for the consideration of estrogen use perioperatively or prior to a pessary trial.

The exam is typically continued with evaluation of levator ani muscle integrity and strength, muscle tone, and trigger points. The palpation of the pelvic floor muscles yields information on tone and pain. We recommend starting palpation with the contralateral finger starting on the puborectalis, extending to the iliococcygeus and internal obturator muscles, and finishing with palpation of the coccygeus muscle, repeating this bilaterally. Asking patients specifically if they feel pain or pressure during palpation can help to identify patients with high-tone pelvic floor dysfunction; some patients can interpret pressure as pain unless specifically educated on the difference. Asking patients whether the pain on exam is similar to their pain with intercourse or prolonged standing is helpful in guiding diagnosis. Then, muscle strength is at minimum assessed by asking the patient to squeeze an examiner's finger inserted in the vagina and to hold the contraction as long as possible without help from simultaneous thigh or buttocks contraction. Muscle strength is rated either by the Oxford scale 0 to 5 or by a more extensive validated rating scale called PERFECT scheme introduced by Laycock (Table 9.5).[16–18] The advantage of PERFECT assessment is ability to lay a foundation for a patient-specific exercise program which is practicable within the context of the individual patient.

A bimanual exam can be performed at this point to assess for size, position, and mobility of the uterus as well as any adnexal masses or tenderness on palpation. These findings guide surgical management and can provide information about potential impact on urinary symptoms (i.e., an enlarged fibroid uterus can externally compress the bladder and worsen incontinence). A bivalve speculum examination is carried out to assess the vaginal walls and cervix or vaginal cuff.

A half speculum examination is indispensable in systematically assessing the vaginal walls for prolapse as demonstrated in Video 9.1. The goal of speculum examination is to assess and grade the prolapse in anterior, apical, and posterior compartment (Fig. 9.1).

Anterior wall: The speculum is split in half and first introduced with finger retraction of the posterior vaginal wall to allow direct visual assessment of any anterior vaginal wall prolapse or defects. Vaginal masses, diverticula, urethral hypermobility, and paravaginal detachment can also be discovered during this maneuver. The extent of anterior vaginal wall prolapse will be evident at this point if it is present at rest. The patient should be asked to strain (Valsalva) to observe the extent of the vaginal wall descent under increased

TABLE 9.5

Muscle Strength Assessment: PERFECT Scheme

PARAMETER	DESCRIPTION
P: Power (or pressure)	Power is measured on a modified Oxford scale.
E: Endurance	Endurance is expressed as the length of time, up to 10 s, that contraction can be sustained before the strength is reduced by 35% or more. Breath holding should be discouraged.
R: Repetitions	The number of repetitions is recorded, allowing 4 s rest between each contraction. The purpose of the PERFECT assessment is to determine the number of contractions necessary to overload the muscle to develop a practical exercise program.
F: Fast contractions	Patient is instructed to "contract relax" as quickly and strongly as possible, in her own time, until the muscles fatigue, and that should be the number practiced by patient on a daily basis.
ECT: Every contraction timed	Reminds the examiner to time and record the above sequence of events

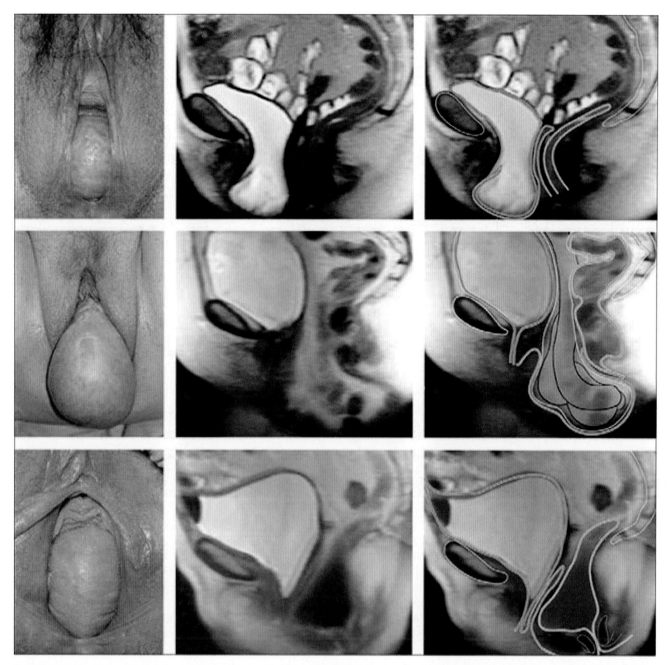

FIGURE 9.1 Photographs in lithotomy position and sagittal MRI showing vaginal wall prolapse. Prolapse might include (**top to bottom**): anterior wall, vaginal apex, or posterior wall. Color codes include *purple* (bladder), *orange* (vagina), *brown* (colon and rectum), and *green* (peritoneum). (Reprinted from *The Lancet*, Jelovsek JE, Maher C, Barber MD. Pelvic organ prolapse. *Lancet* 2007;369[9566]:1028, with permission from Elsevier.)

abdominal pressure.[19] This portion of exam also allows visual assessment of urethral hypermobility.[20]

Posterior wall: Next, examination of the posterior vaginal wall can be performed in a similar fashion after the half speculum is removed, flipped over, and re-introduced in the vagina against the anterior wall (see Video 9.1). Posterior vaginal wall abnormalities will be evident at this point, and the extent of posterior wall prolapse can be assessed. In the upper third of the vagina, the peritoneum covers the surface of the rectovaginal fascia, whereas in the middle third of the vagina, the rectovaginal

fascia is in contact with and loosely attached just underneath the posterior vaginal wall. Posterior vaginal wall prolapse results from a tearing of the rectovaginal fascia that allows the rectal muscularis or even intestinal loops to push upward against the vaginal epithelium with no intervening visceral fascia. The appearance and size of the posterior bulge does not allow the adequate diagnosis of the descending organ behind the vaginal epithelium: It could be rectum or intestinal loops; hence, the use of terms such as *rectocele* and *enterocele* is not advisable to describe the posterior vaginal wall defect.

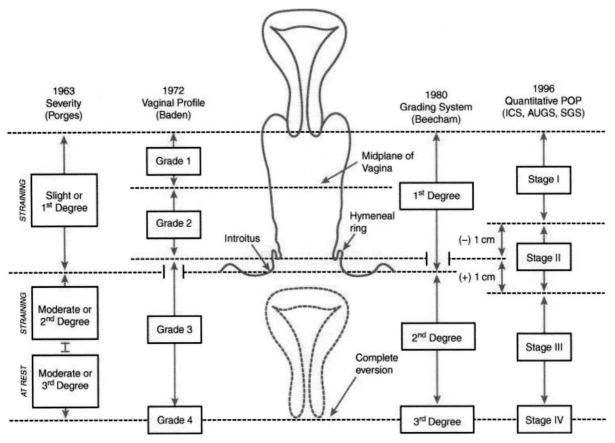

FIGURE 9.2 Comparison of prolapse grading systems. (Reprinted from Mouritsen L. Classification and evaluation of prolapse. *Best Practice Res Clin Obstet Gynaecol* 2005;19[6]:895–911, with permission from Elsevier.)

Vaginal apex: Finally, apical descensus (cervix, or vaginal cuff for women who have had a hysterectomy) is assessed by withdrawing the speculum partially out of the vagina. Failure to execute this maneuver can create artificial correction of apical prolapse with the speculum and apical prolapse can be missed. The diagnosis of apical prolapse is crucial in management; missing it can severely alter the success of surgical outcomes. For example, the risk of anterior wall prolapse recurrence increases if apical prolapse is not addressed in the surgical intervention. If a patient's complaints are consistent with prolapse, but no prolapse is evident on examination, the effort should be made to examine the patient in the standing position. Frequently, this maneuver yields a more accurate assessment of prolapse severity, especially in regard to the apex. It also can be useful if the observed prolapse in the lithotomy position does not match patient-reported symptoms; that is, the vaginal wall is not passing the introitus on exam in the lithotomy position, but the patient reports a large bulge coming outside of her vagina.

The extent of prolapse of the vaginal walls can be reported with descriptive terms, or using measurement systems such as the Pelvic Organ Prolapse Quantification (POP-Q) system, or Baden-Walker scale.[21,22] Other systems of describing prolapse and quantifying it in terms of grade or degree as opposed to staging were used in the past.[23,24] You can find the comparison of them in Figure 9.2.

The POP-Q system is an internationally validated and widely accepted measurement system of prolapse severity. It has significant intraobserver and interobserver reliability among urogynecologists but can be cumbersome to learn and interpret by other professionals.

The POP-Q system assesses the vaginal canal and pertinent external genitalia with a scoring system that both maps and confers severity of prolapse. The hymen serves as a reference point to assess the extent of prolapse of each of the vaginal walls. All measurements, with the exception of total vaginal length, should be obtained under Valsalva to measure the full extent of the prolapse. Measurements are taken in centimeters in increments of 1 cm with positive and negative measurements indicating prolapse distal or proximal to the hymen, respectively.

The six vaginal wall points are defined in Table 9.6.

TABLE 9.6

Mapping Points for POP-Q

POINT	DEFINITION
Aa	A point that represents 3 cm proximal from the external urethral meatus along the midline anterior vaginal wall; values can range from −3 to +3.
Ba	A point that represents the distal portion of the anterior vaginal wall from Aa to the vaginal cuff or anterior vaginal fornix; values can range from −3 to the most prolapsed portion of vagina past the hymen.
C	A point that represents the most distal edge of the cervix or vaginal cuff
Ap	A point that represents 3 cm proximal from the hymen along the midline posterior vaginal wall; values can range from −3 to +3.
Bp	A point that represents the distal portion of the posterior vaginal wall from Ap to the vaginal cuff or posterior vaginal fornix; values can range from −3 to the portion of the vagina posterior to the hymen.
D	A point that represents the posterior fornix if a cervix is present; this is not an applicable measurement if a cervix is not present.

TABLE 9.7

Reference Points for Prolapse Staging as Calculated from Mapping Points Listed in Table 9.6

Stage 0	No prolapse; points Aa, Ba, Ap, and Bp are all −3, and points C or D are within 2 cm of the TVL.
Stage 1	The most distal portion of the prolapse is at least 1 cm proximal to the hymen; POP-Q values are greater than and not equal to −1.
Stage 2	The most distal portion of the prolapse is within 1 cm proximal or distal to the hymen; POP-Q values range from and include −1 to +1.
Stage 3	The most distal portion of the prolapse is >1 cm distal from the hymen but <2 cm of the TVL; POP-Q values range from ≥ +2 to < TVL −2.
Stage 4	The most distal portion of the prolapse is within 2 cm of the TVL; POP-Q values ≥ TVL −2.

The additional POP-Q measurements are defined as follows:

- TVL: This is a measurement of the total vaginal length which is taken by reducing points C or D to their normal position.
- GH: This is a measurement of the genital hiatus from the midurethra to the posterior midline hymen.
- PB: This is a measurement of the perineal body from the posterior midline hymen to the midanal opening.

A staging system allows for a more generalized description of the severity of the prolapse and is defined in Table 9.7.

This animated model is a useful tool that can be used to understand how POP-Q measurements are taken and their correlation with anatomic presentation of prolapse (Fig. 9.3).[25]

POP-Q, although widely accepted, has some shortcomings. It provides granular detail on the anterior and posterior vaginal walls, apex, genital hiatus, and perineal body but does not address all defects. Paravaginal defects can be observed on examination of the anterior vaginal wall by using ring forceps to elevate the lateral vaginal walls. If that maneuver leads to a resolution of the anterior prolapse, a paravaginal detachment defect may be the primary cause of the anterior wall prolapse.

Conversely, an absence of vaginal rugae especially in premenopausal women with anterior wall prolapse can be indicative of a central defect. This difference is not well captured in the POP-Q system.

The other type of defect not described by POP-Q is a perineal descent or detachment—a rarely reported phenomena that is confirmed by noting perineal descent greater than 2 cm past the level of the ischial tuberosities during a Valsalva maneuver. Indirectly, perineal descent can be inferred from increase in GH and PB values with straining. Normally, the perineum is concave because the intact perineal body is attached to the sacrum by the uterosacral ligaments and rectovaginal fascia. Any significant break along this continuity results in an outward bulging of the perineal body as well as its descent far below its normal position. If confirmed, it can present a significant challenge in surgical management. For instance, in patients with a perineal descent who are undergoing a sacrocolpopexy with mesh, the mesh might need to be attached to the perineal body in order to adequately correct the defect.

The Baden-Walker Halfway Scoring System represents a more generalized way to characterize POP. It describes prolapse of each anatomic compartment of the vagina (anterior wall, posterior wall, apex) while the patient is straining. The only anatomic reference is the hymen; therefore, it lacks the ability to convey a detailed assessment of prolapse offered by the POP-Q system.

The pelvic examination can include a rectal examination. The value of the rectal examination varies greatly based on the main presenting symptom. For example, for patients with stress incontinence as their primary complaint, it yields little value. However, for patients with defecatory dysfunction, prolapse, and fecal

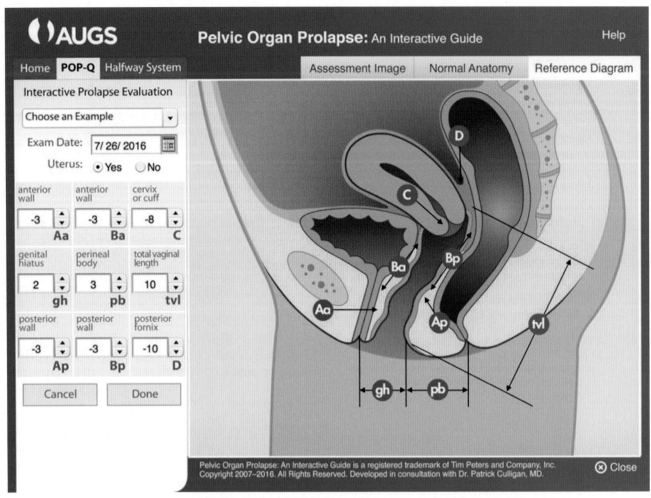

FIGURE 9.3 Interactive POP-Q tool available on web and as phone app. (From POP-Q tool. American Urogynecologic Society. Accessed January 16, 2022. https://www.augs.org/patient-services/pop-q-tool/, with permission.)

incontinence, it is useful to assess for rectal resting tone, squeeze strength, rectovaginal wall laxity, and coexisting conditions such as rectal prolapse. Occasionally, careful inspection reveals peristaltic movements beneath the vaginal epithelium and loops of bowel can be palpated on rectovaginal examination between the rectal and vaginal fingers. Rectovaginal examination in a patient with normal support allows the examiner to appreciate the limits on downward (inferior) movement of the perineal body. The perineal body is thickened and broad between the anus and vaginal introitus. As the finger moves through the anal canal toward the rectum, the examiner should appreciate the pyramidal shape of the perineal body as the examining fingers palpate the close approximation of the rectum with the middle and upper portions of the vagina. The apex of the perineal body is found at the level of the lower third and middle third of the vagina. During a rectal examination, the lateral attachments, the posterior attachment, the uterosacral ligaments, and the lower attachments to the perineal body can be felt as well as other pathologies such as rectal prolapse. Patients with

rectal prolapse usually demonstrate a rectal mass and skin excoriation or irritation of anus. Inspection of the rectal mass will reveal the appearance of the protruded rectum which is distinctly different from hemorrhoids. In case of doubt, it is helpful to ask the patient to strain on the commode and repeat the exam afterward. The other, often underreported, benefit of the rectal examination is its ability to serve as an alternative route to assess for pelvic floor spasm. Transanal levator ani palpation, although not the most preferred route, is especially useful for patients with limited vaginal access, such as those whose prior surgery limits their vaginal length.

The pelvic portion of examination can be concluded with a cough stress test and collection of a catheterized specimen to quantify PVR. Ideally, PVR should be obtained shortly after the patient voids. It can be measured directly by inserting a catheter in the bladder or indirectly with a bladder scanner or more sophisticated ultrasound equipment. PVRs less than 100 mL are generally reassuring. Larger PVRs require clinical correlation with symptoms and may potentially trigger

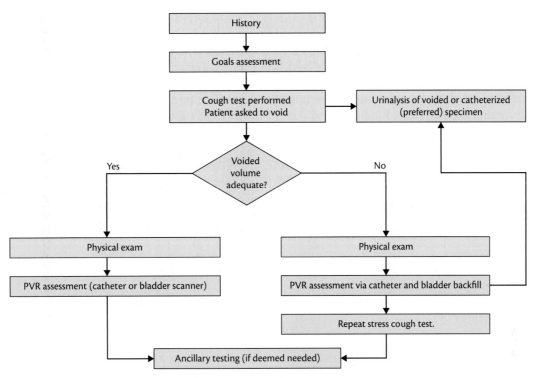

FIGURE 9.4 Flow algorithm for basic evaluation of POP and UI.

assessment of the upper renal tract. Although most studies demonstrate high accuracy of PVR using trans-abdominal point-of-care ultrasound or bladder scanners with automated measurement of bladder volume,[26–29] other recent studies have brought their accuracy into question.[30,31] Abnormal tests should be repeated because the reliability of a single determination is poor.[32]

The cough stress test should be attempted prevoid or via bladder backfilling.[3] It is imperative to ensure that the bladder is relatively full during the cough test. The patient is asked to cough while the examiner directly observes the urethral meatus for signs of leakage. If a cough test is attempted with a naturally filled bladder, the patient should be asked to void afterward and the voided volume should be measured. If the voided volume is inadequate (generally inadequate considered to be less than 200 mL), the stress cough test can be a false negative test and should be repeated after bladder backfill. If a cough test is performed via backfill (instilling up to 300 mL of sterile water or saline in the bladder), methylene blue dye can be added to the irrigant fluid to enhance visualization of the leak. Prolapse should be reduced with procto cotton swab during the stress cough test to assess for occult SUI.

Urinalysis (UA) is considered to be a routine part of POP and UI evaluation and is required by the majority of evaluation algorithms for pelvic floor dysfunction.[5,33,34] UA screens for UTI, a potential modifiable cause of UI. Hematuria should prompt further investigation, and glucose and ketones can be indicative of underlying diabetes or dehydration. UA can be performed as point-of-care testing (dipstick) or core laboratory testing on the specimen collected during voiding or catheterization. The urine dipstick is effective in ruling out UTI: Although a negative test indicates no UTI, a positive one correlates with a positive culture in only one-third of cases.[35–37] A specimen obtained via catheterization generally provides more precise assessment as it decreases contamination of urine which is prevalent especially in patients with prominent prolapse.

For general flow of evaluation, see Figure 9.4.

ANCILLARY TESTS

Usually, a thorough history and physical exam is adequate to completely assess a woman's pelvic floor and provide information to determine a management plan for her incontinence and/or prolapse. Occasionally, additional tests and procedures can further increase the accuracy of evaluation and management. These tools include a voiding diary, urodynamics, magnetic resonance imaging (MRI) defecography, or other imaging.

Voiding diary: Ultimately, regardless of the type of incontinence, a voiding diary is an indispensable tool to obtain more detailed information regarding voiding patterns, volumes of fluid intake and urine output, and severity of incontinence and associated triggers. A 3-day voiding diary can be collected by providing the patient with a measuring hat to collect urine and simple instructions about completing the diary. Information collected should include times of intake and voids, amount of intake and voids, episodes of leakage, and any associated urgency or activity. The diary helps to assess voiding patterns: Voiding up to seven times per day in the waking hours is considered normal,[38] with a micturition volume of 250 to 300 mL per void (although the volume is typically higher with the first morning void). The voiding diary also helps to pinpoint modifiable causes of UI: bladder irritants consumption or large fluid volume intake. Calculation of nighttime to daytime urine production ratio along with assessment of voided volumes can help differentiate nocturnal enuresis due to urine overproduction versus leakage due to urgency incontinence and overactive bladder: The latter is typically associated with small nighttime voids and less than 30% of overall urine production attributed to the nighttime voids.

Pad test: The weight of the absorbent pad worn by the patient at the perineum for 24 hours can provide information for the patients who cannot complete the bladder diary due to the physical impairment (blindness or inability to write due to arthritis) or dementia. A positive pad test is defined as a weight increase of more than 1 g over a 1-hour test or more than 4 g for a 24-hour test. The pad test is a useful indicator of UI severity and can be used to monitor treatment outcomes.

Pyridium pad test: Phenazopyridine hydrochloride (Pyridium) can be given orally, and urinary leakage can be assessed by observation of orange-stained urine on a pad. This may be useful in differentiating between vaginal discharge and urinary leakage but is not considered a

TABLE 9.8

Findings during the Basic Evaluation that Require Further Evaluation

CATEGORY	FINDING	POSSIBLE EVALUATION
History	Recurrent UTIs	Cystoscopy and upper renal imaging (IVP or ultrasound)
	Previous pelvic floor treatments: pelvic radiation or surgery (radical hysterectomy, anti-incontinence, and prolapse repair procedures)	Obtaining more detailed notes and operative reports, cystoscopy, and multichannel urodynamics
	Numerous complex vaguely described voiding symptoms: urgency and frequency, incomplete bladder emptying, painful frequent voids, hesitancy, slow or intermittent stream, spraying of stream or straining to void, leakage with positional changes, positional voiding without clear etiology established during clinical evaluation	Cystoscopy and multichannel urodynamics
	Continuous leakage	Oral Pyridium, backfilled methylene blue with pad test and cystoscopy to rule out fistula
	Neurologic disease suspected of contributing to pelvic floor symptoms	Referral to neurologist if diagnosis is unclear. For example, triad of idiopathic normal-pressure hydrocephalus includes gait and cognitive disturbances along with UI.
	Symptoms of obstructed defecation	Anorectal manometry and defecating proctography or MRI defecography
Pelvic examination	Vagina with obvious urine	Oral Pyridium, backfilled methylene blue with pad test and cystoscopy to rule out fistula
	Suburethral tender mass	Cystoscopy/radiographic study to rule out diverticulum
	Large pelvic mass	Transvaginal ultrasound and age-appropriate workup
Testing	Extremely large voided volumes or urine output of more than 4,000 mL/24 h	Voiding diary and possible endocrine evaluation for diabetes insipidus
	Absence of urethral hypermobility in patient with stress incontinence symptoms	Multichannel urodynamics
	Elevated PVR of >150 mL	Multichannel urodynamics; consider ultrasound in the presence of a history of an anti-incontinence procedure to assess bladder neck for obstruction.
	Hematuria on UA in the absence of UTI	Cystoscopy and upper renal tract imaging

IVP, intravenous pyelogram.

sensitive test for UI.[39] Further, the bladder can be back-filled with methylene blue and pad staining investigated and a vaginal/speculum exam performed to evaluate for fistula. Presence of orange fluid indicates ureterovaginal fistula, whereas blue dye would suggest a lower connection; that is, vesicovaginal or urethrovaginal fistula.

Cotton swab test: Insertion of cotton swab in the urethra can be considered in cases when visual assessment of urethral hypermobility via observation of the anterior vaginal wall produces nonconvincing results. A sterile cotton swab is lubricated with water-based surgical lubricant or lidocaine gel to minimize discomfort and is inserted into the bladder through the urethra. Then, it is gently pulled back, ensuring that the head of the cotton swab sits at the bladder neck. The patient is asked to Valsalva. Observation for cotton swab deflection of greater than 30° confirms urethral hypermobility. Generally, the test is not very well tolerated due to discomfort and has largely been displaced in favor of direct visualization of anterior vaginal wall mobility on exam, or on video urodynamics. It is largely reserved for complicated cases, such as incontinence in patients with prior history of anti-incontinence procedure who are contemplating repeat surgical correction.[40,41]

Multichannel urodynamic evaluation comprises a group of tests that evaluate the function of the urinary tract in terms of storage and evacuation. These tests include cystometrogram, uroflowmeter, electromyography, pressure–flow studies, and urethral pressure profile. Urodynamics can be useful in nonsimple UI (i.e., prior surgery, mixed incontinence, incontinence refractory to treatment) or to assist in evaluation of prolapse or voiding dysfunction. Urodynamic studies are not generally useful if conservative management of uncomplicated UI is planned. Similarly, in patients with clinically diagnosed predominant SUI, no POP, and a PVR volume of less than 150 mL, surgical success rates are not improved in those undergoing urodynamic studies before surgical treatment.[42] Please refer to Chapter 12 for more information.

Various imaging modalities are used to evaluate prolapse and defecatory dysfunction but are not routinely part of the evaluation of POP and UI. Most helpful are transvaginal ultrasound, transperineal ultrasound, and MRI defecography. Please refer to Chapters 13 and 14 for more information.

Thorough history taking and physical exam with some judiciously selected ancillary tests leads to establishing diagnosis in the majority of patients with POP and UI. Table 9.8 lists findings which can trigger more extensive testing considerations.

CONCLUSION

Meticulous systematic clinical evaluation during an office visit yields the majority of information needed to diagnose and plan the initial steps in the treatment of POP

and UI. The patient-centered approach requires integrating goals and expectation assessment at early stages. Ancillary tests can be used to further clarify the diagnosis and guide future management in the small subset of complicated cases when etiology of the condition is unclear or treatment outcome depends on testing results.

References

1. Rortveit G, Subak LL, Thom DH, et al. Urinary incontinence, fecal incontinence and pelvic organ prolapse in a population-based, racially diverse cohort. *Female Pelvic Med Reconstr Surg* 2010;16(5):278–283.

2. Abrams P, Andersson K-E, Apostolidis A, et al. 6th International Consultation on Incontinence. Recommendations of the International Scientific Committee: EVALUATION AND TREATMENT OF URINARY INCONTINENCE, PELVIC ORGAN PROLAPSE AND FAECAL INCONTINENCE. *Neurourol Urodyn* 2018;37(7):2271–2272.

3. American Urogynecologic Society, American College of Obstetricians and Gynecologists. Committee opinion: Evaluation of uncomplicated stress urinary incontinence in women before surgical treatment. *Female Pelvic Med Reconstr Surg* 2014;20(5):248–251.

4. Gutman RE, Ford DE, Quiroz LH, et al. Is there a pelvic organ prolapse threshold that predicts pelvic floor symptoms? *Am J Obstet Gynecol* 2008;199(6):683.e1–683.e7.

5. Jette AM, Davies AR, Cleary PD, et al. The Functional Status Questionnaire: Reliability and validity when used in primary care. *J Gen Intern Med* 1986;1(3):143–149. Erratum in: *J Gen Intern Med* 1986;1(6):427.

6. Aoki Y, Brown HW, Brubaker L, et al. Urinary incontinence in women. *Nat Rev Dis Primers* 2017;3:17042. Erratum in: *Nat Rev Dis Primers* 2017;3:17097.

7. Marshall HJ, Beevers DG. Alpha-adrenoceptor blocking drugs and female urinary incontinence: Prevalence and reversibility. *Br J Clin Pharmacol* 1996;42(4):507–509.

8. Ghoniem G, Stanford E, Kenton K, et al. Evaluation and outcome measures in the treatment of female urinary stress incontinence: International Urogynecological Association (IUGA) guidelines for research and clinical practice. *Int Urogynecol J Pelvic Floor Dysfunct* 2008;19(1):5–33.

9. Ellerkmann RM, Cundiff GW, Melick CF, et al. Correlation of symptoms with location and severity of pelvic organ prolapse. *Am J Obstet Gynecol* 2001;185(6):1332–1337.

10. Burrows LJ, Meyn LA, Walters MD, et al. Pelvic symptoms in women with pelvic organ prolapse. *Obstet Gynecol* 2004;104 (5 Pt 1):982–988.

11. Barber M, Walters MB, Bump R. Association of the magnitude of pelvic organ prolapse and presence and severity of symptoms. *J Pelvic Med Surg* 2003;9:208.

12. Tan JS, Lukacz ES, Menefee SA, et al. Predictive value of prolapse symptoms: A large database study. *Int Urogynecol J Pelvic Floor Dysfunct* 2005;16(3):203–209.

13. de Sam Lazaro S, Nardos R, Caughey AB. Obesity and pelvic floor dysfunction: Battling the bulge. *Obstet Gynecol Surv* 2016;71(2):114–125.

14. Hullfish KL, Bovbjerg VE, Steers WD. Patient-centered goals for pelvic floor dysfunction surgery: Long-term follow-up. *Am J Obstet Gynecol* 2004;191(1):201–205.

15. Mamik MM, Rogers RG, Qualls CR, et al. Goal attainment after treatment in patients with symptomatic pelvic organ prolapse. *Am J Obstet Gynecol* 2013;209(5):488.e1–488.e5.

16. Bø K, Sherburn M. Evaluation of female pelvic-floor muscle function and strength. *Phys Ther* 2005;85:269–282.

17. Laycock J, Jerwood D. Pelvic floor muscle assessment: The PERFECT scheme. *Physiotherapy* 2001;87(12):631–642.

18. Navarro Brazález B, Torres Lacomba M, de la Villa P, et al. The evaluation of pelvic floor muscle strength in women with pelvic floor dysfunction: A reliability and correlation study. *Neurourol Urodyn* 2018;37(1):269–277.

19. Orejuela FJ, Shek KL, Dietz HP. The time factor in the assessment of prolapse and levator ballooning. *Int Urogynecol J* 2012;23(2):175–178.

20. Mattison ME, Simsiman AJ, Menefee SA. Can urethral mobility be assessed using the pelvic organ prolapse quantification system? An analysis of the correlation between point Aa and Q-tip angle in varying stages of prolapse. *Urology* 2006;68(5):1005–1008.

21. Bump R, Mattiasson A, Bø K, et al. The standardization of terminology of female pelvic organ prolapse and pelvic floor dysfunction. *Am J Obstet Gynecol* 1996;175(1):10–11.

22. Baden WF, Walker TA. Genesis of the vaginal profile: A correlated classification of vaginal relaxation. *Clin Obstet Gynecol* 1972;15(4):1048–1054.

23. Porges RF. A practical system of diagnosis and classification of pelvic relaxations. *Surg Gynecol Obstet* 1963;117:769–773.

24. Beecham C. Classification of vaginal relaxation. *Am J Obstet Gynecol* 1980;136(7):957–958.

25. POP-Q tool. American Urogynecologic Society. Accessed January 16, 2022. https://www.augs.org/patient-services/pop-q-tool/

26. Hvarness H, Skjoldbye B, Jakobsen H. Urinary bladder volume measurements: Comparison of three ultrasound calculation methods. *Scand J Urol Nephrol* 2002;36(3):177–181.

27. Bent AE, Nahhas DE, McLennan MT. Portable ultrasound determination of urinary residual volume. *Int Urogynecol J Pelvic Floor Dysfunct* 1997;8(4):200–202.

28. Ouslander JG, Simmons S, Tuico E, et al. Use of a portable ultrasound device to measure post-void residual volume among incontinent nursing home residents. *J Am Geriatr Soc* 1994;42(11):1189–1192.

29. Park YH, Ku JH, Oh S-J. Accuracy of post-void residual urine volume measurement using a portable ultrasound bladder scanner with real-time pre-scan imaging. *Neurourol Urodyn* 2011;30(3):335–338.

30. Mainprize TC, Drutz HP. Accuracy of total bladder volume and residual urine measurements: Comparison between real-time ultrasonography and catheterization. *Am J Obstet Gynecol* 1989;160(4):1013–1016.

31. Alnaif B, Drutz HP. The accuracy of portable abdominal ultrasound equipment in measuring postvoid residual volume. *Int Urogynecol J Pelvic Floor Dysfunct* 1999;10(4):215–218.

32. Scotti RJ, Myers DL. A comparison of the cough stress test and single-channel cystometry with multichannel urodynamic evaluation in genuine stress incontinence. *Obstet Gynecol* 1993;81(3):430–433.

33. Smith A, Bevan D, Douglas HR, et al. Management of urinary incontinence in women: Summary of updated NICE guidance. *BMJ* 2013;347:f5170.

34. Thüroff JW, Abrams P, Andersson K-E, et al. EAU guidelines on urinary incontinence. *Eur Urol* 2011;59(3):387–400.

35. Buchsbaum GM, Albushies DT, Guzick DS. Utility of urine reagent strip in screening women with incontinence for urinary tract infection. *Int Urogynecol J Pelvic Floor Dysfunct* 2004;15(6):391–393.

36. Hessdoerfer E, Jundt K, Peschers U. Is a dipstick test sufficient to exclude urinary tract infection in women with overactive bladder? *Int Urogynecol J* 2011;22(2):229–232.

37. Wong HF, Lee LC, Han HC. Cost-effective screening for urinary tract infections in urogynaecological patients. *Int Urogynecol J Pelvic Floor Dysfunct* 2008;19(5):671–676.

38. Haylen BT, de Ridder D, Freeman RM, et al. An International Urogynecological Association (IUGA)/International Continence Society (ICS) joint report on the terminology for female pelvic floor dysfunction. *Neurourol Urodyn* 2009;29:4–20.

39. Wall LL, Wang K, Robson I, et al. The Pyridium pad test for diagnosing urinary incontinence. A comparative study of asymptomatic and incontinent women. *J Reprod Med* 1990;35(7):682–684.

40. Walters MD, Shields LE. The diagnostic value of history, physical examination, and the Q-tip cotton swab test in women with urinary incontinence. *Am J Obstet Gynecol* 1988;159(1):145–149.

41. Meyer I, Szychowski JM, Illston JD, et al. Vaginal swab test compared with the urethral Q-tip test for urethral mobility measurement: A randomized controlled trial. *Obstet Gynecol* 2016;127(2):348–352.

42. Nager CW, Brubaker L, Litman HJ, et al. A randomized trial of urodynamic testing before stress-incontinence surgery. *N Engl J Med* 2012;366:1987–1997.

CHAPTER 10

Office Evaluation of Pelvic Floor Disorders

Ralph Raymond Chesson, Jr. • Nia Thompson Jenkins

Introduction

Currently, there is no generalized consensus statement or guidelines addressing the evaluation of patients presenting with pelvic floor complaints, including but not limited to, urinary and fecal incontinence, pelvic organ prolapse, fistulas, and vulvovaginal pathology. Various medical specialties ranging from female pelvic medicine and reconstructive surgeons, gynecologists, urologists, colorectal surgeons, and general practitioners may approach patient evaluation differently. Over the years, improvements have been made in the standardization of terminology prompting uniformity in the evaluation and diagnosis amongst practitioners. As it pertains to incontinence in the female, there are published studies; however, none examine the relationship between recommendations and therapeutic outcomes. Given the varying range of invasive and noninvasive therapeutic options for pelvic floor disorders, it is crucial that a practitioner can reliably establish the correct diagnosis. This chapter discusses the utilization of a detailed history, physical exam components, laboratory studies, and in office studies for the evaluation of patients with pelvic floor disorders.

BACKGROUND

The Agency for Health Care Policy and Research (AHCPR), American College of Obstetricians and Gynecologists (ACOG), International Continence Society (ICS), and American Urologic Association (AUA)/Society of Urodynamics, Female Pelvic Medicine & Urogenital Reconstruction (SUFU), and Female Pelvic Medicine & Reconstructive Surgery (FPMRS) have all published documents outlining guidelines for the evaluation of the incontinent female or pelvic floor disorders. In 1992 (modified in 1996), the AHCPR first published their guidelines detailing the suggested workup of urinary incontinence.[1] Their consensus was that a basic evaluation included a thorough history with voiding diary, physical examination, postvoid residual (PVR), and urinalysis. These guidelines were drafted by a panel of experts and targeted for use by primary care practitioners. The inclusion of a PVR was the major change in their recommendations.

In 1996, the Pelvic Organ Prolapse Quantification System (POP-Q) was introduced by the American Urogynecologic Society as a standardized tool used to assess and stage pelvic organ prolapse in females.[2] This also was adopted by the International Urogynecological Association (IUGA), ICS, and eventually the National Institutes of Health. Numerous systems were previously used to stage prolapse; however, the POP-Q was the only system that used objective values to quantify prolapse.[3]

Since then, ACOG has published both practice bulletins and committee options targeted for use by the gynecologic provider. In 2017, a reaffirmed committee opinion on the evaluation of complicated stress urinary incontinence in women before surgical treatment recommended a history, urinalysis, physical examination with assessment for pelvic organ prolapse, cough stress test, assessment of urethral mobility, and measurement a PVR prior to placement of a retropubic midurethral sling for treatment of stress urinary incontinence.[4] To provide better guidance, ACOG also published a practice bulletin on urinary incontinence in 2018 recommending a history, physical exam, symptom severity assessment, goals for treatment, screening for urinary tract infection (UTI), PVR, and cough stress test as key components in the office evaluation.[5] Additionally, the document suggested the use of validated questionnaires could be helpful to aid in thorough and accurate assessment of symptoms. There are six different questionnaires that a provider may choose to use to guide their treatment of a patient: Urogenital Distress Inventory, Incontinence Impact Questionnaire, Questionnaire for Urinary Incontinence Diagnosis, Incontinence Quality of Life Questionnaire, Incontinence Severity Index, and International Consultation on Incontinence Questionnaire. Encompassing the spectrum of pelvic floor disorders, a practice bulletin on the evaluation and treatment of fecal incontinence was released in 2019.[6] Clinical practice guidelines for the treatment of pelvic organ prolapse also issued in 2019.[7] Unlike previously published recommendations, these documents were tailored to the scope of gynecologists and offered more guidance for the initial office evaluation and in the preoperative setting.

The sixth international consultation on incontinence published their detailed guidelines in 2017.[8] Subsections focused on evidence-based findings as it related to physiology, treatment of urinary incontinence in both men and women, treatment of prolapse and fecal incontinence, and painful bladder syndrome. Unfortunately, the published findings reviewed the available treatment options and does not cover any specific recommendations for evaluation except for painful bladder syndrome. Although the public guidelines offer exceptional insight into the available clinical evidence, it is limited in its use for evaluation pelvic floor disorders.

The AUA/SUFU also have guidelines for the evaluation for overactive bladder (OAB) and female stress urinary incontinence (Table 10.1). In 2014, their recommendations for the evaluation of OAB included a detailed medical history, history of bladder symptoms, assessment of fluid intake, medications, degree of bother, Mini-Mental Status Exam, and urinalysis. It notes that urine culture, and PVR, and other validated questionnaires are reasonable to use for unclear diagnoses.[9] In 2017, their recommendations for initial evaluation prior to treatment for female stress incontinence included history, assessment of bother, physical examination including a pelvic examination, demonstration of stress urinary incontinence with a comfortably full bladder, PVR urine, and urinalysis.[10]

OFFICE EVALUATION

A data collection tool as modified from a form that originated from Emory University is a good example of a useful tool for patients presenting with pelvic floor dysfunction (Fig. 10.1). Given the variation among consensus statements, the following four-page tool encompasses a detailed depiction of what is reasonable to collect during the basic office evaluation. This form can assist in the evaluation of a large array of problems with a comprehensive review of systems affecting pelvic floor complaints. It also acts as a guide for a comprehensive physical exam, including the use of the POP-Q. The tool is a useful guide to ensure the collection of important data and is helpful for the experienced FPMRS as well as the teaching of learners at all levels in the evaluation of pelvic floor dysfunctions.

History of Present Illness and Patient History

Often, patients presenting for initial workup may have more than one pelvic floor complaint. Close proximity of the bowel, bladder, and reproductive organs often leads to a constellation of symptoms that can make a diagnosis or diagnoses challenging. It is crucial for the provider to

TABLE 10.1		
Current Recommendations by Society/Organization		
	OVERACTIVE BLADDER/INCONTINENCE	**STRESS INCONTINENCE**
ACOG	2018 • Medical history • Physical exam • Symptom severity assessment • Goals for treatment • UTI screening • PVR • Cough stress test	2017 • Medical history • Physical exam with assessment for pelvic organ prolapse and urethral mobility • Symptom severity assessment • Goals for treatment • Urinalysis • PVR • Cough stress test
AUA/SUFU	2014 • Medical history • History of bladder symptoms • Assessment of fluid intake • Medications • Urinalysis • Degree of bother • Mini-Mental Status Exam	2017 • Medical history • Physical examination with pelvic examination • Degree of bother • Demonstration of stress urinary incontinence with a comfortably full bladder • PVR • Urinalysis

UROGYNECOLOGY DATA BASE
DEPT. OBGYN LSU

Name_____ Date_____
Date of Birth_____ Age_____ S   M   SEP   DIV   WID
Race_____ Parity____-____-____-____ Referring MD_____
Evaluated by_____

CHIEF COMPLAINT:
_____

HISTORY OF THE PRESENT ILLNESS:
_____
_____
_____
_____
_____
_____
_____

PREVIOUS TREATMENT?   No   Yes: (Describe)
_____

WORST SYMPTOM: Incontinence(non-specific)   Stress Incontinence   Urge Incontinence   Frequency
Urgency   Nocturia   Nocturnal Enuresis   Dysuria   Bladder Pain   Lack of Bladder Sensation
Voiding Difficulty(Non-specific)   Hesitancy   Straining to Void   Poor Flow   Intermittent Stream
Incomplete Emptying Prolapse bulge Other:_____

FREQUENCY:_____times/day or every_____hours. **NOCTURIA** up to _____times/night

INCONTINENCE: Yes   No   Don't Know   Not Applicable
Describe a typical leaking episode:
_____
Number of incontinent episodes_____per day _____per week _____per month
Stress incontinence? No Sometimes Often Always Don't Know Not Applicable
Urge incontinence? No Sometimes Often Always Don't Know Not Applicable
Incontinence provoked by: Coughing Laughing Sneezing Lifting Standing Up Walking
Exercise(type):_____
Running Water Putting a Key in a Door Sexual Intercourse Other:_____
Typical amount of leakage: Damp Wet Soaked
Worst amount of leakage: Damp Wet Soaked
Do you wear pads for protection? No Yes Sometimes Always
        Type: Tissues only Mini-pads Tampons Regular menstrual pads   Heavy incontinence pads
        Pad changes____per day _____per week Underwear changes_____
        When you change your pads are they usually: Damp Wet Soaked
Have you changed or restricted your activities because of the bladder leakage? No Yes
Example:_____
Do you wet the bed in your sleep? No Yes--How often?_____
Were you a bed-wetter as a child? No Yes--Age at which you stopped:_____

BLADDER SENSATION:
Aware of fullness? Yes No Don't Know Not Applicable
Aware of wetness? Yes No Don't Know Not Applicable
Dysuria?   No Sometimes Often Only with infection
Bladder pain?   No Sometimes Often Don't Know
        Is the pain relieved by Voiding?   No   Yes

FIGURE 10.1 Urogynecology data base for data collection in the clinic. *(continued)*

VOIDING DYSFUNCTION:

Hesitancy	Never	Sometimes	Often	Don't Know	Not Applicable
Straining to void	Never	Sometimes	Often	Don't Know	Not Applicable
Poor flow	Never	Sometimes	Often	Don't Know	Not Applicable
Intermittent stream	Never	Sometimes	Often	Don't Know	Not Applicable
Can interrupt stream	Never	Sometimes	Often	Don't Know	Not Applicable
Incomplete emptying	Never	Sometimes	Often	Don't Know	Not Applicable
Post-micturition dribble	Never	sometimes	Often	Don't Know	Not Applicable

Acute urinary retention?   No   Yes(Details):_____

INFECTION AND STONES:

Previous UTI?   No   Yes   _____in past year   Don't know

Previous pyelonephritis?   No   Yes   Details_____

Previous IVP?   No   Yes   Don't Know   Findings:_____

History of kidney stones or urinary bladder stones?   No   Yes   Don't know Details:_____

HEMATURIA:

Are you passing blood in your urine now?   No   Yes   Sometimes Details:_____

Have you ever passed blood in your urine in the past?   No   Yes   Details:_____

BOWEL FUNCTION:

Frequency of stool: _____per day   _____per week   _____per month

Laxatives? Suppositories? Enemas? Manual pressure? Fiber? Disimpaction?

Incontinent of gas?	No	Sometimes	Often	Don't Know
Incontinent of liquid stool?	No	Sometimes	Often	Don't Know
Incontinent of solid stool?	No	Sometimes	Often	Don't Know

GYNECOLOGIC HISTORY:

Menarche_____LMP_____PMP_____Cycle_____

Bladder symptoms related to menstrual periods?   No   Yes:_____

Contraception?   No   Yes:_____

Last pap smear_____Previous abnormal smear?   No   Yes:_____

Sexually transmitted diseases?   No   Yes:_____

SEXUAL FUNCTIONING:

Sexually active?   No Widow Impotent No Partner   Yes   _____times/day-week-month

Dyspareunia?   No   Yes   Superficial   Deep   Both   Occasional   Always

Incontinent with intercourse? No   Yes   w. penetration w. orgasm   w. both

OBSTETRICAL HISTORY:

Vaginal deliveries_____   Forceps_____   Cesarean_____

Significant tears or lacerations?   No   Yes:_____

FAMILY HISTORY:

Breast cancer?   No   Yes:_____

Kidney/bladder disease?   No   Yes:_____

PAST MEDICAL HISTORY:

Neurological history?   No   Yes:_____

Low Back problems_____No   Yes_____

Diabetes?   No   Yes:_____How long_____

Chronic lung disease?   No   Yes:_____

Smoker?   No   Yes:_____Packs/day for _____years   Quit_____

Alcohol?   No   Yes:_____

Drug abuse?   No   Yes:_____

Psychiatric history   No   Yes:_____

Previous Mammogram?   No   Yes:_____

Hypertension?   No   Yes:_____

FIGURE 10.1 *(Contiued)*

PAST SURGICAL HISTORY:

_____

_____

_____

CURRENT MEDICATIONS:

_____

_____

ALLERGIES:_____

PHYSICAL EXAMINATION

Weight_____Height____   Blood Pressure_____Pulse_____Other_____

General: _____

Mobility:5-Mobile 4-Uses cane/walker   3-Can stand-unassisted 2-Confined to wheelchair 1-Bedridden

Thyroid: Normal _____

Back: Normal Other_____

Lungs: Normal Other_____

Heart: Normal Other:_____

Abdomen: Normal Other:_____

Neurological: Normal Other:_____

PELVIC EXAMINATION:

Perineum: Perineal Sensation Normal   Other:_____

Anal Wink Reflex   Normal   Absent   Equivocal

Bulbocavernosus Reflex   Normal   Absent   Equivocal

Cough Reflex   Normal   Absent   Equivocal

Vulva: Normal   Atrophic   Other:_____

Levator Contractions: 5/5   4/5   3/5   2/5   1/5   0/5   Valsalva

Bartholin's Glands: Normal   Other:_____

Urethra: Normal   Caruncle   Tender   Induration   Other:_____

Bladder Neck: Normal   Fixed Tender Other:_____Q-Tip____Resting_____strain

Cystocele? None Above Hymen To Hymen Beyond Hymen Defect? Lateral R L Central/Superior

Rectocele? None Above Hymen To Hymen Beyond Hymen Defect? PB R L Central   Superior

Enterocele or Vaginal Vault Prolapse? None   Above Hymen   To Hymen   Beyond Hymen

Vagina: Normal   Atrophic   Other:_____

       Capacity: Normal   Adequate   Reduced   Obliterated

       Mobility: Normal   Adequate   Reduced   Obliterated

       Vaginal Discharge?   No Yes:_____

Cervix: Round Os   Parous Absent   Other:_____

Uterus: Normal   Absent   Enlarged to _____weeks size Comments:_____

       Uterine Descent: None   Above Hymen   To Hymen Beyond Hymen Comments:_____

Adnexal Exam: Normal   Abnormal:_____

Rectovaginal Exam: Confirms   Other:_____

Anal Sphincter Tone: Normal Increased Decreased Flaccid Ability to augment 0-5___

Puborectalis ability to augment 0-5_____

Stool: Heme Negative   Heme Positive   Not tested

IS STRESS INCONTINENCE DEMONSTRATED?   Yes   No

       Marked Incontinence(Copious leak with single cough or minimal exertion)

       Slight leak(Leakage only with multiple coughs or significant exertion)

       Multiple leaks demonstrated   Leakage with empty bladder

       Leaks demonstrated: Erect Dorsal lithotomy   Other:_____

VOLUME VOIDED:_____

POST VOID RESIDUAL:_____

FIGURE 10.1 _(Contiued)_

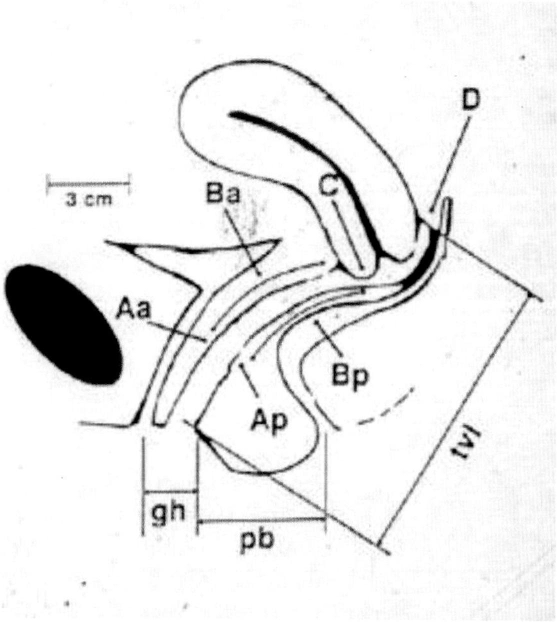

Aa(Anterior wall 3cm from hymen(-3 to +3)_____
Ba(most dependent anterior wall (-3 to TVL) _____
C(cervix or vaginal cuff(±TVL) _____
D(posterior fornix (if no hysterectomy)(±TVL____
Ap(posterior wall 3 cm. from hymen(-3 to +3)__
Bp(most dependent posterior wall(-3 to TVL)_____
GH(genital hiatus-mid urethra to PB) no limit_____
PB(perineal body(PB to mid anus)(no limit) _____
TVL(total vaginal length non straining)(no limit)__
Stage 0=Aa, Ba,Ap,Bp all =-3 and C or D≤(TVL-2)
Stage 1=Leading edge<-1,
Stage 2=Leading edge≥-1but≤+1
Stage 3=Leading edge>+1 but <+(TVL-2)
Stage 4=Leading edge≥+(TVL-2)

POPQ Graph

+8	+6	+4	+2	0	-2	-4	-6	-8	-10

IMPRESSION:_____
_____
_____
_____
_____

PLAN:_____
_____
_____
_____

Urinalysis obtained   Date:_____
Urine Culture Obtained   Date:_____
Patient given bladder chart and plastic hat   Date:_____
Urodynamics scheduled(if indicated) for   Date:_____

_____ **, MD**
          Signature/**name stamp**

FIGURE 10.1 *(Contiued)*

obtain a detailed history and solicit answers to the appropriate questions for efficient and accurate diagnosis.

Upon initial presentation, the history of present illness as well as previous treatments should first be established. Given that patients may have multiple complaints, it is pertinent to define the most bothersome symptom. This symptom could be broken up into categories such as nonspecific incontinence, stress incontinence, urge incontinence, frequency, urgency, nocturia, nocturnal enuresis, dysuria, bladder pain, lack of bladder sensation, voiding difficulty, hesitancy, straining to void, poor flow, intermittent stream, incomplete emptying, prolapse, bulge, or any other unnamed symptom. It is also helpful to establish the degree of bother. After the identification of the most bothersome symptom, it is important to systematically address complaints within the categories of incontinence, voiding dysfunction, bowel function, history, and medications.

*Urinary frequency: **Increased daytime frequency*** is the complaint by the patient who considers that he or she voids too often by day (ICS 2016).

Specifically, the patient should be questioned about how many times a day they void, and if frequently, it is best to break it down into how many times per hour(s). Although voiding patterns may vary, a healthy adult should void approximately six times per day.[11,12] Next, the patient should be questioned about how many times they void at night. *Nocturia* is the complaint that the individual has to wake at night one or more times to void (ICS 2016). This question should be posed as a statement in which the patient is awakened from sleep, voids, and immediately returns to sleep. It should not include voids where the patient is awake at night or does not return to sleep. Awakening three or more times at night is usually indicative of moderate or severe bother for most patients.[13] Occasionally, a voiding diary is necessary to evaluate this component of the history. Most of the voiding diaries are too complex and want too much information. Measuring urine output in a measuring hat in the toilet is more accurate in understanding volume output than trying to figure out dietary intake which is not a precise measurement. We need to know how often and how much they void and possible how many wet pads they have. They need to be given a measuring hat to measure their voids. Three days would be ideal, but in 24 to 48 hours, you will know their intake by measuring their output. Overactive bladder patients will have frequent small voids.

*Urinary incontinence: **Urinary incontinence*** is the complaint of any involuntary leakage of urine (ICS 2016).

In order to establish the appropriate etiology of a patient's incontinence, ideally, a series of questions should be asked in the following order. It is often useful to first ask a patient to describe a typical leaking episode. This should be followed by how many incontinent episodes the patient has per day, per week, or per month if they are less frequent. ***Stress urinary incontinence*** is the complaint of involuntary leakage on effort or exertion, on sneezing, or coughing (ICS 2016). Specifically, the patient should be asked about the presence of stress incontinence and, if present, whether it occurs sometimes, often, always. The same series of questions should be asked regarding urgency incontinence. ***Urge urinary incontinence*** is the complaint of involuntary leakage accompanied by or immediately preceded by urgency (ICS 2016). Many patients will have a combination of both symptoms; therefore, it is also important to ask whether the incontinence is provoked by coughing, laughing, sneezing, lifting, standing up walking, keys in the door, running water, or intercourse. ***Mixed urinary incontinence*** is the complaint of involuntary leakage associated with urgency and also with exertion, effort, sneezing, or coughing (ICS 2016). Further delineation of when the patient leaks is helpful for determining whether the patient has stress or urge incontinence or rather a mixture of the two. Keys in the door and running water would be suggestive of urgency incontinence and not stress incontinence. It is critical to discuss the typical amount of leakage that occurs with episodes of incontinence. Small volumes would be indicative of stress incontinence, whereas large volumes are more concerning for urgency incontinence. Whether or not the patient wears incontinence pads for protection or requires clothing or underwear is also important to ask. A patient who must change their clothing is likely to have larger volume incontinent episodes. Evaluating whether there is limitation in normal activities or change their lifestyle secondary to the incontinence can assess the degree of bother. Lastly, it is very important to discuss nocturnal enuresis and whether this was an issue as a child. If so, details of age and treatment should be reviewed. Again, a bladder diary may help when there are questions regarding this area.

Bladder sensation

Because it relates to bladder sensation and neurourology, it is important to determine if the patient is aware of their bladder fullness and aware of wetness if they have issues with incontinence. Absence of these findings would be concerning for a neurologic etiology that should prompt a different evaluation. Neurologic signs such as abnormalities of the nervous system detected by physical examinations may reflect an underlying neurologic disease such as multiple sclerosis, strokes, or injury. Examples of abnormal signs may include altered sensation, muscle tone, or reflexes. If present, the patient should be referred for a full neurologic examination (Joint terminology 2020). The presence of dysuria should also be discussed. If a patient endorses this symptom, one should discern whether this is in the absence or presence of an infection. It is also pertinent to ask about bladder pain. If the patient endorses pain, the most important factor is to determine whether this pain is relieved by voiding. Pain, in the absence of infection, with frequent voiding would suggest an etiology such as painful bladder syndrome. *Painful bladder syndrome* is the complaint of suprapubic pain related to bladder filling, accompanied by other symptoms such as increased daytime and nighttime frequency, in the absence of proven urinary infection or other obvious pathology. *The ICS believes this to be a preferable term to "interstitial cystitis." Interstitial cystitis (IC) is a specific diagnosis and requires confirmation by typical cystoscopic and histologic features. In the investigation of bladder pain, it may be necessary to exclude conditions such as carcinoma in situ and endometriosis (ICS 2016).*

Voiding dysfunction

Voiding patterns and habits are critical to the appropriate diagnosis. The patient should be asked about hesitancy, straining to void, poor flow, intermittent stream, the ability to interrupt their stream, incomplete emptying, postmicturition dribble, and acute urinary retention. Each one of these categories should be explained in detail to the patient for an appropriate response.

Infections and stones/hematuria

A history of previous UTIs and how many have occurred within the last calendar year should be discussed. It is also important to ask about pyelonephritis isolated from pregnancy, previous intravenous pyelogram (IVP), and history of kidney stones or urinary bladder stones. If the patient endorses any of these, the details and findings should be discussed. Briefly, the patient should be asked whether or not they are actively passing blood in their urine or have seen blood in their urine before. For completeness, it is helpful to ask if a provider has been concerned about blood in their urine.

Bowel function

Shared neurovasculature and proximity of the bowel and bladder can lead to an overlap in pelvic floor disorders. The patient should be questioned about how many times per day they have a bowel movement. If bowel movements are not daily, it should be broken down by week and/or month if less frequently than once per week. The use of laxatives, suppositories, enemas, manual pressure, fiber, and disimpaction should also be discussed. Brief descriptions of the type of stool are sometimes helpful, and the use of the Bristol scale is covered in Chapter 56. Patient should also be asked about incontinence of gas, liquid stool, or solid stool.

Personal history

Gynecologic history, sexual functioning, obstetric history, family history, and medical history should be discussed in detail with the patient. First, it should be established whether the patient is menopausal or not. If not, menarche, last menstrual cycle, cycle length, flow, and contraceptive use should be discussed. If the patient is experiencing bladder symptoms, it is important to know whether or not the symptoms are related to the menstrual cycle. Timing and results of the last Pap smear and previous history of an abnormal Pap smear should be discussed.

Sexual functioning

Sexual activity and the frequency should be reviewed. If the patient is not sexually active, intention of future sexual activity is important to discuss especially when considering surgical options for the treatment of prolapse. Evaluation should include questions about dyspareunia and the categorization of this pain as superficial, deep, both, and occasional or always. Lastly, coital incontinence should be discussed; if present, note whether it is with penetration, orgasm, or both.

Obstetric history

As with any standard obstetric history, parity and the mode of delivery should be discussed. If the patient had a vaginal delivery, it is important to ask if forceps were used and whether the patient experienced any significant lacerations or episiotomy with the delivery. If a cesarean delivery, the reason and when in the labor process (failure to progress, failure of descent, distress, etc.) the decision was made for the cesarean delivery.

Family history

Briefly, the patient should be asked about a history of breast cancer, kidney, urogenital malignancies, or bladder disease.

Past medical history

There are many conditions that can affect a patient's voiding habits as well as contribute to patterns of incontinence. It is important to openly discuss what medical history the patient may have. Specifically, as it relates to urogynecology, it is important to ask the patient about neurologic history, back problems, diabetes and time since diagnosis, chronic lung disease, glaucoma, alcohol abuse, drug abuse, psychiatric history, hypertension, and heart disease. Notably, many neurologic conditions such as multiple sclerosis, recent history of cerebrovascular event, or Parkinson's disease may initially present with urinary symptom manifestations. It is very important for practitioners to keep this in mind when establishing a diagnosis. For example, a diagnosis of Parkinson's disease can be associated with a neurogenic bladder. Thus, a thorough review of history and symptoms is necessary especially in patients with multisystem complaints or atypical presentation. It is also critical to ask the patient about current and former tobacco use as well as environmental exposures.

Past surgical history

Previous surgeries especially those of gynecologic, bowel, or colorectal in nature should be discussed with the patient.

Current medications along with the dosage and timing of administration should be discussed. This is of most importance for diuretics, antihypertensive, and anticholinergic medications. Reviewing medications is an optimal time to ensure that no critical diagnoses such as glaucoma have been missed during the medical history section.

Bladder/voiding diary

Diaries recorded over 3 to 7 days that detail fluid intake, urgency, type of fluid, and volumes voided can be helpful. Patients are provided with a diary and a "top hat" that is placed inside the toilet to measure the volume of each void. Some literature has demonstrated that 3 days is just as effective as 7 days and patients are more likely to be compliant with a shorter duration.[9,14,15] This tool is useful for patients who are poor historians or those who have difficulty describing their intake. Additionally, if there is a high suspicion that symptoms are secondary to personal behavior and/or intake, review of a diary is helpful before initiation of treatment. Review of diaries can also be helpful to trend treatment progress. Not all diaries require the use of recorded volumes. Specifically, review of the voided volume allows the practitioner to assess for polyuria versus pathologic OAB symptoms. This often is cumbersome to complete and 24 to 48 hours of data is sufficient (Fig. 10.2).[9]

Physical Examination

In accordance with any general physical examination, the patient's height, weight and vitals should be reviewed. Additionally, the patient's mental and mobility status should be evaluated. Regarding general physical exam findings, the thyroid, back, lungs, heart, abdomen, and brief neurologic assessment should be performed.

For patients presenting with pelvic floor disorder complaints, the pelvic examination is the most crucial part of the exam. After a detailed history, the practitioner can develop a differential diagnosis and assess for associated symptoms on physical examination. To ensure that a thorough physical exam is completed, it should be carried out in a systematic fashion. First, the perineal sensation should be assessed followed by

3-Day Voiding Diary					
Time of day circle bedtime and wake up times below; also fill in events at right in the time slots when they occurred	**Fluid intake** write down amount of liquid you drank–in oz–from one toileting event to next	**Toilet urinations** write down oz urinated into urinary hat sitting inside toilet seat each time you urinate	**Amount of urine drained via a catheter** if using a catheter, record amount in oz, mL, or cc; indicate if this was catheter [C] residual [R]	**Leaks** place check mark in column if you leaked urine before making it to toilet	**Pad changes** at each toileting event, write "D" if pad is dry or if wet, write down amount: small, mod., large
7 am					
8 am					
9 am					
10 am					
11 am					
noon					
1 pm					
2 pm					
3 pm					
4 pm					

FIGURE 10.2 Example of 3-day voiding diary.

TABLE 10.2		
Detailed Guide for Grading Pelvic Floor Muscle Strength on Physical Exam		
SCORE	**LIMB MUSCLES**	**LEVATOR ANI**
0/5	No movement	No contraction
1/5	Trace of contraction	Flicker, barely perceptible
2/5	Active movement when gravity eliminated	Loose hold, 1–2 s
3/5	Active movement against gravity only	Firmer hold, 1–2 s
4/5	Active movement against resistance but not normal	Good squeeze, 3–4 s, pulls fingers in and up loosely
5/5	Normal strength	Stronger squeeze, 3–4 s, pulls in and up snugly

examination for presence of an anal wink reflex, bulbocavernosus reflex, and cough reflex. Second, the vulva itself should be assessed for atrophy or lesions. Evaluation of tenderness of the hymenal ring to the light touch of a cotton swab is suggestive of a diagnosis of vulva vestibulitis. This is commonly a finding in painful bladder syndrome. Working from external anatomy to internal, the practitioner should assess levator contraction strength on a scale of 0/5 for no contractility to 5/5 for excellent augmentation (Table 10.2).[16] Both the Bartholin and Skene glands can be evaluated for any abnormal findings. Next, the urethra should be assessed for caruncle, prolapse, tenderness, mobility, swelling suggestive of urethral diverticulum, and induration. This should easily transition to examination of the bladder neck specifically commenting on tenderness or whether it is fixed. If there are concerns about urethral mobility, this would be the appropriate time to perform a urethral cotton swab test, especially if there is no hypermobility. Without performing a POP-Q exam at this point, the practitioner should be able to visually recognize whether there is a presence of a cystocele and rectocele and its location in regard to the hymen. Next, the integrity of the vaginal epithelium should be evaluated, and the practitioner should comment on the vaginal capacity and presence or absence of vaginal discharge. The cervix, uterus, and adnexa should all be assessed. The size and appearance of the cervix and uterus should be commented on. Last, the rectovaginal examination should be performed. This would be an appropriate time to examine for an enterocele. The anal sphincter tone and ability to augment the anal sphincter are very important to note.

Supine stress test

Ideally, the patient should have a full bladder, approximately 300 mL or greater during the examination.[4] The patient can then be instructed to cough and Valsalva to determine if urinary incontinence can be demonstrated. If leakage is present on examination, the amount should be noted. If the patient endorsed a history of leakage and does not demonstrate urinary incontinence in the dorsal supine position, she can be instructed to stand erect. To perform the test in the standing position, have the patient stand at the end of the examination table and place one leg on the step. The practitioner should bend to see the labia or urethral meatus. The patient should be instructed to both cough and Valsalva. If leakage is not seen in the dorsal or standing position, the bladder can be retrograde filled with 300 mL or until the patient feels a sensation of fullness and the test can then be repeated.

Pelvic organ prolapse quantification system

The POP-Q is a standardized tool used to assess and stage pelvic organ prolapse in females. In 2016, IUGA/ICS published a joint report that defined and explained all of the components of the POP-Q system.[2] The quantification system is composed of six defined points and three other landmarks.[2,3] For many years, there have been many systems such as the Baden-Walker used to quantify prolapse; to date, the POP-Q creates a standardized context to quantify prolapse. Information on the Baden-Walker system is in Chapter 9 for those practitioners who find POP-Q too difficult to understand. The measurements should be taken and recorded. The measurements can then be demonstrated on the POP-Q graph as suggested by Dr. Bernard Schussler well more than two decades ago. This is then used as a tool for both documentation and patient counseling and can also be used to show progression of prolapse over time. Figure 10.3 demonstrates the use of the POP-Q graph. The points are plotted out and a simple configuration is drawn. This is both an excellent tool for clinic documentation and patient counseling.

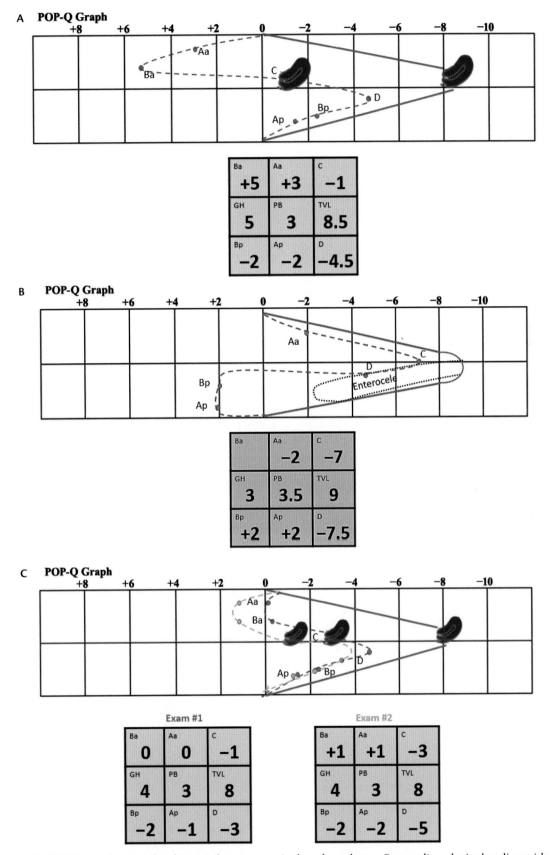

FIGURE 10.3 **A:** POP-Q graph example of incomplete uterovaginal vault prolapse. *Orange lines* depict baseline with no prolapse and the *dotted blue lines* depict prolapse based on the POP-Q measurement. **B:** POP-Q graph example of posthysterectomy vaginal vault with rectocele and enterocele on examination. **C:** POP-Q graph demonstrating the progression of uterovaginal prolapse from the *blue dotted line* during the first examination and 6 months later with the *green dotted line*.

Additional Evaluation

Cotton swab test

The mobility of the urethrovesical junction (UVJ) can be assessed by the Q-tip or cotton swab test.[17,18] Less commonly, ultrasonography, point Aa on the POP-Q examination, and visualization have all been used for assessment.[19–21] The presence of urethral hypermobility is important with assessing for the feasibility of anti-incontinence surgery. Women with minimal or no urethral mobility are more likely to have complicated stress incontinence and have poor results after the placement of a midurethral sling.[22] To perform the test, the urethral meatus must first be cleansed. A local anesthetic jelly can be inserted into the urethra or a lubricated sterile cotton swab in a local anesthetic is gently inserted to the bladder neck. There is a decrease in resistance when the cotton swab enters the bladder, indicating that the tip is past the location of the UVJ. Resting angle can be measured with a goniometer. The patient should then be asked to Valsalva and cough. The excursion of the cotton swab from the resting angle should be measured. A change of greater than 30° from the baseline measurement is defined as urethral hypermobility (Fig. 10.4).[4,23]

Postvoid residual

A PVR should be measured immediately after a patient spontaneously voids. It can be measured by performing a bladder scan or collected by an in and out catheterization. This is also a chance to obtain a sterile specimen for culture. There is varying data on cutoff values for a normal residual volume. Historically, a PVR of less than 100 to 150 mL is considered normal.[9] Elevated PVRs are suggesting of overflow incontinence with etiologies that range from obstruction secondary to prolapse, voiding dysfunction, and neurologic diagnoses. Elevated PVRs should be repeated, and clinical correlation should be considered.

Simple cystometrogram

A simple cystometrogram is not routinely recommended for initial evaluation; however, it is useful in the diagnosis of stress and urge incontinence. This test has the ability to assess bladder capacity, detrusor overactivity, and stress urinary incontinence. The urethral meatus is cleaned with an antiseptic solution, and a Foley catheter is inserted. First, the bladder is drained, and a 60-mL catheter tip syringe is attached to the end of the Foley catheter. The plunger is removed, and the syringe is positioned 10 to 15 cm above the pubic symphysis while the patient is standing or in dorsal lithotomy (Fig. 10.5). The bladder is then backfilled in 60-mL increments until the patient cannot tolerate any more filling. Any rise or fall in the meniscus of the fluid would indicate detrusor overactivity. After the bladder is filled to capacity, the patient can be instructed to cough and Valsalva to assess for stress urinary incontinence.

Urodynamics considerations

When considering an anti-incontinence procedure, additional testing in addition to the office evaluation can be considered. For those with uncomplicated stress incontinence demonstrable on examination, additional testing may not be necessary.[4] In particular circumstances, urodynamic testing should be considered when there is

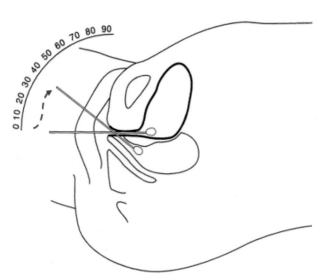

FIGURE 10.4 Demonstration of urethral hypermobility. *Red arrow* demonstrates at least 30° of deviation from baseline.

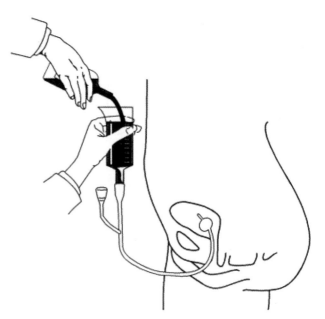

FIGURE 10.5 Simple eyeball cystometrogram in the standing position.

a history of prior pelvic organ prolapse surgery, previous anti-incontinence surgery, voiding dysfunction, urgency, or OAB that has not responded to medications. Other reasons such as incomplete emptying/elevated PVR, discordance between subjective symptoms and objective measures, unconfirmed stress incontinence, and neurogenic-associated lower urinary tract disorders should have urodynamic testing.[10]

Office cystoscopy

In-office cystoscopy may be performed for assessment of the lower urinary tract. Use of the flexible cystoscope (16 or 17 French) has increased the frequency of in-office procedures as they are better tolerated than rigid cystoscopes.[24] Concomitant use of a lubricating gel and transurethral local anesthetic is also recommended. If there are questions about previous surgery with mesh, microscopic or gross hematuria, or indications to remove an indwelling stent, a brief office cystoscopy is essential. A urinalysis and culture should be obtained prior to the procedure to prevent microbial dissemination. In accordance with the AUA, prophylactic antibiotics are not indicated for diagnostic in office cystoscopy except for risk factors.[25] Risk factors necessitating prophylaxis are advanced age, anatomic anomalies of the urinary tract, chronic corticosteroid use, colonized endogenous or exogenous material, distant coexistent infection, immunodeficiency, poor nutritional status, prolonged coexistent infection, and smoking history. Contraindications include acute UTI, intolerance to discomfort or pain, and severe urethral stricture.[24]

Imaging

Imaging is not included in the initial workup for pelvic floor disorders; however, it could be considered prior to definitive surgical management. The reproductive status should be assessed during the detailed history and physical exam. It is reasonable to consider imaging in the form of pelvic and/or abdominal ultrasound if the patient endorses postmenopausal bleeding prior to any uterine-sparing surgical procedure. Additionally, it is reasonable to consider imaging for patients high risk for endometrial hyperplasia in the setting of a uterine-sparing procedure or hysterectomy. For patients with concerning findings on physical examination, the appropriate imaging in the form of ultrasound, computed tomography (CT) scan, or magnetic resonance imaging (MRI) should be ordered. For women suspected to have a urethral diverticulum on exam, pelvic MRI is the most sensitive test to aid with diagnosis.[26] Furthermore, for those presenting with gross hematuria or nephrolithiasis, a CT urogram and/or renal ultrasound is reasonable to order.

Fistula diagnosis

There are many forms for genitourinary fistulas ranging from rectovaginal, vesicovaginal, urethrovaginal, ureterovaginal, colovaginal, peritoneovaginal, and vesicoendometrial fistula. In-office diagnosis of a fistula tract involving the bladder, vagina, and ureter can be diagnosed with a methylene blue or Pyridium test.[16,27,28] This involves instilling a dilute solution of methylene blue into the bladder and watching for extravasation into the vagina. If there is a high suspicion for a vesicovaginal or a vesicoendometrial fistula, and no blue solution is seen in the vagina, a tampon is inserted in the vagina, and the patient is instructed to ambulate assessing for blue fluid on the tampon. If this testing is negative or if a ureterovaginal fistula is suspected, 200 mg of Pyridium can be administered orally. The examiner should wait approximately 30 to 45 minutes and then assess for extravasation of orange solution into the vagina. This test can be performed with or without a tampon in the vagina. Alternatively, indigo carmine is again available and can be given intravenously with less time to see results. Vesicoendometrial fistulas can be challenging to diagnose and often require in-office cystoscopy and imaging. A rectovaginal fistula is more likely to be evident on physical examination. It is important to remember that there should be an assessment for inflammatory bowel disease prior to surgical repair of a rectovaginal fistula. More complicated fistula such as colovaginal fistula often require a vaginal fistula gram; injection of contrast dye in the vagina with a 40-mL balloon Foley looking for extravasation to the bowel that must be completed by radiology.

Chronic interstitial cystitis/painful bladder syndrome

Diagnosis of IC/painful bladder syndrome is one of exclusion and patient management can be very challenging. The AUA guidelines, last updated in 2014, are a resourceful tool for the diagnosis and treatment of these patients.[29] In contrast to patients with OAB, patients with IC void frequently to avoid pain. Usually, these patients have been seen by numerous physicians, treated for numerous UTIs despite negative cultures. Patient with frequency, nocturia, and dyspareunia for at least 6 weeks with negative cultures and negative workup likely has IC. Furthermore, the presence of vulvar vestibulitis to the light touch of a cotton swab test may suggests an angry urethra or bladder, chronic cystitis, urethritis, IC, or incorrectly placed midurethral sling. Inflammation or unstable microbiome of the bladder secondary to atrophic urethritis and lack of *Lactobacillus* in the bladder has been shown to make IC worse.[30] The first step for the treatment of IC involves following a strict diet. Since 2012, the Interstitial Cystitis Network has published a food list that is available as a downloadable application on most electronic devices. If unsure of the diagnosis or poor response to therapy, then cystoscopy with hydrodistension under anesthesia is useful for both diagnosis and treatment, but the response to hydrodistension is poorly understood. Long-term nitrofurantoin is dangerous, and narcotics should be avoided. Step 1 in the AUA guidelines is diet; patient compliance with the diet is predictive of response, and if not compliant, their symptoms will not improve.

Chronic infective cystitis

Chronic cystitis is often diagnosed in older patients and is usually associated with atrophic vaginitis.[30] The lack of estrogen will not allow the *Lactobacillus* bacteria in the vagina, and coliform bacteria will predominate in the vagina. The first step is a small dose of vaginal estrogen. In a breast cancer patient, a very small dose of dehydroepiandrosterone (Intrarosa) will help. If no improvement, then D-Mannose will help in prevention instead of the traditional methenamine (Hiprex), cranberry and trimethoprim suppression.[31]

Vulvar pathology

Finally, it is common to see a significant amount of vulvar pathology. There is large prevalence of lichen sclerosis and lichen planus. Lichen sclerosis diagnosis requires a biopsy to rule out vulvar cancer. Some chronic vulvar conditions may be associated with Sjögren's syndrome and systemic lupus. This pathology is characterized by atrophic changes that do not respond to hormones and responds well to steroids. In younger patients with lichen sclerosis that desire to remain sexually active, some of these adhesions may require dilation and lysis under anesthesia.

More difficult to manage is lichen planus which is characterized by adhesions of vulvar structures with loss of anatomy around the clitoris and the labia minora. If neglected, the entire introitus may scar closed. Also, the variation of erosive lichen planus of the vaginal apex is characterized by erythema and tenderness of the vaginal apex and will also respond to vaginal steroids. If allowed to progress, the potential urinary retention may occur requiring an indwelling Foley or suprapubic catheter.

Microscopic hematuria

Clinicians should define microhematuria as 3 or more red blood cells per high-power field on microscopic evaluation of a single, properly collected urine specimen. A dipstick positive for hemoglobinuria should prompt a microscopic evaluation to define the presence of hematuria and number of red blood cells per high-power field. The newest treatment algorithm recommended by the AUA is based on risk stratification (Table 10.3).

Low risk: In low-risk patients with microhematuria, clinicians should engage patients in shared decision-making to decide between repeating urinalysis within 6 months or proceeding with cystoscopy and renal ultrasound (moderate recommendation; evidence level: grade C).

Initially low risk with hematuria on repeat urinalysis: Low-risk patients who initially elected not to undergo cystoscopy or upper tract imaging and who are found to have microhematuria on repeat urine testing should be reclassified as intermediate or high risk. In such patients, clinicians should perform cystoscopy and upper tract imaging in accordance with recommendations for these risk strata (strong recommendation; evidence level: grade C).

Intermediate risk: Clinicians should perform cystoscopy and renal ultrasound in patients with microhematuria categorized as intermediate risk for malignancy (strong recommendation; evidence level: grade C).

High risk: Clinicians should perform cystoscopy and axial upper tract imaging in patients with microhematuria categorized as high risk for malignancy (strong recommendation; evidence level: grade C).

Options for upper tract imaging in high-risk patients: If there are no contraindications to its use, clinicians should perform multiphasic CT urography (including imaging of the urothelium) (moderate recommendation; evidence level: grade C).

TABLE 10.3

Microhematuria Risk Stratification in Accordance with the AUA Guidelines Published in 2020[32,33]

LOW (PATIENT MEETS ALL CRITERIA)	INTERMEDIATE (PATIENT MEETS ANY ONE OF THESE CRITERIA)	HIGH (PATIENT MEETS ANY ONE OF THESE CRITERIA)
• Women age <50 y; men age <40 y • Never smoker or <10 pack-years • 3–10 RBC/HPF on a single urinalysis • No risk factors for urothelial cancer	• Women age 50–59 y; men age 40–59 y • 10–30 pack-years • 11–25 RBC/HPF on a single urinalysis • Low-risk patient with no prior evaluation and 3–10 RBC/HPF on repeat urinalysis • Additional risk factors for urothelial cancer	• Women or men age ≥60 y • >30 pack-years • >25 RBC/HPF on a single urinalysis • History of gross hematuria

RBC, red blood cells; HPF, high-power field.

If there are contraindications to multiphasic CT urography, clinicians may use magnetic resonance urography (moderate recommendation; evidence level: grade C).

If there are contraindications to multiphasic CT urography and magnetic resonance urography, clinicians may use retrograde pyelography in conjunction with noncontrast axial imaging or renal ultrasound (expert opinion).

Clinicians should perform white light cystoscopy in patients undergoing evaluation of the bladder for microhematuria (moderate recommendation; evidence level: grade C).

In patients with persistent or recurrent microhematuria previously evaluated with renal ultrasound, clinicians may perform additional imaging of the urinary tract (conditional recommendation; evidence level: grade C).

References

1. U.S. Department of Health and Human Services. Managing acute and chronic urinary incontinence. *J Am Acad Nurse Pract* 1996;8(8):390–403.

2. Haylen BT, Maher CF, Barber MD, et al. An International Urogynecological Association (IUGA)/International Continence Society (ICS) joint report on the terminology for female pelvic organ prolapse (POP). *Int Urogynecol J* 2016;27(4):655–684.

3. Persu C, Chapple CR, Cauni V, et al. Pelvic Organ Prolapse Quantification System (POP-Q)—A new era in pelvic prolapse staging. *J Med Life* 2011;4(1):75–81.

4. American Urogynecologic Society, American College of Obstetricians and Gynecologists. Committee opinion: Evaluation of uncomplicated stress urinary incontinence in women before surgical treatment. *Female Pelvic Med Reconstr Surg* 2014;20(5):248–251.

5. ACOG Practice Bulletin No. 155: Urinary incontinence in women. *Obstet Gynecol* 2015;126(5):e66–e81.

6. ACOG Practice Bulletin No. 210: Fecal incontinence. *Obstet Gynecol* 2019;133(4):e260–e273.

7. Pelvic organ prolapse: ACOG Practice Bulletin, Number 214. *Obstet Gynecol* 2019;134(5):e126–e142.

8. Abrams P, Andersson K-E, Apostolidis A, et al. 6th International Consultation on Incontinence. Recommendations of the International Scientific Committee: EVALUATION AND TREATMENT OF URINARY INCONTINENCE, PELVIC ORGAN PROLAPSE AND FAECAL INCONTINENCE. *Neurourol Urodyn* 2017;37(7):2271–2272.

9. Gormley EA, Lightner DJ, Burgio KL, et al. Diagnosis and treatment of overactive bladder (non-neurogenic) in adults: AUA/SUFU guideline. *J Urol* 2012;188(6 Suppl):2455–2463.

10. Kobashi KC, Albo ME, Dmochowski RR, et al. Surgical treatment of female stress urinary incontinence: AUA/SUFU guideline. *J Urol* 2017;198(4):875–883.

11. Burgio KL, Engel BT, Locher JL. Normative patterns of diurnal urination across 6 age decades. *J Urol* 1991;145(4):728–731.

12. van Haarst EP, Heldeweg EA, Newling DW, et al. The 24-h frequency-volume chart in adults reporting no voiding complaints: Defining reference values and analysing variables. *BJU Int* 2004;93(9):1257–1261.

13. Tikkinen KAO, Johnson TM II, Tammela TLJ, et al. Nocturia frequency, bother, and quality of life: How often is too often? A population-based study in Finland. *Eur Urol* 2010;57(3):488–496.

14. Konstantinidis C, Kratiras Z, Samarinas S, et al. Optimal bladder diary duration for patients with suprapontine neurogenic lower urinary tract dysfunction. *Int Braz J Urol* 2016;42(4):766–772.

15. Dmochowski RR, Sanders SW, Appell RA, et al. Bladder-health diaries: An assessment of 3-day vs 7-day entries. *BJU Int* 2005;96(7):1049–1054.

16. Walters MD, Karram MM. *Urogynecology and reconstructive pelvic surgery*, 4th ed. Pensylvania: Elsevier, 2015.

17. Karram MM, Bhatia NN. The Q-tip test: Standardization of the technique and its interpretation in women with urinary incontinence. *Obstet Gynecol* 1988;71(6 Pt 1):807–811.

18. Crystle CD, Charme LS, Copeland WE. Q-tip test in stress urinary incontinence. *Obstet Gynecol* 1971;38(2):313–315.

19. Dalpiaz O, Curti P. Role of perineal ultrasound in the evaluation of urinary stress incontinence and pelvic organ prolapse: A systematic review. *Neurourol Urodyn* 2006;25(4):301–307.

20. Dietz HP, Wilson PD. The 'iris effect': How two-dimensional and three-dimensional ultrasound can help us understand anti-incontinence procedures. *Ultrasound Obstet Gynecol* 2004;23(3):267–271.

21. Mattison ME, Simsiman AJ, Menefee SA. Can urethral mobility be assessed using the pelvic organ prolapse quantification system? An analysis of the correlation between point Aa and Q-tip angle in varying stages of prolapse. *Urology* 2006;68(5):1005–1008.

22. Richter HE, Litman H, Lukacz ES, et al. Demographic and clinical predictors of treatment failure one year after midurethral sling surgery. *Obstet Gynecol* 2011;117(4):913–921.

23. Walters MD, Shields LE. The diagnostic value of history, physical examination, and the Q-tip cotton swab test in women with urinary incontinence. *Am J Obstet Gynecol* 1988;159(1):145–149.

24. Engelsgjerd JS, Deibert CM. *Cystoscopy*. Florida: StatPearls Publishing, 2020.

25. Wolf JS Jr, Bennett CJ, Dmochowski RR, et al. Best practice policy statement on urologic surgery antimicrobial prophylaxis. *J Urol* 2008;179(4):1379–1390.

26. Chou C-P, Levenson RB, Elsayes KM, et al. Imaging of female urethral diverticulum: An update. *Radiographics* 2008;28(7):1917–1930.

27. Deshmukh AS, Bansal NK, Kropp KA. Use of methylene blue in suspected colovesical fistula. *J Urol* 1977;118(5):819–820.

28. O'Brien WM, Lynch JH. Simplification of double-dye test to diagnose various types of vaginal fistulas. *Urology* 1990;36(5):456.

29. Hanno PM, Burks DA, Clemens JQ, et al. AUA guideline for the diagnosis and treatment of interstitial cystitis/bladder pain syndrome. *J Urol* 2011;185(6):2162–2170.

30. Abernethy MG, Rosenfeld A, White JR, et al. Urinary microbiome and cytokine levels in women with interstitial cystitis. *Obstet Gynecol* 2017;129(3):500–506.

31. Lenger SM, Bradley MS, Thomas DA, et al. D-Mannose vs other agents for recurrent urinary tract infection prevention in adult women: A systematic review and meta-analysis. *Am J Obstet Gynecol* 2020;223(2):265.e1–265.13.

32. Barocas DA, Boorjian SA, Alvarez RD, et al. Microhematuria: AUA/SUFU guideline. *J Urol* 2020;204(4):778–786.

33. Grossfeld GD, Wolf SS Jr, Litwan MS, et al. Asymptomatic microscopic hematuria in adults: Summary of the AUA best practice policy recommendations. *Am Fam Physician* 2001;63(6):1145–1154.

CHAPTER 11

STANDARDIZATION OF TERMINOLOGY, VALIDATED QUESTIONNAIRES, AND OUTCOME ASSESSMENTS

Joseph Kim-sang Lee • Bernard T. Haylen

STANDARDIZATION OF TERMINOLOGY

Standardized terminology, as used in communications by scientifically focused societies such as the International Continence Society (ICS) and the International Urogynecological Association (IUGA), is as basic and important as a dictionary is to the wider society.[1] Terminology documents, carefully prepared by experts in a long, consensus-based process, provide a valuable reference for society members and others wishing to publish in the different relevant journals. More importantly, everyone is "speaking the same language" both in their clinical practices and when presenting their research endeavors at scientific meetings and in any written form. Since February 2019, all the relevant terms (1,455 as of February 2021) from both the earlier-mentioned societies are instantaneously available, with their reference documents in a digital format, the ICS Glossary[2]—https://www.ics.org/glossary.

History of Standardization

International Continence Society (1972 to 2008)

In 2020, the ICS completed 50 years of Standardization Committee history.[2] Standardization was an early priority of the early ICS with the first Standardization Committee formed in 1972 under the chairmanship of Tage Hald with committee members Patrick Bates, Hansjorg Melchior, Art Sterling, David Rowan, Derek Griffiths, and Eric Glen (Fig. 11.1). Between 1972 and 1980, there were three reports of the terminology for lower urinary tract (LUT) dysfunction (1974—Annual General Meeting (AGM) Mainz, 1976, 1980). A fourth report was produced in 1983, adding Torsten Sundin, David Thomas, Michael Torrens, Richard Turner-Warwick, and Norman Zinner to the authors of the 1980 report.[2]

The original committee (1980 report) retired in 1983 with Jens Thorup Andersen (1983 to 1991) taking over as chair. Anders Mattiasson (1991 to 1998) followed by Derek Griffiths (1998 to 2000), and Philip van Kerrebroeck (2000 to 2007).

The 1998 LUT report[3] collated the six LUT/pelvic floor reports till that time. Other documents leading up to 2002 LUT report include (1) technical aspects of urodynamic equipment,[4] (2) LUT rehabilitation techniques,[5] (3) pelvic organ prolapse (POP) and pelvic floor dysfunction (PFD),[6] (4) LUT function: pressure-flow studies,[7] (5) standardization of outcome studies: general principles,[8] (6) outcome measures in adult women with symptoms of LUT dysfunction,[9] (7) standardization of definitions of LUT dysfunction in children,[10] (8) neurogenic LUT dysfunction,[11] (9) standardization of urodynamic ambulatory monitoring,[12] (10) treatment of males with symptoms of LUT dysfunction,[13] (11) nocturia,[14] and four ICS outcome reports.

The 2002 ICS terminology for LUT dysfunction report[15] incorporated male and female terminology and became the most referenced terminology document in ICS and LUT dysfunction history (by 2020, more than 11,000 citations in two journals). Standardization documents between 2002 and 2010 include (1) good urodynamic practices[16] and (2) pelvic floor muscle function and dysfunction.[17] Figure 11.2 shows the past and present ICS standardization chairs.

International Urogynecological Association (1999 to 2008)

Although the early history of the IUGA Terminology and Standardization (T & S) Committee is not so well documented, it is commonly accepted that the original chair was Professor Ulf Ulmsten from Sweden. The committee was set up under the guidance of Dr. Harold Drutz from Canada, president and chairman of IUGA committees in 1999 to 2000. Early members included

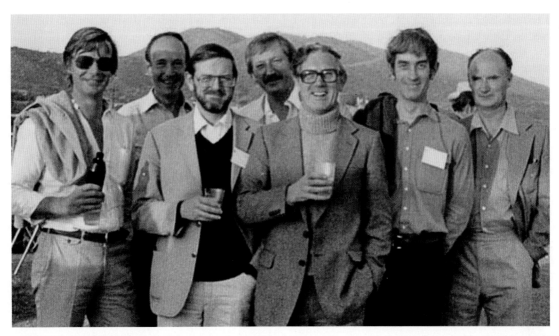

FIGURE 11.1 The first Standardization Committee formed in 1972 under the Chairmanship of Tage Hald with Committee Members: Patrick Bates, Hansjorg Melchior, Art Sterling, David Rowan, Derek Griffiths and Eric Glen. (Courtesy of Internal Archives of the International Continence Society.)

Peter Sand (United States), Bob Freeman (United Kingdom), and Eckhard Petri (Germany), all of whom were to become IUGA presidents. This perhaps indicates the importance of this committee within IUGA.

As noted earlier, around 2000 to 2002, the ICS was developing a report on "The Standardization of Terminology of Lower Urinary Tract Function,"

encompassing terminology for men, women, and children in the one document.[15] Ulf Ulmsten, as T & S chair and a coauthor of the ICS document,[15] would have been updating the IUGA T & S committee on its development, publication, and implementation. Bob Freeman took over the chair from 2003 to 2005, at which time there would have been no particular incentive for IUGA to seek

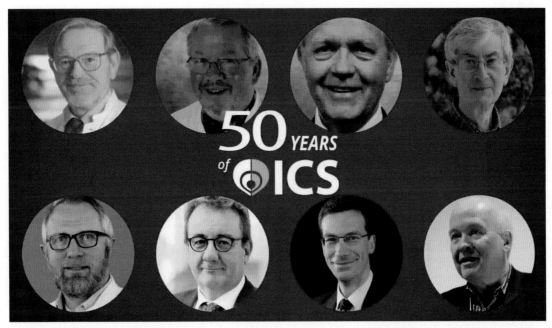

FIGURE 11.2 ICS Standardization Committee chairs. **Top (from left to right):** Tage Hald, Jens Andersen, Anders Mattiassen, and Derek Griffiths. **Bottom (from left to right):** Philip van Kerrebroeck, Dirk de Ridder, Marcus Drake, and Bernie Haylen. (Courtesy of Internal Archives of the International Continence Society.)

alternative terminology documents. Steven Swift (United States) served as IUGA T & S chair from 2006 to 2008. At that time, the Pelvic Organ Prolapse Quantification (POP-Q) system from 1996 was viewed as somewhat complex.[6] An emphasis of the chair was to abridge the questionnaire and create a simplified POP-Q.[18]

International Continence Society-International Urogynecological Association (2007 to 2017)

In 2007, an excellent working relationship developed between ICS Standardization Steering Committee Chair (2007 to 2010) Dirk de Ridder and the IUGA T & S Committee Chair (2008 to 2014) Bernard Haylen, which led to the publication of the IUGA-ICS terminology for PFD,[19] the most cited IUGA terminology publication (second most cited ICS publication—more than 3,800 citations), in January 2010. This female-specific text[20] notably added three "most common" diagnoses (bladder oversensitivity, recurrent urinary tract

infections, and voiding dysfunction) to the three existing female diagnoses in the 2002 report (urodynamic stress incontinence, detrusor overactivity, POP). The terminology for PFD,[19] the initial product of that IUGA-ICS collaboration, was published simultaneously in the *International Urogynecology Journal* and *Neurourology and Urodynamics* in January 2010. Its value in consolidating the definitions for symptoms, signs, investigations, imaging, and the six most common diagnoses have seen it become the core female PFD terminology document. This document is most commonly cited to confirm compliance in *Neurourology and Urodynamics* and the *International Urogynecology Journal* publications with IUGA-ICS terminology. It was the forerunner to further joint IUGA-ICS publications and a template for other ICS publications.

The IUGA-ICS standardization and terminology relationship was maintained till 2017 with seven other joint documents initiated: (1) complications for prostheses and grafts (Fig. 11.3),[21] (2) reporting outcomes of surgical procedures for POP,[22] (3) complications

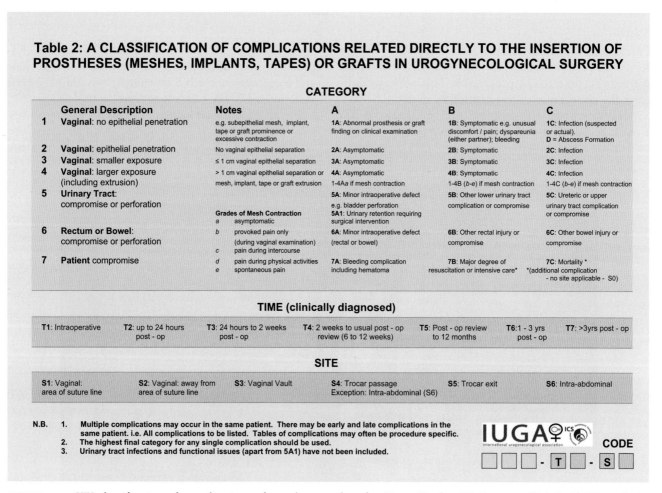

FIGURE 11.3 CTS classification of complications of prostheses and grafts. (From Haylen BT, Freeman RM, Swift SE, et al. An International Urogynecological Association [IUGA]/International Continence Society [ICS] joint terminology and classification of the complications related directly to the insertion of prostheses [meshes, implants, tapes] and grafts in female pelvic floor surgery. *Neurourol Urodyn* 2011;30[1]:2–12.)

of native tissue surgery,[23] (4) POP,[24] (5) conservative and nonpharmacologic management of female PFD,[25] (6) female anorectal dysfunction,[26] and (7) sexual health in women with PFD.[27]

Complications related to the insertion of prostheses and grafts in pelvic floor surgeries[21] was a timely document, published in January 2011, to acknowledge the widespread clinical issues arising from the greatly expanded use of synthetic products in prolapse surgeries, in particular from around 2005. A category, time, and site (CTS) classification, as noted in Figure 11.3, was created. This is the third most cited (626) IUGA document with the POP document (774),[24] the second most cited. Its native tissue equivalent[23] was published in April 2012, along with the important document on definitions, standardized outcome measures, and how to present results of prolapse surgeries.[22] This should be used in all intervention studies of prolapse surgeries.

There were two non–IUGA-ICS documents between 2010 and 2016 when Marcus Drake (2000 to 2016) was Standardization Steering Committee chair: (1) update on good urodynamic practice[28] (2016) and (2) chronic pelvic pain[29] (2017). Figure 11.4 shows the past and present IUGA T & S chairs.

The ICS-IUGA partnership now has a collection of eight key terminology documents. These have allowed tremendous interactions between members of the working groups and between the two societies. All chairs will attest to the different "labors of love" in producing these documents. Both societies are in a strong position going forward in regard to terminology and standardization. Ongoing principles are that (1) documents be of the highest quality, contemporary, interesting, and a valuable contribution to the academic wealth of the respective organizations; and (2) definitions be accurate, concise, and—unless there is good cause.

International Continence Society (2017 to 2020)

Under ICS Standardization Chair Bernard Haylen (2016 to 2020), the emphasis was to update male-specific terminology while initiating further female-specific and other projects. Adult neurogenic LUT dysfunction[30] and nocturnal LUT function[31] were brought to completion. The first core male terminology for LUT and pelvic floor symptoms[32] and dysfunction was published in February 2019 with 390 definitions of which 211 (54%) were new. In February 2019, following the completion of the male terminology paper, the ICS Glossary (https://www.ics.org/glossary) was launched (Haylen—compiler and Glossary Editor). In 2020, published documents added a further 321 new definitions to the ICS Glossary[33] (1,455 total). These include those for

(1) single-use absorbent pads,[34] (2) female pelvic floor fistula,[35] and (3) male LUT surgery.

How Has the Terminology for Female Lower Urinary Tract Dysfunction Progressed?

The 2002 ICS Terminology Report[15] was the first and last to combine female and male terminology in a single document. It has been certainly heavily cited (more than 11,000). The missing diagnoses, voiding dysfunction, recurrent urinary tract infections, and bladder oversensitivity[20] were a problem; there had been a natural male bias to terminology because a majority of authors were urologists. Overall, male diagnoses are oriented toward sensory and voiding dysfunctions including detrusor overactivity and bladder outlet obstruction. Leading female diagnoses are urodynamic stress incontinence, POP, and voiding dysfunction. Only with a female-only core terminology report[19] could eight related areas be properly addressed. These include the terminology for prostheses and grafts[21] and native tissue surgeries,[23] surgical outcomes,[22] POP,[24] anorectal dysfunction,[25] conservative and nonpharmacologic management,[26] sexual health,[27] and pelvic floor fistulas.[35] In turn, it has provided the model for revising male terminology,[32] the benefits of which will be the update of the core female terminology document[19] and exploring specialty male areas beginning with LUT surgery. The availability of the ICS Glossary means that there is no excuse for using incorrect terminology. This is particularly relevant in rating verbal or written research presentations.

Where Is Standardization Heading?

Standardization, overall, is going from strength to strength. Both ICS and IUGA have, over time, provided an example to other societies and other specialties the importance of defining as much of the areas relevant to the society as possible. This has only been possible firstly by a culture that standardization is one of the most important aspects of the society. It relies on the dedication of those chairs and members of the ICS/IUGA Standardization Steering Committees and members of working groups over the last 50 years. Each chair and the members of each committee have provided a legacy for those who follow. Although excellent cooperation has occurred in developing reports, strong debate hasn't been omitted along the way. "The standardization reports are living documents and modification and change is always possible in the future," as reported in the 40-year ICS anniversary report. They have enhanced the stature of the ICS and IUGA as well as the citation index of its two journals, *Neurourology and Urodynamics* and the *International Urogynecology Journal*.

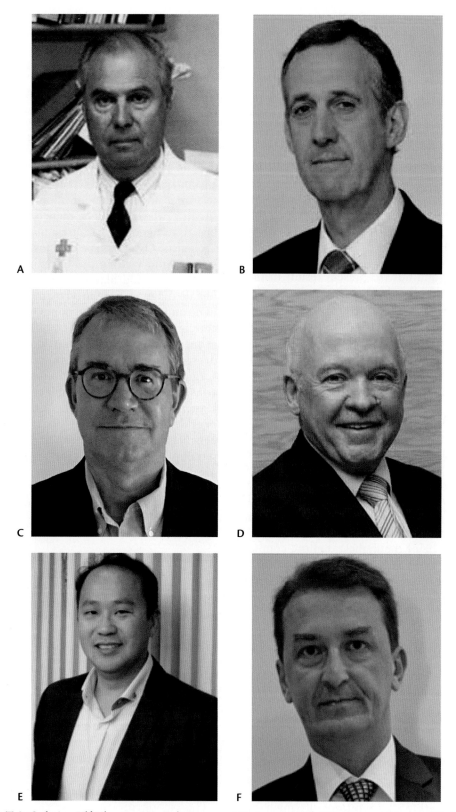

FIGURE 11.4 IUGA T & S chairs: Ulf Ulmsten (**A**), Bob Freeman (**B**), Steven Swift (**C**), Bernard Haylen (**D**), Joseph Lee (**E**), and Renud de Tayrac (**F**). (Reprinted by permission Springer: Haylen BT, Lee JKS, Freeman RM, et al. IUGA terminology and standardization: Creating and using this expanding resource. *Int Urogynecol J* 2017;28[11]:1613–1616.)

VALIDATED QUESTIONNAIRES

The ICS defined symptom as "any morbid phenomenon or departure from normal in structure, function or sensation, possibly indicative of a disease or health problem. Symptoms are either volunteered by, or elicited from the individual, or may be described by the individual's partner or caregiver."[36] Traditionally, clinician obtain the patient's history to understand the patients' symptoms in relation to their health condition. However, traditional history taking usually fails to assess the perception and impact that the patient's condition has in his or her daily activities and is at risk of clinician's bias when interpreting the severity of these symptoms. Urogynecologic symptoms, as perceived by patients, do not always provide a definitive diagnosis. Through a standardized method of data collection, patient-reported outcomes (PRO) provide clinicians with a more objective rather than subjective clinical review of patients' experiences of their symptoms.

Why Use Questionnaires?

PRO, a term introduced by the U.S. Food and Drug Administration (FDA), is any report of the status of a patient's health condition that comes directly form the patient, without interpretation of the patient's response by a clinician or anyone else.[37,38] In the United Kingdom, it is sometimes known as patient-reported outcome measures (PROM). In clinical trials, a PRO instrument or PRO questionnaire can be used to measure the impact of an intervention on one or more aspects of patient's health status (PRO concepts), ranging from purely symptomatic (e.g., vaginal bulge) to more complex concepts (e.g., ability to carry out activities of daily living), to extremely complex concepts such as quality of life, which is widely understood to be a multidomain concept with physical, psychological, and social components. Data generated by a validated PRO instrument can provide evidence of a treatment benefit or risk from the patient perspective, thereby informing the relative effectiveness and quality of treatment. The use of PRO helps provide a framework to agree on treatments and its goals as well as to inform decisions about treatment options and assess treatment outcomes.

The growing prominence of PRO is a shift in focus from clinical outcomes often related solely to survival and complications to outcomes that included the patient's perspective. PRO tools could bridge the disconnect that sometimes occur between what the observer deemed important versus what the patient considers important with regard to symptom management and the balance between relief and quality of life. The PRO's importance is evident in the wide recognition they received by major health care providers and organization, such as the FDA.

Psychometric Properties of Questionnaires

A PRO questionnaire needs to be psychometrically robust, in being able to measure the concepts it claims to measure, with a consistent measuring process and is able to depict change in health status when change had happened. The appropriately selected PRO tool would be applicable to the particular clinical problem of interest as well as to the appropriate population. It should ideally be acceptable and feasible, being not too lengthy and easy to administer, usually confirmed by pilot testing. Most PRO tools are usually designed to be self-administered through pen/paper or Web-based electronic format,[39] although telephone interviews[40] were sometimes used. An additional aspect worth considering before deciding on which questionnaire to use is the recall period (period of time patients are asked to consider in responding to a PRO item) that allows factors to affect the patients' memory. Shorter recall periods may underestimate symptom burden, especially if symptoms have diurnal or day-to-day fluctuation, placing undue burden on patients. Longer recall periods are at risk for either over- or underestimating the health state. Further, parts of certain questions from the PRO should not be used alone, or in modification, or in changing the order or content because the psychometric properties may alter the response, invalidating its score.[41]

Validated PRO instruments must demonstrate robust psychometric properties which includes reliability, validity, and responsiveness.[42] *Reliability* refers to the ability of a measure to produce similar results when assessments are repeated. Reliability is critical to ensure that change detected by the measure is due to the treatment or intervention and not due to measurement error. It reflects its ability to provide reproducible results, free from random errors of measurement. One measure of reliability is the questionnaire's *internal consistency*, which indicates how well individual items within the same domain correlate. Cronbach's alpha assesses internal consistency, with higher alphas indicating greater correlation, with Cronbach's alpha greater than 0.7 generally indicating good internal consistency.[42] *Test–retest reliability* or reproducibility or repeatability indicates how well results can be reproduced with repeated testing. It demonstrates stability of scores over time when no change is expected in the concept of interest. The Spearman correlation of coefficient and intraclass correlation coefficient are used to demonstrate reproducibility, with either correlation coefficient of at least 0.7 would indicate good test–retest reliability.[42] *Inter-rater reliability* indicates how well scores correlate when a measure is administered by different interviewers or when multiple observers rate the same phenomenon. Demonstration of inter-rater reliability is not necessary for self-administered questionnaires but is required for instruments based on observer ratings or using multiple interviewers. A correlation of at least 0.8 between raters indicate good inter-rater reliability.

Validity is the ability of an instrument to measure what it was intended to measure.[42] A measure should be validated for the specific condition or outcome for which it will be used. An instrument designed to assess stress incontinence would not be valid for overactive bladder (OAB) unless it were specifically validated in patients with OAB symptoms. Content validity, convergent validity, discriminant validity, and criterion validity are required to validate a questionnaire. *Content validity* is a qualitative assessment of whether the questionnaire captures the range of the content it is intended to measure. For example, does a measure of symptom severity capture all the symptoms that patients with a particular condition have, and if so, is the measure capturing the items in a manner meaningful to patients in a language patients can understand? To obtain content validity, patients review the measure and provide feedback as to whether the questions are clear, unambiguous, and comprehensive. Construct validity is made up of convergent and discriminant validity. Construct validity is the appropriateness of inferences made on the basis of observations or measurements, for example, test scores, specifically whether a test measures the intended construct. It examines whether the intended measures behave like the theory says a measure of that construct should behave. It is evidence that relationships among items, domains, and concepts conform to an a priori hypothesis concerning logical relationships that should exist with measures of related concepts or scores produced in similar or diverse patient groups. *Convergent validity* is a quantitative assessment of whether the questionnaire measures the theoretical construct it was intended to measure. It refers to the degree to which two measures of the constructs that theoretically should be related are in fact related. Convergent validity indicates whether a questionnaire has stronger relationships with similar concepts or variables. Stronger relationships should be seen with the most closely related constructs and weaker relationships seen with less-related constructs. *Discriminant validity* indicates whether the questionnaire can differentiate between known patient groups (e.g., those with mild, moderate, or severe disease). Generally, measures that are highly discriminative are also highly responsive. It tests whether concepts or measurements that are supposed to be unrelated are in fact unrelated. *Criterion validity* reflects the correlation between the new questionnaire and an accepted reference, or gold standard. If the gold standard measure is not available, criterion validity cannot be established. Concurrent and predictive validity are two types of criterion-related validity. Concurrent validity applies to validation studies in which two measures are administered simultaneously or approximately at the same time,[43] whereas in predictive validity,[44] one measure occurs earlier and is meant to predict a later measure. When criterion validity can be established with an existing measure, the correlation should be 0.40 to 0.70; correlations approaching 1.0 indicate that the new questionnaire may be too similar to the gold standard measure and therefore redundant.

Responsiveness is the ability of an instrument to detect change over time in the construct to be measured. An aspect of responsiveness is determining not only whether the measure detects (statistically significant) change but whether the change is meaningful to the patient. The *minimally important difference* (MID) is the smallest change in a PRO questionnaire score that would be considered meaningful or important to a patient.[45] MIDs for a given PRO measure may vary across populations, so the specific context in which the MID was established should be considered.[46] Thus, the MID score could vary, depending on population or context (e.g., conservative or surgical intervention). Determining the MID is an iterative process that involve two methodologies—the anchor-based approach and distribution-based approach. The anchor-based approach involves using an external indicator, or anchor, to classify individuals into groups according to degree and direction of change. Through an appropriate anchor, individuals are classified as having experienced no change, small change (positive or negative), or large change (positive or negative). The MID is estimated as the mean difference in PRO score that is derived from patients in the small change groups. The most commonly used anchor is patient-reported global rating of change. The distribution-based approach for estimation of MID is determined by statistical distribution of the data, using analyses such as effect size, one-half standard deviation, and standard error of measurement. It is at best an indirect method of estimating MID and is typically used when the anchor-based approach is not possible. An important disadvantage of the distribution-based method is that it does not allow direct calculation of MID, but a standardized mean difference of about 0.5 (i.e., a half standard deviation) is likely to be at least the MID,[47] which corresponds to the widely accepted criterion of a medium effect size.[48] Ideally, MIDs are established using both anchor-based (with multiple clinical and patient-based anchors) and distribution-based methods. Nevertheless, the anchor-based approach has been recommended to produce primary evidence for MID and the distribution-based approach be used to provide secondary or supportive evidence for that MID.[46]

PRO questionnaires are often used in a number of different populations and settings, but these instruments and their psychometric properties may not necessarily be transferable. Linguistic and cultural adaptation of a questionnaire can occur during the development phase before validation, or it can be done after validation in its original language. Affirmation of a PRO instrument's linguistic and cultural validity is important for its use in multinational clinical trials, not to mention during lumping of data during a meta-analysis. Linguistic and cultural adaptation of a PRO instrument generally involve two forward translations, followed by quality control procedures such as backward translation into the original language, adjudication of all translated versions with discussion by an expert panel to ensure clarity of the translated questionnaire, and followed by testing the translated instrument in monolingual or bilingual patients to ensure it measures the same concepts as the original instrument.[49]

Questionnaires Types

PRO instruments are broadly divided into generic or condition-specific questionnaires. *Generic questionnaires* are multidimensional and are designed to attribute to a broad range of population because they tend to assess physical, social, and emotional dimensions of life. Because they do not focus on specific effects of the evaluated therapeutic approach, they lack sensitivity to measure clinically important changes in patients, but they do enable assessment of health gains beyond dimensions captured by condition-specific instruments. Generic questionnaires are applicable to the widest range of patients and can facilitate comparisons between disease and nondisease states as well as comparisons across different patient populations. *Condition-specific questionnaires* ask questions that are sensitive to changes in health status that are related to a given disease, disability or surgery. By design, they are able to detect small changes in health or functional status and therefore be more precise at evaluating the efficacy of treatment specific to the target condition. In addition, questionnaires can be divided into additional five other categories, namely screening questionnaires; symptom questionnaires that measure presence intensity discomfort and impact of specific symptoms; quality-of-life questionnaires; sexual function questionnaires; and measures of the patient's satisfaction, expectations, goal achievements, or work productivity measures. Clinicians often use a range of complementary questionnaires to fully capture different aspects of the patient's experiences of PFD. Some of the more commonly used questionnaires are listed in Table 11.1, together with their respective MIDs.

Screening or Detection

Screeners or screening questionnaires that may be used to detect patients who might have POP or PFD before a clinical examination has its origin in 1989 when the World Health Organization (WHO) conducted a meeting to develop specific questions about chronic obstetric morbidities.[68] These final seven questions could identify 80% to 90% of moderate to severe vaginal prolapse.

- Do you feel anything coming out of your vagina?
- Do you have pain or difficulty in urinating?
- Is it uncomfortable down below?

- Do you have a feeling of heaviness?
- Do you feel any swelling down below when you urinate or move your bowels?
- Do you need to manipulate it to urinate or defecate?
- Do you have any difficulty with intercourse?

A single question screening[69] "Do you have a bulge or something falling out that you can see or feel in your vaginal area?" has a 96% sensitivity and 79% specificity for prolapse beyond level of hymen. The Epidemiology of Prolapse and Incontinence Questionnaire[70] screens well for pelvic floor disorders, including prolapse, stress incontinence, OAB, and anal incontinence. Its positive and negative predictive value for prolapse is 76% and 97%, respectively; stress incontinence 88% and 87%, respectively; OAB 77% and 90%, respectively; and anal incontinence 61% and 91%, respectively. Nevertheless, these screening tools should not be misinterpreted as diagnostic tools even when their cutoff scores were met.

Symptom Questionnaires

Symptom questionnaires generally sought to assess the presence, severity, and bother of a particular pelvic floor symptom or groups of pelvic floor symptoms. Commonly used symptom questionnaires for specific LUT symptoms, those covering multiple domains including prolapse, as well as bowel symptoms are described in the following text.

Lower urinary tract patient-reported outcomes

Bladder diary is a record of patient-completed information regarding urinary and voiding habits. It is known as frequency volume chart when it provides information on frequency of micturition and void volumes only. Bladder diary generally includes information from the frequency volume chart as well as additional insights including urgency and incontinence episodes as well as type and amount of fluid intake completed prospectively. Some diaries incorporate severity of urgency symptoms, nature of events at the time of leakage (rushing to toilet or physical exertion), as well as pads usage. A further unstandardized nature of bladder diary is its length of record. In general, reproducibility improves as the duration of self-reporting increases, although patient compliance tends to also decrease with longer diary duration. Reliability of a 24-hour diary is generally poor. In patients with OAB, a 7-day diary has better reproducibility than a 3-day diary, whereas a 3-day diary has similar reproducibility to a 7-day diary in patients with stress incontinence. The electronic diary has some advantages over the paper diary, including patient prompt or reminder and automated calculation of some parameters. Accurately completed bladder diary contains quantifiable urinary symptoms, and they offer

TABLE 11.1

Frequently Used Patient-Reported Outcomes in Urogynecology and Their Minimally Important Differences

PELVIC FLOOR PRO	CONTEXT	MID
ICIQ-UI SF[50]	Nonsurgical treatment UI	−4
ICIQ-UI SF[51]	MUS treatment 12 mo/24 mo	−5/−4
OAB-q subscale[52]	OAB medication treatment	−10
POP-SS[53]	Prolapse surgery	−1.5
APFQ[54]	Bladder domain for MUS surgery	1.3
APFQ[54]	Prolapse domain for LSC	1.0
PFDI[55]	♀ Pelvic floor symptoms	45 or 15%
UDI[56]	Nonsurgical SUI treatment	−11
UDI[57]	Urge-dominant treatment	−35
UDI[58]	Continence surgery	−30 to −14
	Pelvic floor surgery	−22 to −16
	Vaginal support pessary	−28
POPDI[58]	Pelvic floor surgery	−44 to −21
	Vaginal support pessary	−16
CRADI[58]	Pelvic floor surgery	−37 to −14
	Vaginal support pessary	−25
CRADI[59]	Treatment for fecal incontinence	−11
CCFIS[60] or Wexner	♀ With bowel leakage, PFMT	−3 to −2
SMIS[60] or Vaizey	♀ With bowel leakage, PFMT	−5 to −3
ABLE[61]	♀ With bowel leakage	−0.20
FIQL[60]	♀ With bowel leakage, PFMT	1.1−1.2
PFIQ[55]	♀ Pelvic floor symptoms	36 or 12%
UIQ[56]	Nonsurgical SUI treatment	−16
UIQ[58]	Continence surgery	−28 to −14
	Pelvic floor surgery	−37 to −31
	Vaginal support pessary	−17
POPIQ[58]	Pelvic floor surgery	−40 to −27
	Vaginal support pessary	−29
CRAIQ[58]	Pelvic floor surgery	−34 to −6
	Vaginal support pessary	−31
CRAIQ[59]	Treatment for fecal incontinence	−18
Short Form 6 Dimension (SF-6D)[62]	♀ Pelvic floor surgery/PFMT	0.026
EQ-5D[62]	♀ Pelvic floor surgery/PFMT	0.025
VAS[63,64]	Non traumatic- and/or traumatic pain	9−13 mm
FSFI[65]	♀ Sexual dysfunction	26.55
PISQ[66]	♀ OAB and ♀ POP/UI surgery	6
PISQ-IR[67]	♀ Sexual dysfunction	2.68

UI, urinary incontinence; MUS, midurethral sling; LSC, laparoscopic sacrocolpopexy; PFMT, pelvic floor muscle training.

important PRO that are commonly reported in OAB drug trials.

The use of PROM in urinary incontinence might well be the most standardized among pelvic floor disorders. In recognition of the need for a simple universal questionnaire to measure PRO across populations with different pelvic floor disorders, the ICS developed the International Consultation on Incontinence Modular Questionnaire (ICIQ) in 1998, with instruments assessing LUT symptoms, vaginal symptoms, bowel symptoms, and urinary incontinence.

The *ICIQ-Urinary Incontinence Short Form* (ICIQ-UI SF)[71] is a validated, self-administered, responsive questionnaire that includes an unscored self-diagnostic item to assess perceived cause of urinary leakage and three scored items that evaluate the frequency, severity, and impact of quality of life on urinary incontinence, with a total score ranging from 0 to 21, divided into four categories of severity: slight (1 to 5), moderate (6 to 12), severe (13 to 18), and very severe (19 to 21). Its brevity makes ICIQ-UI SF an ideal research and audit tool. It is intended for continence research, providing robust measures at baseline and follow-up in prevalence and investigative studies, and commonly used as a complement to other surgical pelvic floor outcome data. The recommended MID for ICIQ-UI SF was −4 for women undergoing nonsurgical treatments[50] for urinary incontinence, −5 and −4 for women who underwent surgery[51] for their stress incontinence postoperatively at 12 months and 24 months, respectively.

Incontinence Severity Index (ISI) is a simple severity index with only two questions,[72] with the total score created by multiplying the score of reported frequency (four levels) by the amount of leakage (two levels). The reliable and sensitive ISI has been validated against pad weighing as a gold standard, used in epidemiologic surveys, as well as routine clinical practice. Although the ISI and ICIQ-UI SF have a high degree of correlation between themselves,[73] both evaluate frequency and volume of leakage, ICIQ-UI SF assesses impact on quality of life, whereas the ISI does not.

Overactive Bladder Questionnaire (OAB-q) is self-administered 33-item questionnaire that assesses symptom bother and health-related quality-of-life impact of OAB.[74] Its 8-item symptom bother scale includes frequency, urgency, nocturia, and incontinence symptoms. Its 25 items of health-related quality-of-life impact of OAB domains include coping, concern/worry, sleep, and social interaction. Each question corresponds to a 6-point Likert scale from "none of the time" to "all the time," with total score for each domain ranging from 0 to 100. The OAB-q has two versions of 4-week and 1-week recall. The OAB-q is a reliable valid responsive instrument that discriminates between normal and clinically diagnosed continent and incontinence OAB patients. The MID for OAB-q[52]

was recommended to be 10 points for all OAB-q subscales. Its validated short form (Overactive Bladder Questionnaire Short Form[75] has 13 items and may be more practical for clinical use.

The *Patient Perception of Bladder Condition* (PPBC) questionnaire[76] is a widely used single-item questionnaire that evaluate the patients' global subjective impression of their current urinary problems, rating it on a 6-point Likert scale ranging from "no problems at all" to "many severe problems." The PPBC has good test–retest reliability and construct validity and is responsive to change. Used in several drug trials to evaluate treatment effect, the typical PPBC score change the baseline score typically ranges from −2 to +2, with negative values indicating improvement. Nevertheless, the PPBC reflects a single time point, can be open to the patients' interpretation of their "problems," and no MID was identified.

Urgency is the principal symptom of OAB, and therefore, assessing the symptom and its impact is important. One potential reason why measuring urgency is challenging is the difficulty in distinguishing a normal desire to urinate (urge) and the difficulty to postpone the need to urinate (urgency).[77,78] Sometimes, this compulsion to urinate may be sudden and could be accompanied by fear of leakage or pain but not universally so. Further, some OAB patients are unaware of their urge related incontinence. Nevertheless, *Patient Perception of Intensity of Urgency Scale* (PPIUS) was developed as a single-item tool[79] to evaluate female patient perception of urgency intensity, using a 5-point scale. PPIUS has good test–retest reliability and convergent validity and is responsive.[80] Despite being useful, PPIUS might be inconvenient because it requires records of more than 3 to 7 days to assess degree of urgency at each micturition.

The O'Leary-Sant *Interstitial Cystitis Symptom Index* (ICSI) and the Interstitial Cystitis Problem Index (ICPI) measure urinary and pain symptoms and assess how problematic symptoms are for patients with interstitial cystitis.[81] It contains 4 items that measures severity of day–night frequency, urgency, and bladder pain over the past month, with a score ranging from 0 to 20. Scores of 0 to 6, 7 to 14, and 15 to 20 are indicative of mild, moderate, and severe symptoms, respectively. It has good psychometric properties, including test–retest reliability, internal consistency, construct validity, and sensitivity to change.[82] Despite ICSI's high sensitivity, its low specificity undermines its performance as a diagnostic tool, and the reliability of its 1-month recall has not yet been tested. Nevertheless, ICSI and ICPI can be used to grade baseline symptom severity and monitor response to treatment.

Defined as waking to pass urine during the main sleep period, nocturia is among the most bothersome LUT symptoms, owing to its sleep interruption. Given that the perception of the impact of nocturia can vary among individuals and may not correlate with symptom severity, assessing patients' perspectives is therefore an important component of measuring treatment efficacy. The *Impact of Nighttime Urination* (INTU) was developed as a 10-item questionnaire that assesses the impacts of nocturia on health and functioning.[83] It has a same-day recall period and includes six items that assess the effects of nocturia on daytime activities and four items that measure the nighttime impact of nocturia. It was shown to be psychometrically robust, with concurrent criterion validity measured against the Pittsburgh Sleep Quality Index as well as Nocturia Quality of Life. A 14-point reduction[84] in INTU appears to be meaningful to patients reporting a reduction of at least one nocturia episode.

Female voiding dysfunction is characterized by abnormally slow and/or incomplete micturition based on abnormally slow urine flow rates and/or abnormally high postvoid residuals which often needs to be repeated for confirmation. Abnormal voiding symptoms are common in women without objective voiding difficulties, with several screening tools[85] generally lacking sufficient sensitivity in prediction of female voiding dysfunction. Nevertheless, the most widely used instrument to measure patient-reported female voiding is the *International Prostate Symptom Score* (IPSS). The IPSS was based on the seven original questions of the American Urological Association Symptom Index (AUASI) plus an additional bother score.[86] It assesses severity of LUT symptoms, including incomplete bladder emptying, frequency of urination, intermittency, urgency, weak stream, straining, and nocturia, with each question rated from 0 (not at all) to 5 (almost always) and grading the severity as mild (0 to 7), moderate (8 to 19), and severe (20 to 35). The bother score, rated from 0 (delighted) to 6 (terrible), was not included in the analysis. The self-administered IPSS has a recall period of 4 weeks and was validated by the multidisciplinary measurement committee of American Urological Association on men, and the MID was thought to be 3.1 as it fell within the 95% confidence interval of the group who expressed they hadn't experienced any change in symptoms, although a recent study[87] recommended an MID of 5.2. The IPSS was deemed to be psychometrically robust in women,[88] given its excellent internal consistency, good constructive validity, as well as being responsive, with a mean reduction of 4 points[89] on drug trials. A voiding-to-storage ratio (IPSS-V/S)[90] of ≥1.33 was found to have a high negative predictive value (97.4%) for female voiding dysfunction.

Prolapse patient-reported outcomes

Optimal evaluation of a patient with vaginal prolapse requires a comprehensive review of her pelvic floor symptoms and an assessment of how these symptoms affect her quality of life.[91] The most valid way of measuring the presence, severity, and impact of pelvic floor symptoms on a patient's activities and well-being is through the use of psychometrically robust self-administered questionnaires.

Pelvic Organ Prolapse Symptom Score (POP-SS)[92] was developed to assess prolapse symptoms before and after treatment, consisting of 7 items each with a 5-point Likert response ranging from 0 (never) to 4 (all the time) to allow reporting on how often patient report their symptoms. It has good internal consistency and construct validity and is sensitive to change, being able to detect changes in patients undergoing pelvic floor muscle training and surgical intervention for prolapse, with the varying magnitude of changes dependent on the actual intervention and MID of 1.5 considered to best correspond to the patients' satisfaction.[53]

Although reported symptom of vaginal prolapse is most commonly the sensation of a bulge, many patients also report combined symptoms of multiple pelvic floor disorders. Even if individual bowel, bladder, or prolapse symptoms were mild, their combination could have a profound cumulative effect on a patient's quality of life. The *Australian Pelvic Floor Questionnaire* (APFQ) has wide coverage because it assesses presence, bother, as well as impact on quality of life on all pelvic floor symptoms. It has 42 items divided into four domains of bladder, bowel, prolapse, and sexual function with a 4-point scoring system to assess frequency, severity, and bothersomeness. The self- or interviewer-administered APFQ[93] has robust psychometric properties and a recall period of 4 weeks with a recommended MID of 1.0 in the prolapse domain and 1.3 in the bladder domain following prolapse or continence surgery, respectively.[54] The self-administered version is preferable when evaluating treatment outcomes independently of health care providers.

Symptoms of vaginal prolapse often includes interrelated clinical conditions such as urinary incontinence, fecal incontinence, prolapse, and voiding dysfunction. The *Pelvic Floor Distress Inventory* (PFDI) was developed as a condition-specific PRO tool based on two validated questionnaires, the Urogenital Distress Inventory (UDI) and the Incontinence Impact Questionnaire (IIQ). The PFDI[55] has a total of 46 items from three subscales that consist of UDI, Pelvic Organ Prolapse Distress Inventory (POPDI), and ColoRectal-Anal Distress Inventory (CRADI). Although the PFDI was reliable, reproducible, and responsive, it was time-consuming to complete, taking up to 23 minutes. The short form[94] of PFDI has a total of 20 items consisting of UDI-6, POPDI-6, and CRADI-8 with a recall period of 3 months and is shown in Figure 11.5. Each subscale's questions has a bother score ranging from 1 "not at all" to 4 "quite a bit." The PFDI-20 was validated and correlates well[40] with its long form, and

Pelvic Floor Distress Inventory (PFDI-20)

Instructions: Please answer all of the questions in the following survey. These questions will ask you if you have certain bowel, bladder, or pelvic symptoms and, if you do, **how much they bother you**. Answer these by circling the appropriate number. While answering these questions, please consider your symptoms over the last 3 months. The PFDI-20 has 20 items and 3 scales of your symptoms. All items use the following format with a response scale from 0 to 4.

Symptom scale: 0 = not present 1 = not at all 2 = somewhat 3 = moderately 4 = quite a bit

	NO	YES
Pelvic Organ prolapse Distress Inventory 6 (POPDI-6) *Do you*		
1. Usually experience pressure in the lower abdomen?	0	1 2 3 4
2. Usually experience heaviness or dullness in the pelvic area?	0	1 2 3 4
3. Usually have a bulge or something falling out that you can see or feel in your vaginal area?	0	1 2 3 4
4. Ever have to push on the vagina or around the rectum to have or complete a bowel movement?	0	1 2 3 4
5. Usually experience a feeling of incomplete bladder emptying?	0	1 2 3 4
6. Ever have to push up on a bulge in the vaginal area with your fingers to start or complete urination?	0	1 2 3 4
Colorectal-Anal Distress Inventory 8 (CRAD-8) *Do you*	**NO**	**YES**
7. Feel you need to strain too hard to have a bowel movement?	0	1 2 3 4
8. Feel you have not completely emptied your bowels at the end of a bowel movement?	0	1 2 3 4
9. Usually lose stool beyond your control if your stool is well formed?	0	1 2 3 4
10. Usually lose stool beyond your control if your stool is loose?	0	1 2 3 4
11. Usually lose gas from the rectum beyond your control?	0	1 2 3 4
12. Usually have pain when you pass your stool?	0	1 2 3 4
Urinary Distress Inventory 6 (UDI-6) *Do you*	**NO**	**YES**
15. Usually experience frequent urination?	0	1 2 3 4
16. Usually experience urine leakage associated with a feeling of urgency, that is, a strong sensation of needing to go to the bathroom?	0	1 2 3 4
17. Usually experience urine leakage related to coughing, sneezing or laughing?	0	1 2 3 4
18. Usually experience small amounts of urine leakage (that is, drops)?	0	1 2 3 4
19. Usually experience difficulty emptying your bladder?	0	1 2 3 4
20. Usually experience pain or discomfort in the lower abdomen or genital region?	0	1 2 3 4

Scoring the PFDI-20

Scale Scores: Obtain the mean value of all of the answered items within the corresponding scale (possible value 0 to 4) and then multiply by 25 to obtain the scale score (range 0 to 100). Missing items are dealt with by using the mean from answered items only.

PFSI-20 Summary Score: Add the scores from the 3 scales together to obtain the summary score (range 0 to 300).

FIGURE 11.5 The PFDI-20 and its scoring.[55]

its summary score could also be converted to PFDI. Depending on the target population as well as context, the recommended MID for PFDI-20 (a change of ≥45 points or 15%) and its subscales were listed in Table 11.1. Designed specifically for women with POP, PFDI-20 is the most commonly used PRO tool in studies assessing prolapse treatments, whether surgical or conservative, given its coverage of urinary, colorectal, and prolapse domains. Each subscale of PFDI-20 has also been validated individually and can be used separately. This flexibility allows evaluation of POP interventions with subgroup comparisons of women with or without urinary incontinence and with or without bowel dysfunction as well as assessing postoperative de novo urinary or bowel symptoms.

UDI is a validated, reliable, sensitive, 19-item questionnaire that assesses the presence of irritative, obstructive discomfort, and stress incontinence symptoms and their degree of bother on a 4-point scale.[95] It was not only designed to evaluate urinary incontinence but has also been used for assessment of LUT symptoms in women with prolapse. Within the PFDI, 9 additional questions related to LUT symptoms were added to the original 19 items from UDI. UDI-6 has a high correlation with its longer form and much easier to administer given it has only 6 items.[96] It is responsive to change

in women who underwent surgery for incontinence or prolapse.[97] Both forms of UDI have compromised validity for women with urinary incontinence without a urodynamic diagnosis. Depending on context, the MIDs[56-58] for UDI were listed in Table 11.1.

Anorectal patient-reported outcomes

Used as a medical aid, the *Bristol Stool Chart* is a pictorial chart[98] that classify feces into seven consistencies. It has widespread recognition and face validity despite not being validated as an outcome measure. Its reported change in category may not represent sufficient degree of precision. A *bowel diary* encourages patients to prospectively record their anorectal symptoms, although there is no consensus on what ought to be included. Nevertheless, it could include frequency of bowel movements or anal incontinence episodes, fecal urgency, amount and consistency of fecal incontinence, flatal incontinence, passive staining or soiling, pad changes and their degree of soiling, straining or assisted measures to defecate, laxative use, as well as diet and fluid intake. Unstandardized bowel diaries may not capture[99,100] all anorectal symptoms and underscores the importance of patient-centered measures that capture the full range of symptoms from women.

Also known as the Wexner Score, the *Cleveland Clinic Florida Incontinence Score* (CCFIS) was initially developed as a clinical aid and became one of the most widely used severity index[101] for both fecal incontinence and constipation. It contains five items pertaining to frequency of incontinence with different stool consistencies, use of a pad, and lifestyle alteration. The incontinence score ranges from 0 to 20, whereas the constipation score ranges from 0 to 30, with values >15 defining constipation's presence. Easily understood by patients, the CCFIS can be gathered quickly during consultation to quantify anorectal symptoms and is useful for measurement of treatment efficacy. However, it fails to capture the symptom of fecal urgency, volume of leakage, or impact on quality of life.[102]

The *St. Mark's Incontinence Score* (SMIS), also known as Vaizey Score, not only incorporates the same five questions of CCFIS but also captures the symptoms of urgency as well as quantifying the impact of constipation medications on symptoms of incontinence, in its 7-item questionnaire.[103] The SMIS defines fecal urgency as less than 15 minutes to reach the toilet, but most healthy women reported being able to defer for 5 to 9 minutes, weakening its construct validity. The SMIS is reliable and used to evaluate treatment outcomes related to fecal incontinence and constipation. The estimated MID for CRADI[59] is -11, CCFIS is -3 to -2 and -5 to -3 for SMIS, as shown in Table 11.1.[60] It should be noted both CCFIS and SMIS were developed without patient input, running the risk of not capturing all symptoms that are important to patients.

The Fecal Incontinence Severity Index (FISI)[104] is a reliable tool used in evaluation of treatment for fecal incontinence, assesses severity in four domains of gas leakage, mucous, liquid, and solid stool. Its weighted summary score reflects a combination of surgeon and patients' results, making scoring cumbersome and sometimes difficult to interpret. The FISI does not characterize urgency or volume of leakage. The FISI also does not have some measure of impact, unlike CCFIS or SMIS which also captures use of pads, lifestyle alteration. The Fecal Incontinence and Constipation Assessment[105] is one of the most comprehensively validated instruments for evaluating fecal incontinence. It captures volume of stool leakage, severity of incontinence, fecal urgency, constipation, as well as quality of life in its 98-item questionnaire, which makes it impractical for routine clinical use. It incorporates the Bristol Stool Scale, which may be useful as a surrogate for colonic testing and is also able to distinguish functional constipation and constipation predominant irritable bowel syndrome. Its responsiveness has not been evaluated. The *Accidental Bowel Leakage Evaluation* (ABLE)[106] is a psychometrically robust, validated 18-item questionnaire that captures patient-centered bowel leakage symptoms, including predictability, awareness, control, emptying, and discomfort, in addition to volume, frequency, severity of leakage, as well as urgency. Its recommended MID[61] is -0.20.

Health-Related Quality of Life Questionnaires

Health-Related Quality of Life (HRQoL) refers to a person's total sense of well-being and usually has multiple dimensions including their physical, social, and emotional health. It is an individual's perception of their position in life, within the context of the culture and value systems in which they live in, in relation to their concerns, standards, goals, and expectations. HRQoL instruments generally have domains related to various aspects of a patient's life, including physical health, sleep, energy, emotions, work life, sex life, and social life. Individual pelvic floor symptoms could have distinct impact on HRQoL, and objective improvement pelvic floor interventions may not necessarily come with improvement in HRQoL, underscoring the importance of HRQoL as an important outcome measure for pelvic floor interventions. HRQoL is either generic or condition specific. OAB-q and INTU are earlier described examples of condition-specific symptoms questionnaires that have incorporated HRQoL domains.

The *Medical Outcomes Study Questionnaire Short Form–36* (SF-36)[107] has been used extensively for quality-of-life assessment of men and women across a variety of health conditions. The SF-36 has eight domains pertaining to physical conditioning, bodily pain, role limitations due to physical health problems, role limitations due to personal or emotional problems, general mental health, social functioning, energy/fatigue, and general health perceptions. Notably, the SF-36 does not address sexual functioning. SF-12 also includes eight concepts, whereas SF-6 has six concepts, namely physical and social functioning, role limitation, pain, mental health, and vitality. Although SF surveys are often used as a gold standard for HRQoL measures, it is generally not responsive to change in women with pelvic floor disorders.

The *EuroQol 5 Dimensional Questionnaire* (EQ-5D) is a disease-unspecific, preference-based instrument[108] that measures a patient's health status. It has a descriptive HRQoL scale with five domains of mobility, self-care, usual activities, pain/discomfort, and anxiety/depression, with each subscale graded on a 3-point (EQ-5D-3L)[108] or 5-point (EQ-5D-5L) Likert severity scale giving rise to 243 health states for EQ-5D-3L or 3,125 health states for EQ-5D-5L. Figure 11.6 shows the EQ-5D-3L. EQ-5D has a second part, which is a 20-cm vertical visual analog scale (VAS) that values health status from optimal (100 points) to worst (0 points). Valuation algorithms exists for several countries or regions that generate society-specific preferences that reflect how health is valued. These value sets

EQ-5D-3L – Health Questionnaire

Instructions: By placing a checkmark in one box in each group below, please indicate which statements best describe your own health state today.

1. Mobility:	☐ I have no problems in walking about
	☐ I have some problems in walking about
	☐ I am confined to bed
2. Self-Care:	☐ I have no problems with self-care
	☐ I have some problems washing or dressing myself
	☐ I am unable to wash or dress myself
3. Usual Activities (e.g. work, study, housework, family, or leisure activities):	☐ I have no problems with performing my usual activities
	☐ I have some problems with performing my usual activities
	☐ I am unable to perform my usual activities
4. Pain/Discomfort:	☐ I have no pain or discomfort
	☐ I have moderate pain or discomfort
	☐ I have extreme pain or discomfort
5. Anxiety/Depression:	☐ I am not anxious or depressed
	☐ I am moderately anxious or depressed
	☐ I am extremely anxious or depressed

Best Imaginable
Health State
100
90
80
70
60
50
40
30
20
10
0
Worst Imaginable
Health State

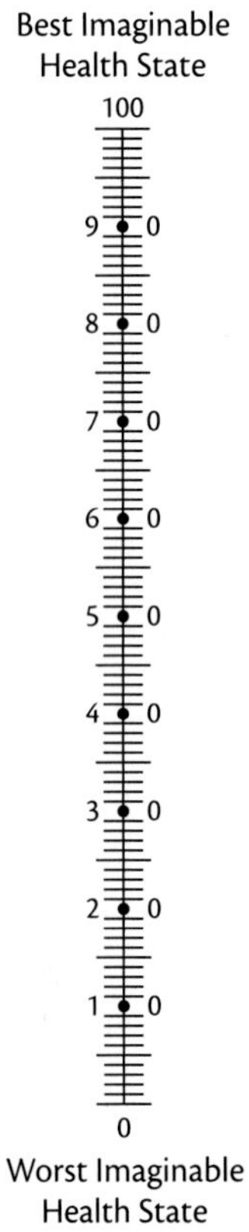

To help people say how good or bad a health state is, we have drawn a scale (rather like a thermometer) on which the best state you can imagine is marked 100 and the worst state you can imagine is marked 0.

We would like you to indicate on this scale how good or bad your own health is today, in your opinion. Please do this by drawing a line from the box below to whichever point on the scale indicates how good or bad your health state is today.

6. Your own Health State Today:	

FIGURE 11.6 The EQ-5D-3L.

are used to convert an individual's EQ-5D health state (their EQ-5D score) to a single summary index value that is weighted to societal preferences, with 1 being optimum health and 0 being death. By having EQ-5D scores before and after treatment, EQ-5D is a utility preference score designed to measure quality-adjusted life years (QALY), by combining its utility score (summary index weighted to societal preferences) with life expectancy, and can thus be used to quantify benefits of any given treatment. EQ-5D is a valid measure of HRQoL in women with prolapse and urinary incontinence. Its recommended MID[62] is a difference in utility score of 0.03.

The VAS is a simple, reproducible, single-item continuous scale originally developed for pain but recently adopted by gynecologists[109] to assess severity and bother of prolapse. When used as a PRO tool for assessing pain, it entails either a 0 to 10 numeric rating scale or 100-mm horizontal visual scale, with those ≤30 mm having mild pain, 31 to 69 mm having moderate pain, ≥70 mm having severe pain,[110] and an MID[63,64] estimated to be 9 to 13 mm irrespective of sex, age, or cause of pain. VAS has a poor correlation between subjective degree of incontinence measured on 10 cm VAS and urine leakage measured by pad testing.[111] Although VAS cannot be directly compared with

complex validated PRO that investigates a wide range of pelvic floor symptoms, it was used to assess the subjective impact of prolapse symptoms because VAS was found to be correlated with prolapse grade[112] on clinical examination and ultrasound. Nevertheless, VAS's sensitivity to change in regard to prolapse bother as well as its MID has not been determined.

Due to its inherent design, a generic questionnaire mandates nonspecific questioning and its scoring systems are applicable to widely varying states of health and therefore lack sensitivities when applied to women with non–life-threatening conditions like urinary incontinence or prolapse. Condition-specific questionnaires overcome this issue by assessing, with greater complexity and accuracy, the impact of specific medical complaints.

The *Pelvic Floor Impact Questionnaire* (PFIQ) was developed together with PFDI, based on two validated questionnaires, the UDI and the IIQ. The PFIQ long form has 93 items from its three subscales that consists of Urinary Impact Questionnaire (UIQ), Pelvic Organ Prolapse Impact Questionnaire (POPIQ), and ColoRectal-Anal Impact Questionnaire (CRAIQ),[55] whereas its short form PFIQ-7 has 21 items across the three identical domains.[94] Their conversion formula showed excellent goodness of fit. Within the PFIQ, 1 additional question was added to IIQ's original 30 items, regarding the effect of bladder bowel, or vaginal symptoms on the patient's relationship with her partner. Both forms of PFDI and PFIQ are designed to be companion questionnaires. Both forms of PFIQ have a recall period of 3 months and are valid, reliable, and responsive instruments that evaluate impact in HRQoL of prolapse-related symptoms. A change of ≥36 points (12%) has been suggested as MID for PFIQ.[55] Depending on context, the MIDs for the three subscales of PFIQ-7 were listed in Table 11.1.

Designed to evaluate psychosocial impact of urinary incontinence in women, the IIQ[95] has 30 items and four subscales of physical activity, travel, social relationships, and emotional health, with mild, moderate, and severe levels of urinary incontinence defined when IIQ is <50, 50 to 70, and >70, respectively.[113] The patient responds to each item based on the degree to which their urinary incontinence affects each activity or feeling from not at all to greatly. Its short form, IIQ-7 has 7 items. Both forms are psychometrically robust and are often used as companion tools to UDI. IIQ-7 is responsive to change in women who underwent surgery for incontinence or prolapse.[97] The MIDs for UIQ, a modified form of IIQ within PFIQ, depending on context are listed in Table 11.1.

The *Fecal Incontinence Quality of Life Scale* (FIQL) has 29 items over four domains pertaining to lifestyle, coping behavior, depression and self-perception, and embarrassment. Developed by a panel of researchers and colorectal surgeons as a project of American Society of Colon Rectal Surgeons (ASCRS), and sometimes known as the ASCRS or Rockwood questionnaire,[114] it is a popular instrument to measure the effect on quality of life of treatment for individuals with fecal incontinence. It has good internal consistency, good discriminant validity, satisfactory test–retest reliability, and significant correlation with SF-36 subscales. The FIQL has not been tested in asymptomatic controls, restricting its capability as a screening tool. The FIQL has an estimated MID[60] 1.1 to 1.2 and is generally regarded as the preferred quality-of-life instrument for patients with fecal incontinence.

Sexual Function Questionnaires

Defined by the WHO as a state of physical, emotional, mental, and social well-being in relation to sexuality and sexual function[115] is not merely the absence of disease, dysfunction, or infirmity; female sexual health is a reflection of the patient's global well-being. Given its complexity, especially when various aspects such as psychological, social, and physiological are involved, female sexual dysfunction (FSD) can be difficult to diagnose. There could be differences in perceptions between clinicians and patients when discussing sexual outcomes. Aspects of sexuality of importance to patients may not be easily communicated to clinicians, and those that are more comfortable for discussion may not have an important influence on true change in sexual outcomes. Validated sexual PRO instruments can provide a means to monitor outcomes following pelvic floor interventions.

Developed by a panel of experts and initially validated in female sexual arousal disorder (FSAD) population, the *Female Sexual Function Index* (FSFI)[116] is a 19-item generic sexual questionnaire across six domains of arousal, desire, lubrication, orgasm, pain, and satisfaction. It is a psychometrically sound sexual function instrument that has demonstrated reliability and validity in a variety of populations, including female orgasmic disorder (FOD), hypoactive sexual desire disorder (HSDD), women with chronic pelvic pain, and postmenopausal women. With a cutoff value of 26.55 that could differentiate women with or without sexual dysfunction,[65] the FSFI could help clinicians understand if pelvic floor interventions contribute to FSD and identify FSD postoperatively. It is widely used as a screening tool and outcome measure for FSD and could also detect patients with FSAD, FOD, or HSDD, given a cutoff score of 5 was established on the desire domain to differentiate women with and without HSDD.[117] However, its questions are only applicable for women with a current sexual partner and not meant to be administered to women not sexually active. Further, the response of "not having intercourse" does not include possible reason; therefore, the FSFI might not detect patients that did not have sexual intercourse for non–FSD-related reasons, including partners sexual problems. Despite its quantifiable measure of clinical sexual dysfunction, it is not a clinically diagnostic tool because it has no measure of distress that provide insight into degree and type of sexual dysfunction, not to mention diagnosis of FSD also needs to rule out other medical diagnoses and medications that can impact sexual functioning. The diagnostic criteria of *Diagnostic and Statistical Manual of Mental Disorders*[118] and International Classification of Diseases[119] require sexual complaints to be associated with significant amount of distress over a representative period of usually 6 months or several months, whereas the recall period of FSFI is 4 weeks. Despite its existing strengths, there is some missing psychometric information on FSFI,[120] including measurement error, responsiveness, and cross-cultural validity; running the risk, it may not be possible to ensure FSFI could be interpreted similarly in different cultures, although its responsiveness[121] was later confirmed.

Designed to evaluate sexual functioning in sexually active heterosexual women with POP and/or urinary incontinence and their impact on sexual function, both long[122] and short[123] forms of *Pelvic Organ Prolapse/Urinary Incontinence Sexual Questionnaire* (PISQ) are psychometrically robust. Scores of 12-item short-form PISQ-12 predicts scores of its longer 31-item PISQ. Both versions cover behavioral, emotional, physical, and partner domains with Likert scale from 0 (always) to 4 (never), with higher scores indicating better sexual functioning, and its MID[66] was recommended to be 6. The PISQ-12 is often the companion questionnaire for PDFI and PFIQ. Both forms of PISQ excluded women who are not sexually active (penetrative intercourse), irrespective of whether that's due to lack of partner or their PFD, and they are not validated in women with anal incontinence. Further, it is not suitable for women in a same-sex relationship, does not screen for other sexual activity, and may not comprehensively capture important surgery-specific sexual dysfunction.

Designed to address the limitations of PISQ, the Pelvic Organ Prolapse/Urinary Incontinence Sexual Questionnaire IUGA-Revised (PISQ-IR)[124] is a condition-specific, psychometrically robust, validated questionnaire suitable for women with urinary incontinence, anal incontinence, and POP who are sexually active as well as those who are not. Sexually active women answer 21 questions in six domains, whereas nonsexually active women answer 12 questions in four domains. Figure 11.7 shows the PISQ-IR. The particularly distinctive features of PISQ-IR include questions for sexually inactive women, who can additionally indicate reasons for sexual inactivity. It allows researchers to analyze patients who are sexually active but without a partner and incorporates gender-neutral questions. The PISQ-IR Summary Score can be calculated only for sexually active women because criterion validity was not met[125] in the nonsexually active group. PISQ-IR Summary Score of 2.68 was determined to be the optimal cutoff for distinguishing[67] between dysfunctional and nondysfunctional women. Possibly due to its user-friendly, uncomplicated scoring system, FSFI is more commonly used at present; although it is designed as a screening tool, it is useful for measuring outcomes. PISQ-IR has a more complicated scoring system, but its responsiveness applies to both sexually active and inactive women, not to mention it is designed and validated as a condition-specific PRO instrument, reaffirming the principle that condition-specific questionnaires have higher sensitivity to change compared to generic questionnaires.

Satisfaction Expectation Questionnaires

It is the patient's perspective, regarding their health status, that drives contact with the medical field or intervention. The PRO instrument on patient's expectations and satisfaction directly evaluates patient's perception regarding effectiveness of their treatments and whether their therapeutic goals has been fulfilled. Patient's expectations could include positive goals of symptom alleviation, improved quality of life, as well as negative fears of de novo symptoms, prolapse recurrence, or surgical complications. Divergence of the patient's stated expectations from what can be reasonable achieved

from medical interventions, could be mitigated against through careful counseling, given that the patient's satisfaction is the bottom line. All patient-centered outcomes are combined in Expectations, Goal Setting, Goal Achievement, and Satisfaction, which has been suggested to become the fourth dimension[126] for the assessment of PFD along with the physical findings, symptoms, and quality-of-life outcomes.

Goal Attainment Scaling (GAS)[127] is a technique for measuring goal achievement after treatment, commonly used in psychiatry but has recently been applied to pelvic floor disorders,[128] with a focus on improvement in quality of life and where success is subjective and highly individualized. Through goal setting, the patient's expectation from treatment were listed together with their relative degree of importance. Subsequent clinician patient interaction could eliminate unrealistic goals and potentially modifying the initial treatment plans, tailored to suit the particular individual. Evaluation of goal achievement after treatment can be measured through VAS or similar Likert type ratings. GAS is specifically tailored for individuals, evaluating only what is important to the patient and could supplement other standardized instruments, which may contain questions unadjusted for the specific individual patient. However, the application of GAS to therapeutic trials for pelvic floor disorders is fraught with challenges. The heterogenous nature of patient's selected goals, including potential large differences in number, magnitude, and characteristics, imposes statistical challenges, especially calculation of the summary score. It could at least be used as a complementary outcome measure.

Patient satisfaction is the subjective, individual evaluation of treatment effectiveness, achieved when results of therapeutic intervention are aligned with the patient's expectations, therefore allowing clinicians to ascertain appropriateness of treatment. Many factors could potentially influence a patient's determination of their satisfaction, including the treatment's efficacy, side effects, cost, availability of information on the condition, general information giving, availability of resources, continuity of care, accessibility/convenience, as well as pleasantness of surroundings or facilities. Patient satisfaction is commonly used as an anchor to determine MIDs for PRO tools.

Validated on OAB drug trials, the Benefit Satisfaction Willingness (BSW)[129] is a generic questionnaire consisting of 3 items designed to capture the patient's perception of effect of treatment, with regard to relative benefit, satisfaction, and their willingness to continue. The BSW showed a reduction of −2.21 micturitions per 24 hours is perceived to be of "much benefit" to women undergoing treatment for OAB. The generic Treatment Satisfaction Questionnaire for Medication has a longer initial version of 55 items and a later shorter version[130] with 31 items covering four domains including side effects, effectiveness, convenience, and global satisfaction.

Prolapse/Incontinence Sexual Questionnaire – IUGA revised (PISQ-IR)

Q1 Which of the following best describes you:

Not sexually active at all   1 □ → Go to item   Q2 (Section 1)
Sexually active with or without a partner   2 □ → Skip to item   Q7 (Section 2)

Q2 The following are a list of reasons why you might not be sexually active, for each one please indicate how strongly you agree or disagree with it as a reason that you are not sexually active.

	Strongly agree	Somewhat agree	Somewhat disagree	Strongly disagree
a. No partner	□ 1	□ 2	□ 3	□ 4
b. No interest	□ 1	□ 2	□ 3	□ 4
c. Due to bladder or bowel problems (urinary or fecal incontinence) or due to prolapse (a feeling of or a bulge in the vaginal area)	□ 1	□ 2	□ 3	□ 4
d. Because of my other health problems	□ 1	□ 2	□ 3	□ 4
e. Pain	□ 1	□ 2	□ 3	□ 4

Q3 How much does the fear of leaking urine and/or stool and/or a bulging in the vagina (either the bladder, rectum or uterus falling out) cause you to avoid or restrict your sexual activity?

Not at all	A little	Some	A lot
□ 1	□ 2	□ 3	□ 4

Q4 For each of the following, please circle the number between 1 and 5 that best represents how you feel about your sex life.

	Rating					
a. satisfied	.. 1 ..	.. 2 ..	.. 3 ..	.. 4 ..	.. 5 ..	dissatisfied
b. adequate	.. 1 ..	.. 2 ..	.. 3 ..	.. 4 ..	.. 5 ..	inadequate

Q5 How strongly do you agree or disagree with each of the following statements:

	Strongly agree	Somewhat agree	Somewhat disagree	Strongly disagree
a. I feel frustrated by my sex life	□ 1	□ 2	□ 3	□ 4
b. I feel sexually inferior because of my incontinence and/or prolapse	□ 1	□ 2	□ 3	□ 4
c. I feel angry because of the impact that incontinence and/or prolapse has on my sex life	□ 1	□ 2	□ 3	□ 4

Q6 Overall, how bothersome is it to you that you are not sexually active?

Not at all	A little	Some	A lot
□ 1	□ 2	□ 3	□ 4

End of Items for Not Sexually Active

The remaining items in the survey are about a topic that one is not often asked to report on in a survey please answer as honestly and clearly as you possibly can

Q7 How often do you feel sexually aroused (physically excited or turned on) during sexual activity?

Never	Rarely	Sometimes	Usually	Always
□ 1	□ 2	□ 3	□ 4	□ 5

Q8 When you are involved in sexual activity, how often do you feel each of the following:

	Never	Rarely	Sometimes	Usually	Always
a. Fulfilled	□ 1	□ 2	□ 3	□ 4	□ 5
b. Shame	□ 1	□ 2	□ 3	□ 4	□ 5
c. Fear	□ 1	□ 2	□ 3	□ 4	□ 5

Q9 How often do you leak urine and/or stool with any type of sexual activity?

Never	Rarely	Sometimes	Usually	Always
□ 1	□ 2	□ 3	□ 4	□ 5

Q10 Compared to orgasms you have had in the past, how intense are your orgasms now?

Much less intense	Less intense	Same intensity	More intense	Much more intense
□ 1	□ 2	□ 3	□ 4	□ 5

Q11 How often do you feel pain during sexual intercourse? (If you don't have intercourse check this box □ and skip to the next item.)

Never	Rarely	Sometimes	Usually	Always
□ 1	□ 2	□ 3	□ 4	□ 5

Q12 Do you have a sexual partner?

1 □   Yes → Go to Q13
2 □   No → Skip to Q15

Q13 How often does your partner have a problem (lack of arousal, desire, erection, etc.) that limits your sexual activity?

All of the time	Most of the time	Some of the time	Hardly ever/Rarely
□ 1	□ 2	□ 3	□ 4

Q14 In general, would you say that your partner has a positive or negative impact on each of the following:

	Very positive	Somewhat positive	Somewhat negative	Very negative
a. Your sexual desire	□ 1	□ 2	□ 3	□ 4
b. The frequency of your sexual activity	□ 1	□ 2	□ 3	□ 4

Q15 When you are involved in sexual activity, how often do you feel that you want more?

Never	Rarely	Sometimes	Usually	Always
□ 1	□ 2	□ 3	□ 4	□ 5

Q16 How frequently do you have sexual desire, this may include wanting to have sex, having sexual thoughts or fantasies, etc.?

Daily	Weekly	Monthly	Less often than once a month	Never
□ 1	□ 2	□ 3	□ 4	□ 5

Q17 How would you rate your level (degree) of sexual desire or interest?

Very high	High	Moderate	Low	Very low or none at all
□ 1	□ 2	□ 3	□ 4	□ 5

Q18 How much does the fear of leaking urine, stool and/or a bulging in the vagina (prolapse) cause you to avoid sexual activity?

Not at all	A little	Some	A lot
□ 1	□ 2	□ 3	□ 4

Q19 For each of the following, please circle the number between 1 and 5 that best represents how you feel about your sex life.

	Rating					
a. satisfied	.. 1 ..	.. 2 ..	.. 3 ..	.. 4 ..	.. 5 ..	dissatisfied
b. adequate	.. 1 ..	.. 2 ..	.. 3 ..	.. 4 ..	.. 5 ..	inadequate
c. confident	.. 1 ..	.. 2 ..	.. 3 ..	.. 4 ..	.. 5 ..	not confident

Q20 How strongly do you agree or disagree with each of the following statements:

	Strongly agree	Somewhat agree	Somewhat disagree	Strongly disagree
a. I feel frustrated by my sex life	□ 1	□ 2	□ 3	□ 4
b. I feel sexually inferior because of my incontinence and/or prolapse	□ 1	□ 2	□ 3	□ 4
c. I feel embarrassed about my sex life	□ 1	□ 2	□ 3	□ 4
d. I feel angry because of the impact that incontinence and/or prolapse has on my sex life	□ 1	□ 2	□ 3	□ 4

FIGURE 11.7 The PISQ-IR.

The Overactive Bladder Satisfaction (OAB-S)[131] questionnaire is a condition-specific five-domain instrument that evaluates OAB control, expectations, impact on daily living, fulfillment of OAB medication tolerability, and satisfaction. The OAB-S is unique in its design, in being able to address the role of expectations in satisfaction assessment.

The *Patient Global Impression* (PGI) is a single-item 7-point global index that asks an individual to rate the severity of a specific condition (Patient Global Impression of Severity [PGI-S]) or to rate the response of her condition to treatment (Patient Global Impression of Improvement [PGI-I]). The PGI-I is simple, direct, and easy to interpret and provides a single best measure of significance of change from the individual's perspective. The PGI was initially developed during licensing trials of duloxetine[132] for treatment of stress urinary incontinence (SUI) and subsequently validated as a measure for improvement and satisfaction following incontinence and prolapse[133] treatment.

Symptom severity PRO or condition-specific HRQoL PRO often covers targeted symptoms, such as urinary incontinence or prolapse, but other aspects of treatment response, such as de novo incontinence or persistent pain, may not be reflected. PGI-I gives a more overall global overview of treatment success and more likely to encompass the range of harms and benefits of the surgical treatment. Symptom severity, condition-specific HRQoL PRO, and global indices measures different aspects of the patient's experience of their treatment and should ideally all be included in a comprehensive outcome assessment.

OUTCOME ASSESSMENTS

Outcome assessment is crucial in determining the most appropriate treatment intervention for women with pelvic floor disorders. In a comparative study, the primary outcome would be of central interest, being part of the study's primary hypothesis, and also used for sample size determination. Secondary outcomes are often not powered by design because they are not the focus of the main study objectives. Secondary outcomes are the remaining outcome measures within a study that provides additional complementary data that covers multiple domains that are often assessed in pelvic floor disorders. The quality of outcome reporting can be assessed using the Management of Otitis Media with Effusion in Cleft Palate (MOMENT) criteria.[134] The MOMENT criteria evaluates the following six items, each worth 1 point:

- The presence of a primary outcome
- Whether the primary outcome was clearly defined for reproducible measures
- Whether the secondary outcomes were clearly stated

- Whether the secondary outcomes were clearly defined for reproducible measures
- Whether the authors explain the choice of outcome
- Whether the methods that were used were appropriate to enhance the quality of measures

Randomized trials are generally regarded as having higher quality if their MOMENT score was more than 4 points.

Pelvic floor disorders are multidimensional, and therefore, intervention studies should have outcome measures that comprehensively attend to all of its relevant domains. Outcome assessments should be made using the same measure before and after an intervention. Both subjective and objective measures should be included, incorporating improvements or deterioration in function as well as complications of intervention. It should be noted that objective can imply that data is factual, and subjective implying that data are illusory. However, when used in research, the term *subjective* designates a symptom or condition perceived by the patient (not by examiner), whereas the term *objective* indicates a more clinician centric meaning, that the symptom or condition was observed by the clinician. Objective outcomes are more suitable for explanatory trials, that determines which intervention has greater efficacy and also its mechanism of success, whereas subjective outcomes are more suitable for pragmatic trials, which tends to mimic the real-world patient's setting. Given its multidimensional aspects, pelvic floor disorders should have outcome measures that assesses the following domains, as illustrated in Table 11.2:

- The patient's observations or their symptoms (subjective)
- Quantification of symptoms
- The clinician's observations (objective)
- Adverse events including perioperative and surgical complications
- Quality of life, including sexual function and satisfaction
- Socioeconomic measures

Economic analysis of interventions in pelvic floor disorders informs payers/funders of health care and could ultimately influence public policy decisions. Economic analysis compares the (costs) benefit of one treatment over another. A cost of illness (COI) study simply sums up all direct and indirect costs of treatment. Direct costs includes personal- and treatment-related costs, whereas indirect costs includes time loss from work. As they do not measure value, COI studies seldom help payers allocate health care funds. Cost minimization studies assumes that medical benefits are close to equivalent and compares costs of alternative strategies. Decision tree analysis is a type of economic analysis that does not involve "real data" from RCT or studies but through construction of a theoretical model.

TABLE 11.2

Outcome Measures in Pelvic Floor Disorders

	PATIENT SYMPTOMS SUBJECTIVE (S)	QUANTIFY SYMPTOM	PHYSICIAN OBSERVATIONS OBJECTIVE (O)	SEXUAL	EXPECTATIONS SATISFACTION	COMPLICATIONS	CURE OR COMPOSITE	QUALITY-OF-LIFE MEASURES	SOCIOECONOMIC EVALUATIONS
SUI	No leak—self-reported or diary	ICIQ-UI SF ISI UDI/UDI-6 Pad test	CTS or UDS Pad test	PISQ-IR PISQ-12	PGI-S PGI-I	Dindo IUGA ICS CTS OT time Hospital stay Blood loss Abscess Return OT Visceral injury Pain	S + O + No retreatment Dry rate	IIQ or UIQ SF-36 EQ-5D	EQ-5D ICER and willingness to pay for QALY
OAB	Frequency urgency nocturia UUI Bladder pain	OAB-q PPBC PPIUS INTU ICSI/ICPI	Diary data—frequency nocturia UIE, micturition volumes	PISQ-IR PISQ-12	BSW TSQM OAB-S	UTI retention Medication AE ISC rate Implant revision	Diary data Dry rate Symptom reduction PRO	OAB-q IIQ or UIQ INTU SF-36	EQ-5D WTP ICER and willingness to pay for QALY
Voiding	Incomplete emptying Poor stream intermittency	IPSS IPSS-V/S	PVR ISC rates	—	—	Retention ISC rates UTI	—	SF-36	—
Prolapse	Absence of bulge PFDI Q3 UDI Q16 APFQ Q28	PFDI-20 POPDI APFQ POP-SS VAS POP bother	POP-Q or POP past hymen POP-Q points Ba, Bp, C "New prolapse" Stenosis or short-ened TVL	PISQ-IR PISQ-12 FSFI Sexual activity New dyspareunia	PGI-S PGI-I Satisfaction VAS GAS	Dindo IUGA ICS CTS OT time Hospital stay Blood loss Abscess Return OT Visceral injury Reintervention rates Pain Mesh exposure Conversion Fistula hematoma drain	S + O + No retreatment Max vaginal descent <0 cm Ba, Bp, C C <½ TVL No retreatment (surgery or pessary) Time to failure Recurrence rate	PFIQ POPIQ SF-36	EQ-5D ICER and willingness to pay for QALY
Anorectal	Anal incontinence Fecal urgency Constipation Straining Stool chart Bowel diary	CRADI ABLE SMIS CCFIS FISI/FICA	—	PISQ-IR PISQ-12 FSFI Sexual activity	—	—	—	CRAIQ FIQL SF-36	EQ-5D ICER and willingness to pay for QALY

UDS, urodynamic studies; OT, operating theatre; UUI, urgency urinary incontinence; UIE, urgency incontinence episode; TSQM, Treatment Satisfaction Questionnaire for Medication; AE, adverse event; UTI, urinary tract infection; ISC, intermittent self catheterisation; WTP, willingness to pay; PVR, postvoid residual.

It involves assigning mathematical probabilities to chance events, assign outcomes (e.g., QALY), calculates expected utility for each strategy, and test robustness by doing sensitivity analysis to varying inputs to see if the model still holds. The Markov model allows dimension of time to come into decision tree analysis (because decision tree assumes that the chance of events is stable over time).

Cost-effectiveness analysis (CEA) uses a health outcome measure and is called cost utility analysis (CUA) if the chosen health outcome is the QALY. CEA evaluates value of interventions by determining if the health benefit (e.g., QALY) is worth what is paid. QALY is a universal outcome measure that combines gains and losses in both morbidity and mortality. It is a measure of a person's length of life weighted by a valuation of their health-related quality of life. Utility score, such as the EQ-5D, can be combined with life expectancy to calculate QALY. QALYs provide a common currency to assess the extent of the benefits gained from a variety of interventions in terms of health-related quality of life and survival for the patient. One result of a CUA/CEA is the incremental cost-effective ratio (ICER), representing the incremental costs required to produce one additional unit of QALY. Cost-effectiveness threshold is the maximum cost per health outcome that a health system is willing to pay. The use of QALY in resource allocation decision does mean that choices between patient groups competing for medical care are made explicit, sometimes focusing on how much society should be prepared to pay for a QALY. CUA helps decision makers compare value of interventions with very different health benefits.

Lower Urinary Tract Symptoms Outcome Assessment

Use of perineal pads is an objective outcome measure of urinary incontinence, more commonly used in the setting of evaluating different interventions for SUI. Quantification of the volume of urine loss is achieved by weighing perineal pads before and after a specified time period and/or group of activities. Perineal pad testing is the only incontinence severity measures that captures the actual volumes of leakage, although it does not provide clues to the mechanism of urine loss. Although numerous protocols were described, they can generally be either short or long term. Perineal pads using short-term protocols are often done in an office setting, requiring the patient to perform a standardized set of provocative maneuvers that last 10 minutes to 2 hours. The only standardized pad test is the ICS 1-hour pad test,[135] which is easy to do, quick and often used in clinical trials, whereby a change of >1 g is considered positive. However, the 1-hour pad test lacks authenticity because the standardized activities do not necessarily represent activities that results in incontinence in patient's everyday life. Short-term pad tests have false-negative rate as well as considerable test–retest variability. Longer term perineal pads are often done in the patient's own environment and could last 24 to 72 hours, capturing the patient's regular activities. Changes of up to 7 g per 24 hours can occur in healthy continent women. Longer term perineal pad testing has more reproducibility and increases its reliability further when used for a longer period (from 24 to 48 to 72 hours), although at a risk of decreasing patient compliance.

The cough stress test is another objective outcome measure commonly used in evaluation of stress incontinence intervention trials. The cough stress test can be performed with the bladder empty or with the patient's bladder filled up to 300 mL or to a subjective fullness, in the upright or supine position after a series of coughs while observing the external urethral meatus for visible loss of urine coincident with or simultaneous to the cough(s). The standardized ICS cough stress test[136] recommends the patient coughs forcefully one to four times in the supine and lithotomy positions with 200 to 400 mL of fluid in the bladder.

Outcome measures for SUI interventions should ideally encompass domains listed in Table 11.2. There is no widely accepted definition of cure for SUI interventions and can include a subjective patient-reported "no stress leakage," objective proof of a negative cough stress test or negative pad test, or a combination of both. However, the occurrence of perioperative complications (such as chronic pain or mesh exposure) or functional issues (such as de novo urgency or voiding dysfunction or sexual dysfunction) may not be comprehensively captured if outcome measures do not adequately cover relevant domains. Varied definition of cure, can come with varying cure rates, as shown by reports of the UK Tension-Free Vaginal Tape-Burch Colposuspension randomized trial, using multiple definition[137] of cure. The IUGA's recommendation[138] for SUI outcomes does not include a clear definition of cure for SUI, although there is agreement it should include all aspects of the condition, including objective, subjective outcomes, satisfaction, and HRQoL. It has also become increasingly common for intervention trials to report perioperative outcomes, including complications using either the more generic Clavien-Dindo classification[139,140] or the more condition-specific IUGA/ICS complication classification system[21] using CTS. Robust economic analysis, using appropriate methods and validated tools, can help funders evaluate cost-effectiveness of various SUI interventions and to ascertain the net health benefit for the population.

Although the ICIQ-UI SF is one of the most relevant outcome measures for evaluation of SUI intervention efficacy,[141] it is popular among researchers to report composite outcomes, which generally include a combination of subjective, objective outcomes, as well as no retreatment (with varying definition that could include no behavioral programs, no medications, no repeat surgery for complications or recurrence). It is crucially important that only validated PRO tools are chosen, with their MID considered when reporting this aspect of SUI outcomes. It comes as no surprise that there is considerable heterogeneity[142] in outcome reporting of SUI surgical trials, including safety aspects of surgical intervention over long term, which is usually being inconsistently evaluated across most clinical trials.[143] With the importance[144] of having core outcomes being increasingly recognized,[145] a proposal[146] was made for development of a core outcome set for SUI intervention, using methods advocated by the Core Outcome Measures in Effectiveness Trials (COMET) and COnsensus based Standards for the selection of health Measurement INstruments (COSMIN) initiatives.

Overactive Bladder Outcomes

There are multiple domains that should be evaluated in the outcome assessment of OAB. These include bladder diary data, such as micturition frequency, (mean) voided volumes, nocturia episodes, urgency incontinence episodes, as well as PRO measures such as PPIUS and OAB-q that quantify symptom severity as well as HRQoL. Other OAB outcomes include medication-related adverse events (type and rate) as well as sexual function as shown in Table 11.2. Physiologic measures, such as urodynamic parameters, although important for "proof of concept" evaluation, are generally not useful for determining clinical effectiveness. *Cure* is probably not an appropriate term in patients with OAB, rather the term *remission* might be preferable. Treatment response[147] or treatment success,[148] defined by ≥50% reduction in all baseline OAB symptoms including urgency and urgency incontinence, was proposed, given it was associated with clinically meaningful improvement in condition-specific HRQoL, especially among those with neurogenic OAB and urge urinary incontinence. Such definition of treatment response was commonly used when considering suitability of sacral neuromodulation in patients with refractory OAB. Given the significant costs of OAB management, and a lack of universally agreed standardized outcome metrics, efforts were invested to develop a core outcome set for OAB,[149] to assist value based therapeutic decision.

Prolapse Outcome Assessment

Like all pelvic floor disorders, POP is a multidimensional phenomenon, and therefore, its outcome assessment should attend to all its important domains. Given the symptom of vaginal bulge correlates[150,151] well with prolapse of all compartments, it is part of not only a clinical definition of prolapse but also an important

subjective outcome measure. Definitions of subjective success generally include absence of (awareness of) vaginal bulge, with this information extracted from commonly used PRO, such as PFDI-20 (question 3), UDI (question 16), or APFQ (question 28). Women presenting with bothersome POP often have concurrent pelvic floor symptoms,[152] including urinary incontinence, urinary urgency, voiding dysfunction, as well as anorectal symptoms, underscoring the value of using multiple domain PRO instruments such as PFDI or APFQ. PRO instruments measure patient perceptions in regard to symptom severity, functioning (including urinary, bowel, and sexual) as well as general health perceptions (including HRQoL, satisfaction, health utility) as shown in Table 11.2.

Objective outcomes of POP interventions are generally defined by the anatomy of various defects in the anterior, apical, and posterior compartments of vagina. Anatomic outcomes can be assessed by physical examination or radiologic studies, although the latter lack standardization, validation, and universal availability. In an effort to accurately describe the topographic anatomy of the pelvic floor and vaginal support, the POP-Q system[6] was introduced jointly by the American Urogynecologic Society and Society of Gynecologic Surgeons in 1996. The POP-Q system has widespread adoption, proven reproducibility, as well as relative precision in its nine sites measurements with 1-cm increments, despite not accounting for vaginal caliber, status of paravaginal support, pelvic floor descent, or urethral mobility. Reporting of anatomic outcomes generally involves not only the dependent points of the POP-Q (Ba, C, Bp) but also, increasingly, the total vaginal length (TVL, to determine vaginal shortening), presence or absence of vaginal stenosis, together with detail of patient position, their bladder fullness, and method for full descent. The dependent points of POP-Q can be presented as average values or categorized to stages depending on how far above or below they are relative to the hymen. Blinded assessment, using an independent clinician, can mitigate against observer bias.[153] The original definition of anatomic success[154] stipulates that the POP-Q dependent points are >1 cm proximal to the hymen, although most authorities have now adopted the hymen[155] being the threshold for anatomic success, given women with prolapse beyond it have more pelvic floor symptoms and are more likely to report a vaginal bulge. These anatomic definitions of success may not be applicable to the apical support, with some researchers using a descent of more than one-third or one-half of TVL as failure.[156]

Table 11.2 details other important aspects of prolapse outcome assessments, including complication profiles of prolapse interventions,[157] which can be reported using the more generic Clavien-Dindo classification[139] or the more condition-specific IUGA/ICS complication

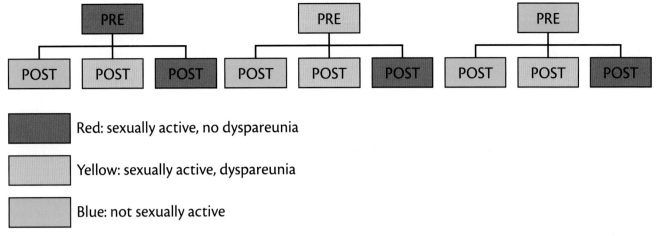

Red: sexually active, no dyspareunia

Yellow: sexually active, dyspareunia

Blue: not sexually active

FIGURE 11.8 Sexual activity, pre- and post-POP intervention.

classification system using CTS for those involving grafts[21] or just native tissue.[23] Economic analysis, using ICER and society's willingness to pay for QALY, can determine the most cost-effective treatment pathways.[158]

Defining success or cure in POP interventions is challenging because there is no single best outcome measure given that anatomic restoration without favorable subsequent urinary, bowel, or sexual function cannot be regarded as cure, especially from a patient's perspective. Despite avoiding the definition of success or failure, the joint report of IUGA and ICS recommended that the following outcomes be reported in studies of POP surgery[22]:

- Objective (e.g., POP-Q)
- PRO (especially presence or absence of vaginal bulge symptoms)
- Satisfaction
- Quality of life
- Perioperative data (e.g., operative time, hospital stay)

Together with a careful report of short- and long-term complications to facilitate weighing the risk–benefit ratio of each POP intervention, this joint report also clarified definitions of reintervention, an important outcome for POP surgery, as shown in Table 11.3. Figure 11.8 illustrates the rate of sexual activities before and after POP intervention.[22] In recognition of the importance of having standardized outcomes for better value-based comparison between prolapse interventions, interim core outcome sets were proposed for POP surgery that deals with anterior,[159] apical,[160] and posterior[161] compartments.

TABLE 11.3

International Urogynecological Association/ International Continence Society Standardized Terminology on Definitions of Reoperation

Primary surgery for POP is the first procedure required for the treatment of POP in any compartment.

Further surgery gives a global figure for the number of subsequent procedures the patient undergoes directly or indirectly relating to the primary surgery. This is subdivided into the following.

- *Primary prolapse surgery/different site*: a prolapse procedure in a new site/compartment following previous surgery in a different compartment (e.g., anterior repair following previous posterior repair)
- *Repeat surgery*: a repeat operation for prolapse arising from the same site. Where combinations of procedures arise, for example, new anterior repair plus further posterior repair, these should be reported separately, that is, repeat posterior repair and primary anterior repair.
- *Surgery for complications*: for example, mesh exposure or extrusion or pain or patient compromise (e.g., hemorrhage) (see complications section)
- *Surgery for nonprolapse conditions*: for example, subsequent surgery for stress urinary incontinence or fecal incontinence

References

1. Haylen BT, Lee JK, Freeman RM, et al. IUGA terminology and standardization: Creating and using this expanding resource. *Int Urogynecol J* 2017;28:1613–1616.
2. Haylen BT. 50 Years of standardisation. Accessed Feb 21, 2021. https://www.ics.org/news/1080
3. Abrams P, Blaivas JG, Stanton SL, et al. ICS 6th report on the standardization of terminology of lower urinary tract function. *Neurourol Urodyn* 1998;7:403–426.
4. Rowan D, James ED, Kramer AEJL, et al. Urodynamic equipment: Technical aspects. ICS Working Party on Urodynamic Equipment. *J Med Engin Tech* 1987;11:57–64.
5. Andersen JT, Blaivas JG, Cardozo L, et al. ICS 7th report on the standardization of terminology of lower urinary tract function: Lower urinary tract rehabilitation techniques. *Neurourol Urodyn* 1992;11:593–603.

6. Bump RC, Mattiasson A, Bø K, et al. The standardization of terminology of female pelvic organ prolapse and pelvic floor dysfunction. *Am J Obstet Gynecol* 1996;175(1):10–17.

7. Griffiths D, Höfner K, van Mastrigt R, et al. Standardization of terminology of lower urinary tract function: Pressure-flow studies of voiding, urethral resistance, and urethral obstruction. International Continence Society Subcommittee on Standardization of Terminology of Pressure-Flow Studies. *Neurourol Urodyn* 1997;16(1):1–18.

8. Mattiasson A, Djurhuus JC, Fonda D, et al. Standardization of outcome studies in patients with lower urinary tract dysfunction: A report on general principles from the Standardisation Committee of the International Continence Society. *Neurourol Urodyn* 1998;17(3):249–253.

9. Lose G, Fantl JA, Victor A, et al. Outcome measures for research in adult women with symptoms of lower urinary tract dysfunction. *Neurourol Urodyn* 1998;17(3):255–262.

10. Noorgard JP, Van Gool JD, Hjalmas K, et al. Standardization and definitions in lower urinary tract function in children. *Brit J Urol* 1998;81(suppl 3):1–16.

11. Stohrer M, Gospel M, Kondo A, et al. ICS report on the standardization of terminology in neurogenic lower urinary tract dysfunction. *Neurourol Urodyn* 1999;18(2):139–158.

12. van Waalwijk van Doorn E, Anders K, Khullar V, et al. Standardisation of ambulatory urodynamic monitoring: Report of the Standardisation Sub-Committee of the International Continence Society for ambulatory urodynamic studies. *Neurourol Urodyn* 2000;19(2):113–125.

13. Nordling J, Abrams P, Ameda K, et al. Outcome measures for research in treatment of adult males with symptoms of lower urinary tract dysfunction. *Neurourol Urodyn* 1998;17(3):263–273.

14. van Kerrebroeck P, Abrams P, Chaikin D, et al. The standardisation of terminology in nocturia: Report from the Standardisation Sub-committee of the International Continence Society. *Neurourol Urodyn* 2002;21(2):179–183.

15. Abrams P, Cardozo L, Fall M, et al. The standardisation of terminology of lower urinary tract function: Report from the Standardisation Sub-Committee of the International Continence Society. *Neurourol Urodyn* 2002;21(2):167–178.

16. Schäfer W, Abrams P, Liao L, et al. Good urodynamic practices: Uroflowmetry, filling cystometry, and pressure-flow studies. *Neurourol Urodyn* 2002;21(3):261–274.

17. Messelink B, Benson T, Berghmans B, et al. Standardization of terminology of pelvic floor muscle function and dysfunction: Report from the pelvic floor clinical assessment group of the International Continence Society. *Neurourol Urodyn* 2005;24(4):374–380.

18. Swift S, Morris S, McKinnie V, et al. Validation of a simplified technique for using the POPQ pelvic organ prolapse classification system. *Int Urogynecol J Pelvic Floor Dysfunct* 2006;17(6):615–620.

19. Haylen BT, de Ridder D, Freeman RM, et al. An International Urogynecological Association (IUGA)/International Continence Society (ICS) joint report on the terminology for female pelvic floor dysfunction. *Int Urogynecol J* 2010;21:5–26. *Neurourol Urodyn* 2010;29(1):4–20.

20. Haylen BT, Chetty N. International Continence Society 2002 terminology report: Have urogynecological conditions (diagnoses) been overlooked? *Int Urogynecol J Pelvic Floor Dysfunct* 2007;18(4):373–377.

21. Haylen BT, Freeman RM, Swift SE, et al. An International Urogynecological Association (IUGA)/International Continence Society (ICS) joint terminology and classification of the complications related directly to the insertion of prostheses (meshes, implants, tapes) and grafts in female pelvic floor surgery. *Int Urogynecol J* 2011;22(1):3–15. *Neurourol Urodyn* 2011;30(1):2–12.

22. Toozs-Hobson P, Freeman R, Barber M, et al. An International Urogynecological Association (IUGA)/International Continence Society (ICS) joint report on the terminology for reporting outcomes of surgical procedures for pelvic organ prolapse. *Int Urogynecol J* 2012;23(3):527–535. *Neurourol Urodyn* 2012;31(4):415–421.

23. Haylen BT, Freeman RM, Lee J, et al. An International Urogynecological Association (IUGA)/International Continence Society (ICS) joint terminology and classification of the complications related to native tissue female pelvic floor surgery. *Int Urogynecol J* 2012;23(5):515–526. *Neurourol Urodyn* 2012;31(4):406–414.

24. Haylen BT, Maher CF, Barber MD, et al. An International Urogynecological Association (IUGA)/International Continence Society (ICS) joint report on the terminology for female pelvic organ prolapse (POP). *Int Urogynecol J* 2016;27(4):655–684. *Neurourol Urodyn* 2016;35(2):137–168.

25. Sultan AH, Monga A, Lee J, et al. An International Urogynecological Association (IUGA)/International Continence Society (ICS) joint report on the terminology for female anorectal dysfunction. *Int Urogynecol J* 2017;28(1):5–31. *Neurourol Urodyn* 2017;36(1):10–34.

26. Bo K, Frawley H, Haylen BT, et al. International Urogynecological Association (IUGA)/International Continence Society (ICS) joint report on the terminology for the conservative and non-pharamacological management of female pelvic floor dysfunction. *Int Urogynecol J* 2017;28(1):191–213. *Neurourol Urodyn* 2017;36(1):10–34.

27. Rogers RG, Pauls RN, Thakar R, et al. An International Urogynecological Association (IUGA)/International Continence Society (ICS) joint report on the terminology for the assessment of sexual health of women with pelvic floor dysfunction. *Int Urogynecol J* 2018;29(5):647–666. *Neurourol Urodyn* 2018;37(4):1220–1240.

28. Rosier PFWM, Schaefer W, Lose G, et al. International Continence Society good urodynamic practices and terms 2016: Urodynamics, uroflowmetry, cystometry, and pressure-flow study. *Neurourol Urodyn* 2017;36:1243–1260.

29. Doggweiler R, Whitmore KE, Meijink JM, et al. A standard for terminology in chronic pelvic pain syndromes: A report from the chronic pelvic pain working group of the International Continence Society. *Neurourol Urodyn* 2017;4(4):984–1008.

30. Gajewski JB, Schurch B, Hamid R, et al. An International Continence Society (ICS) report on the terminology for adult neurogenic lower urinary tract dysfunction (ANLUTD). *Neurourol Urodyn* 2018;37(3):1152–1161.

31. Hashim H, Blanker MH, Drake MJ, et al. International Continence Society (ICS) report on the terminology for nocturia and nocturnal lower urinary tract function. *Neurourol Urodyn* 2019;38(2):499–508.

32. D'Ancona C, Haylen B, Oelke M, et al. The International Continence Society (ICS) report on the terminology for adult male lower urinary tract and pelvic floor symptoms and dysfunction. *Neurourol Urodyn* 2019;38(2):433–477.

33. ICS Glossary. Accessed February 21, 2021. https://www.ics.org/glossary

34. Fader M, Cottenden A, Chatterton C, et al. An International Continence Society (ICS) report on the terminology for single-use body worn absorbent incontinence products. *Neurourol Urodyn* 2020;39(8):2031–2039.

35. Goh J, Romanzi L, Elneil S, et al. An International Continence Society (ICS) report on the terminology for female pelvic floor fistulas. *Neurourol Urodyn* 2020;39(8):2040–2071.

36. ICS Glossary. Symptom. Accessed February 21, 2021. https://www.ics.org/glossary/symptom/symptom?q=symptom

37. McLeod LD, Coon CD, Martin SA, et al. Interpreting patient-reported outcome results: US FDA guidance and emerging methods. *Expert Rev Pharmacoecon Outcomes Res* 2011;11(2):163–169.

38. Center for Drug Evaluation and Research, Center for Biologics Evaluation and Research, Center for Devices and Radiological Health. Guidance for industry: Patient-reported outcome measures: Use in medical product development to support labeling claims: Draft guidance. *Health Qual Life Outcomes* 2006;4:79.

39. Handa VL, Barber MD, Young SB, et al. Paper versus web-based administration of the Pelvic Floor Distress Inventory 20 and Pelvic Floor Impact Questionnaire 7. *Int Urogynecol J Pelvic Floor Dysfunct* 2008;19(10):1331–1335.

40. Barber MD, Chen Z, Lukacz E, et al. Further validation of the short form versions of the Pelvic Floor Distress Inventory (PFDI) and Pelvic Floor Impact Questionnaire (PFIQ). *Neurourol Urodyn* 2011;30(4):541–546.

41. Coyne K, Sexton C. Patient-reported outcomes: From development to utilization. In: Cardozo L, Staskin DR, Ed. *Textbook of female urology and urogynaecology.* 4th ed. Boca Raton: CRC Press; 177.

42. Revicki DA, Osoba D, Fairclough D, et al. Recommendations on health-related quality of life research to support labeling and promotional claims in the United States. *Qual Life Res* 2000;9(8):887–900.

43. Gelhorn HL, Coyne KS, Sikirica V, et al. Psychometric evaluation of health-related quality-of-life measures after pelvic organ prolapse surgery. *Female Pelvic Med Reconstr Surg* 2012;18(4):221–226.

44. Suskind AM, Dunn RL, Morgan DM, et al. The Michigan Incontinence Symptom Index (M-ISI): A clinical measure for type, severity, and bother related to urinary incontinence. *Neurourol Urodyn* 2014;33(7):1128–1134.

45. Jaeschke R, Singer J, Guyatt GH. Measurement of health status. Ascertaining the minimal clinically important difference. *Control Clin Trials* 1989;10(4):407–415.

46. Revicki D, Hays RD, Cella D, et al. Recommended methods for determining responsiveness and minimally important differences for patient-reported outcomes. *J Clin Epidemiol* 2008;61(2):102–109.

47. Norman GR, Sloan JA, Wyrwich KW. Interpretation of changes in health-related quality of life: The remarkable universality of half a standard deviation. *Med Care* 2003;41(5):582–592.

48. Cohen J. *Statistical power analysis for the behavioral sciences.* 2nd ed. Hillsdale: Lawrence Erlbaum Associates; 1988:8–13.

49. Herdman M, Fox-Rushby J, Badia X. A model of equivalence in the cultural adaptation of HRQoL instruments: The universalist approach. *Qual Life Res* 1998;7:323–335.

50. Lim R, Liong ML, Lim KK, et al. The minimum clinically important difference of the International Consultation on Incontinence Questionnaires (ICIQ-UI SF and ICIQ-LUTSqol). *Urology* 2019;133:91–95.

51. Sirls LT, Tennstedt S, Brubaker L, et al. The minimum important difference for the International Consultation on Incontinence Questionnaire-Urinary Incontinence Short Form in women with stress urinary incontinence. *Neurourol Urodyn* 2015;34(2):183–187.

52. Coyne KS, Matza LS, Thompson CL, et al. Determining the importance of change in the Overactive Bladder Questionnaire. *J Urol* 2006;176(2):627–632.

53. Hagen S, Glazener C, Cook J, et al. Further properties of the Pelvic Organ Prolapse Symptom Score: Minimally important change and test-retest reliability. *Neurourol Urodyn* 2010;29(6):1055–1056.

54. Baessler K, Mowat A, Maher CF. The minimal important difference of the Australian Pelvic Floor Questionnaire. *Int Urogynecol J* 2019;30(1):115–122.

55. Barber MD, Kuchibhatla MN, Pieper CF, et al. Psychometric evaluation of 2 comprehensive condition-specific quality of life instruments for women with pelvic floor disorders. *Am J Obstet Gynecol* 2001;185(6):1388–1395.

56. Barber MD, Spino C, Janz NK, et al. The minimum important differences for the urinary scales of the Pelvic Floor Distress Inventory and Pelvic Floor Impact Questionnaire. *Am J Obstet Gynecol* 2009;200(5):580.e1–580.e7.

57. Dyer KY, Xu Y, Brubaker L, et al. Minimum important difference for validated instruments in women with urge incontinence. *Neurourol Urodyn* 2011;30(7):1319–1324.

58. Chan SS, Cheung RY, Lai BP, et al. Responsiveness of the Pelvic Floor Distress Inventory and Pelvic Floor Impact Questionnaire in women undergoing treatment for pelvic floor disorders. *Int Urogynecol J* 2013;24(2):213–221.

59. Jelovsek JE, Chen Z, Markland AD, et al. Minimum important differences for scales assessing symptom severity and quality of life in patients with fecal incontinence. *Female Pelvic Med Reconstr Surg* 2014;20(6):342–348.

60. Bols EM, Hendriks HJ, Berghmans LC, et al. Responsiveness and interpretability of incontinence severity scores and FIQL in patients with fecal incontinence: A secondary analysis from a randomized controlled trial. *Int Urogynecol J* 2013;24(3):469–478.

61. Rogers RG, Bann CM, Barber MD, et al. The responsiveness and minimally important difference for the Accidental Bowel Leakage Evaluation questionnaire. *Int Urogynecol J* 2020;31(12):2499–2505.

62. Harvie HS, Honeycutt AA, Neuwahl SJ, et al. Responsiveness and minimally important difference of SF-6D and EQ-5D utility scores for the treatment of pelvic organ prolapse. *Am J Obstet Gynecol* 2019;220(3):265.e1–265.e11.

63. Kelly AM. Does the clinically significant difference in visual analog scale pain score differ with age, gender or cause of pain? *Acad Emerg Med* 1998;5(11):1086–1090.

64. Kelly AM. The minimum clinically significant difference in visual analogue scale pain score does not differ with severity of pain. *Emerg Med J* 2001;18(3):205–207.

65. Wiegel M, Meston C, Rosen R. The Female Sexual Function Index (FSFI): Cross-validation and development of clinical cut-off scores. *J Sex Marital Ther* 2005;31:1–20.

66. Mamik MM, Rogers RG, Qualls CR, et al. The minimum important difference for the Pelvic Organ Prolapse-Urinary Incontinence Sexual Function Questionnaire. *Int Urogynecol J* 2014;25(10):1321–1326.

67. Grzybowska ME, Futyma K, Wydra D. Identification of the Pelvic Organ Prolapse/Incontinence Sexual Questionnaire-IUGA Revised (PISQ-IR) cutoff scores for impaired sexual function in women with pelvic floor disorders. *J Clin Med* 2019;9(1):13.

68. World Health Organization. *Measuring reproductive morbidity: Report of a technical working group.* Geneva, Switzerland: Division of Family Planning; 1989.

69. Barber MD, Neubauer NL, Klein-Olarte V. Can we screen for pelvic organ prolapse without a physical examination in epidemiologic studies? *Am J Obstet Gynecol* 2006;195(4):942–948.

70. Lukacz ES, Lawrence JM, Buckwalter JG, et al. Epidemiology of Prolapse and Incontinence Questionnaire: Validation of a new epidemiologic survey. *Int Urogynecol J Pelvic Floor Dysfunct* 2005;16(4):272–284.

71. Avery K, Donovan J, Peters T, et al. ICIQ: A brief and robust measure for evaluating the symptoms and impact of urinary incontinence. *Neurourol Urodyn* 2004;23(4):322–330.

72. Sandvik H, Seim A, Vanvik A, et al. A severity index for epidemiological surveys of female urinary incontinence: Comparison with 48-hour pad-weighing tests. *Neurourol Urodyn* 2000;19(2):137–145.

73. Klovning A, Avery K, Sandvik H, et al. Comparison of two questionnaires for assessing the severity of urinary incontinence: The ICIQ-UI SF versus the Incontinence Severity Index. *Neurourol Urodyn* 2009;28(5):411–415.

74. Coyne K, Revicki D, Hunt T, et al. Psychometric validation of an overactive bladder symptom and health-related quality of life questionnaire: The OAB-q. *Qual Life Res* 2002;11(6):563–574.

75. Coyne KS, Thompson CL, Lai JS, et al. An overactive bladder symptom and health-related quality of life short-form: Validation of the OAB-q SF. *Neurourol Urodyn* 2015;34(3):255–263.

76. Coyne KS, Matza LS, Kopp Z, et al. The validation of the Patient Perception of Bladder Condition (PPBC): A single-item global measure for patients with overactive bladder. *Eur Urol* 2006;49(6):1079–1086.

77. Lee UJ, Scott VC, Rashid R, et al. Defining and managing overactive bladder: Disagreement among the experts. *Urology* 2013;81(2):257–262.

78. Drake MJ. Do we need a new definition of the overactive bladder syndrome? ICI-RS 2013. *Neurourol Urodyn* 2014;33(5):622–624.

79. Cartwright R, Srikrishna S, Cardozo L, et al. Validity and reliability of the patient's perception of intensity of urgency scale in overactive bladder. *BJU Int* 2011;107(10):1612–1617.

80. Notte SM, Marshall TS, Lee M, et al. Content validity and test-retest reliability of Patient Perception of Intensity of Urgency Scale (PPIUS) for overactive bladder. *BMC Urol* 2012;12:26.

81. O'Leary MP, Sant GR, Fowler FJ Jr, et al. The Interstitial Cystitis Symptom Index and Problem Index. *Urology* 1997;49(5A suppl):58–63.

82. Lubeck DP, Whitmore K, Sant GR, et al. Psychometric validation of the O'Leary-Sant Interstitial Cystitis Symptom Index in a clinical trial of pentosan polysulfate sodium. *Urology* 2001;57(6 suppl 1):62–66.

83. Bennett JB, Gillard KK, Banderas B, et al. Development of a new patient-reported outcome (PRO) measure on the Impact of Nighttime Urination (INTU) in patients with nocturia—Psychometric validation. *Neurourol Urodyn* 2018;37(5):1678–1685.

84. Cohn JA, Kowalik CG, Reynolds WS, et al. Desmopressin acetate nasal spray for adults with nocturia. *Expert Rev Clin Pharmacol* 2017;10(12):1281–1293.

85. Cartwright R, Cox P, Cardozo L, et al. Screening tools for voiding for voiding difficulties in women: A comparison of the ICIQ-FLUTS and the modified IPSS questionnaires. *Neurourol Urodyn* 2009;28:652–653.

86. Barry MJ, Fowler FJ Jr, O'Leary MP, et al. The American Urological Association symptom index for benign prostatic hyperplasia. The Measurement Committee of the American Urological Association. *J Urol* 1992;148(5):1549–1564.

87. Blanker MH, Alma HJ, Devji TS, et al. Determining the minimal important differences in the International Prostate Symptom Score and Overactive Bladder Questionnaire: Results from an observational cohort study in Dutch primary care. *BMJ Open* 2019;9(12):e032795.

88. Okamura K, Nojiri Y, Osuga Y, et al. Psychometric analysis of international prostate symptom score for female lower urinary tract symptoms. *Urology* 2009;73(6):1199–1202.

89. Zhang HL, Huang ZG, Qiu Y, et al. Tamsulosin for treatment of lower urinary tract symptoms in women: A systematic review and meta-analysis. *Int J Impot Res* 2017;29(4):148–156.

90. Hsiao SM, Lin HH, Kuo HC. International Prostate Symptom Score for assessing lower urinary tract dysfunction in women. *Int Urogynecol J* 2013;24(2):263–267.

91. de Boer TA, Gietelink DA, Vierhout ME. Discrepancies between physician interview and a patient self-assessment questionnaire after surgery for pelvic organ prolapse. *Int Urogynecol J Pelvic Floor Dysfunct* 2008;19(10):1349–1352.

92. Hagen S, Glazener C, Sinclair L, et al. Psychometric properties of the Pelvic Organ Prolapse Symptom Score. *BJOG* 2009;116(1):25–31.

93. Baessler K, O'Neil SM, Maher CF, et al. Australian Pelvic Floor Questionnaire: A validated interviewer-administered pelvic floor questionnaire for routine and research. *Int Urogynecol J* 2009;20(2):149–158.

94. Barber MD, Walters MD, Bump RC. Short forms of two condition-specific quality-of-life questionnaires for women with pelvic floor disorders (PFDI-20 and PFIQ-7). *Am J Obstet Gynecol* 2005;193(1):103–113.

95. Shumaker SA, Wyman JF, Uebersax JS, et al. Health-related quality of life measures for women with urinary incontinence: The Incontinence Impact Questionnaire and the Urogenital Distress Inventory. Continence Program in Women (CPW) research group. *Qual Life Res* 1994;3(5):291–306.

96. Uebersax JS, Wyman JF, Shumaker SA, et al. Short forms to assess life quality and symptom distress for urinary incontinence in women: The Incontinence Impact Questionnaire and the Urogenital Distress Inventory. Continence Program for Women Research Group. *Neurourol Urodyn* 1995;14:131–139.

97. FitzGerald MP, Kenton K, Shott S, et al. Responsiveness of quality of life measurements to change after reconstructive pelvic surgery. *Am J Obstet Gynecol* 2001;185(1):20–24.

98. Lewis SJ, Heaton KW. Stool form scale as a useful guide to intestinal transit time. *Scand J Gastroenterol* 1997;32(9):920–924.

99. Manning AP, Wyman JB, Heaton KW. How trustworthy are bowel histories? Comparison of recalled and recorded information. *Br Med J* 1976;2:213–214.

100. Bharucha AE, Seide BM, Zinsmeister AR, et al. Insights into normal and disordered bowel habits from bowel diaries. *Am J Gastroenterol* 2008;103(3):692–698.

101. Jorge JM, Wexner SD. Etiology and management of fecal incontinence. *Dis Colon Rectum* 1993;36(1):77–97.

102. Norton NJ. The perspective of the patient. *Gastroenterology* 2004;126(1 suppl 1):S175–S179.

103. Vaizey CJ, Carapeti E, Cahill JA, et al. Prospective comparison of faecal incontinence grading systems. *Gut* 1999;44(1):77–80.

104. Rockwood TH, Church JM, Fleshman JW, et al. Patient and surgeon ranking of the severity of symptoms associated with fecal incontinence: The fecal incontinence severity index. *Dis Colon Rectum* 1999;42(12):1525–1532.

105. Bharucha AE, Locke GR III, Seide BM, et al. A new questionnaire for constipation and faecal incontinence. *Aliment Pharmacol Ther* 2004;20(3):355–364.

106. Rogers RG, Sung VW, Lukacz ES, et al. Accidental bowel leakage evaluation: A new patient-centered validated measure of accidental bowel leakage symptoms in women. *Dis Colon Rectum* 2020;63(5):668–677.

107. McHorney CA, Ware JE Jr, Raczek AE. The MOS 36-Item Short-Form Health Survey (SF-36): II. Psychometric and clinical tests of validity in measuring physical and mental health constructs. *Med Care* 1993;31(3):247–263.

108. EuroQol Group. EuroQol—A new facility for the measurement of health related quality of life. *Health Policy* 1990;16(3):199–208.

109. Lukacz ES, Lawrence JM, Burchette RJ, et al. The use of Visual Analog Scale in urogynecologic research: A psychometric evaluation. *Am J Obstet Gynecol* 2004;191(1):165–170.

110. Collins SL, Moore RA, McQuay HJ. The visual analogue pain intensity scale: What is moderate pain in millimetres? *Pain* 1997;72(1–2):95–97.

111. Frazer MI, Haylen BT, Sutherst JR. The severity of urinary incontinence in women. Comparison of subjective and objective tests. *Br J Urol* 1989;63(1):14–15.

112. Ulrich D, Guzman Rojas R, Dietz HP, et al. Use of a visual analog scale for evaluation of bother from pelvic organ prolapse. *Ultrasound Obstet Gynecol* 2014;43(6):693–697.

113. Corcos J, Behlouli H, Beaulieu S. Identifying cut-off scores with neural networks for interpretation of the Incontinence Impact Questionnaire. *Neurourol Urodyn* 2002;21:198–203.

114. Rockwood TH, Church JM, Fleshman JW, et al. Fecal Incontinence Quality of Life Scale: Quality of life instrument for patients with fecal incontinence. *Dis Colon Rectum* 2000;43(1):9–17.

115. World Health Organization. Defining sexual health: Report of a technical consultation on sexual health, 28–31 January 2002. Accessed April 13, 2022. https://www.who.int/teams/sexual-and-reproductive-health-and-research/key-areas-of-work/sexual-health/defining-sexual-health

116. Rosen R, Brown C, Heiman J, et al. The Female Sexual Function Index (FSFI): A multidimensional self-report instrument for the assessment of female sexual function. *J Sex Marital Ther* 2000;26(2):191–208.

117. Gerstenberger EP, Rosen RC, Brewer JV, et al. Sexual desire and the Female Sexual Function Index (FSFI): A sexual desire cutpoint for clinical interpretation of the FSFI in women with and without hypoactive sexual desire disorder. *J Sex Med* 2010;7(9):3096–3103.

118. American Psychiatric Association. *Diagnostic and statistical manual of mental disorders*. 5th ed. Washington: American Psychiatric Publishing, 2013.

119. Reed GM, Drescher J, Krueger RB, et al. Disorders related to sexuality and gender identity in the ICD-11: Revising the ICD-10 classification based on current scientific evidence, best clinical practices, and human rights considerations. *World Psychiatry* 2016;15(3):205–221.

120. Neijenhuijs KI, Hooghiemstra N, Holtmaat K, et al. The Female Sexual Function Index (FSFI)—A systematic review of measurement properties. *J Sex Med* 2019;16:640–660.

121. Grzybowska ME, Wydra D. Responsiveness of two sexual function questionnaires: PISQ-IR and FSFI in women with pelvic floor disorders. *Neurourol Urodyn* 2021;40(1):358–366.

122. Rogers RG, Kammerer-Doak D, Villarreal A, et al. A new instrument to measure sexual function in women with urinary incontinence or pelvic organ prolapse. *Am J Obstet Gynecol* 2001;184(4):552–558.

123. Rogers RG, Coates KW, Kammerer-Doak D, et al. A short form of the Pelvic Organ Prolapse/Urinary Incontinence Sexual Questionnaire (PISQ-12). *Int Urogynecol J Pelvic Floor Dysfunct* 2003;14(3):164–168.

124. Rogers RG, Rockwood TH, Constantine ML, et al. A new measure of sexual function in women with pelvic floor disorders (PFD): The Pelvic Organ Prolapse/Incontinence Sexual Questionnaire, IUGA-Revised (PISQ-IR). *Int Urogynecol J* 2013;24(7):1091–1103.

125. Constantine ML, Pauls RN, Rogers RR, et al. Validation of a single summary score for the Prolapse/Incontinence Sexual Questionnaire-IUGA revised (PISQ-IR). *Int Urogynecol J* 2017;28(12):1901–1907.

126. Lowenstein L, FitzGerald MP, Kenton K, et al. Patient-selected goals: The fourth dimension in assessment of pelvic floor disorders. *Int Urogynecol J Pelvic Floor Dysfunct* 2008;19(1):81–84.

127. Kiresuk T, Sherman R. Goal Attainment Scaling: A general method for evaluating community mental health programs. *Commun Mental Health J* 1968;4(6):443–453.

128. Hullfish KL, Bovbjerg VE, Steers WD. Patient centered goals for pelvic floor dysfunction surgery: Long-term follow-up. *Am J Obstet Gynaecol* 2004;191(1):201–205.

129. Pleil AM, Coyne KS, Reese PR, et al. The validation of patient-rated global assessments of treatment benefit, satisfaction, and willingness to continue—The BSW. *Value Health* 2005;8(suppl 1):S25–S34.

130. Atkinson MJ, Kumar R, Cappelleri JC, et al. Hierarchical construct validity of the Treatment Satisfaction Questionnaire for Medication (TSQM version II) among outpatient pharmacy consumers. *Value Health* 2005;8(suppl 1):S9–S24.

131. Piault E, Evans CJ, Espindle D, et al. Development and validation of the Overactive Bladder Satisfaction (OAB-S) questionnaire. *Neurourol Urodyn* 2008;27(3):179–190.

132. Yalcin I, Bump RC. Validation of two global impression questionnaires for incontinence. *Am J Obstet Gynecol* 2003;189(1):98–101.

133. Srikrishna S, Robinson D, Cardozo L. Validation of the Patient Global Impression of Improvement (PGI–I) for urogenital prolapse. *Int Urogynecol J* 2010;21(5):523–528.

134. Harman NL, Bruce IA, Callery P, et al. MOMENT—Management of Otitis Media with Effusion in Cleft Palate: Protocol for a systematic review of the literature and identification of a core outcome set using a Delphi survey. *Trials* 2013;14:70.

135. Krhut J, Zachoval R, Smith PP, et al. Pad weight testing in the evaluation of urinary incontinence. *Neurourol Urodyn* 2014;33(5):507–510.

136. Guralnick ML, Fritel X, Tarcan T, et al. ICS educational module: Cough stress test in the evaluation of female urinary incontinence: Introducing the ICS-Uniform Cough Stress Test. *Neurourol Urodyn* 2018;37(5):1849–1855.

137. Hilton P. Trials of surgery for stress incontinence—Thoughts on the 'Humpty Dumpty principle.' *Br J Obstet Gynaecol* 2002;109(10):1081–1088.

138. Ghoniem G, Stanford E, Kenton K, et al. Evaluation and outcome measures in the treatment of female urinary stress incontinence: International Urogynecological Association (IUGA) guidelines for research and clinical practice. *Int Urogynecol J Pelvic Floor Dysfunct* 2008;19(1):5–33.

139. Dindo D, Dimartines N, Clavien P. Classification of surgical complications: A new proposal with evaluation in a cohort of 6336 patients and results of a survey. *Ann Surg* 2004;240(2):205–213.

140. Mitropoulos D, Artibani W, Biyani CS, et al. Validation of the Clavien-Dindo grading system in urology by the European Association of Urology Guidelines Ad Hoc Panel. *Eur Urol Focus* 2018;4(4):608–613.

141. Lim R, Liong ML, Leong WS, et al. Which outcome measures should be used in stress urinary incontinence trials? *BJU Int* 2018;121(5):805–810.

142. Cheung FY, Farag F, MacLennan S, et al. Is there outcome reporting heterogeneity in trials that aim to assess the effectiveness of surgical treatments for stress urinary incontinence in women? *Eur Urol Focus* 2021;7(4):857–868.

143. Doumouchtsis SK, Pookarnjanamorakot P, Durnea C, et al. A systematic review on outcome reporting in randomised controlled trials on surgical interventions for female stress urinary incontinence: A call to develop a core outcome set. *BJOG* 2019;126(12):1417–1422.

144. Khan K. The CROWN Initiative: Journal editors invite researchers to develop core outcomes in women's health. *BJOG* 2014;121(10):1181–1182.

145. Duffy JMN, Ziebland S, von Dadelszen P, et al. Tackling poorly selected, collected, and reported outcomes in obstetrics and gynecology research. *Am J Obstet Gynecol* 2019;220(1):71.e1–71.e4.

146. Rada M, Pergialiotis V, Betschart C, et al. A protocol for developing, disseminating, and implementing a core outcome set for stress urinary incontinence. *Medicine* 2019;98(37):e16876.

147. Payne CK, Kelleher C. Redefining response in overactive bladder syndrome. *BJU Int* 2007;99(1):101–106.

148. Campbell JD, Gries KS, Watanabe JH, et al. Treatment success for overactive bladder with urinary urge incontinence refractory to oral antimuscarinics: A review of published evidence. *BMC Urol* 2009;9:18.

149. Foust-Wright C, Wissig S, Stowell C, et al. Development of a core set of outcome measures for OAB treatment. *Int Urogynecol J* 2017;28(12):1785–1793.

150. Swift SE, Tate SB, Nicholas J. Correlation of symptoms with degree of pelvic organ support in a general population of women: What is pelvic organ prolapse? *Am J Obstet Gynecol* 2003;189(2):372–379.

151. Cunkelman J, Mueller E, Brubaker L, et al. Defining pelvic organ prolapse: Correlation of symptoms with vaginal topography. *Neurourol Urodyn* 2001;30:1046–1048.

152. Ellerkmann RM, Cundiff GW, Melick CF, et al. Correlation of symptoms with location and severity of pelvic organ prolapse. *Am J Obstet Gynecol* 2001;185(6):1332–1338.

153. Antosh DD, Iglesia CB, Vora S, et al. Outcome assessment with blinded versus unblinded POP-Q exams. *Am J Obstet Gynecol* 2011;205(5):489.e1–489.e4.

154. Weber AM, Abrams P, Brubaker L, et al. The standardization of terminology for researchers in female pelvic floor disorders. *Int Urogynecol J Pelvic Floor Dysfunct* 2001;12(3):178–186.

155. Barber MD, Brubaker L, Nygaard I, et al. Defining success after surgery for pelvic organ prolapse. *Obstet Gynecol* 2009;114(3):600–609.

156. Meister MR, Sutcliffe S, Lowder JL. Definitions of apical vaginal support loss: A systematic review. *Am J Obstet Gynecol* 2017;216(3):232.e1–232.e14.

157. Diwadkar GB, Barber MD, Feiner B, et al. Complication and reoperation rates after apical vaginal prolapse surgical repair: A systematic review. *Obstet Gynecol* 2009;113(2 pt 1):367–373.

158. Wang R, Hacker MR, Richardson M. Cost-effectiveness of surgical treatment pathways for prolapse. *Female Pelvic Med Reconstr Surg* 2021;27:e408–e413.

159. Durnea CM, Pergialiotis V, Duffy JMN, et al. A systematic review of outcome and outcome-measure reporting in randomised trials evaluating surgical interventions for anterior-compartment vaginal prolapse: A call to action to develop a core outcome set. *Int Urogynecol J* 2018;29(12):1727–1745.

160. de Mattos Lourenço TR, Pergialiotis V, Durnea C, et al. A systematic review of reported outcomes and outcome measures in randomized controlled trials on apical prolapse surgery. *Int J Gynaecol Obstet* 2019;145(1):4–11.

161. Lourenço TRM, Pergialiotis V, Durnea CM, et al. A systematic review of reported outcomes and outcome measures in randomized trials evaluating surgical interventions for posterior vaginal prolapse to aid development of a core outcome set. *Int J Gynaecol Obstet* 2020;148(3):271–281.

CHAPTER 12

URODYNAMICS

Gunnar Lose • Niels Klarskov

Introduction

Urodynamics (UDS) comprise all the measurements that assess the function and dysfunction of the lower urinary tract (LUT) by *any appropriate method*.[1] Consequently, UDS can be subdivided into the following:

- **Invasive UDS**, which are tests that involves insertion of one or more catheters or any other transducer into the bladder and/or other body cavities, or the insertion of probes or needles, for example, for electromyography (EMG) recording.[1]
- **Noninvasive UDS** are those tests performed without insertion of catheters, needles, or probes into the bladder and/or other body cavities, for example, micturition diary, uroflowmetry, or postvoid residual (PVR) measurement by ultrasonography.[1]

UDS testing provides an objective description of LUT function and dysfunction in terms of qualitative and quantitative variables during: (1) *bladder filling and storage* and (2) *bladder emptying*.

Urodynamic investigations and terms are *standardized*.[1,2] The International Urogynecological Association (IUGA)/International Continence Society (ICS) terminology report highlights the need to base diagnoses for female pelvic floor dysfunction on the correlation between a woman's symptoms, signs (Table 12.1), and any relevant diagnostic test including UDS.[2]

UDS tests have gradually been developed and implemented clinically since the 1950s. The mantra has been, *"If urodynamics is not very useful clinically, it is not important to understand how the LUT functions in order to treat it"* (Derek Griffiths).

The rational for the development and use of UDS testing stems from consistent clinical findings showing a weak correlation between symptoms and the underlying dysfunction documented by UDS. Furthermore, it has turned out that only a minor fraction (about one-third) of women urodynamically tested before surgery for stress urinary incontinence (SUI) can be classified as "uncomplicated" SUI. It has been reported that up to 40% of uncomplicated SUI women will have their symptomatic diagnosis changed versus 75% of those classified as complicated after invasive UDS.[3] Thus, even in women with symptomatic pure SUI, invasive UDS may unveil detrusor overactivity (DO) and/or unsuspected voiding dysfunction (VD). Consequently, a history of pure SUI yields a positive predictive value and a negative predictive value of the order 70% in predicting only urodynamic SUI.[4] Hence, a normal invasive UDS does not exclude the diagnosis of SUI.

Between 2009 and 2017, several retrospective and prospective studies and one small randomized controlled trial have demonstrated that UDS can guide appropriate decision-making in female SUI. However, it has not been possible, so far, to establish robust evidence regarding the clinical value of UDS before stress incontinence surgery.[5] Three recent randomized controlled trials (VUSIS-I/II and VALUE study)[6-8] have unfortunately had major conceptual flaws first and foremost breach in the principle of good urodynamic practice (GUP) but also in the choice of UDS, quality, expertise, lack of clear definition of urodynamic entities, and lack of relationship between the result of the urodynamic question and the treatment strategy. The VALUE study (referred to as "high-quality evidence") has obtained "landmark" status, although the study does not follow the principles of GUP by asking a urodynamic question before the investigation and most remarkably the result of the UDS testing had little or no weight in the decision regarding treatment approach (in both the invasive UDS group and the office group, 93% had the same treatment namely a midurethral sling). *If you do not use the result of a test, you cannot evaluate its usability!*

However, altogether, accumulative evidence indicates that UDS can reduce the dangers of empiric management in female LUTs.[5]

GOOD URODYNAMIC PRACTICE

GUP was defined by the ICS in 2002.[9] GUP comprises three main elements:

1. A clear indication for and appropriate selection of relevant test measurements and procedures
2. Precise measurement with data quality control and complete documentation
3. Accurate analysis and critical reporting of results

TABLE 12.1

Examples of Lower Urinary Tract Diagnoses

	SYMPTOMS	SIGN	URODYNAMIC INVESTIGATION
Urodynamic stress (urinary) incontinence	Complaint of involuntary loss of urine on effort or physical exertion, on sneezing, or on coughing	Observation of involuntary leakage from the urethra synchronous with effort or physical exertion, on sneezing, or on coughing	Involuntary leakage during filling cystometry, associated with increased intra-abdominal pressure, in the absence of a detrusor contraction
DO	Urinary urgency, usually accompanied by frequency and nocturia, with or without urgency urinary incontinence, in the absence of urinary tract infection or other obvious pathology		Involuntary detrusor muscle contractions during filling cystometry

NOTE: The diagnoses of female pelvic floor dysfunction are based on the correlation between a woman's symptoms, signs, and any relevant diagnostic investigation.
From Haylen BT, de Ridder D, Freeman RM, et al. An International Urogynecological Association (IUGA)/International Continence Society (ICS) joint report on the terminology for female pelvic floor dysfunction. *Int Urogynecol J* 2010;21(1):5–26, with permission.

The aim of clinical UDS is to reproduce the patient's symptoms while making precise measurements in order to identify the underlying causes for the symptoms and to quantify the related pathophysiologic processes. By doing so, it should be possible to establish objectively the presence of a dysfunction and understand its clinical implication.

Thus, we may either confirm a diagnosis and/or give a new specifically urodynamic diagnosis that might alter diagnosis or treatment. For example, symptomatic SUI may turn out to be caused by DO or the general diagnosis (urodynamic SUI) may be correct, but additional urodynamic findings (DO, bladder outflow obstruction [BOO], or detrusor underactivity [DU]) mandate therapeutic considerations.

Thus, GUP implies a urodynamic "question" followed by an "answer," and treatment guided accordingly.

In 2017, an updated ICS GUP 2016 version was published which provides evidence-based specific recommendations for routine clinical urodynamic testing and includes expert consensus where evidence is lacking. This rapport has newly or more precisely defined more than 30 terms and provides standards for practice, quality control, interpretation, and reporting of UDS.[1]

The *reporting* of UDS in medical journals may be unclear and ambiguous. For example, in some papers, UDS means invasive UDS. In other papers "homemade" definitions are used. UDS should be reported in a clear meaningful way, which implies clear definition of the urodynamic tests used, following the principles of GUP and sticking to IUGA/ICS standardization and terminology.[10]

INDICATION FOR URODYNAMICS

Basic assessment of women with urinary incontinence or VDs aims to identify patients with complicated symptomatology and findings (signs). ICS (working group) suggests, as a minimum, all ICS standard urodynamic test data, that is, (1) a clinical history (should include valid symptom[s] and bother score[s] and medication list), (2) relevant clinical examination, (3) (3-day) bladder diary (rule out polyuria >20 mL/kg/24 h), and (4) representative uroflowmetry with PVR.[1] Clinical examination may also include a cough stress test (detect leakage = sign) and pad testing (quantification of leakage).

The indication of invasive UDS in terms of transurethral cystometry and pressure–flow study (PFS) is still a matter of debate. According to the ICS, "standard urodynamic protocol"[1] cystometry and pressure flow is routinely recommended. However, the indication depends on the urodynamic question. The gain is dubious in uncomplicated women with predominantly SUI and a normal uroflowmetry and PVR.

The indication for invasive UDS, however, is strong, especially before surgery in the following:

1. "Complicated" patients (e.g., recurrent incontinence after surgery, voiding symptoms, or previous pelvic surgery)
2. Urgency predominant mixed urinary incontinence

3. Unclear type of urinary incontinence
4. Abnormal uroflowmetry (decreased maximum flow rate and/or abnormal flow curve configuration) and/or increased PVR

The challenge is when choosing UDS to find an appropriate balance between reducing the danger of empiric management and the drawbacks of especially invasive UDS.

Although UDS generally is well tolerated, there are drawbacks. UDS testing is time-consuming and costly, and it may evoke discomfort and anxiety. Invasive tests may be painful, and catheterization of the bladder carries a small risk of introducing infection (<5%). There are other issues such as technically challenging, burdensome, prone to methodologic errors (artefacts), and the issue of reimbursement.

An explanatory leaflet about UDS may be helpful for both patients and the staff.

Patients with Pelvic Organ Prolapse

Noninvasive UDS may show signs on voiding difficulties in terms of decreased flow rate or abnormal flow curve and/or increased PVR especially in women with a large pelvic organ prolapse (POP).

The risk of de novo urinary incontinence after POP surgery is in average about 15%.[11] A variety of preoperative tests have been tried to uncover occult SUI, but no reliable test has been identified so far. Conversely, women with combined SUI and POP may have their incontinence improved or cured after POP surgery. Currently, however, there is no consensus about the role of UDS before POP surgery, but it is important that patients undergoing POP surgery is informed of the risk of de novo incontinence.

TABLE 12.2		
Urodynamic Examinations Divided into Invasive and Noninvasive and Filling versus Emptying Phase Tests		
	NONINVASIVE	**INVASIVE**
Filling phase	Bladder diary	Cystometry
	Pad weight test	Filling urethrocystometry
		Urethral pressure profilometry
		ALPP
		UPR
		Ice water test
		Bethanechol supersensitivity test
Emptying phase	Uroflowmetry	PFS
	PVR volume	EMG

Urodynamic Examinations

The LUT has two opposite functions: (1) *bladder filling and storage* where the bladder pressure is low while the bladder distends and the urethral pressure is relatively high and (2) *bladder emptying* where the urethral pressure drops to a pressure close to zero followed by a detrusor pressure increase. Urodynamic tests can be divided into those that evaluate the LUT in the filling phase and in the emptying phase. A filling phase test cannot uncover pathology during bladder emptying and vice versa. For example, a high urethral pressure measured during storage is not indicative of bladder outlet obstruction. The urodynamic tests can be divided into a 2 × 2 table based on if it is a filling or emptying phase test and if it is an invasive or noninvasive test (Table 12.2).

NONINVASIVE TEST OF BLADDER FILLING

Bladder Diary

The woman measures and notes the time and amount of voided volume and fluid intake. The bladder diary often includes the incontinence episodes and degree of incontinence, urgency episodes, pad usage, and activities during or immediately preceding the leakages. The ideal duration of the bladder diary has not yet been established. A short duration increases patient compliance, although the more days recorded, the better the spectrum or variation is recorded. A diary should at least cover 24 hours, but 2 to 3 days will generally provide more useful clinical data. A 7-day bladder diary might be used in clinical studies. The bladder diary should be representative for the patients daily living and the woman should perform her normal daily activities during the registration period. Table 12.3 shows the information which can be obtained from a bladder diary.

The bladder diary is mandatory as initial assessment of patients with LUT syndrome. Unfavorable amount and timing of fluid intake can be disclosed, and the diary may be therapeutic as it provides insight into behavior and can be used to monitor the treatment during follow-up.

Polyuria should be addressed before further UDS. Figure 12.1 shows an example of a bladder diary.

Pad Test

The pad test is a diagnostic method for detection and quantification of urine leak based on weight gain in absorbable pads. The pads are weighted before and after the test, and the weight gain is the results of the test. The tests can be divided into office-based and home-based tests.

The office-based tests are short tests from 20 minutes to 2 hours. The bladder volume, fluid intake, and physical

TABLE 12.3

Information Obtained with a Bladder Diary and the Definitions of the Entities

BLADDER DIARY INFORMATION	DEFINITION[a]
Daytime urinary frequency	Number of voids by wakeful hours including last void before sleep and first void after waking
Nocturnal frequency/nocturia	Number of times sleep is interrupted by the need to micturate. Each void is preceded and followed by sleep.
24-h frequency	Total number of daytime voids and episodes of nocturia during a specified 24-h period.
24-h urine production	Summation of all urine volumes voided in 24 h
Maximum voided volume	Highest voided volume recorded
Average voided volume	Summation of volumes voided divided by the number of voids
Median functional bladder capacity	Median maximum voided volume in everyday activities
Polyuria	Over 40 mL/kg body weight during 24 h (2.8 L urine for a woman weighing 70 kg)
Nocturnal urine volume	Cumulative urine volume from voids after going to bed with the intention of sleeping to include the first void at the time of waking with the intention of rising
Nocturnal polyuria	Excess (>20%–30% age dependent) proportion of urine excretion (nocturnal voided volume/total 24 h voided volume × 100%) occurring at night (or when the patient is sleeping)

[a]From Haylen BT, de Ridder D, Freeman RM, et al. An International Urogynecological Association (IUGA)/International Continence Society (ICS) joint report on the terminology for female pelvic floor dysfunction. *Int Urogynecol J* 2010;21(1):5–26, with permission.

Bladder diary				
Time	**Drink (ml)**	**Voided Urine (ml)**	**Leakage**	**Comments**
8–9		250		
9–10	250			
10–11				
11–12				
12–13	250	200		
13–14				
14–15				
15–16	300			
16–17				
17–18	200	150		
18–19				
19–20				
20–21	400	250		
21–22				
22–23	250			
23–24	150	200		Went to bed
24–1				
1–2		200		
2–3				
3–4	100	250	x	Pad 100 g
4–5				
5–6				
6–7				
7–8		300		
total	1850	1800		

FIGURE 12.1 A bladder diary from a woman with nocturia and nocturnal enuresis. Nocturnal urine volume is 200 + 250 + 300 + 100 (from the pad) = 850 mL, which is 45% of the 24-hour urine production; thus, the woman has nocturnal polyuria. The woman drinks 800 mL in the evening and 100 mL during the night which explains the nocturnal polyuria. The woman had fluid restriction during the evening which cured her symptoms.

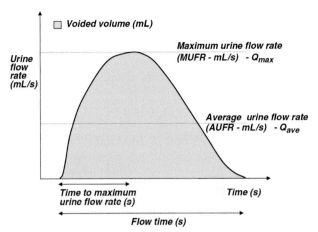

FIGURE 12.2 A schematic representation of urine flow over time. (From Haylen BT, de Ridder D, Freeman RM, et al. An International Urogynecological Association [IUGA]/ International Continence Society [ICS] joint report on the terminology for female pelvic floor dysfunction. *Int Urogynecol J* 2010;21[1]:5–26, with permission.)

activity can be standardized during the test. The home-based tests are conducted under circumstances as close as possible to the woman's standard daily life with normal activities often combined with a bladder diary. The test typically lasts 24 hours, but tests up to 72 hours have been tried; however, the longer test only increases the sensitivity slightly but decreases the patient compliance.

The pad test cannot be used to diagnose the type of incontinence and the reproducibility is generally low. The home-based test has higher sensitivity in detecting urinary incontinence compared to the office-based test.

A small group of women have the unusual complain of incontinence unassociated with symptom of stress or urgency incontinence. The leakage is not associated with urgency or increased abdominal pressure and is often described as continuously leaking despite that the woman often only uses few panty liners per day. Incontinence cannot be demonstrated objectively at stress test or during a cystometry. In these cases, vaginal discharge or sweat might be suspected rather than urinary incontinence. Urinary incontinence can be verified or refuted by coloring the urine during the pad test. The urine can be colored bright yellow by an oral intake of a high dose of vitamin B_2 (riboflavin).

NONINVASIVE TEST OF BLADDER EMPTYING

Uroflowmetry is a noninvasive test that produces flow rate of the external urinary stream as volume per unit time in milliliter per second (Fig. 12.2).

The patient voids into a flowmeter in privacy, in her preferred position, when the bladder is reasonably full, and a normal sensation of voiding. The patient should confirm that the voiding is representative.

The urine flow is continuously measured and demonstrated graphically (see Fig. 12.2). Maximum flow rate (Q_{max}) is the measured value of the maximum flow rate correcting for artefacts. Uroflowmetry minimally reports Q_{max} and volume voided. Total voided volume, shape of the flow curve, Q_{max}, and average flow (Q_{ave}) (voided volume/voiding time) are typical variables used for assessing the bladder emptying function (see Fig. 12.2). If the uroflowmetry values are not normal, it is appropriate to repeat examination to ensure reproducibility. Normal Q_{max} depends on the voided volume which appears from the Liverpool nomogram (Fig. 12.3).

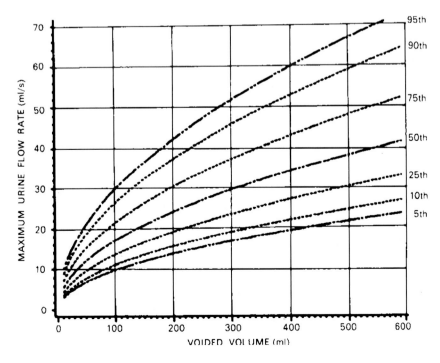

FIGURE 12.3 Liverpool Nomogram for maximum urine flow rate in women. (From Haylen BT, Yang V, Logan V. Uroflowmetry: Its current clinical utility for women. *Int Urogynecol J Pelvic Floor Dysfunct* 2008;19[7]:899–903, with permission.)

When voided volume is greater than 150 mL, a Q_{max} greater than 15 mL/s is normal.

The flow curve describes the interaction of the detrusor/bladder function and the urethra function. Uroflowmetry can be used as screening for voiding difficulties. Thus, decreased flow rate and/or long-lasting flow indicates either a weak detrusor and/or urethral obstruction. An intermittent flow curve (Fig. 12.4A) indicates the use of Valsalva during voiding and/or obstruction/weak detrusor or eventually detrusor/sphincter dyssynergia. The specificity of flow rate and pattern regarding the underlying dysfunction is low. In a case of abnormal findings, the test should be repeated to confirm consistency before a diagnosis is confirmed. When a reproducible low Q_{max} or abnormal flow-curve shape is present, voiding cystometry (pressure/flow study) is indicated to distinguish between obstruction or DU.

Postvoid Residual Volume

PVR is the remaining intravesical fluid volume determined directly after completion of the voiding. It can be measured either by a transurethral catheter or by ultrasonic scanning.

PVR reading may be erroneously elevated by delayed measurement due to renal input (1 to 14 mL/min) into bladder volume. Upper normal limit "immediate" (e.g., transvaginal ultrasound) has been reported to be 30 mL, whereas studies using urethral catheterization (up to 10 minutes delay) quote upper limits between 50 and 100 mL.

Abnormal PVR requires repeated measurement for confirmation.

The indication for PVR measurement follows uroflowmetry; however, women may have severe VD without an abnormal PVR.[12]

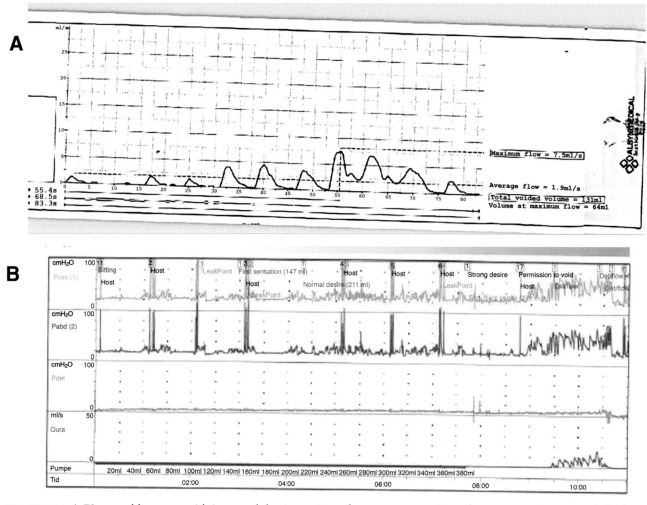

FIGURE 12.4 A 72-year-old woman with increased daytime urinary frequency, nocturia, and recurrent urinary tract infections. The Q_{max} at the free flow is 7.5 mL/s (**A**), average flow 1.9 mL/s, total voided volume is 131 mL, and the curve shows an intermittent pattern. The PVR urine was 230 mL. *DU* was demonstrated at the PFS (**B**), and the patient was treated with clean intermittent catherization.

Decreased Q_{max}, Q_{ave}, and/or increased PVR and/or Valsalva have been reported to be risk factors for VD following midurethral sling placement. However, there is no consensus regarding cutoff levels for the variables.

INVASIVE TEST OF BLADDER FILLING

Cystometry

Cystometry is a measure of the pressure–volume relationship during bladder filling. The aim is to asses bladder sensation, capacity, compliance, and detrusor activity and associated incontinence episodes during bladder filling. Two catheters are placed in the bladder (one double-lumen catheter or two separate catheters). The bladder is filled with saline solution (or x-ray contrast in case of cideo urodynamics) through one of the lumens, and the intravesical pressure is measured through the other. The abdominal pressure is preferably measured in the rectum; however, it can be measured in the vagina or in a stoma if it is not possible in the rectum. The detrusor pressure is calculated by subtracting the abdominal pressure from the intravesical pressure.

The bladder filling rate should be standardized as it affects the results of the cystometry.[1] It should be slow enough to be representative for normal bladder filling and fast enough for the examination time to be acceptable. A filling rate in the range of 30 to 50 mL/min is often suitable. GUP 2016[1] recommend that the pressure is measured with a fluid-filled external transducer, with the transducer placed at the upper edge of the symphysis pubis. If microtip catheters or air-filled catheters are used, it is important to recognize that the measured pressure is not interchangeable with the water-perfused system.

Before the examination

The urodynamic question should be clear, and the examiner should review the bladder diary in order to know which bladder capacity should be expected during the cystometry. The cystometry is not representative for the patient if the cystometric capacity is much lower than the voided volume on the diary.

Quality control

It is important to test the signals and eventually correct them before the test is started. The abdominal pressure depends on the position and size of the patient. Normal ranges of different position are as follows: supine, 5 to 20 cm H_2O; sitting, 15 to 40 cm H_2O; and standing, 30 to 50 cm H_2O. The detrusor pressure is 0 to 6 cm H_2O in 80% of cases and seldom up to 10 cm H_2O.[9] The abdominal and intravesical pressure trace should be "live" and reflecting the woman's breath or talk, whereas the detrusor curve should be "silent." The woman is asked to cough to ensure that the intravesical and abdominal pressure are measured equally (Fig. 12.5).

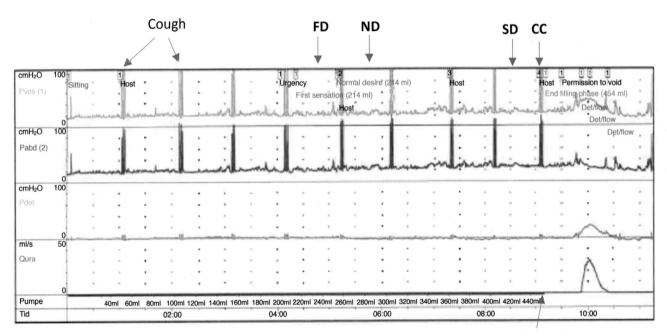

FIGURE 12.5 Normal sitting filling and voiding cystometry. Resting P_{abd} / P_{ves} = 20 cm H_2O. The woman is asked to cough at the beginning of the examination to make sure that the vesical *(upper blue line)* and the abdominal *(middle red line)* pressures are measured correctly. No pressure change is seen in the detrusor pressure *(lower green line)* during the cough which indicate that the vesical and abdominal catheters are placed and calibrated correctly. No incontinence or DO are seen during the examination. FD, first desire to void; ND, normal desire to void; SD, strong desire to void; CC, cystometric capacity.

Bladder sensation

The bladder sensation during cystometry are standardized.[2] The sensation is assessed by questioning the women about the fullness during the filling. The following is noted: The woman's first sensation of bladder filling, first desire to void, normal desire to void, strong desire to void, and if the woman has urgency during the examination. The parameters are demonstrated in Figure 12.5. There are no limits which define when the bladder sensation is abnormal; however, the woman has increased or reduced bladder sensation if she has the above sensations at low or high volumes, respectively. If she reports no bladder sensation during filling, she has absent bladder sensation. The cystometric capacity is the bladder volume at the end of filling. The woman's sensation at cystometric capacity should be noted, for example, normal desire to void or strong desire to void. The maximum cystometric capacity (MCC) is the bladder volume when she can no longer delay micturition.

The measured bladder capacity should be adjusted for diuresis and any incontinence during the examination; thus, the true cystometric capacity is the voided volume plus any residual volume during the following pressure/flow study. The bladder volume at the different sensation is subject to variation in both healthy women and in women with overactive bladder (OAB).

The most reproducible parameter is the MCC.[9,13] A tendency toward higher bladder volumes has been noted if the cytometry is repeated. The mean MCC in healthy women has been reported to be around 570 mL, range 388 to 1,362 mL.[13] Tables 12.4 and 12.5 show normal values and demonstrates test–retest variability.

Incontinence and detrusor function

Provocative maneuvers are made during filling to reproduce the patient's symptoms. The patient is asked to cough forcefully, for example, three times for each 50 mL infused into the bladder in order to detect urodynamic SUI (Fig. 12.6). In rare cases the cough induces a detrusor contraction and the patient leaks; however, this is per definition not urodynamic stress incontinence as this is defined as involuntary leakage during filling cystometry, associated with increased intra-abdominal pressure, in the absence of a detrusor contraction.

Other provocations as postural changes or hand-washing can be made to provoke DO. The detrusor function is normal if no pressure change is registered during the filling cystometry despite provocative maneuvers. The patient has DO if an involuntary detrusor contraction is noted during the filling cystometry, which can be with or without incontinence. The DO may be phasic or terminal (Fig. 12.7). It can be difficult to discriminate between fluctuations in the detrusor curve and DO.

TABLE 12.4		
Results of Duplicate Cystometry in 30 Healthy Women		
	FIRST MEASUREMENT (MEAN AND RANGE)	**SECOND MEASUREMENT (MEAN AND RANGE)**
First desire (mL)	171 (43–508)	205 (79–799)
Normal desire (mL)	284 (182–576)	351 (145–1,123)
Maximum cystometric capacity (mL)	572 (338–1,016)	570 (367–1,362)
Voided volume (mL)	651 (341–1,381)	633 (364–1,448)
Q_{max} (mL/s)	25 (8.1–51.9)	26 (11.7–64.3)
$Q_{average}$ (mL/s)	12 (2.9–29.2)	13 (3.6–24.0)
T_Q, flow time (s)	67 (24–179)	58 (27–138)
$P_{det (open)}$ (cm H_2O)	22 (4–51)	21 (4–44)
$P_{det (Qmax)}$ (cm H_2O)	30 (10–55)	29 (8–61)
$P_{det (max)}$ (cm H_2O)	46 (22–81)	53 (23–95)
$P_{ves (open)}$ (cm H_2O)	29 (10–75)	26 (9–44)
$P_{ves (Qmax)}$ (cm H_2O)	32 (17–71)	38 (13–154)
Unstable detrusor contractions (no. of patients)	4	1

From Haylen BT, de Ridder D, Freeman RM, et al. An International Urogynecological Association (IUGA)/International Continence Society (ICS) joint report on the terminology for female pelvic floor dysfunction. *Int Urogynecol J* 2010;21(1):5–26, with permission.

TABLE 12.5

Comparison of Values in Consecutive Cystometric and Pressure–Flow Studies in 30 Healthy Women

	MEAN OF DIFFERENCES OF THE TWO MEASUREMENTS (BIAS)	95% CONFIDENCE INTERVAL OF BIAS	WILCOXON SIGNED RANKS TEST (P)	LIMITS OF AGREEMENT
First desire (mL)	34	6–62	0.02*	÷104–+172
Normal desire (mL)	51	16–86	0.006**	÷124–227
Maximum cystometric capacity (mL)	÷1.8	÷28–+24	0.94	÷131–+128
Voided volume (mL)	÷11	÷48–25	0.62	÷189–+166
Q_{max} (mL/s)	1.6	÷0.7–+3.8	0.13	÷9–+12
$Q_{average}$ (mL/s)	0.1	÷1.2–+1.3	0.58	÷6–+6
T_Q, flow time (s)	÷5	÷12–+2	0.22	÷38–+28
$P_{det (open)}$ (cm H_2O)	÷2.6	÷5.7–+0.5	0.11	÷16–+11
$P_{det (Qmax)}$ (cm H_2O)	÷2.3	÷5.6–+1.0	0.17	÷14–+10
$P_{det (max)}$ (cm H_2O)	÷8	÷5–+21	0.12	÷42–+58
$P_{ves (open)}$ (cm H_2O)	÷6	÷11–÷1	0.006**	÷28–+16
$P_{ves (Qmax)}$ (cm H_2O)	÷0.5	÷4.9–+5.9	0.98	÷20–+21

*Significant at 5% level.
**Significant at 1% level.
From Haylen BT, de Ridder D, Freeman RM, et al. An International Urogynecological Association (IUGA)/International Continence Society (ICS) joint report on the terminology for female pelvic floor dysfunction. *Int Urogynecol J* 2010;21(1):5–26, with permission.

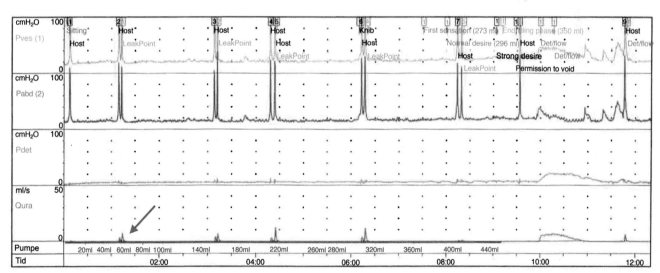

FIGURE 12.6 A 68-year-old woman with the symptoms: mixed incontinence and urgency. She had a positive stress test, the maximum voided volume on the bladder diary was 200 mL, and a pad test showed a leakage of 193 mL/24 h. The free flow was bell shaped with a Q_{max} of 36 mL/s. Mixed incontinence was suspected due to the combination of a positive stress test and the urgency symptom, the large leakage in the pad test, and the low maximum voided volume in the diary. The voiding cystometry showed large leakages during coughing, first time with 50 mL in the bladder (marked with an *arrow*). She lost 103 mL during filling cystometry which is compatible with the pad test. No DO was detected during the examination, and 453 mL was filled into the bladder; however, to calculate the cystometric capacity, the volume lost during the examination shall be subtracted from the infused volume (453 – 103 = 350 mL). The Q_{max} was only 8 mL/s at a detrusor pressure at 20 cm H_2O; however, no voiding disorder was suspected as she had a normal free flow before the examination and no voiding symptoms. The urodynamic diagnosis was *SUI* and she had a midurethral sling.

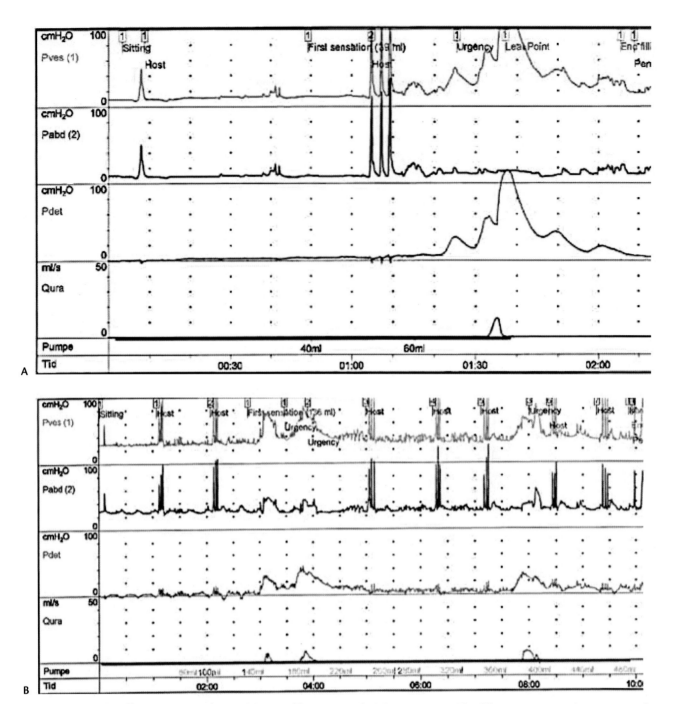

FIGURE 12.7 **A:** Filling cystometry from a 23-year-old woman with OAB symptoms. The filling cystometry shows terminal DO with incontinence. **B:** Phasic DO in a filling cystometry from an 83-year-old woman with urgency incontinence. Both women were successfully treated with intravesical botulinum toxin injection.

No formal definition exists on how large the amplitude in order to be defined as DO. Generally, the amplitude will be lower if the patient has incontinence during the DO as the resistance from the urethra will be low, which is opposed to DO without incontinence where the resistance is infinity. A cutoff value of 5 to 10 cm H_2O for DO without incontinence is often used in studies, whereas some still use the old ICS definition of 15 cm H_2O. The filling cystometry cannot diagnose a neurologic origin per se, but if a patient with DO has a relevant neurologic cause, then she has neurogenic DO per definition; otherwise, she has idiopathic DO.

The bladder compliance describes the relation between the bladder volume and detrusor pressure. It is calculated by dividing the volume change by the change in detrusor pressure and is measured as milliliter per centimeters of water. Compliance less than 20 mL/cm H_2O is abnormal low and can be a result of radiation therapy, neurologic condition, or chronic infection.

The test–retest variation of the filling volumes is around 10% to 15%, and the sensitivity and specificity of the storage symptoms is around 60% to 70% when compared to the filling cystometry. The symptom of SUI is better correlated to the finding of urodynamic SUI than the correlation between urgency and DO. The sensitivity of the cystometry depends on the position of the patient. DO is detected consistently at a higher rate in the upright position compared to the supine position; thus, the more upright the patient is, the more likely the test is to reproduce the patient's symptoms. Supine examinations are generally not recommended, and a sitting cystometry can be followed by an examination in the upright position if the first cystometry does not reproduce the patient's symptoms.

The cystometry ends when the woman is given permission to void.

Urethral Function during Filling Phase

The urethral pressure is defined as the fluid pressure just needed to open the closed urethra.[14] The urethral pressure increases as the bladder is filled due to reflex activation of the striated muscle. The voiding phase starts with a pressure drop in the urethra followed by the detrusor contraction. Urethral pressure drops might be present during urgency episodes in the filling phase as well. During the filling phase, the urethral pressure should be high enough to resist urinary leakage. Different tests can assess the urethral function.

The urethral pressure can be measured with water-perfused catheters, air-charged catheters, and microchip catheters. Microtip catheters can measure fast pressure changes as during a cough but are prone to significant artefacts due to interaction between the sensor and the urethral wall if the catheter is bending relative to the urethra; the catheter should therefore be as flexible as possible ideally as cooked spaghetti. The challenge with the artificial interaction between a stiff catheter and the urethra can be overcome if the microtip transducer is surrounded by a waterfilled balloon. The balloon should be as short as possible as the measured pressure is a mean of the urethral pressure along the length of the balloon, the same is true for the air-charge catheters. The following circumstances have impact on the measured pressure and should therefore be specified: catheter size; orientation of catheter eye or transducer and method for pressure measurement; bladder volume; position of subject; and if the subject is at rest, straining, squeezing, or coughing.

Filling Urethrocystometry

The urethral pressure can be measured with one or more sensors in the urethra during the filling cystometry. This examination may have a role in the identification of the chronologic sequence of bladder and urethral pressure changes in order to differentiate between potential different pathophysiologic entities. However, the examination is prone to artefacts as small movements of the urethral catheter can cause large pressure changes.

Urethral Pressure Profilometry

A pressure profile of the urethra can be measured by withdrawing a catheter from the bladder through the urethral lumen. A series of parameters can be deduced from the pressure profile (Fig. 12.8). The main parameter is the maximum urethral closure pressure (MUCP), which is the maximum pressure measured at the profile minus the bladder pressure. The profile can be carried out while the woman is instructed to squeeze, perform Valsalva maneuver, or while the woman is asked to cough regularly. If a Valsalva or cough profile is made, the pressure transmission can be calculated (change in urethral pressure during Valsalva or cough × 100% / change in vesical pressure during Valsalva or cough) (Fig. 12.9). The reproducibility of the parameters is generally poor, especially the dynamic parameters and if microtip transducers are used.[15] A large variation in MUCP is reported in different studies. The variation is both the results of different patient populations but also variations in the used technique, catheter size, etc. The mean MUCP is lower in groups of SUI patients compared to continent women; thus, weighted averaging mean values in SUI woman and continent women have been calculated to 39 and 54 cm H_2O, respectively; however, the overlap between the two groups are large (standard deviation: 25 cm H_2O). The MUCP declines as a function of age in the order of 1 cm H_2O per year and a very low MUCP (below 20 cm H_2O) seems to be a risk factor for persistent/recurrence of SUI after surgery[16]; however, the clinical utility of urethral pressure profilometry remain unclear.[13]

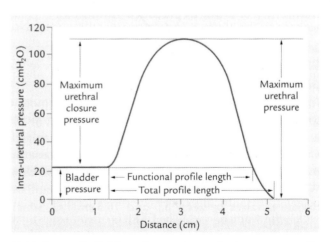

FIGURE 12.8 Definition of terms in urethral pressure profilometry. (From Lose G. Urethral pressure measurements. In: Cardozo L, ed. *Textbook of female urology and urogynecology.* United Kingdom: Informa Healthcare, 2006:251–264.)

FIGURE 12.9 Urethral pressure profiles at rest (**A**) and during coughs (**B**) in a continent woman: 7 French dual sensor tip transducer catheter, supine position, 200-mL bladder volume. p_{ura}, urethral pressure; p_{ves}, vesical pressure; PTR, pressure transmission ratio ($[\Delta p_{ura} / \Delta p_{ves}] \times 100$ %). (From Lose G. Urethral pressure measurements. In: Cardozo L, ed. *Textbook of female urology and urogynecology*. United Kingdom: Informa Healthcare, 2006:251–264.)

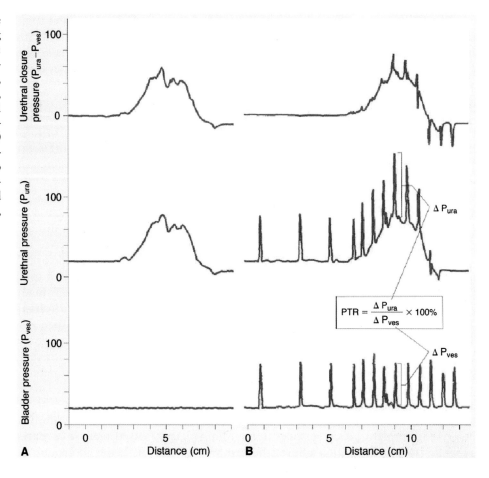

Abdominal Leak Point Pressure

Two types of leak point pressure exist: abdominal and detrusor leak point pressure. The detrusor leak point pressure is a test to assess the risk of upper urinary tract damage in patients with neurologic disease affecting the bladder, and this test will not be described further in this chapter. The abdominal leak point pressure (ALPP) is defined as the lowest value of the intentionally increased intravesical pressure that provokes urinary leakage in the absence of a detrusor contraction.[2] No value can be obtained from continent women as the test implies leaks during the measurement. The ALPP is significantly influenced by a range of circumstances which therefore should be standardized. The abdominal pressure can be increased by Valsalva maneuver at different intensities (Valsalva leak point pressure [VLPP]) or by coughing at different intensities (cough leak point pressure [CLPP]). Often, women do not leak during Valsalva maneuver, which implies that the test must be done during a cough; however, as cough induces fast pressure changes, it is difficult to measure the exact pressure at which the woman leaks. The CLPP is often higher than the VLPP, so the method for increasing the abdominal pressure cannot be used interchangeably and should be stated. The ALPP can be measured with a urethral catheter in situ or without. The urethral catheter will

affect the ALPP per se, and the larger the cross-sectional area of the urethral catheter is, the larger the ALPP will be. A test without a urethral catheter is more physiologic; however, it implies that a detrusor contraction during the test cannot be ruled out. The more volume the woman has in her bladder during the test, the lower the ALPP is. Lowest ALPP is found at MCC. The ALPP will often be lower if the woman is standing compared to sitting during the examination. The leakage can be detected visually optionally on a video recording or in a flowmeter. The test has significant test–retest variation, and the ALPP cannot predict the outcome of SUI surgery. Arbitrary limits of 60 and 90 cm H_2O has been used to discriminate between "intrinsic sphincter deficiency" and "urethral hypermobility"; however, there are no evidence to support that ALPP can reveal the urethral pathology. The clinical value of ALPP is, therefore, questionable.[17]

Urethral Pressure Reflectometry

Urethral pressure reflectometry (UPR) is a method for measuring the urethral function (Fig. 12.10). A thin and very flexible plastic bag is placed in the urethra. The cross-sectional area of the entire length of the plastic bag is continuously measured with acoustic reflectometry. The system is air filled, and a pump can increase

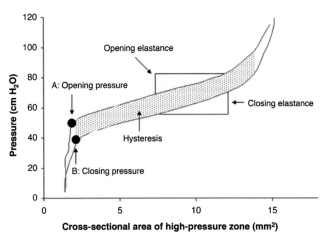

FIGURE 12.10 A UPR measurement of the urethral high-pressure zone of a 47-year-old woman with a midurethral sling. The different parameters which can be obtained from the measurements are shown on the figure. (Reprinted with permission from Saaby M-L, Klarskov N, Lose G. Urethral pressure reflectometry before and after tension-free vaginal tape. *Neurourol Urodyn* 2012;31[8]:1231–1235.)

and decrease the pressure in the system and thereby open and close the plastic bag and thus also the urethra. Measurements can be carried out while the woman relaxes her pelvic floor and during squeezing and straining. Figure 12.11 shows the different parameters which can be obtained. UPR has been used by the pharmaceutical industry to test new drugs with potential effect on SUI,[18,19] and UPR measurements during straining can predict SUI after prolapse surgery.[20] UPR is still not commercially available.

INVASIVE TEST OF BLADDER EMPTYING

PFS is an investigation of micturition. When the filling cystometry is completed, "permission to void" is given, and uroflowmetry, intravesical (P_{ves}), abdominal (P_{abd}), and detrusor ($P_{det} = P_{ves} - P_{abd}$) pressures are measured simultaneously.

The position of the patient, the catheter sizes, and the pressure and flow recording technique should be specified.[1] The parameters measured are standardized (see Fig. 12.11).[2]

The aim of PFS is to sort out symptoms and/or voiding abnormalities found by spontaneous uroflowmetry and PVR measurement, especially to distinguish between BOO or underactive detrusor (DU) function.

"Normal values" have been reported; they depend on the technique and the women population studied (Table 12.4), which lead to large/significant intersite variability, which adds to the inherent test–retest variation (Table 12.5).

According to the IUGA/ICS, **VD**, a diagnosis by symptoms and urodynamic investigations, is defined

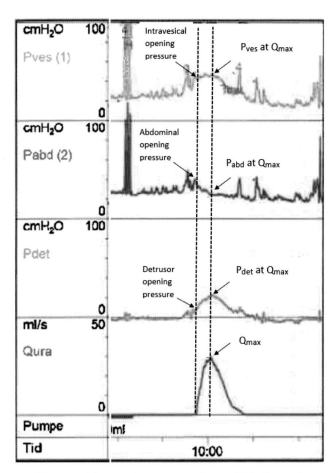

FIGURE 12.11 Most used parameters from a PFS. Q_{ura}, urinary flow.

as abnormally slow and/or incomplete micturition. Abnormally, slow urine flow rates and abnormally high PVRs, the bases of this diagnosis, are outlined in uroflowmetry and PVR (urine volume). The diagnosis should be based on repeated measurement to confirm abnormality. Further evaluation, PFSs are indicated to evaluate the cause of any VD.[2]

VD is not uncommon in women especially among the elderly. Thus, urodynamic VD is a frequent finding either alone or in combination with other entities.

VD symptoms such as hesitancy, slow stream, intermittency, straining to void, and feeling of incomplete (bladder) emptying may cause patients to seek treatment. These symptoms are unspecific, and the correlation to urodynamic VD is unclear. Furthermore, urodynamic VD (increased PVR and/or decreased flow rate) may be asymptomatic or an occasional finding, for example, when assessing women with SUI and/or DO.

If noninvasive urodynamic testing detects abnormalities, invasive pressure flow study, possibly in terms of videocystography (video-UDS) or in combination with EMG of the PFM/striated sphincter, is the gold standard to distinguish between BOO, DU, dysfunctional voiding, or detrusor sphincter dyssynergia (DSD).

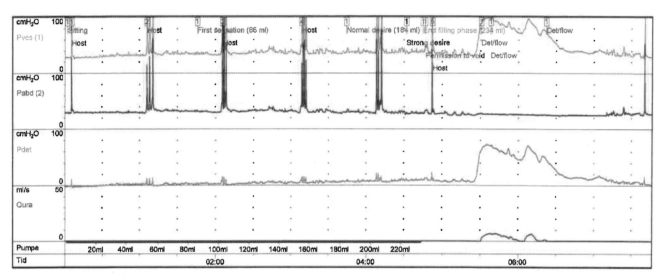

FIGURE 12.12 Filling cystometry and PFS from a 57-year-old woman complaining of slow stream during voiding. She has had a midurethral sling 5 years before, and the stream has gradually become slower over the years. She had a Q_{max} of 7 mL/s on the free flow. The maximum detrusor pressure during voiding is 76 cm H_2O (Q_{max} 7 mL/s); thus, the urodynamic diagnosis is moderate obstruction.

According to ICS/IUGA, **BOO** is the generic term for obstruction during voiding. Urodynamically, BOO is characterized by reduced urine flow rate and/or presence of a raised PVR and an increased detrusor pressure. Common causes are higher degrees of POP, urethral stricture, or obstructed voiding after stress incontinence procedures (Fig. 12.12).

BOO urodynamic is well established in males; however, there is no universally accepted precise diagnostic criterion of BOO in women.

Pressure–flow data from women volunteers are available (see Table 12.4); however, values depend on the technique and the age of women population. Various nomograms (Fig. 12.13) and numbers based on pressure–flow

data and free flows have been suggested.[9,21] Cutoff values to detect BOO (from intubated PFS) varies between Q_{max} less than 12 to 15 mL/s and P_{det}/Q_{max} greater than 20 to 30 cm H_2O with various sensitivities and specificities (Table 12.6). In all studies, there are significant overlap in voiding parameters between normal women and those with VD.

Blaivas and Groutz[21] have described a nomogram to classify BOO into four categories based on videourodynamic studies (see Fig. 12.13). BOO was *defined* as a free Q_{max} less than 12 mL/s combined with a P_{det}/Q_{max} of greater than 20 cm H_2O at the PFS or obvious radiographic evidence of BOO in the presence of a sustained detrusor contraction of at least 20 cm H_2O and poor Q_{max}, regardless of free Q_{max}, or inability to void with the transurethral catheter in place despite a sustained detrusor contraction of at least 20 cm H_2O. This nomogram has been frequently reported.

Elevated PVR is only weakly related to BOO and possibly more indicative of detrusor failure. Thus, normal PVR values at PFS does not exclude BOO.[12]

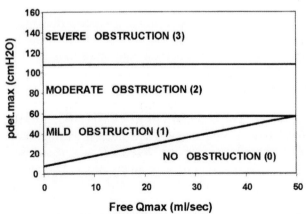

FIGURE 12.13 Bladder outlet obstruction nomogram for women. (From Blaivas JG, Groutz A. Bladder outlet obstruction nomogram for women with lower urinary tract symptomatology. *Neurourol Urodyn* 2000;19[5]:553–564, with permission.)

TABLE 12.6			
Examples from the Literature of Cutoff Values of Q_{max} and P_{det}/Q_{max} to Detect BOO			
Q_{MAX} (mL/s)	**P_{DET}/Q_{MAX} (cm H_2O)**	**SENSITIVITY**	**SPECIFICITY**
12	25	68%	68%
<15	>20	74%	91%
≤15	≥30	82%	94%

According to IUGA/ICS, **DU** is defined as "detrusor contraction of reduced strength and/or duration, resulting in prolonged bladder emptying and/or failure to achieve complete bladder emptying within a normal time span" (Fig. 12.4B).

The diagnosis requires a PFS. Key symptoms of DU have not yet been defined, and there is no consensus regarding the precise urodynamic finding (diagnosis). Various parameters have been suggested. Based on PFS, cutoff values for detection DU of P_{det}/Q_{max} 10 cm H_2O or less and Q_{max} less than 12 mL/s combined with significant P_{abd} rise (25 to 82 cm H_2O) have been proposed.[22] Other authors have defined "impaired contractility" as a P_{det} less than 20 cm H_2O associated with a flow less than 20 mL/s and no radiographic evidence of obstruction or an unsustained detrusor contraction resulting in poor emptying.[23]

Many diseases and disorders may cause DU. Thus, the etiology may be neurogenic, myogenic, and iatrogenic.

Dysfunctional voiding and **DSD** have also been defined.[2] These diagnoses require expert assessment and special tests such as videocystourethrography and sphincter EMG.

NEUROGENIC LOWER URINARY TRACT DYSFUNCTIONS

Cystometry and PFS are used in patients with neurogenic lesions to determine the level of injury, extend of the injury, and the derived lower urinary tract dysfunction.

Injuries in different anatomical locations in the central and peripheral nervous systems cause various urodynamic findings which can be diagnostic for the level of injury. The injuries are divided into upper motor neuron lesions (suprapontine, pontine, suprasacral spinal cord) and lower motor neuron lesions (sacral and subsacral lesions) (Fig. 12.14).

Suprapontine Lesions

The lesion is located above the pontine micturition center and can lead to loss of tonic inhibition of the pontine micturition center, which can lead to DO. The micturition is normally coordinated as the pontine micturition center and the nerve system distally are intact. However, depending on the insults the voluntary initiation of voiding, sensation during filling and voiding may be impaired as well.

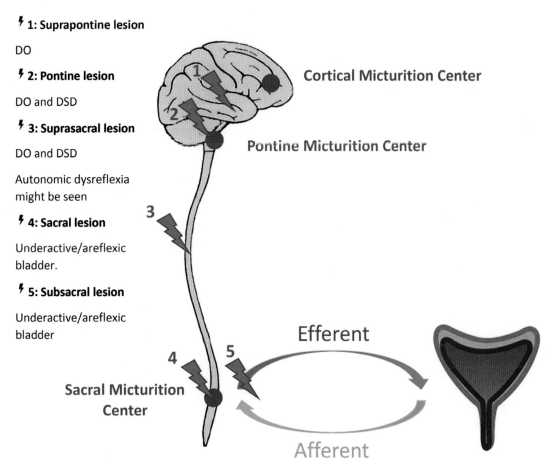

⚡ **1: Suprapontine lesion**

DO

⚡ **2: Pontine lesion**

DO and DSD

⚡ **3: Suprasacral lesion**

DO and DSD

Autonomic dysreflexia might be seen

⚡ **4: Sacral lesion**

Underactive/areflexic bladder.

⚡ **5: Subsacral lesion**

Underactive/areflexic bladder

Cortical Micturition Center

Pontine Micturition Center

Efferent

Sacral Micturition Center

Afferent

FIGURE 12.14 Schematic drawing of the micturition centers in the central nerve system and the typical urodynamic findings. Injuries are divided into suprapontine, pontine, suprasacral, sacral, and subsacral lesions. (Courtesy of Marlene Elmelund.)

Pontine Lesions

The pons is critical in homeostatic and physiologic functions and lesions in the pons are therefore often lethal. In the rare cases where the patient survives the insult, the urodynamic findings may be DO and DSD as the micturition center is placed in pons.

Complete Suprasacral Lesions

An autonomous caudal segment of the spinal cord called distal autonomous cord is formed when the spinal cord is transected at a level above conus medullaris (L1/L2). The LUT is regulated by reflex activity without coordination as the distal autonomous cord does not communicate with the pontine micturition center. Thus, neurogenic DO and DSD are seen on invasive urodynamic tests. Low compliance is often seen years after the injury due to bladder fibrosis.

An important feature in the distal autonomous cord is autonomic dysreflexia, which can be potentially lethal. It is only seen in patients with suprasacral lesions above T6 as the condition is provoked by a sympathetic stimulus in the distal autonomous cord above T6 (e.g., bladder filling). Vasoconstriction is seen in the area supplied by the distal autonomous cord; thus, blood is squeezed to the circulation above this area resulting in significant hypertension in the region above the spinal cord lesion. Baroreceptors in the region with hypertension precipitate bradycardia and vasodilatation in the area above the lesion but not at the area below, which leads to a characteristic appearance of vasoconstriction in the skin below the lesion and vasodilation above.

> It is important to abort the examination and empty the bladder if the patient has symptoms of *autonomic dysreflexia* (hypertension, bradycardia, sweating, goose bumps, blurred vision, headache, or seizure). If the autonomic dysreflexia does not resolve when the bladder is emptied, the condition can be treated with sublingual nitrates or oral hydralazine.

Incomplete Suprasacral Lesions

Variable bladder and sphincter functions are seen depending on the position and extend of the lesion, thus the following can both be present and absent: neurogenic DO, bladder sensation, and DSD.

Sacral Lesions

The patient can have an areflexic bladder if the parasympathetic region is involved in the lesion and a paralytic urethral sphincter if the Onuf nucleus is involved leading to neurogenic SUI.

Subsacral Lesions

Lesions in the cauda equina or peripheral nerves can lead to both parasympathetic and somatic motor function impairment. Thus, the detrusor can be underactive or areflexic and the urethral sphincter and pelvic floor musculature may be paralyzed. The patient may have some pain and filling sensation do to an intact sympathetic hypogastric nerve, which enter in the thoracic roots of the spinal cord.

Some extra urodynamic tests can be added to the examination of the patients with neurogenic lesions.

EMG registration from the urethral sphincter is often added to the examination to detect DSD.

Ice water test: Temperature receptors in the mucosa of the bladder elicit a reflex contraction of the detrusor; however, the reflex is inhibited by supraspinal centers. An upper motor neuron lesion will interrupt the inhibitory fibers resulting in a manifest reflex, whereas the reflex is not present in lower motor neuron lesions and in neurologically intact women. The reflex is provoked by injecting cold water into the bladder, and the test is positive if it results in a detrusor contraction. The sensitivity and specificity to discriminate if the lesion is an upper or lower motor neuro lesion has been debated. The test may have pathophysiologic value in women with multiple sclerosis as the test can discriminate between cerebral and spinal origin of neurogenic DO. As the ice water test is unphysiologic it should not precede other urodynamic tests as it can significantly bias subsequent tests.

Bethanechol supersensitivity test is a test to discriminate between neurologic and myogenic etiology in an acontractile bladder. An organ develops hypersensitivity to the excitatory neurotransmitters when it is deprived of its nerve supply; thus, a muscarinic agonist (bethanechol) given to a patient with a denervated bladder should theoretically provide a strong detrusor contraction, although the detrusor contraction should be weaker in patients with a neurologic intact bladder. The bethanechol supersensitivity test is positive if the detrusor pressure increases more than 15 cm H_2O in response to subcutaneous administration of 2.5-mg bethanechol; however, the reliability of the test has been debated.

Urodynamics Challenges and Errors (Artefacts)

UDS have the direct disadvantages of the inconvenience of the examination and risk of urinary tract infection and dysuria if a catheter is used. However, of more importance are false-positive and false-negative results and misinterpretation due to artefacts, which might lead to an ineffective or harmful treatment or deprive the patient of an effective treatment.

Stress incontinence: It is well known that it can be difficult to reproduce the patients stress incontinence during a stress test or during a cystometry. This can especially be difficult in young women who only leak during sport activity. However, the opposite might also be true where, especially older women, leak during a forceful cough with full bladder. She might not be bothered of stress incontinence as she does not cough regularly, and other LUT symptoms might have led her to seek medical care. Thus, an effective treatment for stress incontinence might not relieve the elderly patient from her real bother.

DO: The absence of DO during a cystometry might be a false-negative test result as well as demonstration of DO can be a false-positive result. Some labs routinely make provocative maneuvers like letting the water run; however, some women might need other circumstances to provoke their DO. Studies on healthy women without OAB syndrome have shown DO in 5% to 10% (see Table 12.4). The DO might be falsely provoked by the bladder catheters, by the infused water, or by the test circumstances per se.

PFS: VDs can, almost with certainty, be excluded if the patient has normal flow without straining; however, a pathologic flow or straining during the test is common in women without VD as it is difficult for the women to void on command during test circumstances. It is, therefore, important to ask the woman if the urination felt consistent with her normal voiding as only a test during normal voiding has value.

EMG: The electrodes can very easily register activity from other muscles especially if surface electrodes are used and the signal can be absent if the electrode has poor contact with the patient or is placed incorrectly.

Artefacts: The possible artefacts are countless. A systematic description can be found in "Urodynamic Features and Artefacts" by Stephen Hogan et al.,[24] but it is beyond the scope of this chapter to discuss them all. However, a few artefacts should be mentioned as they might be misinterpreted and therefore lead to a wrong conclusion.

Cough-induced DO: It is a relatively uncommon condition where a cough induces a detrusor contraction. The patient often has the symptoms of mixed incontinence, but the urodynamic diagnosis is pure DO incontinence. The condition is therefore important to acknowledge. A relatively common artefact mimics cough-induced DO. In the "erroneous cough-induced DO," the increased pressure on the detrusor curve is due to a decrease in the abdominal pressure and not due to an increased bladder pressure. The artefact is due to incorrect calibration of the abdominal catheter, movement of the anal catheter, or relaxation of the rectum after the cough. The patient will often have the symptom stress incontinence or mixed incontinence and the urodynamic diagnosis correspond to this if the artefact is recognized. Figure 12.15 shows examples of both the real and the artificial cough-induced DO.

Low compliance bladder: The detrusor pressure increases when the bladder is filled in the low

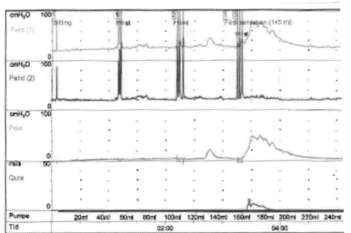
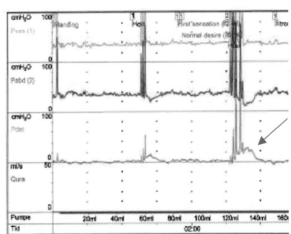

FIGURE 12.15 A: A 38-year-old woman with the symptom SUI. She has had a midurethral sling with no effect. The cystometry showed *cough-induced DO* incontinence but no SUI which can explain the lack of effect of the midurethral sling. **B:** A 48-year-old woman with the symptom SUI. A pressure increase is seen on the detrusor curve *(arrow)*, which could be misinterpreted as true cough-induced DO; however, the *artificial* increase in detrusor pressure is due to a pressure drop in the abdominal pressure *(red curve)*, and no pressure increase is seen in the bladder pressure *(blue curve)*. Large pressure increases are seen in at the detrusor curve *(green curve)* during the cough, which indicates that the abdominal catheter not measure correctly.

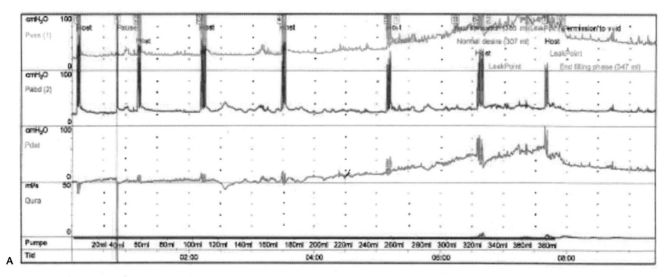

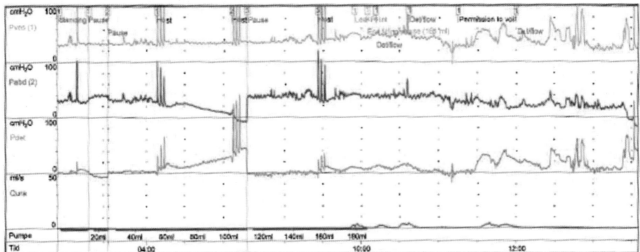

FIGURE 12.16 **A:** A 73-year-old woman with the symptom SUI. She had radiation therapy 16 years before due to cervical cancer. The detrusor pressure *(green line)* increases when more than 200 mL is infused into the bladder due to *decreased compliance*. When 320 mL is infused into the bladder, the detrusor pressure is 50 cm H_2O (compliance: 6.4 mL/cm H_2O) and she leaks during coughing. She was advised to void more frequently so the bladder volume was kept under 250 mL. **B:** A 65-year-old woman with OAB symptoms. The detrusor pressure increases rapidly. In this patient, however, it is an *artefact* because of decreasing abdominal pressure and not an increasing vesical pressure. The pressure drop in the abdominal tracing is due to a leaking tube. The examination is paused, the problem is corrected, and the examination is completed. The cystometry shows *DO* with incontinence and *normal compliance*.

compliance bladder. The patient often has a history with radiation therapy, has a chronic infection, or has a spinal cord injury. A leak from the rectal catheter can mimic a low compliance bladder, but the tracing will show a decreasing abdominal pressure instead of an increasing bladder pressure. Figure 12.16 shows examples of both a low compliance bladder and a cystometry with a leaky rectal catheter. The urodynamic examination should generally be easy to read; otherwise, an artefact should be suspected.

As false-positive and false-negative results and artefacts might lead to the wrong diagnosis, the patient might end up with an inferior treatment compared to if she did not have a urodynamic investigation. To prevent this from happening, it is important to follow the principles of good urodynamic practice.

References

1. Rosier PF, Schaefer W, Lose G, et al. International Continence Society Good Urodynamic Practices and Terms 2016: Urodynamics, uroflowmetry, cystometry, and pressure-flow study. *Neurourol Urodyn* 2017;36(5):1243–1260.
2. Haylen BT, de Ridder D, Freeman RM, et al. An International Urogynecological Association (IUGA)/International Continence Society (ICS) joint report on the terminology for female pelvic floor dysfunction. *Int Urogynecol J* 2010;21(1):5–26.
3. Serati M, Topazio L, Bogani G, et al. Urodynamics useless before surgery for female stress urinary incontinence: Are you sure? Results from a multicenter single nation database. *Neurourol Urodyn* 2016;35(7):809–812.
4. Agur W, Housami F, Drake M, et al. Could the National Institute for Health and Clinical Excellence guidelines on urodynamics in urinary incontinence put some women at risk of a bad outcome from stress incontinence surgery? *BJU Int* 2009;103(5):635–639.

5. Finazzi-Agro E, Gammie A, Kessler TM, et al. Urodynamics useless in female stress urinary incontinence? Time for some sense—A European expert consensus. *Eur Urol Focus* 2020;6(1):137–145.

6. Nager CW, Brubaker L, Litman HJ, et al. A randomized trial of urodynamic testing before stress–incontinence surgery. *N Engl J Med* 2012;366(21):1987–1997.

7. van Leijsen SAL, Kluivers KB, Mol BWJ, et al. The value of preoperative urodynamics according to gynecologists and urologists with special interest in stress urinary incontinence. *Int Urogynecol J* 2012;23(4):423–428.

8. van Leijsen SAL, Kluivers KB, Mol BWJ, et al. Value of urodynamics before stress urinary incontinence surgery: A randomized controlled trial. *Obstet Gynecol* 2013;121(5):999–1008.

9. Schäfer W, Abrams P, Liao L, et al. Good urodynamic practices: Uroflowmetry, filling cystometry, and pressure-flow studies. *Neurourol Urodyn* 2002;21(3):261–274.

10. Lose G, Dwyer PL, Riss P. The standardization of urodynamic reporting in the *International Urogynecology Journal*. *Int Urogynecol J* 2016;27(7):979–980.

11. Khayyami Y, Elmelund M, Lose G, et al. De novo urinary incontinence after pelvic organ prolapse surgery—A national database study. *Int Urogynecol J* 2020;31(2):305–308.

12. Khayyami YN, Klarskov N, Lose G. Post-void residual urine under 150 ml does not exclude voiding dysfunction in women. *Int Urogynecol J* 2016;27(3):467–473.

13. Brostrom SP, Jennum P, Lose G. Short-term reproducibility of cystometry and pressure-flow micturition studies in healthy women. *Neurourol Urodyn* 2002;21(5):457–460.

14. Lose G, Griffiths D, Hosker G, et al. Standardisation of urethral pressure measurement: Report from the Standardisation Sub-Committee of the International Continence Society. *Neurourol Urodyn* 2002;21(3):258–260.

15. Weber AM. Is urethral pressure profilometry a useful diagnostic test for stress urinary incontinence? *Obstet Gynecol Surv* 2001;56(11):720–735.

16. Moe K, Schiotz HA, Kulseng-Hanssen S. Outcome of TVT operations in women with low maximum urethral closure pressure. *Neurourol Urodyn* 2017;36(5):1320–1324.

17. Rosier P. Urodynamic testing. In: Abrams P, Cardozo L, Wagg A, et al, eds. *Incontinence*, 6th ed. United Kingdom: International Continence Society, 2017:599–670.

18. Klarskov N, Scholfield D, Soma K, et al. Measurement of urethral closure function in women with stress urinary incontinence. *J Urol* 2009;181(6):2628–2633.

19. Klarskov N, Van Till O, Sawyer W, et al. Effect of a 5-HT$_{2c}$ receptor agonist on urethral closure mechanism in healthy women. *Neurourol Urodyn* 2019;38(6):1700–1706.

20. Khayyami Y, Lose G, Klarskov N. The urethral closure mechanism is deteriorated after anterior colporrhaphy. *Int Urogynecol J* 2018;29(9):1311–1316.

21. Blaivas JG, Groutz A. Bladder outlet obstruction nomogram for women with lower urinary tract symptomatology. *Neurourol Urodyn* 2000;19(5):553–564.

22. Gotoh M, Yoshikawa Y, Ohshima S. Pathophysiology and subjective symptoms in women with impaired bladder emptying. *Int J Urol* 2006;13(8):1053–1057.

23. Carlson KV, Fiske J, Nitti VW. Value of routine evaluation of the voiding phase when performing urodynamic testing in women with lower urinary tract symptoms. *J Urol* 2000;164(5):1614–1618.

24. Hogan S, Gammie A, Abrams P. Urodynamic features and artefacts. *Neurourol Urodyn* 2012;31(7):1104–1117.

CHAPTER 13

Magnetic Resonance and Fluoroscopic Imaging of the Pelvic Floor

Bahar Mansoori • Suzanne L. Palmer • Gaurav Khatri

Introduction

Magnetic resonance imaging (MRI) and fluoroscopic imaging are widely used imaging modalities for evaluation of patients with pelvic floor disorders. They provide information regarding pelvic floor function during strain and defecation, and MRI, in particular, provides detailed anatomic evaluation due to its high-contrast resolution. This chapter focuses on relevant anatomy of the pelvic floor as seen on MRI, indications for imaging, MRI and fluoroscopic imaging techniques, and imaging findings on MR and fluoroscopic defecography (FD) in patients with pelvic floor dysfunction.

PELVIC FLOOR ANATOMY

Knowledge of pelvic floor anatomy is essential in understanding and imaging disorders of the pelvic floor. For anatomic and functional evaluation, the pelvic floor in females is divided into three distinct compartments: anterior, apical, and posterior. Because the pelvic floor structures are closely interrelated, concomitant dysfunction of more than one compartment is common.[1,2] The anterior compartment of the female pelvic floor includes the bladder and urethra; the apical compartment contains the uterus, cervix, and vagina; and the posterior compartment consists of the rectum and anal canal. Three layers of fascial/ligamentous and muscular structures provide support and integrity to the pelvic floor from superior to inferior: the endopelvic fascia, the pelvic diaphragm, and the urogenital diaphragm.[3,4] These pelvic muscles and fascial/ligamentous structures provide active and passive support of the pelvic floor, respectively. The interaction between the endopelvic fascia and pelvic diaphragm maintains the pelvic organs in place. When the levator ani muscles function as intended, the pelvic floor tone is maintained and there is low tension on ligaments and fascia. However, unrepaired defects, tears, or sustained relaxation of levator ani result in chronic strain on the pelvic ligaments and may eventually result in ligament damage.

Subsequently, chronic deficiency of the levator musculature and pelvic ligaments places increased stress on the connective tissue/endopelvic fascia which may eventually fail to support the pelvic organs.[5]

Endopelvic Fascia

The endopelvic fascia is a connective tissue structure which comprises the most superior layer of support in pelvic floor. It attaches to the lateral pelvic side wall bilaterally at the arcus tendinous levator ani (ATLA), providing lateral support for pelvic organs (Fig. 13.1). Different components of the endopelvic fascia are named based on their anatomic locations (e.g., pubovaginal/pubocervical, rectovaginal, parametrium, and paracorpium fascia). A few identifiable components of the endopelvic fascia on MRI include the urethral ligaments, perineal body, cardinal, and uterosacral ligaments.[3] Because the majority of endopelvic fascia is not directly visualized on imaging, the intact status of the fascia is inferred by normal appearance of the pelvic organs. Defects in various levels of the endopelvic fascia manifest as deformity of the vaginal and/or paravaginal structures on imaging.

Pelvic Diaphragm

The pelvic diaphragm is formed by levator ani muscles and coccygeus muscle. The levator ani is a striated muscle group, constantly in contraction, providing resting tone to the pelvic floor. Further contraction and relaxation of the levator ani muscles plays an important role in pelvic floor function. The levator ani comprises three components: puborectalis, pubococcygeus, and iliococcygeus muscles. Anteriorly, these muscles attach to the posterior aspect of the pubic symphysis and inferior pubic ramus, laterally extend along the tendinous attachment of obturator internus muscle (arcus tendinous), and posteriorly attach to the coccyx. The levator plate (anococcygeal ligament) is the tendinous insertion of the levator ani muscle to the coccyx and

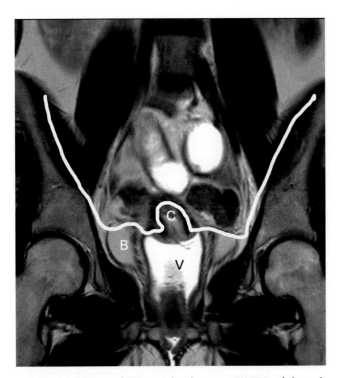

FIGURE 13.1 Coronal T2-weighted image (T2WI) of the pelvis from magnetic resonance defecography. The *white line* denotes the location of the endopelvic fascia which attaches to the lateral pelvic side wall on either side, providing lateral support for pelvic organs. B, bladder; C, cervix; V, vagina.

is a near-horizontally oriented structure parallel to the posterior wall of the rectum (Fig. 13.2A). The levator ani muscles demarcate the urogenital hiatus, where the urogenital apparatus resides. The puborectalis muscle is the interiormost muscle in the levator ani group and is a U-shaped sling that extends from the posterior aspect of the pubic symphysis wrapping around the anorectum and forms the margins of the pelvic floor hiatus (Fig. 13.2B). The levator hiatus has a mean area of 11 cm^2 at rest and 14 cm^2 on maximal strain in nulliparous women.[6] The effect of hiatal enlargement on pelvic organ prolapse (POP) is discussed in the following sections. The puborectalis is the main muscle that maintains the anorectal angle (ARA) and therefore fecal continence. Puborectalis muscle relaxation results in widening of the ARA and pelvic floor hiatus. Furthermore, the puborectalis provides additional support to the periurethral ligaments. The pubococcygeus arises from the superior pubic ramus and attaches to the levator plate posteriorly. The iliococcygeus functionally supports the vagina and appears as a sheet-like muscle arising from the arcus tendineus laterally and inserts upon the levator plate posteriorly. It appears as a slightly convex structure superiorly on coronal images (Fig. 13.2C). The coccygeus muscle is the most posterior aspect of the pelvic diaphragm and extends from the ischial spine to the midline coccyx.

Urogenital Diaphragm (Perineal Membrane)

The urogenital diaphragm is a fibromuscular layer of connective tissue located below the pelvic diaphragm (see Fig. 13.2C). It has a triangular shape and extends horizontally from the ischium on either side to the perineal body in the midline with attachment anteriorly to the pubic symphysis. The perineal body comprises the thick connective tissue in the perineum centrally between the anal verge and anterior urogenital triangle and is an attachment site for multiple pelvic floor structures such as perineal musculature, external anal sphincter, and rectovaginal fascia. In the female pelvis, the urethra and vagina traverse the urogenital diaphragm.[3,7,8]

Effect of Levator Ani Avulsion on Pelvic Organ Prolapse

The etiology for POP is multifactorial. For years, it was speculated that vaginal deliveries contribute to development of POP. Levator ani avulsion which is defined as detachment of the muscle from the pubic insertion occurs in about 10% to 30% of vaginal deliveries. Several studies have demonstrated presence of macroscopic and microscopic abnormalities in the levator ani after childbirth. Replacement of muscle with fibrosis in women with stress urinary incontinence (SUI) and/or POP has been validated on postmortem studies.[9–11] More recent studies have shown that avulsion of the levator ani, resulting in muscle weakness and widening of the levator hiatus, predisposes to POP years later.[12–16] In evaluation of 423 women with vaginal delivery, Handa et al.[15] found 64 (15%) women experienced some degrees of levator ani avulsion. Compared to the control group, these women had larger dimensions of the levator hiatus; the odds of POP were increased by approximately 50% for every 5-cm^2 increase in the levator hiatus area. Furthermore, in this group, pelvic floor muscle strength (measured during voluntary pelvic muscle contraction with a perineometer) was inversely and significantly associated with the odds of prolapse. Imaging abnormalities of levator ani avulsion have been described on MRI and translabial three-dimensional ultrasound (US).[13,17,18] The pertinent imaging findings on US are discussed in Chapter 14. Levator muscle defects on MRI may manifest as absence or detachment of the muscle or scarring (Fig. 13.3). DeLancey et al.[13] showed injury to the levator ani frequently involves the pubovisceral portion of the muscle that arises from the inner surface of the pubic bone just lateral to the vagina but also involves the iliococcygeal muscle.[19] In evaluation of a small cohort of primiparous women 6 to 7 weeks after normal vaginal delivery, Shi et al.[20] demonstrated that majority

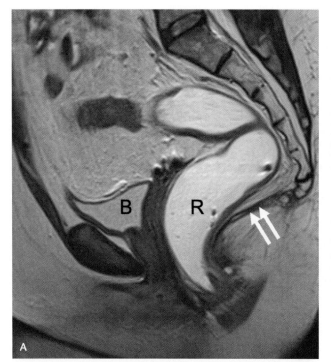

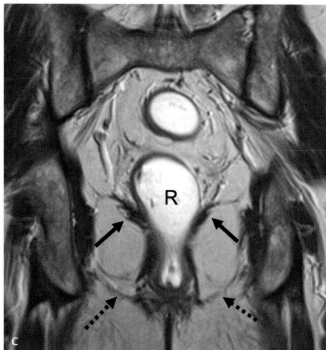

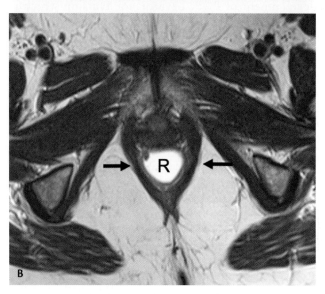

FIGURE 13.2 **A:** T2-weighted image (T2WI) through the mid-sagittal plane of the pelvis. The levator plate (anococcygeal ligament) is the tendinous insertion of the levator ani muscle to the coccyx and is a near-horizontally oriented structure parallel to the posterior wall of the rectum *(arrows in **A**)*. **B:** Axial T2WI demonstrates the normal symmetric puborectalis sling *(solid arrows in **B**)* outlining the urogenital or levator hiatus. **C:** Coronal T2WI shows levator ani muscle with superior convexity *(solid arrows in **C**)* and the urogenital diaphragm (also known as the perineal membrane) inferiorly extending from the ischial tuberosities laterally to the perineal body in the midline *(dashed arrows)*. B, bladder; R, rectum.

of levator ani avulsions occurred at the origin. The tears of the pubococcygeus were located at the pubic origin. The tears of the iliococcygeus were located at or near the fascia of the obturator internus. All tears of the pubococcygeus were associated with focal pubic bone marrow edema. However, in a few cases, bone marrow edema was not accompanied by associated tears. Both MRI and US can provide valuable information about puborectalis muscle tears; however, the origin and insertion of the iliococcygeus are better evaluated on MRI. Therefore, in cases of suspected severe injury to the puborectalis, MRI may be preferred to evaluate any associated injury to the iliococcygeus muscle.[21]

INDICATIONS FOR PELVIC FLOOR IMAGING

Initial assessment of patients with pelvic floor disorders starts with clinical evaluation. Pelvic floor imaging is typically obtained as an adjunct to clinical evaluation particularly when the physical examination is limited or when clinical findings are discordant with or do not fully explain patient symptoms. Clinical evaluation may underestimate severity of POP or extent of involvement in 45% to 90% of cases.[2] Specifically, physical examination can be limited in assessment of patients with evacuation disorders and conditions that clinically could be occult, such as concomitant presence of enterocele or peritoneocele.

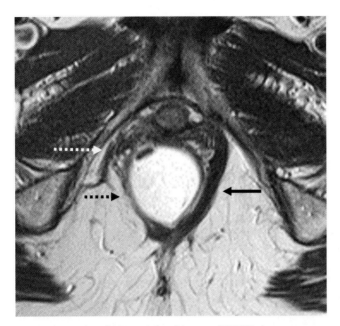

FIGURE 13.3 Axial T2-weighted image (T2WI) demonstrates normal puborectalis muscle on the left *(solid arrow)* and torn atrophic puborectalis muscle on the right *(short dashed arrow)* with anterior detachment and scarring *(long dashed arrow)*.

Failure to identify and address occult defects during the initial procedure has been shown in approximately 40% of the cases which needed reoperation.[22,23] The most common indications for pelvic floor imaging include (1) suspected multicompartmental dysfunction to assess severity and identify clinically occult defects, (2) preoperative assessment to confirm clinical findings and determine the most appropriate surgical approach in patients with suspected pelvis floor disorders, (3) differentiating etiologies of defecatory dysfunction, (4) postoperative evaluation in patients with recurrent pelvic floor dysfunction, and (5) postoperative evaluation in patients with suspected postsurgical complications.[5]

ROLE OF VARIOUS IMAGING MODALITIES

Among the available imaging modalities, computed tomography (CT) has limited role in evaluation of pelvic floor disorders, largely due to lack of soft tissue contrast compared to MRI as well as lack of dynamic imaging capability. Nevertheless, imaging findings of severe pelvic floor weakness may be identified incidentally on the routine CT scans performed for other purposes (Fig. 13.4). Traditionally, fluoroscopy has been the imaging modality of choice for evaluation of patients with pelvic floor disorders. Fluoroscopy can allow assessment of pelvic floor dysfunction in all three compartments in a physiologic upright position; however, it is limited in the evaluation of pelvic floor anatomy. More recently, MRI has become a frequently used modality for evaluation of pelvic floor dysfunction due to its ability to provide detailed anatomic in addition to functional information, lack of ionizing radiation, and ubiquitous availability of MR machines. In this chapter, we provide an overview on role of both MRI and fluoroscopy in evaluation of pelvic floor abnormalities. Pelvic floor US is an emerging modality for assessment of pelvic floor anatomy and function; the role of US in pelvic floor imaging is discussed in Chapter 14.

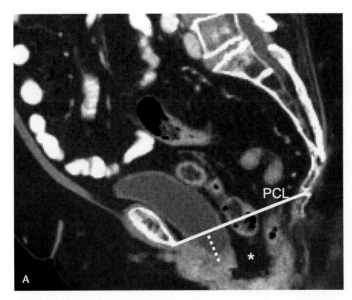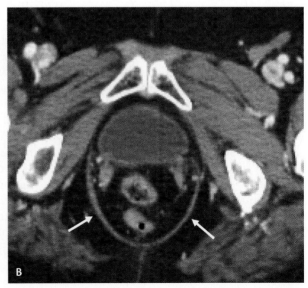

FIGURE 13.4 **A:** Sagittal CT image shows cystocele—descent of the bladder *(dashed line)* below the pubococcygeal line (PCL), a landmark drawn from the inferior tip of the symphysis pubis to the last coccygeal joint. There is also increased fat extending below the PCL and widening the rectovaginal space *(asterisk)*. **B:** Axial CT image shows ballooning of the puborectalis *(arrows)* and widening of the levator hiatus.

MAGNETIC RESONANCE DEFECOGRAPHY

MRI has excellent soft tissue contrast resolution and provides detailed anatomic information on pelvic organs as well as the muscular and ligamentous structures of the pelvic floor. The ability to acquire dynamic imaging during pelvic floor maneuvers such as Kegel, Valsalva, and defecation as part of an MR defecography examination provides additional value in comprehensive evaluation of all three compartments simultaneously. By incorporating anatomic and functional information, MR defecography can provide a roadmap for a tailored individualized surgical approach for each patient and has been shown to alter surgical management in up to 67% of patients.[24]

Patient Positioning and Preparation

Patient preparation for MR defecography starts with patient education. Prior to the examination, the referring physicians should explain the procedure, discuss the importance of adequate patient effort, and alleviate any concerns that patients might have about defecating during an imaging examination. Radiology personnel should ease patient anxiety by explaining clearly the instructions used during the image acquisitions and addressing any concerns patients might have upon arrival to their imaging appointments. MR defecography can be performed with the patient in sitting or supine positions. Imaging in sitting position most closely mimics physiologic positioning during defecation; however, it requires open magnets, which are not readily available at most institutions. Most centers perform MR defecography in the supine position. The patients typically lie on their back on the MRI table with a pillow or wedge under their knees for comfort and to help promote defecation.[25,26] Patients are asked to evacuate the rectal gel on command into an MR compatible enema ring and/or with physical barriers such as absorbable pads covering the surface of the MRI table. Several studies have shown comparable results of MR defecography in supine versus sitting/upright position.[27,28] Kumar and colleagues[29] showed that supine MR defecography demonstrated significantly higher prevalence and degree of cystocele and urethral hypermobility as compared to upright voiding cystourethrogram (VCUG). In preparation for the examination, contrast is instilled in the rectum. Although various institutions used different types and volume of contrast, approximately 120 to 180 mL of US gel is generally recommended.[26,30] Some patients may need a larger volume to induce the sensation of rectal fullness for defecation (particularly in patients presenting with impaired defecation). Administration of vaginal contrast is optional. It may be helpful if there is history of prior surgery such as urethral sling or vaginal mesh, although

routine use is not typically recommended.[26] Many institutions ask patients to drink a standardized volume (e.g., 16 oz) of water, 15 to 20 minutes before the examination to ensure some bladder filling. However, overdistention of the bladder should be avoided because it may prevent prolapse of other compartments.

Magnetic Resonance Defecography Protocol

Although specific sequences and parameters may differ between institutions, in general, static sequences include T2-weighted images (T2WI) in three planes (sagittal, axial, coronal) and, in many cases, a T1-weighted sequence in at least a single plane. These images are used for evaluation of pelvic anatomy including the pelvic organs, muscles, osseous structures, as well as pelvic floor ligaments and fascia. Dynamic imaging is typically performed while the patient evacuates the rectal gel or during other maneuvers (e.g., Kegel) using T2-weighted or balanced steady-state sequences acquired at the rate of approximately one image per second through a single midsagittal plane. This results in a series of images that can be viewed in cine mode to assess change in location of the organs during the maneuvers. Additional similar cine images may be acquired in axial or coronal planes to assess for paramedian pathologies (e.g., lateral rectocele). Each dynamic sequence should be acquired for approximately 30 seconds, and at minimum, three defecation acquisition should be acquired; ideally, the defecatory sequence should be repeated until complete rectal emptying to ensure adequate patient effort. If the patient is unable to fully evacuate on the defecatory phase, he or she may be asked to complete evacuation in a restroom prior to returning to the machine for postdefecation cine images with maximal Valsalva maneuver which may demonstrate more severe dysfunction.[4]

Magnetic Resonance Defecography Interpretation

Anatomic assessment

The first step in interpretation of MR defecography is evaluation for anatomic defects, which may underlie functional abnormalities of the pelvic floor. The anatomic evaluation is performed primarily using the three-plane T2WI. There is wide variability in normal anatomy of the pelvic floor even in asymptomatic women. For instance, the puborectalis may be thinner on the right than on the left when viewed in the axial plane[31,32]; however, substantial differences in levator muscle volume, shape, and integrity can be seen in women with incontinence and pelvic prolapse.[4,24] Thus, any asymmetry (thickening or atrophy), focal tear, scarring, ballooning, or focal eventration of levator ani should be noted.[33] Additional anatomic

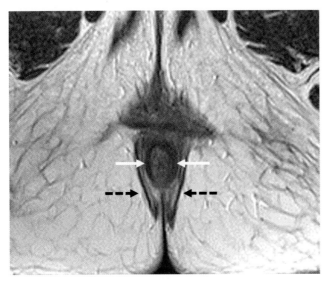

FIGURE 13.5 Axial T2-weighted image (T2WI) demonstrates thick circular internal anal sphincter *(solid arrow)* and thinner more hypointense external anal sphincter muscle *(dashed arrow)*.

abnormalities may include distortion of the vaginal morphology or urethral and periurethral structures which may indicate defects of the various levels of the endopelvic fascia. In patients with fecal incontinence or defecatory dysfunction, the anal sphincter complex should be evaluated for integrity and thickness on axial and coronal images. The sphincter complex consists of the internal sphincter

(smooth muscle which shows intermediate signal intensity on T2WI) and the external sphincter (striated muscle with low signal intensity on T2WI) (Fig. 13.5). Although internal anal sphincter tears are best assessed on endoanal US, MRI can evaluate the external sphincter for presence of tear, scar tissue, atrophy, and fatty replacement.[5] The evaluation of fat spaces (ischiorectal, retropubic, perivesical, perivaginal) is essential in patents with history of prior pelvic floor repair (e.g., placement of mesh/sling).

Functional assessment

Functional assessment of pelvic floor dysfunction is performed relative to anatomic landmarks and reference lines. The most commonly used reference line, the puboccygeal line (PCL), is drawn from the inferior aspect of symphysis pubis to the last coccygeal joint (Figs. 13.4 and 13.6). Prolapse is measured as extension of the various organs below the level of this line during defecation. The H line determines the AP (anteroposterior) diameter of the pelvic hiatus and extends from the inferior aspect of the pubic symphysis to the posterior rectal wall at the anorectal junction (ARJ) (see Fig. 13.6). The normal H line at rest measures less than 6 cm. The M line is a perpendicular line from the PCL to the posteriormost aspect of the H line at the ARJ (see Fig. 13.6). The normal M line at rest measures less than 2 cm. Widening of the pelvic hiatus (increased H line) and descent of ARJ (increased M line) are seen in patients with pelvic floor relaxation.

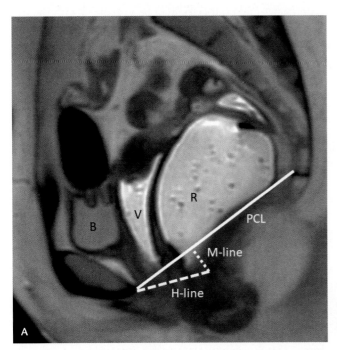

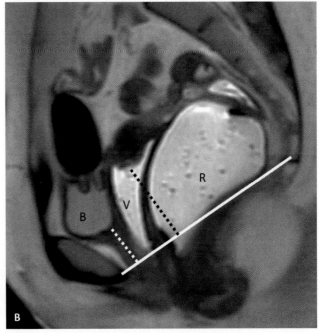

FIGURE 13.6 Midsagittal T2-weighted image (T2WI). **A:** Pubococcygeal line (PCL) is drawn from the inferior aspect of pubic symphysis to the last coccygeal joint *(solid line)*. The H line extends from the inferior aspect of the pubic symphysis to the posterior rectal wall at the anorectal junction *(dashed line)*. M line *(dotted line)* is a perpendicular line from the PCL to the posterior-most aspect of the H line. **B:** Perpendicular lines from reference points in the anterior (bladder—*white dotted line*) and apical (cervix—*black dotted line*) pelvic compartments to the PCL at rest. B, bladder; V, vagina; R, rectum.

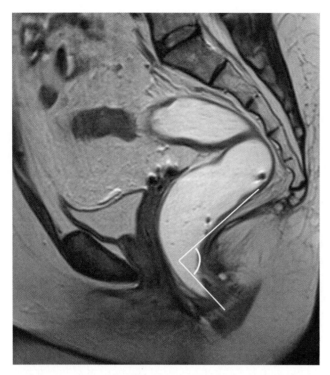

FIGURE 13.7 Sagittal T2WI demonstrated the ARA between the posterior rectal wall and the axis of the anal canal in this patient at rest.

The midpubic line (MPL) is defined as a line extending through the long axis of the pubic bone; however, it is used less commonly than the PCL. The ARA (Fig. 13.7) is measured between levator plate or posterior rectal wall and axis of the anal canal. The normal resting ARA is between 108° and 127°, should narrow by 15° to 20° during Kegel maneuver due to contraction of puborectalis, and widen by 15° to 20° during Valsalva/defecation due to relaxation of puborectalis.[34]

FLUOROSCOPIC DEFECOGRAPHY

FD was the original imaging examination of choice for evaluation of patients with pelvic floor disorders. With increased access to MR defecography at most institutions, FD is used most commonly to evaluate patients with symptoms of obstructed defecation especially when MRI findings are discordant with or do not fully explain patient symptoms. Pathology that is most frequently identified include rectocele, cul-de-sac hernias, intussusception/prolapse, perineal descent, and dyssynergia,[35] although with proper technique, the examination can also be used to assess anterior or apical compartment disorders. FD is the preferred test in some centers because it is most closely mimics the physiologic process and position during defecation given that it is performed in an upright sitting position. Moreover, compared to MRI, it is a relatively inexpensive study and simple to perform.[36] In contrast to MRI, FD uses ionizing radiation.

Patient Positioning and Preparation

Findings on defecography are dependent on patient effort; therefore, patient preparation starts with careful patient education. The patient should understand how and why the study is performed as well as its benefits and limitations. There may be significant patient anxiety when asked to defecate under direct observation and constant reassurance may be necessary. Patient coaching should continue throughout the entire examination to assure maximum effort and optimal visualization of pathology.[37] One of the advantages of FD over MR defecography is that patients are imaged sitting upright on a fluoroscopic commode, which more closely resembles the act of natural defecation. There is no consensus on bowel cleansing/enema prior to FD; however, many centers encourage an enema the morning of the exam as rectal stool may obscure findings and hamper interpretation.[38] The most commonly used rectal contrast for FD is barium paste. The volume instilled is variable but typically ranges from 120 to 240 mL or until the patient reports an urge to defecate. Digital rectal exam (DRE) is not mandatory but should be performed if there is any difficulty inserting the rectal catheter. The examination is commonly performed with administration of vaginal contrast (aqueous gel mixed with barium or iodinated contrast). Vaginal contrast may serve as a landmark for detection of other abnormalities such as rectocele, cystocele, and cul-de-sac hernia.[35,37] Small bowel and bladder contrast may add anatomic detail; however, there is no consensus on their routine use as enteroceles and cystoceles may be visualized with the use of vaginal contrast alone.[37] A perineal marker should be placed as a visible landmark for the purpose of localization and measurement of the pelvic floor.[35,37,39]

Fluoroscopic Defecography Imaging Protocol

Single-exposure radiographs and/or cine imaging are acquired during preevacuation (Kegel and Valsalva), evacuation, and postevacuation (Valsalva) phases. Pelvic landmarks are used to identify and measure anatomic and physiologic abnormalities; therefore, all images should include the pubic symphysis, sacrum/coccyx, and adequate field of view inferiorly to include the perineal region during Valsalva and defecation (Fig. 13.8).[35] Valsalva is omitted in patients with incontinence to reduce the risk of unintentional loss of rectal contrast. Normal defecation takes less than 30 seconds. If there is incomplete emptying, the effort should be repeated and the patient should be asked to use maneuvers they use at home to achieve complete rectal emptying (e.g., changing sitting position, digital manipulation). If patients fail to defecate, they are asked to evacuate in the rest room. After complete rectal emptying, a spot image is obtained during maximum strain to look for pathology that may have been masked by residual rectal contrast.

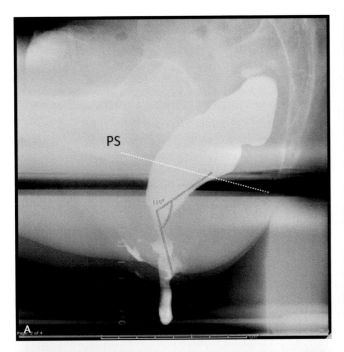

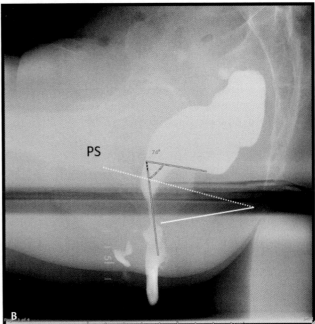

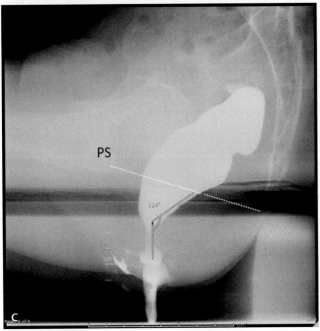

FIGURE 13.8 A 64-year-old woman with chronic constipation. Lateral images acquired during rest (**A**), Kegel maneuver (**B**), and strain/Valsalva (**C**). Pubococcygeal line (PCL) *(dotted lines)* serves as a landmark for assessment of prolapse; if the pubic symphysis is poorly visualized, the ischiococcygeal line (ICL) *(solid line)* may be used as a substitute. There is normal pelvic floor elevation and narrowing of the anal canal during the Kegel maneuver with an expected decrease in the ARA of >20° (from 110° at rest to 74°). During strain/Valsalva, the ARA becomes more obtuse and pelvic floor returns close to resting position. PS, pubic symphysis.

Image Interpretation

Similar to MR defecography, functional assessment of the pelvic floor is performed relative to anatomic landmarks and reference lines. The PCL, as defined previously in the MR defecography section, also serves as a reference landmarks for assessment of POP on FD (see Fig. 13.8).[40] If the pubis symphysis is poorly visualized, the ischiococcygeal line (ICL), drawn from the inferior margin of the ischium to the last coccygeal joint, may substitute for the PCL. The ARJ is the point where a line parallel to the central axis of the anus intersects with the line parallel to the posterior rectal wall. The ARA is created by the intersection of these lines. There is a wide range of normal in FD,[41] and in many instances, visualization of absolute or relative movement of pelvic organ is more helpful than the measurements based on the fixed landmarks. When compared to rest, normal pelvic floor contraction should move the ARJ anteriorly and superiorly with a decrease in the ARA. During strain or Valsalva, the ARJ should descend a few centimeters below the PCL and ARA return to resting configuration. During defecation, the ARJ moves posteroinferiorly with associated increase in ARA and opening of the anal canal. There should be no retention of contrast in the rectum at the end of evacuation.[35]

IMAGING FINDINGS

Anterior Compartment

Cystocele

Cystocele is defined as descent of the bladder greater than 1 cm below the PCL. Cystocele size is measured using a perpendicular line extending inferiorly from the PCL (Fig. 13.9). Cystoceles are directly visible on MRI; however, they can be directly visualized on FD only if iodinated contrast is instilled in the bladder. In the absence of bladder contrast, cystoceles can be inferred on FD by mass effect on the anterior vaginal wall and increased separation of the vagina from the pubic symphysis. This indirect visualization requires instillation of radiopaque vaginal contrast. Large cystoceles may efface the anterior vaginal wall and cause vaginal eversion as well as cause kinking of the urethra and lead to urinary obstruction. In some circumstances, the bladder may occupy the entire pelvic floor hiatus and obscure defects in other compartments. Therefore, in the presence of large cystocele and absence of any other organ prolapse, performing postvoid maneuvers (e.g.,

Valsalva) is crucial to prevent underestimation of apical or posterior defects.[4] Conversely, overdistention of rectum with contrast should be avoided because it can decrease sensitivity for cystoceles.

Stress urinary incontinence (urethral hypermobility and intrinsic sphincter deficiency)

SUI is defined as urinary incontinence associated with increased intra-abdominal pressure as can be seen with coughing. The normal urethra is typically vertical in orientation. SUI may be caused by loss of urethral support resulting in rotational descent of the bladder neck and proximal urethra at times of increased intra-abdominal pressure (urethral hypermobility) (see Fig. 13.9). Urinary incontinence occurs as the poorly supported posterior urethra continues to descend away from the better supported anterior urethra, and the urethrovesical junction opens and descends causing incontinence.[42] MRI provides valuable information regarding integrity of the levator ani, periurethral ligaments, and vaginal attachments. SUI may also be caused by foreshortening or

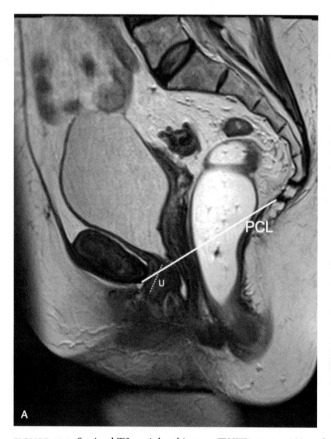 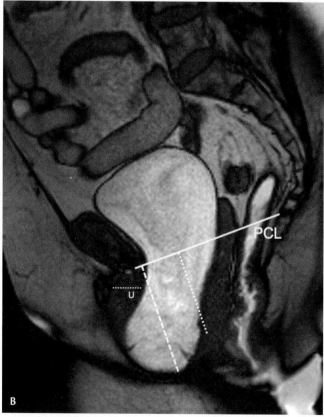

FIGURE 13.9 Sagittal T2-weighted image (T2WI) at rest (**A**) and sagittal True fast imaging with steady state precession (TrueFISP) image during defecation (**B**) show significant drop of the bladder and uterus below the PCL during defecation. The size of the cystocele and uterine prolapse can be measured using a perpendicular line relative to the PCL (*dashed* and *dotted lines*, respectively, in **B**). Note also the urethral axis (*dotted line* labeled *U*) which has a more vertical orientation at rest (**A**) and rotates into a horizontal orientation during defecation (in **B**) consistent with urethral hypermobility.

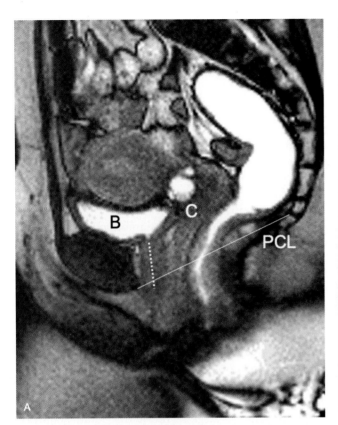 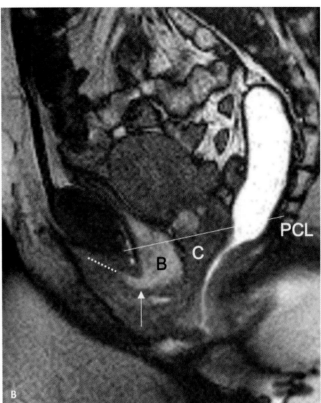

FIGURE 13.10 Sagittal True fast imaging with steady state precession (TrueFISP) images at rest (**A**) and defecation (**B**) demonstrate prolapse of the bladder (B) and cervix (C) below the PCL *(solid lines)* during defecation. The urethral axis *(dotted lines)* rotates from vertical to past the horizontal axis during defecation consistent with urethral hypermobility. In addition, there is widening of the bladder neck and proximal urethra during defecation consistent with funneling *(arrow* in **B**).

thinning of the urethral sphincter muscle manifested as bladder neck widening/funneling which is indirect sign for sphincter insufficiency and incontinence (Fig. 13.10).[43]

Bladder outlet obstruction

Surgical interventions for SUI (anti-incontinence procedures such as autologous slings, Burch suspension, Marshall-Marchetti-Krantz procedure, pubovaginal slings, transvaginal needle suspension, and synthetic urethral slings) are responsible for 1% to 33% of the bladder outlet obstruction cases.[44] Additional causes include POP and severe urethral hypermobility with kinking of the urethra or primary bladder neck obstruction by benign and malignant masses. Anatomic causes such as masses can be directly visualized on MRI and urethral kinking and hypermobility are apparent on MR defecation or Valsalva sequences as described previously. The majority of the cases of bladder outlet obstruction present with lower urinary tract symptoms. Rarely, urinary retention requires catheterization. Bladder outlet obstruction is best evaluated on urodynamic studies. On anatomic MRI, trabeculated and thickened bladder wall are secondary signs of bladder outlet obstruction as are advanced stages of POP.[45]

Apical Compartment

Cervical/vaginal prolapse

Cervical/vaginal prolapse is defined as descent of the cervix or vaginal apex below the PCL. Size of apical prolapse is measured by a perpendicular line from the PCL to the anterior lip of the cervix or vaginal apex (in cases of prior hysterectomy) (see Fig. 13.9). The normal "H shape" appearance of vagina should be present on axial T2-weighted MRI. Abnormal configuration or flattening of the vagina is suggestive of loss of paravaginal support (Fig. 13.11). In severe cases, the vagina may be completely everted, and the uterus or cervix may be prolapsed outside the vaginal introitus. Apical compartment prolapse is a common cause for underestimation of simultaneous defects in the anterior and posterior compartments and a leading cause for failed surgeries.[4] Long-standing prolapse stretches the pelvic hiatus, inducing weakness over time of both the endopelvic fascia and pelvic diaphragm.[46] As the vagina is not directly visualized on FD, the modality is limited for assessment of paravaginal defects. Nonetheless, cervical/vaginal prolapse can be diagnosed on fluoroscopy if there is contrast in the vaginal canal. In the absence of vaginal contrast, mass-like separation of rectum from the pubis is an indirect sign of prolapse.[47]

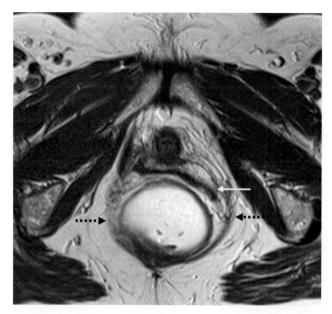

FIGURE 13.11 Axial T2WI demonstrates asymmetric posterior drooping of the vagina on the left *(solid arrow)* due to loss of paravaginal support structures. Note the bilateral thinning and ballooning of the puborectalis muscle *(dashed arrows)*.

Posterior Compartment

Cul-de-sac hernia (enterocele/peritoneocele/sigmoidocele)

A cul-de-sac hernia is defined as herniation of peritoneal contents below the PCL and into the rectovaginal septum. The size is measured as the distance from the inferior extent of cul-de-sac hernia to the PCL.[48] Surgeons may also find it helpful to know the distance of the hernia below the level of the vaginal apex. The type of cul-de-sac hernia is defined based on the contents of the hernia sac: small bowel (enterocele) (Fig. 13.12), peritoneum (peritoneocele), and/or sigmoid colon (sigmoidocele) (Fig. 13.13). The contents of the hernia sac are readily differentiated on MR defecography; however, it may not be discernable on FD unless oral contrast is administered to opacify the small bowel. One of the utilities of pelvic floor imaging with MR defecography or FD is to differentiate cul-de-sac hernia from rectocele as a cause of posterior vaginal bulge as these two entities may not be distinguishable on physical examination and may frequently coexist. Importantly, cul-de-sac hernias typically manifest on imaging at the end of defecation and require complete or near-complete rectal emptying. Thus, a large rectocele that retains contrast may obscure a cul-de-sac hernia.

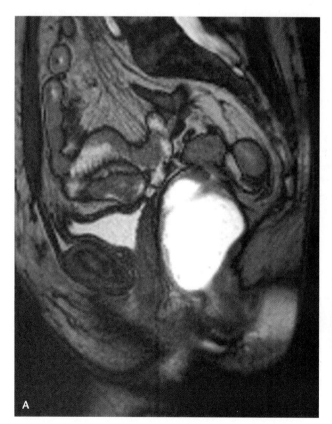
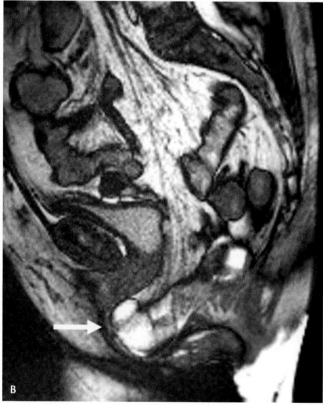

FIGURE 13.12 Sagittal True fast imaging with steady state precession (TrueFISP) images at rest (**A**) and defecation (**B**) demonstrate normal position of the bowel loops at rest (in **A**), but a cul-de-sac hernia containing small bowel loops consistent with enterocele on defecation images causing a bulge along the posterior vaginal wall and perineum *(arrow in **B**)*.

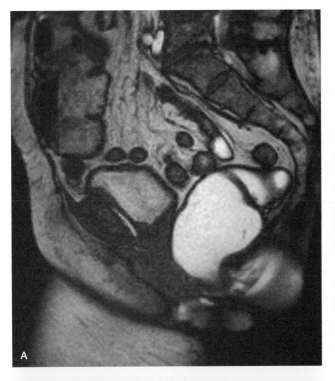

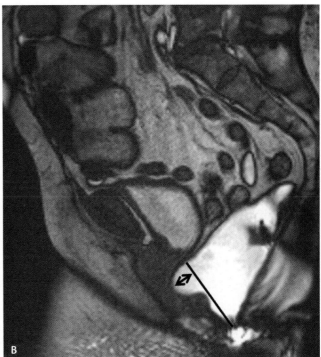

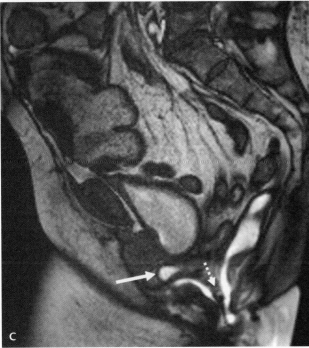

FIGURE 13.13 Sagittal True fast imaging with steady state precession (TrueFISP) images at rest (**A**), early defecation (**B**), and late defecation (**C**) demonstrate an anterior rectocele during early defecation which is measured in AP (anteroposterior) dimension (*double-headed arrow* in **B**) relative to the plane of the anal canal (*solid vertical line* in **B**). Upon continued rectal emptying, there is extension of the sigmoid colon into a cul-de-sac hernia consistent with a sigmoidocele (*solid arrow* in **C**) as well as telescoping of the rectum into the upper portion of the anal canal consistent with intra-anal rectal intussusception (*dashed arrow* in **C**).

Rectocele

Rectocele is defined as an outpouching of the rectal lumen along the anterior rectal wall and is best seen during early defecation phase with maximum strain. If a rectocele is large enough, it presents clinically as bulging of the posterior wall of the vagina. On MRI and FD, anterior rectocele is quantified by measuring the anteroposterior extent of the outpouching from a line drawn through the plane of the anterior wall of the anal canal (Fig. 13.14). Although physical exam may detect the majority of rectoceles, MRI and FD provide information regarding size of the rectocele, clinical significance of the finding (ability to empty on defecatory phase vs. contrast retention), and presence of coexistent abnormalities.[4,5] As described previously, one of the indications for MR defecography and FD is to differentiate

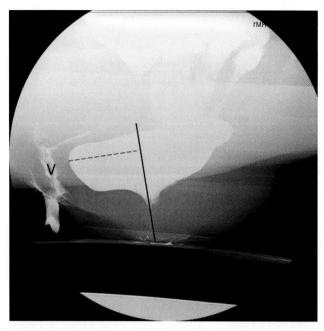

FIGURE 13.14 Anterior rectocele is measured along a line extending anterior from the plane of the anterior rectal wall *(solid line)* to the anterior wall of the rectum *(dashed line)*. This patient manually evacuated the retained contrast at the end of defecation. V, vagina.

rectoceles from cul-de-sac hernias because both these entities can result in posterior vaginal bulges and may not be distinguishable on physical examination. A large rectocele with contrast retention may be an etiology for clinical defecatory dysfunction.

Rectal intussusception

Chronic, incomplete evacuation may be associated with rectal intussusception. Rectal intussusception is defined as invagination of rectal wall during straining and ranges from partial thickness mucosal infolding to full-thickness rectal intussusception. The intussusception usually originates 6 to 8 cm above the anal canal and can be categorized/graded based on the location of the apex of the intussusceptum: intrarectal (within the rectal ampulla), intra-anal (within the anal canal), and external or extra-anal, which is also termed complete rectal prolapse.[48,49] Rectal intussusception can be visualized on both MR defecography and FD and is best seen on end-defecation or postevacuation strain images (Fig. 13.15). It is important to correlate the imaging findings to clinical symptoms because rectal intussusception has been reported on imaging in 50% of asymptomatic volunteers.[48] Rectal intussusception may be a cause of defecatory dysfunction and obstructed defecation, and intrarectal and intra-anal intussusception may or may not be clinically apparent.

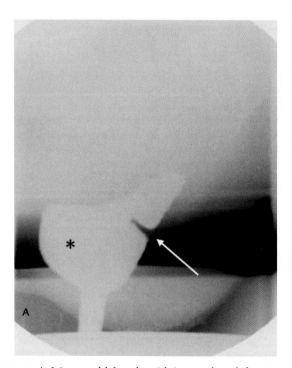
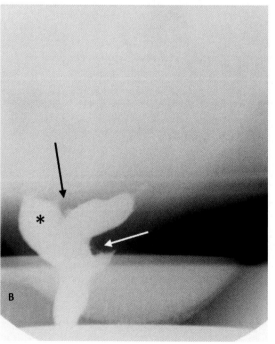

FIGURE 13.15 A 36-year-old female with incomplete defecation requiring manual disimpaction. Lateral cine spot image during early defecation (**A**) demonstrates a moderate size, anterior rectocele *(asterisk)*, and posterior intrarectal intussusception *(arrow)*; late defecation image (**B**) demonstrates anterior and posterior intrarectal intussusception *(arrows)* to the level of the rectocele *(asterisk)*.

Spastic pelvic floor/dyssynergia/anismus

Patients with pelvic floor dyssynergia present with prolonged and incomplete evacuation of the rectal contents as well as delay between the opening of the anal canal and initiation of defecation.[50,51] Dyssynergia is caused by involuntary paradoxical contraction of the pelvic floor musculature during defecation or Valsalva. Imaging findings include failure of the ARA to widen and anal sphincter to relax leading to prolonged or incomplete rectal evacuation. The puborectalis muscle may be hypertrophied, best seen on MRI. Patients with spastic pelvic floor are prone to develop rectocele and infralevator herniation of the anorectum (Figs. 13.16 and 13.17).[35,52] Frequently, dyssynergia is diagnosed or suspected based on clinical evaluation with anal manometry. MR defecography or FD is obtained for confirmation and to exclude other anatomic causes of defecatory dysfunction such as rectocele or rectal intussusception. In contrast to anatomic defects which are treated surgically, pelvic floor dyssynergia is a functional disorder and treated with biofeedback therapy. Dyssynergia may coexist with anatomic defects and is important to treat prior to surgical intervention.

Rectal/anal incontinence

In many cases, the rectal/anal incontinence is the result of sphincter complex injury. MRI provides valuable information on integrity of the internal and external sphincters.

It has been shown that MR defecography findings may change surgical approach in up to 67% of the patients undergoing for surgery for incontinence.[24] Because the sphincter complex is not directly visualized on FD and the difficulty of retaining rectal contrast at rest in patients with incontinence, MRI is the recommended study in patients with incontinence.

Descending perineum syndrome (pelvic floor relaxation)

Descending perineum syndrome (DPS) is one of the indicators of poor prognosis due to complete pelvic floor decompensation. Although there is poor agreement on its definition, DPS is most often defined as excessive ballooning of the perineum due to pelvic floor laxity and is associated with various symptoms including a sensation of incomplete rectal emptying, incontinence, and pelvic discomfort/pain.[53] The definition of abnormal descent on imaging varies; however, descent of the ARJ during strain of greater than 2 cm relative to the pubococcygeal line (PCL) is considered to be the threshold.[37,53] Clinically significant perineal descent has been described as a distance of at least 2 to 3.5 cm.[48,54–56] On MRI, findings include widening of H line (hiatus widening), elongation of M line (descent), and caudal angulation of levator plate.[4,5] Perineal descent can be associated with multiple abnormalities including rectocele, intussusception, and multiorgan prolapse (Fig. 13.18).

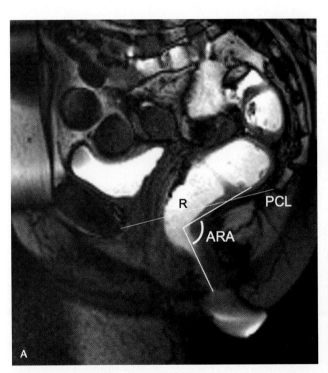 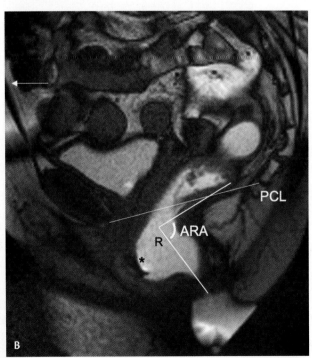

FIGURE 13.16 Sagittal TrueFISP images at rest (**A**) and attempted defecation (**B**) demonstrate no rectal emptying and paradoxical narrowing (rather than widening) of the ARA during defecation (in **B**) compared to rest (**A**). Anterior bulging of the abdominal wall (*arrow* in **B**) and descent of the rectum *(R)* below the PCL during attempted defecation suggest that patient is in fact bearing down and increasing intra-abdominal pressure during image acquisition. Note also small rectocele during defecation *(asterisk)*.

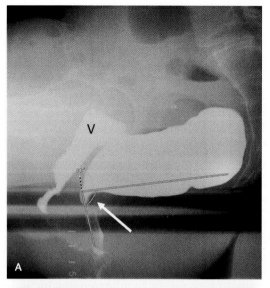

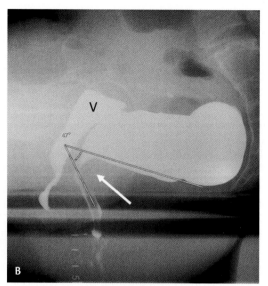

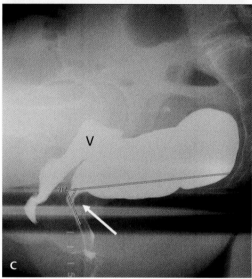

FIGURE 13.17 A 27-year-old female with difficulty in evacuation. Lateral images acquired during rest (**A**), Kegel maneuver (**B**), and straining (**C**) demonstrate expected narrowing of the ARA during Kegel (in **B**) but deep impression of the puborectalis sling on the posterior rectal wall with persistently acute ARA even during straining (in **C**). Despite multiple attempts, evacuation was incomplete. The patient was asked to evacuate in a private bathroom. Upon return, the rectal contrast had been evacuated (image not included). The *arrows* point to the ARA. V, vagina.

FIGURE 13.18 Descending perineum syndrome (DPS) with loss of support due to denervation of the pelvic floor muscles. Patient presents with pelvic discomfort and feeling of incomplete rectal emptying. BL, cystocele; V, vagina; SB, enterocele; *asterisk*, rectocele; *arrow*, anus; *dashed curve*, perineum; *dashed line*, PCL.

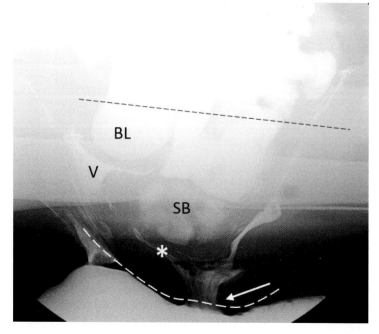

COMPLICATIONS OF PELVIC FLOOR SURGICAL REPAIR

Imaging may play a role in evaluation of postoperative complications associated with pelvic floor repair. The most commonly employed imaging techniques to evaluate for such complications include US and MRI. Although MR defecography can be used if there is concern for recurrent pelvic floor prolapse or other defects, anatomic sequences without defecation are adequate to assess for complications of the prior surgical repair. FD is not a test of choice for this indication because synthetic materials related to the repair and soft tissue anatomy of the pelvic floor is not directly visualized. This section discusses complications of pelvic floor repair as seen on MRI.

Urethral Bulking Agents

Bulking agents (e.g., bovine collagen, silicone, calcium hydroxyapatite) can be injected transurethrally using a minimally invasive technique to improve the coaptation of the urethral mucosa and treat SUI caused by intrinsic sphincter deficiency. Bulking agents expand the urethra and are seen best on T2WI surrounding the urethral lumen. The signal intensity of bulking agents varies depending on the specific material used; however, most tend to be intermediate to slightly high signal intensity on T2WI. Potential complications of

bulking agents include migration outside the urethral wall, which may result in recurrent incontinence or migration into the lumen of the urethral or bladder neck which can result in obstructed voiding. Migration can also lead to granulomatous, inflammatory or infectious processes, which may be seen on MRI. Patients may present with recurrent infection or bladder irritative symptoms.

Midurethral Sling

Midurethral sling surgeries have been the most extensively researched and highly effective treatment for SUI.[57] Of late, synthetic slings are more commonly used than traditional autologous slings or anterior vaginal wall suspension sutures. Synthetic slings are made of polypropylene mesh material and are seen as hypointense bands on T2WI. Depending on the particular types of sling, they may be visualized in the paraurethral space with extension anteriorly into the retropubic space (Fig. 13.19), whereas others may be seen extending laterally into the obturator foramen. Imaging may be obtained to confirm presence of sling material in patients with unclear surgical history or persistent symptoms despite prior history of resection. MRI is the superior modality to show the sling in the retropubic space; however, US is the modality of choice to demonstrate slings in the suburethral space between the urethra and vagina.[58] Potential complications

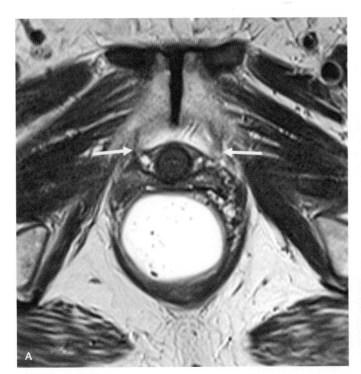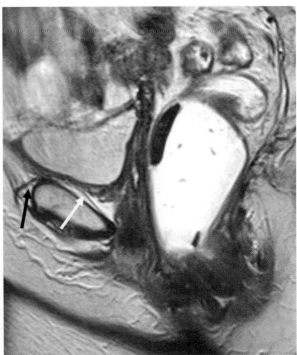

FIGURE 13.19 Retropubic midurethral sling. Axial (**A**), sagittal (**B**), and coronal (**C**) T2-weighted image (T2WI) demonstrate "U-shaped" sling looping behind the urethra (*arrows* in **A**). The sling traverses the retropubic space seen on sagittal and coronal images (*solid arrows* in **B** and **C**) between the bladder and pubic bone. *(continued)*

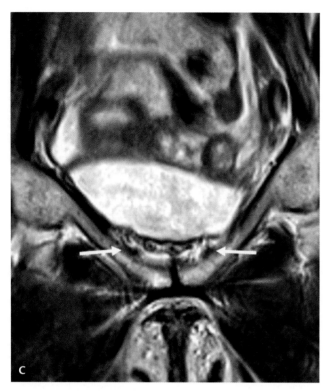

FIGURE 13.19 *(Continued)*

of synthetic midurethral slings include hematoma or infection in the retropubic space, malpositioning of sling, erosion, or extrusion of implanted material into the urethral or vaginal walls or into the urinary bladder.[59] Early erosion or extrusion of sling material can be challenging to identify on imaging. Exuberant

granulation tissue or scar related to indwelling sling material or after removal can be difficult to differentiate from actual sling remnants on MRI.

Transvaginal and Sacrocolpopexy Mesh

Transvaginal mesh placed along the anterior and posterior vaginal walls to treat prolapse may be visualized as linear low signal intensity bands on T2WI. Various transvaginal mesh products with different configurations of arms extending in the obturator foramen, sacrospinous ligament, or ischiorectal fossa have been placed over the last number of years; however, nearly all have lost U.S. Food and Drug Administration approval in the United States more recently. Nonetheless, patients with previously placed transvaginal mesh may present with complications such as erosion/extrusion, infection or fistula formation which can be visualized on MRI (Fig. 13.20). In contrast to transvaginal mesh, sacrocolpopexy mesh is placed transabdominally and is the gold standard treatment for vaginal apex or uterocervical prolapse. It extends from the sacral promontory to the vaginal apex. Due to the smaller field of view of US imaging, MRI is the modality of choice for evaluation of sacrocolpopexy mesh integrity or associated complications. Normal sacrocolpopexy mesh exhibits low signal intensity on T2WI. Some complications of sacrocolpopexy mesh that may be detected on MRI include erosion/extrusion into the vagina, bladder (Fig. 13.21), or other structures; infection; or tearing of the mesh with recurrent prolapse. Functional evaluation with MR defecography should be obtained if there is concern for recurrent prolapse after mesh repair.

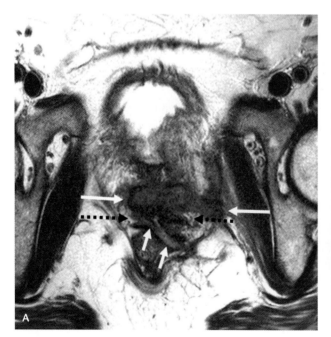
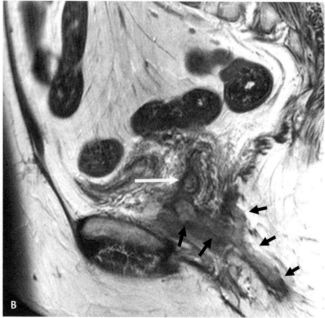

FIGURE 13.20 A 57-year-old female with vaginal mesh erosion. Axial (**A**) and sagittal (**B**) T2-weighted image (T2WI) demonstrate severely thickened vaginal/perivaginal tissues *(long solid arrows)* with suspected vaginal mesh *(dashed arrows* in **A**), as causing a fistula from the posterior vaginal wall *(short arrows* in **A**). Note the branching pattern of complex fistula tract(s) extending into the ischiorectal fossa *(short arrows* in **B**).

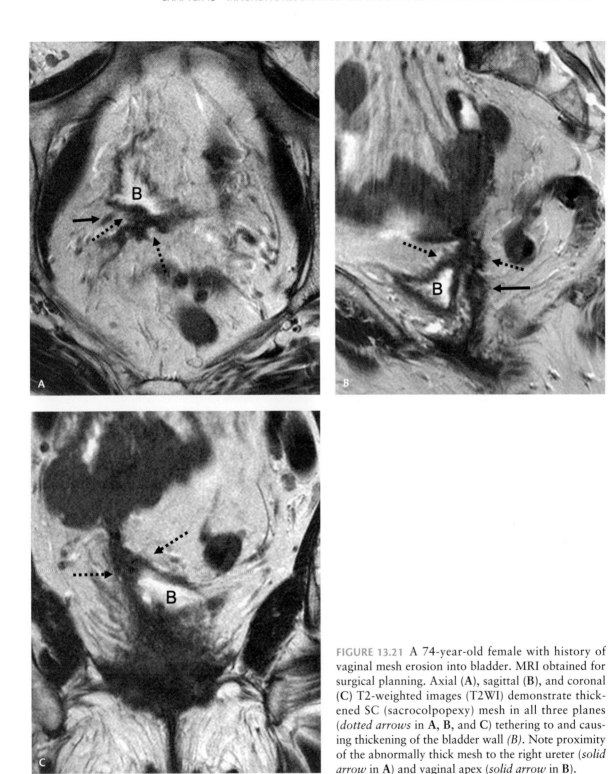

FIGURE 13.21 A 74-year-old female with history of vaginal mesh erosion into bladder. MRI obtained for surgical planning. Axial (**A**), sagittal (**B**), and coronal (**C**) T2-weighted images (T2WI) demonstrate thickened SC (sacrocolpopexy) mesh in all three planes (*dotted arrows* in **A**, **B**, and **C**) tethering to and causing thickening of the bladder wall *(B)*. Note proximity of the abnormally thick mesh to the right ureter (*solid arrow* in **A**) and vaginal apex (*solid arrow* in **B**).

CONCLUSION

Imaging of pelvic floor conditions serves as an adjunct to clinical evaluation. MR defecography and FD are both imaging modalities that are able to provide functional evaluation of the pelvic floor. Patient education prior to the examination to promote adequate patient effort and imaging during defecation are key components of these examinations and are necessary to appropriately evaluate for pelvic floor defects in the various compartments—anterior, apical, and posterior. In addition to functional evaluation, MRI also provides anatomic evaluation of the pelvic organs and muscles/ligaments/fascia that provide support to the pelvic floor as well as synthetic materials used for pelvic floor repair and their complications such as infection, erosion/extrusion, and failure resulting in recurrent dysfunction.

References

1. Healy JC, Halligan S, Reznek RH, et al. Patterns of prolapse in women with symptoms of pelvic floor weakness: Assessment with MR imaging. *Radiology* 1997;203(1):77–81.

2. Maglinte DD, Kelvin FM, Fitzgerald K, et al. Association of compartment defects in pelvic floor dysfunction. *AJR Am J Roentgenol* 1999;172(2):439–444.

3. Khatri G. Magnetic resonance imaging of pelvic floor disorders. *Top Magn Reson Imaging* 2014;23(4):259–273.

4. Khatri G, de Leon AD, Lockhart ME. MR Imaging of the pelvic floor. *Magn Reson Imaging Clin N Am* 2017;25(3):457–480.

5. Shaaban AM. Diagnostic imaging gynecology. In: Shaaban AM, ed. *Diagnostic imaging gynecology*, 2nd ed. Philadelphia: Elsevier, 2015:8–30.

6. Lammers K, Prokop M, Vierhout ME, et al. A pictorial overview of pubovisceral muscle avulsions on pelvic floor magnetic resonance imaging. *Insights Imaging* 2013;4(4):431–441.

7. Brandão AC, Ianez P. MR imaging of the pelvic floor: Defecography. *Magn Reson Imaging Clin N Am* 2013;21(2):427–445.

8. Woodfield CA, Krishnamoorthy S, Hampton BS, et al. Imaging pelvic floor disorders: Trend toward comprehensive MRI. *AJR Am J Roentgenol* 2010;194(6):1640–1649.

9. Dimpfl T, Jaeger C, Mueller-Felber W, et al. Myogenic changes of the levator ani muscle in premenopausal women: The impact of vaginal delivery and age. *Neurourol Urodyn* 1998;17(3):197–205.

10. Hanzal E, Berger E, Koelbl H. Levator ani muscle morphology and recurrent genuine stress incontinence. *Obstet Gynecol* 1993;81(3):426–429.

11. Koelbl H, Strassegger H, Riss PA, et al. Morphologic and functional aspects of pelvic floor muscles in patients with pelvic relaxation and genuine stress incontinence. *Obstet Gynecol* 1989;74(5):789–795.

12. Caudwell-Hall J, Kamisan Atan I, Martin A, et al. Intrapartum predictors of maternal levator ani injury. *Acta Obstet Gynecol Scand* 2017;96(4):426–431.

13. DeLancey JO, Kearney R, Chou Q, et al. The appearance of levator ani muscle abnormalities in magnetic resonance images after vaginal delivery. *Obstet Gynecol* 2003;101(1):46–53.

14. Dietz HP, Lanzarone V. Levator trauma after vaginal delivery. *Obstet Gynecol* 2005;106(4):707–712.

15. Handa VL, Roem J, Blomquist JL, et al. Pelvic organ prolapse as a function of levator ani avulsion, hiatus size, and strength. *Am J Obstet Gynecol* 2019;221(1):41.e1–41.e7.

16. Handa VL, Blomquist JL, Roem J, et al. Levator morphology and strength after obstetric avulsion of the levator ani muscle. *Female Pelvic Med Reconstr Surg* 2020;26(1):56–60.

17. Dietz HP, Bernardo MJ, Kirby A, et al. Minimal criteria for the diagnosis of avulsion of the puborectalis muscle by tomographic ultrasound. *Int Urogynecol J* 2011;22(6):699–704.

18. Dietz HP. Ultrasound imaging of the pelvic floor. Part II: Three-dimensional or volume imaging. *Ultrasound Obstet Gynecol* 2004;23(6):615–625.

19. Chen L, Ashton-Miller JA, Hsu Y, et al. Interaction among apical support, levator ani impairment, and anterior vaginal wall prolapse. *Obstet Gynecol* 2006;108(2):324–332.

20. Shi M, Shang S, Xie B, et al. MRI changes of pelvic floor and pubic bone observed in primiparous women after childbirth by normal vaginal delivery. *Arch Gynecol Obstet* 2016;294(2):285–289.

21. Yan Y, Dou C, Wang X, et al. Combination of tomographic ultrasound imaging and three-dimensional magnetic resonance imaging-based model to diagnose postpartum levator avulsion. *Sci Rep* 2017;7(1):11235.

22. Clark AL, Gregory T, Smith VJ, et al. Epidemiologic evaluation of reoperation for surgically treated pelvic organ prolapse and urinary incontinence. *Am J Obstet Gynecol* 2003;189(5):1261–1267.

23. Olsen AL, Smith VJ, Bergstrom JO, et al. Epidemiology of surgically managed pelvic organ prolapse and urinary incontinence. *Obstet Gynecol* 1997;89(4):501–506.

24. Hetzer FH, Andreisek G, Tsagari C, et al. MR defecography in patients with fecal incontinence: Imaging findings and their effect on surgical management. *Radiology* 2006;240(2):449–457.

25. El Sayed RF, Alt CD, Maccioni F, et al. Magnetic resonance imaging of pelvic floor dysfunction—Joint recommendations of the ESUR and ESGAR Pelvic Floor Working Group. *Eur Radiol* 2017;27(5):2067–2085.

26. Lalwani N, Khatri G, El Sayed RF, et al. MR defecography technique: Recommendations of the Society of Abdominal Radiology's disease-focused panel on pelvic floor imaging. *Abdom Radiol (NY)* 2021;46(4):1351–1361.

27. Bertschinger KM, Hetzer FH, Roos JE, et al. Dynamic MR imaging of the pelvic floor performed with patient sitting in an open-magnet unit versus with patient supine in a closed-magnet unit. *Radiology* 2002;223(2):501–508.

28. Pannu HK, Scatarige JC, Eng J. Comparison of supine magnetic resonance imaging with and without rectal contrast to fluoroscopic cystocolpoproctography for the diagnosis of pelvic organ prolapse. *J Comput Assist Tomogr* 2009;33(1):125–130.

29. Kumar NM, Khatri G, Christie AL, et al. Supine magnetic resonance defecography for evaluation of anterior compartment prolapse: Comparison with upright voiding cystourethrogram. *Eur J Radiol* 2019;117:95–101.

30. Khatri G, Bailey AA, Bacsu C, et al. Influence of rectal gel volume on defecation during dynamic pelvic floor magnetic resonance imaging. *Clin Imaging* 2015;39(6):1027–1031.

31. Fielding JR, Dumanli H, Schreyer AG, et al. MR-based three-dimensional modeling of the normal pelvic floor in women: Quantification of muscle mass. *AJR Am J Roentgenol* 2000;174(3):657–660.

32. Hoyte L, Schierlitz L, Zou K, et al. Two- and 3-dimensional MRI comparison of levator ani structure, volume, and integrity in women with stress incontinence and prolapse. *Am J Obstet Gynecol* 2001;185(1):11–19.

33. Pannu HK, Genadry R, Gearhart S, et al. Focal levator ani eventrations: Detection and characterization by magnetic resonance in patients with pelvic floor dysfunction. *Int Urogynecol J Pelvic Floor Dysfunct* 2003;14(2):89–93.

34. Colaiacomo MC, Masselli G, Polettini E, et al. Dynamic MR imaging of the pelvic floor: A pictorial review. *Radiographics* 2009;29(3):e35.

35. Palmer SL, Lalwani N, Bahrami S, et al. Dynamic fluoroscopic defecography: Updates on rationale, technique, and interpretation from the Society of Abdominal Radiology Pelvic Floor Disease Focus Panel. *Abdom Radiol (NY)* 2021;46(4):1312–1322.

36. Faccioli N, Comai A, Mainardi P, et al. Defecography: A practical approach. *Diagn Interv Radiol* 2010;16(3):209–216.

37. Paquette I, Rosman D, El Sayed R, et al; and the Expert Workgroup on Fluoroscopic Imaging of Pelvic Floor Disorders. Consensus definitions and interpretation templates for fluoroscopic imaging of defecatory pelvic floor disorders: Proceedings of the consensus

meeting of the Pelvic Floor Consortium of the American Society of Colon and Rectal Surgeons, the Society of Abdominal Radiology, the International Continence Society, the American Urogynecologic Society, the International Urogynecological Association, and the Society of Gynecologic Surgeons. *Dis Colon Rectum* 2021;64(1):31–44.

38. Jorge JM, Habr-Gama A, Wexner SD. Clinical applications and techniques of cinedefecography. *Am J Surg* 2001;182(1): 93–101.

39. Gonçalves AN, Sala MA, Bruno RC, et al. Defecography by digital radiography: Experience in clinical practice. *Radiol Bras* 2016;49(6):376–381.

40. Kim AY. How to interpret a functional or motility test— Defecography. *J Neurogastroenterol Motil* 2011;17(4):416–420.

41. Hainsworth AJ, Solanki D, Hamad A, et al. Integrated total pelvic floor ultrasound in pelvic floor defaecatory dysfunction. *Colorectal Dis* 2017;19(1):O54–O65.

42. Macura KJ, Genadry RR. Female urinary incontinence: Pathophysiology, methods of evaluation and role of MR imaging. *Abdom Imaging* 2008;33(3):371–380.

43. Li N, Cui C, Cheng Y, et al. Association between magnetic resonance imaging findings of the pelvic floor and de novo stress urinary incontinence after vaginal delivery. *Korean J Radiol* 2018;19(4):715–723.

44. Dmochowski RR. Bladder outlet obstruction: Etiology and evaluation. *Rev Urol* 2005;7(suppl 6):S3–S13.

45. Bai SW, Park SH, Chung DJ, et al. The significance of bladder trabeculation in the female lower urinary system: An objective evaluation by urodynamic studies. *Yonsei Med J* 2005;46(5):673–678.

46. Fielding JR. Practical MR imaging of female pelvic floor weakness. *Radiographics* 2002;22(2):295–304.

47. Reiner CS, Weishaupt D. Dynamic pelvic floor imaging: MRI techniques and imaging parameters. *Abdom Imaging* 2013;38(5):903–911.

48. Shorvon PJ, McHugh S, Diamant NE, et al. Defecography in normal volunteers: Results and implications. *Gut* 1989;30(12):1737–1749.

49. Cariou de Vergie L, Venara A, Duchalais E, et al. Internal rectal prolapse: Definition, assessment and management in 2016. *J Visc Surg* 2017;154:21–28.

50. Halligan S, Bartram CI, Park HJ, et al. Proctographic features of anismus. *Radiology* 1995;197(3):679–682.

51. Reiner CS, Tutuian R, Solopova AE, et al. MR defecography in patients with dyssynergic defecation: Spectrum of imaging findings and diagnostic value. *Br J Radiol* 2011;84(998):136–144.

52. Mortele KJ, Fairhurst J. Dynamic MR defecography of the posterior compartment: Indications, techniques and MRI features. *Eur J Radiol* 2007;61(3):462–472.

53. Chaudhry Z, Tarnay C. Descending perineum syndrome: A review of the presentation, diagnosis, and management. *Int Urogynecol J* 2016;27:1149–1156.

54. Ambrose S, Keighley MR. Outpatient measurement of perineal descent. *Ann R Coll Surg Engl* 1985;67(5):306–308.

55. Ho YH, Goh HS. The neurophysiological significance of perineal descent. *Int J Colorectal Dis* 1995;10(2):107–111.

56. Parks AG, Porter NH, Hardcastle J. The syndrome of the descending perineum. *Proc R Soc Med* 1966;59(6):477–482.

57. Ford AA, Rogerson L, Cody JD, et al. Mid-urethral sling operations for stress urinary incontinence in women. *Cochrane Database Syst Rev* 2017;(7):CD006375.

58. Schuettoff S, Beyersdorff D, Gauruder-Burmester A, et al. Visibility of the polypropylene tape after tension-free vaginal tape (TVT) procedure in women with stress urinary incontinence: Comparison of introital ultrasound and magnetic resonance imaging in vitro and in vivo. *Ultrasound Obstet Gynecol* 2006;27(6):687–692.

59. Khatri G, Carmel ME, Bailey AA, et al. Postoperative imaging after surgical repair for pelvic floor dysfunction. *Radiographics* 2016;36(4):1233–1256.

CHAPTER 14

ULTRASOUND IMAGING OF THE PELVIC FLOOR

Hans Peter Dietz

Introduction

Ultrasound is the most-used medical imaging technology in general and by far the most popular technique used in obstetrics and gynecology. This is primarily due to easy availability, limited cost, and innate physical properties such as the lack of ionizing radiation and high temporal resolution, resulting from an absence of heavy moving parts. The main downside of diagnostic ultrasound is the rapid attenuation of signals in tissues and the reflection of ultrasound waves by bone and gas. As a result, indications are limited to situations where an external or intracavitary transducer can be brought close to the tissues in question. The pelvis tends to fulfill those criteria. The deeper pelvic organs are reached by endovaginal or endoanal transducers, and the pelvic floor is within the 5 to 7 cm depth covered by the frequency range of modern abdominal and obstetric transducers. The development of three-dimensional (3D) capable transducers in the 1990s allowed access to the axial plane, which previously was only possible with endocavitary probes, and four-dimensional (4D) technology using either mechanical oscillating sectors or, more recently, solid-state matrix probes, have greatly increased temporal resolution.

It is not surprising that there is increasingly widespread uptake of this technology in pelvic floor medicine, even if its speed varies with the availability of equipment and teaching resources, with the adequacy of remuneration by health care funders, and with the extent of regulatory interference. In some jurisdictions with heavy-handed state regulation of medical technology, ultrasound imaging can only be provided in a research setting; in others, professional jealousies have impeded progress. Fortunately, after a decade of efforts, there finally has been a modicum of international standardization,[1] and there is standardized online teaching under the auspices of the International Urogynecological Association.[2]

In this chapter, the author intends to give an overview of what is possible with current technology both in research and in clinical practice, summarize the available literature, and provide an outlook of what is to be expected in this field in the near to medium term.

INSTRUMENTATION AND METHODOLOGY

Two-Dimensional Imaging

Translabial pelvic floor ultrasound at a basic level requires a B-mode capable two-dimensional (2D) ultrasound system with cine loop function, a 3.5- to 6-MHz curved array transducer, and a video printer; all technology that has been available since the mid-1980s. A midsagittal view of the pelvis can be obtained by placing a transducer on the perineum (Fig. 14.1), after covering the transducer with a probe cover such as a glove, condom, or plastic wrap for hygienic reasons. Powdered or coated gloves may impair imaging quality; hence, it is recommended to test probe covers before use to make sure they do not affect image quality. Air between probe and probe cover will cause acoustic artefacts, shadowing, and reverberations and need to be avoided especially when using 3D/4D transducers as bubbles lateral to the main transducer plane may be invisible during acquisition. Sterilization is usually considered unnecessary, with mechanical cleaning and alcoholic wipes used between patients.

Imaging is generally undertaken with the patient in dorsal lithotomy, hips flexed and abducted, or in the standing position. Heels placed close to the buttocks result in an improved pelvic tilt due to reduced lordosis. Scanning is usually done after bladder emptying to allow the determination of residual urine volume and make the patient more relaxed about the risk of leakage of urine on Valsalva. A full rectum sometimes necessitates a repeat assessment after defecation because a full rectum can obscure other structures. Parting of the labia often improves image quality, especially if the labia are hirsute. Imaging conditions are best in pregnancy and poorest in the senium due to tissue hydration. Vaginal scar tissue and mesh implants may also impair visibility, but obesity virtually never is a problem.

Transducer placement between the clitoris and anus can be quite firm, unless there is vulval dermatitis or marked atrophy. The field of view includes the symphysis pubis anteriorly, the urethra and bladder neck, trigone, vagina, cervix, rectum, and anal canal (see Fig. 14.1). The anorectal angle indicates the location of

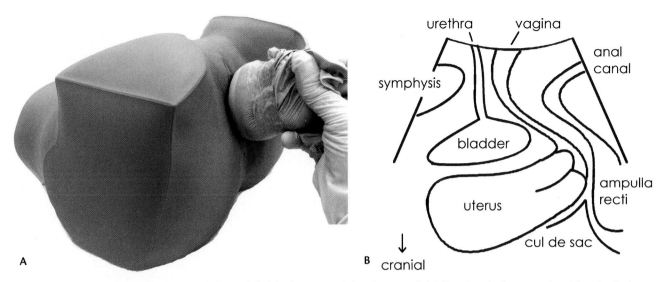

FIGURE 14.1 Transducer placement (**left**) and field of vision (**right**) for translabial/perineal ultrasound, midsagittal plane. (Reprinted from Dietz HP. The role of two- and three-dimensional dynamic ultrasound in pelvic organ prolapse. *J Minim Invasive Gynecol* 2010;17:282–294. Copyright © 2010, with permission from Elsevier.)

the levator plate in the midline. The cul-de-sac may also be visible, filled with anechoic intraperitoneal fluid, echogenic intraperitoneal fat, and peristalsing small bowel or sigmoid.[3]

Three-Dimensional/Four-Dimensional Imaging

The introduction of 3D imaging has given access to the axial plane which is particularly important for pelvic floor medicine as this plane previously was only accessible to sonography through the use of intracavitary transducers. The physical dimensions of transducers designed for prenatal imaging are, rather fortuitously, perfect for pelvic floor imaging. A volume data set obtained with field of vision and acquisition angles of ≥70° will include the entire levator hiatus at rest. Four-dimensional imaging, that is, the continuous acquisition of dozens of volumes at 0.5 to 4 Hz during a Valsalva or Kegel (pelvic floor muscle contraction [PFMC]) maneuver literally adds another dimension to our diagnostic capabilities.[4]

Optimally, the system should allow volume data imaging with field of vision and acquisition angles of ≥80° and store ≥5 seconds of data at 0.5 to 5 Hz. The result are "cine loops" of blocks of imaging data that can be manipulated to allow the examination of any arbitrarily defined plane and changes in that plane during maneuvers.

Display Modes

Figure 14.2 shows both main display modes used on modern ultrasound systems, i.e., sectional orthogonal planes (Fig. 14.2A–C) and rendering (Fig. 14.2D). For pelvic floor imaging, the orthogonal planes are defined as midsagittal

(top left), coronal (top right), and axial (bottom left) planes, although the location and angulation of these planes relative to the main transducer axis can be varied arbitrarily to enhance the visibility of a given structure, either during acquisition or for offline analysis at a later time. The levator ani muscle, for example, requires an axial plane that is tilted, with the direction and degree of this tilt varying between the resting state and maneuvers such as Valsalva or pelvic floor contraction.

These three conventional orthogonal planes are complemented by a "rendered volume," that is, a semitransparent representation of all volume pixels ("voxels") in a "region of interest" (ROI) that again can be varied arbitrarily. Such an ROI is shown in Figure 14.2D with the render direction from caudally to cranially, showing the levator hiatus and the puborectalis component of the levator ani. The ROI thickness is set to 1 to 2 cm for optimal imaging of the muscle and hiatus.

The real-time acquisition of volume ultrasound data at a temporal resolution of several Hertz, especially during maneuvers such as Valsalva and PFMC, makes this technology clearly superior to magnetic resonance imaging (MRI). Assessment of maneuvers by MRI requires ultrafast acquisition and the reliance on predetermined planes,[5] which will not allow optimal resolutions and often result in suboptimal slice location. In addition, it is very difficult to ensure proper performance of maneuvers because observation in real time is virtually impossible. Most women will not perform a proper pelvic floor contraction when asked without biofeedback teaching.[6] A Valsalva is frequently confounded by concomitant levator activation, or a full bladder or rectal gas stops the patient from performing a proper push.[7] Without real-time imaging, confounders are very difficult to control for, explaining the dearth of MR studies

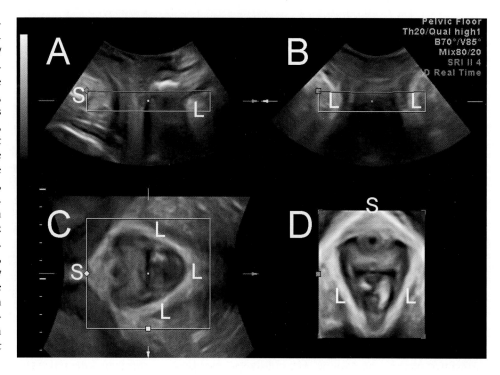

FIGURE 14.2 Standard representation of 3D pelvic floor ultrasound. The usual acquisition/evaluation screen on Voluson-type systems shows the three orthogonal planes: sagittal (**A**), coronal (**B**), and axial (**C**) as well as a rendered volume (**D**), which is a semitransparent representation of all grayscale data in the rendered volume (i.e., the box visible in **A–C**). S, symphysis pubis; L, levator ani. (Republished with permission of McGraw Hill, from Dietz HP. Pelvic floor ultrasound. In: Fleischer AC, Toy EC, Lee W, et al, eds. *Sonography in obstetrics & gynecology: Principles and practice*, 7th ed. New York: McGraw-Hill, 2010:17–23, permission conveyed through Copyright Clearance Center, Inc.)

in prolapse and urinary incontinence. Another advantage is the availability of offline analysis software that is much more powerful than what is available with Digital Imaging and Communications in Medicine (DICOM) viewer software on a set of single-plane MRI images.

Functional Assessment

Valsalva

The Valsalva maneuver, that is, forced expiration against closed glottis and contracted abdominal muscles and diaphragm, is useful in revealing signs of pelvic organ prolapse and to demonstrate distensibility ("ballooning") of the levator hiatus. During Valsalva, one observes a dorsocaudal displacement of urethra and bladder neck that can be quantified against the inferoposterior symphyseal margin (Fig. 14.3).[5] At the same time, there is caudad movement of the bladder, uterus, rectal ampulla, and abdominal contents as well as lateral and caudad distension of the levator hiatus, the largest potential hernia portal in the human body. It is important for the operator to avoid impeding downward movement of pelvic organs and perineum; there should be only enough pressure exerted by the transducer to avoid loss of contact, visible by the appearance of acoustic artifact. A Valsalva should last at least 6 seconds.[8] Intra-abdominal pressure, on the other hand, may not have to be standardized.[9] In women with a strong levator muscle, a Valsalva may be confounded by levator activation.[7] Three consecutive coughs seem sufficient for the assessment of anterior and posterior compartments.[10] At times, it is necessary to repeat

imaging in the standing position in order to avoid false-negative findings, which are most common in the central compartment.[11]

Pelvic floor muscle contraction

A PFMC can be quantified on imaging as a cranioventral shift of pelvic organs and/or a reduction in hiatal diameters.[12] Co-contraction of rectus abdominis and other muscles of the abdominal wall commonly results in an unwanted increase in intra-abdominal pressure which is visible as a dorsocaudal shift of the bladder neck as during a Valsalva maneuver. This is prevented by having the patient place one hand on the abdomen during a PFMC and asking her to keep the abdominal muscles soft while trying to act as if she wanted to stop the escape of gas or urine. Asking the patient to observe the effect of maneuvers on the monitor may provide for visual biofeedback.[13] Reflex pelvic floor activity can be observed on coughing.[14]

CLINICAL CONDITIONS

Urinary Incontinence

Imaging of pelvic floor structures is increasingly employed in the investigation of both stress and urge urinary incontinence. In stress urinary incontinence (SUI), there usually is a moderate degree of cystocele in the sense of a rotatory descent of the bladder and urethra. The commonest observations include opening of the retrovesical angle, rotation of the urethra by 60° or more, and funneling of the internal urethral meatus as shown

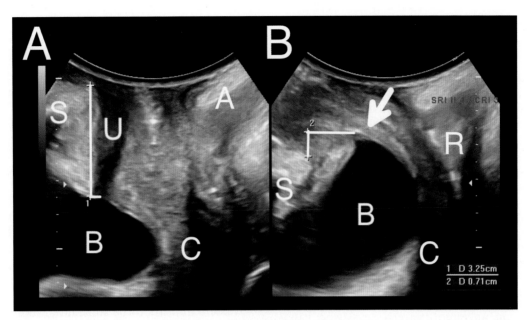

FIGURE 14.3 The midsagittal plane at rest (**A**) and on maximal Valsalva (**B**). Bladder neck descent is measured against the inferoposterior margin of the symphysis pubis: 3.25 − −0.71 = 3.96 cm. The horizontal and vertical distances between inferoposterior margin and bladder neck *(arrow)* are indicated by *white lines*. In practice, only the vertical distances are measured for bladder neck descent. S, symphysis pubis; U, urethra; B, bladder; A, anal canal; C, cervix; R, rectal ampulla.

in Figure 14.3. These findings are not truly diagnostic of urodynamic stress incontinence and can most certainly not be used to posit what is a urodynamic diagnosis.[15] However, such finding will be of help in women with exercise-related urodynamic stress incontinence (USI) in whom urodynamic testing frequently yields a false-negative result, especially in younger women with good urethral closure. Urge urinary incontinence is associated with detrusor hypertrophy, that is, a detrusor wall thickness (DWT) of 5 mm or more.[16] DWT is measured in the midsagittal plane, on the bladder dome, and is unreliable at bladder volumes over 50 mL due to distension of the detrusor. Unfortunately, the association between DWT and detrusor overactivity is too weak to serve as a diagnostic criterion.[17] A markedly thickened DWT should raise a suspicion of obstruction, either mechanical (Fig. 14.4) or due to neuropathic bladder dysfunction. Such findings are, however, quite uncommon and rarely found in older women with clinical voiding dysfunction.

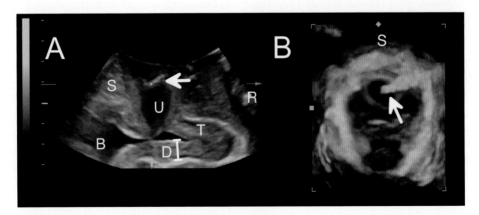

FIGURE 14.4 Hypertrophic detrusor *(D)* in a young woman, measured at over 10 mm, with outflow obstruction due to urethral stenosis in the context of tension-free vaginal tape (TVT) perforation. **A** (midsagittal plane) shows a markedly thickened detrusor muscle and trigone *(T)*, a wide urethra *(U)*, and an irregular echogenicity suggestive of implant material and/or scarring. The cause is evident in the rendered volume, axial plane (**B**). After partial removal, a large TVT remnant has perforated the urethra *(arrows)*. The implant was visible on urethroscopy. S, symphysis pubis; B, bladder; R, rectum.

Pelvic Organ Prolapse

Cystocele

Clinical examination by the Pelvic Organ Prolapse Quantification System (POP-Q)[18] is necessarily limited to quantifying changes in surface anatomy. A view of deeper structures with imaging is highly useful because it will identify urethral diverticula or Gartner cysts that can mimic cystocele. In addition, imaging allows to distinguish between cystourethrocele (usually with good urine flow rates and urodynamic stress incontinence, as in Fig. 14.3), and a cystocele with intact retrovesical angle (associated with poor voiding due to urethral kinking).[19] A cutoff of descent to 10 mm or more below the symphysis pubis has been suggested for the definition of "significant cystocele," that is, a degree of bladder descent that is likely to cause prolapse symptoms,[20] equivalent to a Ba of −0.5 cm on POP-Q.[21] In women after colposuspension, an anterior enterocele may occasionally mimic cystocele, easily diagnosed due to peristalsis and the iso- to hyperechoic nature of small bowel.

Uterine descent

Clinical assessment for prolapse sometimes produces false-negative results, and these seem to be most common in the central compartment.[11] Clearly, uterine supports need more time to distend than those of the anterior and central compartments. The uterus can also be harder to identify on imaging, especially if retroverted and/or atrophic, as the isoechoic echotexture

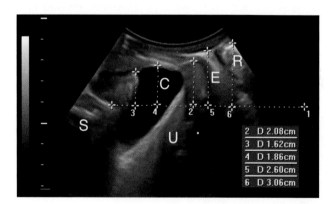

FIGURE 14.5 Three compartment prolapse on maximal Valsalva, midsagittal plane. Organ descent is measured against a horizontal reference line placed through the inferoposterior margin of the symphysis pubis. *Vertical lines* demonstrate cystocele, uterine prolapse, enterocele, and rectocele descent. Measurement 3 is descent of the bladder neck to 16.2 mm below the symphysis, the bladder (measurement 4) reaches 18.6, the uterus (measurement 2) 20.8 mm below. To the left (i.e., dorsal) of the cervix is a small enterocele (measurement 5) to 26 mm below, and the rectal ampulla (measurement 6) reaches to 30.6 mm below the symphysis. S, symphysis pubis; C, cystocele; U, uterus; E, enterocoele; R, rectal ampulla.

of the cervix is similar to vaginal wall. Provided it is not high or obscured by stool or bowel gas in a rectocele, the leading edge of the cervix often shows as a fine hyperechogenic (specular) line, and Nabothian follicles can also act as a marker (Fig. 14.5). An anteriorized cervix and an enlarged, retroverted uterus may impair bladder emptying as occasionally occurs in pregnancy. On the other hand, descent of an anteverted uterus can result in symptoms of obstructed defecation due to compression of the anorectum and/or intussusception. The descending uterus seems to cause prolapse symptoms at a higher station than anterior or posterior vaginal wall, suggesting that clinical staging used in conjunction with the POP-Q needs revision.[22] Consistent with such findings, a sonographically determined position of 15 mm above the symphysis on maximal Valsalva seems to be the optimal cutoff for the definition of "significant uterine descent."[23]

There appears to be substantial interethnic variations regarding uterine descent which may be more common in East Asians.[24] In Caucasians, uterine prolapse is associated with cystocele and levator trauma, but uterine retroversion also seems to be a risk factor. The known high rates of uterine prolapse in Nepalese, for example, may largely be due to retroversion, which seems very common in Nepalese women.[25]

Vault prolapse

In women after hysterectomy, the vault may be identified as the cranial aspect of hypoechoic vaginal walls, sometimes separated by iso- or hyperechogenic echoes that will be more evident after a vaginal examination. Identification of the vault can be helped by depositing a small amount of ultrasound gel in the vagina. Often, however, the vault is obscured by rectocele or enterocele causing acoustic shadowing. As an aside, vault descent to a given position seems to be just as likely to cause symptoms of prolapse than equivalent descent of the cervix.[26]

Posterior compartment

Imaging is most useful in the posterior compartment, not least due to the high prevalence of obstructed defecation in women, a symptom group strongly associated with several distinct forms of vaginal prolapse. In Caucasians, the clinical observation of a "rectocele," that is, descent of the posterior vaginal wall, seems to be most commonly due to a true or "radiologic" rectocele, that is, a defect of the rectovaginal septum or Denonvilliers fascia (associated with symptoms of prolapse, incomplete bowel emptying, and straining at stool).[27] However, an abnormally distensible, intact rectovaginal septum (associated only with prolapse symptoms); a combined rectoenterocele (less common); an isolated enterocele (uncommon); a rectal intussusception (uncommon); or just a deficient perineum may also be diagnosed as rectocele on clinical examination if the latter is limited to the observation of surface anatomy.[28] Hence, this term should probably be avoided and replaced with *posterior compartment descent* unless a true rectocele is diagnosed by imaging or rectal examination on Valsalva.[29] Figure 14.6 shows four of the most common abnormalities associated with clinical prolapse of the posterior vaginal compartment, in descending order of prevalence: true rectocele (Fig. 14.6A), rectoenterocele (Fig. 14.6B), isolated enterocele (Fig. 14.6C), and rectal intussusception (Fig. 14.6D).

Rectocele

A "true" rectocele is due to an anterior diverticulum of the rectal ampulla, which develops into the vagina, more obvious on Valsalva and easily observed on imaging (see Fig. 14.6A). Posterior and lateral rectoceles are rare and associated with more severe anatomical abnormalities such as intussusception or herniation through the iliococcygeus muscle.

The pocket or diverticulum formed by a rectocele mostly contains iso- to hyperechoic feces and bowel gas, causing acoustic artefacts such as shadowing, specular (mirror-like) echoes, and reverberations. Large rectoceles can necessitate repeat assessment after bowel emptying as they will obscure a large part of the field of vision and create a conical area of acoustic shadowing that may even impede imaging of the levator hiatus. If there is no stool in the ampulla, a rectocele may appear much smaller. Appearances can vary considerably from one day to the other making posterior compartment descent less reproducible than other imaging findings.[30]

A rectocele is quantified relative to the symphyseal margin for descent as usual for any other form of prolapse and by measuring the depth of the diverticulum against a baseline drawn through the anterior aspect of the internal anal sphincter (see Fig. 14.6A). "Significant descent of the posterior compartment" is diagnosed if the rectal ampulla or a diverticulum of the ampulla ("true rectocele") reaches to at least 15 mm below the symphysis pubis regardless of the presence of a diverticulum or true rectocele.[20] Attempts at producing a cutoff for significant true rectocele have been unsuccessful likely due to multiple confounding factors.[31] Findings on translabial ultrasound are comparable to those obtained by defecation proctography, provided the evaluation is produced using similar diagnostic criteria (see Dietz and Cartmill[32] for an overview). Finally, it should be pointed out that rectocele can very likely be congenital,[33] that it is less strongly associated with childbirth than just about any other form of prolapse,[34] and that it is the one form of prolapse that is clearly linked to obesity.[35]

Enterocele

An enterocele is imaged as descent of small bowel or any other abdominal contents dorsal to the (anechoic) bladder and ventral to the (hyperechogenic) rectal ampulla and anal canal (see Fig. 14.6B). There often is peristalsis, and intraperitoneal fluid may outline the most caudal point of an enterocele. Small bowel has a ground-grass–like or irregularly iso- to hyperechogenic appearance without acoustic shadowing and can easily be distinguished from stool in the ampulla or a rectocele. Enteroceles often occur in combination with rectocele (see Fig. 14.6B), commonly after hysterectomy

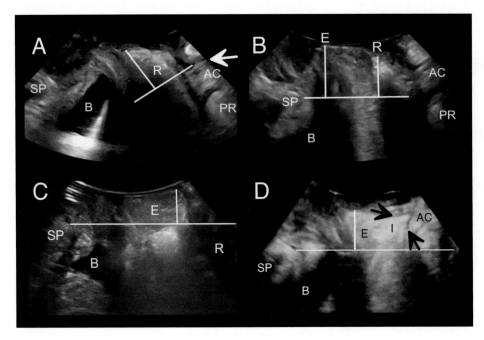

FIGURE 14.6 The four most common anatomical observations in significant posterior compartment descent: true rectocele (**A**), rectoenterocele (**B**), isolated enterocele (**C**), and rectal intussusception (**D**). The reference *line* in **A** shows the measurement of rectocele depth against a reference *line* placed through the internal anal sphincter *(white arrow)*, the *lines* in B–D demonstrate the measurement of organ descent against a horizontal reference *line* placed through the symphysis pubis. SP, symphysis pubis; B, bladder; R, rectal ampulla; AC, anal canal; PR, puborectalis muscle; E, enterocele; I, intussusception *(black arrows)*.

and in the form of vault prolapse where they can be isolated (see Fig. 14.6C), but occasionally, an enterocele may develop anteriorly, that is, between bladder and vault. Enterocele is often only visible after bladder emptying regardless of its type.

In a minority of women with a clinical rectocele, imaging will show a rectal intussusception, a condition that is found in about 4% of our patients and rarely diagnosed clinically. It is clearly associated with symptoms of obstructed defecation.[36] The main diagnostic feature of this underdiagnosed condition is splaying of the (normally tubular) anal canal, while the anterior rectal muscularis (and sometimes the posterior as well) is inverted into the anal canal (see Fig. 14.6D). This inversion is propelled by abdominal contents such as small bowel or sigmoid, omentum, or uterus, the latter termed a "colpocele." Interestingly, rectal intussusception is strongly associated with hiatal ballooning.[37]

Visual biofeedback, that is, demonstrating the effect of straining on anorectal anatomy to the patient, can help in modifying defecatory behavior. One may also be able to demonstrate the mechanism of anismus which is evident as an inability to relax the levator ani, producing a reduction in anteroposterior hiatal diameters on Valsalva. Translabial ultrasound seems to be a simple, inexpensive alternative to radiologic imaging methods.[32]

POSTOPERATIVE FINDINGS

Slings

Due to the high echogenicity of polypropylene threads, synthetic suburethral slings are easily visible on translabial ultrasound as linear hyperechogenic structures between the urethral rhabdosphincter and vaginal muscularis.[38] They act by dynamic compression of the urethra under load, which is easily demonstrated on imaging, with the sling changing from a linear to a c shape.[39] This is likely to be most effective if compression occurs at the locus of maximal urethral pressures, that is, at the midurethra. The type of sling, that is, whether it is a retropubic or a transobturator tape, can be determined in the axial plane, but with some experience, this distinction can also be made on 2D imaging either by placing the transducer in a transverse plane or by following the sling in parasagittal planes. Figure 14.7 demonstrates typical appearances of a transobturator tape in midsagittal, axial, and parasagittal planes. A transobturator tape will reach the levator ani and sometimes perforate its most caudal aspects,[40] a retropubic sling curves ventrally to enter the space of Retzius.

Complications such as urinary retention or worsened/de novo urgency and/or urge incontinence often turn out to be due to a tightly curled, excessively tensioned sling which leaves too small a gap between the implant and the symphysis pubis, especially on Valsalva. This "sling–pubis gap" (Fig. 14.8) seems to be the most useful measure of "sling tightness," with a gap of 8 to 14 mm on maximal Valsalva being rated as "normal."[41] An implant that is close to the urethra, with a low sling–pubis gap of less than 8 mm, will suggest either dilatation/stretching of the sling if identified within the first week or 10 days or a sling division.

Some slings may be detected close to the external meatus or the bladder neck, and there clearly is a large margin of safety regarding placement.[42] The larger the incision, the higher the sling will be found on imaging; if a sling is inserted through an incision contiguous with a colpotomy for anterior repair, it may well come to rest under the trigone, creating appearances similar to after a colposuspension. In this situation, as evident in Figure 14.9, the sling–pubis gap is often very wide, and recurrence of stress incontinence is very likely due to an absence of dynamic compression.

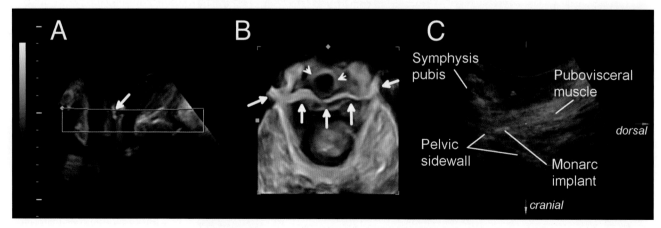

FIGURE 14.7 Suburethral sling in the midsagittal plane (**A**), a rendered volume in the axial plane (**B**) and in an oblique parasagittal plane (**C**). The sling or tape is indicated by *large arrows* in **A** and **B**, the urethra with the circular rhabdosphincter by *small arrows* in **B**. As is evident in **B**, this is a typically placed, fully functional transobturator sling. Transobturator tapes often perforate the caudal aspects of the puborectalis muscle as shown in **C**.

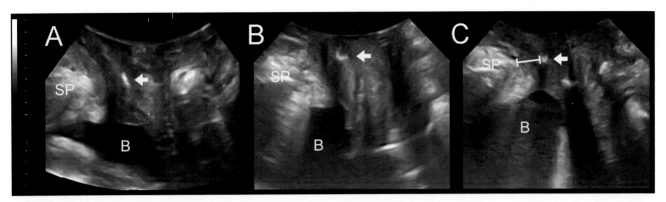

FIGURE 14.8 Appearance of a typical suburethral sling *(arrow)* in the midsagittal plane at rest (**A**), on submaximal Valsalva (**B**), and on maximal Valsalva (**C**). The *line* in **C** demonstrates measurement of the sling–pubis gap. SP, symphysis pubis; B, bladder.

In some instances, slings seem to be "tethered," that is, placed deep to the fascia of the rhabdosphincter, i.e., through the striated urethral muscle rather than outside it. This is not uncommon and indicates suboptimal surgical technique. Occasionally, imaging will suggest perforation and/or stenosis (see Fig. 14.4). Sling division, a minor procedure that can be performed under local anesthetic, results in a 5- to 10-mm gap between sling arms. Rarely, suboptimal sling insertion will result in perforation and ultimately transection of the urethra; eventually, the implant may be found in the space of Retzius (Fig. 14.10).

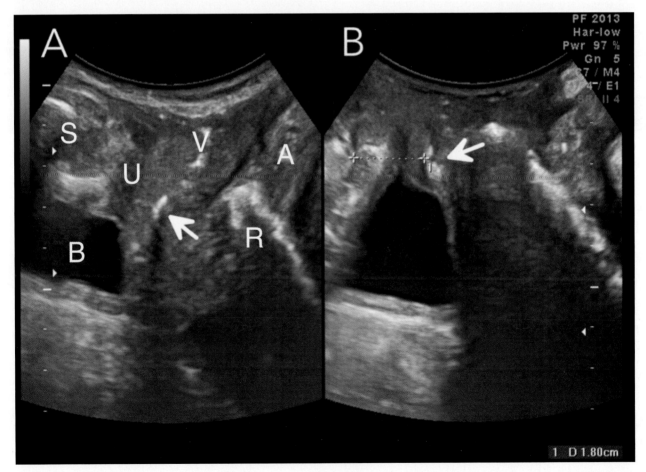

FIGURE 14.9 Abnormally high tension-free vaginal tape as shown in the midsagittal plane, at rest (**A**) and on Valsalva (**B**). It is evident that the sling at rest is situated at the proximal third of the urethra. On Valsalva, the appearances are those of a poor colposuspension, with the sling under the trigone. The abnormally high sling–pubis gap of 18 mm suggests a lack of dynamic compression. This patient had recurrent USI. The sling is indicated by *arrows*. S, symphysis pubis; U, uterus; A, anal canal; B, bladder; R, rectal ampulla.

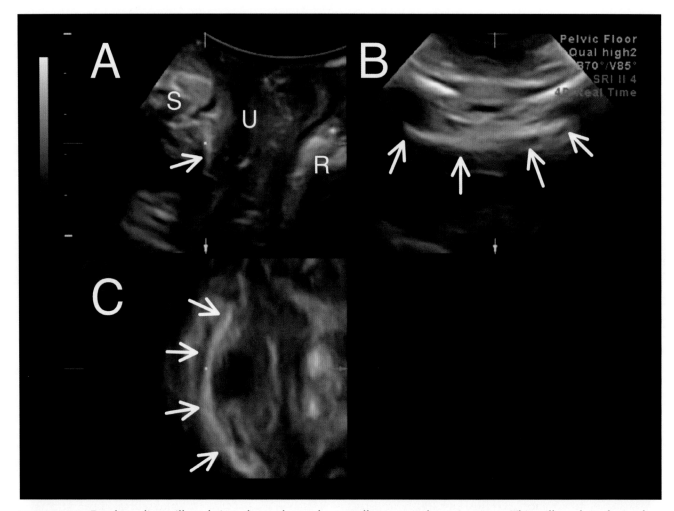

FIGURE 14.10 Rarely, a sling will erode into the urethra and eventually transect the entire organ. This will result in the implant being found in the space of Retzius rather than dorsal to the urethra. In this instance, after several years of symptoms of voiding dysfunction following transobturator tape implantation, the patient felt a sudden sensation of release, after which voiding was much improved. There was no recurrent stress incontinence. **A** shows the implant *(arrows)* ventral to the urethra *(U)* with irregular hyperechogenicity in the area of a urethral scar. Both the coronal (**B**) and the axial plane (**C**) demonstrate a transobturator implant which in **C** is clearly ventral to the urethra. S, symphysis pubis; R, rectum.

Mesh Implants

From 2005 onward, there was a worldwide trend toward the use of woven polypropylene mesh in prolapse surgery, especially for recurrent cystocele. However, by now, the medicolegal environment in Western societies has resulted in the disappearance of most prolapse meshes, especially those that were most effective. Further optimization of patient selection and mesh technology has become largely impossible. This is a pity because some forms of prolapse are virtually impossible to permanently correct by conventional means.[43] Unfortunately, social media attention and litigation have largely arrested development which means that several bioengineering issues remain unresolved. Due to complications such as chronic pain, erosion and recurrence, imaging specialists are increasingly asked to assess such meshes, which presents distinct challenges.

Polypropylene meshes such as the Perigee, Prolift, Avaulta, and Apogee are highly echogenic as seen in Figure 14.11,[44] although imaging may be affected by recurrent prolapse and distance from the transducer. Hyperechogenic linear vaginal echoes may be artefactual; hence, imaging in orthogonal planes is required to demonstrate mesh in three dimensions (Fig. 14.12). Implant position and mobility on Valsalva can be determined as well as anchoring failure and recurrence of prolapse. Polypropylene meshes do not commonly shrink in vivo, as has been claimed.[45,46] Surgical technique is important in determining mesh location and efficacy as well as the likelihood of postoperative de novo or worsened SUI.[44] Anchoring matters, as shown by the universal failure of nonanchored mesh ("overlay techniques"), and transobturator mesh arms appear to be more effective than plastic anchors in providing midvaginal support.[47]

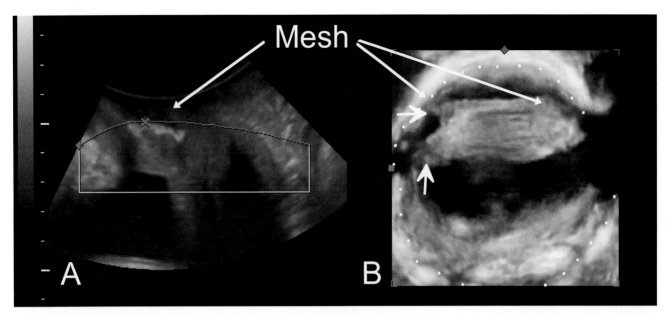

FIGURE 14.11 Perigee anterior compartment mesh in the midsagittal plane (**A**) and in a rendered volume (**B**), the latter showing the entire central aspect of the mesh and the two transobturator arms on the patient's right. The left-hand arms are invisible due to asymmetry. Ballooning indicated by dotted circumference, mesh arms indicated by *short arrows*. (From Dietz HP. Pelvic floor ultrasound. *Aust Soc Ultrasound Med Bull* 10:17–23, with permission [Australian Society for Ultrasound Medicine].)

Three distinct forms of cystocele recurrence after anterior compartment mesh have been described (Fig. 14.13), two of which are more likely in women with major pelvic floor trauma and/or hiatal overdistension.[47] In patients with recurrent prolapse, imaging may show the implant to be an asset rather than a liability. An "anterior recurrence" requires surgical fixation of the prolapsing bladder neck to the inferior margin of an otherwise intact and functional mesh, whereas an apical recurrence suggests an apical suspension procedure. Mesh removal is likely to result in recurrence, especially in women with an abnormal pelvic floor.

Although anterior compartment mesh is often effective in curing prolapse and may in fact be the only realistic option in some women with major levator trauma (see following text),[48] the situation is different for the posterior compartment.[49] Posterior mesh (posterior Prolift, Apogee, etc.) is found anterior to the rectal ampulla, frequently extending to the perineal body and often less mobile than anterior mesh on Valsalva. Recurrence can take several appearances: an enterocele anterior to a well-anchored mesh, or posterior to the mesh as intussusception, or as a true rectocele behind the mesh, developing into the perineum as seen in Figure 14.14.[50] Sonography is however of limited utility in complications such as pain and erosion, apart from determining the presence, type, and mechanical effect of the implant.

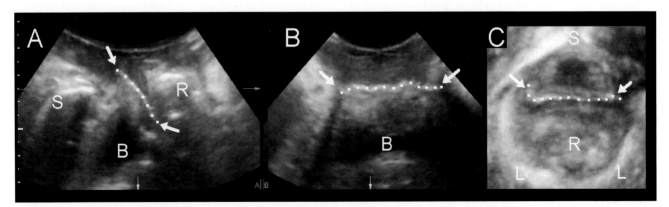

FIGURE 14.12 Identification of anterior compartment mesh on Valsalva: midsagittal plane (**A**), coronal plane (**B**), and axial plane (**C**). *Arrows* show mesh length in the midsagittal (**left**) and the coronal plane (**center** and **right**). S, symphysis pubis; B, bladder; R, rectal ampulla; L, levator ani. (Reprinted from Dietz HP, Erdmann M, Shek KL. Mesh contraction: Myth or reality? *Am J Obstet Gynecol* 2011;204[2]:173.e1–173.e4. Copyright © 2011, with permission from Elsevier.)

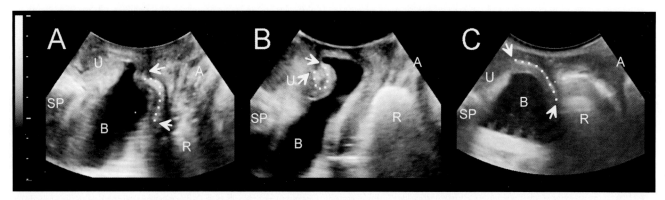

FIGURE 14.13 Recurrence of anterior compartment prolapse can follow at least three different patterns: anterior recurrence ventral to a well-anchored mesh (**A**), apical recurrence after detachment of apical anchoring structures (**B**), and global recurrence after loss of all anchoring (**C**). *Arrows* indicate cranial and caudal mesh margins; the *dotted line* shows the extent of the mesh. SP, symphysis pubis; U, urethra; A, anal canal; B, bladder; R, rectal ampulla.

HIATAL DIMENSIONS

As pelvic organ prolapse is invariably a hernia through the levator hiatus, the triangular gap between the V-shaped sling of the puborectalis muscle and the inferior pubic rami, it makes very good sense to determine the size of this largest potential hernial portal in the human body. Often, excessive distensibility of the hiatus is due to "avulsion" (see following text), but there are women with a highly abnormal pelvic floor muscle without visible tears. Abnormal biomechanical properties of the levator ani may be congenital[51] or the result of overdistension in childbirth, with the latter termed "microtrauma."[52] High congenital hiatal distensibility may have some advantages in vaginal childbirth.[53,54]

Figure 14.15 illustrates the identification of the plane of minimal hiatal dimensions, both in a rendered volume and in a single axial plane. The minimal distance between the posterior contour of the symphysis pubis and the anorectal angle defines the axial plane of minimal dimensions. As this plane is often warped, especially in women with marked overdistension,[55] it is appropriate to measure hiatal dimensions in a thick slice of 1 to 2 cm in thickness (rendered volume; see Fig. 14.15).[56]

Such measures of hiatal dimensions are repeatable[57] and strongly correlated with measurements on MRI.[58] Hiatal distension on Valsalva to >25 cm² on Valsalva

is termed *ballooning* on the basis of normative data in young nulliparous women and receiver operator characteristics statistics.[59] Figure 14.11 shows a case of severe ballooning in a patient with bilateral avulsion after mesh placement. Ballooning can in fact be determined clinically by measuring the distance between urethra and anus (genital hiatus and perineal body), which is part of the POP-Q examination for pelvic organ prolapse.[60] Ballooning is associated with symptoms of prolapse and objective prolapse on examination[59] including rectal intussusception[37] and prolapse recurrence after surgical treatment.[61] Together with avulsion, hiatal dimensions can be used to estimate the likelihood of recurrence.[48]

MATERNAL BIRTH TRAUMA

Levator Avulsion

Until recently, the term *maternal birth trauma*, if interpreted as somatic rather than psychological trauma, was meant to encompass perineal tears and anal sphincter tears (obstetric anal sphincter injury or OASI). Since about 2004, it has become evident that, firstly, major tears of the levator ani muscle (avulsion) are common in vaginally parous women[4] and that, secondly, such tears are usually occult, that is, invisible in delivery suite,

FIGURE 14.14 Rectocele *(large arrow)* developing behind well-supported posterior compartment mesh *(small arrows)*. The pocket is outlined by *dots*. **A** is at rest; **B** at maximal Valsalva. R, rectal ampulla; A, anal canal; L, levator ani. (Reprinted from Dietz HP. Ultrasound in the assessment of pelvic organ prolapse. *Best Pract Res Clin Obstet Gynecol* 2019;54:12–30. doi:10.1016/j.bpobgyn.2018.06.006. Copyright © 2018, with permission from Elsevier.)

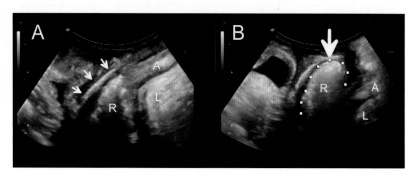

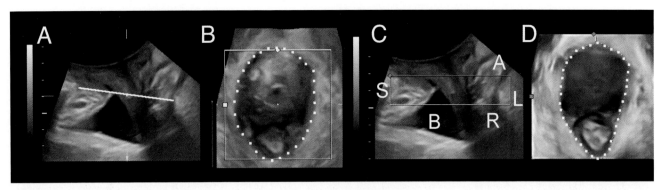

FIGURE 14.15 Measuring hiatal dimensions as shown in an oblique single axial plane (**A** and **B**) and a rendered volume (**C** and **D**). The midsagittal plane on the left (**A**) demonstrates a line indicating the minimal sagittal diameter of the hiatus, that is, the location of the oblique axial plane shown in **B**. The ROI box in **C** (approximately 1.8 cm deep) is located between the symphysis pubis and the levator ani posterior to the anorectal angle. **D** represents a semitransparent view of all pixels in the ROI box on the left. S, symphysis pubis; B, bladder; R, rectal ampulla; A, anal canal. (Adapted from Dietz HP, Wong V, Shek KL. A simplified method for the determination of levator hiatal dimensions. *Aust NZ J Obstet Gynaecol* 2011;51:540–543, with permission [Wiley Blackwell].)

because the vaginal skin and muscularis are more elastic than the underlying muscle.[62] This implies that imaging is essential for diagnosis, especially as palpation requires considerable skill.[63–65] Figure 14.16 shows a comparison of clinical findings, translabial ultrasound and MRI in a patient with a full right-sided levator avulsion after normal vaginal delivery at term.[62] Avulsion is visible on 2D ultrasound on oblique parasagittal views (Fig. 14.17),[66] but tomographic representations (Figs. 14.18 and 14.19) are likely to be more repeatable[67] and have become the international standard over the last 10 years.[1] The first step always is the identification of the plane of minimal dimensions in the midsagittal or "A" plane as shown in Figure 14.15, but for levator

integrity, we use volume data obtained on PFMC, not on Valsalva (Fig. 14.20). If an PFMC cannot be obtained, volume data produced at rest may be used,[68] although image quality may be inferior. In women with a very strong contraction, one may want to use a submaximal PFMC because this avoids the muscle being pulled so high that some aspects of it will be in the acoustic shadow of the inferior pubic rami.

Once the plane of minimal dimensions is identified in the midsagittal (A) plane of an orthogonal representation of volume data obtained at PFMC, this plane is rotated anticlockwise until the minimal distance between the posterior margin of the symphysis pubis and the anterior aspect of the anorectal angle is horizontal (see Fig. 14.20).

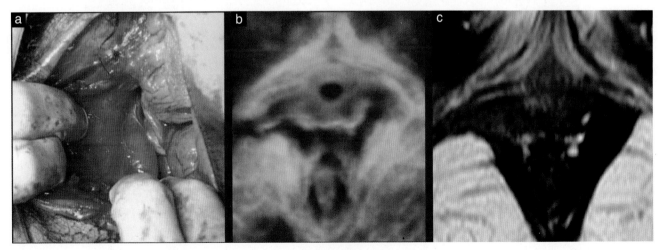

FIGURE 14.16 Typical right-sided levator avulsion injury as diagnosed in the delivery suite after a normal vaginal delivery at term (**left**), on 3D ultrasound (**center**), and on MRI (**right**) 3 months postpartum. This patient was asymptomatic apart from deep dyspareunia. (From Dietz HP, Gillespie A, Phadke P. Avulsion of the pubovisceral muscle associated with large vaginal tear after normal vaginal delivery at term. *Aust NZ J Obstet Gynaecol* 2007;47:341–344, with permission [Wiley Blackwell].)

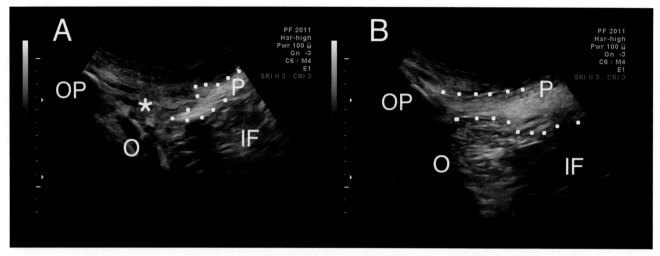

FIGURE 14.17 Parasagittal views of complete right-sided (**A**) and partial left-sided (**B**) avulsion. It is evident that in **A**, there is complete detachment (see *asterisk*) of the hyperechogenic puborectalis from the os pubis *(OP)*, whereas in **B**, there is continuity between the puborectalis *(P)* and the *OP* of about 50% of the muscle. O, obturator foramen; IF, ischiorectal fossa.

The corresponding axial plane slice, the "plane of minimal hiatal dimensions,"[51] in the "C" plane is then used to construct a tomographic set of C-plane slices, centered on the plane of minimal dimensions, with an interslice interval of 2.5 mm.[69] For convenience, the C plane is rotated 90° clockwise to obtain an orientation akin to seeing the recumbent patient's pelvis from below, the "gynecologist's view." Adjustment of the appearance of the symphysis pubis allows highly reproducible slice placement (see Fig. 14.18) and determination of the levator–urethra

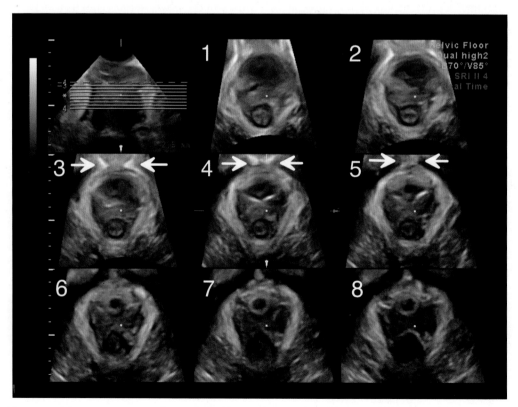

FIGURE 14.18 Tomographic representation of an intact puborectalis muscle, obtained on PFMC, with 2.5-mm interslice interval. The central slice *(4)* represents the plane of minimal hiatal dimensions as identified in the midsagittal plane. The three middle slices *(3–5)* are adjusted to show the symphysis pubis open (**left**), closing (**center**), and closed, that is, no longer visible, on the right *(arrows)*.

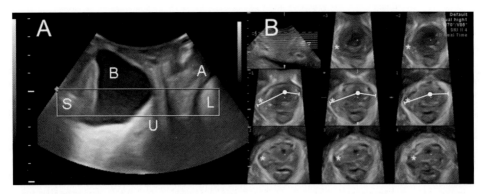

FIGURE 14.19 Midsagittal plane (**A**) and tomographic imaging of a typical right-sided avulsion in a patient with cystocele and mild uterine prolapse shown in **A. B** shows a large right-sided avulsion indicated by *asterisk* and shown on the left-hand aspect of eight axial plane slices placed at 2.5-mm intervals. The *oblique lines* indicate the levator–urethra gap (LUG) which can be helpful in equivocal cases. In a situation as obvious as in this patient, LUG measurement is plainly redundant however. S, symphysis pubis; B, bladder; U, urethra; A, anal canal; L, levator ani.

gap (see Fig. 14.19) may help in difficult cases.[70] The diagnosis of avulsion with this method correlates well with MR findings.[71] A full avulsion is diagnosed if a minimum of three central slices show an abnormal insertion. Figure 14.19 demonstrates a typical combination of findings: a complete right-sided avulsion (Fig. 14.19B) in a patient with cystocele and uterine descent (Fig. 14.19A).[69] Trauma that falls short of those "minimal criteria," that is, "partial" avulsion, seems to be less strongly associated with prolapse.[72]

There surely are other factors influencing the integrity of the levator ani muscle, such as microtrauma or altered biomechanics of otherwise intact muscle, but avulsion likely constitutes a large part of the "missing link" between vaginal childbirth and prolapse postulated in epidemiologic studies (see Dietz et al.[73] for an overview). Neuropathy is unlikely to play a major role.[74] Avulsion enlarges the levator hiatus,[75] the largest potential hernial portal in the human body, reduces pelvic floor muscle function by about one-third,[76,77] and is clearly associated with pelvic organ prolapse,[76,78] especially cystocele and uterine prolapse.[79] Urinary and anal continence are likely to be less affected.[80,81] Levator defects may well be the most important independent risk factor for prolapse recurrence.[61]

Avulsion defects can be detected by digital vaginal palpation which however does require significant teaching and seems less repeatable than imaging.[82] The primary risk factor for avulsion is the obstetric forceps (see Dietz[83] for an overview), with vacuum being much less dangerous.

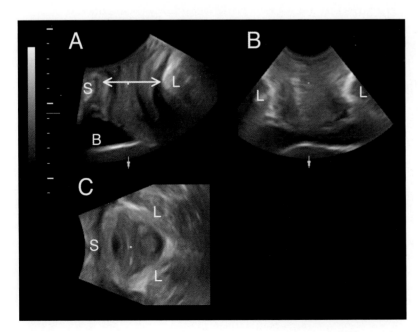

FIGURE 14.20 Once a contraction is obtained on 4D imaging, the most appropriate volume is selected and represented in sectional planes as shown here. This allows the identification of the plane of minimal dimensions *(double-sided arrow)* in the **A** plane which is rotated anticlockwise until the plane of minimal dimensions is horizontal and central. The levator is also visible in the coronal plane (**B**). The associated C plane (**C**) is then selected for tomographic imaging of the puborectalis muscle as in Figure 13.18. S, symphysis pubis; B, bladder; L, levator ani.

Other potential risk factors include the length of the second stage of labor, birthweight, maternal age, head circumference, and perineal/vaginal tears.[52,84-87] Levator trauma seems to largely be limited to the first vaginal birth,[88,89] and substantial improvement over time is unlikely.[90] First attempts at prevention by altering the biomechanical properties of the muscle have been unsuccessful.[91]

In women with a high risk of recurrence due to avulsion or ballooning, surgical reattachment of the puborectalis muscle to the inferior pubic ramus[92] or hiatal reduction have been proposed,[93] with both approaches currently the subject of surgical trials.

Anal Sphincter Trauma

Conceptually, anal sphincter imaging is more complex than the imaging of levator trauma. The latter is very rarely diagnosed and never repaired intrapartum, implying that imaging findings are directly representative of the trauma suffered at crowning of the baby's head. Although a large proportion of OASI are never diagnosed and repaired, in many women, appearances are altered by a primary repair procedure. This can lead to substantial distortion of tissue planes and influences the association between trauma and symptoms. In addition, OASI affects not just one structure but two, that is, both internal and external anal sphincters (EAS). It is not surprising, therefore, that the association between imaging findings and symptoms is often less clear than it is for levator trauma, especially in postmenopausal women in whom other aetiological factors predominate. On the other hand, the latency between trauma and symptoms seems less for OASI, with about half of all women diagnosed and repaired in the delivery suite showing symptoms 5 years after the event.[94]

The anal sphincters are usually imaged with endoanal ultrasound[95] and MRI,[96] sometimes with endocoils.[97] Techniques involving internal probes are more stressful for the patient and inevitably distort the anatomy, which is one reason why textbook illustrations often seem rather unrealistic.

Exoanal ultrasound of the sphincters was first described by Peschers et al.[98] in 1997 and is now widely used to image the anal sphincter using either endovaginal or transabdominal probes.[1] Exoanal sphincter imaging with 4D probes allows tomographic representation of the anal canal and can identify structures never described on endoanal imaging, such as the fascial plane between EAS and levator ani, and distinct subdivisions of the EAS as well as the perineum itself. As a result, highly reproducible tomographic imaging has become feasible.[99,100] Normal values for internal and external sphincter have recently been published.[101] The method has been compared to endoanal imaging, with fair to good agreement demonstrated.[102,103]

Conveniently, the same transducers as for pelvic floor imaging can be used for the sphincters, the only difference being transducer placement. A curved array abdominal/obstetric volume transducer is rotated 90° clockwise and steeply inclined from ventrocaudal to dorsocranial for a coronal view of the anal canal; see Figure 14.21. This results in a representation of orthogonal planes as in Figure 14.22, and tomographic imaging as shown in Figures 14.23 to 14.27. Application of additional gel in the midline may be needed to fill the labial fold, and hirsute labia need to be parted. Imaging is preferably performed on PFMC which seems to enhance the definition of muscular defects; however, imaging at rest is acceptable.[104] Contrary to tomographic imaging of the levator, the interslice interval is adjusted

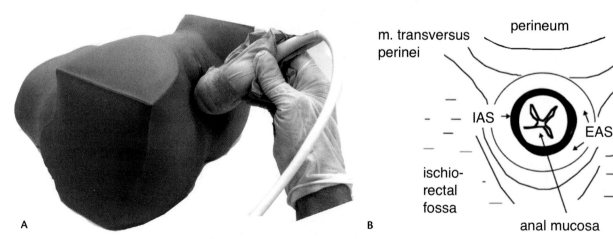

FIGURE 14.21 Transducer placement after rotation of a midsagittally placed volume transducer by 90° clockwise (**A**) and resulting schematic view of structures (**B**). The best tissue discrimination is reached by keeping the transducer surface 0.5 to 1.5 cm from the ventral contour of the EAS, which also allows for imaging of the perineum. IAS, internal anal sphincter. (Adapted from Dietz HP. Pelvic floor ultrasound. In: Fleischer AC, Abramowicz JS, Gonçalves LF, et al, eds. *Sonography in obstetrics and gynecology: Textbook and teaching cases*, 8th ed. New York: McGraw-Hill, 2016:1162, permission conveyed through Copyright Clearance Center, Inc.)

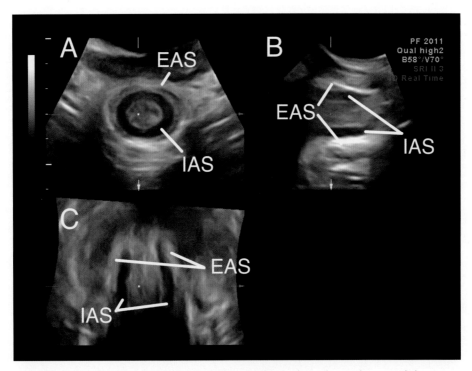

FIGURE 14.22 Imaging of the anal sphincters in orthogonal planes. The **A** plane shows the typical donut appearance of the EAS (hyperechogenic) and internal anal sphincter (IAS) (hypoechoic) in the coronal plane. The standard midsagittal orientation is given in the **B** plane, providing proof that the entire EAS is included in the volume. An oblique axial view is represented in the **C** plane and demonstrates that the anal canal is properly centered in the volume, that is, seen as vertical in C. (Republished with permission of McGraw Hill, from Dietz HP. Pelvic floor ultrasound. In: Fleischer AC, Abramowicz JS, Gonçalves LF, et al, eds. *Sonography in obstetrics and gynecology: Principles and practice*, 8th ed. New York: McGraw-Hill, 2016, permission conveyed through Copyright Clearance Center, Inc.)

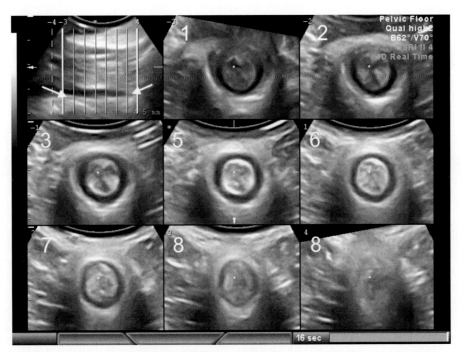

FIGURE 14.23 Tomographic imaging of normal external and internal anal sphincters. The reference plane at the top left shows the midsagittal plane. *Vertical lines* indicate the location of eight coronal slices given on this figure. The most cranial slice (**center top**) is located above the EAS (*left thick line* in the reference image), and the most caudad (**bottom right**) is placed below the internal anal sphincter (*right thick line*) in the reference image. As a result, the entire EAS should be covered in this tomographic representation. (Reprinted by permission from Springer: Shek KL, Della Zazzera V, Kamisan Atan I, et al. The evolution of transperineal ultrasound findings of the external anal sphincter during the first years after childbirth. *Int Urogynecol J* 2016;27[12]:1899–1903. doi:10.1007/s00192-016-3055-z, with permission [Springer].)

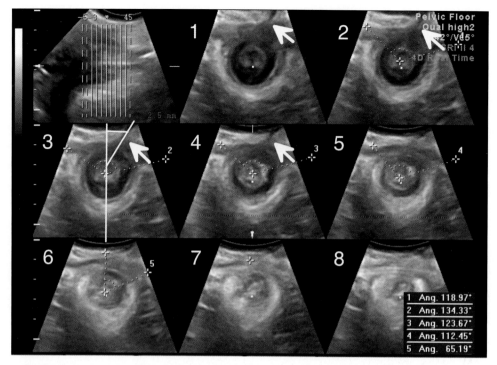

FIGURE 14.24 Overlooked, unrepaired 3B tear with well-repaired episiotomy. The angle measurements illustrate quantification of this tear which measures well over 30° in 5/6 slices. It is also evident that the episiotomy *(arrow)* was started "contralaterally," that is, on the wrong side of the midline, and was cut too steep, that is, toward the anal canal rather than away from it, as indicated by the *lines* in slice 3. Ang., angle. (Adapted from Dietz HP. Pelvic floor ultrasound. In: Fleischer AC, Abramowicz JS, Gonçalves LF, et al, eds. *Sonography in obstetrics and gynecology: Textbook and teaching cases*, 8th ed. New York: McGraw-Hill, 2016:1164, with permission.)

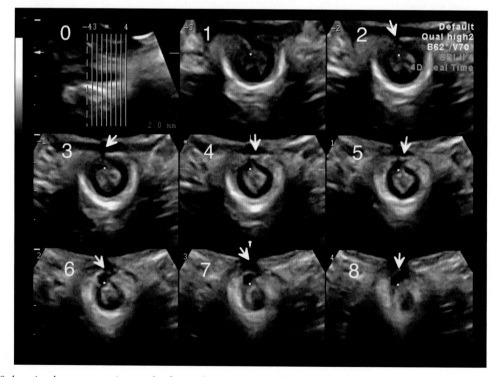

FIGURE 14.25 Suboptimal reconstructive result after end-to-end repair of a 3C tear after forceps delivery. The residual defect is indicated by *arrows*. There are several echogenic foci indicating suture material 10 weeks after primary repair with polydioxanone.

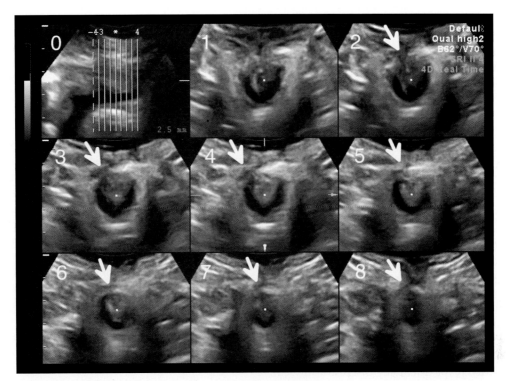

FIGURE 14.26 Status after overlap repair of a 3C tear, showing substantial distortion and a marked perineal scar *(arrows)*. After overlap, there often is a less visible defect of the EAS as here in slices *2, 3,* and *4.*

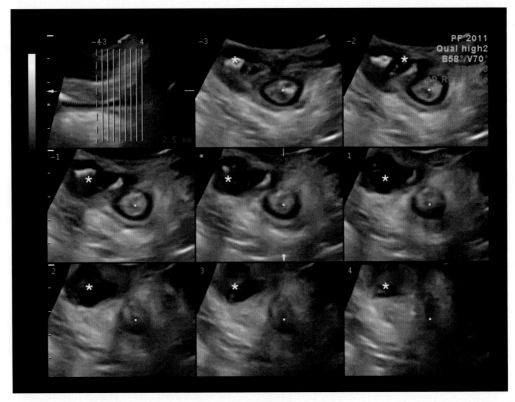

FIGURE 14.27 Distortion and "defect" of both external and internal anal sphincters in a patient with symptomatic perianal abscess prior to surgical intervention *(stars)*. Haemorrhoids also appear as anechoic masses, but they are smaller and usually show a cleaner contour without significant extension into the perianal space.

for each individual patient in order to place slice 1 above the external sphincter (see Figs. 14.22 and 14.23) and slice 8 below the internal sphincter; see location of *arrows* in the midsagittal reference plane provided in Figure 14.23.

EAS defects detected with this methodology are associated with anal incontinence, both after OASI repair[94,105] and later in life.[106] To quantify the degree of trauma, the number of affected slices may be determined, with ≥4/6 abnormal slices defined as a "residual defect." Another approach is to measure the defect angle as in Figure 14.24, with a cutoff empirically set at 30°. Unfortunately, the association between single slice defect angles and anal incontinence does not seem to be sufficiently strong to allow validation of the 30° cutoff,[107] which may partly be due to the confounding effect of attempts at repair.

This methodology lends itself not just to use in research but also in clinical practice. Although pain, edema, and suture material can make imaging difficult over the first postpartum week, follow-up after 2 to 3 months allows an audit of both diagnosis and primary repair. Even the adequacy of episiotomy can be assessed,[108] see Figure 14.24 for an example of an unrecognized and unrepaired 3B perineal tear after an episiotomy that was begun in the wrong place and cut too steeply, in essence aiming for the sphincter rather than away from it. The inclusion of imaging in "perineal clinics" will allow both anal sphincter and levator trauma to be documented as key performance indicators of obstetric services.[109] This seems important in view of the substantial morbidity due to intrapartum pelvic floor and anal sphincter trauma, some of which is plainly due to inadequate diagnosis or poor primary repair.[110]

Figures 14.24 to 14.26 show different forms of residual anal sphincter trauma after vaginal delivery. In Figure 14.24, there is evidence of a missed 3B tear after episiotomy (see *arrow*). Figure 14.25 shows suboptimal reconstruction after end-to-end repair of a 3C tear with residual defects in all slices except 4 and 5 and some bright foci due to suture material, whereas Figure 14.26 shows reasonable results after an overlap repair of a 3C tear. It may be unrealistic to expect much better appearances after 3C tears as defects of the internal sphincter seem to be particularly difficult to reconstruct. Not surprisingly, imaging appearances are associated with anal incontinence after primary repair.[94,105,106] Although this association is weaker in older women due to the prevalence of other etiological factors.[111] Plainly, there remains much opportunity for practice improvement.

On a final note, exoanal sphincter imaging sometimes demonstrates other abnormalities, which can interfere with identification of landmarks, as evident in Figure 14.27 showing a perianal abscess altering the contours of both internal and EAS.

CONCLUSION

The widespread use of sonographic imaging has the potential to substantially influence the management of urinary and anal incontinence, pelvic organ prolapse, and related conditions. Even in units and locations where the required technology is not easily accessible, insights provided by real-time imaging will enhance diagnostic and therapeutic capabilities. It is now evident that clinical examination in women presenting with urogynecologic conditions should include digital palpation of the levator ani muscle for defects as well as determination of the genital hiatus and perineal body on Valsalva. Women with symptoms of obstructed defecation and posterior compartment prolapse should, if imaging is unavailable, be examined per rectum during a Valsalva maneuver, allowing the digital detection of rectocele and intussusception.

Understanding the levator hiatus as hernial portal, and prolapse as a hernia, should enable new therapeutic approaches in women whose condition has been difficult to treat. Because the hiatus cannot possibly be obliterated as, for example, in umbilical hernia, the aim has to be reduction rather than obliteration, a bioengineering challenge that on principle appears surmountable with current technology. Once we learn how to reduce the distensibility of the levator hiatus without interfering with intercourse, voiding, and defecation, we may find that a range of difficult clinical problems will become much easier to resolve.

The development of noninvasive tomographic imaging of maternal birth trauma holds out the potential for the establishment of new key performance indicators for both obstetric practice and research. Currently, up to 80% of all major maternal birth trauma is not diagnosed, and even if diagnosed, often poorly repaired. Clearly, there are very substantial opportunities for practice improvement worldwide.

References

1. AIUM/IUGA practice parameter for the performance of urogynecological ultrasound examinations: Developed in collaboration with the ACR, the AUGS, the AUA, and the SRU. *Int Urogynecol J* 2019;30(9):1389–1400.
2. Dietz H. Pelvic floor imaging online course: IUGA; 2019. Accessed January 13, 2022. https://www.iuga.org/education/pfic/pfic-overview
3. Dietz H. Ultrasound imaging of the pelvic floor: Part I: two-dimensional aspects. *Ultrasound Obstet Gynecol* 2004;23:80–92.
4. Dietz H. Ultrasound imaging of the pelvic floor: Part II: three-dimensional or volume imaging. *Ultrasound Obstet Gynecol* 2004;23(6):615–625.
5. Dietz HP, Haylen BT, Broome J. Ultrasound in the quantification of female pelvic organ prolapse. *Ultrasound Obstet Gynecol* 2001;18(5):511–514.
6. Bo K, Larson S, Oseid S, et al. Knowledge about and ability to do correct pelvic floor muscle exercises in women with urinary stress incontinence. *Neurourol Urodyn* 1988;7:261–262.

7. Ornö A, Dietz H. Levator co-activation is a significant confounder of pelvic organ descent on Valsalva maneuver. *Ultrasound Obstet Gynecol* 2007;30:346–350.

8. Orejuela F, Shek K, Dietz H. The time factor in the assessment of prolapse and levator ballooning. *Int Urogynecol J* 2012;23:175–178.

9. Mulder F, Shek K, Dietz H. The pressure factor in the assessment of pelvic organ mobility. *Aust NZ J Obstet Gynaecol* 2012;52:282–285.

10. Pacquee S, Weeg N, Caudwell Hall J, et al. Clinical assessment of pelvic organ prolapse on coughing. *Int Urogynecol J* 2020;54(Suppl 1):Epub ahead of print.

11. Sathasivam N, Kamisan Atan I, Dietz H. False negative prolapse assessment is most likely to occur in the central compartment. *Ultrasound Obstet Gynecol* 2015;46(Suppl 1):132.

12. Dietz HP, Jarvis SK, Vancaillie TG. The assessment of levator muscle strength: A validation of three ultrasound techniques. *Int Urogynecol J Pelvic Floor Dysfunct* 2002;13(3):156–159.

13. Dietz HP, Wilson PD, Clarke B. The use of perineal ultrasound to quantify levator activity and teach pelvic floor muscle exercises. *Int Urogynecol J Pelvic Floor Dysfunct* 2001;12(3):166–169.

14. Dietz H, Erdmann M, Shek K. Reflex contraction of the levator ani in women symptomatic for pelvic floor disorders. *Ultrasound Obstet Gynecol* 2012;40(2):215–218.

15. Dietz H, Nazemian K, Shek K, et al. Can urodynamic stress incontinence be diagnosed by ultrasound? *Int Urogynecol J* 2012;24(8):1399–1403.

16. Liversidge K, Shek K, Guzman-Rojas R, et al. Negative urodynamic testing in women with stress incontinence. *Aust NZ J Obstet Gynaecol* 2013;55:76–80.

17. Lekskulchai O, Dietz H. Detrusor wall thickness as a test for detrusor overactivity in women. *Ultrasound Obstet Gynecol* 2008;32:535–539.

18. Bump RC, Mattiasson A, Bo K, et al. The standardization of terminology of female pelvic organ prolapse and pelvic floor dysfunction. *Am J Obstet Gynecol* 1996;175(1):10–17.

19. Eisenberg V, Chantarasorn V, Shek K, et al. Does levator ani injury affect cystocele type? *Ultrasound Obstet Gynecol* 2010;36:618–623.

20. Dietz HP, Lekskulchai O. Ultrasound assessment of prolapse: The relationship between prolapse severity and symptoms. *Ultrasound Obstet Gynecol* 2007;29:688–691.

21. Dietz H, Kamisan Atan I, Salita A. The association between ICS POP-Q coordinates and translabial ultrasound findings. *Ultrasound Obstet Gynecol* 2016;47(3):363–368.

22. Dietz H, Mann K. What is 'clinically relevant prolapse'? An attempt at defining cutoffs for the clinical assessment of pelvic organ descent. *Int Urogynecol J* 2014;25(4):451–455.

23. Shek K, Dietz H. What is abnormal uterine descent on translabial ultrasound? *Int Urogynecol J* 2015;26(12):1783–1787.

24. Cheung R, Chan S, Shek K, et al. Pelvic organ prolapse in Caucasian and East Asian women: A comparative study. *Ultrasound Obstet Gynecol* 2019;53:541–545.

25. Turel F, Caagbay D, Dietz H. Pelvic organ prolapse in a Nepali gynecology clinic: A prospective observational study. *Int Urogynecol J* 2018;29:Epub ahead of print.

26. Trutnovsky G, Robledo K, Shek K, et al. Definition of apical descent in women with and without previous hysterectomy: A retrospective analysis. *PLoS One* 2019;14(3):e0213617.

27. Dietz HP, Korda A. Which bowel symptoms are most strongly associated with a true rectocele? *Aust NZ J Obstet Gynaecol* 2005;45:505–508.

28. Dietz HP, Steensma AB. Posterior compartment prolapse on two-dimensional and three-dimensional pelvic floor ultrasound: The distinction between true rectocele, perineal hypermobility and enterocele. *Ultrasound in Obstet Gynecol* 2005;26:73–77.

29. Rachaneni S, Kamisan Atan I, Guzman-Rojas R, et al. Digital rectal examination in the evaluation of rectovaginal septal defects. *Int Urogynecol J* 2017;28(9):1401–1405.

30. Tan L, Shek K, Kamisan Atan I, et al. The repeatability of sonographic measures of functional pelvic floor anatomy. *Int Urogynecol J* 2015;26(11):1667–1672.

31. Dietz H, Zhang X, Shek K, et al. How large does a rectocele have to be to cause symptoms? A 3D/4D ultrasound study. *Int Urogynecol J* 2015;26(9):1355–1359.

32. Dietz H, Cartmill J. Imaging in patients with obstructed defecation. *Tech Coloproctol* 2013;17:473–474.

33. Dietz H, Clarke B. The prevalence of rectocele in young nulliparous women. *Aust NZ J Obstet Gynaecol* 2005;45:391–394.

34. Dietz HP, Steensma AB. The role of childbirth in the aetiology of rectocele. *Br J Obstet Gynaecol* 2006;113:264–267.

35. Young N, Atan I, Rojas R, et al. Obesity: How much does it matter for female pelvic organ prolapse? *Int Urogynecol J* 2018;29(8):1129–1134.

36. Perniola G, Shek K, Chong C, et al. Defecation proctography and translabial ultrasound in the investigation of defecatory disorders. *Ultrasound Obstet Gynecol* 2008;31:567–571.

37. Rodrigo N, Shek K, Dietz H. Rectal intussusception is associated with abnormal levator structure and morphometry. *Tech Coloproctol* 2011;15:39–43.

38. Dietz HP, Barry C, Lim YN, et al. Two-dimensional and three-dimensional ultrasound imaging of suburethral slings. *Ultrasound Obstet Gynecol* 2005;26(2):175–179.

39. Dietz H, Wilson P. The 'Iris effect': How two-dimensional and three-dimensional volume ultrasound can help us understand anti-incontinence procedures. *Ultrasound Obstet Gynecol* 2004;23(3):267–271.

40. Greenland H, Dietz H, Barry C, et al. An independent assessment of the location of the transobturator tape (Monarc) in relation to the levator ani muscle using 3 dimensional scanning techniques. *Int Urogynecol J* 2005;16(Suppl 2):S59.

41. Chantarasorn V, Shek K, Dietz H. Sonographic appearance of transobturator slings: Implications for function and dysfunction. *Int Urogynecol J* 2011;22:493–498.

42. Dietz HP, Mouritsen L, Ellis G, et al. Does it matter where you put your tape? 2002;13:S17.

43. Dietz H. Female pelvic organ prolapse—a review. *Aust Fam Physician* 2015;44(7):446–452.

44. Shek C, Rane A, Goh JTW, et al. Imaging of the Perigee transobturator mesh and its effect on stress incontinence. *Ultrasound Obstet Gynecol* 2007;30(4):446.

45. Dietz H, Erdmann M, Shek K. Mesh contraction: Myth or reality? *Am J Obstet Gynecol* 2011;204(2):173.e1–173.e4.

46. Svabik K, Martan A, Masata J, et al. Ultrasound appearances after mesh implantation—evidence of mesh contraction or folding? *Int Urogynecol J* 2011;22(5):529–533.

47. Shek K, Dietz H, Rane A. Transobturator mesh anchoring for the repair of large recurrent cystocele. *Neurourol Urodyn* 2006;26:554.

48. Rodrigo N, Wong V, Shek K, et al. The use of 3-dimensional ultrasound of the pelvic floor to predict recurrence risk after pelvic reconstructive surgery. *Aust NZ J Obstet Gynaecol* 2014;54(3):206–211.

49. Gillor M, Langer S, Dietz H. Long-term subjective, clinical and sonographic outcomes after native-tissue and mesh-augmented posterior colporrhaphy. *Int Urogynecol J* 2019;30(9):1581–1585.

50. Dietz H. Mesh in prolapse surgery: An imaging perspective. *Ultrasound Obstet Gynecol* 2012;40:495–503.

51. Dietz H, Shek K, Clarke B. Biometry of the pubovisceral muscle and levator hiatus by three-dimensional pelvic floor ultrasound. *Ultrasound Obstet Gynecol* 2005;25:580–585.

52. Shek K, Dietz H. Intrapartum risk factors of levator trauma. *Br J Obstet Gynaecol* 2010;117:1485–1492.

53. Balmforth J, Toosz-Hobson P, Cardozo L. Ask not what childbirth can do to your pelvic floor but what your pelvic floor can do in childbirth. *Neurourol Urodyn* 2003;22(5):540–542.

54. Lanzarone V, Dietz H. Three-dimensional ultrasound imaging of the levator hiatus in late pregnancy and associations with delivery outcomes. *Aust NZ J Obstet Gynaecol* 2007;47(3):176–180.

55. Kruger J, Heap S, Murphy B, et al. Evidence for the non-Euclidean nature of the plane of minimal dimensions. *Neurourol Urodyn* 2009;28(S1):675–676.

56. Dietz H, Wong V, Shek KL. A simplified method for determining hiatal biometry. *Aust NZ J Obstet Gynaecol* 2011;51:540–543.

57. Hoff Braekken I, Majida M, Ellstrom Engh M, et al. Test-retest and intra-observer repeatability of two-, three- and four-dimensional perineal ultrasound of pelvic floor muscle anatomy and function. *Int Urogynecol J Pelvic Floor Dysfunct* 2008;19:227–235.

58. Kruger J, Heap X, Murphy B, et al. Pelvic floor function in nulliparous women using three-dimensional ultrasound and magnetic resonance imaging. *Obstet Gynecol* 2008;111:631–638.

59. Dietz H, De Leon J, Shek K. Ballooning of the levator hiatus. *Ultrasound Obstet Gynecol* 2008;31:676–680.

60. Khunda A, Shek K, Dietz H. Can ballooning of the levator hiatus be determined clinically? *Am J Obstet Gynecol* 2012;206(3):246.e1–246.e4.

61. Friedman T, Eslick G, Dietz H. Risk factors for prolapse recurrence: Systematic review and meta-analysis. *Int Urogynecol J* 2018;28(1):13–21.

62. Dietz H, Gillespie A, Phadke P. Avulsion of the pubovisceral muscle associated with large vaginal tear after normal vaginal delivery at term. *Aust NZ J Obstet Gynaecol* 2007;47:341–344.

63. Dietz HP, Hyland G, Hay-Smith J. The assessment of levator trauma: A comparison between palpation and 4D pelvic floor ultrasound. *Neurourol Urodyn* 2006;25(5):424–427.

64. Dietz H, Shek K. Repeatability of digital palpation for the detection of levator trauma. *Int Urogynecol J* 2007;18(S1):S156.

65. Kruger J, Budgett S, Dietz H. Comparison between transperineal ultrasound and digital detection of levator ani trauma. Can we improve the odds? *Neurourol Urodyn* 2014;33(3):307–311.

66. Dietz HP, Shek KL. Levator defects can be detected by 2D translabial ultrasound. *Int Urogynecol J Pelvic Floor Dysfunct* 2009;20:807–811.

67. Dietz H. Quantification of major morphological abnormalities of the levator ani. *Ultrasound Obstet Gynecol* 2007;29:329–334.

68. Dietz H, Pattillo Garnham A, Guzmán Rojas R. Diagnosis of levator avulsion: Is it necessary to perform TUI on pelvic floor muscle contraction? *Ultrasound Obstet Gynecol* 2017;49:252–256.

69. Dietz H, Bernardo M, Kirby A, Shek K. Minimal criteria for the diagnosis of avulsion of the puborectalis muscle by tomographic ultrasound. *Int Urogynecol J* 2011;22(6):699–704.

70. Dietz H, Abbu A, Shek K. The levator urethral gap measurement: A more objective means of determining levator avulsion? *Ultrasound Obstet Gynecol* 2008;32:941–945.

71. Zhuang R, Song Y, Chen Q, et al. Levator avulsion using a tomographic ultrasound and magnetic resonance–based model. *Am J Obstet Gynecol* 2011;205:232.e1–232.e8.

72. Dietz HP, Low GKK. All or nothing? A second look at partial levator avulsion. *Int Urogynecol J* 2021.

73. Dietz H, Wilson P, Milsom I. Maternal birth trauma: Why should it matter to urogynaecologists? *Curr Opin Obstet Gynecol* 2016;28(5):441–448.

74. Dietz H, Habtemariam T, Williams G. Does obstructed labour in women with urogenital fistula lead to atrophy of the levator ani muscle? *J Urol* 2012;188(5):1772–1777.

75. Abdool Z, Shek K, Dietz H. The effect of levator avulsion on hiatal dimension and function. *Am J Obstet Gynecol* 2009;201:89.e1–89.e5.

76. DeLancey J, Morgan D, Fenner D, et al. Comparison of levator ani muscle defects and function in women with and without pelvic organ prolapse. *Obstet Gynecol* 2007;109(2):295–302.

77. Dietz HP, Shek C. Levator avulsion and grading of pelvic floor muscle strength. *Int Urogynecol J Pelvic Floor Dysfunct* 2008;19(5):633–636.

78. Dietz HP, Steensma AB. The prevalence of major abnormalities of the levator ani in urogynaecological patients. *BJOG* 2006;113(2):225–230.

79. Dietz H, Simpson J. Levator trauma is associated with pelvic organ prolapse. *Br J Obstet Gynaecol* 2008;115:979–984.

80. Dietz H, Kirby A, Shek K, et al. Does avulsion of the puborectalis muscle affect bladder function? *Int Urogynecol J Pelvic Floor Dysfunction* 2009;20:967–972.

81. Chantarasorn V, Shek K, Dietz H. Sonographic detection of puborectalis muscle avulsion is not associated with anal incontinence. *Aust NZ J Obstet Gynaecol* 2011;51(2):130–135.

82. Dietz HP, Shek KL. Validity and reproducibility of the digital detection of levator trauma. *Int Urogynecol J Pelvic Floor Dysfunct* 2008;19:1097–1101.

83. Dietz H. Forceps: Towards obsolescence or revival? *Acta Obstet Gynecol Scand* 2015;94(4):347–351.

84. Shek K, Chantarasorn V, Dietz H. Can levator avulsion be predicted antenatally? *Am J Obstet Gynecol* 2010;202(6):586.e1–586.e6.

85. Valsky DV, Lipschuetz M, Bord A, et al. Fetal head circumference and length of second stage of labor are risk factors for levator ani muscle injury, diagnosed by 3-dimensional transperineal ultrasound in primiparous women. *Am J Obstet Gynecol* 2009;201:91.e1–91.e7.

86. Chan S, Cheung R, Yiu A, et al. Prevalence of levator ani muscle injury in Chinese primiparous women after first delivery. *Ultrasound Obstet Gynecol* 2012;39(6):704–709.

87. Shek K, Green K, Hall J, et al. Perineal and vaginal tears are clinical markers for occult levator ani trauma: A retrospective observational study. *Ultrasound Obstet Gynecol* 2016;47(2):224–227.

88. Horak A, Guzman-Rojas R, Shek K, et al. Pelvic floor trauma: Does the second baby matter? *Int Urogynecol J* 2012;23(S2):S175–S176.

89. Kamisan Atan I, Lin S, Herbison P, et al. It is the first birth that does the damage: a cross-sectional study 20 years after delivery. *Int Urogynecol J* 2018;29(11):1637–1643.

90. Shek K, Chantarasorn V, Langer S, et al. Does levator trauma 'heal'? *Ultrasound Obstet Gynecol* 2012;40(5):570–575.

91. Kamisan Atan I, Shek K, Langer S, et al. Does the EPI-No® prevent pelvic floor trauma? A multicentre randomised controlled trial. *BJOG* 2016;123(6):995–1003.

92. Dietz H, Shek K, Daly O, et al. Can levator avulsion be repaired surgically? *Int Urogynecol J* 2013;24:1011–1015.

93. Dietz H, Korda A, Benness C, et al. Surgical reduction of the levator hiatus. *Neurourol Urodyn* 2012;31(6):872–873.

94. Turel F, Langer S, Shek K, et al. Long-term follow-up of obstetric anal sphincter injury. *Dis Colon Rectum* 2019;62(3):348–356.

95. Sultan AH. The role of anal endosonography in obstetrics. *Ultrasound Obstet Gynecol* 2003;22(6):559–560.

96. Meriwether K, Lockhart M, Meyer I, et al. Anal sphincter anatomy prepregnancy to postdelivery among the same primiparous women on dynamic magnetic resonance imaging. *Female Pelvic Med Reconstr Surg* 2019;25(1):8–14.

97. Stoker J, Rociu E, Wiersma TG, et al. Imaging of anorectal disease. *Br J Surg* 2000;87(1):10–27.

98. Peschers UM, DeLancey JO, Schaer GN, et al. Exoanal ultrasound of the anal sphincter: Normal anatomy and sphincter defects. *Br J Obstet Gynaecol* 1997;104(9):999–1003.

99. Dietz H. Exoanal imaging of the anal sphincters: A pictorial introduction. *J Ultrasound Med* 2018;37(1):263–280.

100. Turel F, Subramaniam N, Bienkiewicz J, et al. How repeatable is the assessment of external anal sphincter trauma by exoanal 4D ultrasound? *Ultrasound Obstet Gynecol* 2019;53:836–840.

101. Magpoc Mendoza J, Turel F, Atan I, et al. Normal values of anal sphincter biometry by 4-dimensional translabial ultrasound: A retrospective study of pregnant women in their third trimester. *J Ultrasound Med* 2019;38(10):2733–2738.

102. Stuart A, Ignell C, Orno A. Comparison of transperineal and endoanal ultrasound in detecting residual obstetric anal sphincter injury. *Acta Obstet Gynecol Scand* 2019;98(12):1624–1631.

103. Taithongchai A, van Gruting I, Volloyhaug I, et al. Comparing the diagnostic accuracy of 3 ultrasound modalities for diagnosing obstetric anal sphincter injuries. *Am J Obstet Gynecol* 2019;221(2):134.e1–134.e9.

104. Subramaniam N, Robledo K, Dietz H. Anal sphincter imaging: Better done at rest or on pelvic floor muscle contraction? *Int Urogynecol J* 2020;31(6):1191–1196.

105. Shek K, Guzman-Rojas R, Dietz H. Residual defects of the external anal sphincter following primary repair: An observational study using transperineal ultrasound. *Ultrasound Obstet Gynecol* 2014;44:704–709.

106. Guzman-Rojas R, Shek K, Langer S, et al. Prevalence of anal sphincter injury in primiparous women. *Ultrasound Obstet Gynecol* 2013;42(4):461–466.

107. Subramaniam N, Dietz H. What is a significant defect of the anal sphincter? *Ultrasound Obstet Gynecol* 2020;55:411–415.

108. Hill MC, Rifkin MD, Tessler FN. Ultrasound evaluation of the anal sphincter in fecal incontinence. *Ultrasound Quarterly* 1999;14(4):209–217.

109. Dietz H, Pardey J, Murray H. Maternal birth trauma should be a key performance indicator of maternity services. *Int Urogynecol J* 2015;26:29–32.

110. Andrews A, Sultan A, Thakar R, et al. Occult anal sphincter injuries—myth or reality? *BJOG* 2006;113(2):195–200.

111. Dietz HP, Shek KL. Confounders of the relationship between anal sphincter trauma and anal incontinence. Paper presented at the 46th Annual Meeting of the International Urogynecological Association, Singapore, December 8–11, 2021.

CHAPTER 15

Pelvic Floor Muscle Training With and Without Biofeedback for Urinary Incontinence and Pelvic Organ Prolapse

Kari Bø

THE FEMALE PELVIC FLOOR

The female pelvic floor consists of fascias, ligaments, and the pelvic floor muscles (PFM). The PFM form the base of the abdominal cavity on which the pelvic organs rest and where the urethra, vagina, and rectum pass through. The area surrounding the three openings of the pelvic floor in women (the levator hiatus) is the largest hernia port in the body.[1,2] The PFM comprise three layers of muscles with the different muscles having different origins, insertions, and fiber directions. There is continuous muscle activity of the PFM, except just before and during voiding and defecation.[3] If we were able to contract each muscle of the pelvic floor separately, each muscle would have a different function. However, a voluntary contraction of the PFM implies a mass contraction observed as a squeeze around the openings and a lift of the pelvic floor in a forward and inward (cranial) direction.[4] Unfortunately, several studies have found that more than 30% of women with urge incontinence (UI) are not able to contract the PFM at their first consultation, even after thorough individual instruction.[5] The most common errors are to contract other outer pelvic muscles such as hip adductor, gluteal muscles, and abdominal muscles instead of or in addition to the PFM.[5,6] In addition, Bump et al.[7] found that 25% were straining instead of performing a squeeze or inward lift of the pelvic floor. They also found that among women who were able to contract, only 49% were doing a contraction of enough intensity to influence the urethral closure pressure. To be effective in treatment of UI, it is essential that the women can perform a correct contraction and with adequate strength to make a difference.

In an intact and well-functioning pelvic floor, the connective tissue of the ligaments and facias and the PFM act together to counteract the impact of any increase in intra-abdominal pressure and ground reaction forces, keeping the pelvic organs in place with little downward movements and little or no opening of the levator hiatus area and/or the urethra.[1,2] This is an automatic function, and for women with a well-functioning pelvic floor and no symptoms, there is no need to think about voluntarily contracting the PFM.

If, for some reason, this entity is not working adequately, for example, due to inherited morphologic factors or acquired factors, pelvic floor dysfunctions may occur.[1–3] Pelvic floor dysfunctions include UI, anal incontinence, pelvic organ prolapse (POP), sensory and emptying abnormalities of the lower urinary tract, defecatory dysfunction, sexual dysfunction, and chronic pain syndromes.[2] DeLancey et al.[2] described the integrated lifespan model where they used a graphical tool to integrate pelvic floor function related to pelvic floor disorders in three major phases. These phases are development of functional reserve during an individual's growth; variations in the amount of injury and potential recovery that occur during and after vaginal birth; and deterioration occurring with advancing age. This chapter focuses on PFM training (PFMT) in treatment of stress urinary incontinence (SUI), overactive bladder (OAB) symptoms, and POP.

MECHANISM OF ACTION IN PELVIC FLOOR MUSCLE TRAINING

The PFM are the only muscles in the body with an anatomical location surrounding the levator hiatus and the three pelvic openings in women. Bø et al.[8] described a possible mechanism for how voluntary contraction of the PFM and strength training over time may positively affect PFM function and prevent and treat UI. A single voluntary contraction of the PFM increases urethral closure pressure[9]; causes simultaneous co-contraction of the urethral sphincter[10]; and reduces the levator hiatus area by 25%, from a resting area of 20 cm^2 (95% confidence interval [CI] 17 to 23) to 15 cm^2 (95% CI 13 to 17). The muscle length shortens 21%, from 12.5 cm (95% CI 11.1 to 13.8) to 9.7 cm (95% CI 8.7

to 10.7),[11] and lifts the pelvic floor higher up in the pelvis, stabilizing the pelvic floor.[8] One effective approach, known as "the Knack," is to practice precontraction/co-contraction of the PFM during situations where such contractions are needed to prevent loss of urine.[12] However, it is unknown whether this approach leads to automatic precontraction/co-contraction of the PFM during such situations.

An assessor-blinded randomized controlled trial (RCT) in 109 women with POP and comorbidities such as UI and anal incontinence found that 6 months of PFMT caused permanent morphologic improvements of the pelvic floor. These morphologic changes included elevation of the bladder neck and rectal ampulla by approximately 0.5 cm, narrowing of the hiatal area by 6%, greater muscle thickness by 16%, and reduced muscle length by 4%.[13] In that trial, there was less opening of the hiatal area and less increase in muscle length during straining in the PFMT group, which may indicate automatic function and increased PFM stiffness.[13] Moreover, several randomized trials have found that women who have trained the PFM have significantly less incontinence during running and jumping (without voluntary contraction) than controls, indicating a positive effect on automatic function.[14] Hence, there are rationales related to anatomy, biomechanics, and exercise physiology that support PFMT in the treatment of UI and POP.[8,14]

As the cause of urinary urge incontinence (UUI) in nonneurogenic patients is unknown, the rationale for PFMT in the group of patients with OAB is not as clear as for SUI. However, a voluntary contraction of the PFM has been shown to inhibit the urge to void, detrusor contraction, and urinary leakage.[15] To date, there is no knowledge about how strong this voluntary contraction needs to be to influence urethral closure pressure. It is also unknown whether PFMT over time is needed in addition to the immediate effect of the voluntary contraction during urge to void to treat UUI and other symptoms of OAB.

EVIDENCE FOR PELVIC FLOOR MUSCLE TRAINING ON URINARY INCONTINENCE IN FEMALES

Stress Urinary Incontinence/Mixed Urinary Incontinence

The National Institute for Health and Care Excellence guidelines states that PFMT is just as effective as surgery for around half of women with SUI.[16] Today, there is level 1 evidence (recommendation A) that PFMT should be first-line treatment for UI in females.[16–18] In the general population, women with SUI who do PFMT are 8 times (95% CI 4 to 19; 56% vs. 6%) more likely to be cured than control groups with no or sham treatments.[18] PFMT reduced UI episodes among women with SUI (MD [mean difference] 1.2 episodes per day,

95% CI 0.7 to 1.8) and among women with any type of UI (MD 1.0 episode per day, 95% CI 0.6 to 1.4).[18] On short pad tests, PFMT reduced the amount of urine lost by women with SUI (MD 10 g, 95% CI 1 to 19) and by women with any type of UI (MD 4 g, 95% CI 2 to 5).[18] PFMT also caused women with any type of UI to report significantly better incontinence-related quality of life and reduced UI symptoms than those who did not receive the treatment. Because of substantial heterogeneity among the outcome measures used to assess quality of life, a meta-analysis of this variable was not conducted. PFMT has rare and minor adverse effects.[16–18]

The effects of PFMT are better if it is delivered with regular supervised training (e.g., once a week).[19] Supervised training is defined as a PFMT program taught and monitored by a health professional/clinician/instructor.[20] This means that the physiotherapist teaches each PFM contraction either individually or in a group setting. Thus, if the physiotherapist only provides teaching and assessment at the first consultation, this would not be considered supervised training.[20]

Overactive Bladder

The Cochrane reviews have concluded that PFMT is consistently more effective in women with SUI only than in women with mixed urinary incontinence (MUI) and UUI.[18,19] A recent systematic review of the effects of PFMT in women with only OAB symptoms (including UUI) included 11 randomized trials.[15] The heterogeneity of outcome measures and intervention protocols was substantial, and a meta-analysis of the included studies was not conducted. Approximately half of the studies showed a positive effect of PFMT and half of them did not.[15] Most of the study protocols included regular strength training of the PFM similar to PFMT protocols used for SUI, whereas three of the protocols also included training of a voluntary contraction to inhibit urge to void and detrusor contraction. In a recent clinical trial, Miller et al.[12] randomized 108 women with SUI and MUI to a 15-minute slide show including either a Knack tutorial on how to contract the PFM to inhibit urgency and to contract before and during increase in intra-abdominal pressure or a video containing good diet and exercise advice. Significant improvement was reported by 71% in the Knack tutorial group compared to 25% in the diet/exercise advice group (P < .001). Self-perceived improvement was 21% to 22% higher in the Knack tutorial group (P < .001).

Pelvic Floor Muscle Training in Prevention of Urge Incontinence

In randomized trials involving women with and without UI during pregnancy, PFMT produced a 26% reduced risk (RR [risk ratio] 0.74, 95% CI 0.61 to 0.90) of UI during pregnancy and the mid-postnatal period (RR 0.73, 95% CI 0.55 to 0.97).[21] Moreover, pregnant continent women who exercise the PFM during pregnancy (primary prevention) are 62% less likely (RR for incontinence 0.38, 95% CI 0.20 to 0.72) to experience UI in late pregnancy and have 29% lower risk (RR 0.71, 95% CI 0.54 to 0.95) of UI 3 to 6 months after giving birth.[21]

To date, there is insufficient evidence for a long-term effect of antenatal PFMT beyond 6 to 12 months postpartum.[21] However, long-term studies of any health care intervention are generally difficult to conduct due to loss to follow-up, the ethical demand to offer the control group the active intervention in a reasonable time frame, co-interventions, and competing and recurrent events in the follow-up period.[22,23] This is especially challenging in the peripartum period because many women become pregnant again during the follow-up period.[22]

Evidence for Adding Biofeedback to Pelvic Floor Muscle Training

Biofeedback has been defined as "a group of experimental procedures where an external sensor is used to give an indication on bodily processes, usually in the purpose of changing the measured quality."[24] Biofeedback equipment has been developed within the area of psychology, mainly to measure sweating, heart rate, and blood pressure during different forms of stress. Kegel[4] always based his training protocol on thorough instruction of correct contraction using vaginal palpation and clinical observation. In addition, he combined PFMT with use of a manometer measuring vaginal squeeze pressure as biofeedback during exercise. Today, a variety of biofeedback apparatus are commonly used in clinical practice to assist with PFMT. Moreover, ability to contract the PFM is usually assessed and confirmed by the physiotherapist using one or more assessment methods.

Unfortunately, the term *biofeedback* is often used to classify a method different from PFMT. However, biofeedback is not a treatment by its own. It is an adjunct to training, measuring the response from a single PFM contraction. In the area of PFMT, both vaginal and anal surface electromyography, and urethral and vaginal squeeze pressure measurements have been used to make patients more aware of muscle function and to enhance and motivate patients' effort during training.[25] However, one should be aware that erroneous attempts at PFM contractions (e.g., by straining) may be registered by manometers and dynamometers, and contractions of other muscles than the PFM may affect surface electromyography activity. Therefore, biofeedback other than imaging methods (ultrasound and magnetic resonance imaging) cannot be used to register a correct contraction.

Several RCTs have shown that PFMT without biofeedback is more effective than no treatment for SUI.[16–18] In a Cochrane review, Herderschee et al.[25] found 24 RCTs or quasi-randomized trials comparing PFMT with and without biofeedback. They concluded that use of biofeedback may provide benefit in addition to PFMT. However, none of the studies comparing PFMT with and without biofeedback have used the exact same training dosage in the two groups.[25] When the two groups under comparison receive different dosage of training in addition to biofeedback, it is impossible to conclude what is causing a possible effect. In a recent study, Hagen et al.[26] randomized 600 women with SUI and MUI to the same training dosage and attention of either PFMT with or without use of biofeedback (16 weeks of 6 individual visits + home training). They reported results after 6 months, 1 year, and 2 years. No difference between groups were found in International Consultation on Incontinence Questionnaire UI Short Form scores; participants reported improvement on Oxford grading of PFM strength. Similar percentage had received surgery (12.3% biofeedback, 9.3% PFMT) and an adherence of about 50% to PFMT at 2-year follow-up was reported for both groups. The researchers concluded that use of biofeedback was therefore not cost-effective.

Because PFMT is effective without biofeedback, a large sample size may be needed to show any beneficial effect of adding biofeedback to an effective training protocol. In most published studies comparing PFMT with PFMT combined with biofeedback, the sample sizes are small, and type II error may have been the reason for negative findings.[25] However, in the largest RCTs published, no additional effect was demonstrated from adding biofeedback.[26]

Many women may not like to undress, go to a private room, and insert a vaginal or rectal device to exercise the PFM.[24] On the other hand, some women may find it motivating to use biofeedback to control and enhance the strength of the contractions when training. Any factor that may stimulate high adherence and intensive training should be recommended to enhance the effect of a training program. Therefore, when available, biofeedback can be given as an option for home training, and the physical therapist should use any sensitive, reliable, and valid tool to measure the contraction force at office follow-up.

Long-term Effect

As for any exercise intervention, it is expected that the benefits gained from PFMT need maintenance training for continuing effects.[23,27] A systematic review on the long-term effects of PFMT included 19 studies with follow-up periods of 1 to 15 years; long-term adherence to PFMT varied between 10% and 70%.[22] Among participants who were treated with PFMT and whose UI resolved initially, 5 studies reported sustained success rates (i.e., percentage remaining free of UI at long-term follow-up), which were between 41% and 85%. Surgery rates in the long term varied between 5% and 58%. It was concluded that the short-term benefit of PFMT can be maintained at long-term follow-up without incentives for continued training, although there was high heterogeneity in both interventional and methodologic quality in short-term and long-term PFMT studies.[22]

Group Pelvic Floor Muscle Training

The first RCT assessing the effect of group training of the PFM came from Norway in 1990.[14] Only women with urodynamically proven SUI were included in the study. All women received the same teaching about how to perform a correct PFM contraction, and ability to contract was assessed by visual observation and vaginal palpation. Vaginal resting pressure, PFM strength (maximal voluntary contraction), and endurance were measured by a vaginal manometer (high-precision microtip pressure transducer connected to a vaginal balloon) before randomization.[14]

For the PFMT protocols, both groups were asked to do 3 sets of 8 to 12 contractions per day at home and had follow-up appointments once a month for 6 months with a trained physiotherapist for measurement of PFM variables. In addition to this protocol, the "intensive training group" attended a 1-hour group PFM exercise class once a week. It is worthwhile noting that what was named the "home training group" in this study had more individual visits with a physiotherapist than the intervention group in many other studies (i.e., 7 visits with assessment of PFM variables and motivation for training).[16–18] The participants who received the additional group training improved their PFM strength from a mean 7 (95% CI 4 to 10) to 23 cm H_2O (95% CI 18 to 27), significantly more than the "home training" participants, who improved from a mean of 8 (95% CI 6 to 10) to 15 cm H_2O (95% CI 12 to 19). A pad test with standardized bladder volume including provocative jumping, running, and sit-ups showed that the participants who received the additional group training improved their UI from a mean of 27 (95% CI 9 to 45) to 7 g (95% CI 1 to 13), again significantly better than the home training participants, who improved from a mean of 29 (95% CI 14 to 44) to 22 g (95% CI 9 to 35). The participants who received the additional group training gained further significant benefits: Fewer still had urodynamically proven SUI after treatment, and 60% (vs. 17% in the home training group) reported that they were cured or almost cured, RR 3.53 (CI 1.49 to 8.36).[14] Secondary analyses of those with or without successful outcomes after PFMT found that moderate PFM strength before starting the training was one of four important factors for success.[14] Furthermore, PFM

strength development during the exercise period and maximal strength after treatment each correlated with the reduction in UI.[28]

The PFMT protocol used in the successful arm of that trial (i.e., weekly group training + daily home exercise) has since been used in several controlled trials in Norway with significant effect.[14] Statistically significant benefits have also been found in men following the same group training concept.[14] Surprisingly, one RCT that investigated exactly the same exercise protocol did not find any significant benefits over control in a group exercising from 6 to 8 weeks postpartum to 6 months postpartum.[29] However, this trial specifically aimed at recruiting women with major levator ani defects, and the participating women may therefore not be comparable to women participating in other postpartum studies.

Group versus Individual Pelvic Floor Muscle Training

A Cochrane review[19] concluded that 90% of those who had combined group and individual supervision reported improvement versus 57% of women receiving individual supervision only (RR for no improvement 0.29, 95% CI 0.15 to 0.55). This meta-analysis was based on only three randomized trials, and although the CI was wide, the effect is strong enough to be clearly worthwhile. Because there were differences in health professional contact in those receiving the additional group training and the other PFMT group, it is impossible to separate the effect of the actual additional group training from the extra attention. The Cochrane review[19] found that PFMT was consistently more effective in those receiving more health professional contact. However, attention alone is unlikely to affect UI. In an assessor-blinded randomized trial, Dumoulin et al.[30] compared three different interventions: PFMT and electrical stimulation; PFMT, electrical stimulation, and transverse abdominal training; and the same attention and time spent with a physiotherapist giving them limb massage. The massage group did not show any improvement in any measures of UI but did improve in disease-specific quality of life.

In a recent systematic review comparing the effect of individual and group PFMT, 10 studies involving group training were included.[31] Five of six randomized trials comparing group PFMT with individual PFMT were included in a meta-analysis. The authors found significant risk of bias in many of the studies: random sequence generation, allocation concealment, and blinding of outcome assessment. The conclusion was that there was no significant difference in results between individual and group-based PFMT. There was a huge heterogeneity in outcome measures and exercise protocols between studies, but a more serious bias was the difference in supervision and content of the intervention between the individual and group training protocols within the same study.

In a well-designed, adequately powered, noninferiority, multicenter randomized trial involving women with SUI and MUI, individual PFMT was compared to group training.[32] Both treatment arms contained the same dosage of training and the same contact and attention from the physiotherapist. Furthermore, both groups received the same individual information and underwent assessment and feedback of their ability to contract the PFM before commencing the training period. At 1-year follow-up, the median reduction in the frequency of leakage episodes per week was similar: 70% (95% CI 44 to 89) in the individual group and 74% (95% CI 46 to 86) in the group training group. Furthermore, there were no important differences between the groups in any other outcome measures, and the researchers concluded that group PFMT is not inferior to individual training in treatment of female UI.

Most group training regimens of PFMT include individual teaching of a correct contraction and assessment and feedback of ability to contract.[31] However, in a few studies, group training has been done without such confirmation of the participants' skills. Nevertheless, all these studies found significant improvement in UI after the intervention and no difference between individual or group training.

In a primary prevention study, 169 first-time pregnant women were randomized to either an exercise group including PFMT three times a week or a control group without any intervention.[33] The participants had no evaluation of their ability to perform a correct contraction. The results showed significant differences in incidence, frequency, and amount of UI in favor of the exercise group, accompanied by a benefit on an incontinence-related quality-of-life score with an effect size of 0.8. The results were presented as per protocol analyses only, but it shows that it is possible to do effective PFMT without individual teaching and control of ability to perform a correct contraction in a group of women with no symptoms and injuries to the PFM. However, we do not know whether the effect would have been even higher with additional individual teaching and control of the women's ability to perform a correct contraction.

To perform a correct PFM contraction can be a special challenge after childbirth. Vermandel et al.[34] studied 958 women (mean age 30, SD [standard deviation] 5) within 1 week postpartum. They asked about experience and knowledge of PFMT using a questionnaire and assessed ability to perform a correct PFM contraction by visual observation of the perineum during contraction attempts. Within the study cohort, 26% had no knowledge of the pelvic floor, 52% had trained the PFM, 52% were unable to contract their PFM, 29% showed no movement at all, and 24% showed some movement but no inward displacement. Among those who had trained the PFM and were convinced they were able to contract their

PFM correctly, 45% were not. However, after verbal instructions by a physiotherapist, 74% improved their PFM contraction.

In a Norwegian cohort study of primiparous women PFM strength and endurance were reduced by more than 50% after vaginal birth, with significantly greater deficits for women with instrumental delivery.[35] Primiparous postpartum women with major PFM injuries diagnosed by ultrasound had 47% weaker PFM than those without injury (MD 8 cm H_2O, 95% CI 5 to 10).[36]

EVIDENCE FOR PELVIC FLOOR MUSCLE TRAINING FOR PELVIC ORGAN PROLAPSE

The International Consensus on Incontinence has concluded that there is level 1, recommendation A for PFMT to treat POP and that PFMT should be first-line treatment for POP together with lifestyle interventions.[17] PFMT significantly improved POP symptoms in all trials and/or prolapse stage (anatomical POP) in some studies. All PFMT studies on POP have been conducted after thorough assessment of ability to perform a correct contraction, most with supervised training and all have so far been conducted as individual training.

Morphologic Changes

The RCTs evaluating the effect of PFMT on anatomical POP typically lift the prolapse one stage only.[13] In an RCT comparing 6 months of PFMT with a control group only receiving lifestyle advice including learning the Knack (precontraction of the PFM before increase in intra-abdominal pressure), Braekken et al.[13] found morphologic changes of the pelvic floor only after PFMT. There was a statistically significant increase in thickness of the PFM, elevation of the bladder neck and rectal ampulla, and decrease of the levator hiatus area and length of the PFM compared to the control group. This indicates that PFMT may positively influence anatomical risk factors for POP which may be used as a theoretical rationale for prevention of the condition.

Long-term Effect

McClurg et al.[37] did an 8- to 10-year follow-up of the Scottish branch of their PFMT study and found that, based on hospital data, a significantly lower proportion of the intervention group (43.6%) had received treatment than the control group (52.8%). So far, this is the only long-term follow-up study of PFMT on POP. Again, long-term follow-up studies are challenging because usually women in the control group of the original studies are invited to do PFMT after cessation of the trial and long-term effect most likely need adherence to maintenance training.

Prevention

Obviously, preventing POP to occur would be the best "cure" for POP. Theoretically, this could be achieved with lifestyle adjustments (e.g., avoid obesity and straining on stool and precontract the PFM with increases in intra-abdominal pressure if the person has PFM weakness) and PFMT. However, to study the preventive effect of PFMT on POP, ideally, a group of women at young age and with no POP should be randomized to PFMT or no training and followed for a long period of time to conclude whether POP can be prevented. However, such a trial seems impossible, and to date, there are no RCTs or studies using other designs reporting on primary prevention (to stop prolapse from developing). In a secondary prevention study, Hagen et al.[38] included 407 women (mean age 46.6 years, SD 4.6, median parity 2 (1 to 11), with Pelvic Organ Prolapse Quantification System stages I to III who had not sought treatment for POP, in a 2-year follow-up study. The women were randomized to either lifestyle advice leaflet or five appointments with a physiotherapist over 16 weeks + two 6-week blocks of once-a-week Pilates classes including specific PFMT. They reported a statistically significant, but small, reduction in POP symptoms in the exercise group compared with the control group.

PFMT in Conjunction with POP Surgery

Somewhat counterintuitively to the results earlier, most studies fail to find any effect of adding PFMT to POP surgery.[17] In a small feasibility study, McClurg et al.[39] found benefits in the intervention group who had received one preoperative and six postoperative PFMT sessions over the control group with usual care after surgery in terms of fewer prolapse symptoms at 12 months (mean difference 3.94; 95% CI 1.35 to 6.75; $t = 3.24$, $P = .006$). However, they concluded that the results of the pilot study must be viewed with caution due to a possible selection bias in favor of the PFMT group.

CONCLUSION

There is evidence from RCT and systematic reviews (including meta-analysis) that PFMT is effective in treatment of SUI and MUI in females. The effect is better following supervised training and more effective in women with SUI only. It is possible to maintain continence after cessation of supervised training, but this most likely needs maintenance training. Following individual assessment and feedback of ability to contract, group training is not inferior to individual training and group training is cost-effective. There is evidence to recommend PFMT as primary and secondary prevention of UI during pregnancy and as treatment in the early postpartum period, but long-term effect is not known over 6 months postpartum. There is an urgent need for robust and larger RCTs with high methodologic and interventional quality in the postpartum period. The effect of PFMT on OAB symptoms is contradictive and needs further investigations. A significant effect of PFMT on POP symptoms in women with stage I to III prolapse has been shown in several RCTs, and there is now level 1, recommendation A that PFMT should be first-line treatment of POP. A prerequisite for effect of PFMT in prevention and treatment of any condition is proper teaching and control of ability to perform a correct contraction and supervised training over time.

References

1. Ashton-Miller J, DeLancey JOL. Functional anatomy of the female pelvic floor. In: Bø K, Berghmans B, Mørkved S, et al, eds. *Evidence-based physical therapy for the pelvic floor. Bridging science and clinical practice*, 2nd ed. United Kingdom: Elsevier, 2014:19–34.
2. DeLancey JOL, Low LK, Miller JM, et al. Graphic integration of causal factors of pelvic floor disorders: An integrated life span model. *Am J Obstet Gynecol* 2008;199(6):610.e1–610.e5.
3. Vodušek D. Neuroanatomy and neurophysiology of pelvic floor muscles. In: Bø K, Berghmans B, Mørkved S, et al, eds. *Evidence-based physical therapy for the pelvic floor. Bridging science and clinical practice*, 2nd ed. United Kingdom: Elsevier, 2014:35–42.
4. Kegel AH. Stress incontinence and genital relaxation; a nonsurgical method of increasing the tone of sphincters and their supporting structures. *Ciba Clin Symp* 1952;42(2):35–51.
5. Bø K, Mørkved S. Motor learning. In: Bø K, Berghmans B, Mørkved S, et al, eds. *Evidence-based physical therapy for the pelvic floor. Bridging science and clinical practice*, 2nd ed. United Kingdom: Elsevier, 2014:111–117.
6. Neels H, De Wachter S, Wyndaele JJ, et al. Common errors made in attempt to contract the pelvic floor muscles in women early after delivery: A prospective observational study. *Eur J Obstet Gynecol Reprod Biol* 2018;220:113–117.
7. Bump R, Hurt WG, Fantl JA, et al. Assessment of Kegel exercise performance after brief verbal instruction. *Am J Obstet Gynecol* 1991;165(2):322–329.
8. Bø K. Pelvic floor muscle training is effective in treatment of stress urinary incontinence, but how does it work? *Int Urogynecol J Pelvic Floor Dysfunct* 2004;15(2):76–84.
9. Zubieta M, Carr RL, Drake MJ, et al. Influence of voluntary pelvic floor muscle contraction and pelvic floor muscle training on urethral closure pressures: A systematic review. *Int Urogynecol J* 2016;27(5):687–696.
10. Bø K, Stien R. Needle EMG registration of striated urethral wall and pelvic floor muscle activity patterns during cough, Valsalva, abdominal, hip adductor and gluteal muscle contractions in nulliparous healthy females. *Neurourol Urodyn* 1994;13(1):35–41.
11. Braekken IH, Majida M, Engh ME, et al. Test-retest reliability of pelvic floor muscle contraction measured by 4D ultrasound. *Neurourol Urodyn* 2009;28(1):68–73.
12. Miller JM, Hawthorne KM, Park L, et al. Self-perceived improvement in bladder health after viewing a novel tutorial on knack use: A randomized controlled trial pilot study. *J Womens Health (Larchmt)* 2020;29(10):1319–1327.

13. Braekken IH, Majida M, Engh ME, et al. Morphological changes after pelvic floor muscle training measured by 3-dimensional ultrasonography: A randomized controlled trial. *Obstet Gynecol* 2010;115(2 Pt 1):317–324.

14. Bø K. Physiotherapy management of female urinary incontinence. *J Physiother* 2020;66(3):147–154.

15. Bø K, Fernandes ACNL, Duarte TB, et al. Is pelvic floor muscle training effective for symptoms of overactive bladder in women? A systematic review. *Physiotherapy* 2020;106:65–76.

16. National Institute for Health and Care Excellence. NICE guideline. Urinary incontinence and pelvic organ prolapse in women: Management [NG123]. National Institute for Health and Care Excellence. Published April 2, 2019. Updated June 24, 2019. https://www.nice.org.uk/guidance/ng123

17. Dumoulin C, Adewuyi T, Booth J, et al. Adult conservative management. In: Abrams P, Cardozo L, Wagg A, et al, eds. *Incontinence*, 6th ed. United Kingdom: International Incontinence Society, 2017:1443–1628.

18. Dumoulin C, Cacciari LP, Hay-Smith EJC. Pelvic floor muscle training versus no treatment, or inactive control treatments, for urinary incontinence in women. *Cochrane Database Syst Rev* 2018;10(10):CD005654.

19. Hay-Smith EJC, Herderschee R, Dumoulin C, et al. Comparisons of approaches to pelvic floor muscle training for urinary incontinence in women. *Cochrane Database Syst Rev* 2011;(12):CD009508.

20. Bø K, Frawley HC, Haylen BT, et al. An International Urogynecological Association (IUGA)/International Continence Society (ICS) joint report on the terminology for the conservative and nonpharmacological management of female pelvic floor dysfunction. *Int Urogynecol J* 2017;28(2):191–213.

21. Woodley SJ, Boyle R, Cody JD, et al. Pelvic floor muscle training for prevention and treatment of urinary and faecal incontinence in antenatal and postnatal women. *Cochrane Database Syst Rev* 2017;12(12):CD007471.

22. Bø K, Hilde G. Does it work in the long term? A systematic review on pelvic floor muscle training for female stress urinary incontinence. *Neurourol Urodyn* 2013;32(3):215–223.

23. Herbert RD, Kasza J, Bø K. Analysis of randomised trials with long-term follow-up. *BMC Med Res Methodol* 2018;18:48.

24. Bø K. Pelvic floor muscle training for SUI. In: Bø K, Berghmans B, Mørkved S, et al, eds. *Evidence-based physical therapy for the pelvic floor. Bridging science and clinical practice*, 2nd ed. United Kingdom: Elsevier, 2015:162–178.

25. Herderschee R, Hay-Smith EJC, Herbison GP, et al. Feedback or biofeedback to augment pelvic floor muscle training for urinary incontinence in women. *Cochrane Database Syst Rev* 2011;(7):CD009252.

26. Hagen S, Elders A, Henderson L, et al. Effectiveness and cost-effectiveness of biofeedback-assisted pelvic floor muscle training for female urinary incontinence: A multicenter randomized controlled trial. International Continence Society. http://www.ics.org/2019/abstract/489

27. Garber CE, Blissmer B, Deschenes MR, et al. Quantity and quality of exercise for developing and maintaining cardiorespiratory, musculoskeletal, and neuromotor fitness in apparently healthy adults: Guidance for prescribing exercise. American College of Sports Medicine (ACSM) Position Stand. *Med Sci Sports Exerc* 2011;43(7):1334–1359.

28. Hilde G, Staer-Jensen JS, Siafarikas F, et al. Postpartum pelvic floor muscle training and urinary incontinence: A randomized controlled trial. *Obstet Gynecol* 2013;122(6):1231–1238.

29. Bø K. Pelvic floor muscle strength and response to pelvic floor muscle training for stress urinary incontinence. *Neurourol Urodyn* 2003;22(7):654–658.

30. Dumoulin C, Lemieux MC, Bourbonnais D, et al. Physiotherapy for persistent postnatal stress urinary incontinence: A randomized controlled trial. *Obstet Gynecol* 2004;104(3):504–510.

31. Paiva LL, Ferla L, Darski C, et al. Pelvic floor muscle training in groups versus individual or home treatment of women with urinary incontinence: Systematic review and meta-analysis. *Int Urogynecol J* 2017;28(3):351–359.

32. Dumoulin C, Morin M, Danieli C, et al. Group-based vs individual pelvic floor muscle training to treat urinary incontinence in older women: A randomized clinical trial. *JAMA Intern Med* 2020;180(10):1284–1293.

33. Pelaez M, Gonzalez-Cerron S, Montejo R, et al. Pelvic floor muscle training included in a pregnancy exercise program is effective in primary prevention of urinary incontinence: A randomized controlled trial. *Neurourol Urodyn* 2014;33(1):67–71.

34. Vermandel A, De Wachter S, Beyltjens T, et al. Pelvic floor awareness and the positive effect of verbal instructions in 958 women early postdelivery. *Int Urogynecol J* 2015;26(2):223–228.

35. Hilde G, Stær-Jensen J, Siafarikas F, et al. Impact of childbirth and mode of delivery on vaginal resting pressure and on pelvic floor muscle strength and endurance. *Am J Obstet Gynecol* 2013;208(1):50.e1–50.e7.

36. Hilde G, Staer-Jensen J, Siafarikas F, et al. How well can pelvic floor muscles with major defects contract? A cross-sectional comparative study 6 weeks after delivery using transperineal 3D/4D ultrasound and manometer. *BJOG* 2013;120(11):1423–1429.

37. McClurg D, Hagen S, Berry K, et al. A 10 year data-linkage follow-up study of trial of pelvic floor muscle training for prolapse. International Continence Society. http://www.ics.org/2019/abstract/491

38. Hagen S, Glazener C, McClurg D, et al. Pelvic floor muscle training for secondary prevention of pelvic organ prolapse (PREVPROL): A multicentre randomized controlled trial. *Lancet* 2017;389(10067):393–402.

39. McClurg D, Hilton P, Dolan L, et al. Pelvic floor muscle training as an adjunct to prolapse surgery: A randomised feasibility study. *Int Urogynecol J* 2014;25(7):883–891.

NONSURGICAL MANAGEMENT OF STRESS URINARY INCONTINENCE AND PELVIC ORGAN PROLAPSE: USE OF THE PESSARY

Isuzu Meyer

Introduction

Pelvic floor disorders, such as pelvic organ prolapse (POP), urinary, and fecal incontinence, are highly prevalent and bothersome conditions. One in 4 women report symptoms of at least one of the pelvic floor disorders in the United States.[1] The prevalence of pelvic floor disorders increases with age; 40% in women aged 60 to 79 years and 53% ages 80 years or older suffer from at least one symptomatic disorder.[1] With the rapidly growing aging population (women ages 65 years or older) predicted to double by 2050,[2] it is inevitable that the prevalence and burden of pelvic floor disorders will continue to increase. This chapter focuses on nonsurgical management of stress urinary incontinence (SUI) and POP with pessaries. The epidemiology, pathophysiology, and evaluation of pelvic floor disorders are discussed in separate chapters.

GENERAL PRINCIPLES

For women who desire nonsurgical management of pelvic floor disorders, pessaries can provide symptomatic relief. Of the pelvic floor disorders, pessaries are indicated for POP and urinary incontinence (specifically SUI) as they provide structural support. Particularly for SUI, pessaries have been shown to increase urethral closure pressure and reduce vaginal Q-tip angle on Valsalva.[3-5] Additionally, the treatment of the stress component can sometimes improve urgency associated urinary incontinence symptoms.

Once determined that the patient is symptomatic and desires treatment, counseling and active patient participation in decision making is essential for treatment success. Although surgery is considered definitive management, nonsurgical options, such as pessaries, are not a "secondary" option. Patient counseling on pessaries should include the following:

- Patient selection, indications, and contraindications
- Establishing goals and expectations
- Alternative treatment options
- Proper fitting techniques (not "one-size fits all")
- Education for management and pessary care instructions

PATIENT SELECTION

It is important to determine whether the patient is a good candidate for pessary use by considering indications and contraindications of pessaries.

Indications include the following:

- Symptomatic POP and/or SUI and desire treatment
- Prefer nonsurgical management
- A poor surgical candidate
- Need to delay surgery
- Pregnancy—current or the desire for future fertility, especially there is a paucity of data on the subsequent childbirth following incontinence or prolapse surgery

Contraindications include the following:

- Nonadherence to pessary self-care or unable to follow up
- Active infection in the pelvis
- Foreign body exposure such as synthetic graft

Other Considerations

Women can choose to wear a pessary either at all times or in certain situations (during exercise, rigorous activities, etc.). Furthermore, pessaries can be used for diagnostic purposes which include the following:

- To determine whether urinary retention is associated with advanced prolapse (obstructive voiding) during urodynamic evaluation

  Up to 94% of women with an advanced stage cystocele had the resolution of obstructive voiding on urodynamics evaluation with pessary insertion.[6]

For surgical planning, prolapse reduction by pessary demonstrated positive predictive value of 94% and negative predictive value of 67% in predicting postoperative resolution of urinary retention in patients with cystocele.[7]

- To perform a reduction stress test using pessary

Pessaries can be used to assess occult SUI or de novo SUI after prolapse surgery. However, pessary stress testing may be less predictive for occult SUI compared to using other tools, such as cotton swab, a speculum blade, or ring forceps, because a pessary may provide pelvic floor support and prevent leakage.

ESTABLISHING GOALS AND EXPECTATIONS

Patient acceptance highly depends on appropriate counseling. Based on the current literature, there is a wide range of patient acceptance and duration of pessary use, which declines over time. A prospective study of women with symptomatic POP reported 46% chose pessary compared to 53% surgery.[8] Patient factors associated with declining pessary include younger age (younger than 65 years), lesser degree of prolapse, and concurrent urinary incontinence symptoms.[9] Among those who elected for pessary trial, the rate of successful fitting ranges between 74% and 97%.[10–12] Factors associated with declining pessary trial versus unsuccessful fitting can overlap (Table 16.1). There is conflicting data regarding the association between specific vaginal dimensions and successful pessary fitting. Whereas some studies demonstrated shorter vaginal length, wider

TABLE 16.1
Factors Associated with Unsuccessful Fitting or Declining Pessary
PATIENT CHARACTERISTICS
• Younger age (65 years or younger)
• Obesity
• Sexually active
• Prior pelvic surgery
PELVIC FLOOR DISORDER SYMPTOMS
• POP with concurrent urinary incontinence
• Advanced posterior prolapse associated with incomplete bowel evacuation, needing to splint
ANATOMY
• Short vaginal length (<7–8 cm)
• Wide vaginal introitus (>4 fingerbreadths)

TABLE 16.2
Factors Associated with Discontinuation of Pessary after Successful Fitting
PATIENT FACTORS
• Sexually active
• Prior vaginal reconstructive surgery (*less likely* to discontinue once successfully fit)
• Advanced posterior predominant prolapse
• Presence of surgical scarring (difficult insertion and retention of pessary)
• Inconvenience, social reasons
PESSARY FACTORS
• Space filling type
• Discomfort
• Increased vaginal discharge
• Retained pessary

introitus, and prior hysterectomy as predictors for unsuccessful fitting, others found no such association.[13,14]

Once successfully fit, those who elect not to continue with pessaries will typically do so within the first few weeks of fitting.[15] Short-term continuation rate (within 6 month) ranges 60% to 92%,[8,16,17] midterm continuation (1 to 3 years) ranges 33% to 80%[9,11,12,18–21]; however, the long-term use (longer than 10 years) declines to less than 15%, although very little prospective data exists.[22] The wide range of continuation rates are likely due to the differences in study design (observational vs. clinical trial) as well as patient characteristics (age, prior surgery, the type[s] of pelvic floor disorders present). Factors associated with discontinuation of pessary after successful fitting are noted in Table 16.2.

In addition to symptomatic improvements achieved with pessary use, some studies have demonstrated anatomic changes (regression of prolapse) with pessary use. Reported anatomic changes include reduction in genital hiatus (4.8 ± 1.6 to 3.9 ± 1.1 cm, $P < .001$) after 3 months of pessary use,[23] and a decrease in prolapse stage assessed by the Pelvic Organ Prolapse Quantification system was seen in 25% of patients after 1 year of pessary use.[18] Hydronephrosis can be present in up to 30% of women with prolapse.[24,25] One study demonstrated that successful pessary use of 1 to 3 months resulted in improvement or resolution of hydronephrosis on ultrasound in 77% of women with advanced prolapse.[25]

ALTERNATIVE TREATMENT OPTIONS

Patient counseling should include the discussion of alternative treatment options to pessaries.

Supervised Pelvic Floor Muscle Training versus Pessary

Stress urinary incontinence

A randomized controlled trial[26] demonstrated that women with SUI have greater symptomatic improvement with supervised pelvic floor muscle training plus pessary compared to pessary use alone during the initial 3 months (much better or very much better on the patient Global Impression of Improvement[27]; pessary = 40% vs. combined pessary and pelvic floor muscle training = 49%, P = .006) and satisfaction (on the Patient Satisfaction Questionnaire[28]; pessary = 63% vs. combined = 75%, P = .003); however, differences in improvement and satisfaction were no longer significant at 12 months.[26]

Pelvic organ prolapse

Comparing pessary use versus supervised pelvic floor muscle training in a randomized controlled trial of women with prolapse beyond the hymen, no intergroup difference was noted in overall symptom severity at 24 months, measured by total Pelvic Floor Disorder Inventory-20 (PFDI-20) scores (−3.7 points, 95% confidence interval [CI] −12.8 to 5.3, via intention to treat). However, the pessary group had greater POP-specific symptomatic improvement measured by the Pelvic Oregon Prolapse Distress Inventory 6 (−3.2 points, 95% CI −6.3 to 0.0) over 24 months. Notably, the rate of successful pessary fitting was 57% in this trial.[29] Another randomized trial compared pelvic floor muscle training alone versus pessary plus pelvic floor muscle training in women with symptomatic stage I to III POP. At 12 months, improvement in POP symptoms (measured by the PFDI-20) and impact on quality of life (measured by the Pelvic Floor Impact Questionnaire) was shown to be greater in those with pessary use in combination with pelvic floor muscle training, compared to the pelvic floor muscle exercises alone.[30]

Surgery

Current evidence is somewhat conflicting regarding symptomatic improvement comparing outcomes of pessary versus surgery. Women with stage II to IV POP had symptomatic improvement either with pessary or reconstructive surgery; however, greater improvement at 12 months was observed with surgery measured by the PFDI,[31,32] whereas others reported no difference in symptom severity or impact on quality of life measured by International Consultation on Incontinence (ICIQ) whether undergoing surgery or pessary at 12 months.[8]

PROPER FITTING TECHNIQUES (NOT "ONE SIZE FITS ALL")

Successful fitting includes proper preparation/positioning, examination, selection of appropriate pessary (type/size), insertion techniques, and care instructions.

Preparation and Positioning

1. Empty bladder and assess postvoid residual volume and urinalysis if warranted to exclude urinary retention and urinary tract infection, respectively.
2. Typical position is the dorsal lithotomy position. However, in women with limited range of motion or lower extremity weakness unable to sustain the position in stir-ups, alternative positioning such as "frog-leg" position may be necessary.

Pelvic Examination

Bimanual and speculum examination should be performed to exclude mass, lesion, foreign body, or any other conditions or findings that preclude pessary fitting. Tissue quality should be also examined. The size of the vaginal canal (length, width, introitus size) is assessed to determine appropriate pessary size and type. Vaginal width is determined by the number of fingerbreadths across the vagina canal (Fig. 16.1), also at the introitus; and length is

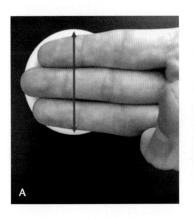
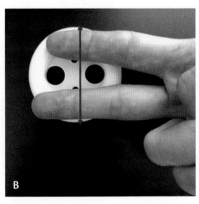

FIGURE 16.1 The size (width) is determined by the number of fingerbreadths across the vaginal canal (**A**) (or between two fingers [**B**]).

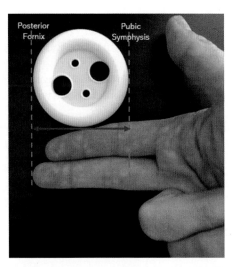

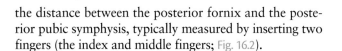

FIGURE 16.2 The size (length) is determined by the distance between the posterior fornix and the posterior pubic symphysis.

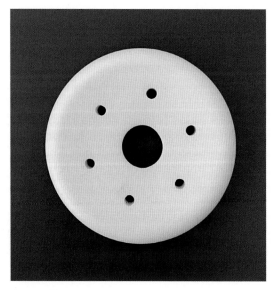

FIGURE 16.4 Shaatz pessary.

the distance between the posterior fornix and the posterior pubic symphysis, typically measured by inserting two fingers (the index and middle fingers; Fig. 16.2).

Selection of Appropriate Pessary (Type, Size)

Most pessaries are made of silicone, nonallergenic, durable, and autoclavable, except for Inflatoballs which contain latex.

Types

The type of pessary is chosen based on examination, indications (POP, SUI, or both), patient preference, and ability for pessary care (self-care vs. removal and insertion by health care providers). Two major types are support versus space filling.

Support pessaries

Support pessaries provide vaginal support using a spring mechanism which rests in the posterior fornix and against the posterior pubic symphysis (two-dimensional). Support pessaries are typically associated with easier insertion and removal and are more comfortable than space-filling pessaries. Support-type pessaries are used for the treatment of both POP and SUI (typically with a knob). Pessaries in this type include ring (most common; Fig. 16.3), Shaatz (Fig. 16.4), and Gehrung (Fig. 16.5).

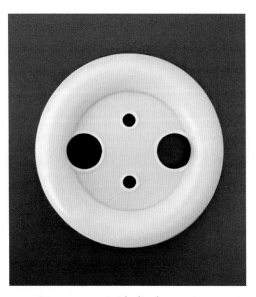

FIGURE 16.3 Ring pessary (with diaphragm "support").

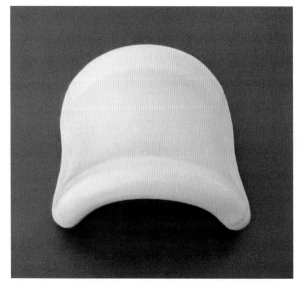

FIGURE 16.5 Gehrung pessary.

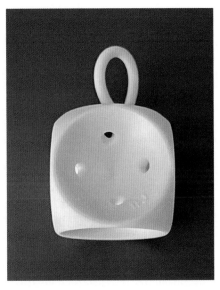

FIGURE 16.6 Cube pessary.

Space-filling pessaries

Space-filling pessaries work by maintaining their position by creating suction between the pessary and vaginal walls (cube; Fig. 16.6), by providing a diameter larger than the genital hiatus (donut; Fig. 16.7), or by both mechanisms (Gellhorn, most common; Fig. 16.8). Space-filling pessaries are indicated for POP.

Most women with prolapse can be successfully fit with either ring or Gellhorn pessaries. In general, a ring pessary is used for stage II to III POP, whereas a Gellhorn is for more advanced stage prolapse. A prospective study demonstrated 100% of women with stage II and 71% stage III prolapse were successfully fit with ring pessaries, whereas most women

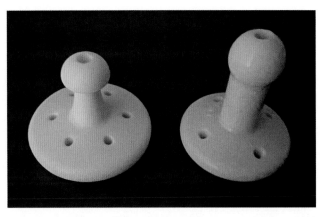

FIGURE 16.8 Short- (**left,** *white*) and long-stem (**right,** *pink*) Gellhorn pessaries.

with stage IV (64%) required Gellhorn pessaries.[33] However, once successfully fit, improvement in prolapse or urinary or bowel symptoms do not appear to depend on the type of pessaries; no differences in pelvic floor symptoms (prolapse, urinary, or bowel) were demonstrated between ring with support versus Gellhorn pessaries in a randomized trial including women with stage II to IV POP.[34]

Size

Pessaries are chosen based on findings on the examination (vaginal length and width, introital size). As fitting is by trial and error, some providers prefer to use a commercially available pessary sizing kit (Fig. 16.9) to determine appropriate pessary size and type before inserting an actual pessary. These fitting kit pessaries recommend they should not be worn longer than 10 to 15 minutes. Size comparison of commonly used pessaries are summarized in Table 16.3. Most commonly used sizes are 3 to 5 for ring pessaries and 2 1/2 to 3 for Gellhorn pessaries.

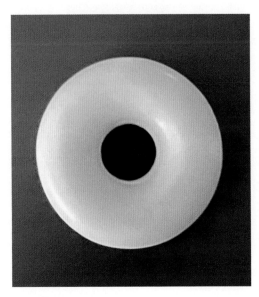

FIGURE 16.7 Donut pessary.

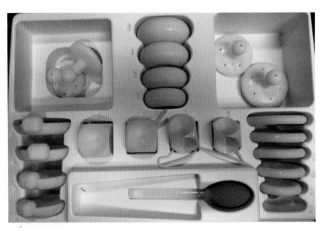

FIGURE 16.9 A pessary fitting kit can be used to determine accurate pessary type and size.

TABLE 16.3

Size Comparison of Commonly Used Pessaries

	RING		INCONTINENCE DISH		CUBE	
SIZE	INCHES	mm	INCHES	mm	INCHES	mm
2	2 1/4	57	2 1/2	65	1 3/8	35
3	2 1/2	64	2 3/4	70	1 1/2	38
4	2 3/4	70	3	75	1 5/8	41
5	3	76	3 1/8	80	1 3/4	44
6	3 1/4	83	—	—	2	51
7	3 1/2	57	—	—	2 1/4	57

GELLHORN		
SIZE	INCHES	mm
2 1/4	2 1/4	57
2 1/2	2 1/2	64
2 3/4	2 3/4	70
3	3	76
3 1/4	3 1/4	83
3 1/2	3 1/2	89
3 3/4	3 3/4	95

NOTE: Gellhorn sizes are in inches. Highlighted: commonly used sizes.

Overview of Pessary Insertion Steps

1. Ensure gloves are dry and compress the tip of the pessary.
2. Use the nondominant hand to separate the labia to open the introitus. Apply a small amount of lubrication at the leading tip of the pessary. Depress the perineal body. Holding the pessary almost parallel to the anterior-posterior axis, the pessary is inserted into the vagina (Fig. 16.10A,B).
3. Ensure proper fit by being able to insert a finger between the vaginal wall and the pessary. Excess pressure can lead to complications including discomfort, bleeding, voiding difficulty, and tissue erosion.
4. After insertion, the patient is asked to cough, perform Valsalva, and other maneuvers to see if the pessary stays in the proper position. She is also asked to ambulate, try different positions, as well as to void and strain while sitting on a toilet. Ask the patient whether there is any discomfort or difficulty urinating.
5. Examine the pessary fit and position both in standing and lithotomy positions.

Pessaries Types and Specific Insertion Tips

Ring pessaries

Ring pessaries, made of silicone and metal, are either with or without support (diaphragm with drainage holes; see Fig. 16.1) and with knob (Fig. 16.11) for stress incontinence. The knob of an incontinence ring should

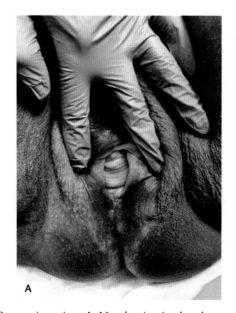
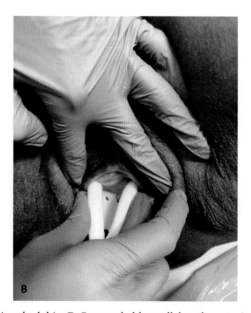

FIGURE 16.10 Pessary insertion. **A:** Nondominating hand separating the labia. **B:** Pessary held parallel to the anterior–posterior axis and inserted into the vagina. The ring pessary is folded in half for easier insertion.

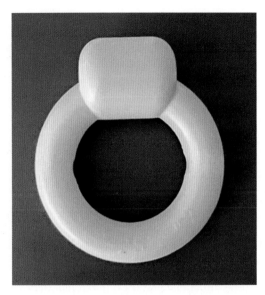

FIGURE 16.11 Incontinence ring pessary (with knob).

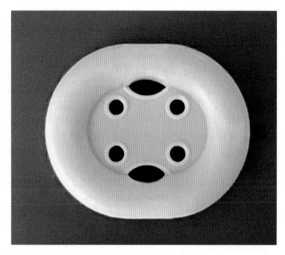

FIGURE 16.13 Oval pessary with support.

fit directly under the urethra for additional urethral support for those with SUI. A ring pessary should be folded in half (bringing sides together, folded edge facing posteriorly) for easier insertion (see Fig. 16.10B). The leading edge should rest in the posterior fornix and the distal edge right behind the pubic symphysis (Fig. 16.12). An oval-shaped pessary is also available (Fig. 16.13).

Shaatz

Shaatz pessary (see Fig. 16.4), made of silicone, is a rigid circular-shaped pessary without the stem of the Gellhorn (see following text). The stiffness of the pessary is thought to provide more support and less likely

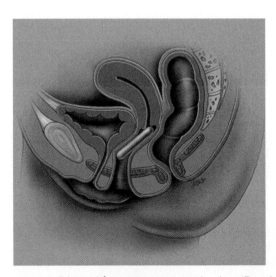

FIGURE 16.12 Ring with support pessary in situ. (Reprinted from Atnip SD. Pessary use and management for pelvic organ prolapse. *Obstet Gynecol Clin North Am* 2009;36[3]:541–563. Copyright [2009] with permission from Elsevier.)

to be displaced or expelled. However, it is more difficult to insert this type of pessary (minimal folding).

Gehrung

U-shaped Gehrung pessary (see Fig. 16.5), made of silicone and metal, has a flexible rim with a rubber diaphragm and can be used to treat cystocele or rectocele. The pessary should be inserted by folding and keeping the heels together. For a cystocele, the diaphragm (convex) part of the curve should be placed against the bulge to support the anterior vaginal wall while the bases (heels) rest on the posterior vaginal wall.

Gellhorn

Gellhorn pessaries, made of silicone, are the most commonly used space-filling pessaries. These pessaries have a broad-base ring with a stem, either short or long (see Fig. 16.8). The circular base is folded in half, away from the stem, and is inserted into the vagina, with the folded side first. The stem should be sitting just inside the introitus (Fig. 16.14). For women with advanced prolapse, a long-stem Gellhorn pessary may be useful.

Cube

Cube pessaries (see Fig. 16.6), made of silicone, provide support by creating suction to the vaginal walls. The cube has holes to allow drainage. A cube pessary is inserted by squeezing the sides and pushed up toward the apex (Fig. 16.15). To facilitate the removal, while gently tugging on the string, break the suction with a fingertip, squeeze the cube, and bring toward the introitus. Because of the suction, this type of pessary is recommended to be removed nightly, cleaned, and should not be reinserted until the following morning

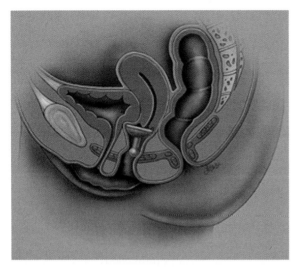

FIGURE 16.14 Gellhorn pessary in situ. (Reprinted from Atnip SD. Pessary use and management for pelvic organ prolapse. *Obstet Gynecol Clin North Am* 2009;36[3]:541–563. Copyright [2009] with permission from Elsevier.)

to prevent vaginal erosion[35] because this can cause potential fistula formation to the surrounding organs, especially if neglected.

Donut

Donut pessaries (see Fig. 16.7), made of silicone, are a thicker and bulkier version of a ring pessary to occupy a larger vaginal space. As it is rigid, the pessary is inserted vertically and rotated horizontally once inside the vaginal canal.

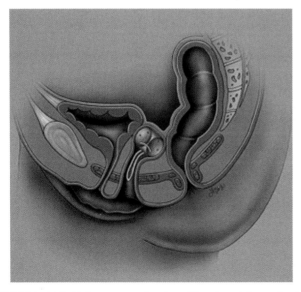

FIGURE 16.15 Cube pessary in situ. (Reprinted from Atnip SD. Pessary use and management for pelvic organ prolapse. *Obstet Gynecol Clin North Am* 2009;36[3]:541–563. Copyright [2009] with permission from Elsevier.)

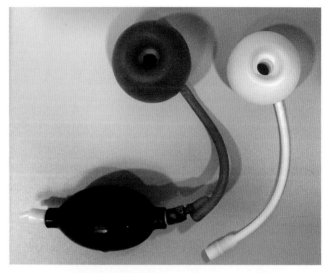

FIGURE 16.16 Inflatable pessaries. Inflatoball (**left**; made of latex) and silicon based (**right**).

Others

Inflatable pessaries

This space-filling pessary has an air-filled ball which is attached to a stem that facilitates insertion and removal. Whereas older inflatable pessaries (Inflatoball) are made of latex, some newer ones are silicon-based with a stem and air pump (Fig. 16.16). The stem can be either left outside the vagina or tucked inside.

Incontinence dish

Similar to incontinence ring pessaries (ring with a knob), an incontinence dish (Fig. 16.17), made of silicone, is another option for women with SUI. Compared to ring pessaries, the dish shape (and more rigid compared to ring) may hold vaginal prolapse better; however, additional benefit is unclear compared to the ring type.

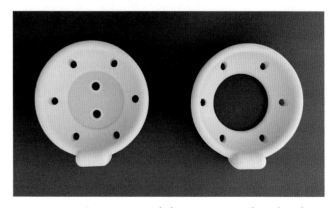

FIGURE 16.17 Incontinence dish pessaries (with and without support).

CARE INSTRUCTIONS AND PATIENT EDUCATION

Patient education regarding management and pessary care instructions is key for successful treatment and patient satisfaction.

Removal

The pessary should be removed on a regular basis, typically nightly to weekly, depending on the pessary type and patient preference. However, current recommendations regarding the frequency of pessary removal are not based on robust data. For easier removal, dental floss can be tied to the pessary (through one of the drainage holes; Fig. 16.18).

Cleaning

Upon removal, the pessary should be washed in mild soap and water and let dry until replaced the following morning.

Follow-up Appointment

There is little consensus on the ideal intervals of pessary care follow-up. After the initial placement, the first return visit may be within 1 to 2 weeks and longer intervals thereafter (3 to 6 months, up to annually) depending on the patient's complaints, vaginal tissue quality, and the type of care required. For patients unable to or unwilling to perform self-care, the pessary can be removed, cleaned, and replaced in a clinical setting typically every 2 to 4 months as indicated. A recent randomized trial demonstrated that an "extended" 24-week outpatient pessary care was noninferior to routine care of every 12 weeks in terms of vaginal epithelial abnormalities, excoriations, or erosions (1.7% extended care vs. 7.4% routine care, difference −5.7, 95% CI −7.4 to −4.7) in women using a ring, incontinence dish, or Gellhorn pessaries. Notably, the majority (74%) of the study subjects were on vaginal estrogen.[36]

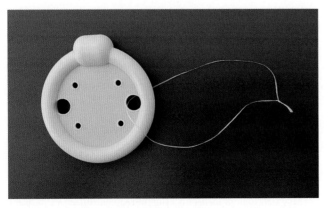

FIGURE 16.18 Dental floss is tied for easy removal.

Complications

Complication rates associated with pessary use of up to 56% have been reported.[22] However, most adverse effects are considered minor.

Minor complications include the following:

- Discomfort: Pessary fit should be assessed. The pessary may need to be decreased in size or changed to a different shape.
- Vaginal discharge: Vaginal discharge either with or without odor is very common and not necessarily due to infection. Pessary use in postmenopausal women can cause changes in bacterial flora due to higher vaginal pH and is associated with a higher rate of bothersome discharge compared to those without pessary (30% pessary use vs. 2% without).[37] However, the discharge was shown to be due to inflammatory responses secondary to pessary use, rather than changes in vaginal flora.[37,38] "Vaginal rest" can be helpful if the symptoms persist.

  Because increased discharge may be related to postmenopausal vaginal changes, low-dose vaginal estrogen is especially helpful in women with bothersome discharge. Vaginal estrogen has been shown to improve tissue quality and lower vaginal pH, and women with vaginal estrogen are more likely to continue pessary use.[39]

  Vaginal estrogen: Vaginal estrogen cream is applied typically twice weekly after pessary removal at night or can be applied along the side of the pessary if unable to remove the pessary. Other estrogen formulations can be used instead of cream. When using an estrogen ring, the estrogen ring is inserted prior to the pessary insertion.

  A pH-lowering product: Some providers recommend a pH-lowering agent, either alone or concurrently with vaginal estrogen. However, no significant benefit has been demonstrated.[40]

- Vaginal spotting, bleeding: Bleeding can be due to vaginal tissue atrophy, trauma from pessary insertion/removal, or vaginal erosion. However, other genital tract pathologies, including malignancy, need to be excluded. Women with a new onset of vaginal bleeding need to be examined to determine the source of bleeding.
- Vaginal erosion: The most common sign of erosion is bleeding with or without vaginal irritation. Erosion is caused by excess pressure from the pessary. Therefore, the pessary should be removed for several weeks ("pessary holiday") while using vaginal estrogen to promote tissue healing. When healed, a smaller and different shape of pessary should be considered. If nightly removal causes frequent vaginal excoriation especially at the introitus, reducing the frequency of pessary removal can be helpful.
- Changes in urinary or bowel symptoms, incomplete emptying: Pessary fit should be assessed and may need to be changed to a different size and/or shape.

Serious complications

Serious complications from pessary use are rare and typically associated with neglect in pessary care and follow-up. These include pessary incarceration, fistula to the surrounding organs (bladder or rectum), urinary or colonic obstruction, and vaginal cancer. Risk factors of serious complications include older age and cognitive impairment. Therefore, patient education (patient, caregivers, family members) is essential in preventing serious pessary related complications. It is helpful to provide a handout with pessary care instructions including frequently asked questions, clinic contact information, and follow-up plans.

Other Considerations

- Sexual intercourse: Pessary removal is not always necessary (typically with support type pessaries) prior to having intercourse if unable to remove or reinsert pessary, as long as it is not uncomfortable for the patient and/or her partner.
- Imaging studies: When undergoing a plain film or magnetic resonance imaging, it is advised to remove the pessary because some pessaries contain metal (see earlier).
- Pessary replacement: A new pessary may be needed when the pessary has a crack, breaks, or the shape is lost. However, pessaries do not "expire."

CONCLUSION

Pessary use is an effective nonsurgical treatment option for POP and/or SUI. Successful treatment with pessaries depends highly on patient counseling to address treatment goals and expectations as well as patient education to ensure treatment adherence and avoid complications.

References

1. Wu JM, Vaughan CP, Goode PS, et al. Prevalence and trends of symptomatic pelvic floor disorders in U.S. women. *Obstet Gynecol* 2014;123(1):141–148.
2. Ortman JM, Velkoff V. An aging nation: The older population in the United States. Accessed November 16, 2020. https://www.census.gov/prod/2014pubs/p25-1140.pdf
3. Bhatia NN, Bergman A, Gunning JE. Urodynamic effects of a vaginal pessary in women with stress urinary incontinence. *Am J Obstet Gynecol* 1983;147(8):876–884.
4. Noblett KL, McKinney A, Lane FL. Effects of the incontinence dish pessary on urethral support and urodynamic parameters. *Am J Obstet Gynecol* 2008;198(5):592.e1–592.e5.
5. Komesu YM, Ketai LH, Rogers RG, et al. Restoration of continence by pessaries: Magnetic resonance imaging assessment of mechanism of action. *Am J Obstet Gynecol* 2008;198(5):563.e1–563.e6.
6. Romanzi LJ, Chaikin DC, Blaivas JG. The effect of genital prolapse on voiding. *J Urol* 1999;161(2):581–586.

7. Lazarou G, Scotti RJ, Mikhail MS, et al. Pessary reduction and postoperative cure of retention in women with anterior vaginal wall prolapse. *Int Urogynecol J Pelvic Floor Dysfunct* 2004;15(3):175–178.
8. Lone F, Thakar R, Sultan AH. One-year prospective comparison of vaginal pessaries and surgery for pelvic organ prolapse using the validated ICIQ-VS and ICIQ-UI (SF) questionnaires. *Int Urogynecol J* 2015;26(9):1305–1312.
9. Powers K, Lazarou G, Wang A, et al. Pessary use in advanced pelvic organ prolapse. *Int Urogynecol J Pelvic Floor Dysfunct* 2006;17(2):160–164.
10. Maito JM, Quam ZA, Craig E, et al. Predictors of successful pessary fitting and continued use in a nurse-midwifery pessary clinic. *J Midwifery Womens Health* 2006;51(2):78–84.
11. Wu V, Farrell SA, Baskett TF, et al. A simplified protocol for pessary management. *Obstet Gynecol* 1997;90(6):990–994.
12. Nemeth Z, Nagy S, Ott J. The cube pessary: An underestimated treatment option for pelvic organ prolapse? Subjective 1-year outcomes. *Int Urogynecol J* 2013;24(10):1695–1701.
13. Markle D, Skoczylas L, Goldsmith C, et al. Patient characteristics associated with a successful pessary fitting. *Female Pelvic Med Reconstr Surg* 2011;17(5):249–252.
14. Nager CW, Richter HE, Nygaard I, et al. Incontinence pessaries: Size, POPQ measures, and successful fitting. *Int Urogynecol J Pelvic Floor Dysfunct* 2009;20(9):1023–1028.
15. Farrell SA, Singh B, Aldakhil L. Continence pessaries in the management of urinary incontinence in women. *J Obstet Gynaecol Can* 2004;26(2):113–117.
16. Moore KH, Foote A, Burton G, et al. An open study of the bladder neck support prosthesis in genuine stress incontinence. *Br J Obstet Gynaecol* 1999;106(1):42–49.
17. Clemons JL, Aguilar VC, Sokol ER, et al. Patient characteristics that are associated with continued pessary use versus surgery after 1 year. *Am J Obstet Gynecol* 2004;191(1):159–164.
18. Handa VL, Jones M. Do pessaries prevent the progression of pelvic organ prolapse? *Int Urogynecol J Pelvic Floor Dysfunct* 2002;13(6):349–352.
19. Friedman S, Sandhu KS, Wang C, et al. Factors influencing long-term pessary use. *Int Urogynecol J* 2010;21(6):673–678.
20. Lone F, Thakar R, Sultan AH, et al. A 5-year prospective study of vaginal pessary use for pelvic organ prolapse. *Int J Gynaecol Obstet* 2011;114(1):56–59.
21. Mao M, Xu T, Kang J, et al. Factors associated with long-term pessary use in women with symptomatic pelvic organ prolapse. *Climacteric* 2019;22(5):478–482.
22. Sarma S, Ying T, Moore KH. Long-term vaginal ring pessary use: Discontinuation rates and adverse events. *BJOG* 2009;116(13):1715–1721.
23. Jones K, Yang L, Lowder JL, et al. Effect of pessary use on genital hiatus measurements in women with pelvic organ prolapse. *Obstet Gynecol* 2008;112(3):630–636.
24. Siddique M, Ingraham C, Kudish B, et al. Hydronephrosis associated with pelvic organ prolapse: A systematic review. *Female Pelvic Med Reconstr Surg* 2020;26(3):212–218.
25. Dancz CE, Walker D, Thomas D, et al. Effect of pessary use on hydronephrosis in women with advanced pelvic organ prolapse: A self-selected interventional trial. *Int Urogynecol J* 2017;28(10):1589–1593.
26. Richter HE, Burgio KL, Brubaker L, et al. Continence pessary compared with behavioral therapy or combined therapy for stress incontinence: A randomized controlled trial. *Obstet Gynecol* 2010;115(3):609–617.

27. Yalcin I, Bump RC. Validation of two global impression questionnaires for incontinence. *Am J Obstet Gynecol* 2003;189(1):98–101.

28. Burgio KL, Goode PS, Richter HE, et al. Global ratings of patient satisfaction and perceptions of improvement with treatment for urinary incontinence: Validation of three global patient ratings. *Neurourol Urodyn* 2006;25(5):411–417.

29. Panman CM, Wiegersman M, Kollen BJ, et al. Effectiveness and cost-effectiveness of pessary treatment compared with pelvic floor muscle training in older women with pelvic organ prolapse: 2-Year follow-up of a randomized controlled trial in primary care. *Menopause* 2016;23(12):1307–1318.

30. Cheung RY, Lee JHS, Lee LL, et al. Vaginal pessary in women with symptomatic pelvic organ prolapse: A randomized controlled trial. *Obstet Gynecol* 2016;128(1):73–80.

31. Sung VW, Wohlrab KJ, Madsen A, et al. Patient-reported goal attainment and comprehensive functioning outcomes after surgery compared with pessary for pelvic organ prolapse. *Am J Obstet Gynecol* 2016;215(5):659.e1–659.e7.

32. Barber MD, Walters MD, Cundiff GW, et al. Responsiveness of the Pelvic Floor Distress Inventory (PFDI) and Pelvic Floor Impact Questionnaire (PFIQ) in women undergoing vaginal surgery and pessary treatment for pelvic organ prolapse. *Am J Obstet Gynecol* 2006;194(5):1492–1498.

33. Clemons JL, Aguilar VC, Tillinghast T, et al. Risk factors associated with an unsuccessful pessary fitting trial in women with pelvic organ prolapse. *Am J Obstet Gynecol* 2004;190(2):345–350.

34. Cundiff GW, Amundsen CL, Bent AE, et al. The PESSRI study: Symptom relief outcomes of a randomized crossover trial of the ring and Gellhorn pessaries. *Am J Obstet Gynecol* 2007;196(4):405.e1–405.e8.

35. Milex. *Patient instructions: Cube and tandem-cube pessary.* Trumbull: CooperSurgical, 2012.

36. Propst K, Mellen C, O'Sullivan DM, et al. Timing of office-based pessary care: A randomized controlled trial. *Obstet Gynecol* 2020;135(1):100–105.

37. Collins S, Beigi R, Mellen C, et al. The effect of pessaries on the vaginal microenvironment. *Am J Obstet Gynecol* 2015;212(1):60.e1–60.e6.

38. Coelho SCA, Giraldo PC, Florentino JO, et al. Can the pessary use modify the vaginal microbiological flora? A cross-sectional study. *Rev Bras Ginecol Obstet* 2017;39(4):169–174.

39. Dessie SG, Armstrong K, Modest AM, et al. Effect of vaginal estrogen on pessary use. *Int Urogynecol J* 2016;27(9):1423–1429.

40. Meriwether KV, Rogers RG, Craig E, et al. The effect of hydroxyquinoline-based gel on pessary-associated bacterial vaginosis: A multicenter randomized controlled trial. *Am J Obstet Gynecol* 2015;213(5):729.e1–729.e9.

CHAPTER 17

SACRAL NEUROMODULATION

Karen L. Noblett • Carly Crowder

Introduction

Sacral neuromodulation (SNM) is a guideline-recommended therapy by both the American Urological Association (AUA) and the American Society of Colon and Rectal Surgeons, with proven long-term success for urinary urgency incontinence (UUI), urinary urgency frequency, nonobstructive urinary retention (NOUR), and fecal incontinence. SNM was first approved for voiding dysfunction in the United States in 1997 (urgency incontinence) and 1999 (urinary urgency frequency and NOUR). In the United States, it took another 12 years before it gained the additional indication for the treatment of fecal incontinence in 2011. Initially, the therapy involved a more invasive surgical approach that included a large cutdown over the sacrum to secure the lead to the periosteum. This initial procedure was performed under general anesthesia and was typically reserved for the most refractory patients. However, early physician-initiated innovation evolved the therapy into a minimally invasive procedure that allowed it to be performed under local anesthesia in an outpatient setting.[1] Historically, there has been only one commercially available SNM device (InterStim, Medtronic, Dublin, Ireland), which is a nonrechargeable neurostimulator with an estimated lifespan of 4.4 years.[2] In late 2019, a second SNM device was approved by the U.S. Food and Drug Administration (FDA) for the bowel and bladder indications listed earlier. The Axonics device (Axonics Modulation Technologies, Irvine, CA) is a miniaturized, rechargeable neuromodulation system qualified to last a minimum of 15 years in the body. In mid-2020, Medtronic also gained FDA approval for InterStim Micro, their miniaturized, rechargeable SNM device, which is also designed to last 15 years. In early 2022, both Axonics and Medtronic received FDA approval for nonrechargeable SNM devices, the Axonics F15 recharge-free SNM system and the Medtronic InterStimX system, respectively. These devices have longer projected life in the body compared to the legacy device. Depending on program settings, the devices are expected to last 10 to 20 years.

This chapter reviews recent advancements in SNM therapy including updates in best practices for implant technique, technological innovations, and the new clinical literature relevant to contemporary practice. This chapter also provides some insight into potential future directions of neuromodulation for pelvic floor disorders.

DEFINITION, INDICATIONS AND MECHANISM OF ACTION

SNM involves placing a quadripolar lead adjacent to a sacral nerve root (typically S3) that is connected to a neurostimulator that delivers nonpainful, electrical pulses to the sacral nerves to modulate the reflexes that influence the bladder, bowels, sphincters, and pelvic floor musculature to improve or restore function (Fig. 17.1).

Currently approved and available devices in the United States include InterStim II, InterStim Micro, and InterStimX (Medtronic, Minneapolis, MN) and the Axonics R15 (rechargeable) and F15 (nonrechargeable) SNM systems (Axonics, Irvine, CA) which are shown in Figure 17.2. The features of these systems are compared in Figure 17.3.

Indications for Sacral Neuromodulation

Although SNM is not considered a first-line therapy for bladder or bowel control disorders, it is a minimally invasive treatment with proven long-term success. Current FDA-approved indications for SNM use include urgency incontinence, urinary urgency frequency, NOUR, and fecal incontinence.

Urinary urgency frequency, urinary urgency incontinence (overactive bladder)

SNM is indicated for patients with overactive bladder (OAB) with and without incontinence who fail conservative therapy and/or medical management, including those who experience intolerable side effects. The AUA guidelines for the treatment of OAB recommend SNM as a third-line therapy; however, a recent update to the guidelines suggests that it is not necessary for all patients to go through each line of treatment in a specific order because there are many factors to consider when deciding on the best treatment option for a particular patient. The AUA

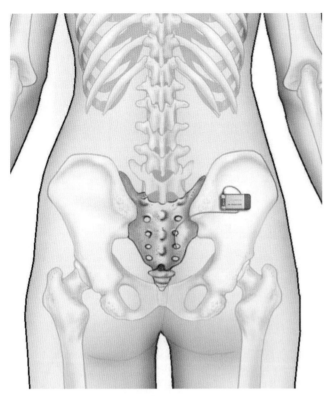

FIGURE 17.1 INS connected to the quadripolar lead at S3. (Courtesy of Axonics, Inc.)

guidelines specifically state, "The patient does not need to proceed through each line of therapy before considering the next. In other words, the lines of therapy, while representing a successive increase in risk or invasiveness, are not intended to represent a strict algorithm." This would suggest that patients with OAB do not necessarily have to trial and fail medications before being offered SNM.[3]

Nonobstructive urinary retention

SNM is also indicated as a treatment option for patients with NOUR.[4] Urinary retention has historically been a challenging condition to manage with few viable treatment options available. Prior to the introduction of SNM, NOUR was typically managed with intermittent or continuous bladder catheterization, both of which can be uncomfortable and are associated with increased risk of bladder infections. SNM has proven to be an effective alternative to catheterization and has been shown to significantly improve the quality of life for this patient population.[4]

Fecal incontinence

SNM is indicated as a second-line therapy for fecal incontinence in patients who have failed conservative therapies. SNM can be ideal and is preferred in patients who have both urinary and bowel disorders. SNM can also be offered to patients with anal sphincter defects and is approved for sphincter defects up to 120°. Generally, 2 weeks of bowel symptoms are documented prior to, and during therapy (e.g., bowel diary), to assess efficacy of SNM treatment. Further anorectal physiology testing may be helpful in comprehensive evaluation of bowel disorders and identification of additional components of dysfunction but has not been shown to be predictive of success with SNM. Although this testing is not necessary prior to SNM, it may prove useful in guiding management.[4]

Further indications

Although considered off-label, other indications that have been treated with SNM include neurogenic bladder, bladder pain syndrome (BPS), chronic pelvic pain, and chronic constipation.

Neurogenic bladder

Although most SNM trials exclude patients with underlying neurologic conditions, there is no data to support this strategy, and, in fact, there is a growing body of evidence to support the use of SNM in this population and that overall safety outcomes are similar for both groups.[5-10] Peters et al.[11] reported OAB responder rates in both neurogenic and nonneurogenic patients. In this study, the test responder rate was similar for both patient populations, with an implantation rate of 89% and 89.6%, respectively, and the long-term therapy responder rate was 86% for neurogenic patients and 63% for nonneurogenic patients. These data suggest that SNM works well for patients with underlying neurologic conditions and also has a similar safety profile.

Bladder pain syndrome/interstitial cystitis

Although not FDA approved for this condition, SNM is an option for BPS/interstitial cystitis (IC) that is refractory to conservative therapies. SNM provides an effective long-term treatment option for refractory BPS.[12] In a study by Maher et al.,[13] 13 of 15 patients (87%) reported a 50% reduction in bladder pain. Similarly, in a study of 17 patients conducted by Comiter,[14] bladder pain was evaluated by visual analogue scale. In this noncontrolled study, patients reported a reduction in pain from 5.8 to 1.6 ($P < .01$), with 87% of patients reporting symptomatic improvement.[14] In another study of 21 patients by Peters and Konstandt,[15] a 36% reduction in morphine dose equivalents was demonstrated in their population, where 22% became narcotic free, and 95% reported moderate to marked reduction in pain. A systematic review and meta-analysis completed in 2017 indicated that SNM may be a safe and effective for treatment of refractory BPS/IC.[16] Overall, 60% to 98% (pooled analysis demonstrated 84%) of patients report

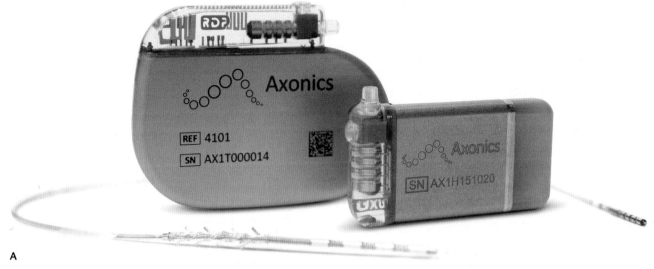

A

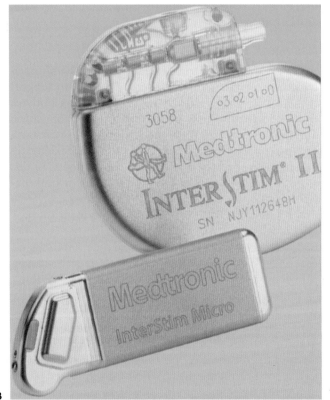

B

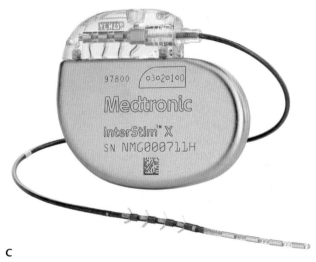

C

FIGURE 17.2 Available SNM devices in the United States. **A:** Axonics R15 INS and Axonics F15 INS. **B:** Medtronic Micro and Interstim II. **C:** Medtronic InterstimX. (**A,** courtesy of Axonics, Inc. **B** and **C,** © 2022 Medtronic. All rights reserved. Used with the permission of Medtronic.)

symptom improvement, and explant rates are reported between 3% and 13%.[16] The AUA endorses SNM in its treatment algorithm for BPS as the consensus of the review panel is that there is adequate data in the literature to support its endorsement.[17]

Constipation

Although off-label in the United States, SNM is approved in Europe for the treatment of chronic constipation for patients with refractory symptoms for over 1 year and no evidence of a mechanically correctable cause. In studies evaluating SNM for use in constipation, it has been shown to induce pan-colonic propagating pressure waves and to increase bowel movement frequency.[18,19] A recent study, evaluating the use of SNM for slow-transit constipation, showed a significant improvement in both colorectal transit time and Cleveland Clinic Constipation Scores at 6 months. However, at 60 months, 48% of patients had the neuromodulator removed.[20] In a review article from 2013 that included 10 prior studies evaluating SNM in the treatment of constipation, a total of 225 SNM trials were performed with 125 going to permanent implant (55.5%).[21] Of those implanted, 89.6% of patients with

Device	Interstim Micro	Axonic R15
Implant life	15 years	15 years
Size Length, Height, Thickness, Volume (L/H/T/V)	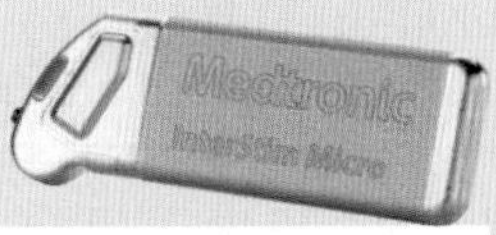 47mm/17mm/5mm/2.8cc	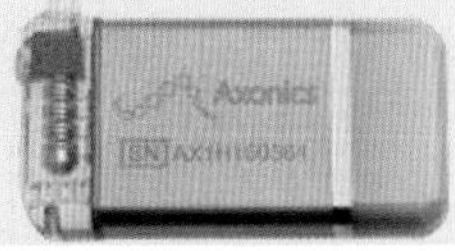 42mm/22mm/6mm/5cc
Device	Interstim X	Axonics F15
Size (L/H/T/V) Length, Height, Thickness, Volume	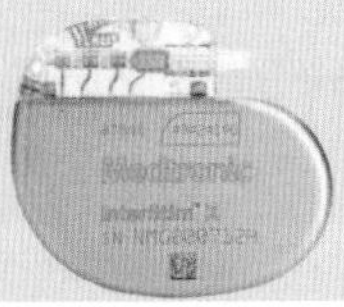 51mm/44mm/7.7mm/12.5cc	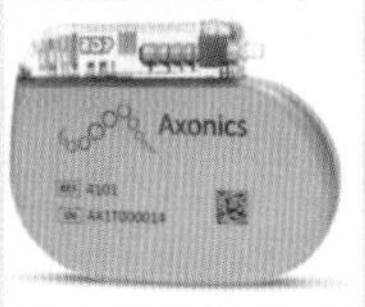 53mm/39mm/6.7mm/10cc
Stimulation Delivery	Constant Current	Constant Current
Full-body MRI	1.5 and 3T	1.5 and 3T
Programming Approach	Standard default programming options	Utilizes programming algorithm based on patient intra-operative responses to find the best program
Patient Remote Control	Samsung Smart Phone plus a Communicator (both require recharging) 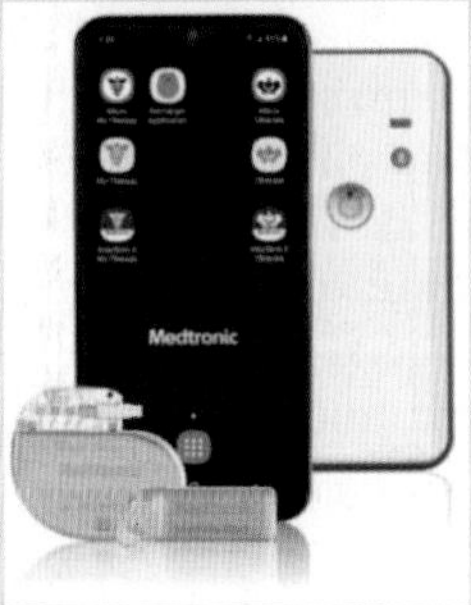	Wireless (no battery replacement or charging required) 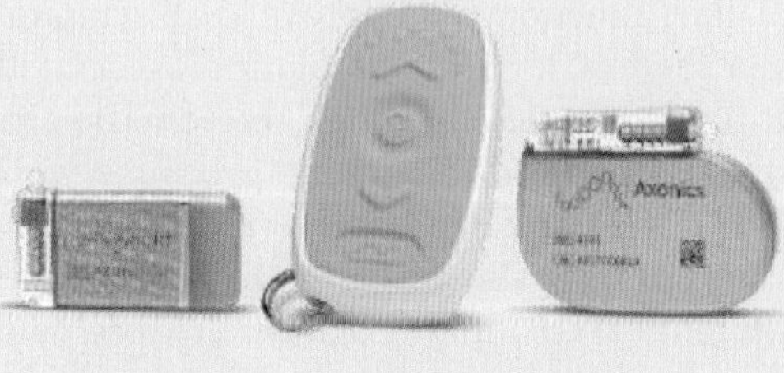
Lead Compatibility	Different leads for Interstim X and Micro	Same lead for Axonics R15 and F15

FIGURE 17.3 Comparison of the available SNM systems. (Courtesy of Axonics, Inc.)

permanent implants reported satisfaction with their SNM device. Overall, data on SNM therapy for constipation is conflicting and further studies to evaluate long-term efficacy are warranted.

Mechanism of Action

Normal voiding

For infants and toddlers who have not yet achieved voluntary control over bladder function, a critical level of bladder distention is required to stimulate the voiding reflex. This sensory input, upon reaching the pontine micturition center, simultaneously allows for a coordinated detrusor contraction and concomitant urethral relaxation, thus facilitating urination. This is a primordial reflex pathway that allows for effective and efficient bladder emptying and prevents the bladder from over distending, causing injury. Gaining voluntary control over, and learning to suppress, this voiding reflex is a complex process that is mediated at a higher level in the cerebral cortex and generally begins to mature around age 2 years and can take as long as 7 years to fully develop. Continence is also maintained via an intact guarding reflex, which is a progressive, involuntary increase in the activity of the external urethral sphincter during bladder filling resulting in increased outlet resistance. Voluntary voiding is facilitated through stimulation of the excitatory efferent pathway, resulting in inhibition of the sympathetic system and pudendal nerve, and activation of the sacral parasympathetics.[22]

The causes of OAB, NOUR, and fecal incontinence can be multifactorial and are not completely understood. SNM treats bladder and bowel dysfunction by electrically modulating neural pathways via stimulation of a sacral nerve root (typically S3). For OAB, SNM most likely functions through two main pathways, with a third pathway that has also been suggested to play a role. These three pathways include the following:

- Spinal reflex pathways that inhibit detrusor overactivity
- Supraspinal areas in the brain that normalize bladder function
- Direct and indirect effects on the urethral sphincter

Taken together, these indicate that SNM most likely works through local reflex pathways that influence bladder activity and also at higher levels in the brain that govern bladder function.

Spinal reflex pathway mechanism of action

In a study by DeGroat and Saum,[23] it was demonstrated that sacral preganglionic outflow to the bladder receives inhibitory input from both somatic and visceral afferents. This suggests that nerves going to the bladder from the sacral nerve roots can be influenced by input from the pudendal nerve before actually affecting the bladder. Thus, activating these somatic afferents can inhibit detrusor/bladder function and improve OAB symptoms.

Given the low level of stimulation associated with SNM, it likely functions through the somatic afferents including the pudendal afferents because we know these nerves depolarize at lower levels than autonomic nerves. Studies have shown that activation of these somatic afferent nerves inhibits bladder sensory pathways and reflex bladder hyperactivity, thereby decreasing symptoms of OAB.[24–28]

Supraspinal pathway mechanism of action

Stimulating the somatic afferent nerves in a sacral spinal root (S3, S4, and/or pudendal) also sends signals to the higher centers in the central nervous system (CNS) that may restore normal communication between the brain and the bladder and thus normal function. SNM appears to normalize brain activity that is responsible for detrusor overactivity, bladder filling sensation, the sense of urge, and timing of micturition. One study using positron emission tomography scans has demonstrated changes in brain activity with SNM stimulation both in the on and off settings in patients with OAB. This study indicates that there is abnormal brain activity in these areas which become normalized with SNM active stimulation.[29]

Activation of the urethral sphincter

Direct activation of motor neurons innervating the striated urethral sphincter can lead to increased outlet resistance which ultimately is inhibitory to bladder reflex activity at the CNS level. In a similar manner, when you have an urge to urinate, if you contract your pelvic floor muscles, this leads to increased resistance/pressure in the urethra. This increased pressure triggers a reflex pathway back to the bladder that promotes bladder relaxation. This is the same concept with SNM. Indirect activation of the urethral sphincter may also occur via activation of afferent projections that influence the sympathetic tone to the urethral striated sphincter, thus promoting bladder relaxation.[30]

IMPLANT PROCEDURE

One of the advantages of SNM is that patients can undergo a test procedure to determine if the therapy is right for them. For surgeons, there is no other existing procedure that offers this advantage. Therapy for SNM is generally completed in two phases: The first phase is when a temporary lead (percutaneous nerve evaluation [PNE] lead) or a tined lead is placed along a sacral nerve root (generally S3) and stimulation of the nerve is conducted for a period of 3 to 14 days depending on the type of trial. Using a shared decision-making model, the patient and physician are able to determine if this therapy is effective and appropriate for their condition. If patients have a ≥50% improvement in symptoms and they are satisfied with their response, they go on to the second phase where the implantable neurostimulator (INS) is implanted. If the trial is inconclusive with a temporary (PNE) trial, patients can go on to a longer tined lead trial, or they may choose to pursue other treatment modalities.

The least invasive trial type is the PNE, also known as a basic evaluation. This type of trial can be completed in an office or surgery center and typically only requires local anesthesia, but monitored anesthesia care is also commonly used. The procedure is completed by placement of a temporary electrode wire in the S3 foramen without or without fluoroscopic guidance and is generally done bilaterally. The wire is then connected to a temporary, external pulse generator and worn by the patient for 3 to 7 days to evaluate if the therapy is effective.[31] The PNE has several benefits including being less costly and less invasive and may require only one trip to the operating room (OR). Limitations of the PNE include lead migration because there is nothing internal to secure the lead, a shorter trial period, and potentially suboptimal wire placement if fluoroscopy guidance is not used. However, a recent randomized clinical trial demonstrated that the outcomes for PNEs performed without fluoroscopy was noninferior to those performed with fluoroscopy arguing against that last point.[32]

The second option for nerve stimulation testing is a staged procedure, where a tined lead is placed parallel to a sacral nerve root, typically S3, under fluoroscopic guidance. The S3 nerve root is the preferred target for

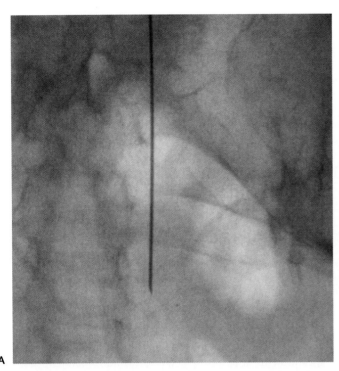

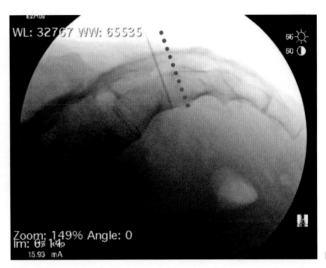

A

B

FIGURE 17.4 Ideal needle placement in AP (**A**) and lateral (**B**) views. In the AP view, a needle is placed parallel and along the medial border of the foramen. In the lateral view, the needle is parallel to the fusion plate of S3 *(red dotted line)* and is approximately 1 cm above and sitting just at the anterior surface of the sacrum.

SNM because S3 is the main contributor to pelvic floor innervation.[33] Patients are positioned prone in the OR to allow visualization of the S3 nerve responses including great toe dorsiflexion and bellows response. General anesthesia with paralytics and regional anesthesia must be avoided in order to visualize these responses.[4]

After identification of the bony landmarks, a 3.5- or 5-inch foramen needle is placed such that it is parallel to the medial border of the foramen on the anteroposterior (AP) image and 1 cm above and parallel to the fusion plate on the lateral image (Fig. 17.4). The needle is only advanced to the anterior surface of the sacrum where the stimulation threshold is tested and considered acceptable if ≤2 mA.[4] If greater than 2 mA, the needle should be redirected to find a better location in the foramen (tip: going back to the AP position on fluoroscopy can be helpful to troubleshoot if not getting the desired response). Once proper response is confirmed, the lead introducer is placed over a directional guide and advanced such that the radiolucent marker is approximately halfway through the bony plate (Fig. 17.5). This can be done under live fluoroscopy or with incremental advancement. Care should be taken not to advance the introducer too deep as this may create a false path for the lead to follow. It is recommended to use the curved stylet when introducing the lead so that it is able to follow the natural path of the nerve. Use of the curved stylet has been shown to have overall less amplitude requirements and is associated with better long-term outcomes as compared to the straight stylet.[34,35] The quadripolar lead, which is self-anchored

via deployable tines, is then placed such that ideal motor responses are achieved on all four electrodes, ideally at less than 2 mA. The length of the staged lead placement trial is generally 7 to 14 days,[4,36] and there has been no evidence demonstrating benefit of performing a bilateral over a unilateral tined lead trial.[37] Patients with at least a 50% improvement in symptoms during the trial period for either PNE or staged lead placement are considered a success and a candidate to progress to implant of the INS. PNE versus a staged trial was evaluated in a prospective trial by Borawski et al.[38] This study showed a significantly

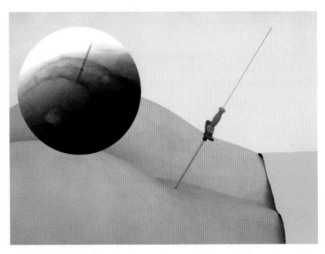

FIGURE 17.5 Passing lead introducer with radiolucent marker halfway through the sacral plate. (Courtesy of Axonics, Inc.)

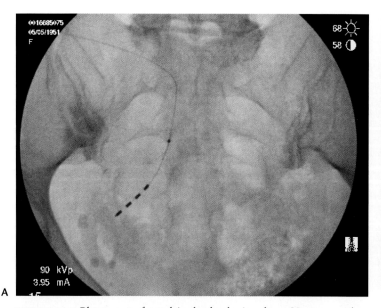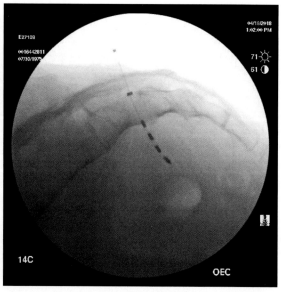

FIGURE 17.6 Placement of quadripolar lead wire along S3 nerve with curved stylet. **A:** AP view. **B:** Lateral view.

increased progression to implant placement with staged procedure versus PNE (88% vs. 46%, P < .02). Banakhar and Hassouna[39] evaluated sensitivity, specificity, and predictive values for a staged implant versus PNE. For PNE, positive and negative predictive values were 99% and 82.1%, respectively, and for staged test were 90% and 92.9%, respectively.[39] This study showed that PNE has a high positive predictive value which, in conjunction with the potential of a simple office-based procedure, may be preferable for certain patients. Although the staged procedure may be more costly and require two OR visits, it has the advantage of a higher conversion rate to implant and potential for a longer trial period. The decision for PNE versus staged procedure should be individualized for each patient and practice model. Preoperatively, patients should be counseled regarding procedure risks including infection, implant site or leg pain, and potential need for revision or reprogramming.[4]

Routine use of intraoperative fluoroscopy is recommended for staged lead positioning in order to optimize lead placement. Both AP and lateral fluoroscopy views should be used to assess needle and final tined lead wire placement. The ideal lead placement in the AP view is shown with the trajectory of the lead curving out from medial to lateral, and on the lateral view having a gentle curvature from cephalad to caudad (Fig. 17.6). Proper lead placement can be confirmed by appropriate sensory and motor responses (Table 17.1). Achieving bellows response before toe flexion at ≤2 mA on all four electrodes is considered ideal.[4]

Best practices recommend perioperative antibiotics given within 60 minutes of skin incision to be targeted to local skin flora and based on the combination of local hospital antibiogram along with patient's allergies.[4] The AUA recommends perioperative antibiotic prophylaxis with a first-generation cephalosporin before placement of the lead wire to cover for skin flora; however, data supporting this recommendation are lacking.[40] A large retrospective cohort analysis of sacral nerve stimulation procedures noted a significant reduction in surgical site

TABLE 17.1

Sacral Nerve Sensory and Motor Responses

SACRAL NERVE ROOT	SENSORY RESPONSE	MOTOR RESPONSE	
		PELVIC FLOOR	**LEG/FOOT**
S2	Generally none, or may have a sensation in the buttocks	Potential clamp response (anterior to posterior contraction of the perineal structures: a clamp-like contraction of the anal sphincter, and in males, a retraction of the penis base)	Rotation of the leg/hip rotation, rotation of the heel, calf contraction
S3*	**Pulling in rectum, extending forward to scrotum or labia**	**Bellows (flattening and deepening of the buttock groove due to lifting and dropping of pelvic floor)**	**Flexing great toe, occasional flexing of other toes**
S4	Pulling in rectum	Bellows	None

*S3 nerve root is the preferred target for SNM.

infections after the implementation of a chlorhexidine wash the night before and the morning of the procedure. The infection rate decreased from more than 7% to 1.7% after the introduction of this intervention. Additionally, 82% of devices that were explanted as a result of an infection were noted to be colonized with methicillin-resistant *Staphylococcus aureus*, which may influence the selection of prophylactic postoperative antibiotics.[41]

The implantable pulse generator (IPG) or INS is typically placed in the lateral upper buttock in the hollow of the ilium and generally no deeper than 2 cm. Fluoroscopy can assist in appropriate placement of the implantable system to reduce risk of patient discomfort (Fig. 17.7). It may be useful to document radiologic views of the final tined lead location in both lateral and AP positions, motor and sensory responses achieved, as well as required stimulus amplitude for troubleshooting in the future.

Postoperatively, patients should be counseled to minimize vigorous activity to reduce lead migration and allow the tined lead to scar into place. There is no data to inform best practices on length of activity restriction and this is left to the discretion of the physician.

Results of Sacral Neuromodulation— Urinary Urgency Frequency (Overactive Bladder), Urgency Incontinence, and Urinary Retention

SNM is currently FDA approved in the United States for UUI, urinary urgency frequency, NOUR, and fecal incontinence. The long-term efficacy and safety of the therapy has been well established. Historically, we have seen therapeutic response rates ranging from 67% to 82% of patients with urge incontinence, 57% to 71% with urge frequency, and 68% to 71% with urinary retention.[42–45]

The InSite trial is the 5-year study evaluating the efficacy and safety of SNM for the treatment of UUI and urinary urgency frequency.[46] This was a postmarket, multicenter prospective trial where participants underwent a staged trial procedure. A total of 340 subjects were initially included and underwent stimulation testing. Of these subjects, 272 (80%) had a ≥50% improvement in symptoms and were considered responders and went on to have a permanent implant. The responders were followed out to 5 years, and the nonresponders exited the

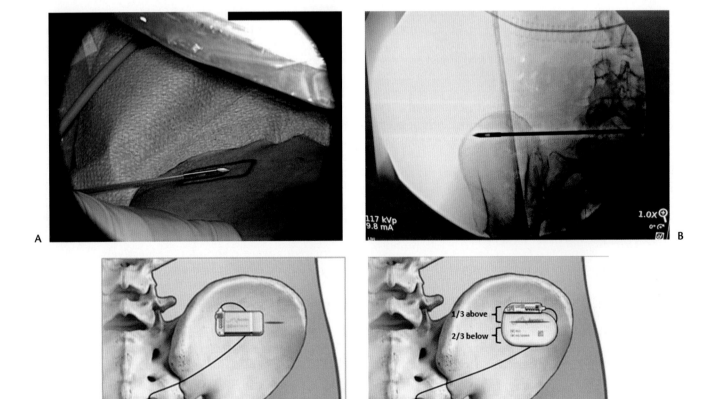

FIGURE 17.7 A: Holding the tunneling tool at the level of the intended IPG/INS pocket. **B:** Radiolucent tunneling tool allows for radiographic confirmation of appropriate IPG/INS placement. **C:** Ideally, this is in the hollow of the ilium, approximately 4 cm below the posterior iliac crest. Make skin incision (depicted by red oval) slightly lateral to IPG/INS pocket. **D:** For the nonrechargeable INS/IPG, make a horizontal incision 4 cm in length in the same location (hollow of the ilium). Create the pocket such that 1/3 is above and 2/3 below the incision and approximately 2-3 in depth. Both incisions should be closed in 2 layers.

study and were not included in the analysis. The therapeutic success rate was 82% in those available for follow-up and 67% in the modified completers analysis (all subjects who received a full system implant and had a baseline and 5-year evaluation or withdrew early due to a device-related adverse event [AE] or lack of efficacy resulting in explant) which is similar to an as-treated analysis. Participants also showed improvement in all quality of life measurements (International Consultation on Incontinence Questionnaire Overactive Bladder Quality of Life [ICIQ-OABqol] measures) which was sustained over time. The overall safety profile was favorable with only one serious device-related adverse event (SADE). Most frequent device-related AEs were undesirable change in stimulation (12%, 32 out of 272); implant site pain (7%, 20 out of 272); and implant site infection (3%, 9 out of 272). Of the 26 events of implant site pain, 13 (50%) required surgical intervention, with only 2 (7.7%) resulting in explant. Ten subjects experienced a surgical site infection, 8 of which required explantation. The overall surgical intervention rate was 13% with the most common reasons being pain at the surgical site (4%), lack/loss of efficacy (4%), and infection (3%).[46]

An additional FDA-approved therapy for UUI is intradetrusor onabotulinumtoxinA (Botox) injections, which is considered a standard third-line therapy for refractory OAB per AUA guidelines.[3] In 2016, Amundsen et al.[47] published the initial results of the Rosetta Trial, a multicenter, randomized clinical trial aimed at assessing whether intradetrusor Botox injections (200-U dose) were superior to SNM for the treatment of refractory UUI. Of the 364 women included in the study, 190 women in the Botox group had significantly less episodes of urgency incontinence than the 174 subjects in the SNM group (−3.9 vs. −3.3) at 6 months. Although this difference was statistically significant, the authors suggested that the clinical importance of this difference is unclear. The Botox group did have higher rates of both urinary tract infections and requirements for intermittent self-catheterization. The rate of SNM device removal or revision was 3%.[47]

Surgical techniques for implantation of SNM systems have evolved over time; the International Continence Society (ICS) has published on best practices for implant technique that have been outlined earlier in this chapter.[4] Recent studies that have adopted these "best practices" techniques have shown higher conversion rates to INS placement and higher longer term success rates.[48–51] In a retrospective study, Adelstein and colleagues[48] evaluated the outcomes in a contemporary cohort undergoing SNM using optimized lead placement technique. A total of 127 patients were included and their primary outcome was successful tined lead trial as determined by progression to implantation of the IPG. Conversion to IPG placement was reported as 89%. Also, through adoption of the optimized lead placement techniques, they were able to achieve motor thresholds in all four electrodes at ≤2 mA in 74% of participants.[48]

The Axonics r-SNM System is one of three currently available SNM systems. The Axonics device is a miniaturized, rechargeable, 1.5 and 3T full-body magnetic resonance imaging (MRI) conditionally safe system designed to function for a minimum of 15 years in the body. Axonics (Axonics, Irvine, CA) has conducted two clinical studies. The Treatment of Refractory Overactive Bladder with the Axonics Sacral Neuromodulation System (RELAX-OAB) study published in 2018 was the first clinical trial evaluating the new rechargeable SNM system (Axonics r-SNM System). A single-staged implant procedure was completed in 51 patients with OAB. Subjects were initially followed at 3 months using bladder diaries and quality of life questionnaires. There were 34 patients who responded to an initial "test" period. At 3-month follow-up, 31 of 34 (91%) patients were therapy responders with at least a 50% reduction in urinary voids or incontinence episodes, and these results were maintained up to 1 and 2 years with a continued success rate of 90% in the test responders and a reported satisfaction with therapy by 93% of subjects.[52–54]

The Axonics Sacral Neuromodulation System for Urinary Urgency Incontinence Treatment - Sacral Neuromodulation (ARTISAN-SNM) study was a single-arm, prospective, multicenter, pivotal study evaluating the safety and efficacy of the Axonics System for the treatment of symptoms of urgency incontinence with the primary endpoint reported at 6-month follow-up. This study included 129 patients with UUI. Each patient was implanted with a tined lead and rechargeable SNM system in a nonstaged procedure (no external trial). Responders were identified as those with at least a 50% improvement from baseline UUI episodes prior to treatment initiation at 1 month. At the 6-month follow-up, 116 out of 129 (90%) were responders with a significant reduction in daily incontinence episodes from 5.6 to 1.3.[49] The 1- and 2-year results have been published in which 89% and 88% of all implanted participants were responders respectively.[50,51] These results reflect an as-treated analysis where all subjects were included in the results. When looking at the completers (those available for follow-up) analysis ($n = 121$) at 2 years, 93% were responders and 82% had a ≥75% reduction in symptoms. All participants were able to recharge their device at 2 years, and 94% reported that the duration and frequency of recharging was acceptable. There were no SADEs at 2 years. These data support the long-term effectiveness and safety of the Axonics r-SNM System. Data from the Axonics Sacral Neuromodulation System for Urinary Urgency Incontinence Treatment (ARTISAN) study at 6, 12, and 24 months are demonstrated in Figure 17.8.[49–51]

Data on the safety and efficacy of the Medtronic Micro is not currently available.

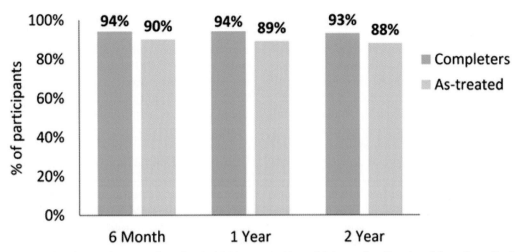

FIGURE 17.8 As-treated and completers analysis for ARTISAN at 6, 12, and 24 months. (Reprinted from Pezzella A, McCrery R, Lane F, et al. Two-year outcomes of the ARTISAN-SNM study for the treatment of urinary urgency incontinence using the Axonics rechargeable sacral neuromodulation system. *Neurourol Urodyn* 2021;40[2]:714–721.)

Results of Sacral Neuromodulation— Fecal Incontinence

SNM has been approved for fecal incontinence since 1994 in Europe and gained FDA approval in the United States in 2011. In 2008, a randomized controlled trial evaluated the efficacy of SNM versus medical therapy in patients with severe fecal incontinence. Mean incontinence episodes decreased from 9.5 to 3.1 in the SNM group without any significant improvement in fecal continence in the medical therapy group.[55] Additionally, 47.2% of patients achieved complete continence and there was a significant improvement in quality-of-life metrics in the SNM group, whereas the medical therapy group demonstrated no significant improvement in quality-of-life metrics.

In 2010, the safety and efficacy of the InterStim SNM system was evaluated for the indication of fecal incontinence.[56] This prospective, single-arm study enrolled 133 participants to undergo test stimulation. Ninety percent (120 out of 133) of subjects ultimately received the SNM implant. At the 1-year follow-up, 83% of participants had greater than 50% reduction in incontinence episodes per week compared to baseline. A 5-year follow-up study was completed that showed sustained benefit.[57,58] Although the combined device revision, explant, or replacement rate was 35.5%, the morbidity and recurrence rate of alternative therapies and surgical treatment for fecal incontinence is high.[59]

Initially, SNM was thought not to be applicable to patients with an anatomic sphincter defect. However, multiple studies have demonstrated efficacy in patients with sphincter defects up to 180°, and the therapy is currently approved for sphincter defects up to 120°.[56,60–63] SNM effectiveness was prospectively evaluated in patients with and without external anal sphincter defects and found to result in similar effectiveness defined by quality-of-life scores and functional outcomes between groups, further supporting use of SNM in patients with sphincter defects.[64] In 2012, a systematic review of the literature was completed to evaluate the clinical efficacy of SNM for fecal incontinence (FI) with the presence of a sphincter defect. Ten studies were included in the review and included 119 patients. The weighted average number of incontinence episodes decreased from 12.1 to 2.3 per week, and the Cleveland Clinic Score decreased from 16.5 to 3.8 after SNM implantation.[65] Efficacy of sphincteroplasty versus SNM in patients with anal sphincter lesions has also been prospectively evaluated with no significant difference in clinical or anorectal manometry parameters posttreatment, providing further support for SNM as a reasonable approach to fecal incontinence with sphincter lesions.[66]

Per a recent best practice statement, SNM should be considered a second-line therapy for fecal incontinence with or without anal sphincter muscle defect. The minimally invasive, safe, and efficacious SNM therapy may be a reasonable alternative option for treatment of fecal incontinence, especially for patients with combined urinary and bowel disorders.[4]

Sacral Neuromodulation in Pregnancy

Although no negative effects of SNM have been reported on the mother (patient), fetus, or SNM device during pregnancy, implantation of a new SNM device during pregnancy is currently contraindicated.[4] A recent study published in 2017 evaluated the effects of SNM in pregnancy and the impact of both vaginal delivery and cesarean section on SNM function.[67] This study included 22 patients (26 pregnancies) with SNM.

In 8 of the pregnancies, the SNM device activation was maintained throughout the pregnancy. The device was deactivated in the other 18 pregnancies (typically in the first trimester). Of these pregnancies with SNM device deactivation, 7 had recurrent urinary tract infections, 1 had pyelonephritis, and 2 patients requested reactivation. Two infants, from the same mother, had pilonidal sinus and motor tic disorder. Of the reported delivery outcomes (25 deliveries), 16 patients underwent cesarean delivery and 9 underwent vaginal delivery (2 with operative vaginal delivery). Regarding the effect on the SNM device, 60% of devices were functioning after delivery. SNM dysfunction was noted in 32% of deliveries; 3 after vaginal delivery and 4 after cesarean section. One episode of lead wire displacement after operative vaginal delivery with recurrence of fecal incontinence was reported. Overall, 4 patients required device reprogramming. The decision to deactivate or maintain SNM device function during pregnancy should be individualized, along with the decision for mode of delivery by weighing the risks and benefits. Although the sample sizes were small, there was no significant difference in SNM dysfunction between vaginal or cesarean deliveries. This limited evidence suggests that SNM during pregnancy may be safe for the mother and fetus. Future studies, ideally a registry to track these cases, may provide further guidance.

Complications

AEs related to SNM are typically not considered serious and are generally treatable. The most common complications include need for revision/reprogramming of device, implant site infection, lead migration, lead fracture, and implant site pain.[46,50,68–70]

Revision, reprogramming, and pain

Revision rates and device-related AEs are now lower (3% to 16%) with the tined lead wire than reported in previous studies.[69,71] In a detailed analysis of the AEs at 1-year follow-up in the InSite trial, the authors reported that device-related AEs occurred in 30% of subjects, with only one considered serious. The most frequent device-related AEs were undesirable change in stimulation at 12%, implant site pain at 7%, and implant site infection at 3%. Of the 26 events of implant site pain, 13 required surgical intervention, with only 2 resulting in explant. The overall surgical intervention rate was 13% with the most common reasons being pain at the surgical site (4%), lack/loss of efficacy (4%), and infection (3%). They concluded that even though an overall 30% complication rate was reported, most AEs were minor and were resolved without surgical intervention.[69] At the 5-year follow-up in the InSite trial, Siegel et al.[46] reported that 22% of patients needed reprogramming

within 5 years of implantation due to decreased efficacy, pain, or change in stimulation. Of all 272 implanted subjects, surgical intervention was performed in 84 subjects (31%) due to an AE, and the permanent explantation rate was 19.1%.[46] Patients with potential device-related pain or efficacy decline should be evaluated in a clinic setting and device interrogation by a health care provider performed.[4] Turning off the device can assist in differentiation between pain at the IPG site versus painful stimulation versus pain from an alternate origin. In the case of painful stimulation, changing the electrode configuration or magnitude of stimulation may prevent the need for lead revision. Patients should try each new program for at least 1 week if tolerable. Patients with persistent pain following reprogramming should undergo radiographic imaging for evaluation of lead migration or fracture. IPG device site pain may require explant or device location revision.[4]

Infection

The most significant surgical complication following SNM device placement is infection. In the case of implant infection, ICS best practices recommend explantation of both lead and IPG along with debridement of the wound.[4] A 3-month waiting period prior to reimplantation should be considered along with reimplant on the contralateral side.[4] Infection rates have been reported to occur between 1% and 10% of cases.[51,68–70] A recent multicenter retrospective case-control study reported an infection rate of 1.97% with the most common causal organism being methicillin-resistant *S. aureus* (38%). Risk factors for infection-related explant were a deep pocket (>3 cm) and postoperative hematomas, which supports the importance of pocket depth of <2.5 cm and intraoperative hemostasis.[72] Preoperative home chlorhexidine washing (CHW) has been shown to significantly reduce the risk of infection, with a reported rate of 7.4% without CHW to 1.7% with CHW.[41] For a staged approach, AUA best practices recommend a first-degree cephalosporin within 60 minutes of incision for both stages 1 and 2 to reduce infection rates.[40] These evidence-based suggestions and procedure techniques have been reported to reduce infection rates to less than 2% in multiple institutions.[40,71]

Cost-effectiveness

SNM has been proven to be a cost-effective method for both urinary disorders and bowel dysfunction. In 2007, a retrospective review compared cost-related treatment of urinary disorders before and after placement of the InterStim SNM implant. After implantation, the mean physician visit number for urinary symptoms decreased by 2.2 visits per year and resulted in a 73% reduction in annual office expenses. Drug costs were also evaluated and were significantly reduced along with costs of therapeutic and diagnostic procedures per patient. Drug expenditures were reduced by 30%, and a total 92% reduction in combined cost of visits and procedures was noted.[73] Efficacy and cost of SNM for treatment of fecal incontinence was studied in the Netherlands in 2012. When added to the surgical algorithm, SNM therapy significantly reduced costs and increased treatment efficacy for fecal incontinence.[74]

Chughtai et al.[74] aimed to compare safety and cost of SNM and onabotulinumtoxinA as third-line therapies for urinary disorders in an all-inclusive, population-based cohort to assess "real-world" performance of both therapies. Although the SNM cohort had significantly lower complication rates (lower number of emergency room visits, urinary retention, urinary tract infection, hematuria), the overall 1- and 3-year cost of SNM was higher.[75] However, this study did not investigate potential long-term cost savings of SNM treatment, which is particularly important given the new 15-year rechargeable SNM devices. Potential cost savings of a rechargeable SNM device over a 15-year horizon have been projected to result in savings of up to 12 billion dollars for the US health care system.[76] Recently, cost savings and outcomes of a single-staged SNM implant procedure have been calculated. The one-stage SNM procedure has been shown to be cost-effective if the conversion rate to long-term implant is greater than 61%. Anger et al.[76] performed an analysis comparing the cost of standard two-stage SNS device placement to that of a combined one-stage placement using a Markov chain model. Their results suggest that in patients and providers with a successful conversion rate greater than 71%, placement of an SNS device in a one-stage procedure would be cost-effective.[77] This is further supported in a study by Lee and colleagues[77] evaluating the single-staged approach. In their study, 15 of 16 (94%) patients had a greater than 50% or greater improvement from baseline and were considered a success for long-term implant which they estimated to provide a total cost savings of $85,366 ($P < .01$) per patient.

This study suggests that a single-staged approach is cost-effective, reasonable, and may have additional benefits of patient satisfaction, along with potential for reduced infection rates and patient time off work.[78] Additionally, in the ARTISAN trial (Axonics) participants underwent a nonstaged procedure, meaning they went onto to full implant without an external trial period. The test responder rate in this study was 88% which is much higher than the 61% to 71% threshold identified as the tipping point for being cost-effective in support of a nonstaged procedure.[49,77,78]

Technological Innovations

Magnetic resonance imaging

One of the biggest unmet needs in SNM was the inability to have a full-body MRI scan. Axonics was the first SNM device to have 1.5 and 3T full-body MRI conditional labeling. Both Axonics R15 and F15 SNM systems have MRI conditional labeling. Medtronic, with the introduction of their SureScan technology, also has 1.5 and 3T full-body conditional labeling for their InterStim II, InterStim Micro, and InterStimX systems. When considering MRI labeling, there are three categories: MRI safe (poses no known hazard in the MRI environment, i.e., a foley catheter), MRI conditional (where conditions need to be met to complete the scan), and MRI unsafe (not approved). A comparison of the Axonics system versus the Medtronic system conditions is summarized in Figure 17.9. Both systems have a maximum continuous scan time of 30 minutes and a wait time of 5 minutes.

Constant current

Implanted neurostimulators can deliver electrical stimulation either as constant voltage (CV) stimulation or constant current (CC) stimulation. With electrical stimulation, the degree of activation of a nerve is related to the applied current, and the use of a CC or CV system

1.5T		Scanner Strength	3T	
Axonics	Medtronic	**Manufacturers**	Axonics	Medtronic
2.0	2.0	**SAR Limit (W/kg)**	1.2	1.4
Not Specified	4.0	**B1+rms Limit (µT)**	1.7	2.0
30 min	30 min	**Allowed Continuous Scan Time**	30 min	30 min
5 min	5 min	**Wait Time**	5 min	5 min

FIGURE 17.9 Whole body scan MRI conditions for the Axonics and Medtronic systems. (Reprinted from Axonics, Inc.)

has different implications on the control and management of the applied stimulation current.[79,80] With a CV system, stimulation voltage is programmed to a set degree, and the current delivered to the patient will vary in response to impedance changes. For example, if the tissue impedance increases, the current delivered to the nerve will decrease based on Ohm law which is voltage equals current × impedance (V = IR). With a CC system, the stimulation current is programmed to a set degree, and when impedance changes occur, the device adjusts voltage automatically, so the current delivered to the patient stays constant.[81,82] Recent literature has suggested that "as electrode impedances change over time, such systems [constant current] may provide more robust efficacy or require less reprogramming than 'constant voltage' systems."[82]

We also know from several studies that impedance increases out to 6 months following placement of a lead for an SNM procedure (InSite, RELAX-OAB, ARTISAN), as summarized in Figure 17.10.[49,51,52]

The Axonics R15 (rechargeable) and F15 (nonrechargeable) SNM systems along with the Medtronic InterStim Micro (rechargeable) are CC systems that automatically change the voltage to overcome tissue impedance changes without the patient having to manually change any parameters on their device. The Medtronic InterStim II is voltage controlled, whereas the InterStimX is constant current controlled. The voltage-controlled InterStim II does not automatically overcome changes in tissue impedance. In this system, as impedance increases, voltage stays the same, and therefore, the amount of current the patient receives decreases. The patient would be required to manually increase the voltage in order to maintain the same current.

An analogy that may make it easier to understand is the cruise control in a car. If you have cruise control and you set the car to a certain speed (current) then when you encounter a hill (impedance) the car will automatically increase the output without having to manually step on the accelerator. This is analogous to a constant current system. In a car that doesn't have cruise control, when it encounters a hill, the driver has to manually step on the gas to maintain the same speed (current). This is analogous to a voltage-controlled system. Since the constant current system automatically increases the voltage when increased impedance is encountered, this infers the potential advantage of being able to avoid patients having to manually adjust the voltage output to maintain the same current, thus keeping them in the therapeutic zone more consistently.

FUTURE DIRECTIONS

Emerging studies show that SNM may be a viable and effective therapeutic option for patients with IC and chronic pelvic pain.[83,84] Targets of neuromodulation are also expanding; specifically, more peripheral nerves have been studied including the pudendal and tibial nerves (via implantable tibial nerve stimulation, eCoin, BlueWind RENOVA, Micron Medical's PROTECT PNS trial).[85] Pudendal neuromodulation has been shown to be potentially even more effective than modulation of the sacral nerve for treatment of urinary urgency/frequency, bowel dysfunction, and pelvic pain.[86] Broadening of nerve targets and indications for neuromodulation creates vast opportunities for improvement in care for patients with pelvic floor disorders.

References

1. Spinelli M, Sievert KD. Latest technologic and surgical developments in using InterStim therapy for sacral neuromodulation: Impact on treatment success and safety. *Eur Urol* 2008;54(6):1287–1296.

2. Cameron AP, Anger JT, Madison R, et al; for Urologic Diseases in America Project. Battery explantation after sacral neuromodulation in the Medicare population. *Neurourol Urodyn* 2013;32(3):238–241.

3. Lightner DJ, Gomelsky A, Souter L, et al. Diagnosis and treatment of overactive bladder (non-neurogenic) in adults: AUA/SUFU guideline amendment 2019. *J Urol* 2019;202(3):558–563.

4. Goldman HB, Lloyd JC, Noblett KL, et al. International Continence Society best practice statement for use of sacral neuromodulation. *Neurourol Urodyn* 2018;37(5):1823–1848.

5. Engeler DS, Meyer D, Abt D, et al. Sacral neuromodulation for the treatment of neurogenic lower urinary tract dysfunction caused by multiple sclerosis: A single-centre prospective series. *BMC Urol* 2015;15:105.

6. Andretta E, Simeone C, Ostardo E, et al. Usefulness of sacral nerve modulation in a series of multiple sclerosis patients with bladder dysfunction. *J Neurol Sci* 2014;347(1–2):257–261.

7. Minardi D, Muzzonigro G. Sacral neuromodulation in patients with multiple sclerosis. *World J Urol* 2012;30(1):123–128.

8. Chaabane W, Guillotreau J, Castel-Lacanal E, et al. Sacral neuromodulation for treating neurogenic bladder dysfunction: Clinical

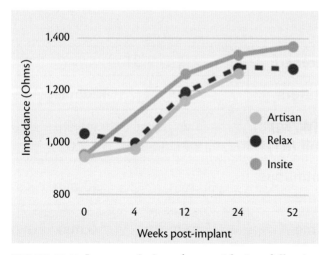

FIGURE 17.10 Increases in impedance with time following implant of an SNM lead. (Courtesy of Axonics, Inc.)

and urodynamic study. *Neurourol Urodyn* 2011;30(4):547–550.

9. Marinkovic SP, Gillen LM. Sacral neuromodulation for multiple sclerosis patients with urinary retention and clean intermittent catheterization. *Int Urogynecol J* 2010;21(2):223–228.

10. Wallace PA, Lane FL, Noblett KL. Sacral nerve neuromodulation in patients with underlying neurologic disease. *Am J Obstet Gynecol* 2007;197(1):96.e1–96.e5.

11. Peters KM, Kandagatla P, Killinger KA, et al. Clinical outcomes of sacral neuromodulation in patients with neurologic conditions. *Urology* 2013;81(4):738–743.

12. Ghazwani YQ, Elkelini MS, Hassouna MM. Efficacy of sacral neuromodulation in treatment of bladder pain syndrome: Long-term follow-up. *Neurourol Urodyn* 2011;30(7):1271–1275.

13. Maher CF, Carey MP, Dwyer PL, et al. Percutaneous sacral nerve root neuromodulation for intractable interstitial cystitis. *J Urol* 2001;165(3):884–886.

14. Comiter CV. Sacral neuromodulation for the symptomatic treatment of refractory interstitial cystitis: A prospective study. *J Urol* 2003;169:1369–1373.

15. Peters KM, Konstandt D. Sacral neuromodulation decreases narcotic requirements in refractory interstitial cystitis. *BJU Int* 2004;93(6):777–779.

16. Wang J, Chen Y, Chen J, et al. Sacral neuromodulation for refractory bladder pain syndrome/interstitial cystitis: A global systematic review and meta-analysis. *Sci Rep* 2017;7(1):11031.

17. Hanno PM, Erickson D, Moldwin R, et al; for American Urological Association. Diagnosis and treatment of interstitial cystitis/bladder pain syndrome: AUA guideline amendment. *J Urol* 2015;193(5):1545–1553.

18. Dinning PG, Fuentealba SE, Kennedy ML, et al. Sacral nerve stimulation induces pan-colonic propagating pressure waves and increases defecation frequency in patients with slow-transit constipation. *Colorectal Dis* 2007;9:123–132.

19. Dinning PG, Hunt LM, Arkwright JW, et al. Pancolonic motor response to subsensory and suprasensory sacral nerve stimulation in patients with slow-transit constipation. *Br J Surg* 2012;99(7):1002–1010.

20. di Visconte MS, Pasquali A, Cipolat Mis T, et al. Sacral nerve stimulation in slow-transit constipation: Effectiveness at 5-year follow-up. *Int J Colorectal Dis* 2019;34(9):1529–1540.

21. Sharma A, Bussen D, Herold A, et al. Review of sacral neuromodulation for management of constipation. *Surg Innov* 2013;20(6):614–624.

22. Chancellor MB, Chartier-Kastler EJ. Principles of sacral nerve stimulation (SNS) for the treatment of bladder and urethral sphincter dysfunctions. *Neuromodulation* 2000;3(1):16–26.

23. DeGroat WC, Saum WR. Synaptic transmission in parasympathetic ganglia in the urinary bladder of the cat. *J Physiol* 1976;256(1):137–158.

24. De Groat WC. Mechanisms underlying recurrent inhibition in the sacral parasympathetic outflow to the urinary bladder. *J Physiol* 1976;257:503–513.

25. De Groat WC, Ryall RW. The identification and characteristics of sacral parasympathetic preganglionic neurones. *J Physiol* 1968;196(3):563–577.

26. De Groat WC, Ryall RW. Recurrent inhibition in sacral parasympathetic pathways to the bladder. *J Physiol* 1968;196(3):579–591.

27. DeGroat WC. Inhibition and excitation of sacral parasympathetic neurons by visceral and cutaneous stimuli in the cat. *Brain Res* 1971;33(2):499–503.

28. DeGroat WC. Changes in the organization of the micturition reflex pathway of the cat after transection of the spinal cord. *Exp Neurol* 1981;71:22.

29. Blok BF, Groen J, Bosch JL, et al. Different brain effects during chronic and acute sacral neuromodulation in urge incontinent patients with implanted neurostimulators. *BJU Int* 2006;98(6):1238–1243.

30. Zhang F, Zhao S, Shen B, et al. Neural pathways involved in sacral neuromodulation of reflex bladder activity in cats. *Am J Physiol Renal Physiol* 2013;304(6):F710.

31. Hassouna MM, Siegel SW, Anyehoult AA, et al. Sacral neuromodulation in the treatment of urgency-frequency symptoms: A multicenter study on efficacy and safety. *J Urol* 2000;163:1849–1854.

32. Gupta A, Kinman C, Hobson DTG, et al. The impact of fluoroscopy during percutaneous nerve evaluation on subsequent implantation of a sacral neuromodulator among women with pelvic floor disorders: A randomized, noninferiority trial. *Neuromodulation* 2020;23(8):1164–1171.

33. Benson JT. Sacral nerve stimulation results may be improved by electrodiagnostic techniques. *Int Urogynecol J Pelvic Floor Dysfunct* 2000;11(6):352–357.

34. Jacobs SA, Lane FL, Osann KE, et al. Randomized prospective crossover study of InterStim lead wire placement with curved versus straight stylet. *Neurourol Urodyn* 2014;33(5):488–492.

35. Vaganée D, Kessler TM, Van de Borne S, et al. Sacral neuromodulation using the standardized tined lead implantation technique with a curved vs a straight stylet: 2-year clinical outcomes and sensory responses to lead stimulation. *BJU Int* 2019;123(5A):E7–E13.

36. Siegel S, Noblett K, Mangel J, et al. Results of a prospective, randomized, multicenter study evaluating sacral neuromodulation with InterStim therapy compared to standard medical therapy at 6-months in subjects with mild symptoms of overactive bladder. *Neurourol Urodyn* 2015;34(3):224–230.

37. Wagner L, Alonso S, Le Normand L, et al. Unilateral versus bilateral sacral neuromodulation test in the treatment of refractory idiopathic overactive bladder: A randomized controlled pilot trial. *Neurourol Urodyn* 2020;39(8):2230–2237.

38. Borawski KM, Foster RT, Webster GD, et al. Predicting implantation with a neuromodulator using two different test stimulation techniques: A prospective randomized study in urge incontinent women. *Neurourol Urodyn* 2007;26(1):14–18.

39. Banakhar M, Hassouna M. Percutaneous nerve evaluation test versus staged test trials for sacral neuromodulation: Sensitivity, specificity, and predictive values of each technique. *Int Neurourol J* 2016;20(3):250–254.

40. Lightner DJ, Wymer K, Sanchez J, et al. Best practice statement on urologic procedures and antimicrobial prophylaxis. *J Urol* 2020;203(2):351–356.

41. Brueseke T, Livingston B, Warda H, et al. Risk factors for surgical site infection in patients undergoing sacral nerve modulation therapy. *Female Pelvic Med Reconstr Surg* 2015;21(4):198–204.

42. Brazzelli M, Murray A, Fraser C. Efficacy and safety of sacral nerve stimulation for urinary urge incontinence: A systematic review. *J Urol* 2006;175(3 pt 1):835–841.

43. van Kerrebroeck PE, van Voskuilen AC, Heesakkers JP, et al. Results of sacral neuromodulation therapy for urinary voiding dysfunction: Outcomes of a prospective, worldwide clinical study. *J Urol* 2007;178(5):2029–2034.

44. Jonas U, Fowler CJ, Chancellor MB, et al. Efficacy of sacral nerve stimulation for urinary retention: Results 18 months after implantation. *J Urol* 2001;165(1):15–19.

45. High RA, Winkelman W, Panza J, et al. Sacral neuromodulation for symptomatic chronic urinary retention in females: Do age and comorbidities make a difference? *Int Urogynecol J* 2020;31(10):2703–2715.

46. Siegel S, Noblett K, Mangel J, et al. Five-year follow-up results of a prospective, multicenter study of patients with overactive bladder treated with sacral neuromodulation. *J Urol* 2018;199(1), 229–236.

47. Amundsen CL, Richter HE, Menefee SA, et al. OnabotulinumtoxinA vs sacral neuromodulation on refractory urgency urinary incontinence in women: A randomized clinical trial. *JAMA* 2016;316(13):1366–1374.

48. Adelstein SA, Lee W, Gioia K, et al. Outcomes in a contemporary cohort undergoing sacral neuromodulation using optimized lead placement technique. *Neurourol Urodyn* 2019;38(6):1595–1601.

49. McCrery R, Lane F, Benson K, et al. Treatment of urinary urgency incontinence using a rechargeable SNM system: 6-month results of the ARTISAN-SNM study. *J Urol* 2020;203(1):185–192.

50. Benson K, McCrery R, Taylor C, et al. One-year outcomes of the ARTISAN-SNM study with the Axonics System for the treatment of urinary urgency incontinence. *Neurourol Urodyn* 2020;39(5):1482–1488.

51. Pezzella A, McCrery R, Lane F, et al. Two-year outcomes of the ARTISAN-SNM study for the treatment of urinary urgency incontinence using the Axonics rechargeable sacral neuromodulation system. *Neurourol Urodyn* 2021;40(2):714–721.

52. Blok B, Van Kerrebroeck P, de Wachter S, et al. A prospective, multicenter study of a novel, miniaturized rechargeable sacral neuromodulation system: 12-month results from the RELAX-OAB study. *Neurourol Urodyn* 2019;38(2):689–695.

53. Blok B, Van Kerrebroeck P, de Wachter S, et al. Three-month clinical results with a rechargeable sacral neuromodulation system for the treatment of overactive bladder. *Neurourol Urodyn* 2018;37(suppl 2):S9–S16.

54. Blok B, Van Kerrebroeck P, de Wachter S, et al. Two-year safety and efficacy outcomes for the treatment of overactive bladder using a long-lived rechargeable sacral neuromodulation system. *Neurourol Urodyn* 2020;39(4):1108–1114.

55. Tjandra JJ, Chan MK, Yeh CH, et al. Sacral nerve stimulation is more effective than optimal medical therapy for severe fecal incontinence: A randomized, controlled study. *Dis Colon Rectum* 2008;51:494–502.

56. Wexner SD, Coller JA, Devroede G, et al. Sacral nerve stimulation for fecal incontinence: Results of a 120-patient prospective multicenter study. *Ann Surg* 2010;251:441–449.

57. Mellgren A, Wexner SD, Coller JA, et al. Long-term efficacy and safety of sacral nerve stimulation for fecal incontinence. *Dis Colon Rectum* 2011;54:1065–1075.

58. Hull T, Giese C, Wexner SD, et al. Long-term durability of sacral nerve stimulation therapy for chronic fecal incontinence. *Dis Colon Rectum* 2013;56:234–245.

59. Madoff RD, Parker SC, Varma MG, et al. Faecal incontinence in adults. *Lancet* 2004;364:621–632.

60. Leroi AM, Parc Y, Lehur PA, et al. Efficacy of sacral nerve stimulation for fecal incontinence: Results of a multicenter double-blind crossover study. *Ann Surg* 2005;242(5):662–669.

61. Hetzer FH, Hahnloser D, Clavien PA, et al. Quality of life and morbidity after permanent sacral nerve stimulation for fecal incontinence. *Arch Surg* 2007;142(1):8–13.

62. Chan MK, Tjandra JJ. Sacral nerve stimulation for fecal incontinence: External anal sphincter defect vs. intact anal sphincter. *Dis Colon Rectum* 2008;51(7):1015–1025.

63. Boyle DJ, Knowles CH, Lunniss PJ, et al. Efficacy of sacral nerve stimulation for fecal incontinence in patients with anal sphincter defects. *Dis Colon Rectum* 2009;52(7):1234–1239.

64. Ratto C, Litta F, Parello A, et al. Sacral nerve stimulation in faecal incontinence associated with an anal sphincter lesion: A systematic review. *Colorectal Dis* 2012;14(6):e297–e304.

65. Ratto C, Litta F, Parello A, et al. Sacral nerve stimulation is a valid approach in fecal incontinence due to sphincter lesions when compared to sphincter repair. *Dis Colon Rectum* 2010;53(3):264–272.

66. Mahran A, Soriano A, Safwat AS, et al. The effect of sacral neuromodulation on pregnancy: A systematic review. *Int Urogynecol J* 2017;28:1357–1365.

67. Wexner SD, Hull T, Edden Y, et al. Infection rates in a large investigational trial of sacral nerve stimulation for fecal incontinence. *J Gastrointest Surg* 2010;14:1081–1089.

68. Noblett K, Benson K, Kreder K. Detailed analysis of adverse events and surgical interventions in a large prospective trial of sacral neuromodulation therapy for overactive bladder patients. *Neurourol Urodyn* 2017;36(4):1136–1139.

69. Siddiqui NY, Wu JM, Amundsen CL. Efficacy and adverse events of sacral nerve stimulation for overactive bladder: A systematic review. *Neurourol Urodyn* 2010;29(suppl 1):S18–S23.

70. Myer ENB, Petrikovets A, Slocum PD, et al. Risk factors for explantation due to infection after sacral neuromodulation: A multicenter retrospective case-control study. *Am J Obstet Gynecol* 2018;219(1):78.e1–78.e9.

71. Aboseif SR, Kim DH, Rieder JM, et al. Sacral neuromodulation: Cost considerations and clinical benefits. *Urology* 2007;70:1069–1073.

72. Pettit P. Current opinion: Complications and troubleshooting of sacral neuromodulation. *Int Urogynecol J* 2010;21(suppl 2):S491–496.

73. van Wunnik BP, Visschers RG, van Asselt AD, et al. Cost-effectiveness analysis of sacral neuromodulation for faecal incontinence in The Netherlands. *Colorectal Dis* 2012;14(12):e807–e814.

74. Chughtai B, Clemens JQ, Thomas D, et al. Real world performance of sacral neuromodulation and onabotulinumtoxinA for overactive bladder: Focus on safety and cost. *J Urol* 2020;203(1):179–184.

75. Noblett KL, Dmochowski RR, Vasavada SP, et al. Cost profiles and budget impact of rechargeable versus non-rechargeable sacral neuromodulation devices in the treatment of overactive bladder syndrome. *Neurourol Urodyn* 2017;36(3):727–733.

76. Anger JT, Cameron AP, Madison R, et al; for Urologic Diseases in America Project. Predictors of implantable pulse generator placement after sacral neuromodulation: Who does better? *Neuromodulation* 2014;17(4):381–384.

77. Lee W, Artenstein D, Tenggardjaja CF, et al. Single institutional experience with single stage sacral neuromodulation: Cost savings and outcomes in a contemporary case series. *J Urol* 2020;203(3):604–610.

78. Lempka SF, Johnson MD, Miocinovic S, et al. Current-controlled deep brain stimulation reduces in vivo voltage fluctuations observed during voltage-controlled stimulation. *Clin Neurophysiol* 2010;121(12):2128–2133.

79. Zander HJ, Graham RD, Anaya CJ, et al. Anatomical and technical factors affecting the neural response to epidural spinal cord stimulation. *J Neural Eng* 2020;17(3):036019.

80. Merrill DR, Bikson M, Jefferys JG. Electrical stimulation of excitable tissue: Design of efficacious and safe protocols. *J Neurosci Methods* 2005;141(2):171–198.

81. Merrill DR, Tresco PA. Impedance characterization of microarray recording electrodes in vitro. *IEEE Trans Biomed Eng* 2005;52(11):1960–1965.

82. Gill G, Gustafson K. Effects of tissue impedance on neural activation using "constant-current" versus "constant-voltage" neuromodulation—benchtop study. Poster presented at: SUFU (Society of Urodynamics, Female Pelvic Medicine & Urogenital Reconstruction) Annual Meeting, 2019.

83. Peters KM. Neuromodulation for the treatment of refractory interstitial cystitis. *Rev Urol* 2002 ;4(suppl 1):S36–S43.

84. Mahran A, Baaklini G, Hassani D, et al. Sacral neuromodulation treating chronic pelvic pain: A meta-analysis and systematic review of the literature. *Int Urogynecol J* 2019;30(7): 1023–1035.

85. Yamashiro J, de Riese W, de Riese C. New implantable tibial nerve stimulation devices: Review of published clinical results in comparison to established neuromodulation devices. *Res Rep Urol* 2019;11:351–357.

86. Peters KM, Feber KM, Bennett RC. Sacral versus pudendal nerve stimulation for voiding dysfunction: A prospective, single-blinded, randomized, crossover trial. *Neurourol Urodyn* 2005;24(7):643–647.

CHAPTER 18

PRINCIPLES OF NEUROPELVEOLOGY

Marc Possover

Introduction

Neuropelveology is a new area in medicine which deals with the diagnosis and treatment of pathologies and dysfunctions of pelvic nerves. Neuropelveology encompasses knowledge that is for the most part already known but scattered in various other specialties. Neuropelveology brings all this knowledge into one. Since the establishment of the International Society of Neuropelveology, this discipline is experiencing a growing interest. In neuropelveology, fields of indications expand from management of pelvic neuropathic pain to pelvic nerve stimulation for management of pelvic organ dysfunctions and loss of functions in spinal cord–injured patients.

The potential novel treatment options not only have therapeutic value but also have preventive advantages, not only in the field of therapeutic medicine but also in preventive medicine with even future applications up to the "Mars mission" project.

The incidence of pelvic nerve pathologies is widely underestimated because of lack of awareness that such lesions may exist, lack of diagnosis and acceptance, and lack of declaration and report of such lesions. The most probable reasons for omission of the pelvic nerves in medicine are the complexity of the pelvic nerve system, the difficulties of etiologic diagnosis, and, probably the main reason, the limitations of access to the pelvic nerves for neurophysiologic explorations and neurosurgical treatments. Neurosurgical procedure techniques are well established in nerve lesions of the upper limb, but pelvic retroperitoneal areas and surgeries to the pelvic nerves are still unusual for neurosurgeons. Few open surgical approaches to the sacral plexus have been described by neurosurgeons for treatment of traumatic pelvic plexopathies, but these approaches are laborious and invasive, offer only limited access to the different pelvic regions, and expose patients to risk of severe vascular complications. Techniques of nerve neuromodulation to control pelvic pain syndromes and dysfunctions are for the same reasons limited to spinal cord and sacral nerve roots stimulation that considerably restrict their indications and effectiveness.

The use of the endoscope in combination with neurofunctional surgical procedures to the pelvic nerves proved to be a decisive advantage in this development,[1-4] and in fact, it was the beginning of a new area in medicine: the neuropelveology.[5-7] This specialty combines the knowledge required for a proper neurologic diagnosis, which is essential for an adapted treatment of intractable pelvic neuropathies. The concept of "neuropelveology," the first medical practice focused on the pathologies of the pelvic nervous system was introduced more than 20 years ago by Possover. Since then, neuropelveology has established itself as a specialty in its own right, promulgated by the creation of the International Society of Neuropelveology in 2014.

Neuropelveology presents three consecutive aspects: the diagnostic stage followed by the therapeutic stage and the posttherapeutic follow-up of the patient.

The effort of neuropelveology focuses on these four major areas:

1. Diagnosis and treatment of pelvic neuropathic pain, with new techniques including laparoscopic pelvic nerves decompression and neurolysis
2. Treatment of pelvic organ dysfunction includes the stimulation of the genital nerves—GNS therapy
3. The technique of Laparoscopic Implantation Of Neuroprothesis to the pelvic nerves—LION procedure—for recovery of lost functions, especially in the spinal cord–injured patients and postsurgery pelvic nerve damage
4. The stimulation of the pelvic autonomic nervous system for prevention and/or treatment of general medical conditions such as osteoporosis, some cardiovascular diseases, or control of sarcopenia—process of aging

The diagnostic stage uses its own instruments and an anamnesis covering many aspects from gynecology, urology, orthopedics, pelvic vessel pathology, and psychology of chronic pain and parapleology. The clinical examination combines the examination of the pelvic organs and their function, the neurologic examination of the musculoskeletal system with a neuropelveologic examination, and the palpation of the pelvic nerves by vaginal or rectal route.[8] Because somatic, neuropathic pain is more specific, neuropelveologic workup typically allows for specific diagnosis of the lesion site in the pelvic nerves.

Neuropelveology employs various medical treatments and surgical treatments of the pelvic nerves.

The latter includes neurosurgical techniques ranging from decompression, neurolysis, reconstruction, and even nerve resection (e.g., sciatic nerve endometriosis) to pelvic neurofunctional surgery.

Because the pelvic nerves contain not only afferent but also efferent fibers involved in sexual function, voiding and storage of the bladder, as well as defecatory function, pelvic nerve damage lead to pelvic organ dysfunctions.

PELVIC NEUROFUNCTIONAL ANATOMY

The innervation of the pelvis is very complex. Sensory and motor nerves are found in the pelvis; the sensory nerve fibers send information to the brain (afferent), or vice versa (efferent), and the motor nerves divide into the following nerves:

- The **somatic** nerves, which innervate the skeletal muscles (voluntary, or red, muscles). These nerves originate in the ventral roots of the spinal cord. The main somatic pelvic nerves involved in pelvic organ functions originate from the sacral plexus and its branches.

- The **autonomic** nerves, which innervate the glands and the smooth muscles (involuntary, or white muscles). These nerves divide into sympathetic nerves (ventral roots of spinal nerves T1–L2) and the parasympathetic nerves (ventral roots of spinal nerves S2–S4/S5).

This division is of great importance in understanding neural anatomy and is essential in understanding management of pelvic pain conditions in neuropelveology. Neuropathic pain as well as functional disorders of the pelvic organs must be considered together. In daily medical practice, the more information there is, the more confusing the situation usually becomes. In neuropelveology, it is exactly the opposite: The more information there is, the easier it is to determine the affected nerve(s) and the anatomical location of the damage. This reminds us of the crucial importance of a thorough history where all the information, even the smallest detail is important.

The sacral plexus (Fig. 18.1) is formed from the lumbosacral trunk and the ventral rami of sacral nerve roots S1–S4/S5. L5 is mainly involved in the dorsal flexion of the ankle (lesion → foot drop), whereas S1 mediates

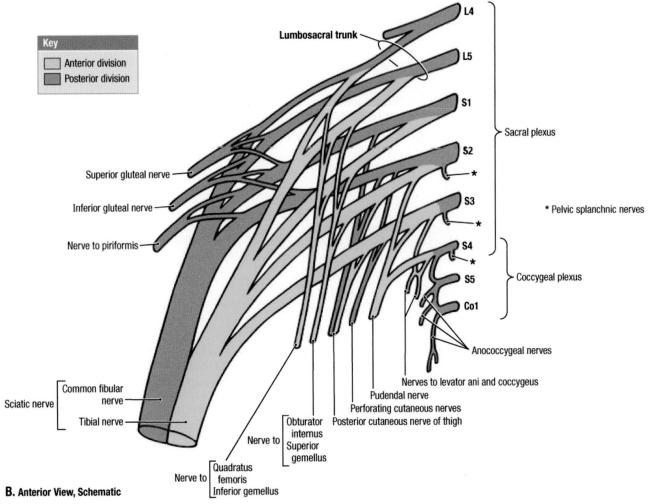

FIGURE 18.1 Sacral plexus. (Reprinted from Agur AM, Dalley AF. *Grant's atlas of anatomy*, 15th ed. Philadelphia: Wolters Kluwer, 2021.)

the plantar flexion of the ankle and consequently the Achilles reflex.

If laparoscopic electrical stimulation of the sacral nerves root is used intraoperatively via laparoscopic neuro-navigation technique, S4 electrical stimulation does not produce any motoric action in the lower extremities, whereas stimulation of S3 nerves is confirmed visually by a deepening and flattening of the buttock groove (bellows reflex/anal wink) as well as a plantar dorsiflexion of the large toe and, to a lesser extent, of the smaller toes. Stimulation of S2 produces an outward rotation of the leg and plantar flexion of the foot as well as a clamp-like squeeze of the anal sphincter from the anterior to the posterior.

The branches of the sacral plexus are:

- The **superior gluteal nerve** emerges from the lumbosacral trunk about 2 cm above the greater sciatic notch and leaves the pelvis through the greater sciatic foramen above the piriformis, accompanied by the superior gluteal artery and the superior gluteal vein. This small nerve is extremely important for the stability of the pelvis because it supplies the gluteus medius, the gluteus minimus, and the tensor fasciae latae muscles.
- The **pudendal nerve** is a sensory and somatic nerve that originates from the ventral rami of the 2nd to 4th (and occasionally 5th) sacral nerve roots. After branching from the sacral plexus just proximal to the sacrospinous ligament, the nerve leaves the pelvis through the greater sciatic notch, reenters the pelvic cavity through the lesser sciatic notch, and finally travels to three main regions: the gluteal region, the pudendal canal, and the perineum. It accompanies the internal pudendal vessels upward and forward along the lateral wall of the ischiorectal fossa, being contained in a sheath of the obturator fascia termed the pudendal canal (Alcock canal). The pudendal nerve gives off three distal branches: the **inferior rectal nerve**, the **perineal nerve**, and the **dorsal nerve of the penis** (in males) or the **dorsal nerve of the clitoris** (in females) (DNP). The pudendal nerve carries sensation from the external genitalia of both sexes and the skin around the anus and perineum as well the motor supply to various pelvic muscles, including the external urethral sphincter and the external anal sphincter. As the bladder fills, the pudendal nerve activates. Contraction of the external sphincter, coupled with that of the internal sphincter, maintains urethral pressure (resistance) higher than normal bladder pressure. The storage phase of the urinary bladder can be switched to the voiding phase either involuntarily (reflexively) or voluntarily.

The pudendal nerve then causes relaxation of the levator ani so that the pelvic floor muscle relaxes. The pudendal nerve also signals the external sphincter to open. The sympathetic nerves send a message to the internal sphincter to contract, resulting in a higher urethral resistance. The pudendal nerve is also known to have a potential modulatory effect on bladder function. Somatic afferent fibers of the pudendal nerve are thought to project on the sympathetic thoracolumbar neurons to the bladder neck and modulate their function. This neuromodulation effect works exclusively at the spinal level and appears to be at least partly responsible for bladder neck competence and urinary continence. Pudendal supply is not significant in the vaginal wall because there is no striated muscle, but efferent supply largely from the pudendal nerve controls the levator muscle that provides support for and influences the function of the lower third of the vagina (Fig. 18.2).

The **pelvic splanchnic nerves (parasympathetic)** (Fig. 18.3): the preganglionic fibers that lead out of the sacral nerve roots S2–S4/S5. The pelvic splanchnic nerves transfix the sacral hypogastric fascia, where they form a meshwork of five to seven smaller nerves after sprouting out from different orientations. A medial group of fibers crosses the pararectal space tangentially and anastomoses to the pelvic plexus at the posterolateral aspect of the rectum. The more lateral fibers are more vertical and anastomose to the pelvic plexus ventrally at the level of the bladder pillar laterally and caudally to the urethrovesical junction. From a surgical point of view, the best way to expose the pelvic splanchnic nerves consists of first exposing sacral nerves S3–S4 laterally to the sacral hypogastric fascia and then following them ventrally until the nerves emerge from the roots. The pelvic splanchnic nerves regulate the emptying of the urinary bladder, control opening and closing of the internal urethral sphincter, influence motility in the rectum, and influence sexual functions such as erection.

Sympathetic pelvic innervation

The sympathetic innervation of the pelvis (Fig. 18.4) originates from:

- The sympathetic trunk which stretches on both sides of the spine as a uniform nerve fiber–ganglion cord. The trunk part of the sympathetic trunk joins up with the lumbar and sacral parts. Both lumbar trunks run directly along the medial insertion of the iliopsoas muscle, ventral to the lumbar veins, and have approximately four associated neural ganglia. Anatomically, the left sympathetic trunk lies beside aorta, whereas the right sympathetic trunk remains hidden behind the inferior vena cava and can only be damaged by a retrocaval lymphadenectomy. Damage to the lumbalis of the sympathetic trunk typically leads to homolateral peripheral vasodilation and a warming up of the homolateral foot. The sacral part of the sympathetic trunk runs along the sacrum medial to the sacral foramens. It normally consists of three sacral ganglia that form fibers ventral to the sacrum of the opposite ganglia and show anastomosis to the inferior hypogastric plexus (IHP).

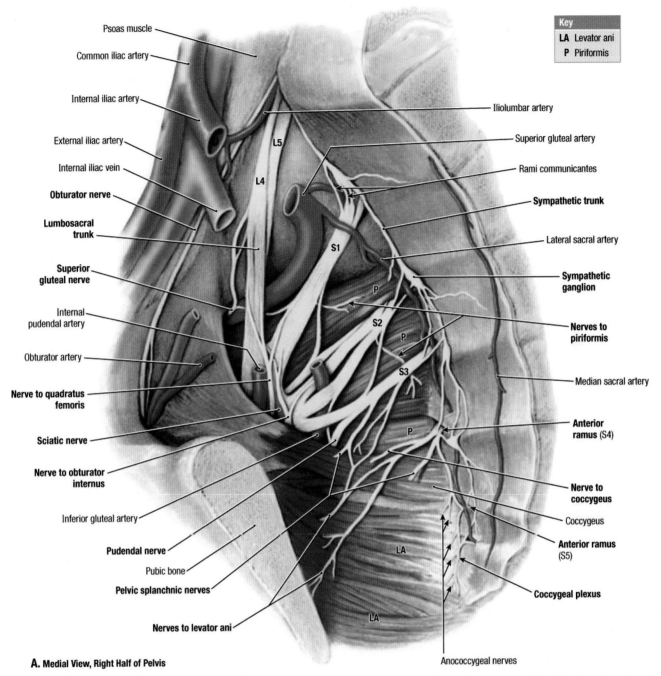

Psoas muscle

Common iliac artery

Internal iliac artery

External iliac artery

Internal iliac vein

Obturator nerve

Lumbosacral trunk

Superior gluteal nerve

Internal pudendal artery

Obturator artery

Nerve to quadratus femoris

Sciatic nerve

Nerve to obturator internus

Inferior gluteal artery

Pudendal nerve

Pubic bone

Pelvic splanchnic nerves

Nerves to levator ani

Iliolumbar artery

Superior gluteal artery

Rami communicantes

Sympathetic trunk

Lateral sacral artery

Sympathetic ganglion

Nerves to piriformis

Median sacral artery

Anterior ramus (S4)

Nerve to coccygeus

Coccygeus

Anterior ramus (S5)

Coccygeal plexus

Anococcygeal nerves

L5

L4

S1

S2

S3

P

P

P

LA

LA

Key
LA Levator ani
P Piriformis

A. Medial View, Right Half of Pelvis

FIGURE 18.2 Pelvic side wall view of sacral and coccygeal nerve plexuses. (Reprinted from Agur AM, Dalley AF. *Grant's atlas of anatomy*, 15th ed. Philadelphia: Wolters Kluwer, 2021.)

- The IHP (or so called plexus pelvicus). Different plexuses originate from the vegetative solar plexus, orientate themselves along the various collaterals of the aorta, and innervate all the abdominal organs. One of these plexuses is the intermesenteric plexus, which runs ventrolaterally to the aorta between both mesenteric arteries and forms the inferior mesenteric plexus. This plexus dispatches branches that partly accompany the mesenteric arteries and branches that run between the inferior mesenteric artery and the aorta. At the level of the 5th lumbar vertebrae or ventral of the promontorium, the superior hypogastric plexus divides into two inferior hypogastric nerves that run downward into the mesorectum, ventral to the Waldeyer fascia. At the level of the pelvis, the sympathetic fibers build on both the rectum and the IHP. The IHP (also known as the knot from Lee, hypogastric knot, or plexus pelvicus) lies deep in the pelvis in the superior pelvirectal space, lateral to the rectum and the craniodorsal part of the vagina. The plexus shows itself as a net of fibers that form a sacrouterine ligament, also called a rectovaginal pillar.

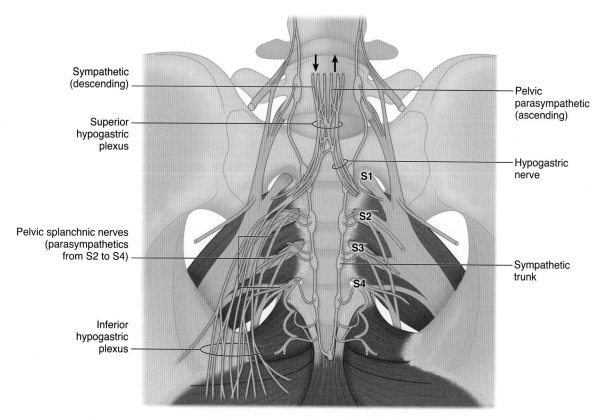

FIGURE 18.3 Pelvic autonomic nervous plexus.

The **lumbar plexus** (Fig. 18.5) is formed by the divisions of the first four lumbar nerves (L1–L4) and from contributions of the subcostal nerve (T12), which is the last thoracic nerve. Additionally, the ventral rami of the 4th lumbar nerve pass communicating branches, the lumbosacral trunk, to the sacral plexus. Several branches of the lumbar plexus run into the pelvis.

- The **iliohypogastric nerve** runs anterior to the psoas major on its proximal lateral border, laterally and obliquely on the anterior side of quadratus lumborum. Lateral to this muscle, it pierces the transversus abdominis to run above the iliac crest. It gives several motor branches to these muscles and a sensory branch to skin of lateral hip. Its terminal branch then runs parallel to the inguinal ligament to exit the aponeurosis of the abdominal external oblique above the inguinal ring, where it supplies the skin above the inguinal ligament with the anterior cutaneous branch.

- The **ilioinguinal nerve** runs on the quadratus lumborum caudally to the iliohypogastric nerve. At the level of iliac crest, it pierces the lateral abdominal wall and runs medially at the level of the inguinal ligament, where it supplies motor branches to the transverse abdominis and sensory branches through the external inguinal ring to the skin over the pubic symphysis and the lateral aspect of the labia majora.

- The **genitofemoral nerve** originates from upper part of the lumbar plexus, pierces the psoas major

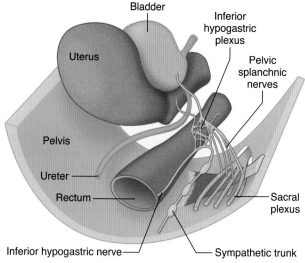

FIGURE 18.4 Sympathic and parasympathetic innervation of the pelvic organs.

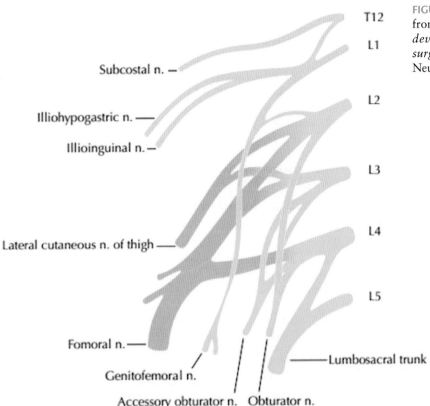

FIGURE 18.5 Lumbosacral plexus. (Reprinted from Possover M. *Neuropelveology: Latest developments in pelvic neurofunctional surgery.* Germany: International Society of Neuropelveology, 2015.)

anteriorly below the iliohypogastric and ilioinguinal nerves, then immediately splits into two branches that run downward on the anterior side of the muscles, lateral to the external iliac artery. The lateral femoral branch is purely sensory and supplies the skin below the inguinal ligament and proximal lateral aspect of the femoral triangle. The genital branch runs in the inguinal canal together with the round ligament. It then sends sensory branches to the skin of the mons pubis and the labia majora.

- The **lateral cutaneous femoral nerve** pierces the psoas major on its lateral side and runs obliquely downward below the iliac fascia. Medial to the anterior superior iliac spine, it leaves the pelvic area through the lateral muscular lacuna. In the thigh, it briefly passes under the fascia lata before it breaches the fascia and supplies the skin of the anterior and lateral aspects of the thigh. Injury to the lateral femoral cutaneous nerve can cause anterior and lateral thigh burning, tingling, and/or numbness that increases with standing, walking, or hip extension.
- The **obturator nerve** descends behind the psoas major, then follows the linea terminalis into the lesser pelvis lateral to the external vessels, and then finally leaves the pelvis through the obturator canal. In the thigh, it sends motor branches mainly to the adductor muscles. The anterior branch contributes a terminal sensory branch, which supplies the skin on the medial distal part of the thigh. Obturator

nerve injury causes loss of thigh adduction. It is commonly injured during retroperitoneal surgeries for malignancies or endometriosis. It presents with sensory loss in the upper medial thigh and motor weakness in the hip adductors. It can also be injured during paravaginal repairs or transobturator sling placement. The anatomical relationship of the obturator nerve to transobturator tapes can be as close as 2.5 cm away from anterior branch.

- The **femoral nerve** is the largest branch of the lumbar plexus. It provides considerable sensory innervation to the anterior aspect of the thigh and knee and motor innervation to the quadriceps muscles. The femoral nerve runs in a groove between the psoas major and iliacus, giving off branches to both muscles, and exits the pelvis through the medial aspect of the muscular lacuna. In the thigh, it divides into numerous sensory and muscular branches and the saphenous nerve, its long sensory terminal branches, which continues down to the foot. Femoral neuropathy is the most common lumbosacral nerve injury at the time of pelvic surgery. Patients typically report falling when attempting to get out of bed after surgery. In addition to difficulty ambulating, they may also report sensory loss over the anteromedial thigh. The femoral nerve commonly can be compressed by self-retaining retractors as it exits from the psoas muscle, and it can be compressed under the inguinal ligament if the thighs are hyperflexed.

Nerve Injuries during Gynecologic Surgeries

Injuries to the lumbosacral plexus can occur up to 2% at the time of gynecologic surgeries. All the approaches of gynecologic surgeries (vaginal/laparoscopic/laparotomy) can cause nerve injury.

Nerve injuries during pelvic surgery can occur due to compression, stretching, and transection.

Compression and stretch injuries can cause mild demyelinating injuries, which recover quickly. They can occasionally result in injury to the nerve fiber or axon. Axonal injuries take longer to recover.

Fortunately, majority of nerve injuries spontaneously resolve. Knowledge of the basic neural anatomy is essential for understanding the nerve injury during surgery (Table 18.1). Nerve fibers are divided into fascicles and are surrounded by loose connective tissue (Fig. 18.6).

TABLE 18.1

Mechanism of Nerve Injury during Gynecologic Procedures

NERVE	ORIGIN	NERVE TYPE	SYMPTOMS	MECHANISM OF INJURY
Ilioinguinal and iliohypogastric	L1	Afferent	• Sensory deficit and pain of skin along the abdominal wall, suprapubic area, and inguinal ligament • Pain in medial groin, labia majora, or inner thigh	• Injury during trocar insertion in laparoscopy • Injury during extended abdominal wall incision • Nerve entrapment during fascial closure
Obturator	L2–L4	Afferent Efferent	• Unable to adduct thigh • Sensory loss in medial thigh	• Prolonged hip flexion • Retropubic and deep pelvic sidewall dissection • Injury during transobturator tape placement • Injury during paravaginal repair
Femoral	L2–L4	Afferent Efferent	• Unable to flex hip • Unable to extend knee • Unable to adduct thigh • Sensory deficit in anterior thigh • Absent patellar reflex • Feeling of knee "giving away" or buckling	• Sidewall retractors during laparotomy • Hyperflexion of the hip during positioning (compression injury) • Hyperextension of the hip during positioning (stretch injury)
Genitofemoral	L1–L2	Afferent Efferent	• Sensory deficit over the anterior thigh below the inguinal ligament and lateral labia • Paresthesia in groin area, over the mons and labia majora	• Injury from retractors • Injury during sling placement for incontinence
Lateral femoral cutaneous	L2–L4	Afferent	• Pain and sensory deficit in anterior lateral thigh to knee • Symptoms increase with standing, walking, or hip extension	• Hip hyperflexion • Abdominal retractors • Tight belt/clothing
Sciatic	L4–S3	Afferent Efferent	• Pain in posterior leg • Unable to extend thigh and flex leg • Sensory loss in posterior thigh, calf, and sole of the foot • Absent Achilles reflex	• Hyperflexion of the hip • Sacrospinous ligament fixation • Sacroiliac fossa hemorrhage
Common peroneal	L4–S2	Afferent Efferent	• Foot drop • Unable to dorsiflex foot • Sensory deficit of lateral leg and foot	• Hip extension and rotation • Lateral pressure of thigh in stirrups
Tibial	L4–S3	Afferent Efferent	• Loss of plantar flexion and inversion of foot • Sensory loss over the sole and heel of the foot	• Compression during positioning
Pudendal	S2–S4	Afferent Efferent	• Pelvic pain • Urinary and fecal incontinence • Sensory loss in vulva, vagina, clitoris, perineum, and rectum	• Vaginal surgery/paravaginal repair • Vaginal birth
Sacral nerve roots	S1–S4	Afferent Efferent	• Sensation of perineum and vagina • Pelvic floor dysfunction, bladder and bowel dysfunction, arousal	• Injury during uterosacral ligament suspension

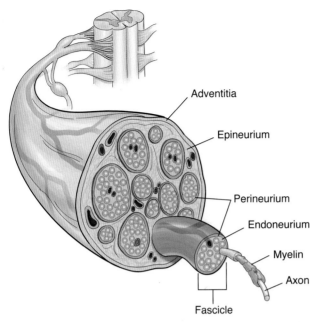

Adventitia

Epineurium

Perineurium

Endoneurium

Myelin

Axon

Fascicle

FIGURE 18.6 Peripheral nerve. (Reprinted from Handa VL, Van Le L. *Te Linde's operative gynecology*, 12th ed. Philadelphia: Wolters Kluwer, 2020.)

Such characteristics along with the elasticity of perineurium protect the nerve fibers from injury caused by compression and stretch forces.

The Seddon classification is used to classify nerve injuries. This classification helps the surgeon to anticipate patient's prognosis and recovery.

- *Neurapraxia (local conduction block)*: The injury is caused by transient nerve ischemia. There is no injury to axons and Schwann cells. This type of injury is similar to when the foot falls asleep. Usually, the resolution is within minutes unless the injury is longer causing demyelination.
- *Axonotmesis (axonal injury with preservation of the protecting Schwann cells)*: It can affect sensory, motor, and autonomic nerves. Wallerian degeneration begins within 1 to 2 days after injury. Axons grow at 1 mm/day, and typically, these injuries take weeks to months until full recovery.
- *Neurotmesis (complete disruption of the axon, Schwann cell, and connective tissue)*: It is caused by complete transection of the nerves. Surgical intervention is required for resolution.

COMMON CONDITIONS

Bladder Hypersensitivity (Increased Bladder Sensation)

Hypersensitive bladder symptoms are defined as increased bladder sensation, usually associated with urinary frequency and nocturia, with or without bladder pain.

Hypersensitivity of the bladder occurs due to an activation of the sensory nerves of the bladder located either in the IHP (which contains afferents fibers originating from the inferior hypogastric nerves and the sympathetic trunks) or in the sacral nerve roots S2–S4, the pudendal nerve, and the DNP. In the first situation, bladder hypersensitivity is associated with visceral pelvic pain, the latter with pelvic somatic pain symptoms.

Pathologies of the inferior hypogastric plexus

The endometriosis of the uterosacral ligaments is a common gynecologic etiology for hypersensitivity of the bladder. Because the disease infiltrates mainly the cranial portion of the IHP that supplies the organs of the pelvis,[2] hypersensitivity of the bladder is associated with visceral pelvic pain, dysmenorrhea, rectal disorders ("irritable colon"), and deep dyspareunia. Because pelvic sympathetic afferent fibers rise upward to the superior hypogastric plexus by crossing the promontory to the solar plexus, pelvic symptoms are associated with ascending back pain and multiple vegetative symptoms affecting the whole vegetative nervous system (Table 18.2). Clinical examination focuses on specific clinical details for vegetative disorders such as pupil dilation, salivation inhibition, and tachycardia.

The second classical etiology, which is widely underestimated, is surgical damage of the IHP secondary to prolapse surgeries, radical pelvic surgery for malignancies, or deeply infiltrating endometriosis.[9–11]

TABLE 18.2	
Visceral versus Somatic Pain: Symptoms	
VISCERAL PAIN	**SOMATIC PAIN**
Pain quality: Vague; poorly localized in the entire lower abdomen with radiation to the lower back; dull in nature	**Pain quality:** Allodynia; similar to an electrical shock; very specific location; precise and clear pain description; lack of vegetative symptoms
+ Vegetative symptoms: Malaise/oppression/syncope Fatigue Irritability Pupil dilation Salivation inhibition Tachycardia Nausea/vomiting Pallor Diaphoresis Anxiety	**+ Caudal radiation to the corresponding dermatome(s)** **+ Pelvic motor dysfunction:** Pelvic organ dysfunctions Sexual dysfunction Locomotion dysfunction

Reprinted from Possover M. *Neuropelveology: Latest developments in pelvic neurofunctional surgery*. Germany: International Society of Neuropelveology, 2015.

Pathologies of the pelvic somatic nerves

Neuropathies of the sacral nerves S2, S3, and S4 and of the pudendal nerve and its branches (especially DNP) may induce pelvic somatic pain with hypersensitivity of the bladder (Fig. 18.7).[12]

In such pelvic neuropathies, neuroanatomical considerations are essential for understanding the combination of symptoms:

- S1 and L5 radiculopathy induces pain in the lower back, the buttock, and the dorsal/external aspect of the leg (dermatomes L5 and S1), without any genitoanal/pudendal pain. With a neurogenic lesion, problems with extension of the foot and motion of the leg can occur as well as gluteal muscle hypotrophy.
- S2 radiculopathy induces pain in the buttock and the dorsal/medial aspect of the leg as well as in the pudendal area (mostly the perianal area) and coccygodynia. Damage to S2 induces difficulties with motion in the toes.

- S3 and S4 radiculopathy induces only pudendal pain (mostly in the perineal and vulvar areas, vulvodynia) without radiation to the buttock or the legs.
- Pudendal neuralgia induces pain in the ventral (vulvodynia), middle (perineal), and dorsal (perianal) pudendal areas combined, without any radiation to the buttock or the leg.

The neuropelveologic approach to such pelvic neuropathies is primarily diagnostic with the application of neurologic principles and an absolute knowledge of the pelvic neurofunctional anatomy. Patient's history is the key with a focus not only on the pain location but also on pain history, irradiation, aggravating factors, and vegetative and somatic symptoms. In somatic pain, it is essential to adopt a "neurologic way of thinking" because location of pain and location of etiology is mostly different. Somatic pain is located superficially at the skin and is described as allodynia or electrical shock, with very specific location, caudal irradiations to the genitoanal areas or to the

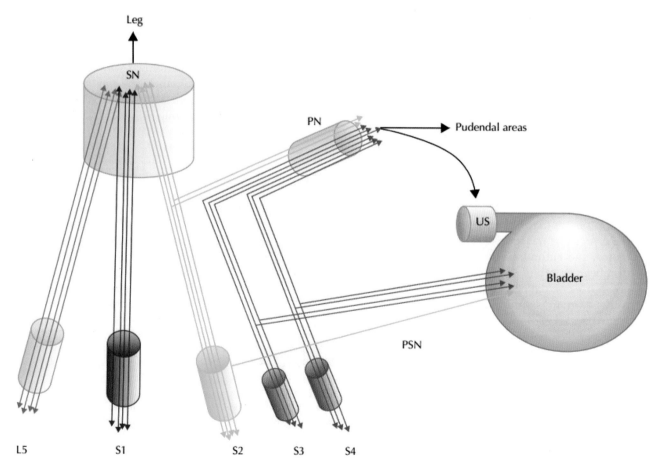

FIGURE 18.7 Neurofunctional anatomy of sacral plexus. SN, sciatic nerve; PN, pudendal nerve; US, urethral sphincter; PSN, pelvic splanchnic nerves. (Reprinted from Possover M. *Neuropelveology: Latest developments in pelvic neurofunctional surgery.* Germany: International Society of Neuropelveology, 2015.)

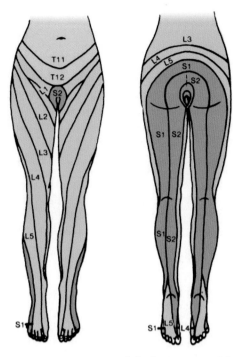

FIGURE 18.8 Dermatome map of the lower extremities. (From Ostergard DR, Bent AK. *Urogynecology and urodynamics: Theory and practice*, 4th ed. Maryland: Lippincott Williams & Wilkins, 1996:682, with permission.)

lower extremities (dermatomes) and lack of vegetative symptoms (Fig. 18.8).

The neuropelveologic workup scheme follows these six steps:

1. Determination of the nerve pathways involved in the relay of pain information to the brain
2. Determination of the location of neurologic irritation/injury (troncular vs. radicular vs. spinal vs. cerebral location)

3. Determination of the type of nerve(s) lesion—irritation versus injury (neurogenic neuropathy)
4. Neurologic confirmation of the suspected diagnosis: The distal branches of the lumbar plexus are accessible for external percutaneous palpation (inguinal palpation of the ilioinguinal and genitofemoral branches), and the pudendal nerve and the sacral nerves (S2–S4) are accessible by vaginal or rectal palpation. Reproduction of the pain (trigger point) in combination with a positive Tinel sign (Tinel, 1905) and an improvement of pain of at least 50% after administration of local anesthesia at the trigger point confirms which nerve is involved.
5. Determination of a potential etiology based on patient history and diagnostic imaging. The most frequent etiologies treated in neuropelveology are the following:
   - Sacral radiculopathy by "vascular or fibrotic entrapment"[13,14]
   - Compression of the sacral plexus by hypertrophy or atypical insertion of the piriformis muscle
   - Deeply infiltrating endometriosis of the sacral plexus and the sciatic nerve[15,16]
   - Tumors of the sacral plexus (Fig. 18.9)[17,18]
   - Postsurgical pelvic neuropathies (Fig. 18.10).[9–11] The surgeon must have a thorough knowledge of pelvic anatomy and must understand the specific nerve damage that each procedure can cause (Table 18.3).
6. Corresponding etiology-adapted therapy. It is absolutely crucial to understand specific nerves that are involved in causing pain and then to assess whether it is a nerve irritation secondary to compression or whether it is an axonal nerve lesion. In the compression case, the neuropelveologic treatment is based

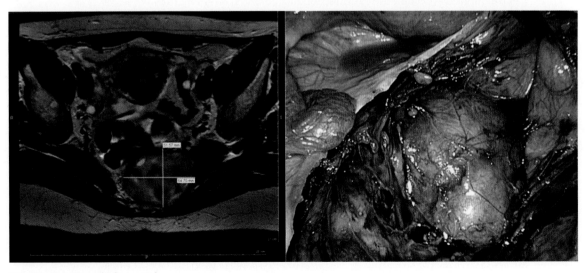

FIGURE 18.9 Sacral Plexus Schwannoma.

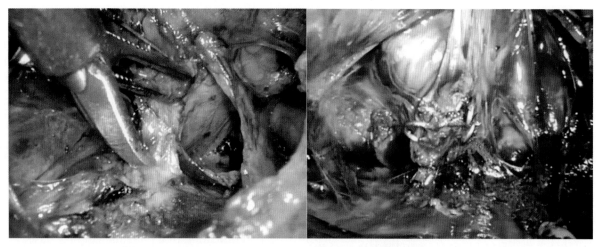

FIGURE 18.10 Lesion of the sacral plexus by suturing (**left**) and helical tack (**right**).

on laparoscopic exploration/decompression of the nerves.[9,19–21] In axonal nerve lesions, treatment is focused on neuromodulation of the affected nerves where electrodes are selectively placed in contact with the pelvic injured nerves for possible control of neuropathic pain and pelvic organ dysfunctions.[22–24]

The remainder of this chapter outlines some of the novel treatments that are in their early stages of development. Even though studies evaluating their long-term outcome are limited at this stage and procedures are often offered by a limited number of surgeons as they are not taught in formal residency and fellowship training programs, the preliminary outcome might be promising to find less invasive solutions in the future for common pelvic floor disorders.

The Sacral LION Procedure for Treatment of Bladder Atony

In the case of motor functional disorders or pelvic neuropathies by nerve damage (neurogenic neuropathies), the laparoscopic exploration of the nerves cannot lead to an improvement in these disorders. Instead, neuromodulation may have a role where electrical stimulation of the nerves can allow the control of troubles of continence/voiding functions or even restoration of a lost function (micturition). Sacral nerve stimulation was the first technique for pelvic nerves stimulation that typically involves electrical stimulation of the sacral nerves (sacral neuromodulation [SNM]) via a dorsal transformational technique of implantation (refer to Chapter 17 for more information regarding SNM).

TABLE 18.3	
Pelvic Surgical Procedures with Corresponding Potential Nerve Injuries	
PROCEDURES	**CORRESPONDING NERVE DAMAGE**
• Pelvic sidewall procedures	Sacral plexus—obturator nerve
• McCall fixation	Sacral nerves S2–S4
• Amreich-Richter fixation	Pudendal nerve, right
• Trans-obturator sling (TOT)/Prolift/episiotomy	Pudendal nerve
• Hip surgeries (prosthesis)	Pudendal nerve; inferior gluteal nerve
• Rectopexy/sacropexy	Sacral nerves S2–S3, right
• Vaginal delivery (forceps, vacuum)	Pudendal nerve
• Herniorrhaphy/lateral trocar by laparoscopy	Ilioinguinal/genitofemoral nerves
• Renal procedures/lithotripsy	Lumbar plexus

Reprinted from Possover M. *Neuropelveology: Latest developments in pelvic neurofunctional surgery.* Germany: International Society of Neuropelveology, 2015.

Some limitations of the SNM has motived the development of the technique of "laparoscopic implantation of neuroprothesis" also called the "LION procedure":

- SNM enables placement of lead electrodes only to the sacral nerve roots, not to all pelvic nerves and plexuses. In contrast, the laparoscopic approach enables exploration of injured nerves with, in turn, a possible etiologic treatment with nerve decompression or reconstruction or, if necessary, the placement of a stimulation's electrode selective and in direct contact to the specific nerve.
- In the classical percutaneous transforaminal technique of implantation, usually, one sacral nerve root can be reached by one implanted electrode while in the LION procedure, as the electrode is placed perpendicular to the sacral plexus, all sacral nerve roots involved on one side (S2–S4/S5) are reached by the electrical field of the electrode (Figs. 18.11 and 18.12).

Some studies show that this might increase the chance of successful neuromodulation in diverse intractable neurogenic bladder dysfunctions even after failure of the classical SNM.[25] The prime indication for the sacral LION procedure is bladder atony secondary to pelvic surgeries, where every stimulated pelvic parasympathetic efferent fiber counts to achieve sufficient bladder function for voiding. The ventral laparoscopic approach provides additional advantages in cases with anatomical anomalies such as spina bifida which the dorsal approach may not be feasible, whereas the endoscopic approach provides access to the nerves.

Efficacy data from both randomized controlled trials and case series studies show that about 70% of the patients who received sacral neuromodulators for bladder dysfunction showed improvement in their main symptoms.[26,27] For the 30% of patients where the SNM shows no improvement, the nonresponse is still a problem of interpretation: As the percutaneous technique is not a direct method of implantation, even when the position of the electrode is radiographically controlled, a "nonresponse" can be due to a "nonresponse" to the stimulation or to a "non-optimal" implantation of the electrode. The laparoscopic approach permits the implantation of the electrode in direct contact to the nerves under direct visualization. Therefore, if postoperatively no improvement is noted, a "non-optimal" implantation of the electrode can be excluded.

Sacral LION procedure is more invasive with higher potential morbidity compared to percutaneous placement of the lead electrodes. A high level of surgical skills is required to perform the procedure. Extensive counseling and patient's involvement in decision making is required to understand the procedure, its anticipated outcome, and the potential complications that may occur.

GNS Therapy for Treatment of Idiopathic Overactive Bladder

The two most frequent pelvic dysfunctions are the idiopathic overactive bladder (IOAB) and erectile dysfunction (ED). One United States-based study demonstrated 16% prevalence of IOAB in men and 16.9% in women.[28] Milsom et al.[29] confirmed these findings in the European population with an estimated prevalence of overactive bladder in 15.6% of men and 17.4% of women on surveys completed by patients older than the

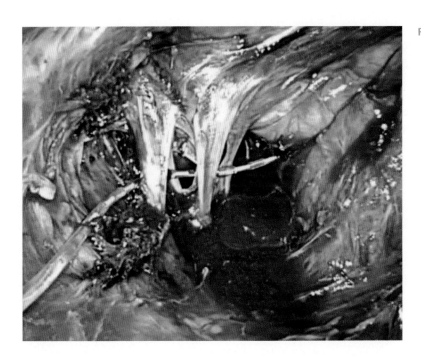

FIGURE 18.11 Sacral plexus LION procedure.

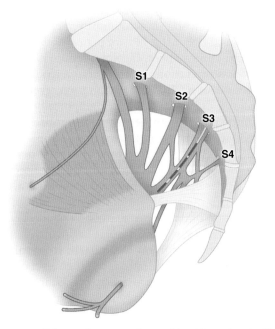
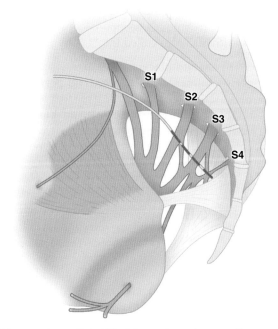

FIGURE 18.12 Schematic comparison of lead location in SNM and LION procedure. (Modified from Agur AM, Dalley AF. *Grant's atlas of anatomy*, 15th ed. Philadelphia: Wolters Kluwer, 2021.)

age of 40 years. Stress and mixed urinary incontinence are more prevalent with advanced age.[30] In addition to the personal, social, and psychological impact, the economic burden of urgency urinary incontinence in the United States is enormous, as it was estimated to approach $76.2 billion dollars in 2015.[31] Sexual dissatisfaction and problems of penile/clitoral dysfunction are also very often rooted in pelvic dysfunctions.

Sacral nerve stimulation was the first technique for S3 root pelvic nerve stimulation that typically involves electrical stimulation of the nerve via a dorsal transformational technique for implantation.

SNM evolved as a widely used treatment for overactive bladder but does not completely resolve symptoms in some of the patients. Stimulation of more distal nerves at other sites might result in a better outcome. Because pudendal nerve stimulation (PNS) can reach more "sphincter-vesico-anal" fibers than SNM, PNS has been proposed for patients who have failed to respond to SNM.[32–34] The good effects of PNS has been reported in neurogenic[35] and in some nonneurogenic disorders.[36] However, implantation of the lead to the pudendal nerve is not easily accomplished either by percutaneous technique or by laparoscopic approach (Fig. 18.13), and the risk for lead migration with implantation below the pelvic floor is increased.

There is definitely a need for a more suitable alternative for neuromodulation treatment to allow easier use by more providers encountering voiding problems. The stimulation of the DNP emerges as a very attractive alternative that might result in great outcome for patients with urinary and fecal disorders.[37] DNP is

extremely interesting because its stimulation effectively increases bladder capacity, inhibits involuntary detrusor contractions and overactive bladder symptoms,[37–39] and may even control idiopathic fecal incontinence.[40] The further crucial role of the DNP in human erectile function is also supported by previous studies.[39] Electrical stimulation of the DNP elicits reflex tonic erections of the penile body and reflex bulbospongiosus muscle activity, flips, and even reflex ejaculatory response.[41]

GNS therapy consists of two phases: a preoperative nonsurgical test phase and a final surgical implantation

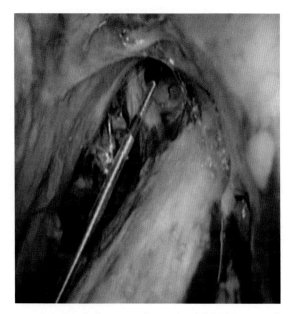

FIGURE 18.13 Lead placement by Pudendal LION procedure.

The effect of stimulation can be tested by the patient in her daily usual environment or can be shown with changes in parameters during urodynamic testing.

After confirmation of effectiveness of GNS, implantation of a permanent neuroprothesis can be planned. The procedure is performed either under general or spinal anesthesia or using only local anesthesia with intravenous sedation as in the classical tension-free vaginal tape (TVT) procedure. The first step of the procedure consists of the introduction of a hollow curve needle applicator (Curve Applicator, NeuroGyn AG, Baar, Switzerland) with a spear from below, behind the pubic bone similar to the classical TVT procedure: A sagittal incision of about 2 mm in length is made approximately 1 cm below the external urethral meatus. The curve needle driver is inserted into the incision. The tip is oriented at an angle of 5° to 10° from the midline, toward the symphysis. The inserter tip is approximately in the 11 o'clock position (1 o'clock on the right side). The curve needle driver is advanced, contacting the inferior edge of the pubic ramus, until it transfixes the urogenital diaphragm, enters into the retropubic space, and comes out through the skin in the suprapubic area (Fig. 18.15).

The passage of the applicator behind and in direct contact with the dorsal aspect of the pubic bone is controlled with two fingers inserted into the vagina. A cystoscopy is performed to make sure the bladder and urethra are intact. The spear of the curve driver needle is removed. A quadripolar lead electrode with an electrode distance of 60 mm is introduced retrograde into the shaft of the curve needle driver; by retraction

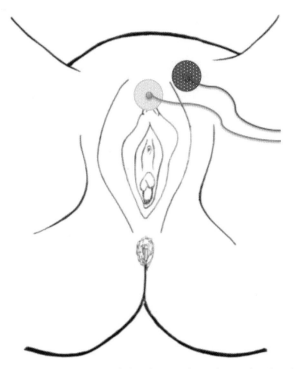

FIGURE 18.14 Position of the skin surface electrodes for the test phase.

of the neuroprothesis. In contrary to the classical technique of stimulation, the GNS test phase does not require any interventional procedure. Considering that the genital nerves are located just few millimeters below the skin, test stimulation can be obtained using skin surface or needle electrode (Fig. 18.14).[42]

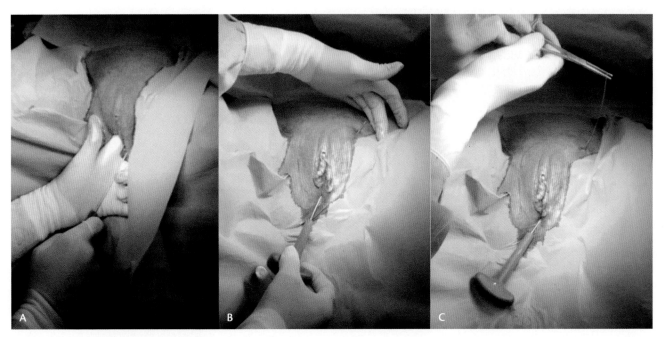

FIGURE 18.15 Introduction of the curve applicator from below, behind the pubic bone (**A** and **B**) and removal of the spear of the curve driver needle (**C**).

FIGURE 18.16 Introduction retrograde of the lead electrode (**A**) and removal of the curve driver needle from below (**B**).

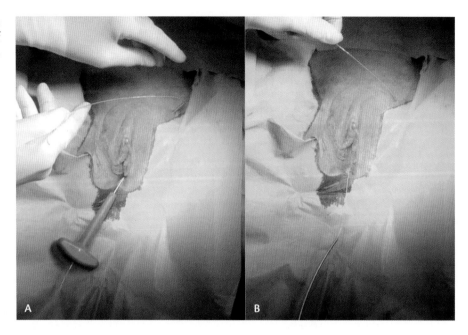

of the curve needle driver, the electrode lead is left in position with the stimulator's pole coming out through the vulvar incision (Fig. 18.16).

Through a second median supravulvar incision, the applicator with the spear is introduced from top to bottom so that it is as deep as possible (ventral to the pubic bone but as close as possible to it in order to assure deep location of the cable electrode) and emerges through the first vulvar incision. After removing the spear, the electrode cable is inserted retrograde into the applicator again (Fig. 18.17).

After removing the applicator, the electrode is in place (Fig. 18.18).

Using the hollow needle driver for retrograde introduction of the lead electrodes enables optimal placement of a lead electrode to the genital nerves without the need for any dissection that, in turn, reduces considerably the risk of bleeding and nerve injury. The last step is then the connection of the lead electrode to the generator, which is finally fixed behind the pubic bone through a suprapubic mini-laparotomy. The fixation of the generator behind the pubic bone

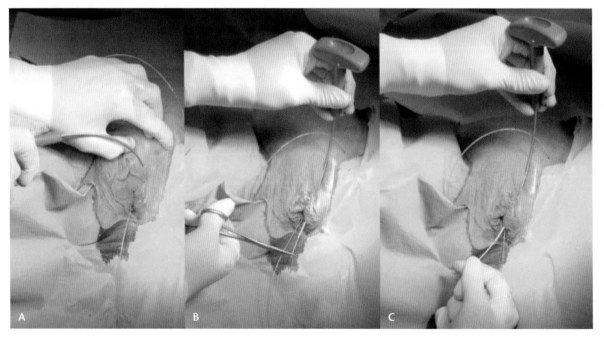

FIGURE 18.17 Second introduction of the curve applicator from above down to the first vaginal incision (**A**), removal again of the spear (**B**), and retrograde introduction once again of the lead electrode (**C**).

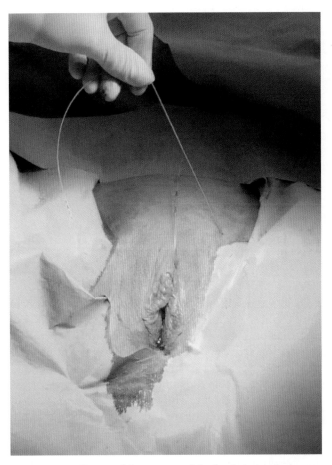

FIGURE 18.18 Retropubic passage of the lead electrode.

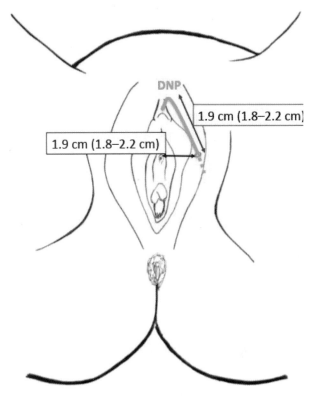

FIGURE 18.19 DNP pathway at the vulva.

protects its damage from external trauma and reduces its dislocation.

In a preliminary study of seven patients affected by IOAB, GNS permitted a reduction of micturition frequency from 25 per day in average (±11.7; 13 to 50) to 10.18 (±2.7; 7 to 15) at 6 months follow-up final evaluation (4 to 8 months). Nocturia decreased from 5.82 (±4.2; 3 to 18) to 2.18 (±1.08; 1 to 5) micturitions per night. Cystometric bladder capacities increased from a mean of 159 mL (±53; 80 to 230 mL) to 312 mL (±104.9; 160 to 500 mL). Mean incontinence episodes at the initial evaluation based on a 3-day voiding diary were 8.1; at final evaluation, six patients were completely dry. Average pads used per day reduced from 7.3 (±4.2) to 1.6 (±2.3).

The GNS technique can easily be performed through percutaneous puncture access. The introduction of the curve needle driver from below is the same as standard urogynecology (TVT procedure). Because the DNP perforates the perineal membrane laterally to the external urethral meatus at an average distance of 2.7 cm (2.4 to 3.0 cm) and then runs along the bulbospongiosus muscle for a distance of 1.9 cm (1.8 to 2.2 cm), before penetrating the pillars of the clitoris (Fig. 18.19), the second passage of the lead electrode in front of the pubis assures direct contact of the electrode to the DNP.[43]

No x-ray screening or neurophysiologic monitoring or stimulation with electromyography electrodes are mandatory during the procedure for a proper implantation. Because the GNS therapy does not need two surgical procedures for both the test and the final implantation but only one for the final implantation, this simple technique allows considerable cost reduction compared to the usual procedures for sacral or pudendal nerve stimulation.

LION Procedure for Spinal Cord Injury

The LION procedure has been used for the treatment of nerve damage and pelvic organ dysfunctions as reported previously, but probably the most impressive indication of this technique is the implantation in patients with spinal cord injuries to allow recovery in walking functions.[44–47] This intervention consists of laparoscopic implantation of fine wire in direct contact with the endopelvic portion of the sciatic/pudendal and femoral nerves for electrical stimulation (Fig. 18.20).

The crucial discovery of this revolutionary technique in patients with spinal cord injury (SCI) is undoubtedly the fact that about 70% of the patients experienced enough recovery of supraspinal control for some leg movement or even standing and walking.[48,49] The mechanism of recovery of walking functions in SCI patients

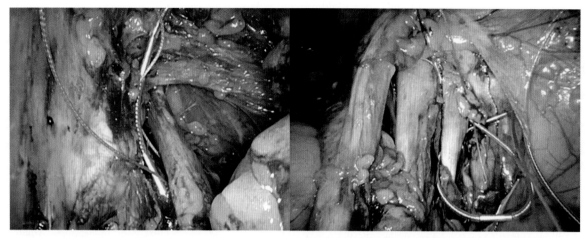

FIGURE 18.20   Placement of lead electrodes to the left sciatic nerve (**left**) and the right femoral nerve (**right**).

after the LION procedure is still unclear. There is emerging increasing evidence to suggest that neuromagnetic/electrical modulation promotes neuroregeneration and neural repair by affecting signaling in the nervous system, but our findings suggest that the information signals to the brain might use not only anatomical nerve pathways but also functional pathways activated by a continuous low-frequency stimulation of the lower motor neurons below the spinal cord lesion.

Beyond the psychological impact and the gaining of some autonomy, the benefits of locomotion include improvement of contractures, prevention of deep venous thrombosis and edema, and amelioration of spasticity.[50] Standing up in combination with gluteal muscle training ("gluteal pads effect") protects patients from decubitus lesions, especially in the buttock.[51] Continuous low-frequency stimulation of the implanted nerves outside periods of training may be advantageous for the reduction of spasticity[52] and regulation of bone density.[53,54] Nerve stimulation has been reported for treatment of arthritis of the legs,[55] but also in vivo studies involving animal models have revealed that electric stimulation of wound healing processes results in more collagen deposition,[56] enhanced angiogenesis,[57] greater wound tensile strength,[58] and a faster wound contraction rate.[59] In addition to these direct cellular actions, electrical stimulation has been shown to improve tissue perfusion and reduce edema formation that results in a significant increase in transcutaneous oxygen pressures.[60] Therefore, the LION procedure to the pelvic nerves is potentially useful in the rehabilitation of patients with spinal cord injuries by reducing the risks of complications.

eBODY-ENS

The development of new technologies to assist patients with paraplegia with their common problems associated with inertia when confined to a wheelchair finds revolutionary applications in preventive medicine and even in the world of space missions. The LION procedure enables a continuous and passive Electrical Nerve Stimulation (ENS) without the need for an external stimulation system. This eBody-ENS may open the door to a whole new area of humanity in which implanted electronics may help the human body to a better performance and a longer life. The process of aging, also called sarcopenia, is characterized by muscle atrophy along with a reduction in muscle tissue quality, characterized by such factors as replacement of muscle fibers with fat, degeneration of the neuromuscular junction leading to progressive loss of muscle function and frailty. Because continuous passive stimulation of the pelvic somatic nerves may reduce this process of muscle atrophy, the "eBody-ENS" can be considered as a preventive treatment for sarcopenia and consequently as an anti-aging treatment. This technique may be appropriate not only in elderly patients who are not capable of active muscle training because of pain, motor limitations, or subcortical pathologies but also in patients confined to bed for long periods of time (prophylaxis of decubitus ulcers).

Due to the fact that there is further evidence of the role of sympathetic innervation of bone tissue and of its role in the regulation of bone remodeling in humans, sympathetic nerve stimulation obtained by stimulation of the pelvic somatic nerves might also open new techniques for the treatment or prevention of osteoporosis not only in patients with SCI as demonstrated in our study but also in elderly people.[53,54] In addition, electrical stimulation has been shown, as reported previously, to improve tissue perfusion and reduce edema formation that results in a significant increase in transcutaneous oxygen pressure.

In addition to this, the eBody-ENS may also find revolutionary applications in the world of space missions. Space is a dangerous, unfriendly place that requires daily exercise to keep muscles and bones from deteriorating. Calf muscle biopsies before flight and after a 6-month mission on the International Space

Station show that even when crew members did aerobic exercise 5 hours a week and resistance exercise 3 to 6 days per week, muscle volume and peak power both still deteriorated significantly. The eBody-ENS by contrast allows muscle mass to be maintained, even while the astronaut is at rest, and provides an extremely effective and time-saving strength-training program. During space flight, crewmembers also lose bone density; the calcium that is released ends up in the urine, which contributes to the increased calcium stone–forming potential. The stone formation if causes obstruction in urinary system can have catastrophic consequences for the astronaut. Due to excruciating pain, affected astronauts could become incapacitated and missions may have to be aborted. Due to the fact that stimulation of pelvic sympathetic nerves may reduce the process of osteoporosis, eBody-ENS may present a potential prophylaxis for kidney stone formation in microgravity.

References

1. Possover M. Laparoscopic exposure and electrostimulation of the somatic and autonomous pelvic nerves: A new method for implantation of neuroprothesis in paralysed patients? *Gynecol Surg* 2004;1:87–90.
2. Possover M, Rhiem K, Chiantera V. The "Laparoscopic Neuro-Navigation"—LANN: From a functional cartography of the pelvic autonomous neurosystem to a new field of laparoscopic surgery. *Minim Invasive Ther Allied Technol* 2004;13(5):362–367.
3. Possover M, Quakernack J, Chiantera V. The LANN technique to reduce the postoperative functional morbidity in laparoscopic radical pelvic surgery. *J Am Coll Surg* 2005;201(6):913–917.
4. Possover M, Chiantera V, Baekelandt J. Anatomy of the sacral roots and the pelvic splanchnic nerves in women using the LANN technique. *Surg Lap Endosc Percutan Tech* 2007;17(6):508–510.
5. Possover M. The neuropelveology: A new speciality in medicine. *Pelviperineol* 2010;29(4):123–124.
6. Possover M, Forman A, Rabischong B, et al. Neuropelveology: New groundbreaking discipline in medicine. *J Minim Invasive Gynecol* 2015;22(7):1140–1141.
7. Possover M, Andersson KE, Forman A. Neuropelveology: An emerging discipline for the management of chronic pelvic pain. *Int Neurourol J* 2017;21(4):243–246.
8. Possover M, Forman A. Neuropelveological assessment of pelvic neuropathic pain. *Gynecol Surg* 2014;11:139–144.
9. Possover M. Laparoscopic management of neural pelvic pain in women secondary to pelvic surgery. *Fertil Steril* 2009;91(6):2720–2725.
10. Possover M, Lemos N. Risks, symptoms, and management of pelvic nerve damage secondary to surgery for pelvic organ prolapse: A report of 95 cases. *Int Urogynecol J* 2011;22(12):1485–1490.
11. Possover M. Pathophysiologic explanation for bladder retention in patients after laparoscopic surgery for deeply infiltration rectovaginal and/or parametric endometriosis. *Fertil Steril* 2014;101(3):754–758.
12. Possover M, Forman A. Voiding dysfunction associated with pudendal nerve entrapment. *Curr Bladder Dysfunct Rep* 2012;7(4):281–285.
13. Possover M, Forman A. Pelvic neuralgias by neuro-vascular entrapment: Anatomical findings in a series of 97 consecutive patients treated by laparoscopic nerve decompression. *Pain Physician* 2015;18(6):E1139–E1143.
14. Possover M, Khazali S, Fazel A. Pelvic congestion syndrome and May-Thurner syndrome as cause for pelvic somatic neuropathic pain: Neuropelveological diagnosis and corresponding therapeutic options. *Facts Views Vis Obgyn* 2021;13(2):141–148.
15. Possover M. Laparoscopic therapy for endometriosis and vascular entrapment of sacral plexus. *Fertil Steril* 2011;95(2):756–758.
16. Possover M. Five-year follow-up after laparoscopic large nerve resection for deep infiltrating sciatic nerve endometriosis. *J Minim Invasive Gynecol* 2017;24(5):822–826.
17. Possover M, Kostov P. Laparoscopic management of sacral nerve root schwannoma with intractable vulvococcygodynia: Report of three cases and review of literature. *J Minim Invasive Gynecol* 2013;20(3):394–397.
18. Possover M, Uehlinger K, Ulrich Exner G. Laparoscopic assisted resection of a ilio-sacral chondrosarcoma: A single case report. *Int J Surg Case Rep* 2014;5(7):381–384.
19. Possover M, Baekelandt J, Flaskamp C, et al. Laparoscopic neurolysis of the sacral plexus and the sciatic nerve for extensive endometriosis of the pelvic wall. *Minim Invasive Neurosurg* 2007;50(1):33–36.
20. Possover M. Laparoscopic management of endopelvic etiologies of pudendal pain in 134 consecutive patients. *J Urol* 2009;181(4):1732–1736.
21. Possover M. New surgical evolutions in management of sacral radiculopathies. *Surg Technol Int* 2010;19:123–128.
22. Possover M, Baekerland J, Chiantera V. The laparoscopic approach to control intractable pelvic neuralgia: From laparoscopic pelvic neurosurgery to the LION technique. *Clin J Pain* 2007;23(9):821–825.
23. Possover M, Baekelandt J, Chiantera V. The laparoscopic implantation of neuroprothesis (LION) procedure to control intractable abdomino-pelvic neuralgia. *Neuromodulation* 2007,10(1):18 23.
24. Possover M. The LION procedure to the pelvic nerves for treatment of urinary and faecal disorders. *Surg Technol Int* 2014;24:225–230.
25. Possover M. The laparoscopic implantation of neuroprothesis to the sacral plexus for therapy of neurogenic bladder dysfunctions after failure of percutaneous sacral nerve stimulation. *Neuromodulation* 2010;13(2):141–144.
26. Schmidt RA, Jonas U, Oleson KA, et al. Sacral nerve stimulation for the treatment of refractory urge incontinence. *J Urol* 1999;162(2):3562–357.
27. Hassouna MM, Siegel SW, Nijeholt AA, et al. Sacral neuromodulation in the treatment of urgency-frequency symptoms: A multicenter study an efficacity and safety. *J Urol* 2000;163(6):1849–1854.
28. Stewart WF, Van Rooyen JB, Cundiff GW, et al. Prevalence and burden of overactive bladder in the United States. *World J Urol* 2003;20(6):327–336.
29. Milsom I, Abrams P, Cardozo L, et al. How widespread are the symptoms of an overactive bladder and how are they managed? A population-based prevalence study. *BJU Int* 2001;87(9):760–766.
30. Sandvik H, Hunskaar S, Seim A, et al. Validation of a severity index in female urinary incontinence and its implementation in an epidemiological survey. *J Epidemiol Community Health* 1993;47(6):497–499.

31. Coyne KS, Wein A, Nicholson S, et al. Economic burden of urgency urinary incontinence in the United States: A systematic review. *J Manag Care Pharm* 2014;20(2):130–140.

32. Tai C, Wang J, Wang X, et al. Bladder inhibition or voiding induced by pudendal nerve stimulation in chronic spinal cord injured cats. *Neurourol Urodyn* 2007;26(4):570–577.

33. Rijkhoff N, Wijkstra H, van Kerrebroeck PE, et al. Urinary bladder control by electrical stimulation: Review of electrical stimulation techniques in spinal cord injury. *Neurourol Urodyn* 1997;16(1):39–53.

34. Possover M. A novel implantation technique for pudendal nerve stimulation for treatment of overactive bladder and urgency incontinence. *J Minim Invasive Gynecol* 2014;21(5):888–892.

35. Spinelli M, Malaguti S, Giardiello G, et al. A new minimally invasive procedure for pudendal nerve stimulation to treat neurogenic bladder: Description of the method and preliminary data. *Neurourol Urodyn* 2005;24(4):305–309.

36. Peters KM, Feber KM, Bennett RC. A prospective, single blind randomized crossover trial of sacral vs pudendal nerve stimulation for interstitial cystitis. *BJU Int* 2007;100(4):835–839.

37. Goldman HB, Amundsen CL, Mangel J, et al. Dorsal genital nerve stimulation for the treatment of overactive bladder symptoms. *Neurourol Urodyn* 2008;27(6):499–503.

38. Oliver S, Fowler C, Mundy A, et al. Measuring the sensations of urge and bladder filling during cystometry in urge incontinence and the effects of neuromodulation. *Neurourol Urodyn* 2003;22(1):7–16.

39. Seftel AD, Resnick MI, Boswell MV. Dorsal nerve block for management of intraoperative penile erection. *J Urol* 1994;151(2):394–395.

40. Giuliano F, Rampin O, Jardin A, et al. Electrophysiological study of relations between the dorsal nerve of the penis and the lumbar sympathetic chain in the rat. *J Urol* 1993;150(6):1960–1964.

41. Pescatori ES, Calabro A, Artibani W, et al. Electrical stimulation of the dorsal nerve of the penis evokes reflex tonic erections of the penile body and reflex ejaculatory responses in the spinal rat. *J Urol* 1993;149(3):627–632.

42. Worsøe J, Fynne L, Laurberg S, et al. Electrical stimulation of the dorsal clitoral nerve reduces incontinence episodes in idiopathic fecal incontinent patients: A pilot study. *Colorectal Dis* 2012;14(3):349–355.

43. Balaya V, Aubin A, Rogez J-M, et al. Le nerf dorsal du clitoris: De l'anatomie a la chirurgie reconstructive du clitoris. *Morphologie* 2014;98(320):8–17.

44. Possover M. The sacral LION procedure for recovery of bladder/rectum/sexual functions in paraplegic patients after explantation of a previous Finetech-Brindley-Controller. *J Minim Invasive Gynecol* 2009;16(1):98–101.

45. Possover M, Schurch B, Henle K-P. New pelvic nerves stimulation strategy for recovery of pelvic visceral functions and locomotion in paraplegics. *Neurourol Urodyn* 2010;29(8):1433–1438.

46. Possover M. The LION procedure to the pelvic nerves for recovery of locomotion in 18 spinal cord injured peoples—A case series. *Surg Technol Int* 2016;29:19–25.

47. Lemos N, Bichuetti DB, Marques RM, et al. Laparoscopic implantation of neuromodulators for treating urinary dysfunctions and improving locomotion in multiple sclerosis patients. *Int Urogynecol J* 2015;26(12):1871–1873.

48. Possover M, Forman A. Recovery of supraspinal control of leg movement in a chronic complete flaccid paraplegic man after continuous low-frequency pelvic nerve stimulation and FES-assisted training. *Spinal Cord Ser Cases* 2017;3:16034.

49. Possover M. Ten-year experience with continuous low-frequency pelvic somatic nerve stimulation for recovery of voluntary walking motion in some patients with chronic spinal cord injuries: A prospective case series of 29 consecutive patients. *Arch Phys Med Rehabil* 2021;102(1):50–57.

50. Figoni SF. Exercise responses and quadriplegia. *Med Sci Sports Exerc* 1993;25(4):433–441.

51. Scremin AM, Kurta L, Gentili A, et al. Increasing muscle mass in spinal cord injured persons with a functional electrical stimulation exercise program. *Arch Phys Med Rehabil* 1999;80(12):1531–1536.

52. Alfieri V. Electrical treatment of spasticity: Reflex tonic activity in hemiplegic patients and selected specific electrostimulation. *Scand J Rehabil Med* 1982;14(4):177–182.

53. Takeda S, Elefteriou F, Levasseur R, et al. Leptin regulates bone formation via the sympathetic nervous system. *Cell* 2002;111(3):305–317.

54. Levasseur R, Sabatier JP, Potrel-Burgot C, et al. Sympathetic nervous system as transmitter of mechanical loading in bone. *Joint Bone Spine* 2003;70(6):515–519.

55. Rettori R, Planchon M, Porte F, et al. Results of epidural electrical stimulation of the spinal cord in 12 cases of arteritis of the legs. *J Mal Vasc* 1989;14(3):267–268.

56. Thawer HA, Houghton PE. Effects of electrical stimulation on the histological properties of wounds in diabetic mice. *Wound Repair Regen* 2001;9(2):107–115.

57. Jünger M, Zuder D, Steins A, et al. Treatment of venous ulcers with low frequency pulsed current (Dermapulse): Effects on cutaneous microcirculation. *Hautartzt* 1997;48(12):879–903.

58. Stromberg B. Effects of electrical currents on wound contraction. *Ann Plast Surg* 1988;21(2):121–123.

59. Mawson A, Siddiqui F, Connolly B, et al. Effect of high voltage pulsed galvanic stimulation on sacral transcutaneous oxygen tension levels in the spinal cord injured. *Paraplegia* 1993;31(5):311–319.

60. Taylor K, Fish DR, Mendel FC, et al. Effect of a single 30-minute treatment of high voltage pulsed current on edema formation in frog limbs. *Phys Ther* 1992;72(1):63–68.

CHAPTER 19

PERIOPERATIVE CARE

Kristina A. Butler

Introduction

All surgical procedures involve risk of complications and the possibility of long-term morbidity, loss of function, or death. These complications may include infection, bleeding, thromboembolism, damage to surrounding structures, and need for additional surgery. Much of the risk to an individual patient is based on the pathology necessitating surgery and her medical comorbidities. Pelvic organ prolapse and urinary and fecal incontinence are disabling conditions with significant burden of disease and loss of function. They are not, however, fatal diseases. Every consideration must be made to weigh the risks of surgery against the natural history of the disease being treated. Many interventions are available to both assess and reduce an individual patient's risk of complications. Additionally, there are some time-honored practices and routines that increase the risk of certain complications. It is every surgeon's responsibility to remain current on the best practices for perioperative care and to advocate for their implementation in an organized fashion in hospital practices and operating rooms. Selecting the appropriate surgery for the patient balancing risk and morbidity is also a surgeon responsibility. Offering a minimally invasive approach when possible provides better outcomes.[1–3]

The goals of perioperative care are to minimize the risk to the individual patient and to maximize the likelihood of a successful surgical outcome and return to normal function. Within this framework are the preoperative medical evaluation, immediate preoperative care, and intraoperative care. The goals of the preoperative medical evaluation are to maximize the functional status of individual patients with known disease and to screen based on history and risk factors for subclinical conditions that may affect their response to surgery. Patients undergoing reconstructive pelvic surgery are often older and have a greater number of comorbidities or risk factors that must be addressed prior to surgery.

Symptoms of pelvic floor dysfunction affect up to 50% of women. The lifetime risk of surgery for pelvic organ prolapse is estimated to be up to 19%.[4] Rates of operative complications and perioperative morbidity are low in benign gynecologic surgery. However, pelvic

reconstructive surgery involves a higher risk due to the extent of procedure and population characteristics. Patients undergoing reconstructive pelvic surgery are often older, undergo lengthy surgeries, and have histories of prior pelvic surgery.[5] All of these are known to increase surgical morbidity and mortality. In addition, patients undergoing reconstructive pelvic surgery often have distorted anatomy that increases the risk of surgical injury. This chapter reviews topics in perioperative care, including preoperative testing and preparations. In addition, intraoperative management is discussed.

PREOPERATIVE CARE

Preoperative Testing

A thorough history and physical exam inclusive of current medications and allergies is necessary for safe surgical care. Baseline laboratory testing in women without systemic disease who are otherwise healthy is not beneficial. The American Society of Anesthesiologists (ASA) recommends patients ASA 1 or 2 not undergo lab testing specifically complete blood count, basic or comprehensive metabolic panel, and coagulation studies when blood loss is expected to be minimal.[6] Preoperative hemoglobin A1c (HgA1c) elevation may be an indication to delay surgery and optimize diabetes management. Diabetes poses significant perioperative risk when poorly controlled and can result in infectious complications (HgA1c >7%), prolonged length of stay (HgA1c >8%), and mortality (HgA1c >9%) following surgery.[7,8] Women without cardiopulmonary disease do not need chest X-ray as only 2% of such images lead to a change in management. Those with chronic stable cardiopulmonary diseases older than age 70 years may benefit if chest radiography has not been performed within 6 months.[9] Similarly, routine 12-lead electrocardiogram is not useful for asymptomatic patients undergoing low-risk surgical procedures.[10] In women with known cardiac disease and asymptomatic, cardiac stress testing and echocardiography provide no advantage when undergoing low or moderate risk noncardiac surgery. These tests do not change the patient's clinical management or outcomes and may result in increased cost and unnecessary additional procedures.[11,12] β-Blockers should be continued in those with preexisting daily use but not started on the day of surgery to avoid harm or cardiovascular instability. Continuation of angiotensin-converting enzyme inhibitors or angiotensin receptor blockers perioperatively is reasonable.[10] Smoking cessation is encouraged to improve cardiopulmonary health.

Pregnancy screening may be safely performed with questionnaire to avoid costs and time associated with laboratory analysis.[13] Alternately, urine pregnancy could be performed. Type and screen antibody testing is costly, and transfusion during pelvic reconstructive surgery is low at 1.26%; therefore, many institutions safely limit its use.[14] Suspected existing infections should be identified and treated prior to elective surgery, for example, urinary tract infection and bacterial vaginosis.[15,16] Additionally, vaginal health improvements gained from topical estrogen use preoperatively in postmenopausal patients have been shown to improve pelvic reconstruction outcomes, although ongoing study continues.[17] Any bleeding in menopausal women prompts evaluation of the cervical, uterine, vulvar, vaginal, and anal areas to screen for malignancy. Pap smear or office biopsy can be performed timely and return results quickly. The uterus can be evaluated with ultrasound or endometrial biopsy.[18]

Preoperative Preparations

Enhanced Recovery after Surgery pathways begin preoperatively with patient education (Table 19.1). The goal is to maintain baseline physiology and patient comfort while providing surgery with improved outcomes, cost savings in reduced hospitalization, and decreased complications. Avoid unnecessary perioperative fasting for elective surgical procedures. Fasting after midnight was thought to reduce pulmonary aspiration; however, data does not support this practice. Prolonged fasting is associated with increased insulin resistance, delayed recovery, and poorer outcomes.[19,20] The ASA and other organizations recommend discontinuing solid food 6 hours before surgery and encourage intake of clear fluids until 2 hours before surgery for improved outcomes and patient satisfaction. Mechanical bowel preparation for pelvic reconstructive surgery is not needed and outcomes are improved without this practice. Return to general diet and hospital dismissal following surgery are significantly improved. Enemas may be used without adverse effect.[21–23] Preoperative showering is encouraged as it aim to reduce the number of microorganisms on the skin near the incision and may reduce the risk of infection.[24] Same-day dismissal to reduce the need for hospitalization and nosocomial infection exposure is safe for women undergoing pelvic floor reconstruction surgery; this can be individualized and does not increase the rate of complications.[25,26]

Pain management begins before the incision is made, and this preemptive strategy has proven to reduce opiate use, nausea and vomiting, impaired bowel function, immobilization, and perioperative morbidity. Medications given may include acetaminophen, nonsteroidal anti-inflammatory agents, and antiemetics. Local injection of an analgesia is also recommended for pain relief. This may be in the form of wound infiltration, using a nerve block, or deep pelvic injection, for example, at the uterosacral ligaments during vaginal surgery.[27]

INTRAOPERATIVE CARE

Preventing hypothermia and maintaining euvolemia during surgery is key. Discussions with the anesthesia team are encouraged on fluid balance and warming devices. Unnecessary costs are accrued from frozen section pathology evaluation if the result will not affect immediate perioperative management.[28] It is preferable to submit the specimen for routine processing and permanent section evaluation if no therapeutic decision for the patient on the day of the surgical procedure is needed.

Antibiotic Use

The use of antibiotics to prevent surgical site infections in hysterectomy patients is well established and used as a quality metric.[29] Surgical site infections are the most common source of health care–associated infections (HAI) in the United States, comprising 22% of all HAI.[30] Prevention and the appropriate use of prophylactic antibiotics has received much attention. The Centers for Disease Control and Prevention (CDC), Centers for Medicare & Medicaid Services, University Health System Consortium, and American College of Surgeons National Surgical Quality Improvement Program have all contributed to guidelines and performance standards aimed at reducing the incidence of surgical quality.

Current guidelines recommend that prophylactic antibiotics be administered within 60 minutes of incision time and be discontinued within 24 hours of surgery. The antimicrobial agent chosen should be active against the likely infectious organisms to be encountered in the surgery performed and should have an appropriate safety profile for the patient.[15,16] For gynecologic surgery, cefazolin is endorsed as appropriate for nonallergic patients. For patients unable to tolerate cephalosporins, alternate regimens are recommended. Immediate hypersensitivity reaction (anaphylaxis, hives, bronchospasm) would be a contraindication to use penicillin or cephalosporin; however, allergy testing is encouraged as time allows because true allergies are not common. Ten percent of the population reports a penicillin allergy; however, research shows that 90% of them are not allergic to penicillin. Patients receiving a penicillin alternate have higher medical costs and longer hospital stays and are more likely to develop complications such as infections with vancomycin-resistant

TABLE 19.1	
Enhanced Recovery after Surgery (ERAS)	
PREOPERATIVE GOALS	
Evaluation	Office or phone evaluation Obtain medical history. Assess for history of sleep apnea or anesthesia complications. Medication reconciliation
Counseling	Provide expectations and goals. Explain ERAS pathway and share documentation. Encourage patient and family collaboration.
Endurance	Recommend walking or exercise prior to surgery, 30 min/d at a minimum.
Diet	Vegetables, fruits, and protein incorporated in daily meals 1–2 wk before surgery Regular diet before midnight the night before surgery Clear liquids ($\leq$12 oz/h) until 2 h prior to surgery Clear liquids include water, soda, tea, juice without pulp and filtered, sports beverages, coffee. Avoid oral bowel preparation; enema may be used.
Wellness	Shower with soap and water the evening before surgery and the morning of surgery. Plan a good night's rest without alcohol or tobacco.
HOSPITAL ARRIVAL	

Perioperative	Maintain intraoperative euvolemia.
	Pain prevention:
	   Acetaminophen 1,000 mg oral once
	   Celecoxib 400 mg oral once (200 mg if age 65 yr or older or weight <50 kg), hold
	      for renal impairment
	Postoperative nausea and vomiting prevention:
	   Before incision ($\pm$30 min): dexamethasone 4 mg IV once, droperidol 0.625 mg
	      IV once
	   Before closure ($\pm$30 min): granisetron 0.1 mg IV once
	   At closure: ketorolac 15 mg IV for patients without contraindications
	Local infiltration with bupivacaine

HOSPITAL CARE AND DISMISSAL	
	Out of bed to chair within 2 h after surgery
	Peripheral IV saline lock when patient has 600 mL oral
	Regular diet
	Scheduled: acetaminophen 1,000 mg oral every 6 h and ibuprofen 600 mg every 6 h ($\pm$3-d use)
	As needed breakthrough opiate use, oxycodone 5 mg every 4 h
	Evaluate for same-day dismissal.

ERAS, Enhanced Recovery after Surgery; IV, intravenous.

Enterococcus and *Clostridium difficile*. Alternate antibiotics have also been shown to be less effective in infection prevention. Allergy skin testing can be performed easily with excellent negative predictive value approaching 100%.[31,32]

Recommendations by the American College of Obstetricians and Gynecologists do not endorse prophylaxis for laparoscopy, cystoscopy, and urodynamics. Antibiotics are repeated when blood loss exceeds 1,500 mL and for lengthy procedures at the appropriate interval, for example, cefazolin is dosed again 4 hours after the first infusion. Antibiotic continuation following surgery is discouraged and has not been shown to provide benefit.[15,16]

Several issues related specifically to reconstructive pelvic surgery are not addressed in the literature.

Clearly, any patient having reconstructive surgery involving a hysterectomy should receive antibiotic prophylaxis. Updated guidelines include antibiotic recommendations for women undergoing colporrhaphy, vaginal sling placement, and laparotomy. Minimally invasive mesh colpopexy is not specifically included for antibiotic use; however, laparoscopic surgeries that include entry into the vagina or bowel are recommended to have prophylaxis. Individualization for each patient at the time of surgery is required to ensure safe practice as we balance the risk of infection and antibiotic stewardship in reducing bacterial resistance.

Venous Thromboembolism Prophylaxis

The risk of venous thromboembolism (VTE) following major gynecologic surgery in patients not receiving prophylaxis is estimated to be between 15% and 40%. Risk factors include increasing age, obesity, previous VTE, and those with clotting disorders.[33] Risk stratification is necessary to determine best preventive management during abdominal-pelvic surgery. Thromboembolism risks are balanced with bleeding risks. Prevention strategies include early mobilization, mechanical intermittent pneumatic compression, and anticoagulation preoperatively and/or postoperatively.[34] Risk scoring is reliably determined using various methods. As an example, Caprini scoring considers key factors including age, surgical duration, and body mass index (BMI). As an example, a typical patient with prolapse may quickly meet high-risk criteria. A patient older than 60 years (2 points), having vaginal hysterectomy colporrhaphy >45 minute surgery (2 points), with BMI >25 (1 point) scores high-risk Caprini score ≥5 prompting the need for dual prophylaxis using pharmacologic and mechanical therapy.

Most trials evaluating VTE prevention initiate prophylactic therapy prior to the surgery start time, including initiating pharmacotherapy preoperatively and mechanical compression prior to gynecologic surgery. Preoperative heparin use does not increase intraoperative bleeding and can be safely used. Use of intermittent pneumatic compression devices is recommended as mechanical prophylaxis for preventing VTE; however, graduated compression stockings should be avoided.[35]

The American College of Chest Physicians and American College of Obstetricians and Gynecologists correlate moderately on their recommendations to reduce thrombosis risk. For low-risk women, early mobilization or mechanical prophylaxis is sufficient. For moderate-risk women mechanical or pharmacologic therapy can be considered. In higher risk categories for thrombosis, dual prophylaxis using pharmacologic and mechanical therapy is recommended and continued during hospitalization. Outpatient pharmacologic prophylaxis can be considered in a highest risk subset for 2 to 4 weeks after discharge. Recent data specific to gynecology surgery does support the safety and improved patient satisfaction of going home with oral anticoagulation prophylaxis.[36]

Chronic anticoagulation is common, and perioperative management may require adjustment. Specific risks have been described for women chronically anticoagulated having prolapse surgery, increased risk is seen in development of vaginal hematoma along with blood transfusion, intensive care unit admission, readmission, and overall complications.[37] Periprocedural bridging anticoagulation may be required and the direct oral anticoagulants are becoming more numerous with varying perioperative recommendations. Online dose adjustment calculators for various anticoagulants are available and recommended for use.[38]

Positioning and Surgical Site Preparation

Patient positioning must provide secure safety while allowing surgical access. Risk factors for positional injury include body habitus at both extremes, patient age, vascular disease, hypotension, and, most importantly, surgery duration. Lithotomy is required often in pelvic reconstruction; therefore, lower extremity safety is a priority to provide support without compression.[39] Boot stirrups provide improved outcomes, although candy cane stirrups are also available.[40] The knees and hips remain flexed at 90° angles, avoiding hip abduction and providing sufficient padding in areas of contact. The arms should also be stabilized in natural positions using similar principles. Retractors are employed to provide visualization of the surgical field while relocating surrounding tissues safely based on the task at hand. Retraction can be handheld or self-retaining and must be implemented to avoid undo tension or pressure on delicate visceral structures, nerves, or vessels. A vaginal pack is an example of soft retraction frequently used. The vaginal Bookwalter is designed specifically for women's care, is reusable, and is secured to the operative bed offering multiple attachments to facilitate stable, self-retaining vaginal access (Fig. 19.1). Robotic surgery also offers stable retraction with instruments functioning actively and passively concurrently. A plethora of high-quality retractors are available based on surgeon's preference and availability.

Site preparation, abdominal or vaginal, is indicated to reduce surgical site infection. Chlorhexidine/isopropyl alcohol solutions offer excellent outcomes in abdominal and vaginal surgery infection reduction and are endorsed by the CDC.[15,16,29,41] Iodine preparations are an alternate and are U.S. Food and Drug Administration approved for use, specifically in the vagina. Removing hair at the surgical site has been associated with an increased rate of surgical site infections because of razor-induced microtrauma. When hair

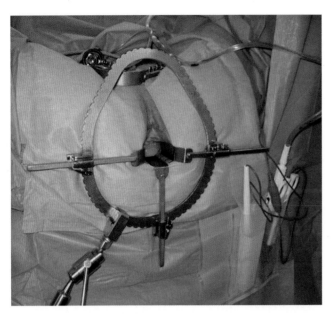

FIGURE 19.1 Vaginal Bookwalter.

removal is necessary, hair at the surgical site should be removed by clipping or depilatory methods. Razor shaving should be avoided.[42]

Cystoscopy and Urinary Care

Urinary tract infection (UTI) occurs in 20% of women following previous urogynecologic surgery.[43,44] As mentioned previously, this is a national quality metric that may impact institutional quality scoring and reimbursement.[45] Preexisting urinary flora have been linked to postoperative UTI risk; therefore, preoperative screening is used at many institutions. Nearly all patients having reconstructive pelvic surgery will have urinary instrumentation during their hospital stay. Catheter care may be needed, and some general principles apply, including aseptic insertion techniques, maintenance of a closed drainage system, and minimizing the duration of catheter usage postoperatively.

Continued or prolonged catheter use is associated with more risk of infection. Management is often complicated in patients undergoing surgery for advanced pelvic organ prolapse or urinary incontinence because of the risk of postoperative urinary retention and the need for voiding trials following surgery. Immediate catheter removal has been shown to be safe following hysterectomy and not inferior to delayed catheter removal.[46] Early catheter removal is seen more commonly in recent years following reconstructive pelvic surgery, with most patients beginning voiding trials the day of surgery or postoperative day 1.[47,48] Patients requiring long-term catheterization are best managed with clean intermittent self-catheterization, although suprapubic catheterization remains an option in selected cases.

There is some evidence to support the use of prophylactic antibiotics to reduce the incidence of UTIs in surgical patients requiring prolonged transurethral catheterization. This limited benefit must be balanced with the concern for antibiotic induced bacterial resistance. Patients managed with clean intermittent catheterization do not require antibiotics. There is also evidence that patients managed with suprapubic catheterization may benefit from prophylactic nitrofurantoin, with reduced rates of UTI at catheter removal. In patients managed by suprapubic catheterization, antibiotic prophylaxis may be warranted.[49]

There is work to be done to discover optimal methods for postoperative urinary care in reconstructive pelvic surgery. The basic principles of a closed drainage system inserted under sterile conditions that remains in place for the shortest duration possible is the standard for appropriate care.

Injury to the bladder or ureter can occur during any pelvic operation. Anti-incontinence procedures and reconstructive surgeries for advanced prolapse increase the risk of such injuries. Unrecognized lower urinary tract injury in gynecologic surgery represents a source of disability to patients and significant litigation risk for surgical teams. This is highlighted by data supporting the low cost of cystoscopy, excellent detection rate for genitourinary injury, and high negative predictive value.[45,50-52] The overall incidence for urinary tract injury in reconstructive pelvic surgery is greater than that of simple hysterectomy. Although data supporting prophylactic culdoplasty during simple hysterectomy to reduce subsequent prolapse risk would further support routine cystoscopy to preclude urinary tract injury.[53] Routine intraoperative cystoscopy is recommended during prolapse surgery and vaginal apex suspension procedures involving the uterosacral ligaments.[5]

Bleeding

Bleeding complications in reconstructive pelvic surgery are uncommon but should be anticipated to expedite response and resolution. Surgical transfusion rates are low and further minimized with minimally invasive surgery. Minimally invasive procedures report a transfusion rate of approximately 1% for incontinence only procedures, minimally invasive sacral colpopexy, and vaginal prolapse repair. Risk factors specific to pelvic reconstruction include anemia, increased ASA class, nonwhite race, Hispanic ethnicity, and concomitant hysterectomy.[14] Interestingly, age and obesity have limited contribution.

Optimizing preexisting conditions prior to surgery can reduce risk of bleeding. Hemorrhage during benign gynecologic surgery is most commonly due to vascular injury. Bleeding can be arterial or venous. Arterial bleeding if identified and localized can be controlled with sutures or clips. Major vascular injury is rare in reconstructive pelvic surgery, but damage to the external iliac artery, obturator vessels, and hypogastric artery can occur even with minimally invasive procedures such as the urethral sling. Venous bleeding presents special challenges because it may be diffuse or profuse, thus making it difficult for identification and ligation of a damaged vein. Several areas at increased risk for significant venous bleeding during reconstructive pelvic surgery include the retropubic and presacral spaces. Each contains a rich venous plexus that is at risk during procedures such as abdominal sacral colpopexy and pubovaginal slings. Careful dissection and awareness of anatomy, individualized variation, and surrounding vasculature is imperative. Cautery will often control bleeding and can be improved with forceps isolation. Packing and manual compression are also effective. Sacral sutures or tacks can be used. Additionally, oxidized cellulose, thrombin preparation, polysaccharide spheres, omental flap, and muscle welding are all modalities to be familiar with.[54] Adequate exposure and lighting and meticulous technique are essential. Injection of epinephrine can provide vasoconstriction, thereby reducing bleeding and this technique can be used vaginally or in the retropubic space.

Postoperative bleeding may be detected in the recovery area and close monitoring of symptoms and vital signs is imperative. Investigation with lab studies and imaging are helpful based on suspicion. Having a low threshold for continued monitoring if any instability is noted may provide safety. Discharge instructions also provide for the patient and family to advocate for themselves once home should their recovery status change. Consideration must always be made toward prevention of such complications and should include attention to anatomy, surgical technique, perioperative care, and patient preparation for surgery.

CONCLUSION

Surgical repair of female pelvic floor disorders is common and is projected to increase in years to come. Along with traditional repairs, multiple minimally invasive approaches are increasingly employed, and techniques are rapidly evolving to benefit women's health care. Adherence to "first do no harm" and expert technique are required to minimize the surgical complications and patient morbidity. Perioperative care must be evidence based and comprehensive, especially in geriatric populations. Health care quality agencies provide and update recommendations, and all surgeons should be familiar with them as they evolve.

Preoperative efforts aim to optimize women for high-quality surgical outcomes while balancing cost-effective strategies to provide value. Intraoperative care aims to minimize complications that may occur. Patients have often had multiple prior surgeries and have distorted anatomy. New procedures will result in new complications. Reconstructive surgeons must be prepared for this and remain ready to handle unforeseen situations. New technology is not a substitute for rigorous surgical training, fundamental principles, and anatomic knowledge. Prevention may indeed be the best medicine, and our patients will also be best served by a rational, evidence-based approach to the adoption of new procedures and technologies.

There is great demand for reconstructive pelvic surgery, and successful outcomes can transform patient's lives. Good surgical outcomes require good preoperative patient preparation and meticulous attention to surgical details to avoid intraoperative complications. This chapter highlights important areas for attention, with specific focus on details relevant to patients and procedures in reconstructive pelvic surgery.

References

1. Committee Opinion No. 701: Choosing the route of hysterectomy for benign disease. *Obstet Gynecol* 2017;129(6):e155–e159.
2. AAGL. AAGL position statement: Robotic-assisted laparoscopic surgery in benign gynecology. *J Minim Invasive Gynecol* 2013;20(1):2–9.
3. Liu H, Lawrie TA, Lu D, et al. Robot-assisted surgery in gynaecology. *Cochrane Database System Rev* 2014;(12):CD008640.
4. Haya N, Feiner B, Baessler K, et al. Perioperative interventions in pelvic organ prolapse surgery. *Cochrane Database Syst Rev* 2018;(8):CD013105.
5. American College of Obstetricians and Gynecologists, American Urogynecologic Society. Pelvic organ prolapse. *Female Pelvic Med Reconstr Surg* 2019;25(6):397–408.
6. Apfelbaum JL, Connis RT, Nickinovich DG, et al. Practice advisory for preanesthesia evaluation: An updated report by the American Society of Anesthesiologists Task Force on Preanesthesia Evaluation. *Anesthesiology* 2012;116(3):522–538.
7. Underwood P, Askari R, Hurwitz S, et al. Preoperative A1C and clinical outcomes in patients with diabetes undergoing major noncardiac surgical procedures. *Diabetes Care* 2014;37(3):611–616.
8. Duggan EW, Carlson K, Umpierrez GE. Perioperative hyperglycemia management: An update. *Anesthesiology* 2017;126(3):547–560.
9. American College of Radiology. ACR Appropriateness Criteria®: Routine admission and preoperative chest radiography. Published 2000. Updated 2011. Accessed September 26, 2020. https://seicat.org/repo/static/public/documentos/ACR_Criteria_Routine_Admission_and_Preoperative_Chest_Radiography.pdf
10. Fleisher LA, Fleischmann KE, Auerbach AD, et al. 2014 ACC/AHA guideline on perioperative cardiovascular evaluation and management of patients undergoing noncardiac surgery: A report of the American College of Cardiology/American Heart Association Task Force on practice guidelines. *J Am Coll Cardiol* 2014;64(22):e77–e137.
11. Sheffield KM, McAdams PS, Benarroch-Gampel J, et al. Overuse of preoperative cardiac stress testing in Medicare patients undergoing elective noncardiac surgery. *Ann Surg* 2013;257(1):73–80.
12. Wijeysundera DN, Beattie WS, Austin PC, et al. Non-invasive cardiac stress testing before elective major non-cardiac surgery: Population based cohort study. *BMJ* 2010;340:b5526.

13. Wyatt MA, Ainsworth AJ, DeJong SR, et al. Implementation of the "Pregnancy Reasonably Excluded Guide" for pregnancy assessment: A quality initiative in outpatient gynecologic surgery. *Obstet Gynecol* 2018;132(5):1222–1228.

14. Pandya LK, Lynch CD, Hundley AF, et al. The incidence of transfusion and associated risk factors in pelvic reconstructive surgery. *Am J Obstet Gynecol* 2017;217(5):612.e1–612.e8.

15. ACOG Practice Bulletin No. 195: Prevention of infection after gynecologic procedures. *Obstet Gynecol* 2018;131(6):e172–e189.

16. Bratzler DW, Dellinger EP, Olsen KM, et al. Clinical practice guidelines for antimicrobial prophylaxis in surgery. *Surg Infect (Larchmt)* 2013;14(1):73–156.

17. Rahn DD, Good MM, Roshanravan SM, et al. Effects of preoperative local estrogen in postmenopausal women with prolapse: A randomized trial. *J Clin Endocrinol Metab* 2014;99(10): 3728–3736.

18. American College of Obstetricians and Gynecologists. The role of transvaginal ultrasonography in evaluating the endometrium of women with postmenopausal bleeding. Published 2018. Accessed April 21, 2021. https://www.acog.org/clinical/clinical -guidance/committee-opinion/articles/2018/05/the-role-of -transvaginal-ultrasonography-in-evaluating-the-endometrium -of-women-with-postmenopausal-bleeding

19. McLeod R, Fitzgerald W, Sarr M. Canadian Association of General Surgeons and American College of Surgeons evidence based reviews in surgery. 14. Preoperative fasting for adults to prevent perioperative complications. *Can J Surg* 2005;48(5):409–411.

20. Brady M, Kinn S, Stuart P. Preoperative fasting for adults to prevent perioperative complications. *Cochrane Database Syst Rev* 2003;(4):CD004423.

21. Kalogera E, Dowdy S. Prehabilitation: Enhancing the Enhanced Recovery after Surgery pathway. *Int J Gynecol Cancer* 2019;29(8):1233–1234.

22. Kalogera E, Bakkum-Gamez JN, Jankowski CJ, et al. Enhanced recovery in gynecologic surgery. *Obstet Gynecol* 2013;122(2 Pt 1): 319–328.

23. Altman AD, Robert M, Armbrust R, et al. Guidelines for vulvar and vaginal surgery: Enhanced Recovery after Surgery society recommendations. *Am J Obstet Gynecol* 2020;223(4):475–485.

24. National Institute for Health and Care Excellence. *Surgical site infections: Prevention and treatment.* London: National Institute for Health and Care Excellence, 2019.

25. Liu L, Yi J, Cornella J, et al. Same-day discharge after vaginal hysterectomy with pelvic floor reconstruction: Pilot study. *J Minim Invasive Gynecol* 2020;27(2):498–503.e491.

26. Lloyd JC, Guzman-Negron J, Goldman HB. Feasibility of same day discharge after robotic assisted pelvic floor reconstruction. *Can J Urol* 2018;25(3):9307–9312.

27. Long JB, Eiland RJ, Hentz JG, et al. Randomized trial of preemptive local analgesia in vaginal surgery. *Int Urogynecol J Pelvic Floor Dysfunct* 2009;20(1):5–10.

28. Taxy JB. Frozen section and the surgical pathologist: A point of view. *Arch Pathol Lab Med* 2009;133(7):1135–1138.

29. Andiman SE, Xu X, Boyce JM, et al. Decreased surgical site infection rate in hysterectomy: Effect of a gynecology-specific bundle. *Obstet Gynecol* 2018;131(6):991–999.

30. Association for Professionals in Infection Control and Epidemiology. U.S. Centers for Medicare & Medicaid Services: Surgical infection prevention proposed rule. Accessed September 26, 2020. http://apic.org/cms/

31. Solensky R. Penicillin allergy as a public health measure. *J Allergy Clin Immunol* 2014;133(3):797–798.

32. Macy E, Contreras R. Health care use and serious infection prevalence associated with penicillin "allergy" in hospitalized patients: A cohort study. *J Allergy Clin Immunol* 2014;133(3):790–796.

33. ACOG Practice Bulletin No. 84: Prevention of deep vein thrombosis and pulmonary embolism. *Obstet Gynecol* 2007;110(2 Pt 1): 429–440.

34. Gould MK, Garcia DA, Wren SM, et al. Prevention of VTE in nonorthopedic surgical patients: *Antithrombotic Therapy and Prevention of Thrombosis*, 9th ed: American College of Chest Physicians evidence-based clinical practice guidelines. *Chest* 2012;141(2 Suppl):e227S–e277S.

35. Kakkos SK, Caprini JA, Geroulakos G, et al. Combined intermittent pneumatic leg compression and pharmacological prophylaxis for prevention of venous thromboembolism. *Cochrane Database Syst Rev* 2016;9(9):CD005258.

36. Guntupalli SR, Brennecke A, Behbakht K, et al. Safety and efficacy of apixaban vs enoxaparin for preventing postoperative venous thromboembolism in women undergoing surgery for gynecologic malignant neoplasm: A randomized clinical trial. *JAMA Netw Open* 2020;3(6):e207410.

37. High R, Kavanagh A, Khavari R, et al. Outcomes in pelvic organ prolapse surgery in women using chronic antithrombotic therapy. *Female Pelvic Med Reconstr Surg* 2017;23(6):372–376.

38. Mayo Clinic. Anticoagulation management (adult): Periprocedural anticoagulation management calculator. Published 2020. Accessed September 28, 2020. https://askmayo expert.mayoclinic.org/topic/clinical-answers/gnt20135224/itt -20137025

39. Bohrer JC, Walters MD, Park A, et al. Pelvic nerve injury following gynecologic surgery: A prospective cohort study. *Am J Obstet Gynecol* 2009;201(5):531.e1–531.e7.

40. Gupta A, Meriwether K, Tuller M, et al. Candy cane compared with boot stirrups in vaginal surgery: A randomized controlled trial. *Obstet Gynecol* 2020;136(2):333–341.

41. Centers for Disease Control and Prevention. Surgical site infection (SSI). Accessed September 26, 2020. https://www.cdc.gov /hai/ssi/ssi.html

42. Tanner J, Norrie P, Melen K. Preoperative hair removal to reduce surgical site infection. *Cochrane Database Syst Rev* 2011;(11):CD004122.

43. El-Nashar SA, Singh R, Schmitt JJ, et al. Urinary tract infection after hysterectomy for benign gynecologic conditions or pelvic reconstructive surgery. *Obstet Gynecol* 2018;132(6):1347–1357.

44. Thomas-White KJ, Gao X, Lin H, et al. Urinary microbes and postoperative urinary tract infection risk in urogynecologic surgical patients. *Int Urogynecol J* 2018;29(12):1797–1805.

45. Erekson EA, Iglesia CB. Improving patient outcomes in gynecology: The role of large data registries and big data analytics. *J Minim Invasive Gynecol* 2015;22(7):1124–1129.

46. Sandberg EM, Twijnstra A, van Meir CA, et al. Immediate versus delayed removal of urinary catheter after laparoscopic hysterectomy: A randomised controlled trial. *BJOG* 2019;126(6):804–813.

47. Carter-Brooks CM, Zyczynski HM, Moalli PA, et al. Early catheter removal after pelvic floor reconstructive surgery: A randomized trial. *Int Urogynecol J* 2018;29(8):1203–1212.

48. Meekins AR, Siddiqui NY, Amundsen CL, et al. Improving postoperative efficiency: An algorithm for expedited void trials after urogynecologic surgery. *South Med J* 2017;110(12):785–790.

49. Marschall J, Carpenter CR, Fowler S, et al. Antibiotic prophylaxis for urinary tract infections after removal of urinary catheter: Meta-analysis. *BMJ* 2013;346:f3147.

50. Anand M, Casiano ER, Heisler CA, et al. Utility of intraoperative cystoscopy in detecting ureteral injury during vaginal hysterectomy. *Female Pelvic Med Reconstr Surg* 2015;21(2):70–76.

51. Practice Bulletin No. 176: Pelvic organ prolapse. *Obstet Gynecol* 2017;129(4):e56–e72.

52. AAGL practice report: Practice guidelines for intraoperative cystoscopy in laparoscopic hysterectomy. *J Minim Invasive Gynecol* 2012;19(4):407–411.

53. Blandon RE, Bharucha AE, Melton LJ III, et al. Risk factors for pelvic floor repair after hysterectomy. *Obstet Gynecol* 2009;113(3):601–608.

54. Hokenstad ED, Occhino JA. Management of presacral bleeding. *Int Urogynecol J* 2020;31(1):215–217.

CHAPTER 20

PRINCIPLES OF VAGINAL SURGERY

Rosanne M. Kho • Surabhi Tewari

Introduction

Vaginal surgery is one of the defining procedures that sets gynecologic surgeons apart from surgeries of other specialties. For hysterectomy for benign indications, the vaginal route remains the most minimally invasive approach. The most recent Cochrane Review in 2015 that involved 47 studies and 5,102 women concluded that the vaginal route is superior to the abdominal, laparoscopic, and robotic-assisted approach due to fewer intraoperative visceral injuries, less major long-term complications of fistula, less pain, fewer urinary/bowel/pelvic floor and sexual dysfunction, faster return to normal activities, greater patient satisfaction, and improved quality of life.[1] The American College of Obstetricians and Gynecologists (ACOG) Committee Opinion (Committee Opinion No. 701) recommends vaginal hysterectomy as the preferred and most cost-effective for benign hysterectomy.[2] ACOG also states that the need to perform adnexectomy should not be considered a contraindication to the vaginal approach. There is evidence that additional patient factors such as obesity, nulliparity, previous cesarean section or laparotomy, or an enlarged uterus should not preclude the patient from benefiting from the vaginal approach.[3]

The safety of vaginal hysterectomies as compared to other approaches has been well investigated. A recent meta-analysis indicated that there is a lower risk of vaginal cuff dehiscence and conversion to laparotomy in vaginal hysterectomy as compared to total laparoscopic hysterectomy.[4] This same analysis found no difference in overall complications, risk of ureter and bladder injuries, and intraoperative blood loss between the two approaches.[4] However, there is a greater risk of severe postoperative complications (Accordion complications grade 3 or higher) in robotic hysterectomy as compared to vaginal hysterectomy.[5] Additionally, vaginal hysterectomy demonstrates lower rates of superficial surgical site infections as compared to total abdominal hysterectomy.[6] These factors demonstrate that vaginal hysterectomy is a safer option with regard to several complications when compared to all other hysterectomy approaches.

Despite the evidence indicating that vaginal hysterectomy is the preferred surgical approach for benign conditions, there has been a decline in the last decade in not only the total number of hysterectomies but also the number of vaginal hysterectomies performed in the United States. The total number of inpatient hysterectomies peaked in 2002 and since then has demonstrated a steady decline as 36.4% fewer hysterectomies were performed in 2010 when compared to 2002.[7] More recent data demonstrates a 12.4% decrease in rate of utilization of hysterectomy between 2010 and 2013.[8] The rates of vaginal hysterectomies have mirrored this decline as the rate of total vaginal hysterectomy decreased from 51% to 13% between 2008 and 2018.[9] In the same 10-year span, rates of total laparoscopic hysterectomy increased from 12% to 68%, making it the most common surgical approach for hysterectomy.[8,9]

With declining numbers in both total hysterectomies and vaginal hysterectomies, training and surgical skills of residents and practicing surgeons are adversely impacted. Previous studies using validated surgery skills assessment tools have demonstrated that an average of 27 vaginal hysterectomies are needed to achieve competency in this procedure.[10] However, the minimum number of required vaginal hysterectomies as determined by the Accreditation Council for Graduate Medical Education is only 15, and the average number of vaginal hysterectomies logged by graduating residents was only 20 (standard deviation [SD] 10.9) in 2018 to 2019.[11] These patterns in training have impacted the level of preparedness of graduated residents when starting fellowship. For example, a 2015 study that surveyed female pelvic medicine and reconstructive surgery fellowship program directors demonstrated that only 20% of first-year fellows could adequately perform a vaginal hysterectomy.[12]

Decreased training in vaginal hysterectomy over the last decade has impacted both operative time and complication rates when using this approach. Traditionally, transvaginal hysterectomy is the fastest approach and was 73 minutes faster than a laparoscopic hysterectomy in 2002.[9] However, in 2018, this difference has declined over the past decade as the transvaginal approach is only 20 minutes faster than the laparoscopic approach.[9] This narrowed time differential can be attributed to both reduced median operating time in total laparoscopic hysterectomies by 37 minutes and increased median operating time for vaginal hysterectomies by 20 minutes between 2002 and 2018.[9] This same analysis noted a decrease in both major (adjusted odds ratio [OR] [95% confidence interval, CI]: 0.813 [0.750 to 0.881] vs. 0.873 [0.797 to 0.957]) and minor (0.723 [0.676 to 0.772] vs. 0.896 [0.832 to 0.964]) complications in total laparoscopic hysterectomy as compared to vaginal hysterectomy, respectively, although these results were not found to be statistically significant.[9] Such changes in classically reported trends in operating time and complication rates may reflect the increasing focus on laparoscopic and robotic surgery in obstetrics and gynecology training rather than demonstrating true changes in the efficacy of vaginal surgery versus laparoscopic surgery.

Surgical volume impacts patient outcomes in benign gynecologic surgery. Studies across various surgical fields have demonstrated that patients operated on by low-volume surgeons or at low-volume hospitals have increased complications, morbidity, and mortality in comparison to those patients operated on by high-volume surgeons.[13,14] These trends are also noted in gynecology as patients operated on by high-volume vaginal surgeons (performing greater than 13 vaginal surgeries a year) are 31% less likely to have an operative injury (OR [95% CI]: 0.69 [0.59 to 0.80]) in comparison to low-volume surgeons (performing less than 5.4 vaginal procedures annually).[15] In addition to decreased preoperative, intraoperative, and postoperative complications, the cost of a vaginal hysterectomy is also decreased by more than $600 when performed by a high-volume vaginal surgeon in comparison to a low-volume vaginal surgeon (parameter estimate [95% CI]: −609 [−664.86 to −554.21]).[15] Another study using the all-payer Maryland Health Services Cost Review Commission database found that 68.2% of general gynecologists are very low-volume surgeons (performing 0 to 5 hysterectomies annually) or low-volume surgeons (performing 6 to 10 hysterectomies annually), and both are associated with increased perioperative complications in comparison to high-volume surgeons (performing at least 21 hysterectomies annually) (adjusted OR [95% CI]: very low volume 1.73 [1.22 to 2.47]; low volume 1.60 [1.11 to 2.23]).[16] The same study found that patients undergoing a procedure performed by a medium-volume surgeon (performing 11 to 20 hysterectomies annually) compared to a high-volume surgeon had a lower likelihood of having a minimally invasive approach (OR [95% CI]: 0.87 (0.78 to 0.97]).[16] These findings indicate that higher-volume surgeons who perform more minimally invasive surgeries, including transvaginal surgeries, have better surgical outcomes and use more cost-effective approaches. Therefore, there is a need to increase both the volume of transvaginal hysterectomies performed and the time spent training in the vaginal approach at both the trainee and provider level.

There is a clear benefit in achieving proficiency in the steps of a transvaginal hysterectomy. Here, we describe and illustrate methods for setup in order to optimize exposure and visualization. Additionally, we provide a step-by-step approach to a transvaginal hysterectomy, including challenges such as entry to the anterior and posterior cul-de-sac, morcellation of a large uterus, and salpingectomy/adnexectomy. We present these steps to provide techniques to those who may have limited experience in transvaginal hysterectomy.

SETUP

Patient Positioning

Patient positioning is a critical first step for a successful vaginal procedure. Care should be taken to balance the need for access to surgical site while ensuring patient safety. It is estimated that 1.8% of patients undergoing gynecologic surgery will develop lower extremity neuropathy.[17] Although the exact incidence of nerve injuries from vaginal surgery is unknown, neuropathies have been reported as both transient and long term, some with pain and/or paresthesias lasting nearly 4 months.[18] Avoidance of compression on the ilioinguinal, femoral, and peroneal nerves with proper positioning is of paramount importance.

Both candy cane and boot stirrups have been employed in vaginal surgery. A recent randomized controlled trial showed that worse physical function at 6 weeks was associated with greater hip abduction at the time of surgery.[19] We prefer the use of candy cane stirrups that allows for the feet and legs to be raised in order to minimize flexion at the hip and knee level. It also minimizes hip abduction while providing ample room for the surgeon and assistant to operate (Fig. 20.1).

Exposure and Visualization

Traditional vaginal surgery often finds the gynecologist and assistants in a nonneutral trunk position with asymmetrical strain on the upper extremities. As such, vaginal surgery is reported as the most common clinical activity to cause back pain among gynecologists.[20] In one study, a large proportion (86.7%) of surveyed vaginal surgeons reported work-related musculoskeletal disorders.[21] Furthermore, surgeons involved in teaching were more likely to have work-related musculoskeletal disorders likely because of the time spent as a retracting bedside assistant.[21] Female surgeons were also reported to have more frequent and severe work-related musculoskeletal disorders than male colleagues.[21]

The use of a camera is integral to endoscopic surgery, whereas table-mounted retractor systems have

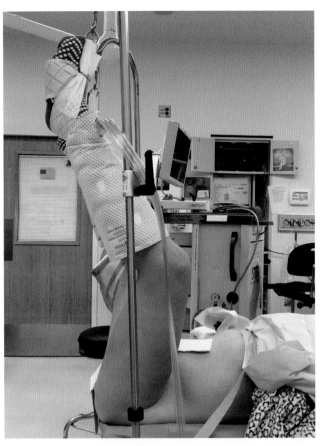

FIGURE 20.1 Patient positioning using candy cane stirrups. Legs are raised the minimize overabduction at hip level and overflexion at knee level.

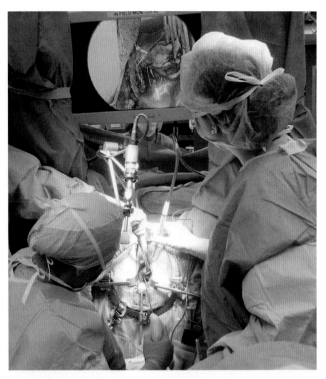

FIGURE 20.2 Camera and vaginal retractor system are mounted to the table to facilitate exposure and visualization. Video for setup is available in Woodburn and Kho.[22]

been used for decades in open surgery. Bringing these two systems to vaginal surgery has been proposed to improve ergonomics and visualization for the entire surgical team.[22] We routinely use a table-mounted vaginal retractor system and camera system and set it up at the beginning of the surgery (Fig. 20.2). Video for setup available in Woodburn and Kho.[22] Depending on the type of surgical table used and patient body habitus, the table post may be attached to the foot of the bed or along the rail on the patient's torso. Once the ring is secured to the surgical table via the post, the retractors are placed as in open abdominal surgery. These retractors are available in varying lengths and configurations and are replaced throughout the surgery.

A table-mounted camera system with a 90° lens is brought in to vaginal surgery to provide magnification, illumination, and concomitant projection of the operative field to external monitors. We prefer to set the camera holding system at the patient's side and the monitor screen situated between the patient's legs. The camera/lens is positioned at approximately 40° from the vaginal field which allows the camera to be out of the surgeon's field of vision while not restricting movements. When the surgeon prefers to stand during vaginal surgery, the camera system can be set up from below the level of the operating field, and to position the camera at the surgeon's chest level. Video monitors are placed strategically so that surgical assistants and other members of the surgical team can visualize the operative field without straining.

STEPS

See Video 20.1.

Initial Incision

Prior to incision, 5 mL of 0.5% bupivacaine with 1:200,000 of epinephrine is injected into the uterosacral ligaments bilaterally for preemptive analgesia.[23] Dilute vasopressin is then injected circumferentially under the vaginal epithelium to minimize bleeding.

When the vaginal introitus is narrow, we perform a superficial relaxing incision on the distal 2 cm of the posterior vaginal mucosa using a monopolar instrument (Fig. 20.3A,B). This allows up to a 2-cm widening of the introitus to facilitate exposure. The incision is closed at the end of the hysterectomy with an absorbable suture in a running manner.

Attention is directed to identify the cervicovesical and cervico-rectal junctions. We use a long knife handle with a #10 blade to make an elliptical incision

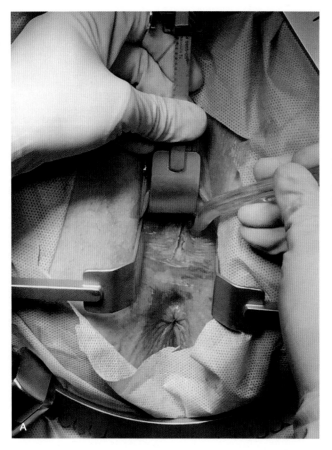

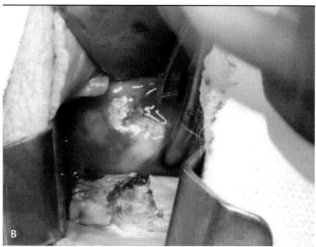

FIGURE 20.3 **A,B:** A superficial relaxing incision (no deeper than 2 to 3 mm) on the distal posterior provides up to 2 cm of additional width to the introitus. This can facilitate greater exposure in patients with narrowing of the introitus.

around the cervix, as opposed to a round circumferential incision. This is preferred in order to achieve a larger culdotomy for lateral access to the vascular pedicles and greater room for morcellation in the case of a large uterus. The anterior vaginal epithelium is sharply dissected off the cervix with heavy Mayo scissors until the vesicouterine space is reached. With blunt dissection, the bladder pillars are pushed superiorly and laterally. No further attempt is made to enter the anterior cul-de-sac especially when there is minimal uterine descensus. Attention is directed to entering into the posterior cul-de-sac.

Entry into the Posterior Cul-de-sac

Entry into the posterior cul-de-sac is best achieved with retraction of the posterior vaginal wall down and deflecting the cervix anteriorly to obtain the correct angle for entry. Sharp incision is made with the heavy Mayo scissors which are placed parallel to the plane of the cervix to avoid inadvertent rectal injury. A long self-retaining posterior blade is repositioned, inserted into the abdominal cavity, and attached to the vaginal ring. The uterosacral ligaments can be clamped, cut, and ligated using the traditional technique of clamps and suture ligation or sealed and divided using the vessel-sealing device. Some studies have shown possible shorter

operative time,[3] less blood loss,[3] and postoperative pain[24] associated with the use of the vessel-sealing device in vaginal surgery. Studies also demonstrate that complication rates in vaginal hysterectomies remain the same as previously reported when using electrothermal bipolar vessel sealing.[25] The same principles regarding the use of energy in minimally invasive surgery such as laparoscopy are applied in vaginal surgery. Advanced vessel-sealing devices deliver bipolar energy that is able to seal vessels up to 7 mm. Because of lateral thermal spread of up to 2 mm, it is important to stay close to the cervix and the uterus and isolate ligaments and the blood vessels to avoid injury to other organs such as the bladder, ureter, or bowel. Because the clamp gets hot during sealing, we use the suction tip to quickly dissipate the heat while retracting nearby structures to prevent lateral thermal injury (Fig. 20.4).

Entry into the Anterior Cul-de-sac

After the uterosacral ligaments are divided, the cardinal ligaments can be clamped, cut, and tied in the traditional manner or sealed and divided using the vessel-sealing device. We prefer to skeletonize and isolate the uterine arteries by dividing the posterior leaf of the broad ligament first. This allows for the isolation of the descending branches of the uterine vessels that can be sealed and

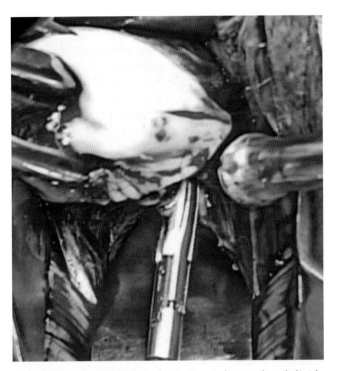

FIGURE 20.4 Vessel-sealing device is used to seal and divide the uterosacral and cardinal ligaments. Suction tip is brought into the operative field to quickly dissipate the heat to minimize thermal injury to nearby structures. It is also used to evacuate smoke to maximize visualization.

divided separately. With further uterine descensus, entry into the anterior cul-de-sac can then be attempted.

The posterior blade is removed to allow maximum dorsal traction of the cervix. The anterior vaginal wall is picked up with forceps, and the bladder is dissected sharply from the anterior cervix using the Metzenbaum scissors. After the vaginal attachments are completely excised from the cervix, we recommend staying parallel to the plane of the cervix which allows for safe entry into the avascular vesicouterine space. The vesicouterine peritoneum should be clearly visualized (Fig. 20.5A,B). Mastering this step is critical to safely enter the anterior cul-de-sac. During this dissection, it is important to note that cutting into the cervix will feel hard against the tips of the scissors, whereas cutting into the softer striated detrusor muscles will manifest with excessive bleeding. The vesicouterine peritoneal fold is identified as a crescent-shaped peritoneal fold that can be lifted and divided for entry. Palpation of this peritoneal fold can aid in identification.

In cases where dense adhesions are encountered such as in patients with previous cesarean sections, entry can be achieved by dissecting from the lateral to medial aspect until a clear adhesion-free space is encountered. Confirmation of entry into the anterior cul-de-sac can be achieved by inserting the back end of a pair of pickups to visualize loops of bowel.

Upon entry into the anterior cul-de-sac, the ascending branches of the uterine vessels can be further sealed and divided.

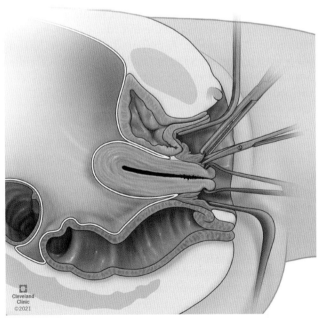
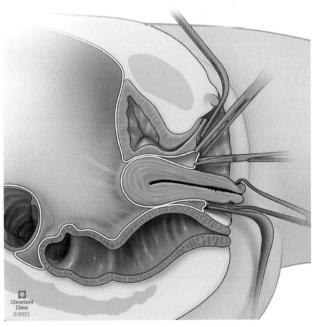

FIGURE 20.5 **A,B:** The vaginal cuff is separated completely off of its attachments to the cervix to enter into the vesicouterine space. Once achieved, the vesicouterine peritoneal fold can be isolated and incised to enter the anterior cul-de-sac. (Reprinted with permission, Cleveland Clinic Foundation © 2022. All Rights Reserved.)

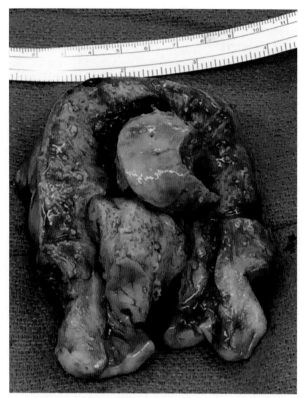

FIGURE 20.6 Morcellation is performed using a series of coring and wedging technique while maintaining the lateral and fundal borders. This technique decreases the risk of injury to extrauterine structures such as loops of bowel, vessels in the lateral pelvic sidewall, and the ureter.

Morcellation of the Large Uterus

We emphasize the need for thorough preoperative evaluation that includes Pap test, endometrial biopsy, and selective imaging to rule out malignant involvement prior to any manual morcellation. In uteri involved with fibroids and/or adenomyosis, manual morcellation is often required in order to decompress the uterus and safely secure the utero-ovarian ligaments. To morcellate, we divide the cervix in half and remove segments of the uterus using a core-and-wedge technique with the use of a long curved knife handle with a #10 blade and double-toothed Schroeder tenaculum (Video 20.2). Traction is placed on each sides of the cervix, and morcellation is conducted to maintain the lateral and fundal borders of the uterus. Keeping this configuration in mind allows the surgeon to stay away from the lateral and superior abdominal and pelvic structures (Fig. 20.6).

After morcellation, the utero-ovarian ligaments can be isolated by placing a finger around the uterine cornua for traction, and a Heaney clamp is used to clamp the ligament. Once clamped, the utero-ovarian pedicle is suture ligated, passing a suture through the middle, and tied and carried around the pedicle as in a modified Heaney suturing technique.

Salpingectomy and Adnexectomy

There is a large body of evidence suggesting that many aggressive epithelial ovarian cancers arise from the distal fallopian tubes. Risk-reducing salpingectomy is therefore offered and recommended at the time of hysterectomy.[26] In a decision analysis model, when a strategy of routine salpingectomy is performed at every vaginal hysterectomy, 1 diagnosis of ovarian cancer per 225 surgeries and 1 death from ovarian cancer per 450 surgeries can be prevented.[27] We advocate the round ligament technique to facilitate access to the distal fallopian tube for its complete removal during vaginal hysterectomy.[28] After the uterus is removed and the utero-ovarian pedicle is suture ligated, the pedicle and ovary are grasped separately with long Allis clamps while the fimbriated end of the fallopian tube is brought down to the operative field with a long Russian forceps. The round ligament is identified from the utero-ovarian complex (that contains the round ligament, the utero-ovarian pedicle, and the proximal fallopian tube) and divided using the monopolar cautery pencil (Bovie). To remove the fallopian tube, a window is created in the mesosalpinx immediately inferior to the proximal tube. A clamp is placed, distal to the ovary, to isolate the utero-ovarian pedicle. The mesosalpinx is subsequently divided using the vessel-sealing device, and the entire fallopian tube is removed.

To remove both the tube and ovary, the long Allis clamp is placed on the ovary and proximal tube. The round ligament is identified and divided as described earlier. The curved ovarian clamp is placed on the ovarian ligament that is proximal to the ovary. This technique allows both the tube and ovarian tissue to be removed in their entirety. It is important not to place the clamp too close to the ovarian tissue in order to prevent ovarian remnant syndrome. A prepared polyglactin ligating loop with a delivery system (such as Surgitie, Covidien Surgical, Dublin, Ireland) suture can be used to secure the pedicle particularly when it is in the pelvic brim.

Completion of Hysterectomy

To ensure hemostasis, a peritoneal suture using 2-0 polyglactin suture is placed to secure the peritoneum to the vaginal cuff in a running fashion between the uterosacral pedicle to the cardinal pedicle bilaterally. We perform prophylactic apical suspension by attaching the vaginal apex to the uterosacral ligaments bilaterally. The posterior vaginal fornix at 4 o'clock is grasped with toothed forceps to delineate the uterosacral ligament. An intermediate length Deaver retractor is then placed into the pelvic cavity at the 3 o'clock position to protect the ureter which would be found coursing in the 2 or 3 o'clock position. With upward traction of the vaginal at the level of the uterosacral ligament, the proximal uterosacral ligament is clearly visualized. Adequate purchase of the uterosacral ligament is obtained with the suture placed 1 to 2 cm below the level of the ischial spine. The contralateral uterosacral ligament is similarly delineated and purchased. This midline modified McCall suture is then brought out through the posterior vaginal wall lateral to the entry stitch and tagged for ligation after the vaginal cuff is closed.

The vaginal cuff is closed in an interrupted fashion with 2-0 polyglactin suture, and the uterosacral ligament suspension suture is tired. These sutures are tagged with a clamp until ureteral patency and absence of bladder injuries are confirmed with cystoscopy. We prefer the use of universal intraoperative cystoscopy at the time of hysterectomy in order to detect most bladder and ureteral injuries prior to the end of the surgery.

CONCLUSION

Vaginal hysterectomy should be incorporated in the surgical armamentarium of minimally invasive surgeons given its many advantages. This chapter describes the step-by-step approach to vaginal hysterectomy and manual morcellation, risk-reducing salpingectomy and adnexectomy, and support of the vaginal apex. Knowledge and familiarity of the anatomy, surgical principles, and new tools and techniques are helpful in overcoming many of the challenges of the vaginal hysterectomy.

References

1. Aarts JW, Nieboer TE, Johnson N, et al. Surgical approach to hysterectomy for benign gynaecological disease. *Cochrane Database Syst Rev* 2015;2015(8):CD003677.
2. Committee Opinion No. 701: Choosing the route of hysterectomy for benign disease. *Obstet Gynecol* 2017;129(6):e155–e159.
3. Jeppson PC, Balgobin S, Rahn DD, et al. Comparison of vaginal hysterectomy techniques and interventions for benign indications: A systematic review. *Obstet Gynecol* 2017;129(5):877–886.
4. Sandberg EM, Twijnstra ARH, Driessen SRC, et al. Total laparoscopic hysterectomy versus vaginal hysterectomy: A systematic review and meta-analysis. *J Minim Invasive Gynecol* 2017;24(2):206.e22–217.e22.
5. Schmitt JJ, Carranza Leon DA, Occhino JA, et al. Determining optimal route of hysterectomy for benign indications: Clinical decision tree algorithm. *Obstet Gynecol* 2017;129(1):130–138.
6. Lake AG, McPencow AM, Dick-Biascoechea MA, et al. Surgical site infection after hysterectomy. *Am J Obstet Gynecol* 2013;209(5):490.e1–490.e9.
7. Wright JD, Herzog TJ, Tsui J, et al. Nationwide trends in the performance of inpatient hysterectomy in the United States. *Obstet Gynecol* 2013;122(2 Pt 1):233–241.
8. Morgan DM, Kamdar NS, Swenson CW, et al. Nationwide trends in the utilization of and payments for hysterectomy in the United States among commercially insured women. *Am J Obstet Gynecol* 2018;218(4):425.e1–425.e18.
9. Luchristt D, Brown O, Kenton K, et al. Trends in operative time and outcomes in minimally invasive hysterectomy from 2008 to 2018. *Am J Obstet Gynecol* 2021;224(2):202.e1–202.e12.
10. Jelovsek JE, Walters MD, Korn A, et al. Establishing cutoff scores on assessments of surgical skills to determine surgical competence. *Am J Obstet Gynecol* 2010;203(1):81.e1–81.e6.
11. Accreditation Council for Graduate Medical Education. Case log statistical reports in obstetrics and gynecology, 2018–2019. Accessed January 3, 2021. https://www.acgme.org/Data-Collection-Systems/Case-Log-Graduate-Statistics
12. Guntupalli SR, Doo DW, Guy M, et al. Preparedness of obstetrics and gynecology residents for fellowship training. *Obstet Gynecol* 2015;126(3):559–568.
13. Birkmeyer JD, Siewers AE, Finlayson EVA, et al. Hospital volume and surgical mortality in the United States. *N Engl J Med* 2002;346(15):1128–1137.
14. Birkmeyer JD, Stukel TA, Siewers AE, et al. Surgeon volume and operative mortality in the United States. *N Engl J Med* 2003;349(22):2117–2127.
15. Rogo-Gupta LJ, Lewin SN, Kim JH, et al. The effect of surgeon volume on outcomes and resource use for vaginal hysterectomy. *Obstet Gynecol* 2010;116(6):1341–1347.
16. Mehta A, Xu T, Hutfless S, et al. Patient, surgeon, and hospital disparities associated with benign hysterectomy approach and perioperative complications. *Am J Obstet Gynecol* 2017;216(5):497.e1–497.e10.
17. Bohrer JC, Walters MD, Park A, et al. Pelvic nerve injury following gynecologic surgery: A prospective cohort study. *Am J Obstet Gynecol* 2009;201(5):531.e1–531.e7.
18. Warner MA, Warner DO, Harper CM, et al. Lower extremity neuropathies associated with lithotomy positions. *Anesthesiology* 2000;93(4):938–942.
19. Gupta A, Meriwether K, Tuller M, et al. Candy cane compared with boot stirrups in vaginal surgery. *Obstet Gynecol* 2020;136(2):333–341.
20. Dolan LM, Martin DH. Backache in gynaecologists. *Occup Med (Lond)* 2001;51(7):433–438.
21. Kim-Fine S, Woolley SM, Weaver AL, et al. Work-related musculoskeletal disorders among vaginal surgeons. *Int Urogynecol J* 2013;24(7):1191–1200.
22. Woodburn K, Kho RM. Vaginal surgery: Don't get bent out of shape. *Am J Obstet Gynecol* 2020;223(5):762–763.
23. Long JB, Eiland RJ, Hentz JG, et al. Randomized trial of preemptive local analgesia in vaginal surgery. *Int Urogynecol J Pelvic Floor Dysfunct* 2009;20(1):5–10.
24. Gizzo S, Burul G, Di Gangi S, et al. LigaSure vessel sealing system in vaginal hysterectomy: Safety, efficacy and limitations. *Arch Gynecol Obstet* 2013;288(5):1067–1074.
25. Clavé H, Clavé A. Safety and efficacy of advanced bipolar vessel sealing in vaginal hysterectomy: 1000 cases. *J Minim Invasive Gynecol* 2017;24(2):272–279.
26. Society of Gynecologic Oncology. SGO Clinical Practice Statement: Salpingectomy for ovarian cancer prevention. Accessed February 5 2021. https://www.sgo.org/clinical-practice/guidelines/sgo-clinical-practice-statement-salpingectomy-for-ovarian-cancer-prevention/
27. Cadish LA, Shepherd JP, Barber EL, et al. Risks and benefits of opportunistic salpingectomy during vaginal hysterectomy: A decision analysis. *Am J Obstet Gynecol* 2017;217(5):603.e1–603.e6.
28. Kho R, Magrina J. Round ligament technique and use of vessel-sealing device to facilitate complete salpingectomy at the time of vaginal hysterectomy. *J Minimal Invasive Gynecol* 2015;22(6):1084–1087.

CHAPTER 21

PRINCIPLES OF LAPAROSCOPY

Megan Cesta • Resad Pasic • Meagan Slate • Ceana Nezhat

Introduction

Conventional video-assisted laparoscopy has challenged the notion that "bigger is better." As surgeons develop novel techniques, using smaller incisions and less invasive approaches, the perspective has undoubtedly shifted to "less is more." It has become clear that we, as surgeons, must continue to push the limits of ingenuity. The wealth of information available to both physicians and patients is remarkable but at times can lead to misguided information or unorthodox requests. Pleas for unconventional treatment often prove to be a blessing in disguise, leading to developments for new surgical techniques (single-site laparoscopy, transvaginal natural orifice transluminal endoscopic surgery [vNOTES]) and new technology. Despite this pivot toward a world of innovation and ingenuity, the beauty of laparoscopy lies in its simplicity of traditional surgical principles.

The most important concepts in laparoscopic surgery focus on two things: the machine and the driver; or better said, the skill of the surgeon and the availability of proper instrumentation. The equipment available in the operating room, or the machine, enhances the surgeon's ability to perform the most complex of cases. This includes having the appropriate laparoscope, adequate pneumoperitoneum, and the correct choice of energy and dissection tool. The other, more important, component is the knowledge and skill of the surgeon. Although advancements in technology continue to evolve, the level to which a surgeon's skill set is enriched by machinery is finite. Knowledge, training, experience, and creativity remain at the forefront of surgical success.

In order to fully understand the benefits of laparoscopic surgery, it is first necessary to review the annals of gynecologic surgery and its roots in the development of endoscopy. Over a century ago, in 1901, George Kelling performed the first endoscopy to examine the effects of pneumoperitoneum on dogs. Soon after, he performed the first human abdominal endoscopy, which he published in 1910.[1] The first gynecologist to use laparoscopy was Karl Fervers who, in 1933, described his technique for lysis of adhesions. Soon after, in 1936, Swiss gynecologist, Boesch, performed a laparoscopic

sterilization using electrocautery of the fallopian tubes. Raoul Palmer, a gynecologist at the Hôpital Broca in Paris, and his wife Elizabeth started to perform laparoscopic procedures in occupied Paris in 1943. In 1980, Hubert Manhes, from Clermont, France, published his laparoscopic approach to ectopic pregnancy.[2] Either tubal aspiration or salpingostomy were used to treat 60 young women diagnosed with ectopic pregnancy; only three cases resulted in laparotomy.[3]

Kurt Semm is known as the father of modern *pelviscopy*, a term he coined to differentiate between gynecologic laparoscopy and procedures in the upper abdomen or liver. He was a German gynecologist with many inventions including an electronic carbon dioxide (CO_2) insufflator, a uterine manipulator, and a tubal patency device.[4] He performed the first laparoscopic appendectomy in 1981. It was the invention of video laparoscopy by Dr. Camran Nezhat in the early 1980s which proved to be the beginning of a surgical renaissance. He presented his technique at American Association of Gynecologic Laparoscopists (AAGL) in 1984 and American Society for Reproductive Medicine in 1985, and he published his experience describing the treatment of stage IV endometriosis with video-assisted laparoscopy.[5] He proposed that with the application of this technique, the majority of laparotomies could be avoided. The major incentive for further advancement of laparoscopic procedures was the first total laparoscopic hysterectomy performed by Dr. Harry Reich in 1989. Dr. Kurt Semm performed the first laparoscopic supracervical hysterectomy which he referred to as the classic intrafascial supracervical hysterectomy in 1992.[6] He described coring the cervix intrafascially without colpotomy and removing the transformation zone of the cervix as prophylaxis against cervical cancer. Introduction of laparoscopy into urogynecology started with Dr. Terry Vancaillie who performed the first laparoscopic modified Burch procedure. Camran Nezhat in the United States and Arnaud Wattiez in Europe were the first to perform the laparoscopic sacrocolpopexy.

When trainees are asked to describe the benefits of laparoscopic surgery, they often give a predictable response. The trainee describes the benefits of minimally invasive procedures with regard to the patient: less pain, shorter recovery time, lower risk of infection, improved cosmetics, and shorter hospital stay. Although all of these factors remain relevant, it is important to remember the benefits to the surgeon. Video augmentation helps surgeons, as one who can see better can do better. In a traditional laparotomy, as the surgeon advances deeper into the pelvis, visualization declines and views of the pelvic structures become diminished. This shortcoming is bypassed with video-assisted laparoscopy. Maintaining the assistant's focus or sharing information with the operating room staff, simply by directing the camera to the task at hand, is a benefit not observed in traditional laparotomy. The laparoscopic surgeon can maintain the same visual distance between the camera and the target organs throughout the case. This provides better ergonomic maneuverability during extensive pelvic dissections. With video laparoscopy, compared with conventional laparoscopy, the entire surgical team is watching the procedure, and can therefore predict the needs of the surgeon. This allows for better preparation and shorter operating times, which benefit both the patient and the surgeon.

The training and technique of the laparoscopic surgeon stems from the belief that knowledge is power. The expert surgeon spends equal amounts of time out of the operating room: preparing for the case, honing their skills, and anticipating any complications that may arise. As visualization during laparoscopy continues to improve, the understanding of pelvic anatomy has blossomed. Structures such as the hypogastric nerve plexus, avascular planes in the space of Retzius, knowledge of embryonic variants, and deviations of the ureteral pathways are key to safe dissection.

It is important to select the appropriate patient for minimally invasive surgery. Relative contraindications to laparoscopic surgery include hemodynamic instability, inability to tolerate pneumoperitoneum, and some of the known metastatic diseases. An unstable patient presenting with hemoperitoneum was previously considered a contraindication to laparoscopy. Over the last decades, though, a palpable shift was noted in residency programs, with particular attention being placed on laparoscopic training. This has resulted in enhanced teaching and surgical experience, and as a result, many young gynecologic surgeons feel comfortable addressing gynecologic emergencies, such as a ruptured ectopic pregnancy or ovarian torsion, using a minimally invasive approach.

The physician must understand the physiologic variations observed in laparoscopic surgery. These focus mainly on respiratory and cardiovascular changes which may restrict adequate Trendelenburg positioning, limit visualization, or create an operative field with inadequate pneumoperitoneum. This is less of a concern in young, healthy patients but can be surgically prohibitive in patients with a history of cardiovascular or pulmonary compromise. Absorption of CO_2 into the systemic circulation can result in hypercarbia, metabolic acidosis, and subsequent changes in myocardial

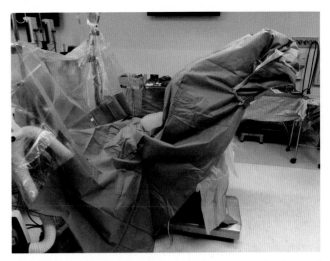

FIGURE 21.1 The Trendelenburg position elevates the feet and places the patient's head down to allow for better visualization of the pelvic organs during gynecologic surgery.

contractility. Intra-abdominal pressure is typically limited to 12 to 15 mm Hg, with an upper threshold of 25 mm Hg. Elevated intra-abdominal pressure compresses the inferior vena cava, resulting in decreased preload and subsequent decrease in cardiac output. Suboptimal oxygenation occurs as a result of the upwardly displaced diaphragm and reduced lung volume observed with a combined pneumoperitoneum and the Trendelenburg position (Fig. 21.1). Also, a temporary decline of urine production is to be expected. This is due to a combination of decreased cardiac output, increased release of renin and antidiuretic hormone, and direct renal compression. Renal function should return to normal after surgery and have no lingering effects.

Prior to the incision, it is the responsibility of the surgeon to ensure that the patient, the operating room, the staff, and the equipment is prepared for the procedure in their respective ways. The patient should be an active participant in preparing for the procedure as well as in the recovery process. Enhanced recovery after surgery actually begins preoperatively, by reviewing expectations and discussing the importance of optimizing a patient's health prior to the procedure. This should begin in the office, where there is sufficient time to discuss weight loss goals, exercise routines, tactics for smoking cessation, and initiation of medications to improve underlying medical conditions.[7] On the morning of surgery, the operating room staff should ensure that the room is cleaned and stocked, with all instruments in working order. Important steps, such as operating room organization, instrument setup, and proper patient positioning, are often overlooked. A team approach to ensure the safest possible environment must be used.

Setting the surgical team up for success starts with a well-thought-out operating room configuration. Laparoscopic instrument movement is limited to fixed ports through the fascia; therefore, proper planning

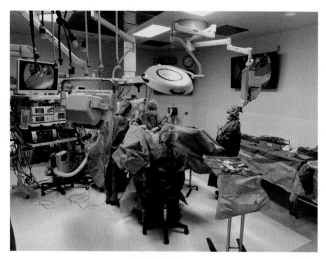

FIGURE 21.2 Operating room setup fully equipped for minimally invasive surgical procedures with ample video monitors and appropriate ergonomics.

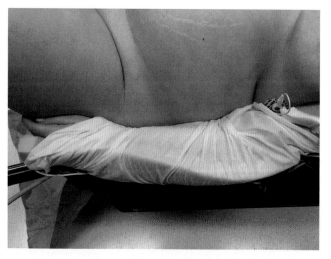

FIGURE 21.3 Arms are tucked during laparoscopic procedures to allow for improved surgical maneuverability and protection against neuropathy.

must occur prior to the procedure beginning. Ideally, the operating table is in the center of the room with surgical lighting directly above. Table mechanics should be in working order to allow for quick adjustments and graduated Trendelenburg position. Special considerations may be necessary for bariatric patients. Video monitors should be positioned directly in front of the surgeon and the assistant, 10 to 20 degrees below eye level to limit neck strain. The table height should be adjusted to maximize the surgeon's comfort and ergonomics as well as reduce operative fatigue (Fig. 21.2). The video monitor tower is positioned opposite of the primary surgeon to provide an unobstructed view of the equipment display panels. Foot pedals are placed comfortably within reach, allowing the surgeon to use energy without removing his or her eyes from the video monitor.

PATIENT POSITIONING

Correct patient positioning is crucial to performing successful laparoscopy. Incorrect positioning can lead to complications such as nerve injury and compartment syndrome. The symptoms present as burning, numbness, and weakness depending on the specific nerve damage, and the deficit is almost always present immediately after surgery. Injury resulting from improper positioning typically occurs from the following common mechanisms: ischemia, stretching, and compression. Common risk factors for injury include low and high body mass index (BMI), immobility, and long operative times.[8] Other surgical factors such as incision type and use of retractors can also lead to nerve injury through various mechanisms. Trocar placement during laparoscopy can injure the ilioinguinal and iliohypogastric nerves. This chapter focuses on nerve injury resulting from surgical positioning.

The patient should be placed caudal on the operating bed to allow vulvar and vaginal access during surgery. The sacrum must be well supported by the operating table. Once positioned appropriately on the table, the patient's arms should be tucked when performing laparoscopy to avoid brachial nerve injury. The brachial plexus arises from the anterior nerve roots of C5–T1. Upper root injury can cause Erb's palsy, whereas lower root injury to C8–T1 will cause Klumpke paralysis. Padding along the medial epicondyle of the arm protects the ulnar nerve, as it is most vulnerable in this location (Fig. 21.3). Care should be taken to wrap or pad any hard surfaces or potential pressure points along any intravenous lines that may rest against the patient. The arms should be placed at the patient's side in a neutral position with the thumb facing up and properly padded. The arms should not be pronated or supinated while tucked. The shoulders should be neutral and pressure points such as the acromioclavicular joint should be padded.[9] Shoulder braces may be placed laterally. However, if placed improperly, it can cause compression of the brachial plexus along the neck.

Next, the legs are positioned in stirrups for laparoscopy. There are different weight tolerances for boots, and the correct weight should be selected based on the patient. Positioning the legs may also be done while the patient is awake to ensure comfort and correct placement. The hip flexors must be positioned with slight flexion to avoid femoral and sciatic compressions and extensions (Fig. 21.4). Flexion should be limited to no more than 90 degrees, and abduction of the hip should not exceed more than 45 degrees. Incorrect placement at this point could lead to lateral femoral cutaneous or obturator nerve injury. Knees must be flexed between 90 and 120 degrees with care taken to ensure the heel is placed firmly and remains in contact with the boot. If the heel is not seated correctly

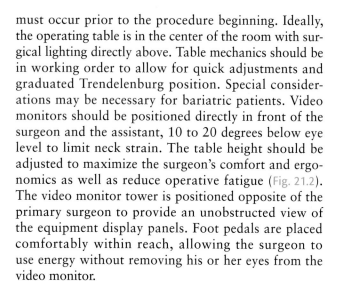

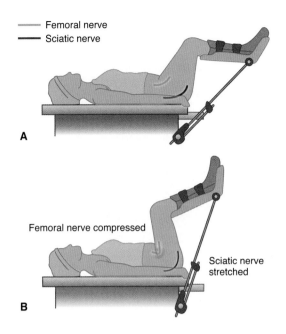

— Femoral nerve
— Sciatic nerve

A

Femoral nerve compressed

Sciatic nerve
stretched

B

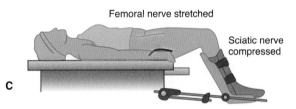

Femoral nerve stretched

Sciatic nerve
compressed

C

FIGURE 21.4 Nerve injury as a result of patient positioning. **A:** Standard lithotomy with neutral positioning. **B:** Incorrect positioning with compression of the femoral nerves and stretching of the sciatic nerves. **C:** Incorrect positioning with stretching of the femoral nerves and compression of the sciatic nerves.

in the boot, the weight of the calf may rest on the top of the boot, creating a pressure point on the common peroneal nerve as it courses along the posterior leg. In extreme cases, compartment syndrome can result from concomitant vascular compression. This can present a challenge when positioning the morbidly obese patient. The surgeon should allow for additional padding to be placed at potential pressure points (Fig. 21.5). The foot should not be dorsiflexed or plantar flexed but should rest evenly on the boot surface. Attention should also be directed at avoiding any compression of the peroneal nerve at the lateral fibular head, which may come in close proximity to the lateral portion of the booted stirrup (Fig. 21.6). Candy cane stirrups should not be used during laparoscopy.

There are many assistive devices when positioning a patient to prevent sliding in the Trendelenburg position. Sliding cephalad on the operating table can lead to patient injury and reduce vaginal access during surgery.[10] Many gynecologic surgeries require steep Trendelenburg and thus patients are at increased risk for slipping. Patients can be placed on a specially designed nonslip foam pad or a gel

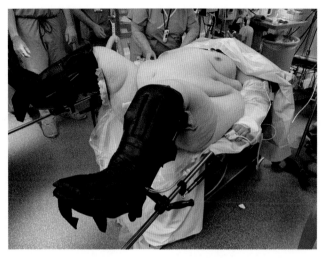

FIGURE 21.5 Additional padding at pressure points with foam pads aids in avoiding nerve injury in the morbidly obese patient.

pad to reduce the amount of weight placed on pressure points.[11] Beanbag systems are commonly used, especially in robotic-assisted laparoscopic surgery (Fig. 21.7). There are also foam restraint systems that may be placed around the neck and shoulders to maintain proper shoulder positioning and minimize risk of brachial plexus injury. Additionally, consider leveling the patient from Trendelenburg or steep Trendelenburg every 3 hours during surgery to decrease risk of neuropathy resulting from positioning.

The surgeon must also be aware of external forces on the patient that can lead to nerve injury or facial edema. Surgical team members should avoid resting their weight, or placing any instruments, on the patient or the stirrups. Instruments should be kept in established drape pockets or on the surgical instrument table. They should not rest freely on the patient when not in use. Finally, the patient should be continuously monitored during surgery for equipment failure or slippage that may require repositioning.

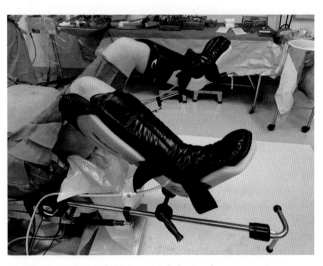

FIGURE 21.6 Booted stirrup used during laparoscopy protects against compression of the peroneal nerve at the posterior knee and lateral fibular head.

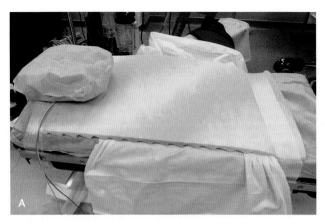
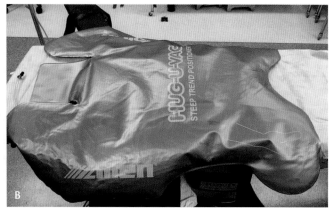

FIGURE 21.7   **A:** Pink pad antislip device. **B:** Hug-U-Vac bean bag in deflated state before patient positioning.

ABDOMINAL ENTRY AND ESTABLISHING PNEUMOPERITONEUM

Site of Entry

There are many options for site of entry in laparoscopy with several key factors playing into the decision-making process, such as the patient's surgical history, body habitus, and the surgeons' experience. No single entry site method is proven to be safer than another.[12] Preparation is required in laparoscopy before establishing the pneumoperitoneum. Pneumoperitoneum is rarely contraindicated but should be avoided in patients with closed-angle glaucoma or elevated intracranial pressure. Intra-abdominal pressure rise is accompanied by an intracranial and intraocular pressure rise, both of which are increased by the Trendelenburg position.[13,14] For gynecologic surgery, the patient must be positioned in the dorsal lithotomy position. A Foley catheter should be placed to drain the bladder and the surgical table must be leveled. An orogastric tube should be placed, especially if the site of entry is in the left upper quadrant (Palmer's point).

The umbilicus is a common site for laparoscopic entry. It is the thinnest point of the abdomen, providing a short distance for the trocar to course before entering the abdomen. All entry techniques can be used at this site. The umbilicus is typically located at the T10 dermatome level. The aorta bifurcates just caudally to this point, near the L4 level. Extremes of BMI can alter the usual location of the umbilicus. Obesity, or extreme weight loss, may displace the umbilicus caudally. Therefore, instead of the recommended 45-degree angle of entry, a 90-degree angle is permissible given that the aortic bifurcation is further away. Prior abdominoplasty can also alter the true location of the umbilicus. When entering at the umbilicus, the surgical table must be level. Placing a patient in Trendelenburg position will bring the umbilicus and the aortic bifurcation closer together, putting them at higher risk for vascular injury. The right common iliac vein is the most commonly injured vessel during umbilical entry. Trocar entry at a 45-degree angle is usually performed in patients with low or normal BMI but may lead to preperitoneal insufflation (Fig. 21.8).[15] Abdominal wall elevation with towel clips or lap cap allows a 90-degree entry, minimizing this risk.

Difficulty entering at the umbilicus can be caused by adhesions from previous surgery, most commonly seen with prior midline vertical laparotomy incision, or in patients who have abdominal mesh. Complications of umbilical entry include injury to bowel and large vessels. Preoperative periumbilical ultrasound-guided saline infusion (PUGSI) is a quick and effective way to diagnose subumbilical adhesions preoperatively. This technique involves tenting the abdominal wall with towel clamps and passing a sterile 19G needle into the peritoneal cavity. Water is then injected, under transabdominal ultrasound monitoring, and fluid loculation indicates the presence of umbilical adhesions (Video 21.1). A positive test would indicate to the surgeon that an alternative port entry site is preferable.[16]

Another common site of laparoscopic entry is Palmer's point. Initially described by Raoul Palmer in the 1970s, the point is located in the left midclavicular line, 2 fingerbreadths below the inferior costal margin (Fig. 21.9). Potential complications of entry at this site include stomach, spleen, liver, or bowel injury. An alternative to Palmer's entry is recommended if the patient has had gastroesophageal surgery or splenectomy. Palmer's is a popular choice for entry if the patient has had previous laparotomies or is pregnant. Although this site of entry is located far from the pelvis with normal pathology, it can be useful in cases with suspected adhesions, enlarged uteri, or ovarian pathology. Multiple entry techniques can be used at this point such as closed entry or direct vision entry.[12]

The right subcostal margin has also been described as a point of entry. It important for the surgeon to note

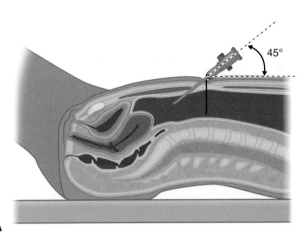

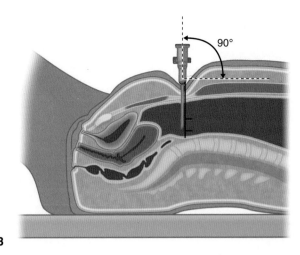

A **B**

FIGURE 21.8 Umbilical entry angles for various BMI. Nonobese patient, Veress entry at 45 degrees. **A:** Overweight patient, Veress entry between 45 and 90 degrees. **B:** Obese patient, Veress entry at 90 degrees.

that the liver and bowel are in close proximity. The subxiphoid region known as the Lee-Huang point, located between the xiphoid and umbilicus point, can also be used. It is imperative that the table be leveled if this entry technique is used.[17] Transuterine insufflation may be helpful in patients who are obese.[18] Finally, the ninth intercostal space may be used as well.

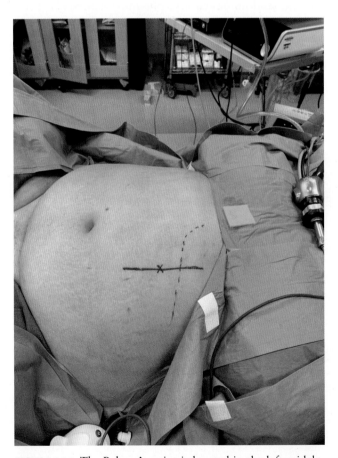

FIGURE 21.9 The Palmer's point is located in the left midclavicular line, 2 fingerbreadths below the inferior costal margin.

Entry Technique

Closed entry by Veress needle insertion is the most common technique used by gynecologists (Fig. 21.10). The needle is used at the umbilicus or in Palmer's point entries. The base of the umbilicus is the thinnest point in the abdomen as there is no muscle or fat between the umbilicus and peritoneum. The Veress needle is punctured through two layers of tissue and the audible click or retraction of the needle tip reinforces that the needle is placed in the correct plane. At the Palmer's point, the Veress enters three tissue planes, and three audible clicks are heard and felt. The three planes here are the aponeuroses of the external and internal oblique, the aponeuroses of the internal oblique and transversus abdominis, and the peritoneum (Video 21.2). To ensure the needle is in the correct plane, the insufflation is connected to the Veress needle and opening pressures below 10 mm Hg usually is an indication of entrance into the intraperitoneal space. If higher pressures are encountered, the Veress needle should be slightly pulled back to make sure that the tip of the needle is not blocked by the omentum. A syringe with the depressor removed may be filled with normal saline and placed on the Veress needle to perform the "water drop" test. If water flows freely, the needle is presumed to be intraperitoneal. False-positive tests can occur if water flows freely into the preperitoneal space. A trocar is then inserted blindly until no resistance is felt or under direct visual entry.

The Hasson technique, or open entry, was first reported by Dr. Harrith Hasson in 1971. This is most commonly performed at the umbilicus. This method of entry is performed with direct visualization as the fascia and peritoneum are grasped and entered sharply. The fascia is then marked with suture on both sides. A blunt trocar is then placed within the incision, and the suture is wrapped to lateral attachments on the port to ensure it does not

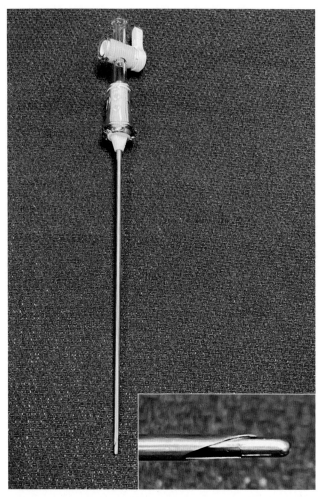

FIGURE 21.10 Veress needle is used in the closed entry technique and allows for insufflation of the abdomen once the peritoneal cavity is entered. **Inset:** Veress needle tip.

move during the procedure (Fig. 21.11) (Video 21.3). This placement enables the surgeon to rapidly establish pneumoperitoneum through the cannula. This technique can be more cumbersome in the presence of larger BMI, umbilical hernias, or periumbilical adhesions.

Direct port placement is another method of entry. This can be performed at the umbilicus. The technique involves grasping the abdominal wall and elevating the tissue. A trocar is then placed in the umbilical incision and then directly inserted into the abdomen until no further resistance is felt. A laparoscope is then inserted to confirm entry and then insufflation can be started. This method of insertion is blind as the trocar is inserted without a camera.

Direct visual entry is performed through specialized trocars that allow for insertion of the laparoscope and visualization as the trocar is passing through the tissue planes. This method of entry is versatile and can be used at the umbilicus or upper abdominal sites. If used in the umbilicus, the trocar is introduced through an umbilical incision and the abdominal wall is held up by hand or with towel clamps. If used at Palmer's point, this method requires no elevation of the abdominal wall as the risk of major vascular injury is miniscule (Video 21.4).

Radially expanding trocars consist of an expandable outer sheath around the Veress needle. It is placed into the abdominal cavity; pneumoperitoneum is obtained, and the inner needle is removed. Radially expanding trocars may cause less fascial defects and may reduce the risk of subsequent hernia formation postoperatively. Next, the desired diameter for the trocar is obtained by serially dilating the tract while gaining access to the abdomen.

FIGURE 21.11 Hasson technique for open entry with fascia incised prior to trocar placement.

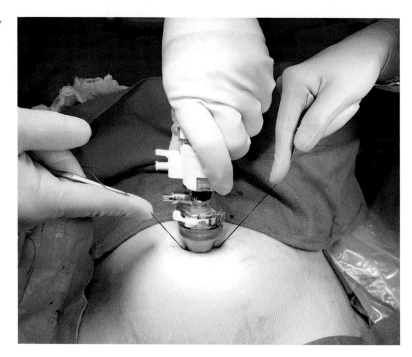

Once initial port placement is established, assistant port placement is safely accomplished under direct visualization to reduce the chance of injury to nearby organs and nerves. The inferior epigastric vessels perforate through the rectus abdominis at the level of the arcuate line. Care must be taken to avoid injury to the superficial epigastric artery which can be visualized with transillumination from the laparoscopy. Additionally, the inferior epigastric artery can be seen on the anterior abdominal wall and is localized to the lateral one-third of the rectus abdominis. Trocars should also be placed carefully to avoid nerve injury which can occur in ilioinguinal and iliohypogastric nerves. These nerves perforate the transversus abdominus near the iliac crest and course medially and inferiorly along the anterior abdominal wall.

Laparoscopies are complicated by port site herniation approximately 1% of the time. Risk factors for hernia development include larger incisions (>10 mm) and the use of Hasson entry technique, pyramidal, and bladed trocar entry. Although herniation at lateral port sites and above the umbilicus is less common, closure of the fascial defect is still recommended. In obese patients, closure of the fascial defect may often be more easily facilitated by using a laparoscopic closure device.

ELECTROSURGERY

Electrosurgical devices provide an alternative to traditional cutting and suturing techniques, allowing surgeons to perform procedures in a more efficient manner. It is important to recognize the difference between electrosurgery and electrocautery. Electrosurgery is the use of kinetic energy in the form of an alternating current, which is transmitted to tissues via radiofrequency. This current raises intracellular temperatures and causes proteins within tissue to denature at different rates. *Coagulation* and irreversible protein denaturation occur at 60°C. *Desiccation* occurs when the cell becomes dehydrated at 90°C and the intracellular fluid evaporates. A rapid increase in temperature to 100°C results in *vaporization*; here, the cell wall ruptures and liquid water turns to steam. *Fulguration* is the charring and carbonization of tissues which occurs when temperatures reach upward of 250°C. Using electrical current to cut tissue requires less force and improves wound healing compared to electrocautery.

Electrosurgery is sometimes referred to as electrocautery; however, they are not synonymous. Cautery, derived from the Greek work Kauterion, or "hot iron," transfers heat from a hot object onto a tissue's surface. The transferred heat raises the temperature within tissue to a level that denatures proteins. In short, electrosurgery dissipates electrical power *directly* to the affected tissue, whereas electrocautery uses electricity to heat an object that is then used to *indirectly* burn tissue, such as a hot wire. Electrocautery is rarely used in the operating room because it requires excess force for cutting and has impaired wound healing compared to electrosurgery.

As a surgeon, it is important to have a sound foundation of knowledge involving the basic laws of physics. Electrical *current* is simply the flow of electrons. The current is determined by the *voltage* (the pushing force on electrons along a circuit) and the *resistance* (opposition to the free flow of electrons), which is defined by Ohm's law (current = voltage / resistance). Of note, resistance is related to the amount of water within the tissue.[19]

The requirements to perform electrosurgery include a generator, an active electrode, and a return electrode. The generator converts electricity from a wall outlet in the operative room (~60 Hz) to a much higher frequency of 200,000 Hz to 3 million Hz (Fig. 21.12). The active electrode delivers modulated energy to the targeted tissue in the appropriate configuration. When using monopolar energy, the dispersive or "return" electrode completes the series once it is placed on the patient's skin. As a result, the patient becomes part of the circuit. At a frequency of 100,000 Hz, electricity can pass through the body without inducing muscle spasms or convulsions (faradic effect); therefore, the conversion from 60 Hz to a frequency of >200,000 Hz is required for operative use.[19,20] The frequency produced by electrosurgical generators overlaps with the range of AM radio waves and is thus referred to as "radiofrequency" (Fig. 21.13). The "ground" was previously part of the circuit, until

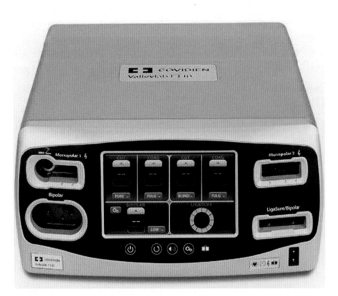

FIGURE 21.12 Electrosurgical unit. (With permission, Cleveland Clinic Foundation © 2022. All Rights Reserved.)

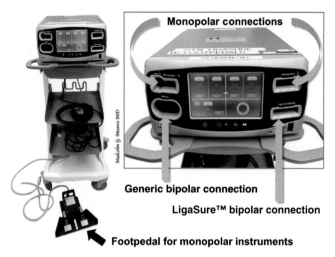

Monopolar connections

Generic bipolar connection

LigaSure™ bipolar connection

Footpedal for monopolar instruments

FIGURE 21.13 Radiofrequency spectrum. The frequency produced by electrosurgical generators overlaps with the range of AM radio waves and is thus referred to as "radiofrequency." (© 2021 Medtronic. All rights reserved. Used with the permission of Medtronic.)

dispersive units via adhesive pads were introduced in the 1960s (Fig. 21.14). These function to disperse the current and reduce the risk of injury by decreasing the *current density* at a localized site. If improperly placed or partially detached, the current density could result in a burn.

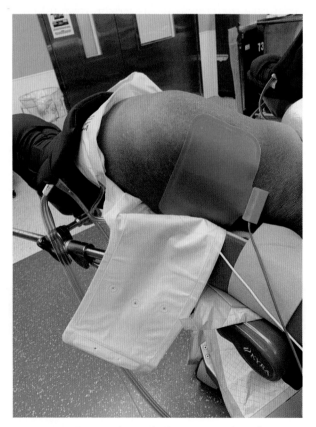

FIGURE 21.14 Return electrode dispersive pad used in monopolar electrosurgery.

Monopolar and Bipolar Energy

The ability to harness monopolar and bipolar circuits has progressively advanced the field of surgery since its development by Dr. William Bovie in the 1920s.[21] Bovie discovered that current will travel through tissues with high water content very fast (muscles, vessels) compared to organs with low water content (bone, fibrous tissue), in which it travels quite slowly. It is important to recognize that as the surgeon coagulates and desiccates (removes water) tissue, resistance will increase. When the electrical current meets tissues with high resistance, it will find alternative pathways, causing the electron's path to become variable. Monopolar circuits place the active electrode and dispersive electrode remote from one another. The electrons travel from the tip of the instrument, through the path of least resistance, and out through the dispersive pad, in essence, "taking the long route." Monopolar energy, therefore, has a less predictable route and electricity must go through the patient to complete the circuit (Fig. 21.15). Bipolar current travels only through the tissue between the active and return electrodes on the instrument, located closely adjacent to one another (Fig. 21.16). It has a more predictable electrical pathway and is overall safer. The only part of the patient involved in the bipolar circuit is the tissue directly between the two electrodes; however, heat can propagate beyond the edges of the instrument, referred to as *lateral thermal spread*.

Monopolar circuits use either continuous or interrupted waveforms of radiofrequency to achieve the desired effect for surgical use.[20] The CUT function delivers continuous low voltage energy to the active electrode. The COAG function delivers high-voltage, interrupted pulses through the active electrode, allowing time for resistance to increase within the tissue as it becomes desiccated and denatures. With COAG, energy is administered only 6% of the time, whereas the remaining 94% of time is spent in a resting phase (Fig. 21.17). When electrosurgical units offer a "BLEND" option, it is the CUT settings which determine the distribution of power; the COAG setting has no impact. Bipolar devices deliver only continuous waveform energy. Excessive bipolar energy results in carbonization or "char" of the tissue. This can increase the risk of thermal spread. Once the tissue is desiccated and has turned white, the end of the vapor phase has been reached, and further application of energy provides no benefit. In addition to avoiding excessive bipolar energy use, the risk of thermal spread can be reduced by using various surgical techniques. These include using irrigation fluid to cool nearby tissues, alternating between incremental desiccation and tissue transection to divide a pedicle, and administering intermittent current rather than continuous energy in a pulsatile fashion.

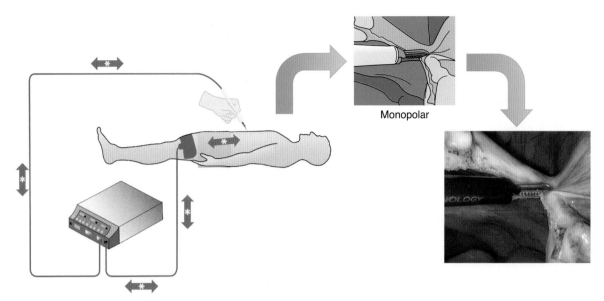

FIGURE 21.15 Monopolar energy circuit. Energy leaves the active electrode, courses through the patient as part of the circuit, and collects at the dispersive electrode. (Modified from Handa VL, Van Le L. *Te Linde's operative gynecology*, 12th ed. Philadelphia: Wolters Kluwer, 2019.)

Tissue Effects

The more important concept to grasp regarding the use of continuous versus interrupted waveforms refers to how each option affects the targeted tissue. The CUT function causes cells to explode and vaporize at 100°C, releasing the heated water from the cell and allowing it to dissipate. This immediate release of dissipated heat reduces thermal spread to nearby tissue. It is important to activate the energy just prior to heating the tissue, and the electrode should avoid direct contact with the tissue. During gynecologic surgery, the CUT function is useful for lysing adhesions or creating a bladder flap by opening the vesicouterine peritoneum. COAG uses a much higher voltage to heat the cell, dehydrate it, and shrink it. This causes proteins to denature, similar to when a cooked egg first begins to turn white. With COAG, it is important to grasp the tissue first before applying energy. It is the optimal choice for achieving hemostasis. There is less precision, and energy is spread wider and deeper. Therefore, COAG is primarily used to achieve hemostasis when transecting the uterine arteries once areolar tissue is dissected and the vessel is adequately exposed.

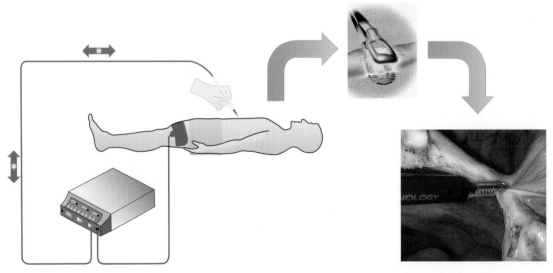

FIGURE 21.16 Bipolar energy circuit. Energy leaves the active electrode and is concentrated on the dispersive electrode which is in close proximity. The patient is not part of the circuit. (Reprinted from Handa VL, Van Le L. *Te Linde's operative gynecology*, 12th ed. Philadelphia: Wolters Kluwer, 2019.)

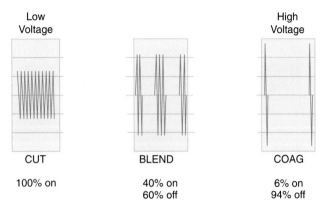

Low Voltage — High Voltage

CUT
100% on

BLEND
40% on
60% off

COAG
6% on
94% off

FIGURE 21.17 Continuous and interrupted waveforms for CUT and COAG, respectively. (Reprinted from Handa VL, Van Le L. *Te Linde's operative gynecology*, 12th ed. Philadelphia: Wolters Kluwer, 2019.)

Advanced Bipolar Energy

The routine use of laparoscopic approach during gynecologic surgery today is largely due to the development of advanced bipolar energy devices. Compared to single function tools such as Kleppinger forceps, the electric hook, or vascular clips, surgeons are able to use these devices to operate more efficiently and to minimize thermal spread. Advanced bipolar instruments combine desiccation and vaporization functions as well as vessel sealing and cutting options within the same device. They also combine various forms of energy, including radiofrequency and ultrasound. This avoids the repetitive exchange of instruments, shortening operative time, and duration of anesthesia. They offer "vessel sealing" capabilities by using pressure and heat to reconfigure collagen fibers within the vessel wall, a concept referred to as *tissue response technology* (Fig. 21.18). Tissue response technology allows an adaptive electrosurgical unit to measure tissue impedance thousands of times per second and discontinue energy delivery when complete tissue effect has been achieved. This reduces thermal spread, minimizes tissue carbonization, and allows for complete sealing and transection of vessels up to 7 mm in diameter. For these reasons, they have widespread application in both laparoscopy and laparotomy.

Ultrasonic Energy

Ultrasonic energy provides an alternative method for dissection, coagulation, and hemostasis. Ultrasonic energy uses piezoelectric crystal as the source of sound waves and generates heat by propagating vibrational and frictional forces (Fig. 21.19). The ultrasonic devices vibrate between 23 kHz and 55 kHz using a linear blade to produce friction.[22] The undulating forces between the blades cause excitation and heating of water molecules. It is important to note that electrical energy does not flow through the patient. High-frequency ultrasonic shears are revered by laparoscopic surgeons, most notably, for their ability to dissect tissue in a precise and efficient manner. There are several factors influencing the function of the device including the power setting, the shape and thickness of the blade, the flexibility of the tissue, and the traction applied to the blade and tissue. When tissue is tightly compressed, the maximum power setting is used, and tissue is lifted or placed on tension, the cutting function will be maximized, whereas the coagulation effects will be minimal. Coagulation is

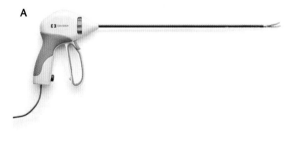

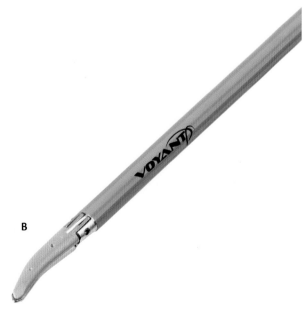

FIGURE 21.18 Advanced bipolar energy. **A:** LigaSure. (© 2021 Medtronic. All rights reserved. Used with the permission of Medtronic.) **B:** Voyant. (© 2019 Applied Medical Resources. All rights reserved.)

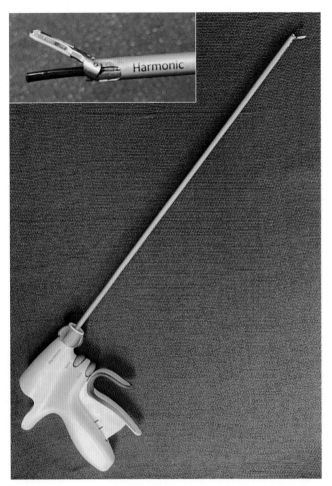

FIGURE 21.19 Ultrasonic energy device. **Inset:** Ultrasonic energy device tip.

maximized when the lowest power setting is used, tension is completely relieved, and the blunt side of the blade is used. A unique function that is particularly helpful with difficult dissection is the ability to "drill" or use the active blade to enter and transect tissue in a similar fashion to a traditional scalpel. This is a function that is unique to ultrasonic scalpels.

Safety Concerns and Avoiding Injury

Understanding the safety principles and judicious use of energy is paramount to sound laparoscopy.[23] The same fundamentals of laparotomy hold true for minimally invasive surgery; however, several differences must be noted. Unintentional energy application can occur within the closed intra-abdominal system and can result in direct coupling, capacitive coupling, or insulation failure. These risks are highest with monopolar energy, when insulation failures allow electric currents to travel through an alternative pathway. *Direct coupling* is when the instruments make direct contact with each other and energy is passed from the active electrode to a conductive instrument. A common example occurs when monopolar scissors contact neighboring bowel graspers; energy from the activated scissors is directly transferred to the unintended site of bowel, resulting in injury. *Capacitive coupling* occurs when energy is transferred from an active electrode to a nearby conductor despite intact insulation. Injury results more commonly with the use of metal trocars, especially when monopolar scissors are passed through the operative channel of the laparoscope (Fig. 21.20). Another common mistake

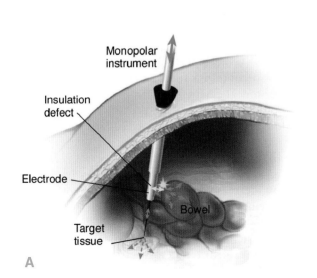
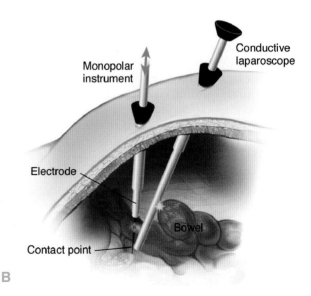

FIGURE 21.20 Monopolar scissors used through an operative laparoscope which acts a capacitor demonstrates capacitive coupling. (Reprinted from Berek JS. *Berek & Novak's gynecology essentials*. Philadelphia: Wolters Kluwer, 2020.)

is looping the Bovie wire through a metal instrument that is secured to the drape as capacitive coupling can cause burn injury or a drape fire. This should never be performed. A plastic holster should be used to secure the Bovie to avoid an operating room fire. *Insulation failure* occurs when a break in the insulation cover allows stray energy to be discharged to unintended organs, most commonly the bowel. This can occur with repeated removal and reinsertion of an instrument, or during cleaning of the instrument.

Thermal injury occurs in 2 to 5 per 1,000 laparoscopic cases. Complications from thermal injury typically present 3 to 7 days postoperatively. Given the life-threatening nature of bowel injury, early recognition and early intervention are crucial to reducing morbidity and mortality. If pale or blanching tissue is noted intraoperatively, the bowel needs to be evaluated for potential deeper injuries, and bowel repair or resection may be necessary.[24]

LAPAROSCOPIC INSTRUMENTATION

Instrumentation varies between conventional laparoscopy and robotic-assisted laparoscopy, but the concepts are the same. Laparoscopy was first performed in the early 1900s using a laparoscope in which the surgeon looked directly through to visualize the target organ. With the advent of video-assisted laparoscopy, the technique became more widely accessible.

The video tower is an essential piece of equipment in video-assisted laparoscopy that consists of a high-resolution video camera, light source, capturing device, and insufflator (Fig. 21.21). In order to transmit light from the source to the patient, a cable is used. The light source for laparoscopy is typically a Xenon lamp light transmitted through fiber-optic cables. The cost-conscious surgeon recognizes the delicate fiberglass can be damaged when bent or rolled over and takes extracaution to prevent these injuries. The camera contains a built-in microprocessor chip and is attached to the laparoscope and to a capturing device that allows for projection of the intra-abdominal image onto the video tower viewing screen. To produce the best quality image most cameras and video screens are high definition (4K LED or 3D). Modern cameras have the ability to adjust the brightness setting or enhance color contrast to improve the image on screen.

Newer sources of light within the operating room are using LED; however, it is mostly in the form of overhead lights in laparotomy. LED uses low energy and has a long operative life while producing no heat. However, laparoscopic use of LED lights is still in its early development.

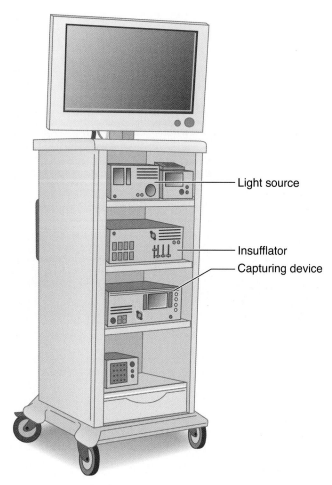

Light source
Insufflator
Capturing device

FIGURE 21.21 The laparoscopic tower consists of a high-resolution video camera, light source, capturing device, and insufflator.

Carbon dioxide (CO_2) can be delivered by way of CO_2 bottles or central insufflators. There are insufflation devices which propel CO_2 into the abdomen measured to a fixed set pressure. The insufflation tubes should also contain a filter to reduce contamination of the peritoneal cavity. The working insufflation pressure should be less than the central venous pressure and is therefore <15 mm Hg. At 20 mm Hg, there are hemostatic effects on the small vessels within the anterior abdominal wall. When the pressure is reduced, bleeding may ensue. High pressure may lead to gas embolism, decreased cardiac outflow, and emphysema. Comanagement with the anesthesiologist will help to reduce the abdominal pressure by reducing the stimulation of skeletal muscles within the abdominal wall. To maintain central temperature, humification of the gas can be used.

The laparoscope diameter usually is 3, 5, or 10 mm (Fig. 21.22). Most commonly, a 0-degree laparoscope is

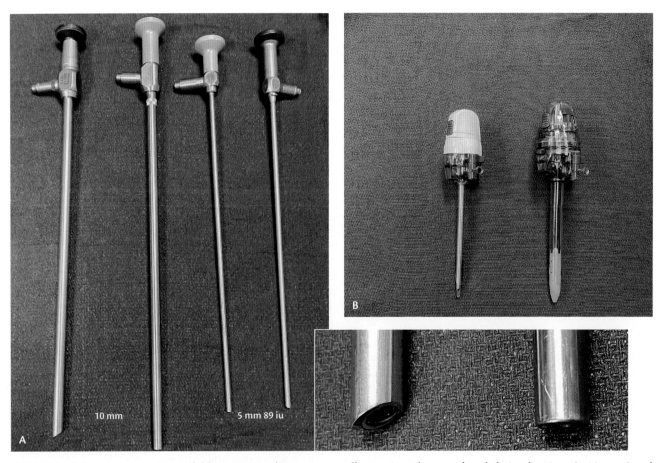

FIGURE 21.22 Laparoscopes are available in various diameters as well as various degrees of angled visualization. **A:** 10 mm 0 and 30 degrees and 5 mm 0 and 30 degrees. **Inset:** Trocar tips. **B:** 10 and 5 mm.

used. This provides a straightforward, linear view of the target anatomy. A 30-degree laparoscope provides an angled view and has many advantages. It provides added visualization around difficult anatomy, such as a large fibroid or dense adhesion. When the pathology cannot be moved either due to adhesions or size, a 30-degree laparoscope is useful to obtain the necessary view allowing the surgeon to look up or down. There is a learning curve with an angled laparoscope as the light cord must be positioned opposite of the desired viewing field. The depth of field determines the quality of the image. The closer the depth of field, the closer the camera is to the target tissue. Smoke and fog can obstruct the image, unless humidifiers and smoke evacuators are used.

Cannulas are available in various lengths and diameters. They are selected according to the patient's body habitus and surgical requirements and come in 3-, 5-, 8-, 10-, 12-, and 20-mm diameters. Five- and 10-mm diameters are most commonly used, and standard instruments are 5 mm. There are sharp versus blunt as well as bladed and nonbladed trocars

(Fig. 21.23) Pyramidal trocars are sharp at the tip. Of the bladed trocars, there are shielded and unshielded types.

New cameras have a light temperature of 6000°K. When the light lamp becomes old, after roughly 500 hours of use, it begins to fade, and the temperature will drop closer to 3000°K. This is when "white balance" is imperative, as it will adjust the color and brightness to an image that is consistent with views at 6000°K. When blood appears black, as opposed to red, this is an indication to change the light bulb or the cord for optimal view.

For many surgeons, the uterine manipulator is one of the most vital components of gynecologic surgery. It can apply countertraction by anteverting, retroverting, and rotating the uterus, helping the surgeon to identify pelvic anatomy and delineate surgical planes (Fig. 21.24). There are numerous types of reusable or disposable uterine manipulators. Some have a cervical cup to help define surgical planes when placed on tension. The cup also helps to maintain pneumoperitoneum after laparoscopic colpotomy. A small balloon may inflate to hold

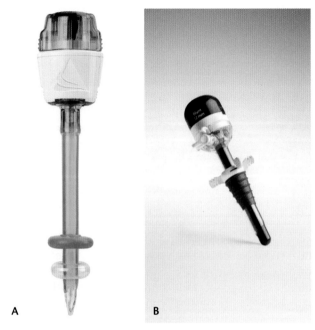

A   B

FIGURE 21.23 Trocars are available in a variety of options including sharp versus blunt as well as bladed and nonbladed. **A:** Balloon trocar. (© 2021 Medtronic. All rights reserved. Used with the permission of Medtronic.) **B:** Hasson trocar. (© 2021 Medtronic. All rights reserved. Used with the permission of Medtronic.)

the manipulator in place, and chromopertubation is usually possible with these instruments. When a uterine manipulator is unable to safely be placed, either due to cervical stenosis, disrupted anatomy, or large obstructing fibroids, a sponge stick can be placed in the vagina. This can help delineate the anterior and posterior fornix during colpotomy. The sponge can be dipped in methylene blue or the instrument can be rotated in a clockwise fashion to help the surgeon identify the proper surgical planes.

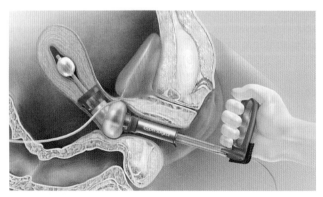

FIGURE 21.24 Uterine manipulators assist the surgeon by applying countertraction during surgery.

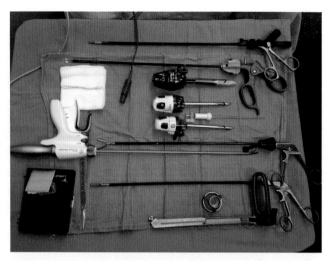

FIGURE 21.25 Instrument setup prior to laparoscopy is simple and involves basic instrumentation, graspers, scissors, trocars, energy source, and uterine manipulator.

Operative laparoscopic instruments can be divided into several categories (Fig. 21.25):

1. Graspers
2. Scissors or cutting instruments
3. Suturing materials
4. Energy and vessel sealing devices
5. Suction-irrigation devices
6. Instruments for tissue extraction

Graspers come in all shapes and sizes. The most common are 5 mm in diameter and 33 cm long; however, longer (44 cm) instruments are available. Atraumatic graspers can be used to elevate, retract, or provide gentle traction. The blunt probe, bowel grasper, and Babcock are considered atraumatic. These can be used to grasp and mobilize delicate structures such as the bowel or fallopian tubes. The laparoscopic tenaculum and biopsy forceps have teeth at the tip to provide a strong hold on dense tissue and are considered traumatic. There are also Crocodile Graspers and Raptor Graspers which have long contoured jaws and tissue herniation channels, allowing for superior grasping capability. The Maryland Dissector and Fenestrated Bipolar Dissector are used to dissect and divide tissue in an atraumatic fashion. Handles are either locking or nonlocking.

Scissor tips vary depending on the type of dissection and may be smooth, serrated, or hooked. They can be disposable or reusable. Regardless of the cutting device available, the most important element to consider is the sharpness of the blade.

Instruments used for laparoscopic suturing can be divided into intracorporeal and extracorporeal. The basic intracorporeal instruments include a needle driver, a suturing needle on a short suture (≤20 cm),

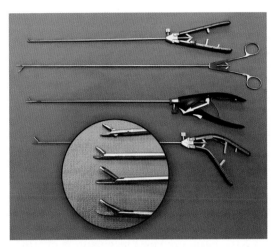

FIGURE 21.26 Laparoscopic needle drivers have various hand grips and locking mechanisms depending on surgeon preference and comfort.

and laparoscopic scissors (Fig. 21.26). There are alternative device systems, such as the Endo Stitch, which simultaneously grasps tissue and threads a suture (Fig. 21.27) (Video 21.5); however, there is only one needle size so it cannot adapt for every type of suturing. The Endoloop is a prefabricated slipknot which comes in a variety of suture materials. Titanium and absorbable clips have been adapted for laparoscopic procedures. Various stapling devices combine hemostasis, suturing, and cutting. The extracorporeal devices include a standard suture and a knot pusher. The needle is introduced into the abdominal cavity through a port, and a needle driver is used to suture the target tissue. A longer (90 cm) suture length is required given that the needle must be removed from the same port, and the knot tied outside of the patient's body. The suture has to be long enough that the surgeon can effectively tie a knot. A knot pusher is then used to cinch the knot in place. Extracorporeal suturing is more robust and provides better tension. It is more commonly used in

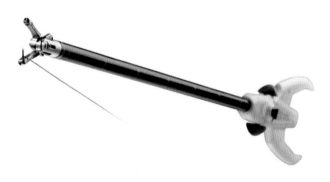

FIGURE 21.27 Endo Stitch. (© 2021 Medtronic. All rights reserved. Used with the permission of Medtronic.)

urogynecology and pelvic floor surgery. Intracorporeal suturing is more delicate and is a useful technique for laparoscopic fallopian tube reanastomosis or enterotomy repair. With the increasing popularity of barbed suture, there are now increasing instances that no longer require knot tying (Video 21.6).

Several multifunctional tools exist which allow for both vessel sealing and dissection, eliminating the need to repetitively switch out instruments and thus shortening operative time. When ligating dense tissue or larger arteries, the vessel sealing capabilities of bipolar energy has allowed for the wide acceptance of new surgical techniques. The LigaSure Sealing System uses an automated system to signal when fusion is achieved. There is minimal smoke, minimal thermal diffusion (<2 mm), and less sticking due to low energy output. It is designed to seal vessels up to 7 mm in diameter. It is important to understand that the device may not perform optimally in damaged atherosclerotic vessels. The surgeon needs to take this into consideration when facing sealing failure and subsequent risk of hemorrhage. The quality of the fusion is superior to bipolar forceps. It produces complete obliteration of the lumen and fusion of the arterial wall, without formation of a thrombosis. The proximity of the various functions allows the surgeon to seal and cut tissue with just the slight drop of a finger. It must also be stated, one of the downfalls with combination devices is the inevitable mistake of cutting the tissue prior to vessel sealing. The LigaSure Advance provides an additional function in which monopolar energy can be applied to the tip of the jaws, and dissection can be performed in a more exact fashion (Video 21.7).

Suction-irrigator devices are necessary to provide a clear visual field by evacuating smoke, blood, ascites, and irrigation fluid. It consists of a vacuum which is connected to a central operating room tower, and a cannula which can be solid or perforated. Its main function is to suction blood, smoke, or bodily fluids to clear the surgical field and provide enhanced visualization. The irrigation system administers fluid to the abdominal cavity and is used to clear debris, evaluate sources of bleeding, and dilute bacterial load. It can also be used to help with tissue dissection, retraction, and application of pressure to a bleeding vessel. Cold irrigation fluid can be used to cool nearby tissue and reduce thermal spread.

Tissue extraction is often the most frustrating step of a surgical procedure. Specimens are often able to be removed from the vagina. During laparoscopic hysterectomy, the initial step often includes placing a stay suture on the cervix prior to uterine manipulator insertion. This allows for traction on the specimen after colpotomy is created.

Specimens may also be removed en bloc by creating a mini laparotomy 4 to 6 cm at the completion of the case. There are a variety of laparoscopic bagging systems available. The most common sizes of endoscopic bag retrieval systems allow for placement into 5-, 10-, or 15-mm port sites. For larger pathologies, there are larger retrieval bags on the order of 14 and 17 cm that can be placed directly through a minilaparotomy incision.

If the specimen is too large to be removed from the vagina, the minilaparotomy site is most often extended at the umbilicus or suprapubically. There is a higher incidence of bladder injury during suprapubic minilaparotomy. The bag is brought through the incision, and the specimen can then be cut and removed. The most common technique is the laparoscopy-assisted minilaparotomy (LAM) technique and has been widely used by different surgical specialties since the early 1990s. Different sizes of disposable wound retractors are available and have a protective effect for the wound while extracting the tissue (Fig. 21.28). Laparoscopic power morcellators also exist. However, with U.S. Food and Drug Administration warnings and potential for iatrogenic, parasitic tissue dissemination of benign or malignant tissues, their popularity of use during hysterectomy or myomectomy has declined.[25] Nonetheless, in the appropriately selected and appropriately counseled patient, this is a useful adjunct to efficiently remove a large specimen. They involve the use of a continued system by placing the specimen in a bag system to avoid spread of aerosolized particles during cutting and extraction.

Although instrument choice, energy source, and knowledge of pelvic anatomy are of utmost importance,

abdominal entry remains the most critical step in laparoscopic surgery. To date, a single, ideal method of entry for all patients has yet to be described. The best approach is individualized and must consider the patient's risk of prior adhesion formation; the possibility of distorted anatomy, size, and contour of the pelvic organs; the patient's body habitus; and the planned surgical approach. Once the first incision has been made, correct port placement is pivotal. The choice of primary port placement location (umbilical vs. nonumbilical) will depend on several factors. There are conditions that can make primary umbilical entry cumbersome such as advanced pregnancy, a large pelvic mass, extensive adhesive disease, prior midline vertical incision, and a prior ventral hernia repair. Once entry is obtained, the remainder of the case will rely on the surgeon's techniques of dissection and laparoscopic suturing, the judicious use of electrosurgical energy, as well as prediction and management of complications.

Patient positioning is one of the most critical steps in preparing for a surgical procedure. Low dorsal lithotomy is necessary to provide adequate visualization when performing a speculum exam, placing a uterine manipulator, and performing vaginal surgery. A gel pad, or other antiskid material, is placed underneath the patient to prevent inadvertent slipping while in steep Trendelenburg. The legs are supported in booted stirrups, with the heels fully supported. Special attention is paid to the angle and rotation of the hip and knee joints to avoid femoral and common peroneal

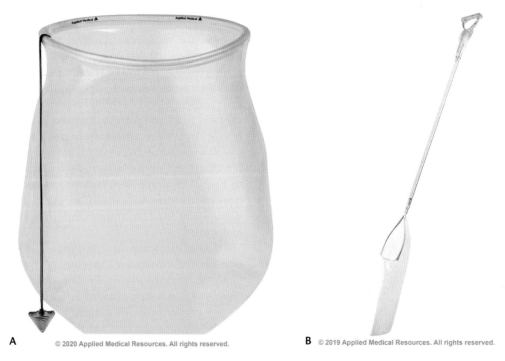

FIGURE 21.28 **A:** Alexis contained extraction system. (© 2020 Applied Medical Resources. All rights reserved.) **B:** Inzii retrieval system. (© 2019 Applied Medical Resources. All rights reserved.)

nerve injury. To prevent brachial plexus injury, hyperflexion of the shoulder is avoided by tucking the arms by the patient's side.

ROBOTIC SURGERY

The first robotic surgery was performed in the 1980s, obtaining stereotactic brain biopsies using the programmable universal manipulation arm (PUMA) robotic system.[26] During the 1990s, the da Vinci platform was used mostly for cholecystectomies, mitral valve replacement, and orthopedic surgery. The first robotic surgery in the gynecology realm was performed in 1998 using the ZEUS robotic system for a fallopian tube reanastomosis. Unlike earlier versions of robot machines, the da Vinci and ZEUS systems depend entirely on the surgeon's activity and movements. Once the robot is docked, there are no preprogrammed or autonomous components. A separate console transmits the surgeon's hand movements to the docked laparoscopic instruments at the patient's bedside. This technology allows for precise, real-time instrumentation inside of the patient, under the direction of the surgeon at the console. The first robotic hysterectomy was documented in 2002.[27]

The da Vinci platform uses a four-armed system with the central arm typically serving as a focal point for the camera (Fig. 21.29). Binocular lenses provide 3D vision. Benefits of robotic surgery are numerous; however, most would argue the top advantage is the surgical instrument's ability to articulate at the wrist, providing seven degrees of freedom. The 3D vision provides enhanced visualization, which is most useful in confined spaces or if microdissection if needed. For a competent laparoscopic surgeon, the seamless adaptation from existing laparoscopic techniques to robotic techniques has allowed for its vast expansion and adoption. In addition to improved ergonomics, a seated position at the console helps to alleviate surgeon fatigue, especially for long cases or multiple surgeries in 1 day. Compared to laparoscopy, robotics permits the presence of a less skilled assistant because the surgeon has complete control of the arms once the robot is docked.

The downsides to robotic surgery include higher cost, long docking times, and lack of training for some laparoscopic surgeons.[28] During the training phase, surgeries can take up to twice as long as conventional laparoscopic technique. This exposes the patient to more anesthesia and requires additional resources, that is, operating room staff. Some of the earlier limitations have been addressed in the Xi system, including setup automation, integrated table motion, multiquadrant access, and streamlined port placement. The da Vinci SP is designed for single-port access. A single arm introduces three multijointed instruments and a freely articulating camera.

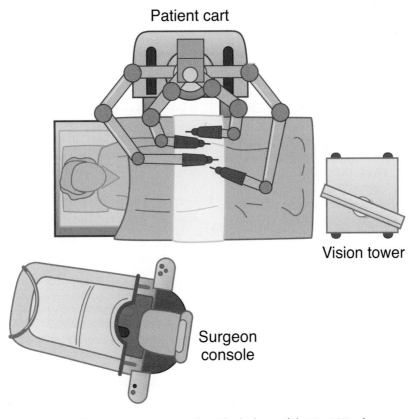

Patient cart

Vision tower

Surgeon console

FIGURE 21.29 Operating room setup for side docking of da Vinci Xi robot.

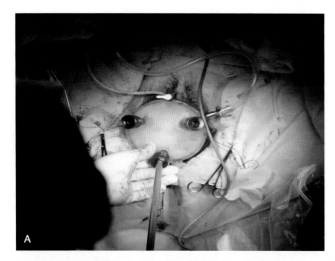 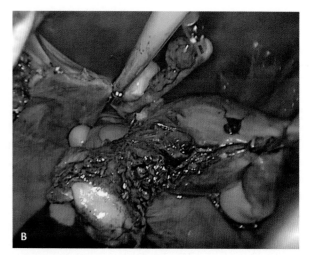

FIGURE 21.30 vNOTES. **A:** Use of GelPOINT V-Path Transvaginal Access Platform which contains Alexis retractor with GelSeal Cap with sleeves (Applied Medical, Rancho Santa Margarita, CA) after dissection of vesicouterine and rectovaginal spaces. **B:** Removal of adnexa using vaginal NOTES approach.

This provides an added level of complexity for the surgeon but leaves the patient with only one incision.

NATURAL ORIFICE TRANSLUMINAL ENDOSCOPY

Natural orifice transluminal endoscopic surgery (NOTES) or transvaginal NOTES (vNOTES) is a novel approach to performing gynecologic surgery, combining both vaginal and laparoscopic techniques (Fig. 21.30). The premise is to use a natural orifice, such as the vagina, to enter the abdominal cavity.[29] Bladder dissection, vesicouterine peritoneum dissection, and anterior colpotomy are completed using traditional vaginal techniques. Once the peritoneum has been entered, a self-retaining sleeve is placed, along with a gelport cap, to allow insufflation of CO_2. Introduction of a laparoscope allows for enhanced endoscopic visualization, and is useful for operating on large, bulky fibroids, or to reach adnexal structures. With the vNOTES approach, all of the advantages of a vaginal hysterectomy are combined with the benefits of endoscopic surgery: less pain, quicker recovery, less incisions, improved cosmesis, more operating space, magnified vision, and ergonomic maneuverability.[30]

COMPLICATIONS

Complications in surgery are inevitable. Recognizing, managing, and correcting surgical complications are skills that all laparoscopic surgeons must cultivate. Some injuries can occur intraoperatively and remain unrecognized until the postoperative period. The most frequently injured organ during laparoscopy is the bowel and at times can be missed intraoperatively. The patient can present with vague symptoms of abdominal pain, malaise, or weakness; however, these complaints may represent a serious or life-threatening condition. These conditions include hemorrhage, infection or abscess formation, bowel or bladder injury, ureteral obstruction, or need for additional surgical procedures. Complications can arise secondary to puncture injury, visceral organ injury, nerve injury, vascular injury, thermal injury, port-site metastasis, or development of abdominal hernias.

Awareness of these possible complications helps surgeons to be more vigilant to minimize the risk of occurrence as well as make attempts to recognize and manage intraoperatively. It is important to note that the surgeon should prepare for possible complications when anticipating a difficult surgery. In patients with a history of extensive intra-abdominal adhesive disease, there are several steps that may reduce the risk of bowel injury, which have been outlined in this chapter. Postoperatively, patients have progressive recovery. Surgeons should be cognizant of potential complications and have a low threshold to evaluate the patient who is not progressing appropriately.

References

1. Hatzinger M, Badawi JK, Häcker A, et al. Georg Kelling (1866-1945): Der Erfinder der modernen Laparoskopie [Georg Kelling (1866-1945): The man who introduced modern laparoscopy into medicine]. *Urologe A* 2006;45(7):868–871.
2. Nezhat C. *Nezhat's history of endoscopy: A historical analysis of endoscopy's ascension since antiquity.* Tuttlingen: Endo Press, 2011.
3. Bruhat MA, Manhes H, Mage G, et al. Treatment of ectopic pregnancy by means of laparoscopy. *Fertil Steril* 1980;33(4):411–414.

4. Mettler L, Semm K. Pelviscopic uterine surgery. *Surg Endosc* 1992;6(1):23–31.

5. Nezhat C, Crowgey SR, Garrison CP. Surgical treatment of endometriosis via laser laparoscopy. *Fertil Steril* 1986;45(6):778–783.

6. Semm K. Endoscopic subtotal hysterectomy without colpotomy: Classic intrafascial SEMM hysterectomy. A new method of hysterectomy by pelviscopy, laparotomy, per vaginam or functionally by total uterine mucosal ablation. *Int Surg* 1996;81(4):362–370.

7. Nelson G, Bakkum-Gamez J, Kalogera E, et al. Guidelines for perioperative care in gynecologic/oncology: Enhanced Recovery After Surgery (ERAS) Society recommendations—2019 update. *Int J Gynecol Cancer* 2019;29(4):651–668.

8. Abdalmageed OS, Bedaiwy MA, Falcone T. Nerve Injuries in gynecologic laparoscopy. *J Minim Invasive Gynecol* 2017;24(1):16–27.

9. Shveiky D, Aseff JN, Iglesia CB. Brachial plexus injury after laparoscopic and robotic surgery. *J Minim Invasive Gynecol* 2010;17(4):414–420.

10. Takmaz O, Asoglu MR, Gungor M. Patient positioning for robot-assisted laparoscopic benign gynecologic surgery: A review. *Eur J Obstet Gynecol Reprod Biol* 2018;223:8–13.

11. Das D, Propst K, Wechter ME, et al. Evaluation of positioning devices for optimization of outcomes in laparoscopic and robotic-assisted gynecologic surgery. *J Minim Invasive Gynecol* 2019;26(2):244–252.

12. Ahmad G, Baker J, Finnerty J, et al. Laparoscopic entry techniques. *Cochrane Database Syst Rev* 2019;(1):CD006583.

13. Arvizo C, Mehta ST, Yunker A. Adverse events related to Trendelenburg position during laparoscopic surgery: Recommendations and review of the literature. *Curr Opin Obstet Gynecol* 2018;30(4):272–278.

14. Sahay N, Sharma S, Bhadani UK, et al. Effect of pneumoperitoneum and patient positioning on intracranial pressures during laparoscopy: A prospective comparative study. *J Minim Invasive Gynecol* 2018;25(1):147–152.

15. Stanhiser J, Goodman L, Soto E, et al. Supraumbilical primary trocar insertion for laparoscopic access: The relationship between points of entry and retroperitoneal vital vasculature by imaging. *Am J Obstet Gynecol* 2015;213(4):506.e1–506.e5.

16. Nezhat C, Cho J, Morozov V, et al. Preoperative periumbilical ultrasound-guided saline infusion (PUGSI) as a tool in predicting obliterating subumbilical adhesions in laparoscopy. *Fertil Steril* 2009;91(6):2714–2719.

17. Lee CL, Huang KG, Jain S, et al. A new portal for gynecologic laparoscopy. *J Am Assoc Gynecol Laparosc* 2001;8(1):147–150.

18. Pasic R, Levine RL, Wolf WM Jr. Laparoscopy in morbidly obese patients. *J Am Assoc Gynecol Laparosc* 1999;6(3):307–312.

19. Brill AI. Electrosurgery: Principles and practice to reduce risk and maximize efficacy. *Obstet Gynecol Clin North Am* 2011;38(4):687–702.

20. Vilos GA, Rajakumar C. Electrosurgical generators and monopolar and bipolar electrosurgery. *J Minim Invasive Gynecol* 2013;20(3):279–287.

21. Goldwyn RM. Bovie: The man and the machine. *Ann Plast Surg* 1979;2:135–153.

22. Devassy R, Hanif S, Krentel H, et al. Laparoscopic ultrasonic dissectors: Technology update by a review of literature. *Med Devices (Auckl)* 2018;12:1–7.

23. Law KS, Abbott JA, Lyons SD. Energy sources for gynecologic laparoscopic surgery: A review of the literature. *Obstet Gynecol Surv* 2014;69(12):763–776.

24. Elbiss HM, Abu-Zidan FM. Bowel injury following gynecological laparoscopic surgery. *Afr Health Sci* 2017;17(4):1237–1245.

25. Lum DA, Sokol ER, Berek JS, et al. Impact of the 2014 Food and Drug Administration warnings against power morcellation. *J Minim Invasive Gynecol* 2016;23(4):548–556.

26. Ghezzi TL, Campos CO. 30 Years of robotic surgery. *World J Surg* 2016;40(10):2550–2557.

27. Diaz-Arrastia C, Jurnalov C, Gomez G, et al. Laparoscopic hysterectomy using a computer-enhanced surgical robot. *Surg Endosc* 2002;16(9):1271–1273.

28. Albright BB, Witte T, Tofte AN, et al. Robotic versus laparoscopic hysterectomy for benign disease: A systematic review and meta-analysis of randomized trials. *J Minim Invasive Gynecol* 2016;23(1):18–27.

29. Yoshiki N. Review of transvaginal natural orifice transluminal endoscopic surgery in gynecology. *Gynecol Minim Invasive Ther* 2017;6(1).1–5.

30. Puisungnoen N, Yantapant A, Yanaranop M. Natural orifice transluminal endoscopic surgery-assisted vaginal hysterectomy versus total laparoscopic hysterectomy: A single-center retrospective study using propensity score analysis. *Gynecol Minim Invasive Ther* 2020;9(4):227–230.

CHAPTER 22

REGENERATIVE MEDICINE APPLICATIONS IN PELVIC RECONSTRUCTIVE SURGERY

Jeffrey L. Cornella

Introduction

The number of clinical consultations for urinary incontinence and pelvic organ prolapse are increasing in the United States. Demographic data has predicted a 35% increase in pelvic floor disorders over a 20-year period ending in 2030.[1] A percentage of these patients will be managed with pelvic reconstructive surgery for symptomatic incontinence and prolapse. A subgroup of those operative patients will require additional surgery for symptomatic recurrence. Wu et al.[2] estimated a cumulative incidence of a subsequent surgery for women aged older than 65 years at 9.9%. The medical cost outlay for procedures related to pelvic floor dysfunction is estimated to be 714,000,000 dollars annually in 2001 dollars.[3] It is predicted that the number of women undergoing stress incontinence surgery will increase 47.2% from 2010 to 2050.[4] It is highly desirable that operations for pelvic floor dysfunction have limited morbidity, restore quality of life, and have a low risk of anatomic recurrence. This chapter discusses how regenerative medicine offers promise in the clinical and surgical response to female pelvic floor dysfunction.

THE LIMITATIONS OF MESH IMPLANTED TRANSVAGINALLY

Recurrent issues of prolapse and incontinence are associated with decreased innervation, weakened tissues, and the effects of aging. An attempt has been made to mitigate these factors and decrease the rate of prolapse recurrence with the use of synthetic mesh. The clinical results have been only partially successful because synthetic materials are not consistent with an optimal homeostasis for biochemistry and biomechanics of pelvic floor tissues. Systematic reviews have shown insufficient evidence for the use of synthetic materials in the apical and posterior compartments.[5] A prospective study comparing native tissue repair with augmented synthetic mesh in the anterior and posterior compartments, showed no benefit in terms of outcomes and demonstrated a cumulative 12% risk of synthetic mesh complications.[6]

Synthetic materials can have deleterious effects on vaginal histomorphologic, biochemical, and mechanical end points when implanted into the vaginal wall. This can include negative effects on collagen, elastin, and smooth muscle.[7,8]

The debacle of complications and associated litigation related to a variety of synthetic materials and their application demonstrates that they are not adequate to fully meet the future medical demands of pelvic floor dysfunction and its sequelae.

VAGINAL HOMEOSTASIS AND THE RISKS OF PELVIC FLOOR DYSFUNCTION

It is important to understand the biochemical and biomechanical pathophysiologic factors predisposing to pelvic floor dysfunction. This understanding is intrinsic to a scientific foundation for regenerative medicine response to adverse tissue factors.

The integrity of the pelvic support tissues is dependent on connective tissue (structural proteins), fibroblasts, matrix, smooth muscle, adhesion molecules, muscle integrity, and innervation. Individuals may have genetic connective tissue deficiencies leading to prolapse.[9] A systematic review reported an association between joint hypermobility and pelvic organ prolapse in women.[10] There been multiple studies assessing tissue proteins and cross-linking enzymes, including lysyl oxidases and fibulins, in patients with prolapse.[11,12] Collagen changes in pelvic organ prolapse show abnormal biochemical composition with fibrils becoming bulkier, more uneven in width, and exhibiting changing ratios of type I to type III collagen.[13] Studies are beginning to assess genes at the transcriptional level and their effects on structural proteins and matrix. Expressions of extracellular matrix remodeling proteins were shown to be altered in the vaginal tissue of premenopausal women with severe pelvic organ prolapse as compared asymptomatic controls.[14]

The authors postulated that dysregulation of matrix metalloproteinases (MMP)/tissue inhibitor of metalloproteinases complexes and protein abnormalities may cause connective tissue defects in pelvic organ prolapse patients. Damaser et al. found that bone morphogenetic protein 1 (BMP1) gene expression was more than twofold higher in women with pelvic organ prolapse compared with controls, regardless of menopausal status (lysyl oxidases require activation by BMP1).[15]

Vaginal delivery, aging, and occupational stresses can increase nerve, muscle, and connective tissue damage. A Swedish nationwide matched cohort study shows an estimated probability of symptomatic prolapse 12 times higher following vaginal delivery as compared to caesarean delivery in patients reaching age 64 years.[16] The interaction between vaginal delivery and aging was the most important factor for the occurrence of symptomatic prolapse.

SECONDARY EFFECTS OF PROLAPSE ON TISSUE BIOCHEMISTRY

In addition to the genetic effects on tissue biochemistry and resultant prolapse, vaginal relaxation itself can result in secondary changes of structural proteins and matrix. This further compounds the difficulty of assessing pelvic tissue pathophysiology.

Kerkhof et al.[17] used premenopausal patients as their own controls comparing biopsies from an isolated cystocele and a well-supported vaginal apex. Results showed a higher amount of collagen III, elastin, and a significant increase of smooth muscle cells at the pelvic organ prolapse site compared to the apex. Apex biopsies were also compared to a control group without prolapse, which showed no histologic or biochemical differences. A similar study in premenopausal patients showed delayed fibroblast-mediated collagen contraction and lower production of MMP-2 at the site the cystocele compared to the supported apex.[18] This implied an acquired rather than an intrinsic tissue defect. There is evidence that mechanical strain induces oxidative stress, promotes apoptosis, and senescence of pelvic support fibroblasts.[19]

There may be a benefit to regenerative medicine intervention in mild to moderate prolapse prior to secondary biochemical changes which further weaken the tissues.

REGENERATIVE MEDICINE OPPORTUNITIES IN FEMALE PELVIC RECONSTRUCTION

Regenerative interventions in pelvic floor dysfunction include tissue-engineered implants, urethral injection, and the use of growth factors, exosomes, nanovesicles, micro ribonucleic acids (miRNAs), and other inducers for injection into tissues to induce desirable substrate changes.

Tissue-engineered three-layered vaginas had been created and implanted in animal models and humans. Atala et al. reported an 8-year follow-up in female patients with vaginal agenesis.[20] The patient cells were taken from vulvar biopsies and seeded onto Surgisis which acted as the scaffolding sized to the patient's estimated pelvic dimensions measured on magnetic resonance imaging. Immunohistochemical analysis confirmed the presence of normal smooth muscle and epithelium in this trilayered structure. This has a benefit over common neovagina constructs which create a structure lacking smooth muscle.

Surgisis is extracellular matrix from porcine subintestinal submucosa. Extracellular matrix–like materials can also be created by nano-spinning or automated three-dimensional printing.[21] Matrix can be seeded with adipose-derived mesenchymal stem cells (AMCs) and nanovesicles, small interfering ribonucleic acids (siRNAs), or miRNAs to create a good manufacturing practice (GMP) hybrid tissue construct that could be implanted into humans.[22]

An example would be the use of the hybrid graft to support attenuated endopelvic fascia between the anterior bladder and vaginal wall.[23] The hybrid scaffold imbedded with growth factors could potentially stimulate local tissues to develop a desirable homeostasis of optimal collagen, smooth muscle, and matrix. AMCs and fibroblasts seeded on the scaffolding would be taken form the individual patient to decrease immune response.

Immune response is highly important for successful implant incorporation into living tissues. There is a strong correlation between early macrophage response to implant materials and the outcome of tissue remodeling.[24] Regenerative medicine interventions can drive a beneficial response via the effects of AMCs and potentially with the use of scaffold containing nanovesicles with specific proinflammatory miRNAs.[25,26]

Mesenchymal stem cells (MSCs) produce a significant amount of bioactive molecules (secretome) that can have anti-inflammatory, proangiogenic, and tropic effects. The MSC secretome includes cytokines, chemokines, growth factors, proteins, hormones, and extracellular vesicles (mesenchymal stem cell derived extracellular vesicles [MSC-EVs]). This has allowed researchers to produce anti-inflammatory and proangiogenic effects without the needs for the mesenchymal cell survival or physical proximity of transplanted cells in tissue.[27] The secretome could be a potential method of promoting myogenesis and the angiogenesis in pelvic floor tissues.[28] Selected paracrine molecules and specific MSC-EVs could be injected into weakened tissues, promoting recovery. The advantages of MSC-EVs are that they cannot proliferate, are simple and easy to transfer, and are easier to produce.[29]

Systemic delivery of MSCs has been shown to have a beneficial effect on sites of tissue injury. Bone marrow–derived mesenchymal stem cells (BMSC) injected into animal models have been shown to maintain urethral function following neuromuscular injury.[30] It is possible that in the future, patients may bank their MSCs prior to parturition with subsequent systemic injection following vaginal delivery. This hypothesis has been assessed in animal model with injection of mesoangioblasts following vaginal delivery.[31] Mesoangioblasts may have the ability to differentiate into both smooth and striated muscle and are attracted to inflammation and injury. The study demonstrated intra-arterial delivery of the cells to injured pelvic tissues with a homogeneous distribution.

Aging plays a significant role in pelvic relaxation and urinary incontinence through changes in fibroblasts, collagen, and innervation. Stem cells can also age and impair their utility in regenerative medicine applications. Factors such as telomerase shortening, oxidative stress, mechanical forces, and aged exosomes can induce stem cell aging.[32] It may be possible to reduce these effects by the regulation of aging related genes and proteins.

Fibroblasts and stem cells harvested from prolapse patients may be able to undergo interventions that reverse senescence. Chen et al. reprogrammed fibroblasts from older women by redifferentiation from induced pluripotent stem cell lines.[33] The new fibroblasts were compared to younger controls, and no differences were found in a senescence activity or mitotic index. Fibroblasts can also undergo reversal of senescence by modulation with extracellular matrix derived from younger cells.[34] These methods can be used to create a younger and stronger construct using the cells of an older patient.

URETHRAL SPHINCTER DEFICIENCY

The female urethra has a length of 3 to 4 cm with inner circular and outer longitudinal muscle layers, surrounded by a thick vascular submucosa.[35] Factors which affect urethral function include innervation, vascularity, muscle integrity, and its relationship to the paravaginal and clitoral structures. An understanding of urethral continence mechanisms and anatomic components lends itself to regenerative medicine intervention.

Researchers have injected a variety of stem cells, muscle precursor cells, and tissue-engineered microspheres into the urethral complex for urinary incontinence.

Silk fibroin microspheres and adipose-derived stem cells (ADSCs) were combined to create a bulking agent that was used successfully in animal model for intrinsic urethral sphincter deficiency.[36]

Chancellor has been one of the early investigators using autologous muscle–derived cells, both in animal models and in humans.[37] Peters et al.[38] reported

a 12-month safety and potential efficacy study of autologous muscle–derived cells in 80 patients. Higher dose groups demonstrated a 50% reduction in stress leaks and pad weight at 12-month follow-up. A large multi-institutional study of urethral autologous muscle cell injection in women will be reported.

Investigators have also used BMSC, AMCs (ADSC), muscle-derived stem cells, and human umbilical cord stem cells for urethral injection.[39]

Future injection into the urethra and associated tissue complexes may result in revitalization of supportive connective tissue, muscle, and angiogenesis of vascularity. Muscle apoptosis leading to decreased urethral pressure may be decreased by injection of growth factors. A recent study assessed injection of exosomes from human adipose–derived stem cells in animal urethral injury model.[40] The study showed that exosomes injection resulted in growth of skeletal muscle and Schwann cells in a dose-dependent manner. Animals in the exosome group had higher bladder capacity and leak point pressures. In addition, there were more striated muscle fibers and peripheral nerves found in the urethras from the intervention group. This suggests that the mesenchymal secretome including exosomes or miRNAs specific for nerve and muscle regeneration could be delivered to the urethra via injection. This could be manufactured as a GMP product which would be free of immunologic reaction.

ANAL SPHINCTER DEFICIENCY

Regenerative medicine techniques have been used for anal incontinence or anal sphincter deficiency. These have included injection of autologous muscle cells, injection of mesenchymal stem cells, and implantation of bioengineered constructs.[41]

A phase 2 randomized placebo-controlled study of intrasphincteric injection of autologous myoblasts was accomplished in humans whose fecal incontinence scores (Cleveland Clinic incontinence) showed clinical benefit at 12 months following injection.[42]

Although histologic assessment reveals labeled myoblasts integrating into animal model external anal sphincter tissue, mesenchymal stem cells do not appear to survive or incorporate but rather show benefit from associated paracrine effects. These effects include improvement in animal model resting anal pressures.[43]

Internal anal sphincter constructs have been generated using biopsies from internal sphincter smooth muscle cells and enteric neural progenitor cells.[44] These bioengineered constructs were used to treat passive fecal incontinence in a large animal model. These intrinsically innervated implants resolved fecal soilage, restored anal resting pressure, and the rectoanal inhibitory reflex within 1 month. The study outcomes were sustained over time and efficacy was demonstrated at least up to 12 months following the intervention.

CONCLUSION

The demand for consultations and medical management for pelvic floor dysfunction is growing at an exponential rate in the United States. Current surgical interventions are limited by the lack of optimal materials and the weakness of anatomic structures affected by injury and aging. Synthetic mesh has limitations and associated risks of complications resulting in corrective surgery. Regenerative medicine through the interventions described in this chapter may prove to be the ultimate solution for these difficult problems.

References

1. Kirby AC, Luber KM, Menefee SA. An update on the current and future demand for care of pelvic floor disorders in the United States. *Am J Obstet Gynecol* 2013;209(6):584.e1–584.e5.

2. Wu JM, Dieter AA, Pate V, et al. Cumulative incidence of a subsequent surgery after stress urinary incontinence and pelvic organ prolapse procedure. *Obstet Gynecol* 2017;129(6):1124–1130.

3. Subak LL, Waetjen LE, van den Eden S, et al. Cost of pelvic organ prolapse surgery in the United States. *Obstet Gynecol* 2001;98(4):646–651.

4. Wu JM, Kawasaki A, Hundley AF, et al. Predicting the number of women who will undergo incontinence and prolapse surgery, 2010 to 2050. *Am J Obstet Gynecol* 2011;205(3):230.e1–230.e5.

5. Sung VW, Rogers RG, Schaffer JI, et al. Graft use in transvaginal pelvic organ prolapse repair: A systematic review. *Obstet Gynecol* 2008;112(5):1131–1142.

6. Glazener CM, Breeman S, Elders A, et al. Mesh, graft, or standard repair for women having primary transvaginal anterior or posterior compartment prolapse surgery: Two parallel-group, multicentre, randomised, controlled trials (PROSPECT). *Lancet* 2017;389(10067):381–392.

7. Jallah Z, Liang R, Feola A, et al. The impact of prolapse mesh on vaginal smooth muscle structure and function. *BJOG* 2016;123(7):1076–1085.

8. Liang R, Zong W, Palcsey S, et al. Impact of prolapse meshes on the metabolism of vaginal extracellular matrix in rhesus macaque. *Am J Obstet Gynecol* 2015;212(2):174.e1–174.e7.

9. Mastoroudes H, Giarenis I, Cardozo L, et al. Prolapse and sexual function in women with benign joint hypermobility syndrome. *BJOG* 2013;120(2):187–192.

10. Veit-Rubin N, Cartwright R, Singh AU, et al. Association between joint hypermobility and pelvic organ prolapse in women: A systematic review and meta-analysis. *Int Urogynecol J* 2016;27(10):1469–1478.

11. Alarab M, Bortolini MAT, Drutz H, et al. LOX family enzymes expression in vaginal tissue of premenopausal women with severe pelvic organ prolapse. *Int Urogynecol J* 2010;21(11):1397–1404.

12. Kow N, Ridgeway B, Kuang M, et al. Vaginal expression of LOXL1 in premenopausal and postmenopausal women with pelvic organ prolapse. *Female Pelvic Med Reconstr Surg* 2016;22(4):229–235.

13. Kim T, Sridharan I, Ma Y, et al. Identifying distinct nanoscopic features of native collagen fibrils towards early diagnosis of pelvic organ prolapse. *Nanomedicine* 2016;12(3):667–675.

14. Alarab M, Kufaishi H, Lye S, et al. Expression of extracellular matrix-remodeling proteins is altered in vaginal tissue of premenopausal women with severe pelvic organ prolapse. *Reprod Sci* 2014;21(6):704–715.

15. Borazjani A, Kow N, Harris S, et al. Transcriptional regulation of connective tissue metabolism genes in women with pelvic organ prolapse. *Female Pelvic Med Reconstruct Surg* 2017;23(1):44–52.

16. Åkervall S, Al-Mukhtar Othman J, Molin M, et al. Symptomatic pelvic organ prolapse in middle-aged women: A national matched cohort study on the influence of childbirth. *Am J Obstet Gynecol* 2020;222(4):356.e1–356.e14.

17. Kerkhof MH, Ruiz-Zapata AM, Bril H, et al. Changes in tissue composition of the vaginal wall of premenopausal women with prolapse. *Am J Obstet Gynecol* 2014;210(2):168.e1–168.e9.

18. Ruiz-Zapata AM, Kerkhof MN, Zandieh-Doulabi B, et al. Functional characteristics of vaginal fibroblastic cells from premenopausal women with pelvic organ prolapse. *Mol Hum Reprod* 2014;20(11):1135–1143.

19. Li BS, Guo WJ, Hong L, et al. Role of mechanical strain-activated PI3K/Akt signaling pathway in pelvic organ prolapse. *Mol Med Rep* 2016;14(1):243–253.

20. Raya-Rivera AM, Esquiliano D, Fierro-Pastrana R, et al. Tissue-engineered autologous vaginal organs in patients: A pilot cohort study. *Lancet* 2014;384(9940):329–336.

21. Murphy SV, De Coppi P, Atala A. Opportunities and challenges of translational 3D bioprinting. *Nat Biomed Eng* 2020;4(4):370–380.

22. Nelson CE, Kim AJ, Adolph EJ, et al. Tunable delivery of siRNA from a biodegradable scaffold to promote angiogenesis in vivo. *Adv Mater* 2014;26(4):607–614.

23. Boennelycke M, Gras S, Lose G. Tissue engineering as a potential alternative or adjunct to surgical reconstruction in treating pelvic organ prolapse. *Int Urogynecol J* 2013;24(5):741–747.

24. Brown BN, Londono R, Tottey S, et al. Macrophage phenotype as a predictor of constructive remodeling following the implantation of biologically derived surgical mesh materials. *Acta Biomater* 2012;8(3):978–987.

25. Huleihel L, Bartolacci JG, Dziki JL, et al. Matrix-bound nanovesicles recapitulate extracellular matrix effects on macrophage phenotype. *Tissue Eng Part A* 2017;23(21–22):1283–1294.

26. Xu R, Zhang F, Chai R, et al. Exosomes derived from pro-inflammatory bone marrow-derived mesenchymal stem cells reduce inflammation and myocardial injury via mediating macrophage polarization. *J Cell Mol Med* 2019;23(11):7617–7631.

27. Sun DZ, Abelson B, Babbar P, et al. Harnessing the mesenchymal stem cell secretome for regenerative urology. *Nat Rev Urol* 2019;16(6):363–375.

28. Eleuteri S, Fierabracci A. Insights into the secretome of mesenchymal stem cells and its potential applications. *Int J Mol Sci* 2019;20(18):4597.

29. Mardpour S, Hamidieh AA, Taleahmad S, et al. Interaction between mesenchymal stromal cell-derived extracellular vesicles and immune cells by distinct protein content. *J Cell Physiol* 2019;234(6):8249–8258.

30. Janssen K, Lin DL, Hanzlicek B, et al. Multiple doses of stem cells maintain urethral function in a model of neuromuscular injury resulting in stress urinary incontinence. *Am J Physiol Renal Physiol* 2019;317(4):F1047–F1057.

31. Mori da Cunha M, Giacomazzi G, Callewaert G, et al. Fate of mesoangioblasts in a vaginal birth injury model: Influence of the route of administration. *Sci Rep* 2018;8(1):10604.

32. Chen Y, Tang L. Stem cell senescence: The obstacle of the treatment of degenerative disk disease. *Curr Stem Cell Res Ther* 2019;14(8):654–668.

33. Wen Y, Wani P, Zhou L, et al. Reprogramming of fibroblasts from older women with pelvic floor disorders alters cellular behavior associated with donor age. *Stem Cells Transl Med* 2013;2(2):118–128.

34. Choi HR, Cho KA, Kang HT, et al. Restoration of senescent human diploid fibroblasts by modulation of the extracellular matrix. *Aging Cell* 2011;10(1):148–157.

35. Faiena I, Koprowski C, Tunuguntla H. Female urethral reconstruction. *J Urol* 2016;195(3):557–567.

36. Shi LB, Cai HX, Chen LK, et al. Tissue engineered bulking agent with adipose-derived stem cells and silk fibroin microspheres for the treatment of intrinsic urethral sphincter deficiency. *Biomaterials* 2014;35(5):1519–1530.

37. Carr LK, Robert M, Kultgen PL, et al. Autologous muscle derived cell therapy for stress urinary incontinence: A prospective, dose ranging study. *J Urol* 2013;189(2):595–601.

38. Peters KM, Dmochowski RR, Carr LK, et al. Autologous muscle derived cells for treatment of stress urinary incontinence in women. *J Urol* 2014;192(2):469–476.

39. Lane FL, Jacobs S. Stem cells in gynecology. *Am J Obstet Gynecol* 2012;207(3):149–156.

40. Ni J, Li H, Zhou Y, et al. Therapeutic potential of human adipose-derived stem cell exosomes in stress urinary incontinence—An in vitro and in vivo study. *Cell Physiol Biochem* 2018;48(4):1710–1722.

41. Gräs S, Tolstrup CK, Lose G. Regenerative medicine provides alternative strategies for the treatment of anal incontinence. *Int Urogynecol J* 2017;28(3):341–350.

42. Boyer O, Bridoux V, Giverne C. Autologous myoblasts for the treatment of fecal incontinence: Results of a phase 2 randomized placebo-controlled study (MIAS). *Ann Surg* 2018;267(3):443–450.

43. Salcedo L, Mayorga M, Damaser M, et al. Mesenchymal stem cells can improve anal pressures after anal sphincter injury. *Stem Cell Res* 2013;10(1):95–102.

44. Dadhich P, Bohl JL, Tamburrini R, et al. BioSphincters to treat fecal incontinence in nonhuman primates. *Sci Rep* 2019;9(1):18096.

Evaluation and Treatment of Lower Urinary Tract Disorders

CHAPTER 23

Overview of Stress Urinary Incontinence

Alexandra Dubinskaya • Jennifer T. Anger

Introduction

Approximately 1 in 3 women will experience stress urinary incontinence (SUI) in their lifetime.[1] SUI affects a woman's quality of life on many levels. Often, this condition is considered to be a normal part of aging, and, unfortunately, the general public is not widely aware of curative treatment options. This chapter describes the anatomy and the mechanisms underlying SUI. Conservative methods, considered to be an initial step in therapy, including pelvic floor muscle (PFM) exercises, incontinence devices, and pessaries are reviewed.

Furthermore, this chapter provides an overview of surgical techniques that have evolved rapidly over time, culminating in the synthetic midurethral sling, along with the outcomes of the most notable trials which consist of successes, failures, and complication rates.[2–4]

ANATOMY AND MECHANISM OF ACTION

Urinary continence in women is achieved by a combination of urethral constriction and urethral support. Several components are required to maintain continence: a healthy urethral mucosa and submucosa, functioning intrinsic urethral smooth muscles and striated sphincter, intact pudendal nerve function, and properly functioning PFM.[5] The urethral mucosal lining produces secretions that increase surface tension. The submucosal layer contains an abundant amount of spongy vascular tissue that contributes to the closure pressure. The sphincteric mechanism controls the urine flow from the bladder to the urethra and contains two parts: an involuntary internal urethral sphincter and a voluntary external urethral sphincter. The internal sphincter consists of smooth muscle and is continuous with the detrusor muscle of the bladder. The external sphincter is located more distally and contains striated muscle: the compressor urethrae (the rhabdosphincter) that passes anteriorly and connects to the ischial rami and the urethrovaginal sphincter that surrounds both the vagina and urethra. In contrast to the compressor urethrae, which constricts just the urethra, the urethrovaginal sphincter constricts both the urethra and vagina. Innervation of the sphincteric mechanism comes from the S2 to S4 nerve roots. Control of the voluntary sphincter is provided by the pudendal nerve and nicotinic receptors. The involuntary sphincter is controlled by the autonomic nervous system via hypogastric nerves and alpha-1 receptors.[6–8]

The anatomic support of the urethra comes from the endopelvic fascia. Because the anterior vaginal wall is fused with the urethra and this connective tissue in turn attaches to the arcus tendinous fascia pelvis (ATFP) this forms the backstop by which the urethra is compressed during increases in intra-abdominal pressure.[9] These attachments prevent the downward movement of the urethra. Damage to these structures is a significant predisposing factor for SUI (Fig. 23.1).[10–12]

According to the integral theory by Petros and Woodman,[13] connective tissue laxity of the vagina and its supporting ligaments are the main cause of pelvic organ prolapse and SUI symptoms. This theory describes intimately dependable relationships between the pelvic organs and suspensory ligaments. According to this theory, the organs are storage containers (bladder stores urine, the bowel holds feces, and the uterus holds the fetus), each of them connected to the outside by a tubelike urethra, anus, or vagina. Muscles pull against the ligaments to close these tubes by compressing them and open them by stretching them. The bladder, vagina, and rectum are connected to the pelvic brim via ligaments, including the bulbourethral, cardinal/uterosacral, and ATFP. Weakening and damage to the suspensory system cause dysfunction that manifests as incontinence, retention, and/or organ prolapse.[13,14] In addition, weakening of the pelvic floor causes the upper part of the urethra to relax and funnel into the bladder, which interferes with equal pressure transmission. This creates a situation in which bladder pressure is higher than urethral pressure, resulting in incontinence.[15,16] This is the theoretical mechanism by which the Burch procedure (retropubic colposuspension) works. The main goal is to bring the urethra back into the pelvis and restore equal distribution of pressure. This is the same way that the traditional bladder neck sling works—by keeping the urethra closed with increased intra-abdominal pressures (Fig. 23.2).

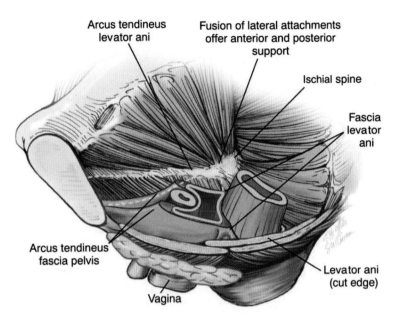

FIGURE 23.1 Sagittal view of lateral pelvis. Also shown are the ATFP, arcus tendineus fasciae rectovaginalis, and ischial spine. (Modified by J. Taylor from illustration by Lianne Krueger Sullivan. From Cundiff GW, Fenner D. Evaluation and treatment of women with rectocele: Focus on associated defecatory and sexual dysfunction. *Obstet Gynecol* 2004;104:1403–1421, erratum in *Obstet Gynecol* 2005;105:222, with permission.)

De Novo Stress Urinary Incontinence

With worsening of vaginal prolapse, SUI tends to "improve" as the urethra becomes progressively "kinked" as the anterior vaginal wall prolapse (cystocele) worsens. Manual reduction of the prolapse or placement of a pessary will trigger the return of incontinence symptoms. This phenomenon is classically present in association with anterior prolapse; however, it can present in cases of severe apical or posterior compartment prolapse causing external compression of urethra.[17]

This phenomenon has been called latent, masked, or occult SUI. In the Colpopexy and Urinary Reduction Efforts (CARE) trial, women without SUI but with pelvic organ prolapse were randomly assigned to undergo abdominal sacrocolpopexy (ASC) alone or ASC with the addition of a Burch procedure in order to prevent possible de novo SUI postoperatively. They demonstrated a significant reduction in postoperative SUI with Burch (32% vs. 57.4%).[18] A 7-year follow-up of this study, reported as eCARE, demonstrated that even

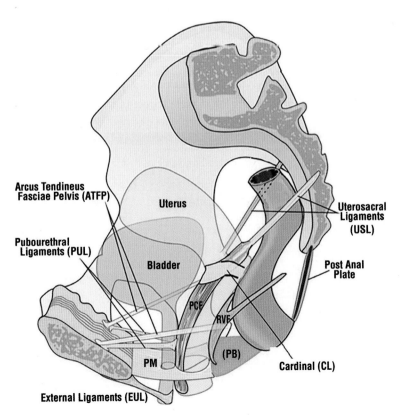

FIGURE 23.2 The integral theory system. Four ligaments suspend the organs from above like a suspension bridge. The perineal body (PB) supports the organs from below. PCF, pubocervical fascia; RVF, rectovaginal fascia; PM, perineal membrane; CL, cardinal ligament; EUL, external urethral ligament. (Reprinted from Petros P. The Integral System. *Cent European J Urol* 2011;64[3]:110–119. doi:10.5173/ceju.2011.03.art1)

though efficacy decreased over time, urethropexy prevented SUI longer than no urethropexy.[19]

Another multicenter randomized controlled trial (RCT), the Outcomes Following Vaginal Prolapse Repair and Mid Urethral Sling (OPUS) trial, randomized women with apical and/or anterior vaginal prolapse to vaginal repair (anterior colporrhaphy, paravaginal repair, colpocleisis, use of allograft, xenograft, or synthetic graft material) with or without a prophylactic midurethral sling placed at the time of surgery. The sling group had significantly lower rates of de novo postoperative SUI at 12 month follow-up (27.6% vs. 43%) but higher rates of adverse events.[20,21]

Performing prophylactic continence procedures, such as a midurethral sling, on preoperatively continent patients remains controversial. It is important to evaluate patients for the presence of occult stress incontinence before surgery, in order to best predict the need for concomitant correction with a midurethral sling. To best assess this, prolapse reduction can be performed using a variety of methods with different rates of success in detection of de novo incontinence: manually 16% (19 of 122), pessary 6% (5 of 88), swab 20% (32 of 158), and speculum 30% (35 of 118).[22] The goal of the prolapse reduction is to simulate the prolapse repair and assess the risk for developing SUI postoperatively. Patients can wear a pessary at home and assess for SUI, or urodynamics can be performed in the office with the prolapse reduced. Of note, it is important to not obstruct the urethra because this would give an inaccurate result.

TREATMENT

The degree of SUI can vary from mild, with urinary leakage during rigorous activity (playing sports, exercising, sneezing, laughing, coughing, or lifting) to moderate and severe leakage, with loss of larger volumes of urine that occurs with low-impact movements such as standing up, walking, or bending over.

Body mass index (BMI) plays an important role in the development and progression of SUI. Excess weight increases intra-abdominal pressure, bladder pressure, and urethral mobility. In fact, Gleicher et al.[23] found the prevalence of SUI to be significantly higher in women with BMI >30 compared to those with BMI <30 (63.4% vs. 36.5%, respectively, $P < .001$). Several epidemiologic studies have demonstrated that an increase in BMI by five units is associated with a 20% to 70% increase in the risk of developing incontinence.[24,25] The opposite is true, weight loss (with exercise or bariatric surgery) improves SUI symptoms.[26] In fact, Subak et al. demonstrated that weight loss of 8.0% of body weight over the 6 months period decreased the frequency of SUI episodes by 47%.[24]

As with most pelvic floor disorders, the treatment strategy should progress from more conservative to less conservative. Depending on the level of symptom bother, patients should first be provided with education on avoiding triggering activities, emptying the bladder before exercise and learning to voluntarily contract the PFMs in situations that would normally cause urinary leakage, such as cough or sneeze.

Pelvic Floor Muscle Therapy

Pelvic floor muscle therapy (PFMT) is training of the levator ani muscles. These include the iliococcygeus, pubococcygeus, and puborectalis muscles. The goal of PFMT exercises is to improve the strength and function of the pelvic floor. The levator ani muscles are predominantly composed of slow-twitch/type I fibers; only one-third of the levator ani muscles fibers are fast-twitch/type II fibers. The slow-twitch muscles provide baseline tonic activity and contribute to the compression of the urethra against the pubic bone. This results in passive continence. The fast-twitch muscle fibers provide continence in the setting of a sudden increase in intra-abdominal pressure. The thickness of the levator ani muscles correlates with their strength.[27]

One of the most common factors adversely impacting pelvic muscle strength is vaginal delivery. In a study of postpartum women who underwent vaginal deliveries, MRI series showed disruption in levator ani muscles.[28] Pelvic muscle strength was significantly affected by vaginal delivery and also by a trial of labor, even if women ultimately underwent cesarean delivery.[29,30]

PFM function can be determined by both their tone at rest and the strength of voluntary contractions. Strength is defined as strong, weak, or absent. There are several grading methods to quantify the strength of the PFMs. The Modified Oxford scale assigns grades of 0 (no discernable PFM contractions) to grade 5 (strong PFM contraction) (Table 23.1) The Brink assessment scale evaluates three PFM contraction variables: vaginal pressure or muscle force, elevation or vertical

---

TABLE 23.1

Modified Oxford Grading Scale of Pelvic Floor Muscle Contraction

OXFORD GRADING SCALE

0	No muscle activity
1	Minor muscle "flicker"
2	Weak muscle activity without a circular contraction
3	Moderate muscle contraction with a circular contraction and elevation of the vagina
4	Good muscle contraction
5	Strong muscle contraction

Reprinted by permission from Springer: Laycock J. Clinical evaluation of the pelvic floor. In: Schussler B, Laycock J, Norton P, et al, eds. *Pelvic floor re-education.* London: Springer-Verlag, 1994:37–101.

TABLE 23.2

Brink Scoring System of Pelvic Floor Muscle Contraction

BRINK SCORING SYSTEM

MUSCLE FUNCTION DIMENSION	SCORE
Squeeze pressure	1 = none
	2 = weak squeeze, felt as a flick at various points along finger surface; not all the way around
	3 = moderate squeeze; felt all the way around finger surface
	4 = strong squeeze; full circumstance of fingers compressed
Muscle contraction duration	1 = none
	2 = less than 1 s
	3 = greater than 1 s; less than 3 s
	4 = greater than 3 s
Vertical displacement	1 = none
	2 = finger bases move anteriorly (pushed up by muscle bulk)
	3 = whole length of fingers moves anteriorly
	4 = whole fingers move anteriorly; are gripped and pulled in
Total	Range = 3–12

From Borello-France DF, Handa VL, Brown MB, et al. Pelvic-floor muscle function in women with pelvic organ prolapse. *Phys Ther* 2007;87(4):399–407, by permission of Oxford University Press

TABLE 23.3

Tips on How to Identify an Ideal Pelvic Floor Muscle Contraction

- Observation of "puckering" of the anus
- Observation of "nodding" of the clitoris
- Patient visualization of contraction through use of handheld mirror
- Palpation of superior movement and muscle tension medial to the ischial tuberosity
- Palpation of a squeeze around a finger inserted into the vagina
- Palpation of a "lift" or anterior movement of the posterior vaginal wall
- Negligible visible activity of the gluteal, adductors, and rectus abdominis
- Slight inward motion of the abdominal wall
- No visible motion of the spine/pelvis
- Maintenance of normal breathing pattern

displacement of the examiner's fingers, and the duration of contraction (Table 23.2). Each of these variables is rated on a 4-point scale and summed together to obtain total score ranging from 3 to 12. Tips on how to identify an ideal PFM contraction listed in Table 23.3.

It is important for providers to assess a patient's PFM strength and ability to recruit the correct muscles while performing PFM exercises. These exercises, known as Kegel exercises, are simple to perform, noninvasive, and are an effective first-line therapy for SUI.[31] In a recent Cochrane review of 31 trials that studied 1,874 women, women in the PFM training groups were more likely to report cure compared to the no-treatment groups.[32,33]

The key to PFMT effectiveness is daily compliance. Different options to promote compliance have been suggested: setting a reminder on one's phone, performing exercises in the car while stopped at a stop sign, and weekly sessions with a nurse practitioner and/or pelvic floor therapist in the office. There are many new

commercial devices available online that facilitate performance of the exercises, with some of them providing feedback about the strength of the contractions and correct muscle use. In fact, the use of mobile apps for PFM training have shown effectiveness and relevant improvement in women with SUI.[34] PFM exercise is also a great option for muscle recovery in the postpartum period.[35] However, women with more severe and long standing leakage are more likely to benefit from surgical treatment, and extensive trials of conservative management may be futile in these women.

Biofeedback

Biofeedback is a technique that involves the use of visual or auditory feedback to help a woman gain control over her PFM. Biofeedback is achieved with one of several methods: electromyography, which monitors the electrical activity of muscles during contraction and relaxation; manometry, which measures pressure generated by muscle contractions; direct palpation by a provider with verbal feedback; or commercial devices with built-in apps that provide feedback. Considered by many to be the father of PFM training, Arnold Kegel implemented a vaginal perineometer as a biofeedback modality for SUI in 1956. He reported a 90.6% success rate with this technique and claimed that correct performance of PFM exercise is crucial to success.[36] Biofeedback use in PFM training has also demonstrated efficacy and improvement of SUI in more recent trials.[37-39]

For those women who have weak PFMs or unable to identify the correct muscle group, adding electrical stimulation to the vaginal probe used for biofeedback might facilitate muscle identification and enhance exercise performance. However, electrical stimulation in women capable of performing muscle contractions provides no additional benefits.[40] Electrical stimulation should be avoided in pregnancy, vaginal infection, an open vaginal or vulvar wound, and recent (within 6 weeks) pelvic surgery.[41] Another option to help with identification of PFMs is a real-time ultrasound. This biofeedback technique helps to visualize the "lift" component of the PFM contraction. Although this tool can be added during exercise instructions, limited studies assess the value of real-time ultrasound versus PFM exercise alone.

Vaginal Inserts

The idea behind the insertion of vaginal cones is to provoke PFM contraction when inserted into vagina. The original set of cones was introduced in 1985 and contained nine different cones with weight between 20 and 100 g.[42] These devices are best used in women with mild SUI and those able to accommodate the device without discomfort. The training starts with the heaviest insert that a patient can retain for 1 minute twice a day. The time holding the insert progressively increases to 15 minutes twice a day. After that, the patient progresses to a higher insert weight. There are commercially available inserts with different weight sets and with extra options for vibration that can be purchased to facilitate at-home PFM training. Most of the trials done with vaginal cones are small. There is a lack of evidence that weighted vaginal cones are better than no active treatment. According to a Cochrane systematic review, cones plus PFMT has not shown improvement over cones alone or PFMT alone in women with SUI.[43]

Pessary

The pessary has been in use for centuries. Most commonly, pessaries are used for pelvic organ prolapse. However, there are pessaries with a specially designed "knob" (additional anterior–posterior width that is placed at the urethrovesical junction) that are predominantly used for SUI. The most commonly used pessaries of this type are a "ring with knob" and "incontinence dish."

A pessary is an effective alternative to surgery in women who have multiple comorbidities preventing them from undergoing surgical treatment safely or for those who simply prefer to avoid surgery. Despite ease of use, finding a comfortable, well-fitted pessary can be a hurdle. There are several factors affecting adherence to pessary use and pessary "fit." A history of prior vaginal surgery, short vaginal length (less than 8 cm), prior hysterectomy, wide vaginal introitus, or a genital hiatus/total vaginal length ratio greater than

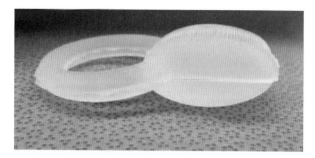

FIGURE 23.3 Final three-dimensional-printed silicone vaginal pessary. Three-dimensional model of a vaginal pessary consisting of a ring and elliptical cylindrical knob. (Reprinted from Barsky M, Kelley R, Bhora FY, et al. Customized pessary fabrication using three-dimensional printing technology. *Obstet Gynecol* 2018;131[3]:493–497.)

0.9 contributes to a pessary fitting failure.[44] Younger age and vaginal atrophy are associated with poor continuation of pessary use.[45] Severe posterior prolapse is also a single predictor of pessary discontinuation. This is likely due to the fact a rectocele is not always reduced adequately with a pessary, which is better at reducing anterior and apical prolapse.[46] A three-dimensional-printed customized pessary for SUI was made and successfully fitted in a 90-year-old woman who strongly desired nonsurgical treatment and was unable to be fitted with standard incontinence pessaries. As we could see on Figure 23.3, this printed pessary had an elongated knob not available with standard SUI pessaries. Future pessary customization could be a feasible option to improve continuation of the pessary use.[47]

Cleaning a pessary can be done in the office or at home. Women who can remove and replace a pessary themselves do not have to be seen in the office more often than annually. Many providers see patients (unable to change their pessary) quarterly for pessary cleaning. A recent RCT demonstrated that routine follow-up at 6 months is noninferior to 3-month follow-up.[48] The main concern with pessary use is vaginal wall erosion and ulcer formation. In order to prevent both, vaginal estrogens are recommended for postmenopausal women using a pessary.

In a multicenter RCT entitled "Ambulatory Treatments for Leakage Associated with Stress (ATLAS) trial," women with SUI or stress-predominant mixed urinary incontinence were assigned to one of three arms: continence pessary (149 women), behavior therapy (146 women), or combined therapy (pessary + behavior therapy) for SUI (151 women). Outcomes were measured at 3, 6, and 12 months. The primary outcomes in this study was subjective improvement as measured by the Urinary Distress Inventory-Short Form (UDI-6) and the Patient Global Impression of Improvement (PGI-I) at 3 months. The secondary outcome measured was the proportion of women with at least a 75% reduction of incontinence episodes based on 7-day voiding diary.

The improvement in the combined group was not different from the behavior group, based on the PGI-I at 3 months, but scores in both the combined and behavior groups were better than the pessary group. UDI scores in the behavior group similarly showed better continence than the pessary group (49% vs. 33%, $P = .006$) but not significantly different from the combined group (49% vs. 44%, $P = .49$). According to the voiding diaries, all groups had about a 50% reduction in their symptoms. Women were more satisfied in the behavior group than in the pessary group. The treatment success at 12 months did not differ between groups on both intention-to-treat and per-protocol analysis. The conclusion based on the ATLAS study was that behavioral therapy was more effective than pessary use alone.[49]

Commercially available vaginal inserts for stress urinary incontinence

An RCT Short-term Uresta Efficacy trial[50] in 2017 demonstrated a reduction in pad use among women using a specialized commercially available device, Uresta (66.7%), versus a sham intravaginal ring (22.2%). The shape of the Uresta is specially designed to compress the urethra and prevent leakage similar to incontinence pessaries. This reusable device comes in different sizes so that women can use the larger size when they need it the most: during physical activity and exercise. Another similar over-the-counter device is Impressa, a tampon-like vaginal insert designed to help with light urinary leakage.

Occlusive Urethral Devices

This group of devices can be divided into two subgroups: external and internal urethral devices. External devices are applied on the urethra externally and stay in place with a proprietary suction mechanism (Fig. 23.4). The suction creates negative pressure that enables coaptation of the urethral wall and provides urethral resistance.[51–53] In a multicenter nonblinded trial, a 97% improvement in pad weight was noted, with 45% improvement in patient's quality of life based on the Incontinence Quality of Life Questionnaire (I-QOL). Irritation and the inability to apply the device correctly were the common complaints causing withdrawal from the study.

Internal devices, such as the urethral plug, the Reliance Urinary Control Insert (UroMed Corp, Needham, MA), Vesiflo (Vesiflo Inc., Redmond, WA), and FemSoft (FemSoft, Stewartville, MN), are inserted into the urethra and function by occluding the urethral lumen. Some of them have an inflatable balloon that helps to stabilize the device at the bladder neck. Women insert these devices themselves and, based on studies, are mostly comfortable and satisfied with the ease and comfort of use. However, a urinary tract infection rate as high as 30% has been reported with these devices.[54–58]

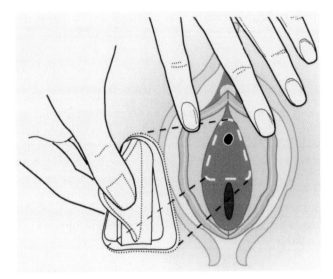

FIGURE 23.4 Proper application of external urethral barrier. (Reprinted from Brubaker L, Harris T, Gleason D, et al. The external urethral barrier for stress incontinence: A multicenter trial of safety and efficacy. *Obstet Gynecol* 1999;93[6]:932–937.)

Medical Therapy

Pharmacologic therapy has not had a significant role in treatment of SUI. Off-label use of estrogen and alpha-adrenergic agonists has been reported but with limited improvement in symptoms. Duloxetine (Irenka, Cymbalta) is a selective serotonin and norepinephrine reuptake inhibitor. Administration of duloxetine leads to an increase in urethral closure forces through stimulation of pudendal motor neuron alpha-1 adrenergic and 5-hydroxytryptamine-2 receptors and resulted in significant dose-dependent reduction of SUI episodes. Among 436 women, the incontinence episode frequency decreased (50% with duloxetine vs. 27% with placebo, $P < .001$). However, discontinuation rate was 24% for duloxetine versus 4% with placebo, with nausea as the most common reason for discontinuation (6.4%).[59–61]

A European multicenter RCT compared the effect of innovative pelvic floor therapy plus oral duloxetine therapy to oral duloxetine alone. The innovative pelvic floor muscle training (iPFMT) included education about PFMs, PFMs training in various positions with a focus on endurance and strength, with regular assessments of performance. At 12 weeks of treatment, a statistically significant difference was observed in the incontinence episode frequency per week (66.7% decrease in weekly incontinence episodes in duloxetine plus iPFMT vs. 50.0% decrease in duloxetine alone, $P < .001$) as well as a decrease in the number of pads used per day (50.0% vs. 22.5%, $P < .001$). The PGI-I score improved significantly (70.8% vs. 65.6%, $P < .01$) along with I-QOL score (19.3% vs. 6.6%, $P < .001$).[62] Despite being used in Europe for the treatment of SUI, the U.S. Food and Drug Administration (FDA) has only approved duloxetine for the management of major depressive disorder and diabetic peripheral neuropathy, not SUI.

Behavior and Lifestyle Interventions

Many women are counseled to decrease their fluid intake or adjust their exercise routine so as not to leak with SUI. However, SUI should not dictate a woman's exercise routine. Instead, we believe in correcting a woman's SUI so that she can enjoy the exercise routine of her choice. We recommend shared decision-making and intervention based on patient choice because SUI is curable, and a large variety of treatment options are available.

Surgical Treatment

Per the 2017 American Urological Association guidelines, the following surgical options can be offered as a surgical treatment of SUI in women: midurethral sling (synthetic), autologous fascia pubovaginal sling, Burch colposuspension, and bulking agents. For historical purposes, it is important to understand the commonly used procedures that preceded these four recommended options.

Kelly plication

In 1913, Howard Kelly placed horizontal mattress suture at the level of urethrovesical junction with intention to narrow the urethra and provide elevation of the bladder neck.[63] The procedure acquired its author's name and is termed the "Kelly plication." Later, this technique was modified by Kennedy and evolved into the modern-day anterior colporrhaphy.[64] Due to low morbidity, the ease of a transvaginal approach, and the simplicity of the procedure, this technique was used for a long time as a primary treatment of SUI. However, recurrent incontinence rates after this procedure were 46.81% at 5 years.[65] Therefore, it is no longer commonly used for the treatment of SUI but still remains a commonly used technique for transvaginal correction of the anterior prolapse.

Anterior urethropexy

Urologist Dr. Victor F. Marshall and gynecologists Andrew A. Marchetti and Kermit E. Krantz developed the method of anterior urethropexy as a treatment of SUI. The Marshall-Marchetti-Krantz (MMK) procedure, first performed in 1944, involves direct fixation of the urethra and bladder to the periosteum of the symphysis pubis.[66,67] Despite a relatively high success rate of 86% at 6 months, the MMK had a long-term failure rate of 36% at 5 years.[68,69] In addition, this procedure did not effectively reduce a cystocele, and periosteal suture placement was associated with osteitis pubis in 2.5% of women.[68] Later, in the 1960s, gynecologist John Burch modified the MMK procedure by using Cooper ligament for suture suspension.[70] The Burch retropubic urethropexy has the benefits of correcting a cystocele while eliminating the risk of osteitis pubis. The success rates are 85% to 90% within the first year and 70% after 5 years (Fig. 23.5).[2,69,71]

A multicenter RCT, the Stress Incontinence Surgical Treatment Efficacy Trial, compared outcomes

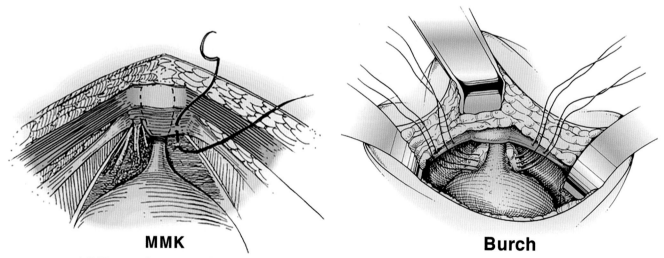

MMK   **Burch**

FIGURE 23.5 MMK procedure versus the Burch procedure. **A:** MMK: Sutures are placed into the endopelvic fascia along the urethra and fixed into the periosteum of the symphysis pubis. **B:** Burch: Sutures are placed at the level of the bladder neck and attached to the Cooper ligament. (A: Reprinted from Jones HW, Rock JA. *Te Linde's operative gynecology,* 11th ed. Philadelphia: Wolters Kluwer, 2015. B: Adapted from Tanagho EA. Colpocystourethropexy: The way we do it. *J Urol* 1976;116[6]:751–753. Copyright © 1976 Wolters Kluwer. With permission.)

of the Burch procedure versus the autologous fascial sling. At 24 months, cure rates, as defined by absence of SUI, were higher among women who underwent a sling procedure than among those who underwent the Burch procedure (66% vs. 49%, $P < .001$). Treatment satisfaction was also significantly higher in the sling group (86% vs. 78%, $P = .02$), however, at a cost of an increased rate of adverse events, including postoperative urgency urinary incontinence and voiding dysfunction (63% vs. 47%, $P < .001$) in the fascial sling group.[21,72,73]

Needle suspension

Another historical technique is the transvaginal needle suspension, first described by Pereyra[74] in 1959. This technique underwent multiple modifications by Pereyra and others, such as Stamey, Raz, and Gittes, in attempt to improve the cure rates and minimize complications.[10] These procedures were abandoned after several comprehensive reviews and randomized trials demonstrated that they were significantly less effective than retropubic colposuspensions and traditional sling procedures.[75]

Urethral bulking agents

The use of injectable material for the treatment of SUI goes back to 1938 when sodium morrhuate was injected into the anterior vaginal wall to produce periurethral scarring. Since then, many other agents including paraffin wax, sclerosing agents, polytetrafluoroethylene (Teflon), autologous fat, ethylene vinyl alcohol (Tegress), and hyaluronic acid/dextranomer copolymer (Zuidex) were trialed and taken off the market due to associated side effects and complications. The ideal agent for urethral bulking should be biocompatible, easily injectable, nonimmunogenic, hypoallergenic, and cause minimal scarring. Several materials that met these criteria underwent FDA approval: calcium hydroxyapatite (Coaptite), carbon coated zirconium (Durasphere), polydimethylsiloxane elastomer (Macroplastique), and most recently polyacrylamide hydrogel (Bulkamid).

The main goal of urethral bulking is to maintain the coaptation of the urethra during the storage phase and also during periods of increased abdominal pressure, without disturbing voiding function. This procedure involves injection of a bulking agent into the submucosal tissues of the urethra. This is done under urethroscopic control and can be performed transurethrally or paraurethrally,[76] although transurethral methods are the preferred method for most providers. This is a relatively quick, easy-to-perform procedure with a low morbidity that can be done in the office under local anesthesia. Urethral bulking procedures are an option for women who have low-volume stress-related urinary leakage or for those who are trying to avoid more invasive surgical procedures, such as women of advanced age with medical comorbidities.

Urethral bulking agents lose their effectiveness over time and often require repeat injections. When success rates were compared between pubovaginal sling and transurethral Macroplastique injections, 81% of women in the pubovaginal sling group had no leakage at 6 months compare to 9% in the injection group.[77,78] According to Herschorn and Radomski, the probability of remaining continent without additional injections was 72% at 1 year, 57% at 2 years, and 45% at 3 years.[2,79] The complication rate of urethral bulking is overall low, with temporary urinary retention, urgency incontinence, and transient hematuria being the most common. Rare complications include outlet obstruction, foreign body granuloma, and urethral mucosal prolapse.[78,80–83]

Sling procedures

The surgical treatment of SUI underwent a rapid evolution over the past century. In 1907, at a surgery convention in Paris, Giordano presented the concept of a sling procedure using a gracilis muscle flap. He was followed by Goebel[84] who in 1910 described the technique of detaching the pyramidalis muscle and suturing it beneath the urethra. Frangenheim[85] modified the technique in 1914 by attaching a vertical strip of rectus fascia to the pyramidalis muscle. The final alteration to this technique was made by Stoeckel in 1917, who added plication of the periuretheral fascia at the vesical neck.[86] This procedure is known as the Goebel-Frangenheim-Stoeckel procedure and includes securing the pyramidalis muscle and the rectus fascia beneath the urethra after plication of the periuretheral fascia.[87] In 1933, Price described a sling made from fascia lata, and later in 1942, Aldridge[88] described the use of rectus fascia to create a sling. He used two strips of rectus fascia that were brought down through the rectus muscle and behind the symphysis pubis. He then sutured them in the midline under the urethra at the urethrovesical junction through a separate vaginal incision. This technique served as a foundation for the modern-day sling.

In 1992, Medicare claims data revealed that the most common surgical procedure for SUI was needle suspension (7,840 procedures, or 2.4 procedures/100 Medicare beneficiaries with a diagnosis of SUI) followed by anterior urethropexy (7,080 procedures). The sling gained popularly and was by far the most commonly performed procedure for SUI in 2001 (17,680) and increased in use since then.[89] This corresponded to a steady decline in procedures like needle suspension and anterior urethropexy.[2] The most common materials for an autologous sling were autologous rectus fascia and fascia lata. Harvesting fascia lata avoids a large abdominal incision, possible lower abdominal hernias, and wound complications. However, the fascia lata harvest can cause thigh hematoma and seroma formation.[90] The primary disadvantage of the autologous sling of either type is increased operating and recovery time.

In order to decrease the operating time and associated morbidity with harvesting the graft, several allograft materials have been explored: cadaveric fascia allograft, cadaveric human acellular dermis, xenograft, nylon, silicone, Mersilene, Gore-Tex, and the latest synthetic mesh sling. Based on the integral theory mentioned earlier, SUI is the result of impairment of urethral support. Petros and Ulmsten[91] developed tension-free vaginal tape (TVT) procedure.

This procedure introduced several new concepts into the sling techniques: placement of the sling at the miduretha versus the bladder neck, the use of a polypropylene mesh sling kit with fine trocars, and placement of the sling without tension ("TVT"). Synthetic slings have multiple advantages, including consistent and durable strength, no potential for infectious disease transmission, reduced morbidity with no fascial harvesting, and decreased operating time.

Although most sling-related complications, such as UTIs, voiding dysfunction, and urgency incontinence, complications unique to mesh include mesh extrusion, mesh erosion, and, rarely, mesh-related pain. Mesh extrusion is mesh exposure through the vagina, usually at the prior incision area. Mesh erosion is erosion of the mesh into an organ (such as bladder or urethra) or surrounded tissue. Both of these mesh-specific complications have decreased in frequency after the introduction of loosely woven, macroporous polypropylene synthetic material. Richter et al.[92] reported the rates of mesh extrusion of 2.7% and mesh erosion of 0.3% for the retropubic sling. Overall, the success rate for different sling materials varies in literature, with mean 12-month cure rates of 87% for the autologous sling, 79% for cadaveric sling material, 82% for xenograft, and up to 90% for synthetic sling.[93–95]

There are currently multiple "TVT-like" slings with varying options of sling material and surgical approaches on the market. Despite a great deal of controversy surrounding the use of vaginal mesh, the midurethral synthetic sling remains the gold standard for surgical correction of SUI.[96]

Another significant milestone in the surgical treatment of SUI was the development of the transobturator tape (TOT) sling that was described by Delorme[97] in 2001. This minimally invasive synthetic sling is placed through an obturator approach and was created to reduce the risk of bladder perforation and eliminate the risk of bowel perforation and major vascular injury. The retropubic sling was compared to the transobturator sling in a multicenter randomized nonblinded equivalence and superiority trial, the Trial of Mid-Urethral Slings (TOMUS). Objective success at 12 months was reported as 80.8% in the retropubic sling group and 77.7% in the transobturator group. Subjective success was 62.2% and 55.8%, respectively. Voiding dysfunction that required surgical correction was 2.7% in the retropubic sling group and 0% in TOT group ($P = .004$). There were no significant differences in postoperative urgency incontinence, satisfaction, or quality of life. At 5 years, treatment success was 7.9% greater after retropubic compared to transobturator (51.3% vs. 43.4%, 95% confidence interval to 1.4%, 17.2%).[98] Urinary symptoms and quality of life worsened over time ($P < .001$). Mesh extrusion were acceptably low and not statistically different between groups.[21,92]

As sling procedures continue to evolve, single-incision or mini-slings were developed (Fig. 23.6). The advantage of this type of sling is a lower risk of bladder, vessel, and obturator nerve injury. Also, mini-slings introduce less foreign material into the body while having

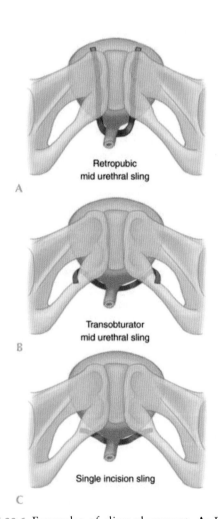

FIGURE 23.6 Examples of sling placement. **A:** Retropubic sling. **B:** Transobturator sling. **C:** Single-incision sling. (Modified from Wound, Ostomy and Continence Nurses Society, Doughty DB, Moore KN. *Wound, Ostomy and Continence Nurses Society core curriculum: Continence management.* Philadelphia: Wolters Kluwer, 2015; and Kovac RS, Zimmerman CS. *Advances in reconstructive vaginal surgery,* 2nd ed. Philadelphia: Lippincott Williams & Wilkins, 2012.)

potentially the same continence properties as the retropubic sling. Clinical trials are ongoing to compare outcomes of the single-incision sling versus retropubic sling.[99] In a multicenter international study, the Altis Single Incision Sling System (SIS) showed similar safety and efficacy to transobturator and retropubic midurethral slings at 12-month follow-up.[100,101] Although more comparative data is needed, the SIS holds promise as the next generation of sling.

CONCLUSION

A wide variety of treatment methods are currently available for SUI. However, the treatment approach should be based on the woman's symptom bother and her desire for treatment. It is reasonable to start from the least invasive options for mild symptoms and progress to the more invasive ones. It is important to recognize that severe SUI is unlikely to benefit from conservative methods, and patients should be counseled appropriately.[2]

References

1. Luber KM. The definition, prevalence, and risk factors for stress urinary incontinence. *Rev Urol* 2004;6(Suppl 3):S3–S9.
2. Anger JT, Weinberg AE, Albo ME, et al. Trends in surgical management of stress urinary incontinence among female Medicare beneficiaries. *Urology* 2009;74(2):283–287.
3. Harding C, Thorpe A. The surgical treatment of female stress urinary incontinence. *Indian J Urol* 2010;26(2):257–262.
4. Richardson ML, Sokol ER. A cost-effectiveness analysis of conservative versus surgical management for the initial treatment of stress urinary incontinence. *Am J Obstet Gynecol* 2014;211(5):565.e1–565.e6.
5. Firoozi F. *Interpretation of basic and advanced urodynamics*. Cham: Springer, 2017.
6. Ahmed DG, Mohamed MF, Mohamed SA. Superior hypogastric plexus combined with ganglion impar neurolytic blocks for pelvic and/or perineal cancer pain relief. *Pain Phy* 2015;18(1):E49–E56.
7. Tong X-K, Huo R-J. The anatomical basis and prevention of neurogenic voiding dysfunction following radical hysterectomy. *Surg Radiol Anat* 1991;13(2):145–148.
8. Sam P, Jiang J, LaGrange CA. *Anatomy, abdomen and pelvis, sphincter urethrae*. Treasure Island: StatPearls Publishing, 2021.
9. Fritsch H, Pinggera GM, Lienemann A, et al. What are the supportive structures of the female urethra? *Neurourol Urodyn* 2006;25(2):128–134.
10. Raz S. Modified bladder neck suspension for female stress incontinence. *Urology* 1981;17(1):82–85.
11. Balgobin S, Jeppson PC, Wheeler T II, et al. Standardized terminology of apical structures in the female pelvis based on a structured medical literature review. *Am J Obstet Gynecol* 2020;222(3):204–218.
12. DeLancey J. Anatomy. In: Cardozo L, Staskin D, eds. *Textbook of female urology and urogynaecology*. London: Isis Medical Media, 2001.
13. Petros PEP, Woodman PJ. The integral theory of continence. *Int Urogynecol J Pelvic Floor Dysfunct* 2007;19(1):35–40.
14. Petros P. The Integral System. *Cent European J Urol* 2011;64(3):110–119.
15. Enhörning G. Simultaneous recording of intravesical and intra-urethral pressure. A study on urethral closure in normal and stress incontinent women. *Acta Chir Scand Suppl* 1961;276:1–68.
16. Blaivas J, Chancellor M, Weiss J, et al. Stress urinary incontinence in women. In: Blaivas J, Chancellor M, Weiss J, et al, eds. *Atlas of urodynamics*, 2nd ed. New York: Wiley, 2007:184–185.
17. Romanzi LJ. Management of the urethral outlet in patients with severe prolapse. *Curr Opin Urol* 2002;12(4):339–344.
18. Brubaker L, Cundiff GW, Fine P, et al. Abdominal sacrocolpopexy with burch colposuspension to reduce urinary stress incontinence. *N Engl J Med* 2006;354(15):1557–1566.
19. Nygaard I, Brubaker L, Zyczynski HM, et al. Long-term outcomes following abdominal sacrocolpopexy for pelvic organ prolapse. *JAMA* 2013;309(19):2016.
20. Wei J, Nygaard I, Richter H, et al. Outcomes following vaginal prolapse repair and mid urethral sling (OPUS) trial—Design and methods. *Clin Trials* 2009;6(2):162–171.
21. Fitzgerald JJ. Landmark FPMRS trials. Accessed October 15, 2020. https://urogyntrials.glideapp.io/
22. Visco AG, Brubaker L, Nygaard I, et al. The role of preoperative urodynamic testing in stress-continent women undergoing sacrocolpopexy: The Colpopexy and Urinary Reduction Efforts (CARE) randomized surgical trial. *Int Urogynecol J Pelvic Floor Dysfunct* 2008;19(5):607–614.
23. Gleicher S, Byler T, Ginzburg N. Association between stress urinary incontinence and the components of metabolic syndrome among females 20–59 years. *Urology* 2020;145:100–105.
24. Subak LL, Richter HE, Hunskaar S. Obesity and urinary incontinence: Epidemiology and clinical research update. *J Urol* 2009;182(6 Suppl):S2–S7.
25. Whitcomb EL, Subak LL. Effect of weight loss on urinary incontinence in women. *Open Access J Urol* 2011;3:123–132.
26. Brown JS, Wing R, Barrett-Connor E, et al. Lifestyle intervention is associated with lower prevalence of urinary incontinence: The Diabetes Prevention Program. *Diabetes Care* 2006;29(2):385–390.
27. Yu H, Zheng H, Zhang X, et al. Association between elastography findings of the levator ani and stress urinary incontinence. *J Gynecol Obstet Hum Reprod* 2021;50(4):101906.
28. Hoyte L, Damaser MS. Magnetic resonance-based female pelvic anatomy as relevant for maternal childbirth injury simulations. *Ann N Y Acad Sciences* 2007;1101(1):361–376.
29. Baytur YB, Deveci A, Uyar Y, et al. Mode of delivery and pelvic floor muscle strength and sexual function after childbirth. *Int J Gynecol Obstet* 2005;88(3):276–280.
30. Davidson MJ, Nielsen PMF, Taberner AJ, et al. Change in levator ani muscle stiffness and active force during pregnancy and post-partum. *Int Urogynecol J* 2020;31(11):2345–2351.
31. Theofrastous JP, Wyman JF, Bump RC, et al. Effects of pelvic floor muscle training on strength and predictors of response in the treatment of urinary incontinence. *Neurourol Urodyn* 2002;21(5):486–490.
32. Dumoulin C, Cacciari LP, Hay-Smith EJC. Pelvic floor muscle training versus no treatment, or inactive control treatments, for urinary incontinence in women. *Cochrane Database Syst Rev* 2018;(10):CD005654
33. Wu Y, Welk B. Revisiting current treatment options for stress urinary incontinence and pelvic organ prolapse: A contemporary literature review. *Res Rep Urol* 2019;11:179–188.

34. Asklund I, Nyström E, Sjöström M, et al. Mobile app for treatment of stress urinary incontinence: A randomized controlled trial. *Neurourol Urodyn* 2017;36(5):1369–1376.

35. Meyer S. Pelvic floor education after vaginal delivery. *Obstet Gynecol* 2001;97(5):673–677.

36. Kegel AH. Stress incontinence of urine in women; physiologic treatment. *J Int Coll Surg* 1956;25(4 Pt 1):487–499.

37. Liu Y-J, Ting SW-H, Hsiao S-M, et al. Efficacy of bio-assisted pelvic floor muscle training in women with pelvic floor dysfunction. *Eur J Obstet Gynecol Reprod Biol* 2020;251:206–211.

38. Nunes EFC, Sampaio LMM, Biasotto-Gonzalez DA, et al. Biofeedback for pelvic floor muscle training in women with stress urinary incontinence: A systematic review with meta-analysis. *Physiotherapy* 2019;105(1):10–23.

39. Richmond CF, Martin DK, Yip SO, et al. Effect of supervised pelvic floor biofeedback and electrical stimulation in women with mixed and stress urinary incontinence. *Female Pelvic Med Reconstr Surg* 2016;22(5):324–327.

40. Huebner M, Riegel K, Hinninghofen H, et al. Pelvic floor muscle training for stress urinary incontinence: A randomized, controlled trial comparing different conservative therapies. *Physiother Res Int* 2011;16(3):133–140.

41. Lee J-Y, Chancellor MB. Using electrical stimulation for urinary incontinence. *Rev Urol* 2002;4(1):49–50.

42. Peattie AB, Plevnik S, Stanton SL. Vaginal cones: A conservative method of treating genuine stress incontinence. *Br J Obstet Gynaecol* 1988;95(10):1049–1053.

43. Herbison GP, Dean N. Weighted vaginal cones for urinary incontinence. *Cochrane Database Syst Rev* 2013;(7):CD002114.

44. Markle D, Skoczylas L, Goldsmith C, et al. Patient characteristics associated with a successful pessary fitting. *Female Pelvic Med Reconstr Surg* 2011;17(5):249–252.

45. Nager CW, Richter HE, Nygaard I, et al. Incontinence pessaries: Size, POPQ measures, and successful fitting. *Int Urogynecol J* 2009;20(9):1023–1028.

46. Maito JM, Quam ZA, Craig E, et al. Predictors of successful pessary fitting and continued use in a nurse-midwifery pessary clinic. *J Midwifery Womens Health* 2006;51(2):78–84.

47. Barsky M, Kelley R, Bhora FY, et al. Customized pessary fabrication using three-dimensional printing technology. *Obstet Gynecol* 2018;131(3):493–497.

48. Propst K, Mellen C, O'Sullivan DM, et al. Timing of office-based pessary care: A randomized controlled trial. *Obstet Gynecol* 2020;135(1):100–105.

49. Richter HE, Burgio KL, Goode PS, et al. Non-surgical management of stress urinary incontinence: Ambulatory Treatments for Leakage Associated with Stress (ATLAS) trial. *Clin Trials* 2007;4(1):92–101.

50. Lovatsis D, Best C, Diamond P. Short-term Uresta efficacy (SURE) study: A randomized controlled trial of the Uresta continence device. *Int Urogynecol J* 2017;28(1):147–150.

51. Bellin P, Smith J, Poll W, et al. Results of a multicenter trial of the CapSure (Re/Stor) continence shield on women with stress urinary incontinence. *Urology* 1998;51(5):697–706.

52. Brubaker L. The external urethral barrier for stress incontinence: A multicenter trial of safety and efficacy. *Obstet Gynecol* 1999;93(6):932–937.

53. Shinopulos NM, Dann JA, Smith JJ III. Patient selection and education for use of the CapSure (Re/Stor) continence shield. *Urol Nurs* 1999;19(2):135–140.

54. Sand PK, Staskin D, Miller J, et al. Effect of a urinary control insert on quality of life in incontinent women. *Int Urogynecol J* 1999;10(2):100–105.

55. Staskin D, Bavendam T, Miller J, et al. Effectiveness of a urinary control insert in the management of stress urinary incontinence: Early results of a multicenter study. *Urology* 1996;47(5):629–636.

56. Miller JL, Bavendam T. Treatment with the Reliance urinary control insert: One-year experience. *J Endourol* 1996;10(3):287–292.

57. Dunn M, Brandt D, Nygaard I. Treatment of exercise incontinence with a urethral insert: A pilot study in women. *Phys Sportsmed* 2002;30(1):45–48.

58. Sirls LT, Foote JE, Kaufman JM, et al. Long-term results of the FemSoft urethral insert for the management of female stress urinary incontinence. *Int Urogynecol J Pelvic Floor Dysfunct* 2002;13(2):88–95.

59. Klarskov N, Cerneus D, Sawyer W, et al. The effect of single oral doses of duloxetine, reboxetine, and midodrine on the urethral pressure in healthy female subjects, using urethral pressure reflectometry. *Neurourol Urodyn* 2018;37(1):244–249.

60. Mizutani H, Sakakibara F, Komuro M, et al. TAS-303, a novel selective norepinephrine reuptake inhibitor that increases urethral pressure in rats, indicating its potential as a therapeutic agent for stress urinary incontinence. *J Pharmacol Exp Ther* 2018;366(2):322–331.

61. Dmochowski RR, Miklos JR, Norton PA, et al. Duloxetine versus placebo for the treatment of North American women with stress urinary incontinence. *J Urol* 2003;170(4 Pt 1):1259–1263.

62. Hagovska M, Svihra J, Breza J, et al. A randomized, intervention parallel multicentre study to evaluate duloxetine and innovative pelvic floor muscle training in women with uncomplicated stress urinary incontinence—The DULOXING study. *Int Urogynecol J* 2021;32(1):193–201.

63. Kelly HA. Incontinence of urine in women. *Urol Cutaneus Rev* 1913;17:291–293.

64. Kennedy WT. Incontinence of urine in the female, the urethral sphincter mechanism, damage of function, and restoration of control. *Am J Obstet Gynecol* 1937;34(4):576–589.

65. Thaweekul Y, Bunyavejchevin S, Wisawasukmongchol W, et al. Long term results of anterior colporrhaphy with Kelly plication for the treatment of stress urinary incontinence. *J Med Assoc Thai* 2004;87(4):357–360.

66. Parnell JP, Marshall VF, Darracott Vaughan E. Primary management of urinary stress incontinence by the Marshall-Marchetti-Krantz vesicourethropexy. *J Urology* 1982;127(4):679–682.

67. Marshall VF, Marchetti AA, Krantz KE. The correction of stress incontinence by simple vesicourethral suspension. *Surg Gynecol Obstet* 1949;88(4):509–518.

68. Mainprize TC, Drutz HP. The Marshall-Marchetti-Krantz procedure: A critical review. *Obstet Gynecol Surv* 1988;43(12):724–729.

69. McCrery RJ, Thompson PK. Outcomes of urethropexy added to paravaginal defect repair: A randomized trial of burch versus Marshall-Marchetti-Krantz. *J Pelvic Med Surg* 2005;11(3):137–143.

70. Burch JC. Urethrovaginal fixation to Cooper's ligament for correction of stress incontinence, cystocele, and prolapse. *Am J Obstet Gynecol* 1961;81(2):281–290.

71. Lapitan MCM, Cody JD, Grant A. Open retropubic colposuspension for urinary incontinence in women. *Cochrane Database Syst Rev* 2005;(3):CD002912.

72. Brubaker L, Richter HE, Norton PA, et al. 5-Year continence rates, satisfaction and adverse events of Burch urethropexy and fascial sling surgery for urinary incontinence. *J Urol* 2012;187(4):1324–1330.

73. Albo ME, Richter HE, Brubaker L, et al. Burch colposuspension versus fascial sling to reduce urinary stress incontinence. *N Engl J Med* 2007;356(21):2143–2155.

74. Pereyra AJ. A simplified surgical procedure for the correction of stress incontinence in women. *West J Surg Obstet Gynecol* 1959;67(4):223–228.

75. Glazener C, Cooper K. Bladder neck needle suspension for urinary incontinence in women. *Cochrane Database Syst Rev* 2017;7(7):CD003636.

76. Schulz JA, Nager CW, Stanton SL, et al. Bulking agents for stress urinary incontinence: Short-term results and complications in a randomized comparison of periurethral and transurethral injections. *Int Urogynecol J Pelvic Floor Dysfunct* 2004;15(4):261–265.

77. Maher CF, O'Reilly BA, Dwyer PL, et al. Pubovaginal sling versus transurethral Macroplastique for stress urinary incontinence and intrinsic sphincter deficiency: A prospective randomised controlled trial. *BJOG* 2005;112(6):797–801.

78. Hussain SM, Bray R. Urethral bulking agents for female stress urinary incontinence. *Neurourol Urodyn* 2019;38(3):887–892.

79. Herschorn S, Radomski SB. Collagen injections for genuine stress urinary incontinence: Patient selection and durability. *Int Urogynecol J Pelvic Floor Dysfunct* 1997;8(1):18–24.

80. Kirchin V, Page T, Keegan PE, et al. Urethral injection therapy for urinary incontinence in women. *Cochrane Database Syst Rev* 2017;(2):CD003881.

81. Lai HH, Hurtado EA, Appell RA. Large urethral prolapse formation after calcium hydroxylapatite (Coaptite) injection. *Int Urogynecol J Pelvic Floor Dysfunct* 2008;19(9):1315–1317.

82. Mayer RD, Dmochowski RR, Appell RA, et al. Multicenter prospective randomized 52-week trial of calcium hydroxylapatite versus bovine dermal collagen for treatment of stress urinary incontinence. *Urology* 2007;69(5):876–880.

83. Crites MA, Ghoniem GM. Bladder mass "collagenoma." *Int Urogynecol J* 2011;22(5):621–623.

84. Goebel R. Zur operativen beseitigung der angelborenen incontinenz vesicae. *Ztsch F Gynak U Urol* 1910;2:187–190.

85. Frangenheim P. Zur operativen Behandlung der Inkontinenz der männlichen Harnröhre. *Verh Dtsch Ges Chir* 1914;43:149–154.

86. Bent AE. Sling and bulking agent placement procedures. *Rev Urol* 2004;6(suppl 5):S26–S46.

87. Ridley JH. Appraisal of the Goebell-Frangenheim-Stoeckel sling procedure. *Am J Obstet Gynecol* 1966;95(5):714–721.

88. Aldridge AH. Transplantation of fascia for relief of urinary stress incontinence. *Am J Obstet Gynecol* 1942;44(3):398–411.

89. Rogo-Gupta L, Litwin MS, Saigal CS, et al. Trends in the surgical management of stress urinary incontinence among female Medicare beneficiaries, 2002-2007. *Urology* 2013;82(1):38–42.

90. Peng M, Sussman RD, Escobar C, et al. Rectus fascia versus fascia lata for autologous fascial pubovaginal sling: A single-center comparison of perioperative and functional outcomes. *Female Pelvic Med Reconstr Surg* 2020;26(8):493–497.

91. Ulmsten U, Petros P. Intravaginal slingplasty (IVS): An ambulatory surgical procedure for treatment of female urinary incontinence. *Scand J Urol Nephrol* 1995;29(1):75–82.

92. Richter HE, Albo ME, Zyczynski HM, et al. Retropubic versus transobturator midurethral slings for stress incontinence. *New Engl J Med* 2010;362(22):2066–2076.

93. Basok EK, Yildirim A, Atsu N, et al. Cadaveric fascia lata versus intravaginal slingplasty for the pubovaginal sling: Surgical outcome, overall success and patient satisfaction rates. *Urol Int* 2008;80(1):46–51.

94. Abdel-Fattah M, Barrington JW, Arunkalaivanan AS. Pelvicol pubovaginal sling versus tension-free vaginal tape for treatment of urodynamic stress incontinence. *Eur Urol* 2004;46(5):629–635.

95. Smith A, Daneshgari F, Dmochowski R. Surgery for urinary incontinence in women. In: Abrahms P, Cordozo L, Koury S, et al, eds. *Third consultation on incontinence.* Paris: Health Publication, 2005:1216.

96. Kobashi KC, Albo ME, Dmochowski RR, et al. Surgical treatment of female stress urinary incontinence: AUA/SUFU guideline. *J Urol* 2017;198(4):875–883.

97. Delorme E. Transobturator urethral suspension: Mini-invasive procedure in the treatment of stress urinary incontinence in women. *Prog Urol* 2001;11(6):1306–1313.

98. Kenton K, Stoddard AM, Zyczynski H, et al. 5-Year longitudinal followup after retropubic and transobturator mid urethral slings. *J Urol* 2015;193(1):203–210.

99. ClinicalTrials.gov. Retropubic vs. single-incision mid-urethral sling for stress urinary incontinence. Accessed October 15, 2020. https://ClinicalTrials.gov/show/NCT03520114

100. Erickson T, Roovers J-P, Gheiler E, et al. A multicenter prospective study evaluating efficacy and safety of a single-incision sling procedure for stress urinary incontinence. *J Minim Invasive Gynecol* 2021;28(1):93–99.

101. White AB, Kahn BS, Gonzalez RR, et al. Prospective study of a single-incision sling versus a transobturator sling in women with stress urinary incontinence: 3-Year results. *Am J Obstet Gynecol* 2020;223(4):545.e1–545.e11.

CHAPTER 24

CYSTOURETHROSCOPY FOR GYNECOLOGISTS

Debjyoti Karmakar • Peter L. Dwyer

Introduction

The techniques for endoscopic evaluation of pelvic organs include laparoscopy, hysteroscopy, cystourethroscopy, and proctocolonoscopy and are essential in evaluating and treating pelvic disorders. Good skills and knowledge of cystourethroscopy and lower urinary tract conditions are critical to all surgeons operating in the pelvis. Although gynecologists were at the forefront of developing cystoscopy with Kelly and Hunner and urethroscopy with Jack Robertson, training in cystoscopy was neglected in gynecology in the 20th century despite being a safe and straightforward procedure. The proximity of the urinary tract to the genital tract and overlap of urogenital conditions and symptoms makes evaluation of both frequently necessary. Gynecologic surgery can result in urinary injuries which are frequently undiagnosed; 70% of ureteric injuries and 30% of bladder injuries are undetected at the time of hysterectomy without cystoscopic assessment.[1]

This chapter describes the technique of cystourethroscopy, the equipment used, indications for, and normal and abnormal lower urinary tract findings frequently found. The terms *cystourethroscope* and *cystoscope* are interchangeable; however, both the bladder and urethra need careful assessment often by different scopes or abnormalities and injuries will be missed. We are using the term *cystourethroscope/cystourethroscopy* throughout this chapter.

THE PROCEDURE AND THE EQUIPMENT

Cystourethroscopy can be done as an outpatient procedure without sedation or general anesthesia for most indications (see following text).

The components of setup include the following:

- A light source
- An endoscopic video system/tower
- A suspending stand for a sterile water bag and related tubing
- A cystourethroscope

The comprising parts are the following:

The sheath: The outermost rigid part protects the interchangeable fragile telescopes. It acts as the conduit for distending media (irrigation) and a channel for instruments. They can vary in size from pediatric (#8 to #12 French) to adult from #17 French to larger caliber for operating devices.

A regular cystoscopic sheath has a fenestrated tip to allow completion of the bladder visualization with 30- and 70-degree scopes.

Urethroscope sheaths (Sachse sheath) are flush at the distal end with no fenestration to allow distention and visualization of the urethral walls important in detecting urethral diverticulum orifices and other pathology (Fig. 24.1).

The obturator is used to introduce the sheath providing a smooth tip for insertion.

The bridge serves as a connection between the scope and the sheath with side arms for instrument placement (Fig. 24.2A,B). It is a water-tight attachment. Some bridges have specialized functions such as providing a channel for biopsy forceps or the Albarran bridge with a defector to allow more accurate ureteric stent placement (Fig. 24.2C,D).

The telescopes carry the illuminating system, extending from the eyepiece to the tip, which provides 70-, 30-, and 0-degree views (Fig. 24.3). The illuminating system uses optical fiber. The 70-degree lens is best for operative cystoscopy and inspection of anterolateral bladder walls and is useful in seeing the ureteric orifices, especially after urethral suspensions or prolapse surgery. The 0-degree scope is used for a complete examination of the urethra.

Rigid or Flexible Scopes

Rigid scopes can be inserted painlessly in women using local anesthetic lubricant and have another channel to insert needles or biopsy forceps for outpatient procedures such as Botox injections. General anesthesia is required when cystoscopy is expected to be painful, for example,

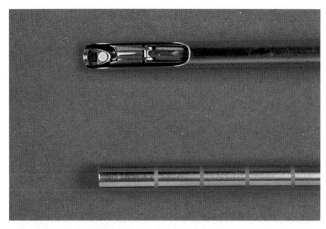

FIGURE 24.1 Urethroscope sheaths. Upper image is a 70 degree cystoscope with a fenestrated introducer. Lower image is a 0 degree urethroscope with a sheath (Sachse sheath) cut flush to distal end with no fenestration so as to allow urethral distension and visualization of urethral walls.

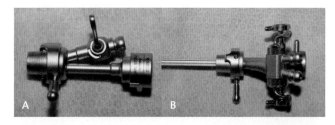

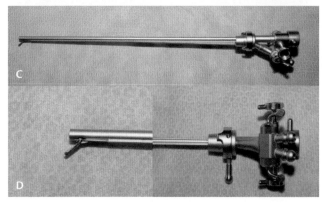

FIGURE 24.2 Cystoscopic bridges. **A,B:** Bridges with single channel (**A**) and dual channels (**B**). **C,D:** Cystoscopic sheath with Albarran lever (**C**) and Albarran bridge (**D**).

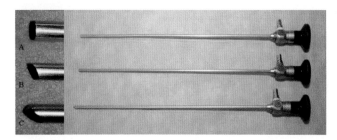

FIGURE 24.3 Cystoscope lenses: 0 degree (**A**), 30 degrees (**B**), 70 degrees (**C**).

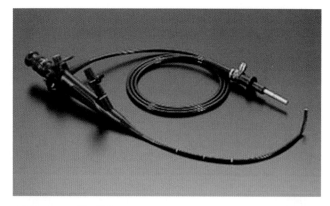

FIGURE 24.4 Flexible cystoscope.

cystodistention in interstitial cystitis (IC), procedures with biopsy or cautery, or when more careful evaluation bladder and vagina for urinary fistulas is needed.

Flexible scopes give excellent 360-degree views of both the bladder and the urethra and are convenient for clinicians and comfortable for patients (Fig. 24.4).

Rigid cystoscopy can be performed with 70-, 30-, or 0-degree scopes

- A 70- or 30-degree lens can be used to carefully evaluate bladder abnormalities, the bladder mucosa for infection or neoplastic change, and the bladder wall for trabeculation and diverticulum. Bladder trabeculation (Fig. 24.5) is muscular hypertrophy of the bladder wall and can be secondary to detrusor overactivity, urethral obstruction, or the ageing process. The ureteric orifices are sited at the most lateral point of the interureteric bar (interureteric ridge) and upper trigone. Their patency can be confirmed by the efflux of urine, which can be enhanced with intravenous dyes such as indigo

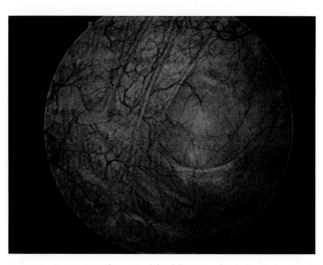

FIGURE 24.5 Moderate bladder trabeculation with diverticulum.

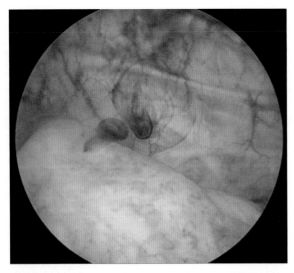

FIGURE 24.6 Indigo carmine efflux confirming right ureteric patency.

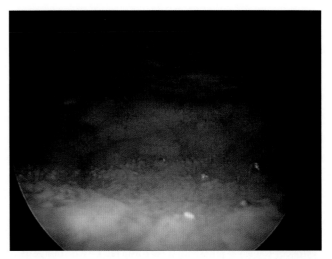

FIGURE 24.7 Squamous metaplasia of the trigone. Common finding and histologic analysis shows stratified squamous epithelium on a background of normal transitional cell mucosa.

carmine (Fig. 24.6) or oral agents such as vitamin B complex and phenazopyridine (Pyridium). Another alternative is to fill the bladder retrogradely with 50% dextrose which creates a difference of specific gravity from urine and any efflux is clearly visualized. We use all of these methods in our unit depending on the availability and surgeon preference.

- The air bubble identifies the dome. Once the ureteric orifices are identified, the trigone is seen between the interureteric bar (interureteric ridge) and bladder neck. Pearly gray-white epithelial patches with irregular borders called squamous metaplasia (Fig. 24.7) are frequently present in the urethra and the trigone. It is the stratified squamous epithelium, a normal variant not needing a biopsy. The epithelium changes from keratinized squamous epithelium at the distal urethra to non-keratinized squamous epithelium to pseudostratified with urethral glands to transitional mucosa in the bladder.

- Cystoscopy is performed in the sitting, lithotomy or supine position with general, regional, or local anesthesia with a size #17 French sheath or a #21 French sheath with an operating channel for the passage of ureteral guidewires, stents, biopsy forceps and scissors (Fig. 24.8), and electrosurgical instruments (Fig. 24.9).

Distention Media

- Can be conductive or nonconductive fluids or gases (carbon dioxide)
- Nonconductive fluids (e.g., glycine and water) should be used when electrocautery is required. Because the risk of fluid absorption is low in diagnostic procedures, we prefer glycine as visualization is better in the presence of active bleeding and hemolysis.
- Monitoring fluid absorption to avoid volume overload and possible hyponatremia is necessary when an operative procedure is performed, such as resecting a bladder tumor.

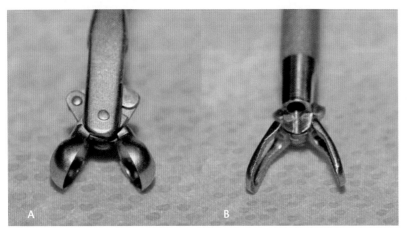

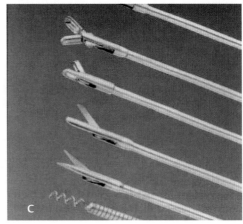

FIGURE 24.8 **A–C:** Cystoscopic instruments including biopsy forceps.

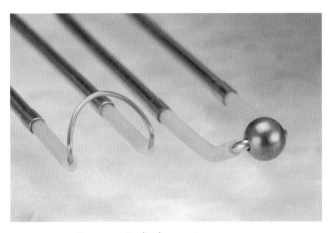

FIGURE 24.9 Cystoscopic diathermy instruments.

PROCEDURE

The patient is positioned in the sitting or dorsal lithotomy position with 1% lignocaine (lidocaine), such as Instillagel (CliniMed Ltd, High Wycombe, United Kingdom), instilled in the urethra for anesthesia and lubrication.

The cystourethroscope is placed into the urethra under direct vision with the scope facing anteriorly to minimize urethral trauma. The urethra should be assessed with a 0-degree scope for any abnormalities, such as diverticulum or tumors, and function (Video 24.1).

Prophylactic oral antibiotics are not routinely recommended except for women at higher risk of urinary tract infection (UTI) with a history of recurrent infection or women with functional or anatomical urinary tract abnormalities. Oral phenazopyridine (Pyridium) preprocedure or postprocedure urinary alkalizer like Ural (Amcal Pharmacy) can alleviate postprocedure dysuria with or without UTI.

INDICATIONS FOR CYSTOURETHROSCOPY IN UROGYNECOLOGY

The broad categories of indications for gynecologists are the following:

1. Urinary tract injury
2. Irritative bladder symptoms, including interstitial cystitis (IC)/bladder pain syndrome
3. Exclude urinary tract cancer
4. Urinary fistula
5. Congenital abnormalities of the urinary tract and anatomical lesions
6. Evaluation of recurrent UTIs
7. Evaluation of voiding difficulty
8. Evaluation of macroscopic/microscopic hematuria
9. Injection of therapeutic agents—bulking agents, botulinum toxin
10. Cystoscopy-guided suprapubic catheter placement
11. Ureteral stent placement

Urinary Tract Injury

Early detection of injury to the ureter, bladder, or urethra intraoperatively will allow any injury to be repaired without significant sequelae such as urinary fistulas or renal failure secondary to ureteric obstruction. Intraoperative detection of injury can be performed by inspecting the urinary tract for injury or urine leakage during and after surgery but is more accurately assessed by endoscopic inspection of the bladder for injury and the ureters for patency immediately after surgery.

Gynecologic surgery accounts for over three-quarters of iatrogenic urinary tract injuries.[1] Presently, only 1 in 10 ureteral injuries and 1 in 3 bladder injuries are detected at the time of surgery without intraoperative cystoscopy.[2] The risk of injury varies with the procedure performed but is common in urogynecology procedures for stress incontinence and prolapse. Gilmour et al.[1] found the ureteric injury rate per 1,000 operations for vaginal hysterectomy was 0.2, subtotal abdominal hysterectomy was 0.6, total abdominal hysterectomy was 1.3, and laparoscopic hysterectomy was 7.8. The most typical cause of ureteric damage during laparoscopic surgery is electrocoagulation, but injury from clamping, misplaced sutures, and trocar entry has been reported. In a prospective study with routine cystoscopy after hysterectomy, Vakili et al.[3] reported a urinary tract injury rate between 4% and 5% in 471 women with a bladder and ureteral injury rate of 3.6% and 1.7%. Ibeanu et al.[4] reported a 2.9% bladder and 1.8% ureteral injury rate in 839 women. The majority of ureteric injuries were only diagnosed on cystoscopy and missed at the time of surgery.[1,5] Cystourethroscopy can identify the presence of trauma to the bladder either by direct vision or by the leakage of fluid to the abdomen/vagina during cystodistention. The cause of the trauma to the bladder (suture/cystotomy/trocar injury) and proximity to ureteric orifices, urethra, and trigone should be documented.

The incidence of bladder perforation at the insertion of a midurethral sling is 1% to 20%. Risk factors are previous Cesarean section and Burch colposuspension, body mass index less than 30 kg/m², rectocele, inexperienced surgeon, and local anesthesia.[6] Cystoscopy is a routine part of tension-free vaginal tape procedures. The common areas for perforation are the lateral corner and dome of the bladder and best seen using a 70-degree cystourethroscope at 11 and 1 o'clock. The risk of bladder injury is less with the transobturator midurethral sling, but urethral perforation is higher, and in our opinion, cystourethroscopy should be performed routinely (Fig. 24.10). Pelvic reconstructive surgery for pelvic organ prolapse (POP) and stress incontinence and major vaginal/abdominal/laparoscopic gynecologic (such as hysterectomy, adnexectomy) surgery carry an inherent risk of urinary tract injury.[1,5,7] The risk of ligation has significantly increased in recent years with pelvic mesh usage, for example, sacrocolpopexy and vaginal repair

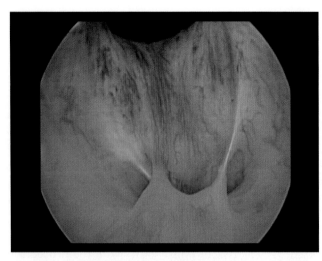

FIGURE 24.10 Urethroscopy of a urethrovaginal fistula caused by inadvertent injury during removal of a midurethral sling.

with mesh and midurethral slings.[8] A frequently asked question by lawyers is whether early diagnosis can prevent the consequences of urinary tract injury (fistula, nonfunctioning kidney)? The answer is often yes.[2]

The rate of missed diagnoses of clinically significant urinary injuries in a systematic review of 17 retrospective studies of women who underwent benign gynecologic surgery with routine intraoperative use of cystoscopy was 0.8 per 1,000 procedures.[9] Devascularization or thermal injuries may not be identifiable by cystoscopy with ischemic necrosis causing a fistula typically occur 10 to 14 days later. Cystourethroscopy and imaging should be performed if bladder symptoms or oliguria and back pain occur in the early postoperative phase to exclude ureteric obstruction, or in the longer term, de novo bladder symptoms can be caused by bladder calculus, an overlooked suture or mesh in the bladder or cancer.[2]

After pelvic floor reconstructive surgery, institutions with a routine cystoscopy policy are likely to have lower rates of urologic injuries. A retrospective cohort study of 2,822 women undergoing hysterectomy for benign indications noted urologic injury rates dropping from 2.6% to 1.8% and delayed urologic injury rates going down from 0.7% to 0.1%, respectively, in the postpolicy group versus the prepolicy group.[10,11]

In a study of Burch colposuspension[7] with routine intraoperative cystoscopy in 925 open colposuspensions, there was one bladder injury detected intraoperatively and two postoperatively. Out of 178 laparoscopic colposuspensions, there were three bladder injuries seen intraoperatively and none postoperatively. There were no cases of ureteric injury in open cases. However, there were three ureteric injuries, two detected intraoperatively, and one postoperatively in the laparoscopic group.

Irritative Bladder Symptoms, including Interstitial Cystitis/Bladder Pain Syndrome

Overactive bladder (OAB) is defined as frequency, urgency, and nocturia with (wet OAB) or without incontinence (dry OAB). Cystoscopy is indicated to exclude lower urinary tract pathology, usually where standard evaluation and first-line pharmacotherapy has not cured the symptoms.[12] The bladder pain syndrome (BPS) is a chronic inflammatory disorder defined by frequency, urgency, and bladder pain relieved by micturition, where no other cause is found. Some experts believe that IC is a more severe form of this bladder disease.[12,13]

Classical cystoscopic appearances of IC are the appearance of cascading petechial hemorrhage seen in 9 out of 10 women with IC/PBS[12,13] following cystodistention with bladder emptying under cystoscopic vision. Less frequently, there are submucosal ecchymoses, mucosal tearing, and Hunner ulcers or whitish patches (5%) (Fig. 24.11), which are tears in the bladder mucosa following cystodistention usually surrounded by hemorrhagic mucosa that bleeds on bladder emptying.[14] Maximum cystoscopic capacity (bladder capacity under anesthesia) should be recorded. The biopsy may exclude other pathologies such as carcinoma in situ, which can have a similar appearance (see Video 24.1). There is no diagnostic histologic picture of IC. However, epithelial ulceration, submucosal oedema and inflammation, and increased submucosal and detrusor mast cell number and activation are seen more often present in severe IC.[14] Cystodistention itself can have a therapeutic benefit (usually transient up to 6 months) in up to 20% to 30% of women with severe OAB/IC.[15]

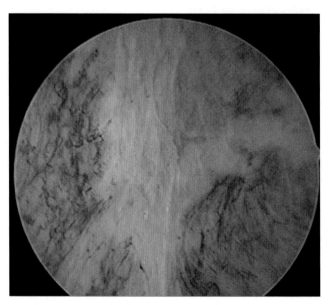

FIGURE 24.11 Hunner ulcer.

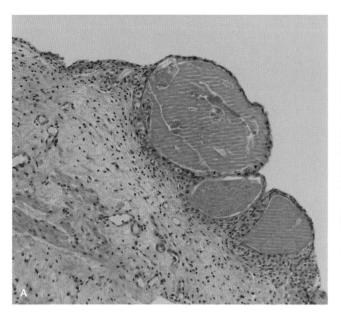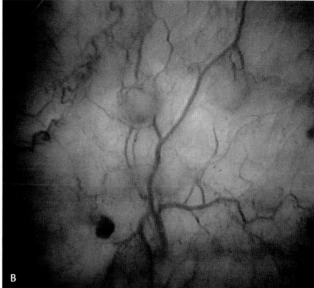

FIGURE 24.12 Cystitis cystica: histology (**A**) and cystoscopic appearance (**B**).

Cystitis cystica is a benign condition where cystic spaces develop within von Brunn nests in the lamina propria form and is frequently seen in women with recurrent UTI (Fig. 24.12). Cystoscopically, the appearance is of rounded clear or yellow 1- to 5-mm submucosal cysts most frequently located in the trigone or anterior bladder wall. Histologically, these are spaces lined by urothelium or cuboidal cells. *Cystitis glandularis* is the histologic term given when columnar cells are lining the spaces within von Brunn nests are of the intestinal type relating to goblet cells and mucin production. The diffuse form is called intestinal metaplasia and is often associated with chronic calculi or chronic catheterization; if extensive, it is a risk factor for adenocarcinoma.

Exclusion of Urinary Tract Cancer

Urinary tract cancer frequently presents with urinary symptoms of bleeding, recurrent infection, and bladder or vaginal pain. Gross hematuria is the presenting symptom in up to 90% of patients with bladder cancer, and therefore, women with gross hematuria are best evaluated by urologists.[16,17] The positive predictive value for cancer associated with asymptomatic microhematuria (defined by American Urological Association as 3 or more red blood cells per high power field on microscopic evaluation of single, properly collected urine specimen) is only 0% to 2%.[16,17] There is an increased incidence of cancer in women with asymptomatic microhematuria over 40 years, smoking (past or current), history of pelvic irradiation/cyclophosphamide use, and exposure to certain dyes and benzenes.[17] In cases of asymptomatic microhematuria in low-risk women (i.e., younger than 40 years), renal ultrasound and urine

cytology may be sufficient testing and cystourethroscopy may be reserved if symptoms arise.

Urologists usually treat urinary tract cancer, so early diagnosis and referral is appropriate. However, many bladder or urethral cancers have minimal symptoms, so a high index of suspicion is needed. Urogynecologists must be aware of the various cystoscopic appearances of transitional cell and invasive carcinoma of the bladder and urethra (Figs. 24.13 and 24.14). Malignancies have been commonly reported in urethral and bladder diverticulum, so careful inspection is needed. Carcinoma in situ may proceed or be associated with invasive cancer and has an appearance similar to a severe infection or IC. Hence, a biopsy is necessary

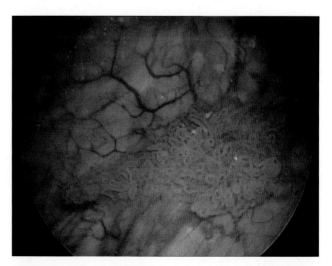

FIGURE 24.13 Superficial noninvasive grade 1 papillary transitional cell carcinoma found on routine cystoscopy following vaginal repair.

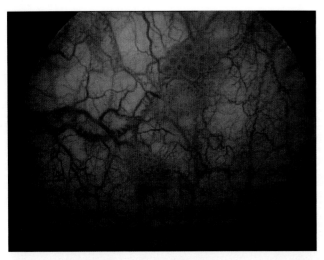

FIGURE 24.14 Papillary and solid muscle-invasive poorly differentiated bladder tumor.

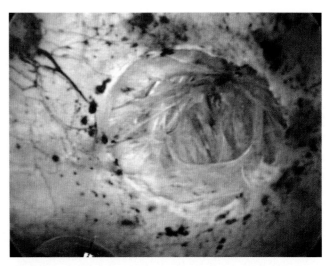

FIGURE 24.16 Detrusor defect due to deep biopsy.

when doubt exists. The histologic appearance of carcinoma in situ is epithelial cells with anaplastic features without invasion of the basement membrane. It appears at cystoscopy as a red velvety patch or a granular lesion of the bladder wall, often associated with the papillary or nodular tumor (Video 24.2). Urine cytology is very accurate in diagnosing high-grade carcinoma (grade 3) and carcinoma in situ but is less helpful in low-grade transitional cell carcinoma and should be done with a biopsy in suspicious cases. Radiation cystitis has a typical appearance of abnormal blood vessels and telangiectasia often present postpelvic irradiation even when symptoms are minor (Fig. 24.15).

Biopsies can be taken using biopsy forceps with either rigid or flexible scopes. The tumor is grasped at its base and removed in a single motion. The biopsy site if bleeding can be cauterized using a flexible electrode or rollerball diathermy. Large tumors require resection

with a resectoscope. Biopsies are frequently deep into the muscular bladder wall, so catheter drainage overnight is wise to avoid perforation, urine leakage, and urinoma formation (Fig. 24.16). If cancer is suspected, have a urologist present at the time of the cystoscopy or take accurate photographs of the tumor endoscopically for a referral.

Urinary Fistula

Cystourethroscopy with vaginal examination under anesthesia is frequently needed for accurate diagnosis and to plan treatment for women with vesicovaginal fistulas (VVF) and urethrovaginal fistulas (see Fig. 24.10).[7] Cystourethroscopy provides information on size, number and location of the fistulas, ureteric location and patency, healing, and presence of infection of the fistula so that surgical management and timing can be decided. Also, on examination under anaesthesia (EUA), accessibility for vaginal or abdominal closure and repair of the VVF can be assessed. The vaginal approach has lower morbidity and cost and is appropriate in majority of cases of fistulas of the bladder and urethra, even when the fistula is at the vaginal vault which is well supported. The VVF can be assessed with good exposure from a Brantley Scott retractor (Lone Star Medical Products Inc.) and downward traction on an inflated catheter placed through fistula and closed with a Latzko procedure.

Other Pathology

Bladder diverticulum are common, frequently associated with bladder trabeculation and may cause incomplete voiding but are usually asymptomatic (Fig. 24.17). This outpouching of the bladder wall can lead to recurrent UTI by acting as a reservoir for bacterial colonization.[18] A urethral diverticulum (Fig. 24.18) may cause

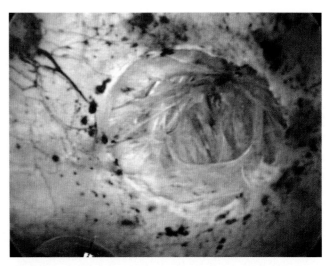

FIGURE 24.15 Radiation cystitis.

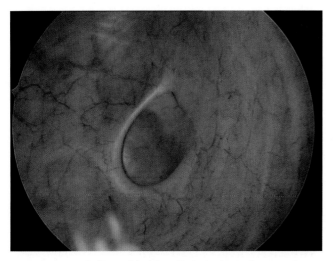

FIGURE 24.17 Solitary bladder diverticulum; frequently asymptomatic but can predispose to urinary stasis and infection.

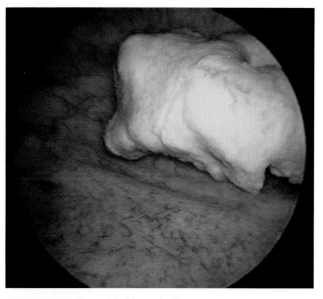

FIGURE 24.19 Large bladder calculus.

recurrent UTIs, dyspareunia, and voiding difficulty/postvoid dribble with or without a suburethral anterior vaginal lump.[19] A diagnostic urethral orifice can frequently be seen on careful inspection using a 0-degree urethroscope on urethral distention (see Chapter 35).

Congenital malformations such as ectopic implantation of the ureter into the urethra, Gartner duct cysts, double ureters, ureteroceles, and congenital fistulas can cause incontinence and urinary symptoms.[20]

Recurrent Urinary Tract Infections

Recurrent UTI is defined as more than three culture-proven UTIs over 1 year or more than two infections within 6 months. Cystourethroscopy is indicated in women with recurrent UTI to identify possible etiologic factors such as calculus (Fig. 24.19), foreign body (suture or mesh; Figs. 24.20 and 24.21), urethral obstruction, fistula, cancer, urethral diverticula, cystocele, and other anatomical abnormalities of the lower urinary tract.[21]

Voiding Difficulty

Cystourethroscopy can detect bladder and urethral anatomical causes for impaired bladder emptying including urethral obstruction from urethral slings and suspensions strictures, tumors, and diverticula and bladder pathology such as diverticulum and ureteroceles (Fig. 24.22).[22]

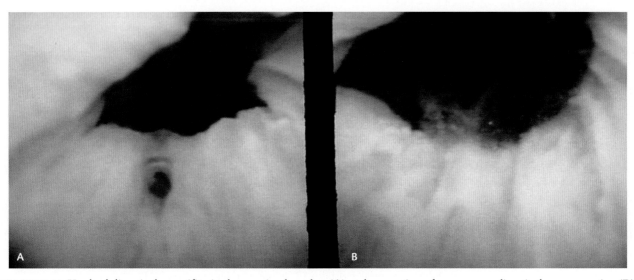

FIGURE 24.18 Urethral diverticulum orifice in the proximal urethra (**A**) and expression of pus seen on diverticular compression (**B**).

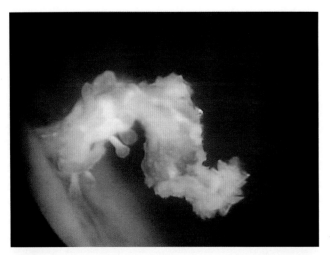

FIGURE 24.20 Intravesical bladder suture with calcification in a woman following Burch colposuspension using Ethibond braided suture.

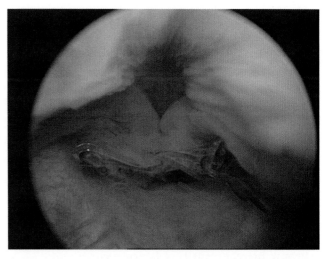

FIGURE 24.21 Misplacement of a transobturator midurethral sling in a woman presenting with voiding dysfunction and recurrent UTI 6 months postoperatively.

Injection of Therapeutic Agents—Bulking Agents, Botulinum Toxin

Urethral bulking agents (Macroplastique, Collagen, Bulkamid) can be injected under urethroscopic guidance either periurethrally or transurethrally to improve urethral coaptation to treat urinary stress incontinence. Success rates have been reported as high as 80%, although the beneficial effect decreases significantly with time and reinjection is often necessary.[23]

A systematic review of the therapeutic efficacy and adverse events of onabotulinumtoxinA for OAB by Mangera et al.[24] showed that Botox improves daily frequency, urgency, and urinary incontinence. However, UTI and urinary retention requiring intermittent self-catheterization are possible risks.[10,24] The toxin is injected at several sites (10 to 30) within the bladder

excluding the trigone area, using a rigid or flexible cystoscope under general or local anesthesia. Most clinicians prefer to use local anesthetic with either a rigid or flexible cystoscope.

Cystoscopy-Guided Suprapubic Catheter Placement

Suprapubic catheters are at times more convenient for patients and enable the accurate assessment of postvoid residual volumes without urethral catheter removal. Suprapubic catheters can be inserted under cystoscopic guidance to allow more precise placement. Long-term suprapubic catheters are mostly reserved for women with chronic retention of the neurologic origin or in the very debilitated elderly when urethral catheters are problematic.

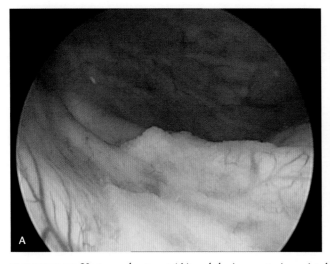

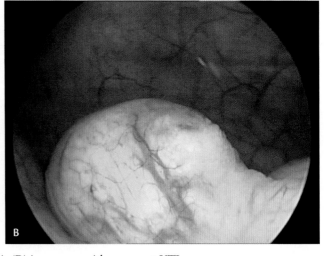

FIGURE 24.22 Ureterocele at rest (**A**) and during ureteric peristalsis (**B**) in woman with recurrent UTI.

Ureteral Stent Placement

This may be done preemptively where complex pelvic surgery is being undertaken where a high risk of ureteric injury is anticipated (Video 24.3) including procedures for severe endometriosis, difficult hysterectomy, and removal of prolapse mesh prosthesis. Urogynecologists should be able to pass a ureteric catheter to exclude ureteric occlusion with the suture or injury when ureteric patency cannot be confirmed.

CONTRAINDICATIONS

Any UTI should be treated before cystoscopy if possible as ascending infection and pyelonephritis can occur.[25] Chronic or recurrent UTI is not a contraindication. Complete urethral occlusion with advanced stricture is not a contraindication but can cause difficulties because the urethra will need to be dilated with urethral dilators and anesthetic gel.

COMPLICATIONS

After cystoscopy, the incidence of UTI is common (2% to 10%), but severe sepsis is rare.[25] Other complications include urethral and bladder trauma, including perforation, but it is very unusual. Small mucosal trauma can be managed by observation, electrocautery, or catheterization. Patients should be advised that if they experience severe pain, fresh and significant bleeding, fever, flank pain, and systemic illness postprocedure, they should seek medical attention.

EDUCATION, CERTIFICATION, AND RECOMMENDATIONS

In the past, the use of cystoscopy by gynecologists has been controversial and not commonly performed. Over the last two decades, this situation has changed considerably with gynecologists increasingly performing cystourethroscopy not only as part of a stress incontinence procedure but also in routine pelvic surgery to diagnose urinary tract injury.

The American College of Obstetricians and Gynecologists[26] (ACOG) Committee Opinion No. 372 in 2007 states that "perhaps the most important indications for cystourethroscopy are to rule out cystotomy and intravesical or intraurethral suture or mesh placement and to verify bilateral ureteral patency during or after specific gynecologic surgical procedures. The procedures with a relatively high risk for these complications (at least 1% to 2%) may benefit from cystourethroscopy." In 2013 ACOG Committee Opinion states that cystoscopy is an essential diagnostic and therapeutic tool.[27] Practicing

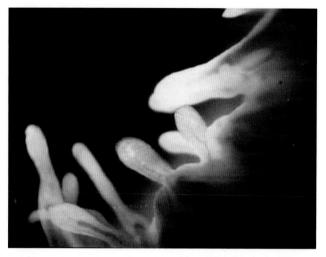

FIGURE 24.23 Benign polyps seen on urethroscopy of the bladder neck and a common finding in asymptomatic women.

gynecologists should become comfortable with the routine performance of the procedure and perform this intraoperatively, at least in all high-risk urinary injury cases.

Although urologic input will be necessary in some cases, we believe all gynecologists should perform cystourethroscopy expertly and be able to diagnose what they see and whether it is normal or abnormal (Fig. 24.23). There are numerous publications available for gynecologists to upgrade their knowledge.[28] Currently, cystourethroscopy training is required by all obstetrics and gynecology residency programs accredited by the Accreditation Council for Graduate Medical Education in the United States[27,29,30] and the obstetrics and gynecology training program in the United Kingdom (Royal College of Obstetricians and Gynaecologists),[17] Australia, and New Zealand (Royal Australian and New Zealand College of Obstetricians and Gynaecologists).[31] We believe colleges should continue to offer various training courses, including cadaver labs and simulation models designed to develop cystoscopy skills.

CONCLUSION

Cystourethroscopy is now an established tool in the armament of gynecologists.

Based on available literature and our experience, we recommend universal cystoscopy be performed at the time of all pelvic organ reconstructive operations where the urinary tract is at risk. This adds only a few minutes to the procedure and very little morbidity. As gynecologists perform cystourethroscopy more frequently, they become more skilled in its use and more familiar with normal and abnormal bladder conditions.

References

1. Gilmour DT, Das S, Flowerdew G. Rates of urinary tract injury from gynecologic surgery and the role of intraoperative cystoscopy. *Obstet Gynecol* 2006;107(6):1366–1372.

2. Dwyer PL. Urinary tract injury: Medical negligence or unavoidable complication? *Int Urogynecol J* 2010;21(8):903–910.

3. Vakili B, Chesson RR, Kyle BL, et al. The incidence of urinary tract injury during hysterectomy: A prospective analysis based on universal cystoscopy. *Am J Obstet Gynecol* 2005;192(5):1599–1604.

4. Ibeanu OA, Chesson RR, Echols KT, et al. Urinary tract injury during hysterectomy based on universal cystoscopy. *Obstet Gynecol* 2009;113(1):6–10.

5. Dwyer PL. In the footsteps of Kelly and Robertson; revival of the art of cystourethroscopy in gynecology. *Int Urogynecol J Pelvic Floor Dysfunct* 2007;18(7):713–714.

6. Stav K, Dwyer PL, Rosamilia A, et al. Risk factors for trocar injury to the bladder during mid urethral sling procedures. *J Urol* 2009;182(1):174–179.

7. Dwyer P, Carey M, Rosamilia A. Suture injury to the urinary tract in urethral suspension procedures for stress incontinence. *Int Urogynecol J* 1999;10(1):15–21.

8. Karmakar D, Dwyer PL. Failure of expectations in vaginal surgery: Lack of appropriate consent, goals and expectations of surgery. *Curr Urol Rep* 2016;17(12):87.

9. Siff LN, Hill AJ, Jallad K, et al. Intraoperative evaluation of urinary tract injuries at the time of pelvic surgery: A systematic review. *Female Pelvic Med Reconstr Surg* 2020;26(11):655–663.

10. Chen J-L, Kuo H-C. Clinical application of intravesical botulinum toxin type A for overactive bladder and interstitial cystitis. *Investig Clin Urol* 2020;61(Suppl 1):S33–S42.

11. Chi AM, Curran DS, Morgan DM, et al. Universal cystoscopy after benign hysterectomy: Examining the effects of an institutional policy. *Obstet Gynecol* 2016;127(2):369.

12. Hanno PM, Landis JR, Matthews-Cook Y, et al. The diagnosis of interstitial cystitis revisited: Lessons learned from the National Institutes of Health Interstitial Cystitis Database study. *J Urol* 1999;161(2):553–557.

13. Han E, Nguyen L, Sirls L, et al. Current best practice management of interstitial cystitis/bladder pain syndrome. *Ther Adv Urol* 2018;10(7):197–211.

14. Rosamilia A, Dwyer PL. Pathophysiology of interstitial cystitis. *Curr Opin Obstet Gynecol* 2000;12(5):405–410.

15. Rosamilia A, Cann L, Scurry J, et al. Bladder microvasculature and the effects of hydrodistention in interstitial cystitis. *Urology* 2001;57(6):132.

16. Barocas DA, Boorjian SA, Alvarez RD, et al. Microhematuria: AUA/SUFU guideline. *J Urol* 2020;204(4):778–786.

17. Foon R, Elbiss H, Moran PA. Cystoscopy for gynaecologists. *Obstet Gynecol* 2006;8(2):78–85.

18. Farhi J, Dicker D, Goldman J. Giant diverticulum of the bladder simulating ovarian cyst. *Int J Gynecol Obstet* 1991;36(1):55–57.

19. Ganabathi K, Leach GE, Zimmern PE, et al. Experience with the management of urethral diverticulum in 63 women. *J Urol* 1994;152(5):1445–1452.

20. Dwyer PL, Rosamilia A. Congenital urogenital anomalies that are associated with the persistence of Gartner's duct: A review. *Am J Obstet Gynecol* 2006;195(2):354–359.

21. Nikpoor P, Dwyer PL. Recurrent urinary tract infections: Management in women. *Med Today* 2020;21(9):14–19.

22. Dmochowski RR. Bladder outlet obstruction: Etiology and evaluation. *Rev Urol* 2005;7(Suppl 6):S3–S13.

23. Maher CF, O'Reilly BA, Dwyer PL, et al. Pubovaginal sling versus transurethral Macroplastique for stress urinary incontinence and intrinsic sphincter deficiency: A prospective randomised controlled trial. *BJOG* 2005;112(6):797–801.

24. Mangera A, Apostolidis A, Andersson KE, et al. An updated systematic review and statistical comparison of standardised mean outcomes for the use of botulinum toxin in the management of lower urinary tract disorders. *Eur Urol* 2014;65(5):981–990.

25. Bavetta S, Olsha O, Fenely J. Spreading sepsis by cystoscopy. *Postgrad Med J* 1990;66(779):734–735.

26. American College of Obstetricians and Gynecologists. ACOG Committee Opinion. Number 372. July 2007. The role of cystourethroscopy in the generalist obstetrician-gynecologist practice. *Obstet Gynecol* 2007;110(1):221.

27. American College of Obstetricians and Gynecologists. *Core curriculum in obstetrics and gynecology*, 10th ed. Washington: American College of Obstetricians and Gynecologists, 2013.

28. Dwyer PL, ed. *Atlas of urogynecological endoscopy*. London: CRC Press, 2007.

29. Bowling CB, Greer WJ, Bryant SA, et al. Testing and validation of a low-cost cystoscopy teaching model: A randomized controlled trial. *Obstet Gynecol* 2010;116(1):85.

30. Hibbert ML, Salminen ER, Dainty LA, et al. Credentialing residents for intraoperative cystoscopy. *Obstet Gynecol* 2000;96(6):1014–1017.

31. Dwyer PL. Training requirements for endoscopy of the urinary tract in female pelvic medicine. In: Dwyer PL, ed. *Atlas of urogynecological endoscopy*. London: CRC Press, 2007:181–184.

CHAPTER 25

OVERACTIVE BLADDER AND URGE INCONTINENCE

Breffini Anglim • Barry A. O'Reilly

Introduction

Overactive bladder (OAB) and associated urinary incontinence (UI) affects 16.5% of the U.S. population as well as a similar percentage of European men and women and poses a significant economic burden on society through direct medical and nonmedical costs, indirect costs and intangible costs, resulting in billions of dollars of health care expenditure on a yearly basis.[1,2] OAB symptoms and urge urinary incontinence (UUI) have more profound effects on quality-of-life measures when compared to symptoms of stress urinary incontinence (SUI) because nocturia can result in significant sleep disturbance and daytime fatigue.[3]

OAB is defined by the International Continence Society (ICS) as a symptom-based condition characterized by urinary urgency, usually with urinary frequency and nocturia, with or without UUI.[4,5] Urgency is defined as the complaint of sudden, compelling desire to pass urine which is difficult to defer. Frequency is defined as the complaint that micturition occurs more frequently during waking hours than previously deemed normal by the woman. Nocturia is defined as the complaint of interruption of sleep one or more times because of the need to micturate. Each void is preceded and followed by sleep.[5] Urge incontinence is defined as the involuntary loss of urine associated urgency.[4] OAB is a symptom-based diagnosis and therefore does not require urodynamic testing or cystometry for confirmation. Self-reporting of UI using validated questionnaires, such as the International Consultation on Incontinence Questionnaire Short Form and International Consultation on Incontinence Questionnaire Female Lower Urinary Tract Symptoms Modules, allows for assessment of both frequency of UI, and perceived bother to the patient. It is important to establish the degree of bother of symptoms because self-reporting of severity of incontinence symptoms alone may not correlate with felt or expressed need for treatment.[6]

Detrusor overactivity (DO) is a urodynamic-based diagnosis characterized by involuntary detrusor contractions during filling cystometry which may be spontaneous or provoked. OAB symptoms such as urgency or urge incontinence may not always occur when DO is observed on filling cystometry, and equally, DO is not always present in women who report OAB symptoms.[7] DO is only confirmed in 44% to 69% of patients with symptoms of OAB.[8,9] Also, up to 50% of patients with DO visible on filling cystometry do not have associated urgency or urge incontinence symptoms.[10] This confirms Jarvis and Millar[11] observation that the "bladder is an unreliable witness."

The coexistence of detrusor hyperreflexia and impaired contractility (DHIC) was first described by Resnick and Yalla[12] in 1987 and was found primarily in elderly patients. This phenomenon consists of DO during the storage phase, but the emptying phase is characterized by detrusor underactivity (DU) resulting in large postvoid residuals. The contractile capabilities of the detrusor are impaired, but it is not possible to distinguish which causative factors (detrusor muscle or detrusor innervation) are compromised. The term detrusor overactivity with detrusor underactivity (DO-DU) is intended by the ICS to supersede DHIC. It is defined as urodynamic DO (on cystometry) in combination with urodynamic DU on pressure–flow studies. DU is typically seen as a low pressure, low flow, and poorly sustained detrusor contractility on urodynamic studies. In a study of urodynamics (UDS) among patients older than the age of 70 years, 6% of women were found to have DO-DU.[13] DU can be seen in combination with DO or SUI in 72% of women with DU.[14,15] Symptoms of underactive bladder may overlap with OAB symptoms including urgency, frequency, nocturia, and incontinence.[16] Treatment of DO-DU can be problematic, and the use of anticholinergics, β_3-agonist or onabotulinumtoxinA injection can pose a higher risk for urinary retention in these women due to DU during the contraction phase of emptying.[17-19] Sacral neuromodulation is considered to be an effective treatment for this patient group because it is thought to modify the afferent pathway by increasing parasympathetic activity and also by acting on the urethral and sphincter complex by triggering the guarding reflex to relax the outlet.[20,21]

OAB symptoms are frequently reported in women with pelvic organ prolapse (POP) and can occur in up to 88% of women.[22] Both OAB and POP prevalence increase with increasing age, which may explain their association.[23,24] There is some evidence that OAB symptoms improve following repair of POP due to an improvement in voiding function; however, other studies have shown de novo OAB symptoms following pelvic floor surgery.[25,26] The pathophysiology of OAB in patients with POP is poorly understood.[25] A study by Frigerio et al.[27] found age, body mass index (BMI), preoperative OAB (based on symptomatic diagnosis not urodynamic evidence of DO), suburethral sling insertion, and postoperative SUI to be independent risk factors for OAB after POP repair. Preoperative OAB and postoperative constipation were significantly associated with persistent OAB following POP surgery. De novo OAB was associated with age, postoperative SUI and voiding symptoms, and concomitant suburethral sling placement.[27] De novo OAB following surgery for pure SUI is reported to be between 5% and 18%.[28,29] It is thought that repeated surgeries at the bladder neck may disrupt the autonomic nerve supply of the bladder and cause OAB symptoms.[28]

PREVALENCE

Several population-based studies have reported on the prevalence and burden of OAB. The National Overactive Bladder Evaluation (NOBLE) program was a population-based, cross-sectional, computer-assisted, telephone interview survey undertaken in the United States. In this study, OAB was estimated to occur in 16.9% of women and 16.0% of men. The age related increase in urge incontinence was significantly higher in women than men and was reported in 19% of women and 9% of men older than the age of 44 years.[1] The epidemiology of lower urinary tract symptoms (LUTS) study was a population-based cross-sectional Internet-based survey carried out in the United States, United Kingdom, and Sweden to update the results of the NOBLE study. ICS definitions of LUTS were also used. Specific to the United States, 20,000 participants aged older than 40 years were included. It showed a prevalence of OAB symptoms at least "sometimes" in 27.2% of men and 43.1% in women. Of this group of women 38.9% were bothered "quite a bit" by their symptoms. In both men and women, prevalence increased with age.[30] The Milsom study was a population-based prevalence study carried out in France, Germany, Italy, Spain, Sweden, and the United Kingdom. A combination of telephone and direct interviews were conducted in 16,776 randomly selected men and women aged older than 40 years. They reported an overall prevalence of OAB symptoms of 16.6%, 17.4%, and 15.6% in males and females, respectively.[31] The EPIC study, a computer-assisted telephone interview of more than 19,000 participants aged older than 18 years across five countries, including Canada, Germany, Italy, Sweden, and the United Kingdom, showed the prevalence of LUTS suggestive of OAB to be 10.8% in men and 12.8% in women. ICS definitions of LUTS and OAB were used to survey the population for symptoms.[32] The incidence of OAB is higher in elderly women, being reported in 45% of women older than 65 years[33] and higher than 80% in institutionalized women.[34]

EFFECT ON QUALITY OF LIFE

Patient perception of bother is important in assessing need for treatment in women with OAB. Both frequency of micturition and amount of urine lost can be used to determine OAB severity, but overall effect on quality of life is essential to determine suitable treatment options. OAB symptoms and UUI can have detrimental effects on a woman's physical, social, and psychological well-being. Commonly used coping mechanisms to avoid incontinence episodes include fluid restriction, awareness of nearby bathroom facilities, and social isolation in order to avoid embarrassment. These factors contribute to a cycle of anxiety and psychological distress and may ultimately result in social isolation. The top 10 items affecting quality of life are listed in Table 25.1.

Health-related quality of life (HRQL) measures can be used to assess the effect of OAB on quality of life. Examples of grade A HRQL measures that exist include Bristol Female Lower Urinary Tract Symptoms Questionnaire, International Consultation on Incontinence Questionnaire Urinary Incontinence Short Form, Overactive Bladder Questionnaire Short Form, The Kings Health Questionnaire, Pelvic Floor Distress Inventory (PFDI), PFDI Short Form (PFDI-20), Pelvic

TABLE 25.1

Top 10 Incontinence-Related Quality-of-Life Items

1. Urinary incontinence psychological, not physical, problem
2. Self-concept
3. Resignation
4. Loss of sleep
5. Lack of predictability
6. Fear of public embarrassment
7. Shame
8. Adaptation of daily routine
9. Lack of self-control
10. Need for preemptive strategies to avert urinary incontinence

Adapted from DuBeau CE, Levy B, Mangione CM, et al. The impact of urge urinary incontinence on quality of life: Importance of patients' perspective and explanatory style. *J Am Geriatr Soc* 1998;46(6):683–692.

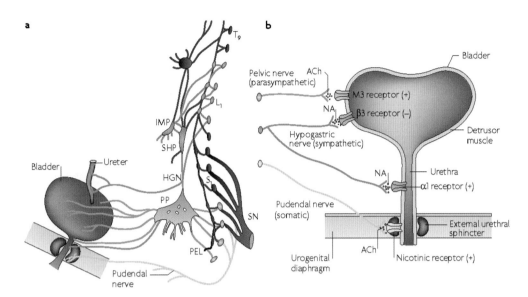

FIGURE 25.1 Efferent pathways of the lower urinary tract. IMP, inferior mesenteric plexus; SHP, superior hypogastric plexus; HGN, hypogastric nerve; PP, pelvic plexus; PEL, pelvic nerves; SN, sciatic nerve; ACh, acetylcholine; NA, noroadrenaline. (Reprinted by permission from Springer: Fowler CJ, Griffiths D, de Groat WC. The neural control of micturition. *Nat Rev Neurosci* 2008;9[6]:453–466.)

Floor Impact Questionnaire (PFIQ), PFIQ Short Form (PFIQ-7). Assessment of symptom bother and overall bother must also be carried out. The Patient Perception of Bladder Condition and the Urogenital Distress Inventory are the only Grade A validated questionnaires that exist which assess symptom bother.

PATHOPHYSIOLOGY

Three basic functions are required for the bladder to fill and empty in a socially acceptable manner. Compliance is required so that the bladder can increase in volume without increasing intravesical pressure. The urothelium must protect the underlying neural and muscular layer from urine as the bladder expands. Finally, there must be a coordinated effort by the bladder muscle wall to contract so that the bladder empties adequately.[35] An intact circuit between the brain, spinal cord, and peripheral ganglia is essential for the bladder to function, and removal of this extrinsic neural input renders the bladder nonfunctional. Switch-like patterns of activity are seen in the bladder unlike other systems, such as the cardiovascular system that are tonically contracted. Micturition is a learnt behavior and requires voluntary control. Urine storage and release are coordinated through integrated somatic and autonomic efferents in the lumbosacral spinal cord (Fig. 25.1).[36]

The pathophysiology of the OAB syndrome and DO is still incompletely understood and is likely to be multifactorial. The lower urinary tract function is dependent on complex central neural networks which can be altered by a variety of neurologic disorders. OAB can be triggered by discreet disease entities including infection, interstitial cystitis, urethrotrigonitis, urolithiasis,

and neoplasia. Idiopathic OAB implies that a causative agent has not been identified and comprises 90% of patients with OAB.[37] Pathologic causes of OAB include cerebrovascular accidents, intracranial lesions, interstitial cystitis, spinal cord injury, obstruction, Parkinson disease, multiple sclerosis, and diabetes.

Women with idiopathic OAB were compared to age-matched controls using neurophysiologic tests and subtracted cystometry. Both patients and controls had normal neurophysiologic tests, and there was no difference in testing between the two groups.[38] The pathophysiology of OAB does not seem to be explained by clinical or subclinical damage of the central nervous system or motor pathways, and other causative theories have been suggested. The complex pathophysiology of OAB is likely related to a combination of four theories: outflow obstruction hypothesis, urothelium-based hypothesis, myogenic hypothesis and neurogenic hypothesis (Fig. 25.2).

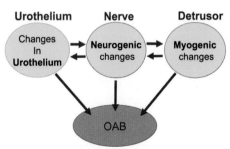

Aberration in the voiding reflex leading to involuntary detrusor contractions

FIGURE 25.2 Mechanisms underlying OAB. (Reprinted from Tyagi P. Pathophysiology of the urothelium and detrusor. *Can Urol Assoc J* 2011;5[5 Suppl 2]:S128–S130.)

Overactive Bladder Due to Outflow Obstruction

The clinical, structural, and neuropathic changes characteristic of DO are caused by bladder outflow obstruction. This can occasionally be seen in women with advanced stage POP or following midurethral sling or bladder neck surgery, leading to increased outflow resistance.[37] Partial ligation of the urethra in rat models has been shown to cause muscle hypertrophy of the detrusor muscle and afferent and efferent neuronal hypertrophy.[39,40] Similar observations have been shown in humans, suggesting development of new spinal circuits after obstruction of the outflow tract. Nerve growth factor which is responsible for regrowth of nerves after injury, and for maintenance of sympathetic and sensory neurons, is responsible for this plasticity.[35] Speakman et al.[41] hypothesized that outlet obstruction and irritative voiding symptoms are as a result of postjunctional supersensitivity, possibly as a result of partial denervation. The sensitivity to electrical stimulation of the detrusor nerve supply is reduced, but it is more sensitive to stimulation with acetylcholine.[42] Brading et al.[43] hypothesized that bladder instability is as a result of smooth muscle change due to a reduction in functional bladder wall innervation.

Urothelial-Based Hypothesis

The urothelium-based hypothesis postulates that enhancement of involuntary contractions is caused by alterations in urothelial receptor function and release of neurotransmitter, in addition to the sensitivity and coupling of the suburothelial interstitial cell network.[44] There is increasing evidence that the response of the urothelial cells and suburothelial fibroblasts to both chemical and mechanical stimuli contributes to regulation of bladder activity through the activation of bladder afferent nerves. Nerve endings of C-fiber afferents are found in the suburothelial layer of the bladder wall and urothelium. Bladder distension has been shown to cause ATP release from the urothelium, which may lead to activation of afferent nerve terminals, resulting in bladder contraction.[45] The urothelium synthesizes prostanoids and nitric oxide which are both release during distension of the bladder.[46,47]

Myogenic Hypothesis

The myogenic hypothesis is based on the concept that uninhibited contractions are generated by changes in the coupling and excitability of smooth muscle cells with interstitial cells or other myocytes.[43,48] It has been hypothesized that partial denervation of the detrusor is a widespread feature in all cases of DO. This may lead to alteration of the smooth muscle properties, resulting in increased excitability of cells, with activity spreading more easily between cells, resulting in a coordinated myogenic detrusor contraction.[43,48] This theory disputes the concept of neurogenic DO as the underlying mechanism of DO in OAB. It is hypothesized that there is a fundamental abnormality at the bladder wall level, including increased electrical cellular coupling due to altered contractile activity and variable detrusor denervation with increased sensitivity to potassium.[49] Another theory is that of cellular hypertrophy. It is thought that increased elastin and collagen are produced in the muscle fascicles, and this combined with a loss of nerves, results in idiopathic and neuropathic bladders.[50] Enhanced, spontaneous contractile activity of the detrusor has been noticed. In vitro studies by Kinder and Mundy[51] showed that muscles from bladders with OAB, regardless of the etiology, spontaneously contract more often and with a greater amplitude than muscles from urodynamically normal bladders. Structural abnormalities have been noted in both neuropathic and nonneuropathic unstable detrusor muscles in the form of narrower junctional gaps between muscle cells as compared with the normal detrusor.[52]

Neurogenic Hypothesis

Central and peripheral nervous system pathways which may contribute to OAB include increase excitatory response in reflex pathways due to axonal sprouting in the spinal cord forming new synaptic connections or enforcing existing ones, reduced bulbospinal inhibition in central or peripheral nervous systems and higher afferent input from the lower urinary tract, and development of bladder reflexes which are resistant to central inhibition.[36] The detrusor muscle has been shown to contract more than a normal detrusor muscle in case of idiopathic DO. These contractions are not nerve-mediated and can be inhibited by vasoactive intestinal polypeptide and activated by increased α-adrenergic activity.[51,53] Cat models with central nervous system lesions noted inhibition of voiding functions by the cerebral cortex.[54] In patients with Parkinson, it is postulated that the loss of dopaminergic receptors is causative of their OAB symptoms because this has been demonstrated in monkey models.[55] Reorganization of reflex correction seems to occur after spinal cord injury, with facilitates C-fiber afferents and elimination of A-fiber afferents, causing OAB symptoms. These axons are sensitive to capsaicin and have been linked to upper motor neuron diseases including spinal cord injury, multiple sclerosis, and Parkinson disease.[56]

The pathophysiology of OAB may never be fully understood because this is likely a convergence of several pathophysiologic processes into one common clinical entity.

CLINICAL PRESENTATION

Patients with OAB present with symptoms of urgency, frequency, nocturia, and urge incontinence. A history of childhood nocturnal enuresis may exist in some patients.[57] It is important to establish if there is a mixed incontinence picture, with OAB coexisting with SUI and to accurately determine if a stressful activity may trigger a detrusor contraction causing urge incontinence. A study by Hashim and Abrams[58] reported that 58.7% of female OAB patients have DO on urodynamic studies. A systematic review and meta-analysis on diagnostic predictability of UI showed that clinical history alone was found to be 0.61 (0.57 to 0.65) sensitive and 0.87 (0.85 to 0.89) specific for the diagnosis of DO.[59] Because the symptoms of OAB overlap with those of other lower urinary tract conditions, a number of other diagnoses must be entertained. Differential diagnoses include urinary tract infection, severe genuine SUI, urethral diverticulum, urinary tract fistula, cystitis, foreign body, bladder tumor and urethritis.

EVALUATION OF OVERACTIVE BLADDER

History

A focused clinical history is fundamental to assessing UI.[4] Some studies have shown that the type of incontinence cannot be accurately determined from history alone.[60,61] However, a systematic review and meta-analyses on diagnostic assessment methods for UI showed that the clinical history alone had a sensitivity of 0.92 (95% confidence interval [CI] 0.91 to 0.93) and specificity of 0.56 (0.53 to 0.60) for diagnosis of urodynamic SUI and a sensitivity of 0.61 (0.57 to 0.65) and specificity of 0.87 (0.85 to 0.89) for diagnosis of DO.[59] Reversible causes of incontinence must be ruled out using the DIAPPERS mnemonic: delirium, infection, atrophy, pharmaceuticals, psychological problems, endocrine problems, restricted mobility, and stool impaction.[12]

A focused history should be taken to include the following:

1. Patient demographics—age, BMI, menopausal status
2. Detailed characterization of OAB symptoms—duration, severity, voiding diary
3. Assessment of quality of life using validated questionnaires
4. Other symptoms such as SUI, POP, incomplete voiding, bowel symptoms
5. Evaluation of urinary tract—recurrent urinary tract infections, bladder calculi
6. Fluid intake including caffeine and alcohol
7. Pad usage
8. Previous treatments and their success
9. Obstetric history—number and mode of deliveries
10. Past medical history—heart failure, diabetes, disc herniation or spinal cord injury, Parkinson disease, multiple sclerosis, dementia, and psychiatric disease
11. Past surgical history—previous midurethral sling, colposuspension, or POP surgery
12. Current medications—diuretics, benzodiazepines, adrenergic blockers, angiotensin-converting enzyme inhibitors
13. Social history—living environment, mobility, falls risk

Physical Examination

The physical examination should include an observation of the patient followed by a focused examination of organ systems that may affect UI.

1. Abdominal examination for scars, masses, hernias, bladder distension
2. Neurologic screen for lower motor neuron lesions to include the bulbocavernosus and anal wink reflexes.
3. Neurologic screen for intrapelvic nerve entrapments as a cause of refractory urgency. Associated symptoms include sciatica with urinary symptoms, gluteal pain with associated perineal or vaginal pain, dysuria, or refractory pelvic and perineal pain.[62]
4. Neurologic screen for upper motor lesions such as Parkinson disease
5. Mental status examination
6. Pelvic examination to assess for genitourinary prolapse which may impair bladder emptying, atrophic vaginitis, vaginal masses, and a cough stress test to assess for SUI
7. A digital rectal examination will determine anal tone, the presence of fecal impaction which may compromise bladder emptying.
8. Assessment of postvoid residual by urethral catheter or bladder ultrasound
9. Urine microscopy and culture to assess for hematuria or infection

Bladder Diary

The patient is also asked to complete a daily diary, as illustrated in Table 25.2. The micturition time chart records time of voiding over a 24-hour period. Another chart used is the frequency-volume chart which captures both the amount voided and the frequency of voiding. The most comprehensive diary is a bladder diary, which may include fluid intake, UI episodes, use of pads, and the sensations and activities preceding the episode of UI. This is usually performed over 2 to 3 days. When a bladder diary is completed properly it will illustrate: day and night time input and output, urine production over 24 hours, maximum and average voided volume, median functional bladder capacity, and polyuria. These charts may not accurately predict the type of UI the patient has,[63,64] and some patients may find it too complex to complete the diary accurately.[65] Measuring the voided volume of urine and recording timing of voids is a minimum, and the only sure way of differentiating between polyuria with large volumes, and a hypersensitive, small-capacity bladder with small volumes.

TABLE 25.2

Bladder Diary

DATE	DRINK		URINE		LEAKAGE		
TIME	TYPE	HOW MUCH (mL)	VOLUME OF URINE (mL)	HOW URGENT 0–3 3 = MOST URGENT	LEAKAGE WITH URGENCY	LEAKAGE WITH ACTIVITIES	PAD CHANGE
0200			200	3	Y		
0700	Mug Coffee	300	300	2			
0800							
0900						Cough	P
1000						Sneeze	
1100	Glass water	300					
1200			200	1			
1300	Glass juice	300					
1400			200	1			
1500							
1600							
1700	Cup of tea	200				Walking	P
1800			200	2	Y		
1900							
2000	Glass water	200					
2100			100	1			
2200							
2300							

Investigations

Advanced testing including UDS, cystoscopy, and renal tract imaging may not be part of the original workup in an uncomplicated OAB presentation. However, it should be considered in refractory patients who do not respond to multiple medication treatments and in patients with hematuria without infection.[66]

Uroflowmetry is a noninvasive measurement of urine flow rate. It allows the maximum flow rate, voided volume, and the flow curve to determine if the patient is emptying their bladder in a normal fashion. It may reveal obstructive voiding patterns secondary to severe genitourinary prolapse or tumor. Traditional multichannel cystometry is considered the gold standard for diagnosis. Provocation maneuvers including coughing (Fig. 25.3), positional change, and running water may help to simulate the circumstances in which OAB or incontinence usually occur.[67] Multichannel cystometry may not always achieve a diagnosis, and alternative diagnostic methods should be performed in this scenario. In a subset of patients, standard urodynamic studies does not adequately verify or exclude a lower urinary tract dysfunction, particularly if the patient's symptoms cannot be reproduced by standard examination. In this cases, ambulatory UDS may be a suitable alternative, as more physiologic conditions can be obtained with patients moving more freely during the recording, thus simulating activities that may usually provoke urinary symptoms.[68] Conflicting results have been demonstrated with ambulatory UDS. One study by Salvatore et al.[69] showed a low rate of DO in asymptomatic women, which was similar to findings in routine laboratory UDS. However, other studies have shown rates of up to 68% of asymptomatic women,[70] and so the clinical role of this procedure is contentious. It is recommended by the ICS as a second-line diagnostic tool when standard office UDS fails to produce a diagnosis. In women with a neurologic history or in those who have had previous

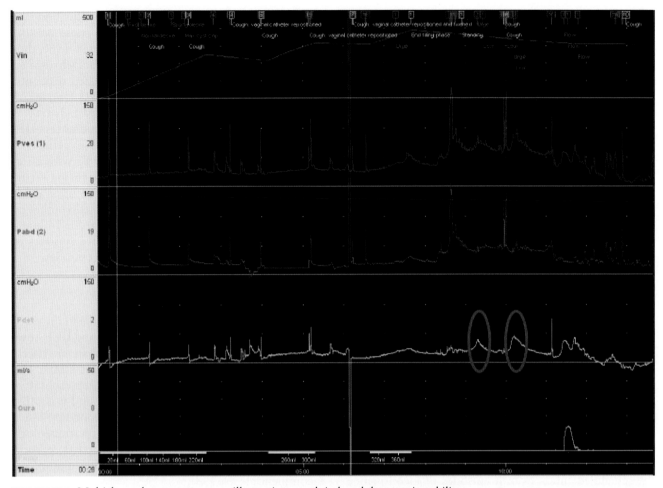

FIGURE 25.3 Multichannel cystometrogram illustrating cough induced detrusor instability.

pelvic surgery, videourodynamic study (VUDS) may be a more suitable test. This allows concurrent screening of the lower urinary tract during filling cystometry and voiding studies. A VUDS combines voiding pressure, urine flow, and imaging studies during the voiding phase and may aid in differentiating dysfunctional voiding from LUTS in women.[71]

TREATMENT OF OVERACTIVE BLADDER

Medical therapies can be commenced based on symptoms of OAB without any invasive investigations. New medical therapies are being developed which have fewer side effects and better patient compliance. Current management options are included in Table 25.3.

Conservative Management

Conservative measures are low cost, noninvasive lifestyle alterations such as altering fluid intake; weight loss; dietary changes; and reduction in caffeine, carbonated beverages, and alcohol consumption. Advice should be given to consume between 1 and 1.5 L in any

TABLE 25.3
Management of Overactive Bladder
Conservative management
Medical
Anticholinergics
Tricyclic antidepressants
Antidiuretic agents
β_3-Adrenoceptor agonists
Local estrogen therapy
Intravesical therapy
Neuromodulation/electrical stimulation
Sacral neuromodulation
Peripheral neuromodulation
Surgical
Augmentation cystoplasty
Bladder denervation

24-hour period. Caffeine and alcohol are known to irritate the bladder, and women should be advised to try to avoid caffeine-based drinks or substitute them with decaffeinated drinks. Obesity has been shown to be associated with OAB in women.[72] Increased chemokines have been found in the bladders of obese women which may suggest a chronic, low-grade inflammation in the bladders of obese women.[73] Weight loss programs have been shown to improve urgency UI symptoms.[74] Bariatric surgery has been shown to substantially improve both urge and SUI in women who are severely obese in the first year postoperatively.[75,76] In a prospective study of women undergoing bariatric surgery, 34% reported symptoms of SUI, 21% reported symptoms of OAB, and 44% reported symptoms of mixed incontinence. The cure rates at 1-year postoperatively for SUI, OAB, and mixed incontinence, were 41%, 38%, and 48%, respectively.[77]

Bladder Training (Timed Voiding)

Bladder retraining principles are based on the capability to suppress the urge to void and gradually extend the intervals between voids. Frequency of urination reduces the bladder capacity and leads to bladder instability. Bladder training aims to break this cycle by requiring the patient to resist urgency and delay voiding until the specified interval is reached. The patient is asked to void at strict voiding intervals and is not allowed to void in between the scheduled times, even if episodes of incontinence occur. Once she is dry, the period between intervals is lengthened. This is repeated and extended until a continence interval of 3 to 4 hours is achieved. Cure rates using conservative bladder retraining alone, without any pharmacologic therapies is 44% to 90%.[11] The combination of pelvic floor exercises with bladder retraining can aid in suppressing symptomatic urinary urgency because the ability to increase pelvic floor muscle tone will increase the patient's ability to prevent urge incontinence caused by strong, involuntary bladder contractions. The treatment is considered successful if the patient achieves a voiding interval of 2.5 to 3 hours and is free of OAB symptoms. A randomized, placebo-controlled trial of 197 women, aged between 55 and 92 years of age with either urge or mixed incontinence were randomized to pelvic floor physiotherapy, immediate release oxybutynin, or placebo. With pelvic floor rehabilitation, there was an 80.7% mean reduction in episodes of incontinence. This was statistically superior to both oxybutynin and placebo.[78]

Behavioral Modification in Elderly Patients

OAB incidence increases with age. The combination of OAB, reduced mobility, and cognitive deficits increase the rates of UI in this population. It is not uncommon for many elderly patients to instinctively reduce their fluid intake for better symptom control. This however can cause chronic dehydration and may cause bladder irritation with resultant highly concentrated urine, thus resulting in worsening symptoms of OAB. Dehydration is particularly common in institutionalized residents, exacerbating both constipation and OAB.[79] Urinary incontinence is associated with a significant falls risk. A recent systematic review including 15 studies reported that the proportion of patients with OAB experiencing at least one fall a year ranged from 18.9%, with a significant number (10.2% to 56%) experiencing recurrent or serious falls.[80] A study of 133 institutionalized women looking at the efficacy of prompted voiding by assisting them to the bathroom every hour for 14 hours a day, showed a reduction of incontinence episodes of 0.6 per day, an overall 26% reduction in episodes.

Medical Management

Medical management has an important role in the management of women with OAB symptoms and UUI; however, all current drugs that we use have systemic effects and none target the urethral and bladder alone. The extensive number or drugs available is representative of the fact that there is no perfect drug, and it is often their systemic effects which result in noncompliance and cessation of medical therapy. The pharmacology of drugs and recommendations for usage has recently been reviewed by the 6th International Consultation on Incontinence (Table 25.4).[81]

Antimuscarinic (anticholinergic) drugs

The innervation of the detrusor is by the parasympathetic nervous system (pelvic nerve), the sympathetic nervous system (hypogastric nerve), and by noncholinergic, nonadrenergic neurons. The pelvic nerve conveys the motor supply via S2, S3, and S4. Acetylcholine is the neurotransmitter at the neuromuscular junction, which acts on muscarinic receptors. Antimuscarinic agents work at the ganglionic receptor to block detrusor contractions in both the normal bladder and the OAB. Antimuscarinic agents also competitively block acetylcholine receptors at postganglionic parasympathetic receptor sites. Contraindications to these medications include urinary retention, impaired gastric emptying, uncontrolled narrow-angle glaucoma. Side effects of this class of medication involve atropine-like side effects, such as dry mouth and dry eyes, gastroparesis, constipation, gastroesophageal reflux, and somnolence, the severity of which are dose dependent. In elderly patients, the lowest dose is prescribed and then gradually titrated to efficacy and tolerability of side effects.

There are five different muscarinic receptor subtypes which have been identified (M_1 to M_5). The urinary bladder, like numerous other tissues, has a mixed

TABLE 25.4

Drugs Used in the Treatment of Overactive Bladder

	LEVEL OF EVIDENCE	GRADE OF RECOMMENDATION
Antimuscarinic drugs		
Atropine, hyoscyamine	3	C
Darifenacin	1	A
Fesoterodine	1	A
Imidafenacin	1	A
Propantheline	2	B
Solifenacin	1	A
Tolterodine	1	A
Trospium	1	A
Drugs with mixed actions		
Oxybutynin	1	A
Propiverine	1	A
Flavoxate	2	D
Drugs acting on membrane channels		
Calcium antagonists	2	D
K-channel openers	2	D
Antidepressants		
Imipramine	3	C
Duloxetine	2	C
α-AR antagonists		
Alfuzosin	3	C
Doxazosin	3	C
Prazosin	3	C
Terazosin	3	C
Tamsulosin	3	C
Silodosin	3	C
Naftopidil	3	C
β-AR antagonists		
Terbutaline ($\beta2$)	3	C
Salbutamol ($\beta2$)	3	C
Mirabegron ($\beta3$)	1	A
PDE-5 inhibitors		
(Sildenafil, taladafil, vardenafil)	1	B

(continued)

TABLE 25.4 (*Continued*)

Drugs Used in the Treatment of Overactive Bladder

	LEVEL OF EVIDENCE	GRADE OF RECOMMENDATION
COX-inhibitors		
Indomethacin	2	C
Flurbiprofen	2	C
Toxins		
Botulinum toxin (neurogenic)[a]	1	A
Botulinum toxin (idiopathic)[a]	1	A
Capsaicin (neurogenic)[b]	2	C
Resiniferatoxin (neurogenic)[b]	2	C
Other drugs		
Baclofen[c]	3	C
Hormones		
Estrogen	2	C
Desmopressin[d]	1	A

[a]Bladder wall.
[b]Intravesical.
[c]Intrathecal.
[d]Nocturia (nocturnal polyuria), caution hyponatremia especially in the elderly.
AR, adrenergic receptor; PDE-5, phosphodiesterase type 5; COX, cyclooxygenase.

population of muscarinic subtypes.[82] The main subtype found within the bladder is the M_2 muscarinic receptor, but there is also a subpopulation of M_3 receptors, with a ratio of 3:1 (M_2:M_3 receptors) present in human bladders.[83] Rat models have shown the M_3-receptor subtype to be the sole mediator of bladder contraction, and the M_2 muscarinic receptor subtype does not have a direct involvement in bladder contraction.[84] The M_3-receptor subtype is also present in salivary glands, and therefore drugs selective for M3 receptors are more likely to cause dry mouth. In vivo cat studies have shown tolterodine, a nonselective muscarinic antagonist, oxybutynin, an M_1- and M_3-receptor antagonist and darifenacin, an M_3-selective antagonist, are equally effective at inhibiting bladder contractions, but tolterodine is more potent at inhibiting bladder contraction than inhibiting salivation. This suggests that selectivity for M_3 over M_2 receptors has a stronger effect on salivation than bladder contraction in vivo.[85,86] Therefore, drugs that are more selective for the M_3-receptor subtype have lower rates of associated anticholinergic side effects such as dry eyes and dry mouth.

Tolterodine

In 1997, tolterodine tartrate was introduced to treat OAB. Available preparations include an immediate-release and a time-release preparation. The immediate-release dose is 2 mg twice daily and the extended-release is 2 to 4 mg once daily. Tolterodine is a competitive muscarinic receptor antagonist with relative functional selectivity for bladder muscarinic receptors. Several placebo-controlled studies have documented the effectiveness of both forms of therapy in terms of significant reduction in urgency, frequency, and number of incontinence episodes.[87,88] A double-blind multicenter trial of 1,234 women comparing immediate- and extended-release (ER) tolterodine and placebo, showed the ER to be significantly more effective.[89]

Oxybutynin

This medication is an anticholinergic with muscle relaxant and local anesthetic properties and acts predominantly on M_3 subtype receptors. The recommended dose is 2.5 to 5 mg three to four times per day with increasing anticholinergic side effects associated with increasing dosages.[87] It can improve symptoms by more than 50%, with up to 61% to 86% improvement in doses of 15 mg per day.[90] A once-daily ER is available which has equivalent efficacy with a lower side effect profile.[91] Oxybutynin is also available in a transdermal form which avoids first-pass metabolism, with equivalent efficacy to immediate-release tolterodine but much less dry mouth (38% for transdermal vs. 94% for immediate release).[92] Dmochowski et al.[93] combined the results of two randomized controlled trials (RCTs) for analysis, showing topical tolterodine to be efficacious and well tolerated with dry mouth occurring rarely (7.0% vs. placebo 5.3%). Pruritus and erythema at the application site occurred in 16.1% and 7%, respectively. A gel formulation of tolterodine was approved by the U.S. Food and Drug Administration (FDA) in January 2009, in an attempt to reduce the skin reactions to transdermal preparations. Staskin et al.[94] reported on a large prospective multicenter, randomized, double-blind placebo-controlled study on the use of oxybutynin gel OAB management in 704 patients. There was a significant reduction in urgency, urge incontinence, day time frequency, and an increase in voided volume compared to the placebo group. Dry mouth occurred more commonly in the treatment arm (6.9% vs. placebo group 2.9%); however, skin reactions were uncommon in both arms (5.4% and 1.0% in the placebo arm).[94] This formulation may present a more tolerable administration of oxybutynin in terms of patient acceptability.

Trospium chloride

Trospium chloride is a quarternary amine compound that acts as competitive antagonist at muscarinic cholinergic receptors. Due to its limited crossing of the blood–brain barrier (BBB), it has less cognitive side effects and might be a more suitable option in elderly patients.[95] A placebo-controlled, randomized, double-blind multicenter trial of trospium has been shown to increase cystometric capacity and bladder volume and first unstable contraction, with comparable adverse events over placebo.[96] It has been shown to be as effective as oxybutynin, with a lower incidence of dry mouth and patient withdrawal.[97]

Solifenacin

Solifenacin succinate is a potent competitive M_3-receptor antagonist, with higher affinity for the bladder smooth muscle over the salivary glands and thus with a lower side effect profile. A multicenter, randomized, double-blind, parallel group, placebo-controlled study of once daily solifenacin 5 mg and 10 mg in patients with OAB showed a statistically significant reduction in frequency with both doses compared to placebo. The higher dose had a larger effect, with side effects leading to discontinuation being dry mouth and constipation, both of which were dose related.[98]

Darifenacin

Darifenacin is a highly selective M_3-receptor antagonist. A review of the pooled darifenacin data from the three multicenter, double-blind clinical trials in patients with OAB showed a significant reduction in urge incontinence episodes per week, which was dose related. Patients had a significant decrease in the frequency and severity of urgency, micturition frequency, urge incontinence, and also an increase in bladder capacity. Side effects included constipation and dry mouth but resulted in few discontinuations.[99]

Fesoterodine

Fesoterodine is a potent antimuscarinic agent that has more recently been developed for the management of OAB. It is a prodrug that shares the same active metabolite as tolterodine, 5-hydroxymethyl tolterodine (5-HMT). 5-HMT is metabolized in the liver to inactive metabolites by the CYP3A4 or CYP2D6 pathway, and a small percentage is excreted unchanged in the urine.[85,100] A phase III randomized placebo-controlled trial comparing fesoterodine 4 and 8 mg with tolterodine ER 4 mg for treatment of OAB in 1,135 patients at 150 sites throughout Australia, New Zealand, South Africa, and Europe showed fesoterodine to be superior to tolterodine in reduction of frequency and urge incontinence episodes.[101] This is further supported by two large phase IV studies, showing fesoterodine to be superior to over tolterodine in terms of efficacy and flexible dosing regimens.[102,103]

β_3-Adrenoceptor agonists

β_3-Adrenoceptor agonists activate adenyl cyclase, followed by the subsequent formation of cyclic adenyl monophosphate which results in bladder relaxation. This drug class has been shown to increase bladder capacity with no change in micturition pressure and residual urine volumes.[104] The proof-of-concept BLOSSOM study, mirabegron (100 and 150 mg mirabegron, BID) showed a significant improvement in frequency and urgency episodes compared to placebo.[105] The dose-ranging DRAGON study (50, 100, 200 mg) showed a dose-dependent decrease in 24-hour frequency, incontinence, urgency and nocturia episodes, which were statistically significantly different between the placebo and 50-, 100-, and 200-mg mirabegron groups.[106] Nitti et al.[107] reported a pooled analysis on the SCORPIO, ARIES, and CAPRICORN studies, with a total of 2,542 patients included. This pooled analysis showed a statistically significant improvement in episodes of UI and frequency episodes per 24 hours. The adjusted mean (95% CI) change from baseline to final visit in the mean number of incontinence episodes per 24 hours was 1.10 (1.23, 0.97), 1.49 (1.63, 1.36), and 1.50 (1.67, 1.34) in the placebo, mirabegron 50 and 100 mg groups, respectively, and 1.20 (1.34, 1.06), 1.75 (1.89, 1.61), 1.74 (1.91, 1.56) for the adjusted mean change from baseline to final visit in the mean number of micturitions per 24 hours.

The pooled analysis by Nitti et al.[107] showed the most common drug-related side effects were hypertension and headache, with a similar incidence to placebo and tolterodine and with no evidence of dose-response relationship. The discontinuation rate due to side effects was low and similar in all groups: placebo (3.3%), mirabegron 25 mg (3.9%), mirabegron 50 mg (3.9%), mirabegron 100 mg (3.7%), total mirabegron (3.8%), and tolterodine ER 4 mg (4.4%).[107] A randomized, placebo, and active-controlled (400 mg moxifloxacin), parallel, crossover heart rate-corrected QT interval (QT/QTc) study in 352 healthy individuals showed no evidence of QTc interval prolongation in doses of 100 mg or lower.[108] In the pooled population from the SCORPIO, ARIES, and CAPRICORN, and 12-month TAURUS study, mirabegron was associated with an increase of ≤1 mm Hg in blood pressure compared with placebo. Hypertension incidence was equal between mirabegron, placebo, and 4-mg tolterodine ER groups.[109] β_3-adrenceptor agonists are as efficacious as antimuscarinics but have a better side effect profile, thus reducing discontinuation rates.

Tricyclic antidepressants

Imipramine

The effects of tricyclic antidepressants on the lower urinary tract are twofold: anticholinergic properties as described previously and α-adrenergic properties to increase tone of the urethra and bladder neck. Imipramine has antimuscarinic, antihistamine, and local anesthetic properties with side effects including antimuscarinic side effects, tremor, and fatigue. Imipramine has been shown to be useful in treatment of nocturnal enuresis[110,111]; however, there are no good quality random controlled trials to show its effectiveness in treatment of DO. The cardiac side effect profile including QTc prolongation, orthostatic hypotension, and ventricular arrhythmias should be considered when prescribing this drug, and the risk and benefits of prescribing this drug in the treatment of OAB have yet to be assessed.

Antidiuretic agents

Desmopressin

Desmopressin (1-desamino-8-D-arginine vasopressin) is a synthetic vasopressin which has been shown to reduce nocturnal urine output by 50% and is used in the treatment of nocturia or nocturnal enuresis.[112] A randomized, double-blind study comparing 0, 25, 50, or 100 μg desmopressin versus placebo showed a dose-related improvement in nocturia, with the lowest dose reaching statistical significance compared to placebo ($P < .05$ vs. placebo).[113] It should be avoided in patients with underlying cardiac conditions such as ischemic heart disease, congestive heart failure, or hypertension. It is associated with hyponatremia and current recommendations are that serum sodium should be checked in the first week following treatment. It has also been shown to be effective in the treatment of OAB.[114]

Local estrogen therapy

Estrogen replacement following menopause can improve physiologic voiding function and reduce OAB symptoms. Animal models have shown estrogen deficiency to affect smooth muscle contraction and contribute to OAB symptoms.[115] In vitro studies in ovariectomized rats showed a reduction in voided volume and higher levels of frequency with an increase in basal and stretch-induced acetylcholine release. This was reversed with estrogen replacement therapy.[116] Based on these findings, estrogen replacement may improve voiding function and reduce OAB symptoms. Given the concerns regarding the use of systemic estrogen replacement therapy, vaginal administration of estrogen may offer a better treatment option. Both the International Menopause Society Writing Group and the North American Menopause Society have deemed local estrogen therapy to be safe.[117,118] It has been shown that shortly after the start of treatment, once the vaginal mucosa has recovered from the atrophic state, systematic absorption of estradiol is minimal. There was no incidence of increased endometrial thickness or endometrial hyperplasia following a years' treatment with 10 μg of vaginal estradiol.[119,120]

Local vagina estrogen in the form of 17β-estradiol tablets (Vagifem) has been shown to improve urgency symptoms.[121] A double-blind, randomized, placebo-controlled trial showed a significant improvement in frequency, urgency, and stress incontinence in women treated with local estrogen therapy; however, no objective urodynamic assessment was performed.[122] It is difficult to ascertain if this subjective improvement in symptoms was due to reversal of urogenital atrophy rather than a direct effect on lower urinary tract function. A meta-analysis of 10 randomized placebo-controlled trials analyzing estrogen in the treatment of OAB showed estrogen to be superior to placebo in management of urge incontinence, frequency and nocturia, and vaginal estrogen was found to be superior to placebo in treatment of urgency symptoms.[123] An open-labeled, single center, prospective study showed vaginal estrogen to significantly improve subjective symptoms of OAB based on the overactive bladder symptom score (OABSS) questionnaire and also showed an objective improvement on urodynamic evaluation with an increase in time to first desire to void and maximum cystometric capacity.[124]

Prescribing in the elderly

Age-related changes in pharmacology include increased absorption due to slower gastric motility and reduction in skin thickness (transdermal preparations), higher concentrations of medication due to decrease in lean body mass and protein binding, reduced hepatic metabolism, and reduced renal clearance. Some UI medication may be effective at lower than normal doses.[125] Low-dose oxybutynin and a combination of low-dose solifenacin and trospium chloride have shown to be effective in older patients.[126,127] Polypharmacy is common in older patients,[128–130] with adverse drug events increasing significantly with increasing number of medications and with increasing age.[131] One must consider if any existing medication are contributing to urinary symptoms prior to commencing and UI medications, as recommended by geriatric prescribing principles of "subtract before adding." The Fit fOR The Aged criteria is a system of lower urinary tract medication prescription for older patients.[132] Levels of appropriateness in terms of UI medications are assigned, and fesoterodine was the only medication categorized as beneficial.

The most common muscarinic receptors in the central nervous system are M_1 receptors and play a key role in executive functions and episodic memory.[133] Memory processing is primarily through M_2 receptors and regulation of acetylcholine levels is through M_4 receptors. Thus, cognitive disturbance and cell death may result from antagonism of these receptors.[134] However, anticholinergics can only cause central effects if they cross the BBB. BBB penetration, as predicted by molecular size, lipophilicity, and polarity, are highest for oxybutynin; lower for solifenacin, darifenacin, and tolterodine, and lowest for trospium chloride and fesoterodine.[135] Oxybutynin is a relatively small (357 kDa) molecule which readily crosses the BBB, unlike tolterodine (475.6 kDa), solifenacin (480.6 kDa), and darifenacin (507.5 kDa) which limits them crossing the BBB.[136] A review by Kay and Ebinger[137] looked at five randomized, double-blind, multiple-dose studies assessing the effects of anticholinergics on cognitive function. Oxybutynin was uniformly associated with cognitive decline (four studies), whereas darifenacin was not shown to be associated with cognitive deficit (three studies). These findings were supported by electroencephalogram and sleep/attention studies.[137] A study by Staskin and Harnett[138] looked at trospium chloride levels in cerebrospinal fluid samples, and it was shown to be undetectable on day 10 of treatment. This was confirmed by memory testing showing no net medication effect on recall or learning. In contrast to anticholinergics, β_3-adrenoceptor agonists did not appear to affect cognitive function. A phase IV placebo-controlled study (PILLAR) assessed the effect of mirabegron on cognitive function in patients ≥65 years using the Montreal Cognitive Assessment as a rapid screening instrument for mild cognitive impairment. Although the follow-up was only 12 weeks, mirabegron did not contribute to drug-related cognitive side effects.[139]

There have been numerous cross-sectional studies which have shown an association between anticholinergic exposure and shorter term cognitive dysfunction including delirium or confusion.[140–145] A systematic review by Ruxton et al.[146] showed an association between antimuscarinics and cognitive impairment, falls and all-cause mortality in older adults. Brain changes comparable to those found in Alzheimer disease have been shown with prolonged anticholinergic treatment, including reduction in cortical volume temporal lobe and global atrophy and increase in ventricular volume.[147,148] A short period of treatment with anticholinergic medication has been associated with cognitive impairment but not dementia. However, with prolonged exposure dementia, not only cognitive impairment, has been proven.[149] It is not known whether discontinuation reverses these effects as conflicting evidence exists.[150,151] Currently, it is believed that a prolonged anticholinergic-free period is required before improvements in cognition are seen. Where prolonged use of anticholinergics is likely to be necessary, medication with a mild anticholinergic load or β_3-antagonists should be considered.[134]

Anticholinergic prescription cannot always be avoided in the geriatric population, and where necessary medications which do not cross the BBB with a mild anticholinergic load should be considered.[134] These medications should be continuously reevaluated, particularly in treatment periods extending beyond 3 months. Oxybutynin and tolterodine have the highest anticholinergic load and oxybutynin the highest BBB permeability in contrast to trospium chloride with the lowest BBB permeability. Alternatives such as onabotulinum toxin or β_3-adrenoceptor agonists should be considered.

Intravesical Therapy

Botulinum toxin type A

Although first described for the treatment of neurogenic DO,[152] there is currently sizeable evidence to support the use of intravesical botulinum toxin type A (onabotulinumtoxinA) in the treatment of idiopathic DO. Botulinum toxin is a neurotoxin produced by *Clostridium botulinum*. There are seven subtypes of botulinum toxin, of which subtype A has the longest duration of action and is therefore clinically most relevant. A phase II, multicenter, randomized, double-blind study of 313 patients with idiopathic OAB and urinary urgency incontinence were given 50, 100, 150, 200, or 300 U intradetrusor onabotulinumtoxinA, or placebo. A sustained efficacy was observed in reduction in urgency and urge incontinence episodes in patients receiving 100 U or more. Doses greater than 150 U were not associated with an added clinical improvement when dose response curves were analyzed. Increase in postvoid residuals and urinary retention requiring self-catheterization was also dose dependent and increased with doses higher than 150 U.[153] Balancing efficacy and risk of urinary retention, a dose of 100 U offered the best balance between efficacy and safety. A further large phase III randomized double-blind placebo-controlled trial of onabotulinumtoxin 100 IU in 557 patients with idiopathic OAB showed significantly decreased levels of incontinence episodes with onabotulinumtoxin when compared to placebo (-2.65 vs. -0.87, $P < .001$) and cure of incontinence in 22.9% versus 6.5% of patients, respectively. The most common adverse event was urinary tract infection (15.5%), and urinary retention occurred in 5.4% of patients; however, half of these patients no longer required intermittent self-catheterization after 6 weeks.[154]

The trigone was traditionally avoided during Botox administration due to its highly dense sensory innervation because there were concerns regarding a higher risk of urinary retention and vesicoureteric reflux. A systematic review and meta-analysis of eight studies (419 participants) showed significantly improved symptom scores, higher complete dryness rates, and lower number of incontinence episodes in patients with trigone-including injections. Trigone-including injections was also associated with lower detrusor pressure and higher volume and first void. There were equal incidences of vesicoureteral reflux, hematuria, general weakness, bladder discomfort, large postvoid residual, and urinary tract infection between intradetrusor and detrusor-sparing groups.[155] A randomized double-blind placebo-controlled trial in 249 women compared onabotulinumtoxin 100 U to antimuscarinic therapy (solifenacin 5 mg escalating to 10 mg and trospium chloride 60 mg). There was no significant difference in reduction in urge incontinence between the onabotulinumtoxin arm and the antimuscarinic arm (3.3 vs. 3.4; $P = .813$) and cure of incontinence was reported in 27% and 13%, respectively ($P = .003$).[156] Onabotulinumtoxin is effective in managing women with refractory OAB symptoms and can be administered under general or local anesthetic.

Neuromodulation

Sacral neuromodulation

In the 1980s, sacral nerve neuromodulation (SNM) was established by Tanagho and Schmidt[157,158] as a treatment option for patients with OAB and neurogenic DO. It is unclear what the exact mechanism of action for neuromodulation is, but the sites of action appear to be at the spinal and supraspinal level.[159] InterStim Therapy (Medtronic, Minneapolis, MN) is licensed by the FDA since 1997 for the treatment of UUI. It has subsequently been approved by the FDA for treatment of pelvic floor dysfunction including urinary frequency, nonobstructive urinary retention, and fecal incontinence.

SNM methods are continuously being improved and placement is now a minimally invasive technique.

The dorsal sacral nerve root is stimulated with a permanent electrode device which is implanted in the S3 sacral foramen. This electrode is connected to an implanted pulse generator which can modulate the sphincter activity and detrusor muscle activity. A test phase is performed which lasts for days to weeks in order to determine if a permanently implanted device will be successful. If the test phase results are successful, the implantable pulse generator is implanted in the upper buttocks. The test phase of SNM can either be with a temporary electrode to perform peripheral nerve evaluation or by a staged implanted of a permanent, tined-lead electrode.[160-162] Historically, SNM used a nonrechargeable implantable pulse generator with an average device lifespan of 4 years. Lead migration and implant site infections were not uncommon causes for surgical revision. More recently new devices with longer battery life or rechargeable implanted pulse generators have been developed and have improved patient satisfaction with SNM.

The RELAX-OAB study was a prospective, multicenter postmarket clinical study of 51 patients which evaluated the safety and efficacy of the Axonics r-SNM System. Device satisfaction based on bladder diary criteria was present in 94% at 1 year, with 84% of patients reporting satisfaction with their r-SNM therapy, and 98% being satisfied with their charging experience. Device adverse events occurred in 21% of subjects, with 20% being due to device discomfort which was resolved with reprogramming in all cases.[163] The InSite trial was a prospective, multicenter study of 272 subjects SNM therapy with the InterStim System. This study showed significant improvement in UI success rates of 77% and 81% in less severe (less than 2 leaks a day) and more severe ($\geq$2 leaks a day) groups. At baseline, the less severe and more severe groups had an average of 9.4 and 15.1 voids per day, respectively, which was reduced to 6.6 and 7.5 voids per day, respectively, at 24 months. At 24 months, the less severe group had an average of 0.4 leaks per day and the more severe group had an average of 1.3 leaks per day.[164]

The Rosetta study compared onabotulinumtoxinA 200 U bladder injections against SNM (InterStim) in refractory OAB patients.[165] Urinary incontinence at baseline was 5.4 and 5.2 in the onabotulinumtoxinA and the SNM group, respectively. The onabotulinumtoxinA group had a significantly higher response than the SNM group and a significantly higher number of patients experience cure (20% vs. 4%) or 75% reduction in UUI episodes (46% vs. 26%). However, the 200 U dose is not the standard dose of onabotulinumtoxinA approved by the FDA. Although SNM is both an invasive and expensive procedure, improvements and technical advances make it a good alternative where patients have failed other medical therapies or as an alternative to botulinum toxin intravesical injection.

Percutaneous posterior tibial nerve stimulation

Percutaneous tibial nerve stimulation (PTNS) was first proposed as a treatment option for urge incontinence in 1983.[166] The tibial nerve contains L4–S3 fibers and originates from the same spinal cord segments as the nerves supply to the bladder and pelvic floor. This procedure is performed by inserting a needle posterior to the tibia and two finger widths above the medial malleolus. This is an outpatient procedure which is usually performed weekly for the first 12 weeks and may be continued on a monthly basis for maintenance, with each session lasting 30 minutes. A prospective, randomized, multicenter study comparing PTNS with tolterodine 4 mg ER in 100 patients showed a 75% of patients with PTNS compared to 55.8% with tolterodine ER.[167]

The SUmiT trial was a multicenter, double-blind, RCT comparing the efficacy of percutaneous tibial nerve stimulation to sham over 12 weeks of therapy. There was a statistically significant improvement in bladder symptoms in the treatment group compared to the sham group, with 54.5% reporting moderately or markedly improved symptoms compared to 20.9% of sham subjects from baseline.[168] A follow on from this study is the sustained therapeutic effects of percutaneous tibial nerve stimulation (STEP) study, wherein 50 participants who met the primary effectiveness end point after 12 weeks were enrolled in this prospective study to assess long-term outcomes with PTNS. Twenty-nine patients completed 36 months of follow-up, receiving a median of 1.1 treatments per month after a 14-week treatment tapering protocol with 77% of patients having a moderate or marked improvement in OAB symptoms at 3 years. Compared to baseline, urinary frequency reduced from 12.0 at baseline to 8.7, nocturia reduced from 2.7 to 1.7 episodes per night, and urge incontinence reduced from 3.3 to 0.3 episodes per day, all of which were significant.[169]

A systematic review of PTNS on treatment of OAB examined 28 studies with a total of 2,461 patients.[170] Included were 12 RCTs and 16 observational studies, with half of the studies adopting 30-minute sessions weekly for 12 weeks as their protocol, and the remainder conducting a different schedule of treatment. PTNS significantly improved daily frequency (mean difference [MD] = −2.48; $P < .001$), daily nocturia episodes (MD = −1.57; $P < .001$), daily urgency episodes (MD = −2.20; $P = .006$), daily UUI episodes (MD = −1.37; $P < .001$), maximum cystometric capacity (MD = 63.76; $P < .001$) and bladder compliance (MD = 7.62; $P = .033$), with an overall response rate of 68% ($P < .001$). The addition of OAB medication to PTNS was examined in 4 studies, with an improvement in OAB symptom management demonstrated in the first 3 studies[171–173] but no additional improvement reported in the last study.[174] There were few, minor side

effects associated with PTNS, with the only major complication being pain at the puncture site.

Although PTNS appears to be a promising treatment option, it does require weekly in-person visits in order to complete the treatment schedule, which may not be logistically convenient for patients. As such, implantable devices have been developed which stimulate the tibial nerve and appear to be safe and effective in the long term[175,176]; however, larger studies are required to establish efficacy and safety. Long-term success has been shown with monthly treatments following the initial treatment schedule.[169] PTNS is a safe, effective treatment option for treatment of OAB and, in refractory cases, may offer an alternative therapeutic option.

Chronic pudendal neuromodulation

An alternative in patients who do not respond to SNM is chronic pudendal neuromodulation (CPNS). Approximately 10% to 25% of patients do not respond to SNM.[177,178] The pudendal nerve innervates the pelvic floor muscles, anal sphincters, external urethra, and pelvic organs, and directly targeting it is a viable alternative to SNM or PTNS. A transgluteal or ischiorectal approach have been described with equivalent safety levels to SNM.[177] A study by Peters et al.[168] reported a 93.2% success in patients (78.6% female) undergoing CPNS for interstitial cystitis or OAB, almost all of which failed SNM. A further route for access to the pudendal nerve and S3 nerve route has been described.[179,180] This involves laparoscopic implantation of electrodes for bilateral neuromodulation inserted into Alcock canal with attachment to the pelvic pectineal line and a further lead placed juxtancurally to S3. The leads were connected to a 16-pole pulse generator which was implanted subcutaneously in the left lower abdomen.[179]

Surgery

Surgery is an option to be considered when all other medical and behavioral therapies have been exhausted or contraindicated. The most commonly performed procedures include enterocystoplasty, urinary diversion, and bladder denervation

Enterocystoplasty

Enlargement or augmentation cystoplasty can be used in intractable OAB cases with decreased functional or organic capacity. A low-pressure reservoir for urine with adequate capacity is created from a segment of bowel. This is rarely performed due to the associated morbidity of the procedure, the associated metabolic and bowel-related sequelae, and the need for self-intermittent catheterization. A preoperative evaluation must consider the presence of neurologic and gastrointestinal disease and previously abdominal surgeries which may complicate surgery due to adhesions. A colonoscopy should be considered in at risk patients prior to proceeding with the procedure. Renal function assessment (serum creatinine and electrolytes) and renal imaging should be performed to rule out obstruction. A cystoscopy should be performed to rule out any intravesical pathology.

The surgical technique involves a midline abdominal incision in order to obtain a well-vascularized mesenteric pedicle of ileum or colon. Usually, a 20- to 40-cm segment is used, and an end-to-end anastomosis is performed with the remaining bowel segments. The bladder is mobilized and a vertical cystotomy is performed and extended from the bladder neck to the bladder base. The bowel segment is then detubularized on the antimesenteric border and refashioned into a U-, S-, or W-shaped pouch, which is anastomosed to the bladder. A Mitrofanoff or Monti technique can be performed to create a continent catheterizable channel if desirable at the time of surgery. A urethral catheter or suprapubic tube are left in situ for 2 to 3 weeks and can be removed once cystography confirms absence of a leak. The renal tract must be monitored with imaging during follow-up and renal function assessed with serum electrolytes and creatinine. The cystoplasty should be irrigated daily to prevent a buildup of mucous and stone formation. Annual cystoscopy to out rule development of adeno or transitional cell carcinoma should be considered.

Early complications include anastomotic leak, postoperative ileus, fistula formation, and abscess formation. Later complications include bowel obstruction, infection and pyelonephritis, stone formation, bladder perforation, and metabolic acidosis. Successful outcomes have been achieved in greater than 80% following surgery, with resultant increased capacity and reduction in spontaneous detrusor contractions in.[181,182]

Urinary diversion

Noncontinent urinary diversion in the form of an ileal conduit was originally described by Seiffert[183] in 1935 and popularized by Bricker[184] in 1950. The ileum has been chosen as a reservoir due to the fact that absorption of electrolytes is reduced in this segment of small bowel.[185] Isolation of 15 to 20 cm of bowel of the terminal ileum 10 to 15 cm from the ileocecal anastomosis is required, and the remaining bowel is reanastomosed. Following transection of the ureters 3 to 4 cm from the bladder, anastomosis to the antimesenteric of the ileal loop or the proximal end of the ileal loop is performed. A stoma on the anterior abdominal wall is created using the ileal loop, and the ureters drain into this. Associated complications include deterioration in renal function, voiding dysfunction, stoma complications, intestinal obstruction, ureteroenteric stricture formation, fistula

formation, metabolic disorders, infectious complications and rarely urolithiasis, and malignant transformation of the ileal loop.[186]

Bladder denervation

A novel technique of selective bladder denervation using radiofrequency ablation of the subtrigone region is a further option in the treatment of refractory OAB. Selective bladder denervation is achieved using a cystoscopically delivered thermal delivery probe. This is placed along the left border of the trigone, 5 mm below the ureteric orifice. Radiofrequency energy was applied following advancement of the electrodes 3 mm below and parallel to the urothelium, and suburothelial ablation was achieved. Treatment success defined as "greatly improved" or "improved" was reported as 79% at 12 weeks.[187]

FUTURE POSSIBILITIES

The Nonadrenergic, Noncholinergic Pathway

P2X₃-receptors and P2X₃-receptor antagonists

Bladder filling causes stretching of the urothelium and release of adenosine 5'-triphosphate (ATP) from the umbrella cells. This stimulates purinergic receptors on suburothelial sensory nerves via mechanotransduction pathways and mediates the bladder filling sensation and triggers the voiding reflex.[188,189] P2X-receptors are ligand-gated ion channels which are expressed in sensory neurons and area activated by ATP. Sensory nerve fibers expressing P2X₃ immunoreactivity are present in the urothelium, detrusor smooth muscle, and lamina propria.[190] Studies have shown that intravesical infusion of ATP can stimulate bladder contraction in rats, thus P2X₃ may play a role in detecting volume changes during bladder filling, and may contribute to lowering the C-fiber activation threshold in disease conditions.[191]

A study of female patients with idiopathic detrusor instability showed an increase in P2X₂-receptors and a decrease in other P2X-receptor subtypes. In contrast to the patients with OAB, a purinergic component of nerve mediated contractions was not evident in the control group.[192] In a study comparing bladder P2X-receptor expression in male patients with DO secondary to outlet obstruction (undergoing prostate surgery), the concentration of P2X₁-receptor per smooth muscle cells was higher in the study compared to the control group. This highlights the increase in purinergic function associated with an unstable detrusor caused by bladder outlet obstruction.[193] A-317491, a selective P2X₃-antagonist has been shown to improve bladder function in rat models with spinal cord injury.[194] This P2X$_3$-antagonist has also been shown to reduce detrusor contractions during bladder filling, reduce frequency, and increase bladder capacity, without affecting the amplitude of voiding contractions. Further studies on humans are needed to determine clinical efficacy.

Transient receptor potential channel antagonists

The transient receptor potential (TRP) superfamily is made up of cation channels that regulate membrane excitability and intracellular calcium levels.[195] These receptors are present in the bladder and act as sensors for mechanosensory transduction and nociception. Animal models of lower urinary tract disorders have reported promising outcomes for these drugs acting on various types of TRP channels, including TRPV1, TRPV2, TRPV4, TRPM4, TRPM8 and TRPA1.[196,197] It has not yet been shown if this research will translate to clinical practice, and further trials will be needed to establish their use in OAB treatment.[198]

CONCLUSION

OAB is a symptomatic diagnosis in patients complaining of frequency, urgency, nocturia, with or without urge incontinence. It has a high prevalence among the general population, affecting 16.5% of the U.S. population. Its prevalence increases with increasing with age and with our aging population will pose a significant economic burden in years to come. There have been many advancements in therapy in recent years, with the addition of β$_3$-adrenoceptor agonists, intravesical therapy, onabotulinumtoxinA, and neuromodulation therapies. Advances are being made in pathways not involving muscarinic or cholinergic pathways which may hold propitious future therapies.

References

1. Stewart E, Van Rooyen J, Cundiff G, et al. Prevalence and burden of overactive bladder in the United States. *World J Urol* 2003;20(6):327–336.
2. Akobundu E, Ju J, Blatt L, et al. Cost-of-illness studies: A review of current methods. *Pharmacoeconomics* 2006;24(9):869–890.
3. Abrams P, Kelleher C, Kerr L, et al. Overactive bladder significantly affects quality of life. *Am J Manag Care* 2000;6(11 Suppl):S580–S590.
4. Abrams P, Cardozo L, Fall M, et al. The standardisation of terminology of lower urinary tract function: Report from the standardisation sub-committee of the International Continence Society. *Neurourol Urodyn* 2002;21(2):167–178.
5. Haylen B, de Ridder D, Freeman R, et al. An International Urogynecological Association (IUGA)/International Continence Society (ICS) joint report on the terminology for female pelvic floor dysfunction. *Neurourol Urodyn* 2010;29(1):4–20.
6. Stach-Lempinen B, Kujansuu E, Laippala P, et al. Visual analogue scale, urinary incontinence severity score and 15 D—Psychometric testing of three different health-related quality-of-life instruments for urinary incontinent women. *Scand J Urol Nephrol* 2001;35(6):476–483.
7. D'Ancona C, Haylen B, Oelke M, et al. The International Continence Society (ICS) Report on the terminology for adult male lower urinary tract and pelvic floor symptoms and dysfunction. *Neurourol Urodyn* 2019;38(2):433–477.
8. Malone-Lee J, Henshaw D, Cummings K. Urodynamic verification of an overactive bladder is not a prerequisite for antimuscarinic treatment response. *BJU Int* 2003;92(4):415–417.
9. Matharu G, Donaldson M, McGrother C, et al. Relationship between urinary symptoms reported in a postal questionnaire and urodynamic diagnosis. *Neurourol Urodyn* 2005;24(2):100–105.
10. Wyndaele J, Van Meel T, De Wachter S. Detrusor overactivity. Does it represent a difference if patients feel the involuntary contractions? *J Urol* 2004;172(5 Pt 1):1915–1918.
11. Jarvis G, Millar D. Controlled trial of bladder drill for detrusor instability. *Br Med J* 1980;281(6251):1322–1323.
12. Resnick N, Yalla S. Detrusor hyperactivity with impaired contractile function. An unrecognized but common cause of incontinence in elderly patients. *JAMA* 1987;257(22):3076–3081.
13. Abarbanel J, Marcus EI. Impaired detrusor contractility in community-dwelling elderly presenting with lower urinary tract symptoms. *Urology* 2007;69(3):436–440.
14. Osman N, Chapple C, Abrams P, et al. Detrusor underactivity and the underactive bladder: A new clinical entity? A review of current terminology, definitions, epidemiology, aetiology, and diagnosis. *Eur Urol* 2014;65(2):389–398.
15. Jeong S, Kim H, Lee Y, et al. Prevalence and clinical features of detrusor underactivity among elderly with lower urinary tract symptoms: A comparison between men and women. *Korean J Urol* 2012;53(5):342–348.
16. Gammie A, Kaper M, Dorrepaal C, et al. Signs and symptoms of detrusor underactivity: An analysis of clinical presentation and urodynamic tests from a large group of patients undergoing pressure flow studies. *Eur Urol* 2016;69(2):361–369.
17. Wagg A, Nitti V, Kelleher C, et al. Oral pharmacotherapy for overactive bladder in older patients: Mirabegron as a potential alternative to antimuscarinics. *Curr Med Res Opin* 2016;32(4):621–638.
18. Chapple C, Siddiqui E. Mirabegron for the treatment of overactive bladder: A review of efficacy, safety and tolerability with a focus on male, elderly and antimuscarinic poor-responder populations, and patients with OAB in Asia. *Expert Rev Clin Pharmacol* 2017;10(2):131–151.
19. Wang C, Lee C, Kuo H. Efficacy and safety of intravesical onabotulinumtoxinA injection in patients with detrusor hyperactivity and impaired contractility. *Toxins (Basel)* 2016;8(3):82.
20. Chancellor M, Chartier-Kastler E. Principles of sacral nerve stimulation (SNS) for the treatment of bladder and urethral sphincter dysfunctions. *Neuromodulation* 2000;3(1):16–26.
21. Hennessey D, Hoag N, Gani J. Sacral neuromodulation for detrusor hyperactivity with impaired contractility. *Neurourol Urodyn* 2017;36(8):2117–2122.
22. Digesu G, Chalihia C, Salvatore S, et al. The relationship of vaginal prolapse severity to symptoms and quality of life. *BJOG* 2005;112(7):971–976.
23. Tegerstedt G, Maehle-Schmidt M, Nyrén O, et al. Prevalence of symptomatic pelvic organ prolapse in a Swedish population. *Int Urogynecol J Pelvic Floor Dysfunct* 2005;16(6):497–503.

24. Lawrence J, Lukacz E, Nager C, et al. Prevalence and co-occurrence of pelvic floor disorders in community-dwelling women. *Obstet Gynecol* 2008;111(3):678–685.

25. de Boer T, Salvatore S, Cardozo L, et al. Pelvic organ prolapse and overactive bladder. *Neurourol Urodyn* 2010;29(1):30–39.

26. Spelzini F, Frigerio M, Manodoro S, et al. Modified McCall culdoplasty versus Shull suspension in pelvic prolapse primary repair: A retrospective study. *Int Urogynecol J* 2017;28(1):65–71.

27. Frigerio M, Manodoro S, Cola A, et al. Risk factors for persistent, de novo and overall overactive bladder syndrome after surgical prolapse repair. *Eur J Obstet Gynecol Reprod Biol* 2019;233:141–145.

28. Cardozo L, Stanton S, Williams J. Detrusor instability following surgery for genuine stress incontinence. *Br J Urol* 1979;51(3):204–207.

29. Langer R, Ron-el R, Newman, M, et al. Detrusor instability following colposuspension for urinary stress incontinence. *Br J Obstet Gynaecol* 1988;95(6):607–610.

30. Coyne K, Sexton C, Vats V, et al. National community prevalence of overactive bladder in the United States stratified by sex and age. *Urology* 2011;77(5):1081–1087.

31. Milsom I, Abrams P, Cardozo L, et al. How widespread are the symptoms of an overactive bladder and how are they managed? A population-based prevalence study. *BJU Int* 2001;87(9):760–766.

32. Irwin D, Milsom I, Hunskaar S, et al. Population-based survey of urinary incontinence, overactive bladder, and other lower urinary tract symptoms in five countries: Results of the EPIC study. *Eur Urol* 2006;50(6):1306–1315.

33. Sexton C, Coyne K, Thompson C, et al. Prevalence and effect on health-related quality of life of overactive bladder in older Americans: Results from the epidemiology of lower urinary tract symptoms study. *J Am Geriatr Soc* 2011;59(8):1465–1470.

34. Starer P, Libow L. The measurement of residual urine in the evaluation of incontinent nursing home residents. *Arch Gerontol Geriatr* 1988;7(1):75–81.

35. Chancellor M, Yoshimura N. Physiology and pharmacology of the bladder and urethra. In: Walsh PC, ed. *Campbell's urology.* Philadelphia: Saunders, 2002:831–886.

36. de Groat W. A neurologic basis for the overactive bladder. *Urology* 1997;50(6A Suppl):36–56.

37. Goldberg R, Sand P. Pathophysiology of the overactive bladder. *Clin Obstet Gynecol* 2002;45(1):182–192.

38. Del Carro U, Riva D, Comi G, et al. Neurophysiological evaluation in detrusor instability. *Neurourol Urodyn* 1993;12(5):455–462.

39. Steers W, Ciambotti J, Etzel B, et al. Alterations in afferent pathways from the urinary bladder of the rat in response to partial urethral obstruction. *J Comp Neurol* 1991;310(3):401–410.

40. Steers W, De Groat W. Effect of bladder outlet obstruction on micturition reflex pathways in the rat. *J Urol* 1988;140(4):864–871.

41. Speakman M, Brading A, Gilpin C, et al. Bladder outflow obstruction—A cause of denervation supersensitivity. *J Urol* 1987;138(6):1461–1466.

42. Sibley G. An experimental model of detrusor instability in the obstructed pig. *Br J Urol* 1985;57(3):292–298.

43. Brading A, Turner W. The unstable bladder: Towards a common mechanism. *Br J Urol* 1994;73(1):3–8.

44. Yoshida M, Masunaga K, Nagata T, et al. The forefront for novel therapeutic agents based on the pathophysiology of lower urinary tract dysfunction: Pathophysiology and pharmacotherapy of overactive bladder. *J Pharmacol Sci* 2010;112(2):128–134.

45. Ferguson D, Kennedy I, Burton T. ATP is released from rabbit urinary bladder epithelial cells by hydrostatic pressure changes—A possible sensory mechanism? *J Physiol* 1997;505(Pt 2):503–511.

46. Maggi C. Prostanoids as local modulators of reflex micturition. *Pharmacol Res* 1992;25(1):13–20.

47. Birder L, Apodaca G, De Groat WC, et al. Adrenergic- and capsaicin-evoked nitric oxide release from urothelium and afferent nerves in urinary bladder. *Am J Physiol* 1998;275(2):F226–F229.

48. Brading A. A myogenic basis for the overactive bladder. *Urology* 1997;50(6A Suppl):57–73.

49. Mills I, Greenland J, McMurray G, et al. Studies of the pathophysiology of idiopathic overactive bladder: The physiological properties of the detrusor smooth muscle and its pattern of innervation. *J Urol* 2000;163(2):646–651.

50. Charlton R, Morley A, Chambers P, et al. Focal changes in nerve, muscle and connective tissue in normal and unstable human bladder. *BJU Int* 1999;84(9):953–960.

51. Kinder R, Mundy A. Pathophysiology of idiopathic detrusor instability and detrusor hyper-reflexia. An in vitro study of human detrusor muscle. *Br J Urol* 1987;60:509–515.

52. Haferkamp A, Dörsam J, Resnick N, et al. Structural basis of neurogenic bladder dysfunction. II. Myogenic basis of detrusor hyperreflexia. *J Urol* 2003;169(2):547–554.

53. Eaton A, Bates C. An in vitro physiological study of normal and unstable human detrusor muscle. *Br J Urol* 1982;54(6):653–657.

54. De Groat W, Booth A, Yoshimura N. Neurophysiology of micturition and its modification in animal models of human disease. In: Maggi CA, ed. *The autonomic nervous system, nervous control of the urogenital system*, Vol. 3. London: Harwood Academic Publishers, 1993:227–290.

55. Yoshimura N, Mizuta E, Kuno S, et al. The dopamine D1 receptor agonist SKF 38393 suppresses detrusor hyperreflexia in the monkey with parkinsonism induced by 1-methyl-4-phenyl-1,2,3,6-tetrahydropyridine (MPTP). *Neuropharmacology* 1993;32(4):315–321.

56. Geirsson G, Fall M, Sullivan L. Clinical and urodynamic effects of intravesical capsaicin treatment in patients with chronic traumatic spinal detrusor hyperreflexia. *J Urol* 1995;154(5):1825–1829.

57. Fitzgerald M, Thom D, Wassel-Fyr C, et al. Childhood urinary symptoms predict adult overactive bladder symptoms. *J Urol* 2006;175(3 Pt 1):989–993.

58. Hashim H, Abrams P. Do symptoms of overactive bladder predict urodynamic detrusor overactivity? *Neurourol Urodyn* 2004;23:484.

59. Martin J, Williams K, Sutton A, et al. Systematic review and meta-analysis of methods of diagnostic assessment for urinary incontinence. *Neurourol Urodyn* 2006;25(7):674–684.

60. Summitt R Jr, Stovall T, Bent A, et al. Urinary incontinence: Correlation of history and brief office evaluation with multichannel urodynamic testing. *Am J Obstet Gynecol* 1992;166(6 Pt 1):1835–1844.

61. Jensen J, Nielsen F Jr, Ostergard D. The role of patient history in the diagnosis of urinary incontinence. *Obstet Gynecol* 1994;83(5 Pt 2):904–910.

62. Lemos N, Possover M. Laparoscopic approach to intrapelvic nerve entrapments. *J Hip Preserv Surg* 2015;2(2):92–98.

63. Holroyd-Leduc J, Tannenbaum C, Thorpe K, et al. What type of urinary incontinence does this woman have? *JAMA* 2008;299(12):1446–1456.

64. Bright E, Drake M, Abrams P. Urinary diaries: Evidence for the development and validation of diary content, format, and duration. *Neurourol Urodyn* 2011;30(3):348–352.

65. Tannenbaum C, Corcos J. Outcomes in urinary incontinence: Reconciling clinical relevance with scientific rigour. *Eur Urol* 2008;53(6):1151–1161.

66. Lightner DJ, Gomelsky A, Souter L, et al. Diagnosis and treatment of overactive bladder (non-neurogenic) in adults: AUA/SUFU guideline amendment 2019. *J Urol* 2019;202(2):558–563.

67. Schäfer W, Abrams P, Liao L, et al; for International Continence Society. Good urodynamic practices: Uroflowmetry, filling cystometry, and pressure-flow studies. *Neurourol Urodyn* 2002;21(3):261–274.

68. Rosario D, MacDiarmid S, Radley S, et al. A comparison of ambulatory and conventional urodynamic studies in men with borderline outlet obstruction. *BJU Int* 1999;83(4):400–409.

69. Salvatore S, Khullar V, Cardozo L, et al. Evaluating ambulatory urodynamics: A prospective study in asymptomatic women. *BJOG* 2001;108(1):107–111.

70. Heslington K, Hilton P. Ambulatory monitoring and conventional cystometry in asymptomatic female volunteers. *Br J Obstet Gynaecol* 1996;103(5):434–441.

71. Everaert K, Van Laecke E, De Muynck M, et al. Urodynamic assessment of voiding dysfunction and dysfunctional voiding in girls and women. *Int Urogynecol J Pelvic Floor Dysfunct* 2000;11(4):254–264.

72. Hunskaar S. A systematic review of overweight and obesity as risk factors and targets for clinical intervention for urinary incontinence in women. *Neurourol Urodyn* 2008;27(8):749–757.

73. Tyagi P, Barclay D, Zamora R, et al. Urine cytokines suggest an inflammatory response in the overactive bladder: A pilot study. *Int Urol Nephrol* 2010;42(3):629–635.

74. Phelan S, Kanaya A, Subak L, et al. Weight loss prevents urinary incontinence in women with type 2 diabetes: Results from the Look AHEAD trial. *J Urol* 2012;187(3):939–944.

75. Whitcomb E, Horgan S, Donohue M, et al. Impact of surgically induced weight loss on pelvic floor disorders. *Int Urogynecol J* 2012;23(8):1111–1116.

76. Bulbuller N, Habibi M, Yuksel M, et al. Effects of bariatric surgery on urinary incontinence. *Ther Clin Risk Manag* 2017;13:95–100.

77. Anglim B, O'Boyle C, O'Sullivan O, et al. The long-term effects of bariatric surgery on female urinary incontinence. *Eur J Obstet Gynecol Reprod Biol* 2018;231:15–18.

78. Burgio K, Locher J, Goode, PS, et al. Behavioral vs drug treatment for urge urinary incontinence in older women: A randomized controlled trial. *JAMA* 1998;280(23):1995–2000.

79. Burgio K. Influence of behavior modification on overactive bladder. *Urology* 2002;60(5 Suppl 1):72–77.

80. Szabo S, Gooch K, Walker D, et al. The association between overactive bladder and falls and fractures: A systematic review. *Adv Ther* 2018;35(11):1831–1841.

81. Abrams P. *Incontinence: 6th International consultation on incontinence*, 6th ed. Tokyo: International Continence Society, 2017.

82. Hedge S, Choppin A, Bonhaus D, et al. Functional role of M2 and M3 muscarinic receptors in the urinary bladder of rats in vitro and in vivo. *Br J Pharmacol* 1997;120(8):1409–1418.

83. Goepel M, Wittmann A, Rübben H, et al. Comparison of adrenoceptor subtype expression in porcine and human bladder and prostate. *Urol Res* 1997;25(3):199–206.

84. Longhurst PA, Leggett RE, Briscoe JA. Characterization of the functional muscarinic receptors in the rat urinary bladder. *Br J Pharmacol* 1995;116(4):2279–2285.

85. Nilvebrant L, Andersson K, Gillberg PG, et al. Tolterodine—A new bladder-selective antimuscarinic agent. *Eur J Pharmacol* 1997;327(2–3):195–207.

86. Gillberg P, Sundquist S, Nilvebrant L. Comparison of the in vitro and in vivo profiles of tolterodine with those of subtype-selective muscarinic receptor antagonists. *Eur J Pharmacol* 1998;349(2–3):285–292.

87. Van Kerrebroeck P, Kreder K, Jonas, U, et al. Tolterodine once-daily: Superior efficacy and tolerability in the treatment of the overactive bladder. *Urology* 2001;57(3):414–421.

88. Appell R, Abrams P, Drutz HP, et al. Treatment of overactive bladder: Long-term tolerability and efficacy of tolterodine. *World J Urol* 2001;19(2):141–147.

89. Swift S, Garely A, Dimpfl T, et al; for Tolterodine Study Group. A new once-daily formulation of tolterodine provides superior efficacy and is well tolerated in women with overactive bladder. *Int Urogynecol J Pelvic Floor Dysfunct* 2003;14(1):50–55.

90. Haylen B, Law M, Frazer M, et al. Urine flow rates and residual urine volumes in urogynecology patients. *Int Urogynecol J Pelvic Floor Dysfunct* 1999;10(6):378–383.

91. Birns J, Lukkari E, Malone-Lee J. A randomized controlled trial comparing the efficacy of controlled-release oxybutynin tablets (10 mg once daily) with conventional oxybutynin tablets (5 mg twice daily) in patients whose symptoms were stabilized on 5 mg twice daily of oxybutynin. *BJU Int* 2000;85(7):793–798.

92. Davila G, Daugherty C, Sanders S; for Transdermal Oxybutynin Study Group. A short-term, multicenter, randomized double-blind dose titration study of the efficacy and anticholinergic side effects of transdermal compared to immediate release oral oxybutynin treatment of patients with urge urinary incontinence. *J Urol* 2001;166(1):140–145.

93. Dmochowski R, Nitti V, Staskin D, et al. Transdermal oxybutynin in the treatment of adults with overactive bladder: Combined results of two randomized clinical trials. *World J Urol* 2005;23(4):263–270.

94. Staskin D, Dmochowski R, Sand P, et al. Efficacy and safety of oxybutynin chloride topical gel for overactive bladder: A randomized, double-blind, placebo controlled, multicenter study. *J Urol* 2009;181(4):1764–1772.

95. Füsgen I, Hauri D. Trospium chloride: An effective option for medical treatment of bladder overactivity. *Int J Clin Pharmacol Ther* 2000;38(5):223–234.

96. Cardozo L, Chapple C, Toozs-Hobson P, et al. Efficacy of trospium chloride in patients with detrusor instability: A placebo-controlled, randomized, double-blind, multicentre clinical trial. *BJU Int* 2000;85(6):659–664.

97. Madersbacher H, Stöhrer M, Richter R, et al. Trospium chloride versus oxybutynin: A randomized, double-blind, multicentre trial in the treatment of detrusor hyper-reflexia. *Br J Urol* 1995;75(4):452–456.

98. Cardozo L, Lisec M, Millard R, et al. Randomized, double-blind placebo controlled trial of the once daily antimuscarinic agent solifenacin succinate in patients with overactive bladder. *J Urol* 2004;172(5 Pt 1):1919–1924.

99. Chapple C, Steers W, Norton P, et al. A pooled analysis of three phase III studies to investigate the efficacy, tolerability and safety of darifenacin, a muscarinic M3 selective receptor antagonist, in the treatment of overactive bladder. *BJU Int* 2005;95(7):993–1001.

100. Cole P. Fesoterodine, an advanced antimuscarinic for the treatment of overactive bladder: A safety update. *Drugs Future* 2004;29:715–720.

101. Chapple C, Van Kerrebroeck P, Jünemann K, et al. Comparison of fesoterodine and tolterodine in patients with overactive bladder. *BJU Int* 2008;102(9):1128–1132.

102. Herschorn S, Swift S, Guan Z, et al. Comparison of fesoterodine and tolterodine extended release for the treatment of overactive bladder: A head-to-head placebo-controlled trial. *BJU Int* 2010;105(1):58–66.

103. Kaplan S, Schneider T, Foote J, et al. Superior efficacy of fesoterodine over tolterodine extended release with rapid onset: A prospective, head-to-head placebo controlled trial. *BJU Int* 2011;107(9):1432–1440.

104. Igawa Y, Yamazaki Y, Takeda H, et al. Relaxant effects of isoproterenol and selective beta3-adrenoceptor agonists on normal, low compliant and hyperreflexic human bladders. *J Urol* 2001;165(1):240–244.

105. Chapple C, Amarenco G, López Aramburu M, et al. A proof-of-concept study: Mirabegron, a new therapy for overactive bladder. *Neurourol Urodyn* 2013;32(8):1116–1122.

106. Chapple C, Dvorak V, Radziszewski P, et al. A phase II dose-ranging study of mirabegron in patients with overactive bladder. *Int Urogynecol J* 2013;24(9):1447–1458.

107. Nitti V, Khullar V, van Kerrebroeck P, et al. Mirabegron for the treatment of overactive bladder: A prespecified pooled efficacy analysis and pooled safety analysis of three randomised, double-blind, placebo-controlled, phase III studies. *Int J Clin Pract* 2013;67(7):619–632.

108. Novara G, Cornu J. Mirabegron as a new class of oral drug for overactive bladder syndrome: Many positive perspectives, some concerns. *Eur Urol* 2013;63(2):306–308.

109. Chapple C, Cardozo L, Nitti V, et al. Mirabegron in overactive bladder: A review of efficacy, safety, and tolerability. *Neurourol Urodyn* 2014;33(1):17–30.

110. Glazener C, Evans J, Peto R. Tricyclic and related drugs for nocturnal enuresis in children. *Cochrane Database Syst Rev* 2003;(3):CD002117.

111. Hunsballe J, Djurhuus J. Clinical options for imipramine in the management of urinary incontinence. *Urol Res* 2001;29(2):118–125.

112. Nørgaard J, Rittig S, Djurhuus J. Nocturnal enuresis: An approach to treatment based on pathogenesis. *J Pediatr* 1989;114(4 Pt 2):705–710.

113. Weiss J, Zinner N, Klein B, et al. Desmopressin orally disintegrating tablet effectively reduces nocturia: Results of a randomized, double-blind, placebo-controlled trial. *Neurourol Urodyn* 2012;31(4):441–447.

114. Hashim H, Malmberg L, Graugaard-Jensen C, et al. Desmopressin, as a "designer-drug," in the treatment of overactive bladder syndrome. *Neurourol Urodyn* 2009;28(1):40–46.

115. Hong S, Yang J, Kim T, et al. Effects of ovariectomy and estrogen replacement on the function an dexpression of Rho-kinase in rat bladder smooth muscle. *BJU Int* 2006;98(5):1114–1117.

116. Yoshida J, Aikawa K, Yoshimura Y, et al. The effects of ovariectomy and estrogen replacement on acetylcholine release from nerve fibres and passive stretch-induced acetylcholine release in female rat bladder. *Neurourol Urodyn* 2007;26(7):1050–1055.

117. The North American Menopause Society. Management of symptomatic vulvovaginal atrophy: 2013 Position statement of The North American Menopause Society. *Menopause* 2013;20(9):888–904.

118. de Villiers T, Pines A, Panay N, et al. Updated 2013 International Menopause Society recommendations on menopausal hormone therapy and preventive strategies for midlife health. *Climacteric* 2013;16(3):316–337.

119. Simon J, Maamari R. Ultra-low-dose vaginal estrogen tablets for the treatment of postmenopausal vaginal atrophy. *Climacteric* 2013;16(Suppl 1):37–43.

120. Notelovitz M, Funk S, Nanavati N, et al. Estradiol absorption from vaginal tablets in postmenopausal women. *Obstet Gynecol* 2002;99(4):556–562.

121. Benness C, Wise B, Cutner A, et al. Does low dose vaginal oestradiol improve frequency and urgency in postmenopausal women. *Int Urogynaecol J* 1992;3(2):281.

122. Eriksen P, Rasmussen H. Low dose 17 beta-oestradiol vaginal tablets in the treatment of atrophic vaginitis: A double-blind placebo controlled study. *Eur J Obste Gynecol Reprod Biol* 1992;44(2):137–144.

123. Cardozo L, Lose G, McClish D, et al. A systematic review of the effects of estrogens for symptoms suggestive of overactive bladder. *Acta Obs Gynecol Scand* 2004;83(10):892–897.

124. Matarazzo M, Caruso S, Giunta G, et al. Does vaginal estriol make urodynamic changes in women with overactive bladder syndrome and genitourinary syndrome of menopause? *Eur J Obstet Gynecol Reprod Biol* 2018;222:75–79.

125. Rochon PA, Anderson G, Tu J, et al. Age- and gender-related use of low-dose drug therapy: The need to manufacture low-dose therapy and evaluate the minimum effective dose. *J Am Geriatr Soc* 1999;47(8):954–959.

126. Bemelmans B, Kiemeney L, Debruyne F. Low-dose oxybutynin for the treatment of urge incontinence: Good efficacy and few side effects. *Eur Urol* 2000;37(6):709–713.

127. Kosilov K, Loparev S, Ivanovskaya M, et al. Comparative effectiveness of combined low- and standard-dose trospium and solifenacin for moderate overactive bladder symptoms in elderly men and women. *Urol Int* 2014;93(4):470–473.

128. Craftman ÅG, Johnell K, Fastbom J, et al. Time trends in 20 years of medication use in older adults: Findings from three elderly cohorts in Stockholm, Sweden. *Arch Gerontol Geriatr* 2016;63:28–35.

129. Moriarty F, Hardy C, Bennett K, et al. Trends and interaction of polypharmacy and potentially inappropriate prescribing in primary care over 15 years in Ireland: A repeated cross-sectional study. *BMJ Open* 2015;5(9):e008656.

130. Nishtala P, Salahudeen M. Temporal trends in polypharmacy and hyperpolypharmacy in older New Zealanders over a 9-Year Period: 2005–2013. *Gerontology* 2015;61(3):195–202.

131. Feinberg M. The problems of anticholinergic adverse effects in older patients. *Drugs Aging* 1993;3(4):335–348.

132. Oelke M, Becher K, Castro-Diaz D, et al. Appropriateness of oral drugs for long-term treatment of lower urinary tract symptoms in older persons: Results of a systematic literature review and international consensus validation process (LUTS-FORTA 2014). *Age Ageing* 2015;44(5):745–755.

133. Sathienluckana T, Unaharassamee W, Suthisisang C, et al. Anticholinergic discontinuation and cognitive functions in patients with schizophrenia: A pharmacist-physician collaboration in the outpatient department. *Integr Pharm Res Pract* 2018;7:161–71.

134. Bishara D, Harwood D, Sauer J, et al. Anticholinergic effect on cognition (AEC) of drugs commonly used in older people. *Int J Geriatr Psychiatry* 2017;32(6):650–656.

135. Kerdraon J, Robain G, Jeandel C, et al. Impact on cognitive function of anticholinergic drugs used for the treatment of overactive bladder in the elderly. *Prof Urol* 2014;24(11):672–681.

136. Kay G, Wesnes K. Pharmacodynamic effects of darifenacin, a muscarinic M selective receptor antagonist for the treatment of overactive bladder, in healthy volunteers. *BJU Int* 2005;96(7):1055–1062.

137. Kay G, Ebinger U. Preserving cognitive function for patients with overactive bladder: Evidence for a differential effect with darifenacin. *Int J Clin Pract* 2008;62(11):1792–1800.

138. Staskin D, Harnett M. Effect of trospium chloride on somnolence and sleepiness in patients with overactive bladder. *Curr Urol Rep* 2004;5(6):423–426.

139. Griebling T, Campbell N, Mangel J, et al. Effect of mirabegron on cognitive function in elderly patients with overactive bladder: MoCA results from a phase 4 randomized, placebo-controlled study (PILLAR). *BMC Geriatr* 2020;20(1):109.

140. Nebes R, Pollock B, Meltzer C, et al. Serum anticholinergic activity, white matter hyperintensities, and cognitive performance. *Neurology* 2005;65(9):1487–1489.

141. Cao Y-J, Mager D, Simonsick E, et al. Physical and cognitive performance and burden of anticholinergics, sedatives, and ACE inhibitors in older women. *Clin Pharmacol Ther* 2008;83(3):422–429.

142. Cancelli I, Gigli G, Piani A, et al. Drugs with anticholinergic properties as a risk factor for cognitive impairment in elderly people: A population-based study. *J Clin Psychopharmacol* 2008;28(6):654–659.

143. Uusvaara J, Pitkala K, Kautiainen H, et al. Detailed cognitive function and use of drugs with anticholinergic properties in older people: A community-based cross-sectional study. *Drugs Aging* 2013;30(3):177–182.

144. Sittironnarit G, Ames D, Bush A, et al. Effects of anticholinergic drugs on cognitive function in older Australians: Results from the AIBL study. *Dement Geriatr Cogn Disord* 2011;31(3):173–178.

145. Lampela P, Lavikainen P, Garcia-Horsman J, et al. Anticholinergic drug use, serum anticholinergic activity, and adverse drug events among older people: A population-based study. *Drugs Aging* 2013;30(5):321–330.

146. Ruxton K, Woodman R, Mangoni A. Drugs with anticholinergic effects and cognitive impairment, falls and all-cause mortality in older adults: A systematic review and meta-analysis. *Br J Clin Pharmacol* 2015;80(2):209–220. Erratum in: *Br J Clin Pharmacol* 2015;80(4):921–926.

147. Swami S, Cohen R, Kairalla J, et al. Anticholinergic drug use and risk to cognitive performance in older adults with questionable cognitive impairment: A cross-sectional analysis. *Drugs Aging* 2016;33(11):809–818.

148. Risacher SL, McDonald B, Tallman E, et al; for Alzheimer's Disease Neuroimaging Initiative. Association between anticholinergic medication use and cognition, brain metabolism, and brain atrophy in cognitively normal older adults. *JAMA Neurol* 2016;73(6):721–732.

149. Cai X, Campbell N, Khan B, et al. Long-term anticholinergic use and the aging brain. *Alzheimers Dement* 2013;9(4):377–385.

150. Gray S, Anderson M, Dublin S, et al. Cumulative use of strong anticholinergics and incident dementia: A prospective cohort study. *JAMA Intern Med* 2015;175(3):401–407.

151. Salahudeen M, Chyou T, Nishtala P. Serum anticholinergic activity and cognitive and functional adverse outcomes in older people: A systematic review and meta-analysis of the literature. *PLoS One* 2016;11(3):e0151084.

152. Schurch B, de Sèze M, Denys P, et al. Botulinum toxin type A is a safe and effective treatment for neurogenic urinary incontinence: Results of a single treatment, randomized, placebo controlled 6-month study. *J Urol* 2005;174(1):196–200.

153. Dmochowski R, Chapple C, Nitti, VW, et al. Efficacy and safety of onabotulinumtoxinA for idiopathic overactive bladder: A double-blind, placebo controlled, randomized, dose ranging trial. *J Urol* 2010;184(6):2416–2422.

154. Nitti V, Dmochowski R, Herschorn S, et al. OnabotulinumtoxinA for the treatment of patients with overactive bladder and urinary incontinence: Results of a phase 3, randomized, placebo controlled trial. *J Urol* 2013;189(6):2186–2193.

155. Jo J, Kim K, Kim D, et al. The effect of onabotulinumtoxinA according to site of injection in patients with overactive bladder: A systematic review and meta-analysis. *World J Urol* 2018;36(2):305–317.

156. Visco A, Brubaker L, Richter H, et al. Anticholinergic therapy vs. onabotulinumtoxina for urgency urinary incontinence. *N Engl J Med* 2012;367(19):1803–1813.

157. Tanagho E, Schmidt R. Bladder pacemaker: Scientific basis and clinical future. *Urology* 1982;20(6):614–619.

158. Tanagho E, Schmidt R, Orvis B. Neural stimulation for control of voiding dysfunction: A preliminary report in 22 patients with serious neuropathic voiding disorders. *J Urol* 1989;142(2 Pt 1):340–345.

159. Mehnert U, Boy S, Svesson J, et al. Brain activation in response to bladder filling and simultaneous stimulation of the dorsal clitoral nerve—An fMRI study in healthy women. *Neuroimage* 2008;41(3):682–689.

160. Leong R, De Wachter S, Nieman F, et al. PNE versus 1st stage tined lead procedure: A direct comparison to select the most sensitive test method to identify patients suitable for sacral neuromodulation therapy. *Neurourol Urodyn* 2011;30(7):1249–1252.

161. Amend B, Khalil M, Kessler T, et al. How does sacral modulation work best? Placement and programming techniques to maximize efficacy. *Curr Urol Rep* 2011;12(5):327–335.

162. Siegel S, Noblett K, Mangel J, et al. Results of a prospective, randomized, multicenter study evaluating sacral neuromodulation with InterStim therapy compared to standard medical therapy at 6-months in subjects with mild symptoms of overactive bladder. *Neurourol Urodyn* 2015;34(3):224–230.

163. Blok B, Van Kerrebroeck P, de Wachter S, et al. A prospective, multicenter study of a novel, miniaturized rechargeable sacral neuromodulation system: 12-month results from the RELAX-OAB study. *Neurourol Urodyn* 2019;38(2):689–695.

164. Noblett K, Berg K, Kan F, et al. Baseline symptom severity and therapeutic success in a large prospective trial of sacral neuromodulation therapy for overactive bladder patients. *Neurourol Urodyn* 2018;37(5):1667–1671.

165. Amundsen C, Richter H, Menefee S, et al. PI-LBA01 Sacral neuromodulation versus onabotulinumtoxinA for refractory overactive bladder. *J Urol* 2016;195(4S):e949–e950.

166. McGuire E, Zhang S, Horwinski E, et al. Treatment of motor and sensory detrusor instability by electrical stimulation. *J Urol* 1983;129(1):78–79.

167. Peters K, Macdiarmid S, Wooldridge L, et al. Randomized trial of percutaneous tibial nerve stimulation versus extended-release tolterodine: Results from the overactive bladder innovative therapy trial. *J Urol* 2009;182(3):1055–1061.

168. Peters K, Carrico D, Perez-Marrero RA, et al. Randomized trial of percutaneous tibial nerve stimulation versus Sham efficacy in the treatment of overactive bladder syndrome: Results from the SUmiT trial. *J Urol* 2010;183(4):1438–1443.

169. Peters K, Carrico D, Wooldridge L, et al. Percutaneous tibial nerve stimulation for the long-term treatment of overactive bladder: 3-year results of the STEP study. *J Urol* 2013;189(6):2194–2201.

170. Wang M, Jian Z, Ma Y, et al. Percutaneous tibial nerve stimulation for overactive bladder syndrome: A systematic review and meta-analysis. *Int Urogynecol J* 2020;31(12):2457–2471.

171. Kizilyel S, Karakeçi A, Ozan T, et al. Role of percutaneous posterior tibial nerve stimulation either alone or combined with an anticholinergic agent in treating patients with overactive bladder. *Turk J Urol* 2015;41(4):208–214.

172. Vecchioli-Scaldazza C, Morosetti C. Effectiveness and durability of solifenacin versus percutaneous tibial nerve stimulation versus their combination for the treatment of women with overactive bladder syndrome: A randomized controlled study with a follow-up of ten months. *Int Braz J Urol* 2018;44(1):102–108.

173. Karademir K, Baykal K, Sen B, et al. A peripheric neuromodulation technique for curing detrusor overactivity: Stoller afferent neurostimulation. *Scand J Urol Nephrol* 2005;39(3):230–233.

174. Iyer S, Laus K, Rugino A, et al. Subjective and objective responses to PTNS and predictors for success: A retrospective cohort study of percutaneous tibial nerve stimulation for overactive bladder. *Int Urogynecol J* 2019;30(8):1253–1259.

175. van Breda H, Martens F, Tromp J, et al. A new implanted posterior tibial nerve stimulator for the treatment of overactive bladder syndrome: 3-month results of a novel therapy at a single center. *J Urol* 2017;198(1):205–210.

176. Dorsthorst MJT, Digesu G, Tailor V, et al. 3-year followup, of a new implantable tibial nerve stimulator for the treatment of overactive bladder syndrome. *J Urol* 2020;204(3):545–550.

177. Spinelli M, Weil E, Ostardo E, et al. New tined lead electrode in sacral neuromodulation: Experience from a multicentre European study. *World J Urol* 2005;23(3):225–229.

178. Peters K, Killinger K, Ibrahim IA, et al. The relationship between subjective and objective assessments of sacral neuromodulation effectiveness in patients with urgency-frequency. *Neurourol Urodyn* 2008;27(8):775–778.

179. Li A, Marques R, Oliveira A, et al. Laparoscopic implantation of electrodes for bilateral neuromodulation of the pudendal nerves and S3 nerve roots for treating pelvic pain and voiding dysfunction. *Int Urogynecol J* 2018;29(7):1061–1064.

180. Possover M. A novel implantation technique for pudendal nerve stimulation for treatment of overactive bladder and urgency incontinence. *J Minim Invasive Gynecol* 2014;21(5):888–892.

181. Reyblat P, Chan K, Josephson D, et al. Comparison of extraperitoneal and intraperitoneal augmentation enterocystoplasty for neurogenic bladder in spinal cord injury patients. *World J Urol* 2009;27(1):63–68.

182. Hasan S, Marshall C, Robson W, et al. Clinical outcome and quality of life following enterocystoplasty for idiopathic detrusor instability and neurogenic bladder dysfunction. *Br J Urol* 1995;76(5):551–557.

183. Die Seiffert L. Darm-siphonblase. *Arch Klin Chir* 1935;102:569–574.

184. Bricker EM. Bladder substitution after pelvic evisceration. *Surg Clin North Am* 1950;30(5):1511–1521.

185. Hautmann R, Abol-Enein H, Hafez K. Urinary diversion. *Urology* 2007;69(1 Suppl):17–49.

186. Amini E, Djaladat H. Long-term complications of urinary diversion. *Curr Opin Urol* 2015;25(6):570–577.

187. Tu LM, De Wachter S, Robert M, et al. Initial clinical experience with selective bladder denervation for refractory overactive bladder. *Neurourol Urodyn* 2019;38(2):644–652.

188. Burnstock G. Purinergic signalling in the urinary tract in health and disease. *Purinergic Signal* 2014;10(1):103–155.

189. Burnstock G. Purinergic signalling in the lower urinary tract. *Acta Physiol (Oxf)* 2013;207(1):40–52.

190. Ford A, Cockayne D. ATP and P2X purinoceptors in urinary tract disorders. *Handb Exp Pharmacol* 2011;(202):485–526.

191. Pandita R, Andersson K. Intravesical adenosine triphosphate stimulates the micturition reflex in awake, freely moving rats. *J Urol* 2002;168(3):1230–1234.

192. O'Reilly B, Kosaka A, Knight G, et al. P2X receptors and their role in female idiopathic detrusor instability. *J Urol* 2002;167(1):157–164.

193. O'Reilly B, Kosaka A, Chang T, et al. A quantitative analysis of purinoceptor expression in the bladders of patients with symptomatic outlet obstruction. *BJU Int* 2001;87(7):617–622.

194. Lu S, de Groat W, Lin A, et al. Evaluation of purinergic mechanism for the treatment of voiding dysfunction: A study in conscious spinal cord-injured rats. *J Chin Med Assoc* 2007;70(10):439–444.

195. Nilius B, Szallasi A. Transient receptor potential channels as drug targets: From the science of basic research to the art of medicine. *Pharmacol Rev* 2014;66(3):676–814.

196. Avelino A, Charrua A, Frias B, et al. Transient receptor potential channels in bladder function. *Acta Physiol (Oxf)* 2013;207(1):110–122.

197. Franken J, Uvin P, De Ridder D, et al. TRP channels in lower urinary tract dysfunction. *Br J Pharmacol* 2014;171(10):2537–2551.

198. Cruz F. Transient receptor potential channel: A reality that still requires many years of scientific efforts. *BJU Int* 2015;115(5):676–677.

CHAPTER 26

Evaluation and Management of Voiding Dysfunction and Urinary Retention

Aqsa Azam Khan • Victor W. Nitti

Introduction

Women with incomplete bladder emptying may experience a number of bothersome lower urinary tract symptoms (LUTS). These may manifest as voiding symptoms, such as urinary hesitancy, slow stream, or a sensation of incomplete bladder emptying, or storage symptoms, such as urinary frequency, urgency, nocturia, or incontinence. They may experience medical issues including urinary tract infections, and in more severe cases can have decompensation of their upper urinary tract function. In order to gain a full understanding of the various potential etiologies for incomplete bladder emptying, knowledge of the anatomy and voiding physiology is essential. In this chapter we aim to review the various etiologies for incomplete bladder emptying and voiding dysfunction in women and to review the diagnosis and management for the various conditions.

DEFINITION AND CLASSIFICATION

LUTS globally refer to the array of symptoms that may be representative of any bladder, urinary outlet, neurologic, pelvic floor, or endocrine abnormalities related to storage of urine and voiding. The International Continence Society (ICS) first developed a report of standardized definitions for LUTS in 1988[1] with the most recent update specifically for female pelvic floor dysfunction in 2010.[2] Definitions as they pertain to retention and bladder emptying disorders are listed in Table 26.1.

Incomplete bladder emptying in women is a relatively poorly understood condition. Part of the reason for this may be due to varying classification systems and definitions to define this accurately and an overall paucity of studies.[3] There is much value in understanding the terminology of lower urinary tract function in order for providers to have a common language and to develop universally applied guidelines and treatment paradigms.

PREVALENCE AND INCIDENCE

In 2005, Irwin et al.[4] conducted the EPIC study, a population-based, cross-sectional telephone survey of 19,165 participants older than 18 years old in 2005 in five countries (Canada, Germany, Italy, Sweden, and the United Kingdom) using the 2002 ICS definitions for frequency, nocturia, urgency, overactive bladder (OAB), urgency urinary incontinence (UUI), stress urinary incontinence (SUI), mixed urinary incontinence (MUI), intermittency, slow stream, straining, terminal dribble, postmicturition dribble, and incomplete emptying. In their cohort, 59.2% of women reported at least one storage symptom (nocturia, urgency, frequency, UUI, MUI, SUI, other urinary incontinence) and 19.5% reported at least one voiding symptom (intermittency, slow stream, straining, terminal dribble).

Subsequently, Coyne et al.[5] conducted a large international cross-sectional population-representative Internet survey of participants aged 40 years or older in the United States, United Kingdom, and Sweden which included over 15,000 women older than the age of 40 years.[5] LUTS were again defined using 2002 ICS definitions and classified into storage (frequency, urgency, nocturia, incontinence [stress, urgency, mixed, coital, insensible]), voiding (weak stream, terminal dribble, hesitancy, straining, intermittency, split stream), postmicturition (incomplete emptying, postmicturition incontinence), and other (bladder pain, dysuria). The questions were asked according to a five-point Likert scale. In this cohort, women reported "sometimes" and "often" having a weak stream (20.1% and 4.4%), split stream (10.2% and 2.4%), intermittency (15.9% and 4%), hesitancy (11.8% and 2.8%), straining (5.9% and 1.4%), terminal dribble (38.3% and 14.5%), sensation of incomplete emptying (27.4% and 7.4%), and postmicturition incontinence (14.9% and 9.4%).

Studies using a postvoid residual (PVR) of 100 mL as the lower limit for voiding dysfunction in women have estimated a prevalence rate of 11%.[6,7]

TABLE 26.1

International Urogynecological Association/International Incontinence Society 2010 Terminology as They Pertain to Urinary Retention and Bladder Emptying Disorders

TERMINOLOGY	DEFINITION
LUTS	Any morbid phenomenon or departure from the normal in structure, function, or sensation experienced by the woman and indicative of disease or a health problem. Symptoms are either volunteered by, or elicited from the individual, or may be described by the individual's caregiver. **Bladder storage symptoms:** frequency, nocturia, urgency, OAB, urgency syndrome **Sensory symptoms:** increased/reduced/absent bladder sensation **Voiding and postmicturition symptoms:** slow stream, spraying, intermittency, hesitancy, straining, feeling of incomplete (bladder) emptying, need to immediately re-void, postmicturition leakage, position-dependent micturition, dysuria, (urinary) retention **Urinary incontinence symptoms:** stress, urgency, postural, nocturnal enuresis, mixed, continuous, insensible, coital **Pelvic organ prolapse (POP) symptoms:** vaginal bulge, pelvic pressure, bleeding/discharge/infection, splinting/digitation, low backache
Normal detrusor function (during voiding cystometry)	Achieved by an initial (voluntary) reduction in intraurethral pressure (urethral relaxation). This is generally followed by a continuous detrusor contraction that leads to complete bladder emptying within a normal time span. Many women will void successfully (normal flow rate and no PVR) by urethral relaxation alone, without much of a rise in detrusor pressure. The amplitude of the detrusor contraction will tend to increase to cope with any degree of bladder outflow obstruction.
Voiding dysfunction	A diagnosis by *symptoms and urodynamic investigations*, defined as abnormally slow and/or incomplete micturition
Detrusor underactivity	Detrusor contraction of reduced strength and/or duration, resulting in prolonged bladder emptying and/or a failure to achieve complete bladder emptying within a normal time span
Acontractile detrusor	One that cannot be demonstrated to contract during urodynamic studies resulting in prolonged bladder emptying and/or a failure to achieve complete bladder emptying within a normal time span
Bladder outflow obstruction	The generic term for obstruction during voiding. It is a reduced urine flow rate and/or presence of a raised PVR and an increased detrusor pressure. It is usually diagnosed by studying the synchronous values of urine flow rate and detrusor pressure and any PVR measurements.
Dysfunctional voiding	Voiding characterized by an intermittent and/or fluctuating flow rate due to involuntary intermittent contractions of the periurethral striated or levator muscles during voiding in neurologically normal women. This type of voiding may also be the result of an acontractile detrusor (abdominal voiding) with EMG or videourodynamics required to distinguish between the two entities.
Detrusor sphincter dyssynergia	Incoordination between detrusor and sphincter during voiding due to a neurologic abnormality (i.e., detrusor contraction synchronous with contraction of the urethral and/or periurethral striated muscles)
Acute retention of urine	A generally (but not always) painful, palpable, or percussible bladder, when the patient is unable to pass any urine
Chronic retention of urine	A nonpainful bladder where there is a chronic high PVR

Adapted from Haylen BT, de Ridder D, Freeman RM, et al. An International Urogynecological Association (IUGA)/International Continence Society (ICS) joint report on the terminology for female pelvic floor dysfunction. *Neurourol Urodyn* 2010;29(1):4–20.

LOWER URINARY TRACT PHYSIOLOGY

Many factors contribute to normal storage of urine and voiding, some which include neurologic, muscular, endocrine, and cognitive components.[8] Figure 26.1 is a simplified schematic of the urinary tract and its neurologic inputs and outputs. Fowler et al.[8] provide an excellent comprehensive and detailed review of lower urinary tract physiology. In order for the bladder to properly empty, it must generate a contraction that is strong enough to overcome the resistance of the outlet.[9] Disorders may develop of the bladder (detrusor dysfunction) or of the outlet (bladder outlet obstruction) that may lead to incomplete bladder emptying and voiding dysfunction.

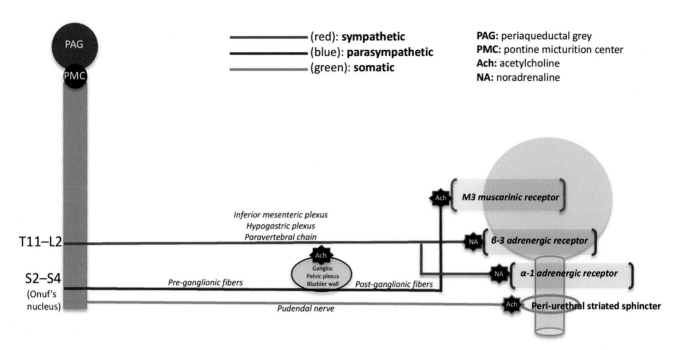

FIGURE 26.1 Physiology of voiding. (Reprinted by permission from Springer: Nitti V, Khan A. Retention and bladder-emptying disorders. In: Heesakkers J, Chapple C, De Ridder D, et al, eds. *Practical functional urology*. Switzerland: Springer International Publishing, 2016:353–370, reprinted with permission [License Number 4933271299074].)

Storage: The primary controller of urinary storage is the sympathetic nervous system, which uses activation of β_3-adrenergic receptors on the detrusor to promote bladder smooth muscle relaxation and α_1-receptors to contract the urethral smooth muscle. The effects on the outlet are reinforced by the somatic motor neurons which pass through the pudendal nerve to innervate the external urethral sphincter striated muscle and allow for a maintained contraction of these muscles.

Voiding: With increased bladder filling, the afferent messaging increases in intensity via pelvic nerves. This in turn stimulates the spinobulbospinal reflex pathway which then activates the pontine micturition center (PMC). The PMC then "flips the switch" and will simultaneously activate the parasympathetic nervous system while reflexively inhibiting the sympathetic and somatic fibers. This allows for relaxation of the outlet (the bladder neck and urethral sphincter) followed by stimulation of the detrusor muscarinic receptors by acetylcholine release. Subsequently, the bladder is able to contract through an open bladder outlet. Ongoing work is being done to learn about the roles of less studied pathways, such as periaqueductal gray matter and cognitive brain centers.

PATHOPHYSIOLOGY

There are many potential causes for incomplete bladder emptying and voiding dysfunction in women (Table 26.2). These causes can further be classified by whether it is due to dysfunction of the bladder (detrusor underactivity) or dysfunction of the bladder outlet (bladder outlet obstruction).

Bladder: Detrusor Underactivity

Primary dysfunction of the bladder now referred to as "detrusor underactivity" is defined as "a contraction of reduced strength and/or duration, resulting in prolonged bladder emptying and/or a failure to achieve complete bladder emptying within a normal time span."[10] Detrusor underactivity has replaced terms such as "impaired detrusor contractility," "detrusor areflexia," "hypotonic bladder," "underactive bladder (UAB)," and "detrusor/bladder failure." The causes for detrusor underactivity are variable and may stem from a variety of causes such as neurologic, pharmacologic, or myogenic etiologies. The clinical syndrome that occurs with detrusor underactivity is difficult to define due to the variability and nonspecific nature of symptoms associated with this condition, unlike with the clinical syndrome that accompanies OAB, but has been gaining attention by the medical community as of recently. One suggested definition by Osman et al.[11] of the clinical syndrome of UAB as "reduced sensation of the need to void (the opposite of urgency) that may be associated with frequency and nocturia or reduced voiding frequency often with a feeling of incomplete bladder emptying and incontinence that may predominate at nighttime." A study by Gammie et al.[12] analyzing their urodynamic database over 28 years identified several symptoms and signs that correlated with detrusor underactivity. Urodynamic criteria to be considered as having detrusor underactivity included a $P_{detQmax}$ <20 cm H_2O, Q_{max} <15 mL/s, <90% bladder volume emptying, and excluding any clinical obstruction. Women with detrusor underactivity compared to women with normal

TABLE 26.2

Causes of Incomplete Bladder Emptying in Women

INCOMPLETE BLADDER EMPTYING					
DETRUSOR UNDERACTIVITY			**BLADDER OUTLET OBSTRUCTION**		
NEUROPATHIC	**PHARMACOLOGIC**	**MYOGENIC**	**FIXED OBSTRUCTION**	**FUNCTIONAL OBSTRUCTION (INCOMPLETE RELAXATION)**	
				BLADDER NECK	**URETHRAL SPHINCTER**
Decentralization Infection Diabetes PD Multiple system atrophy Damage to lower motor neurons	Anticholinergics α-Agonists Narcotics Anesthetics	Overdistension Aging	**Distorted anatomy:** • Pelvic organ prolapse • Ectopic ureterocele **Vaginal/uterine pathology:** • Skene gland cyst/abscess • Retroverted/impacted uterus • Fibroid uterus • Vaginal/pelvic malignancy **Bladder neck/urethral pathology:** • Urethral caruncle • Urethral prolapse • Urethral diverticulum • Urethral stricture • Urethral carcinoma • Meatal stenosis **Iatrogenic:** • Anti-incontinence surgery • Urethral dilation	PBNO	Dysfunctional voiding Detrusor sphincter dyssynergia Fowler syndrome

pressure-flow studies had higher rates of decreased urinary stream, interrupted urinary stream, hesitancy, incomplete bladder emptying, palpable bladder, absent and/or decreased sensation, enuresis, and impaired mobility. Most recently in 2018, the ICS Working Group on UAB released a terminology report in which they define UAB symptoms as being "characterized by a slow urinary stream, hesitancy and straining to void, with or without a feeling of incomplete bladder emptying sometimes with storage symptoms," maintaining their prior ICS definitions for abnormal urodynamic detrusor activity for detrusor underactivity or acontractile detrusor.[13] They further state that UAB occurs in association with diverse pathophysiologies and based on current knowledge there is no single distinguishing symptom.

Neuropathic causes: Certain infections, such as HIV, herpes simplex virus, postinfectious polyneuritis causing Guillain-Barre, and tertiary syphilis have been found to cause neurologic dysfunction leading to impaired detrusor function.[14] Diabetic neuropathy may affect innervation to the detrusor leading to dulled sensory input and altered smooth muscle function.[15] Parkinson disease (PD) typically causes detrusor overactivity but has been found to present with detrusor underactivity or acontractility.[16] Patients that have suffered hemorrhagic or cerebellar infarcts have also demonstrated these findings.[17] Damage to the subsacral

lower motor neurons which exit from the lumbosacral vertebrae may occur through a variety of conditions, some which include trauma, multiple sclerosis, pelvic surgeries, disc herniation, spinal stenosis, myelodysplasia, and spinal arteriovenous malformations.

Pharmacologic causes: The impact of certain medications on the bladder may lead to poor detrusor function or poor relaxation of the bladder outlet. Although antimuscarinics are used for management of LUTS, they can have an effect in some in which the detrusor function is inhibited enough to lead to incomplete bladder emptying. Opioids can have similar effects on the bladder. The study discussed previously by Gammie et al.[12] also found a higher rate of detrusor underactivity on those on antidepressants. α-Agonists, such as phenylephrine, pseudoephedrine,[18] and clonidine, can lead to poor relaxation of the bladder neck.

Myogenic causes: Normal aging has been found to be associated with morphologic changes to the detrusor muscle in which there are decreased ratios of detrusor muscle to collagen.[19] Loss of bladder contractility and voiding efficiency with increasing ages has been demonstrated on urodynamic studies.[20] The insula, which is the region of the brain responsible for sensing visceral sensations, has shown diminished response to bladder filling on magnetic resonance imaging (MRI) in asymptomatic aging people.[21]

Overdistension can lead to reversible and irreversible changes to the detrusor smooth muscle contractile function.[22,23] Bladder outlet obstruction may lead to chronic overdistension that results in reduced blood flow and ischemic damage to detrusor myovesical plexuses and subsequent denervation.[24] There has also been an association found between childbirth and possible overdistension injury. Labor exceeding 700 minutes has shown to have increased risk for postpartum voiding dysfunction,[25] and persistent postpartum urinary retention has an estimated 0.05% incidence in a study that analyzed 8,000 consecutive births.[26] Independent risk factors associated with postpartum urinary retention are cesarean section birth and third- or fourth-degree perineal tearing.[27]

Postoperative urinary retention (PUR) following regional or general anesthesia has been reported in several surgical specialties. Urinary retention and urinary tract infection in patients who underwent hip fracture repair were reported in 39.3% and 24%, respectively,[28] which may have implications for hardware placed in those cases. Factors predictive of PUR include preoperative obstructive symptoms, age older than 50 years, male gender, spinal/epidural anesthesia, greater than 750 mL intraoperative fluids, anesthesia time greater than 2 hours, prolonged postoperative analgesia, and bladder volume greater than 270 mL upon entry to the postanesthesia care unit.[29,30] Extensive pelvic surgeries such as radical hysterectomy may lead to some degree of denervation that may also impact bladder function.[31]

Bladder Outlet Obstruction

Bladder outlet obstruction may be due to a fixed anatomic obstruction, or, less obviously, a failure of the outlet to relax resulting in a *functional* obstruction not due to a structural abnormality. Chronic outlet obstruction has shown association with many morphologic changes of the bladder, including changes to the extracellular matrix, mitochondria, smooth muscle enzymes, and electrical gap junctions.[22,32] It can lead to a rapid growth and hypertrophy of the smooth muscle of the bladder with an increase in collagenous connective tissue[33] but decreased myosin concentrations resulting in a diminished contractility of the bladder.[33,34] It has also been postulated that obstruction may lead to ischemia, which in turn can impact all the components of the bladder that comprise its viscoelastic properties such as the epithelium, connective tissue, vasculature, and smooth muscle. Ultimately, this may lead to acute muscle dysfunction.[33] It is theorized that the degree of muscle dysfunction is related to the degree of hypertrophy of the tissue and not so much the duration of the obstruction.[35] The bladder has shown remarkable regenerative abilities, however, and has shown recovery following some cases of obstruction in as short as 14 days after unobstruction.[36]

Fixed obstruction

There are many potential sources of fixed obstruction that may lead to incomplete bladder emptying in women, including distortion of the normal anatomy, vaginal, uterine, or urethral pathologies, or iatrogenic sources.

Distorted anatomy: There may be abnormal or distorted anatomy that leads to obstruction of the bladder neck or urethra. Some examples of this include an ectopic ureterocele or pelvic organ prolapse. Bladder prolapse in some may lead to kinking of the urethra or there may be extrinsic compression from a large rectocele or enterocele.[37]

Vaginal or uterine pathology: Conditions such as a Skene gland cyst or abscess, Bartholin gland cyst, retroverted or fibroid uterus, or impacted pregnant uterus may also be sources of extrinsic compression on the urethra. Vaginal malignancies or large pelvic malignancies may also cause extrinsic compression.[38,39]

Urethral pathology: Anatomic abnormalities or malignancies of the urethra may act as a fixed obstruction. These include conditions such as urethral diverticulum, urethral caruncle,[40] urethral prolapse, urethral stricture, meatal stenosis, or urethral carcinoma. Urethral stricture are estimated to have a prevalence of less than 1% in women who present with voiding complaints,[41] although they are likely underreported. They may be affiliated with a history of trauma, lichen sclerosis, or transurethral surgeries such as urethral dilations.

Iatrogenic: The most common cause for female bladder outlet obstruction in women is anti-incontinence surgery. Data evaluating PUR have estimated a 2% incidence of obstruction following SUI surgery.[42] This may be an underestimation, however, as it is possible that many women have significant obstructive symptoms due to a subclinical obstruction without significant voiding dysfunction.[43,44] There are varying rates of obstruction depending on which procedure was performed, with reports from greatest to least of 33% after autologous slings, 22% after Burch colposuspension, 20% following retropubic slings, and 7% and 4% for transvaginal needle suspension and tension-free vaginal tape, respectively.[45] Risk factors for obstruction following an anti-incontinence surgery include concomitant pelvic organ prolapse, prior history of anti-incontinence surgery, and preoperative urodynamics findings of a PVR greater than 100 mL, peak flow of less than 20 mL/s, or detrusor acontractility.[44]

Functional obstruction

A functional obstruction occurs due to a failure of relaxation or coordination of the bladder outlet rather than a fixed and structural obstruction. This may occur at the level of the bladder neck or at the urethral sphincter.

Primary bladder neck obstruction (PBNO): Failure of the bladder neck to open adequately during voiding is referred to as PBNO. This diagnosis is based on two general requirements, which are a lack of anatomic obstruction and lack of increased striated sphincter activity during voiding,[46] and is postulated to be due to either underlying neurologic pathology[47] or a failure of mesenchymal elements to properly degrade with subsequent incorporation of connective tissue and hypertrophy of smooth muscle in the region.[48] Recently, there has been an increased recognition of this condition in women,[49,50] although overall there is a paucity of literature and little estimation as to the prevalence of this condition.

Dysfunctional voiding: Poor relaxation of the urethral sphincter and/or pelvic floor in the absence of a neurologic etiology is referred to as dysfunctional voiding. In children, this was coined by Dr. Frank Hinman Jr as the "nonneurogenic neurogenic bladder,"[51,52] and sometimes is also called Hinman syndrome. This condition is thought to develop early in childhood and thought to resolve in most cases after puberty.[52] One theory on its development is a habitual pelvic floor and/or urethral sphincter contraction during micturition in young children with pelvic floor discomfort, such as from constipation or possibly abuse, or in response to urinary urgency.[53] This condition has also been noted in adults, possibly as a compensatory response to detrusor overactivity which leads to habitual urethral sphincter contraction throughout voiding, and is often is associated with a myriad of bothersome storage and voiding symptoms.[52] This dysfunctional voiding is diagnosed when the patient is noted to have variable contractions throughout their void which prevents them from emptying normally.

Fowler syndrome: First described in 1988,[54] Fowler syndrome differs from dysfunctional voiding or detrusor sphincter dyssynergia because these patients are often in retention but asymptomatic at the time of diagnosis.[55] This presents in typically postmenarche young females in the second and third decades of life with chronic inhibition of the detrusor due to a long-standing poorly relaxing external urethral sphincter.[55] An association was made in the original paper with Fowler syndrome and polycystic ovarian syndrome because 14 of the 22 women had this condition while also demonstrating abnormal electromyography (EMG) activity suggesting a possible hormonal contribution,[54] but as of yet, there is poor data to support this claim.[55]

NEUROGENIC LOWER URINARY TRACT DYSFUNCTION AND INCOMPLETE BLADDER EMPTYING

Urine storage and voiding is strongly mediated by the neurologic system. Neurologic insult through trauma or neurologic disease has the potential to manifest as urinary tract dysfunction in multiple ways depending on

where the injury has occurred. For the purposes of lower urinary tract dysfunction, classification of the region of injury can be classified further into cortical lesions (suprapontine), spinal cord lesions (pontine to suprasacral spinal cord), and sacral and peripheral nerve lesions.[56]

Cortical lesions may cause a lack of inhibition to the PMC, which leads to unmodulated output to the sacrum and uninhibited detrusor contractions causing urinary frequency, urgency, and at times incontinence. These lesions do not, however, typically cause incomplete bladder emptying. Spinal cord lesions have a variable impact on lower urinary tract function depending on the location of the lesion and if there is involvement of afferent input or upper or lower motor efferent fibers. If upper motor neurons fibers have been impacted, this has the potential to lead to increased spasticity of the bladder neck or urethral sphincter, which can lead to incomplete bladder emptying. Spinal cord lesions can lead to a failure of coordination of voiding such that the detrusor will contract, and the outlet will not relax or will reflexively also contract. This is called detrusor sphincter dyssynergia, and this can be further classified due to failure of the external sphincter to relax (detrusor external sphincter dyssynergia [DESD]) or the internal sphincter (detrusor internal sphincter dyssynergia [DISD]). It is possible to have concomitant DISD and DESD. DESD can occur from any suprasacral spinal cord lesion, where DISD can occur in lesions above the lower thoracic cord where the sympathetic nerves in the hypogastric nerve exit the spinal cord (see Fig. 26.1). Sacral and peripheral nerve lesions can lead to a nonfunctioning detrusor and a fixed external urethral sphincter, both which also can lead to incomplete bladder emptying with variable symptoms.

EVALUATION

It is important to perform a thorough workup and evaluation if concerned about voiding dysfunction in order to identify those at risk of upper and lower urinary tract decompensation and to offer appropriate therapies in a timely fashion. It is also critical to keep in mind that the patients can present anywhere along the spectrum of LUTS and objective findings; some may have symptoms that are quite debilitating despite limited objective findings; however, others may be relatively asymptomatic and present with upper tract deterioration.[43] The aims for the evaluation should be to define and characterize the LUTS, establish a diagnosis, and to identify those at risk for long-term sequelae or those already with urinary tract changes or dysfunction.

Symptoms and History

Generally, LUTS can be classified into storage (frequency; urgency; nocturia; and stress, urgency, mixed, coital, insensible incontinence), voiding (weak stream, terminal dribble, hesitancy, straining, intermittency, split stream), postmicturition (incomplete emptying, postmicturition incontinence), and other (bladder pain, dysuria). Familiarity with the terminology is important in order to fully understand the patient's condition, in addition to understand the acuity, duration, and level of bother associated with the symptoms.[57]

In patients with urinary retention, it is important to understand if this is an acute issue or has been chronic. Acute distention for a prolonged period of time has been termed "acute prolonged bladder overdistension" (ApBO),[58] defined as "a bladder filling volume at the time of diagnosis of at least 120% of a normal bladder capacity, which has lasted at least 24 hours."[59] This may be a consequence of spinal or epidural anesthesia, prolonged childbirth, or extensive pelvic or orthopedic surgery, and is often asymptomatic which may delay treatment. ApBO often differs from acute distention, which is more often due to an anatomic obstruction and causes significant symptoms.[58]

Surveys can be helpful in understanding patients' symptoms, degree of bother, and also for assessing progress over time. Studies predominantly have used the International Prostate Symptom Score (IPSS) when defining the prevalence of LUTS within a population; however, the IPSS was originally designed in 1992 by the American Urological Association for men.[60] Further studies have found that the survey can be found to be helpful in assess LUTS in women as well[61–63] independent of incontinence.[64] There is an instrument specifically designed for women, the International Consultation on Incontinence Modular Questionnaire on Female Lower Urinary Tract Symptoms which is a scored form derived from the Bristol Female Lower Urinary Tract Symptoms questionnaire. It is designed to assess symptom severity for the female lower urinary tract, impact to quality of life, and outcome effectiveness.[65,66]

A routine history should also be taken including obtaining any history of diabetes, infections, abdominal or pelvic radiation history, prolonged and/or complicated anesthesia or childbirth, trauma, stroke or any other neurologic diagnosis or abdominal, back, gynecologic or pelvic surgery history. Additional information should be obtained about childhood voiding patterns or any history of recurrent urinary tract infections and triggers for infections. Gastrointestinal symptoms of constipation, diarrhea, or fecal incontinence should be elicited. A sexual history is important, including obtaining information about dyspareunia, sexually transmitted diseases, or any history of any abuse. She should be queried for any symptoms of vaginal bulge or pelvic organ prolapse. Any prior evaluations she may have had and their results can be very helpful, and it is prudent to obtain labs, imaging, and operative notes that pertain to urogynecologic symptoms and history. Finally, it is important to understand the patient's functional status and social and home situations because these may have an impact on the treatment choices.

Physical Exam

A routine physical exam should also include particular aspects, including a lower abdominal exam to assess for a palpable or percussible bladder and a back exam to assess for vertebral or costovertebral angle tenderness. Abrams et al. cited the lowest threshold for a suprapubically palpable bladder of 300 mL based on urodynamic findings.[67] In patients with gastrointestinal symptoms, a rectal exam can demonstrate the presence of hard stools, fecal impaction, masses, or weak or loss of anal sphincter tone. Patients with a neurologic history or who relay neurologic symptoms (e.g., weakness in extremities, loss of sensation in the pelvis and perineum, spasticity) should have a basic neurologic exam. The extremities should also be examined for signs of edema or end-stage neuropathic or vascular disease. A pelvic exam is mandatory in women with symptoms of voiding dysfunction. The meatus should be examined for signs of stenosis or mass. The urethra should be palpated to assess for abnormalities, such as presence of foreign body in those who have had prior gynecologic surgeries, widening or expression of discharge that may suggest a urethral diverticulum, or for a mass. The vagina should be examined with a speculum to assess for cysts, masses, foreign bodies, and for pelvic organ prolapse. The position and mobility of the bladder neck and urethra can also be examined at this time. In addition, a palpation of the pelvic floor musculature is prudent to assess for pain or tension.

Labs

A urine dipstick should be obtained to assess for urinary tract infection or microscopic hematuria. If there is concern for any infection, the urine should be sent for culture and sensitivity. If there is microscopic hematuria and there is concern for malignancy in the patient due to their history (e.g., a history of smoking or occupational exposures), a urine cytology may be warranted. The urinalysis may also reveal proteinuria or significant glucosuria in those with early upper tract failure or poorly controlled diabetes. In those that there is concern for any renal dysfunction, a basic metabolic panel should be obtained to assess serum creatinine, electrolytes, and glomerular filtration rate.

Imaging

Routine upper tract imaging is not necessary unless there is concern for upper tract dilation or failure due to poor drainage or vesicoureteral reflux. If a patient has a significantly elevated PVR, complains of flank pain, or has a condition that is associated with impaired bladder compliance, it is reasonable to start by obtaining a renal and bladder ultrasound to assess for hydronephroureterosis, renal cyst, thinning renal parenchyma, renal or upper ureteral stone or mass, ureteral jets, and bladder stones.

Another option to assess for these findings would be a noncontrast computed tomography (CT) scan, and if necessary, a three-phase contrast CT scan can be performed to further elicit information in the entire urinary tract such as a potential source for any microscopic hematuria, enhancing lesions, transition points in the ureter in cases of hydroureter, and any other potential abdominal or pelvic pathology, such as large pelvic masses, colonic dilation or large stool burden, and pelvic floor laxity.

If the patient is unable to get contrast and an ultrasound does not provide sufficient information, a magnetic resonance urogram may be performed. A dedicated pelvic MRI is also an option in looking for pelvic and or urethral pathology such as urethral diverticulum, müllerian duct remnants,[68] or leiomyoma.[69] In patients with low glomerular filtration rate, there are risks of further renal function injury with intravenous contrast and the risk of nephrogenic systemic fibrosis with gadolinium, and any other suitable alternative imaging should be used to avoid these complications.

A voiding cystourethrogram (VCUG) is a study to assess for anatomic abnormalities of the bladder or urethra, such as urethral or bladder diverticulum. It can give some information on bladder capacity and can evaluate for vesicoureteral reflux. It is also very helpful in identifying the level of obstruction if it is present. Combined with multichannel urodynamics, this can be a very helpful tool in identifying the potential cause for incomplete bladder emptying and is discussed further when reviewing urodynamics (Figs. 26.2 to 26.5).

Studies

Cystourethroscopy/vaginoscopy: A cystourethroscopy can provide information on any mucosal or structural abnormalities of the urethra and bladder, such as masses, foreign bodies, potential entry point for the neck of a urethral diverticulum, significant trabeculations, bladder diverticulum, or displaced or abnormal appearing ureteral orifices. A pelvic exam may be performed to follow the cystoscopy if necessary. In some cases, a vaginoscopy at the time of cystoscopy may also help to identify any issues such as fistula or foreign body exposures.

Uroflow: A uroflow is a basic and noninvasive test to evaluate voided volume, peak and average flow rates, voiding time, and for possible straining during voiding. Low voided volumes, slow flows, prolonged voiding time, and a fluctuant or intermittent voiding pattern may all suggest some degree of voiding dysfunction is present.

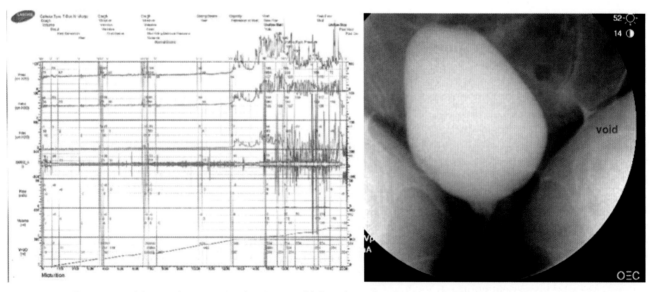

FIGURE 26.2 Detrusor sphincter dyssynergia. A 54-year-old female with a history of relapsing-remitting multiple sclerosis. Symptoms include urinary urgency, frequency, urinary hesitancy, sensation of incomplete bladder emptying, and occasional bilateral flank pain. Physical and pelvic exam, urinalysis, and renal function normal. PVR 165 mL. Renal ultrasound demonstrates bilateral renal scarring. Videourodynamics demonstrates a normal capacity bladder, normal compliance, normal sensation, and no incontinence. On voiding, the patient Valsalva voided and she had an increase in EMG activity resulting in a low flow rate with intermittency and a PVR of 400 mL. Fluoroscopy demonstrates narrowing at the midurethra with voiding. The patient was started on clean intermittent catheterization and is also being managed on an anticholinergic and will undergo annual surveillance.

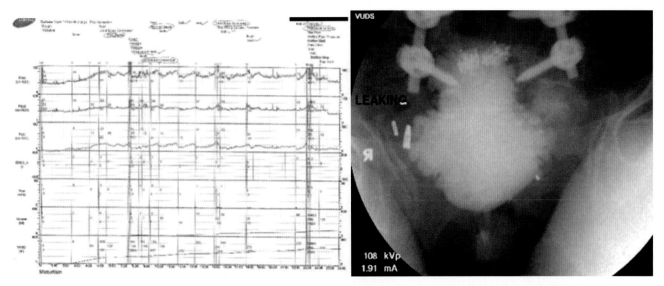

FIGURE 26.3 Impaired contractility. A 77-year-old female with a history of L2–L5 lumbar fusion in 2015 after which she developed UUI and recurrent urinary tract infections. She has failed therapy with four antimuscarinics and elected to undergo therapy with 100 units of onabotulinumtoxinA. Preprocedure PVR was 24 mL, and postprocedure ranged from 300 to 500 mL. Symptoms did not resolve and infections continued. Exam, renal function, and renal ultrasound normal. Videourodynamics demonstrated a small capacity early sensation bladder with mildly impaired compliance (detrusor leak point pressure [DLPP] 15 cm H_2O). She demonstrates detrusor overactivity with filling and detrusor underactivity with voiding (formally known as detrusor hyperreflexia with impaired contractility [DHIC]) with leakage with Valsalva maneuvers. PVR measurement is 227 mL. Fluoroscopy demonstrates a small bladder with multiple saccules and outpouchings and poor funneling of her bladder neck with voiding. The patient is currently performing self-intermittent catheterization (SIC) six times daily and is in discussions for potential lower urinary tract reconstruction.

PVR: A PVR measurement can be performed non-invasively with a bedside bladder scan or ultrasound and can often be the first identifier of incomplete bladder emptying. If these tools are unavailable or if a precise value is needed, a postvoid catheterization may be necessary. Portable ultrasonographic measuring tools have been shown to be comparable to catheterization.[70] There is no set definition for what is an abnormally elevated PVR measurement, but in the literature, a PVR of greater than 100 mL is often quoted.[3] A single site retrospective review study using this definition found an elevated PVR rate of 19% out of 201 charts reviewed, and on multivariate analysis, the independent predictors for an elevated PVR to be age older than 55 years, prior incontinence surgery, history of multiple sclerosis, and stage 2 or greater pelvic organ prolapse.[7] In another study evaluating women with OAB symptoms, those with a PVR greater than 100 mL had urgency and frequency without incontinence in 5% and 10% versus in those with urgency incontinence with an overall incidence of 9%.[6] It is prudent to interpret the PVR measurement in the context of the patient's symptoms and other clinical findings, particularly the urodynamics if available. An elevated PVR in a patient with decreased compliance may have more clinical significant than in the same patient were they to have normal compliance.

Urodynamics: The best and most definitive study to assess for the underlying factors contributing to incomplete bladder emptying is urodynamics.[71] The breadth of information obtained from urodynamics surpasses simple noninvasive tests and can give important details about the storage, voiding, and postvoid phases. Storage phase data includes characterization of lower urinary tract sensations with filling, bladder capacity, compliance, storage pressures, involuntary contractions, and urinary incontinence (stress, urgency, overflow, etc.). Voiding and postvoid phase information includes the same information as one may obtain from a uroflow and PVR measurement, but the distinguishing feature is the measurement of detrusor pressures while voiding. There can also be an assessment of pelvic floor and urethral sphincter activity and for the presence of straining during voiding. Although many variables such as test anxiety and catheter size may impact the results of urodynamics, it still remains the best test available to assess for detrusor contractile dysfunction with simultaneous pressure-flow analysis and quantification of the degree of any outlet obstruction.[43]

As discussed earlier, use of fluoroscopy to perform a VCUG at the time of urodynamics can be very helpful in identifying obstruction and at what level it exists. This is particularly helpful when trying to identify if there is a potential functional cause of the obstruction. In patients who have detrusor sphincter DESD, the classic description is a "spinning top" urethra.[72] In PBNO, there is a failure of the bladder neck to open and funnel

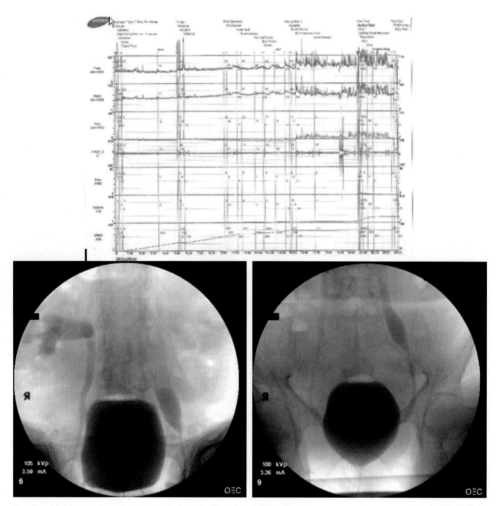

FIGURE 26.4 Neurogenic bladder. A 73-year-old female with a distant history of ovarian cancer status post total hysterectomy, bilateral salpingo-oophorectomy and chemoradiation in 1977. Urinary symptoms include nocturia, UUI, and recurrent urinary tract infections. Cystoscopy demonstrated debris and displaced ureteral orifices with a stadium-like appearance of the ureteral orifices. PVR was 170 mL. Pelvic exam largely unremarkable except she demonstrated severe vulvovaginal atrophy and SUI. Creatinine range of 1.2 to 1.4. CT scan demonstrates severe left hydronephroureterosis to pelvic ureter, right hydronephrosis, and a thickened bladder wall. Renal scan demonstrated 8% function of the left kidney and 92% function of the right kidney. Videourodynamics demonstrated a normal capacity bladder with no incontinence. On fluoroscopy, she demonstrated bilateral high-grade vesicoureteral reflux, and a long ureteral stricture of her distal left ureter is identified. She voided with Valsalva effort and an acontractile bladder with a PVR of 300 mL and no bladder outlet obstruction identified on fluoroscopy. The patient has initiated SIC and is considering urinary diversion with likely removal of her bladder and possibly her left kidney.

at the time of voiding. We have found fluoroscopy is the best identifier for outlet obstruction, independent of detrusor pressures, and maximum flow rates.[72] Additional information may also be obtained, including structural anatomic abnormalities of the bladder (diverticulum, filling defects, trabeculations) and urethra (diverticulum, stricture), and for the presence and grade of vesicoureteral reflux. The case vignettes discussed later show the enormous benefit of including fluoroscopy as part of the urodynamic evaluation (see Figs. 26.2 to 26.5).

A number of nomograms have been developed to define obstruction using data from urodynamics; however, their application is largely used in the evaluation of men. Perhaps because the prevalence and causes of obstruction in women are different, the existing

nomograms do not apply to women. Criteria that have been recommended for women include peak flows of less than 12 mL/s,[73] and 15 mL/s,[74–77] and detrusor pressure at peak flow rates of 20 cm H_2O[76] to greater than 50 cm H_2O.[78] Although it has been shown to overestimate the prevalence of obstruction in women,[79] the Blaivas-Groutz nomogram defines obstruction at a maximum rate of flow less than 12 mL/s in the presence of a sustained detrusor contraction greater than 20 cm H_2O with or without radiographic evidence of obstruction and/or the inability to void.[80] Choi et al.[77] went further and defined "voiding difficulty" as a peak flow rate of less than or equal to 15 mL/s. If the detrusor pressure at peak flow was greater than 20 cm H_2O on urodynamics, they were subclassified as having

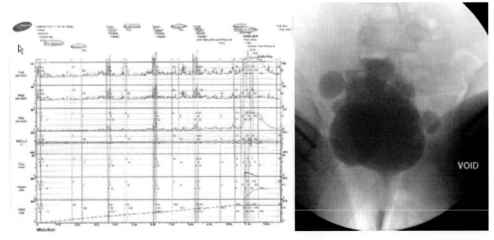

FIGURE 26.5 Dysfunctional voiding. A 29-year-old female with a history of epilepsy, polycystic ovarian syndrome, and endometriosis and a history of cervical conization and laser treatment for cervical dysplasia, with complaints of urgency, urgency and insensate incontinence, fecal incontinence, and bedwetting. Cystoscopy demonstrates significantly distorted bladder architecture with multiple bladder diverticulum. Pelvic exam demonstrates hypertense pelvic floor musculature with pain upon palpation. Renal function and urine testing normal. Videourodynamics demonstrate a very high-pressure flow which resulted in only moderate flow. Fluoroscopy demonstrates bladder neck funneling and some narrowing at midurethra. She demonstrated multiple bladder diverticulum with no evidence of vesicoureteral reflux. PVR measured 200 mL. An MRI of her spine is normal. The patient has begun therapy with PFPT and is trialing an antimuscarinic.

bladder outlet obstruction. If less than 20 cm H_2O, it was defined as detrusor underactivity. Under these criteria, analysis of 1,415 women that presented to urology offices, 12.8% complained of voiding difficulties and were found to have peak flows lower than 15 mL/s. Of these 102 women, 87.2% demonstrated obstruction and 12.8% demonstrated detrusor underactivity. In 1999, we developed the videourodynamics criteria for the diagnosis of obstruction.[72] This essentially states that obstruction is present if there is radiographic evidence of obstruction between the bladder neck and urethral meatus in the presence of a detrusor pressure of any magnitude independent of flow rate. More recently, the Solomon–Greenwell nomogram has been described to diagnose bladder outlet obstruction in women[81] using the videourodynamics criteria as the referent. Presented as a mathematical formula if $P_{detQmax} - 2.2 * Q_{max}$ is <0, there is <10% chance of obstruction, if >5 there is likely obstruction (50%) and if >18 obstruction is almost certain (>90%). Still today, our experience has shown that there can be quite a bit of variability in pressure-flow dynamics in women. We feel that an individualized diagnosis is crucial and favor the use of fluoroscopy for the diagnosis rather than the nomogramic approach when it is critical to diagnosis obstruction.

MANAGEMENT

After a proper evaluation, management options should be based on the patient's risks and bothersome symptoms. In patients with no risk factors who have a normal physical exam, negative urinalysis, acceptably low PVR, and either no or minimally bothersome symptoms, it is very reasonable to simply monitor the patient. In those with concerning history, such as a history of tobacco use, abdominal or pelvic radiation history, or prior urogynecologic surgeries, particularly if an implant was used, further studies may be warranted even if measured to have a low PVR. If a patient has an abnormal urinalysis with demonstration of microscopic hematuria, infection, proteinuria, and/or glucosuria, further testing is warranted. Drainage of the urinary tract is indicated in patients who are found to have any compromise to their renal function and drainage or those with risks of impending future upper tract deterioration. In patients that struggle with clinically significant recurrent urinary tract infections, defined in the 2019 American Urological Association Guidelines as three or more culture-proven infections in 12 months or two or more within 6 months,[82] who have elevated residuals, frequent drainage of the urinary tract is very important. Those patients with an elevated residual who do not have any risks or damage to their renal function and do not struggle with recurrent infections, the guiding factor for management will then be if and what LUTS they experience and the degree of bother they have from them. Figure 26.6 provides an algorithmic approach for the evaluation and management in the patient with concern for incomplete bladder emptying.

When it has been determined that a patient should have drainage of their urine, the next decision is how best to perform the drainage. Often drainage of the bladder via an indwelling catheter or by intermittent

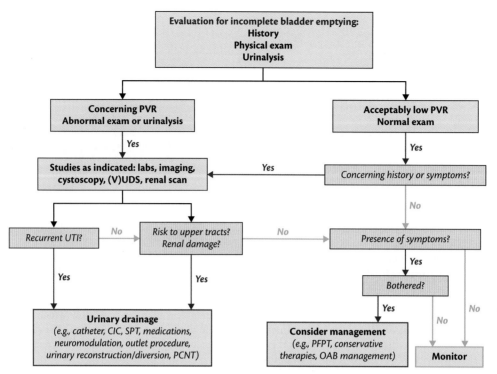

FIGURE 26.6 Approach to incomplete bladder emptying and voiding dysfunction in women. VUDS, videourodynamics; UTI, urinary tract infection; CIC, clean intermittent catheterization; SPT, suprapubic tube; PCNT, percutaneous nephrostomy tube.

catheterization is the first step regardless of the cause of impaired drainage. Patients may also be instructed to double or triple void to maximize their drainage. These are relatively conservative therapies and may be particularly helpful in patients with significant comorbidities that render them poor surgical candidates or in those refusing other medical or surgical interventions. In those that require chronic drainage, it may be preferable to place a suprapubic tube in order to avoid destruction of the bladder neck and/or urethra and for increased comfort and tolerability of the catheter.[83] Strict control of patient comorbidities and fluid management may assist in preventing progression of deteriorating function.

Bladder Dysfunction: Detrusor Underactivity

If a patient is determined to have detrusor underactivity, it is important to determine if there are any reversible causes for their dysfunction. For pharmacologic causes of detrusor dysfunction, exploration of suitable alternatives is warranted. For patients on antimuscarinics, consideration could be made to initiate a β_3-agonist instead, or consider advanced therapies such as neuromodulation. Intradetrusor onabotulinumtoxinA needs to be used cautiously due to its known risk for urinary retention. For those with chronic pain on opiates chronically, it may be prudent to enlist the help of pain medicine specialists to determine if there are nonopiate

options to assist in their management. The degree of dysfunction from medications is largely dependent on the mechanism of action of the drug and the patient's metabolizing and clearance ability and therefore can be quite variable between patients. No established time frame can usually be determined as to if and when the patient may regain bladder function.

General management should also include strict control of comorbidities and appropriate fluid management in order to prevent progression of any deteriorating lower urinary tract function. In patients with a neurologic disorder, early intervention and appropriate management of their condition may assuage progression of detrusor dysfunction, although in some may be unavoidable. It is also important to assess for any potential outlet obstruction that may be present. If it is deemed that there is obstruction, then the patient should be counseled about management options for those as well and also be apprised of the risks such as incontinence. Also, treatment of the outlet may not assist in bladder emptying if the bladder does not regain contractile ability, and the patient may still need to drain with a catheter or other therapies.

Drugs that have been used, although not all that effectively, to stimulate detrusor activity include α-adrenergic antagonists, muscarinic receptor agonists (e.g., bethanechol, carbachol), cholinesterase inhibitors (e.g., distigmine, pyridostigmine, neostigmine), prostaglandin E, and acotiamide.[14,84] Some data exists for support of using combination therapy with 5-mg distigmine with an α-blocker.[85] Unfortunately, many of the medications can cause significant side effects such as nausea, vomiting, diarrhea, sweating, and bronchospasm and are used infrequently in practice.

Patients that experience nonobstructive urinary retention due to a functional cause, such as Fowler syndrome, dysfunctional voiding, or detrusor sphincter dyssynergia, often have bladder hypocontractility or acontractility due to hypertonicity and failure of relaxation of the sphincter thereby leading to a chronic inhibition of detrusor function. In essence, their functional obstruction leads to detrusor dysfunction.

Neuromodulation: Neuromodulation, particularly sacroneuromodulation (SNM), has been extensively studied in animals as early as the 18th century, and over the past century, we have begun to have an understanding of its role in humans. The PMC is thought to provide stimulatory inputs to the sacral micturition reflex pathway. During the process of toilet training, the learned behavior of normal storage and voiding is provided through supraspinal inhibition to the PMC. Stimulation of sacral efferents demonstrates an impact on the reflex between the bladder and the urinary sphincter.[86] SNM can have impacts on both urinary storage and voiding disorders through its mechanisms. In 1999, the U.S. Food and Drug Administration approved its use in nonobstructive urinary retention. In patients in whom the retention is thought to be from nonneurogenic inhibition of sphincteric relaxation, SNM is postulated to have function at the level of the midbrain to allow afferent activity to modulate supraspinal circuitry and turn off the spinal guarding and urethral reflexes.[87-89] This in turn will decrease cortical activity to remove inhibition on the detrusor and allow resumption of bladder contractility.[55] One prospective study compared unilateral and bilateral stimulation in 33 patients with voiding dysfunction and found improved voiding parameters in those with bilateral stimulation but similar improvement in storage symptoms between groups.[90] Generally, however, it is not thought that there is not enough data to suggest a significant role for bilateral stimulation.

Bladder Outlet Obstruction

Table 26.2 reviews possible causes of a fixed and functional obstruction in women. If obstruction is identified early or without allowing chronic overdistension of the bladder, there is a high likelihood that there can be improvement of the retention after removing or bypassing the level of obstruction. If there has been long-standing obstruction, however, there can be irreversible changes to the bladder wall, such as trabeculations, fibrous replacement within bladder walls, or chronic distention

and decreased bladder contractility. On the other hand, some patients will develop detrusor hyperreflexia secondary to their obstruction, and aggressive surgical management can cause significant issues with incontinence following relief of the obstruction. It is important to have a thorough evaluation in order to properly understand the patient's risks and counsel on appropriate treatment choices.

Fixed obstruction

Distorted anatomy: In women with distortion of her anatomy due to conditions such as pelvic organ prolapse causing urethral kinking or extrinsic compression leading to obstruction, options for treatment should be discussed which include placing a pessary or proceeding with surgery. The options for prolapse surgery are vast and include restorative repairs or obliterative repairs. It is important to bear in mind that prolapse surgery in itself has been associated with PUR that may need to be managed long-term.[91,92] A recent retrospective review of 484 patient by Yune et al.[93] found a rate of PUR, defined as a PVR of greater than 150 mL following a retrograde fill voiding trial on the day of discharge of 26.4%, with an odds ratio of 3.26 for transvaginal prolapse repairs compared to robotic sacrocolpopexy.

Vaginal/uterine pathology: extrinsic compression of the bladder outlet by a vaginal mass or retroverted or impacted uterus likely needs to managed surgically, such as removal of a large vaginal cyst, consideration for hysterectomy, or management of any large pelvic or vaginal malignancies if oncologically appropriate.

Bladder neck/urethral pathology: Bladder neck, urethral, or meatal anomalies can cause obstruction due to narrowing of the lumen from intrinsic or extrinsic sources. Intrinsic sources may include large urethral caruncles or prolapse, urethral carcinoma, or urethral stricture or meatal stenosis. Depending on the cause, these may need to be surgically managed. In postmenopausal women, urethral caruncles and/or urethral prolapse can attempt to be managed by the use of topical estrogen therapy[94] but if refractory to therapy or if significantly large or thrombosed may need to be surgically excised. Urethral carcinoma should be managed per oncology guidelines based on the grade and stage of the malignancy. Urethral strictures may be managed with urethral dilation or with urethroplasty and meatal stenosis with meatoplasty. The largest series to date evaluating multi-institutional female urethral stricture management was recently published and reported on 210 patients.[95] At a median follow-up of 14.6 months, 64% of patients remained recurrence-free with the highest rate in those that underwent urethroplasty with either a local or free flap compared to women that underwent urethral dilation (recurrence-free at 12 months 83% and 77%, vs. 68%, respectively).[95]

Iatrogenic: For those that suffer from bladder outlet obstruction secondary to antimanagement, there is a possibility of significant improvement with removal or lysis of the sling or urethrolysis.[96] Gomelsky et al.[42] reported that up to 30% of women that undergo autologous sling may need to undergo sling lysis with 42% needing to perform long-term catheterization and up to 8% needing undergoing urethral dilation. In patients with obstructing transvaginal tape slings, cutting or loosening has shown high rates of restoration of normal voiding with significant improvement in urinary symptoms.[97,98]

Functional obstruction

PBNO: α-Adrenergic blocker medications are typically a low-risk option for PBNO in women.[99] If this fails, consideration could be made for transurethral incision of the bladder neck (TUIBN), but this has potential risks such as urinary incontinence or fistula.[100] The largest series to date for TUIBN is reported by Zhang et al.[101] on 84 women which reported improvement in 84.5% of women at 2-year follow-up. They also reported a 5% risk for fistula and stress incontinence when performing incisions at 5 and 7 o'clock compared to 2 and 10 o'clock.

Dysfunctional voiding: In women in whom they have a failure of sphincteric relaxation during voiding, pelvic floor physical therapy (PFPT) and biofeedback may be employed in order to "relearn" proper voiding coordination.[102] Patients may benefit from psychotherapy as well, particularly in those with a history of abuse.[103] Additional therapies that have been used include muscle relaxers, α-blockers, vaginal and oral benzodiazepine, neuromodulation, and Botox injections into the urinary sphincter.[104,105]

Fowler syndrome: Women with Fowler syndrome are often found to be in retention but are asymptomatic. These patients respond well to neuromodulation, although the other therapies previously discussed may also be considered. De Ridder et al.[106] evaluated 62 women with urinary retention who had SNM implantation of which 30 were diagnosed with Fowler syndrome. The women with Fowler syndrome compared to the idiopathic retention group had less SNM failures and had longer and better benefit over time. Success rates for resumption of spontaneous voiding have been found to be as high as 75%.[107,108]

Detrusor Sphincter Dyssynergia

Patients with a neurologic cause for sphincteric dysfunction need close surveillance to avoid upper tract deterioration. OnabotulinumtoxinA injections into the sphincter have been reported with moderate success but with a side effect of urinary incontinence.[109] Consideration could also be made to perform a sphincterotomy. The risks of this, however, are rendering the patient incontinent. Patients with neurologic conditions have higher risks for having detrusor hyperreflexia and should be counseled about their risks for incontinence following these therapies. In some, SIC may be their best outcome if they have good use of their upper extremities. In those with functional impairment, an indwelling urethral or suprapubic catheter may be preferred. Consideration could be made for urinary tract reconstruction or diversion. Patients with good dexterity of their upper extremities can be considered for a continent urinary diversion.

CONCLUSION

Voiding dysfunction and incomplete bladder emptying in women can be thought of as either a failure of either the detrusor (detrusor underactivity), obstruction of the bladder outlet, or both. They can lead to bothersome storage and voiding symptoms and can cause greater health concerns if developing recurrent infections and/or upper tract injury. There are multiple considerations to take into account when obtaining the history from the patient, and the evaluation should be catered based off those factors. The gold standard study to determine the underlying cause for the incomplete emptying is urodynamics, preferably with fluoroscopy, and should be performed for patients at risk for upper tract involvement or if there is not a clear etiology. After a complete and thorough evaluation, shared decision-making should guide the treatment choices employed. Detrusor underactivity has limited therapies, but a number of investigational therapies are on the horizon, including gene therapy promoting nerve growth factor, a neurotrophic protein important for sensory and sympathetic neuron function,[110,111] skeletal muscle-derived stem cell therapy.[110,112-115] In women with obstruction, determination between a functional and fixed obstruction will be the guiding factor in management.

References

1. Abrams P, Blaivas JG, Stanton S, et al. ICS standardisation of terminology of lower urinary tract function 1988. *Scand J Urol Nephrol Suppl* 1988;114:5–19.
2. Haylen BT, de Ridder D, Freeman RM, et al. An International Urogynecological Association (IUGA)/International Continence Society (ICS) joint report on the terminology for female pelvic floor dysfunction. *Neurourol Urodyn* 2010;29(1):4–20.
3. Robinson D, Staskin D, Laterza RM, et al. Defining female voiding dysfunction: ICI-RS 2011. *Neurourol Urodyn* 2012;31(3):313–316.

4. Irwin DE, Milsom I, Hunskaar S, et al. Population-based survey of urinary incontinence, overactive bladder, and other lower urinary tract symptoms in five countries: Results of the EPIC study. *Eur Urol* 2006;50(6):1306–1315.

5. Coyne KS, Sexton CC, Thompson CL, et al. The prevalence of lower urinary tract symptoms (LUTS) in the USA, the UK and Sweden: Results from the Epidemiology of LUTS (EpiLUTS) study. *BJU Int* 2009;104(3):352–360.

6. Fitzgerald MP, Jaffar J, Brubaker L. Risk factors for an elevated postvoid residual urine volume in women with symptoms of urinary urgency, frequency and urge incontinence. *Int Urogynecol J Pelvic Floor Dysfunct* 2001;12(4):237–240.

7. Milleman M, Langenstroer P, Guralnick ML. Post-void residual urine volume in women with overactive bladder symptoms. *J Urol* 2004;172(5 Pt 1):1911–1914.

8. Fowler CJ, Griffiths D, de Groat WC. The neural control of micturition. *Nat Rev Neurosci* 2008;9(6):453–466.

9. Brucker BM, Nitti VW. Evaluation of urinary retention in women: Pelvic floor dysfunction or primary bladder neck obstruction. *Curr Bladder Dysfunct Rep* 2012;7:222–229.

10. Abrams P, Cardoza L, Fall M, et al. The standardisation of terminology in lower urinary tract function: Report from the standardisation sub-committee of the International Continence Society. *Urology* 2003;61(1):37–49.

11. Osman NI, Chapple CR, Abrams P, et al. Detrusor underactivity and the underactive bladder: A new clinical entity? A review of current terminology, definitions, epidemiology, aetiology, and diagnosis. *Eur Urol* 2014;65(2):389–398.

12. Gammie A, Kaper M, Dorrepaal C, et al. Signs and symptoms of detrusor underactivity: An analysis of clinical presentation and urodynamic tests from a large group of patients undergoing pressure flow studies. *Eur Urol* 2016;69(2):361–369.

13. Chapple CR, Osman NI, Birder L, et al. Terminology report from the International Continence Society (ICS) Working Group on Underactive Bladder (UAB). *Neurourol Urodyn* 2018;37(8):2928–2931.

14. Miyazato M, Yoshimura N, Chancellor MB. The other bladder syndrome: Underactive bladder. *Rev Urol* 2013;15(1):11–22.

15. Yoshimura N, Chancellor MB, Andersson KE, et al. Recent advances in understanding the biology of diabetes-associated bladder complications and novel therapy. *BJU Int* 2005;95(6):733–738.

16. Araki I, Kitahara M, Oida T, et al. Voiding dysfunction and Parkinson's disease: Urodynamic abnormalities and urinary symptoms. *J Urol* 2000;164(5):1640–1643.

17. Burney TI, Senapati M, Desai S, et al. Acute cerebrovascular accident and lower urinary tract dysfunction: A prospective correlation of the site of brain injury with urodynamic findings. *J Urol* 1996;156(5):1748–1750.

18. Shao IH, Wu CC, Tseng HJ, et al. Voiding dysfunction in patients with nasal congestion treated with pseudoephedrine: A prospective study. *Drug Des Devel Ther* 2016;10:2333–2339.

19. Gilpin SA, Gilpin CJ, Dixon JS, et al. The effect of age on the autonomic innervation of the urinary bladder. *Br J Urol* 1986;58(4):378–381.

20. Madersbacher S, Pycha A, Schatzl G, et al. The aging lower urinary tract: A comparative urodynamic study of men and women. *Urology* 1998;51(2):206–212.

21. Griffiths D, Tadic SD, Schaefer W, et al. Cerebral control of the bladder in normal and urge-incontinent women. *Neuroimage* 2007;37(1):1–7.

22. Levin RM, Longhurst PA, Monson FC, et al. Effect of bladder outlet obstruction on the morphology, physiology, and pharmacology of the bladder. *Prostate Suppl* 1990;3:9–26.

23. Levin RM, Levin SS, Zhao Y, et al. Cellular and molecular aspects of bladder hypertrophy. *Eur Urol* 1997;32(Suppl 1):15–21.

24. Drake MJ, Mills IW, Gillespie JI. Model of peripheral autonomous modules and a myovesical plexus in normal and overactive bladder function. *Lancet* 2001;358(9279):401–403.

25. Yip SK, Sahota D, Pang MW, et al. Screening test model using duration of labor for the detection of postpartum urinary retention. *Neurourol Urodyn* 2005;24(3):248–253.

26. Groutz A, Gordon D, Woman I, et al. Persistent postpartum urinary retention in contemporary obstetric practice. Definition, prevalence, and clinical implications. *J Reprod Med* 2001;46(1):44–48.

27. Buchanan J, Beckmann M. Postpartum voiding dysfunction: Identifying the risk factors. *Aust N Z J Obstet Gynaecol* 2014;54(1):41–45.

28. Poh KS, Lingaraj K. Complications and their risk factors following hip fracture surgery. *J Orthop Surg (Hong Kong)* 2013;21(2):154–157.

29. Baldini G, Bagry H, Aprikian A, et al. Postoperative urinary retention: Anesthetic and perioperative consideration. *Anesthesiology* 2009;110(5):1139–1157.

30. Sivasankaran MV, Pham T, Divino CM. Incidence and risk factors for urinary retention following laparoscopic inguinal hernia repair. *Am J Surg* 2014;207(2):288–292.

31. Smorgick N, DeLancey J, Patzkowsky K, et al. Risk factors for postoperative urinary retention after laparoscopic and robotic hysterectomy for benign indications. *Obstet Gynecol* 2012;120(3):581–586.

32. Haefliger JA, Tissières P, Tawadros T, et al. Connexins 43 and 26 are differentially increased after rat bladder outlet obstruction. *Exp Cell Res* 2002;274(2):216–225.

33. Malmqvist U, Arner A, Uvelius B. Contractile and cytoskeletal proteins in smooth muscle during hypertrophy and its reversal. *Am J Physiol* 1991;63(5 Pt 1):C1085–C1093.

34. Sjuve R, Haase H, Morano I, et al. Contraction kinetics and myosin isoform composition in smooth muscle from hypertrophied rat urinary bladder. *J Cell Biochem* 1996;63(1):86–93.

35. Downie JW, Dean DM, Carro-Ciampi G, et al. A difference in sensitivity to alpha-adrenergic agonists exhibited by detrusor and bladder neck of rabbit. *Can J Physiol Pharmacol* 1975;53(4):525–530.

36. Elbadawi A, Meyer S, Regnier CH. Role of ischemia in structural changes in the rabbit detrusor following partial bladder outlet obstruction: A working hypothesis and a biomechanical/structural model proposal. *Neurourol Urodyn* 1989;8:151–162.

37. Florian-Rodriguez ME, Mehta K, Khatri G, et al. Rectal prolapse and urinary retention: A case report of an "anal cystocele." *Case Rep Womens Health* 2019;21:e00100.

38. Yazdany T, Bhatia NN, Nguyen JN. Urinary retention and voiding dysfunction in women with uterine leiomyoma: A case series. *J Reprod Med* 2012;57(9–10):384–389.

39. Kumar S, Sarkar D, Prasad S, et al. Large pelvic masses of obscure origin: Urologist's perspective. *Urol Int* 2012;88(2):215–224.

40. Coban S, Bıyık I. Urethral caruncle: Case report of a rare acute urinary retension cause. *Can Urol Assoc J* 2014;8(3–4):E270–E272.

41. Ackerman AL, Blaivas J, Anger JT. Female urethral reconstruction. *Curr Bladder Dysfunct Rep* 2010;5(4):225–232.

42. Gomelsky A, Scapero HM, Dmochowski RR. Sling surgery for stress urinary incontinence in the female: What surgery, which material? *AUA Update Series* 2003;XXII(Lesson 34):266–276.

43. Dmochowski RR. Bladder outlet obstruction: Etiology and evaluation. *Rev Urol* 2005;7(Suppl 6):S3–S13.

44. Shah S, Nitti VW. Diagnosis and treatment of obstruction following incontinence surgery—Urethrolysis and other techniques. In: Cardoza L, Staskin D, eds. *Textbook of female urology and urogynecology: Surgery for urinary incontinence*, 3rd ed. London: Informa UK, 2010:749–762.

45. Leach GE, Dmochowski RR, Appell RA, et al. Female Stress Urinary Incontinence Clinical Guidelines Panel summary report on surgical management of female stress urinary incontinence. The American Urological Association. *J Urol* 1997;158(3 Pt 1):875–880.

46. Padmanabhan P, Nitti VW. Primary bladder neck obstruction in men, women, and children. *Curr Urol Rep* 2007;8(5):379–384.

47. Awad SA, Downie JW, Lywood DW, et al. Sympathetic activity in the proximal urethra in patients with urinary obstruction. *J Urol* 1976;115(5):545–547.

48. Leadbetter GW Jr, Leadbetter WF. Diagnosis and treatment of congenital bladder-neck obstruction in children. *N Engl J Med* 1959;260(13):633–637.

49. Diokno AC, Hollander JB, Bennett CJ. Bladder neck obstruction in women: A real entity. *J Urol* 1984;132(2):294–298.

50. Axelrod SL, Blaivas JG. Bladder neck obstruction in women. *J Urol* 1987;137(3):497–499.

51. Hinman F Jr. Nonneurogenic neurogenic bladder (the Hinman syndrome)—15 Years later. *J Urol* 1986;136(4):769–777.

52. Allen TD. The non-neurogenic neurogenic bladder. *J Urol* 1977;117(2):232–238.

53. Brucker BM, Fong E, Shah S, et al. Urodynamic differences between dysfunctional voiding and primary bladder neck obstruction in women. *Urology* 2012;80(1):55–60.

54. Fowler CJ, Christmas TJ, Chapple CR, et al. Abnormal electromyographic activity of the urethral sphincter, voiding dysfunction, and polycystic ovaries: A new syndrome? *BMJ* 1988;297(6661):1436–1438.

55. Osman NI, Chapple CR. Fowler's syndrome—A cause of unexplained urinary retention in young women. *Nat Rev Urol* 2014;11(2):87–98.

56. Gajewski JB, Schurch B, Hamid R, et al. An International Continence Society (ICS) report on the terminology for adult neurogenic lower urinary tract dysfunction (ANLUTD). *Neurourol Urodyn* 2018;37(3):1152–1161.

57. Drake MJ. Fundamentals of terminology in lower urinary tract function. *Neurourol Urodyn* 2018;37(Suppl 6):S13–S19.

58. Madersbacher H, Cardozo L, Chapple C, et al. What are the causes and consequences of bladder overdistention? ICI-RS 2011. *Neurourol Urodyn* 2012;31(3):317–321.

59. Hinman F. Editorial: Postoperative overdistention of the bladder. *Surg Gynecol Obstet* 1976;142(6):901–902.

60. Wein AJ, Lee D. Benign prostatic hyperplasia and related entities. In: Wein AJ, Hanno PM, Malkowicz SB, eds. *Penn clinical manual of urology*. Philadelphia: Saunders Elsevier, 2007:479–522.

61. Lepor H, Machi G. Comparison of AUA symptom index in unselected males and females between fifty-five and seventy-nine years of age. *Urology* 1993;42(1):36–41.

62. Chancellor MB, Rivas DA. American Urological Association symptom index for women with voiding symptoms: Lack of index specificity for benign prostate hyperplasia. *J Urol* 1993;150(5 Pt 2):1706–1709.

63. Hsiao SM, Lin HH, Kuo HC. International prostate symptom score for assessing lower urinary tract dysfunction in women. *Int Urogynecol J* 2013;24(2):263–267.

64. Scarpero HM, Fiske J, Xue X, et al. American Urological Association Symptom Index for lower urinary tract symptoms in women: Correlation with degree of bother and impact on quality of life. *Urology* 2003;61(6):1118–1122.

65. Jackson S, Donovan J, Brookes S, et al. The Bristol Female Lower Urinary Tract Symptoms questionnaire: Development and psychometric testing. *Br J Urol* 1996;77(6):805–812.

66. Brookes ST, Donovan JL, Wright M, et al. A scored form of the Bristol Female Lower Urinary Tract Symptoms questionnaire: Data from a randomized controlled trial of surgery for women with stress incontinence. *Am J Obstet Gynecol* 2004;191(1):73–82.

67. Abrams PH, Dunn M, George N. Urodynamic findings in chronic retention of urine and their relevance to results of surgery. *Br Med J* 1978;2(6147):1258–1260.

68. Okur H, Gough DC. Management of müllerian duct remnants. *Urology* 2003;61(3):634–637.

69. Pavlica P, Bartolone A, Gaudiano C, et al. Female paraurethral leiomyoma: Ultrasonographic and magnetic resonance imaging findings. *Acta Radiol* 2004;45(7):796–798.

70. Huang YH, Bih LI, Chen SL, et al. The accuracy of ultrasonic estimation of bladder volume: A comparison of portable and stationary equipment. *Arch Phys Med Rehabil* 2004;85(1):138–141.

71. Nitti VW. Pressure flow urodynamic studies: The gold standard for diagnosing bladder outlet obstruction. *Rev Urol* 2005;7(Suppl 6):S14–S21.

72. Nitti VW, Tu LM, Gitlin J. Diagnosing bladder outlet obstruction in women. *J Urol* 1999;161(5):1535–1540.

73. Defreitas GA, Zimmern PE, Lemack GE, et al. Refining diagnosis of anatomic female bladder outlet obstruction: Comparison of pressure-flow study parameters in clinically obstructed women with those of normal controls. *Urology* 2004;64(4):675–681.

74. Dwyer PL, Desmedt E. Impaired bladder emptying in women. *Aust NZ J Obstet Gynaecol* 1994;34(1):73–78.

75. Stanton SL, Ozsoy C, Hilton P. Voiding difficulties in the female: Prevalence, clinical and urodynamic review. *Obstet Gynecol* 1983;61(2):144–147.

76. Lemack GE, Zimmern PE. Pressure flow analysis may aid in identifying women with outflow obstruction. *J Urol* 2009;163(6):1823–1828.

77. Choi YS, Kim JC, Lee KS, et al. Analysis of female voiding dysfunction: A prospective, multi-center study. *Int Urol Nephrol* 2013;45(4):989–994.

78. Massey JA, Abrams PH. Obstructed voiding in the female. *Br J Urol* 1988;61(1):36–39.

79. Massolt ET, Groen J, Vierhout ME. Application of the Blaivas-Groutz bladder outlet obstruction nomogram in women with urinary incontinence. *Neurourol Urodyn* 2005;24(3):237–242.

80. Blaivas JG, Groutz A. Bladder outlet obstruction nomogram for women with lower urinary tract symptomatology. *Neurourol Urodyn* 2000;19(5):553–564.

81. Solomon E, Yasmin H, Duffy M, et al. Developing and validating a new nomogram for diagnosing bladder outlet obstruction in women. *Neurourol Urodyn* 2018;37(1):368–378.

82. Malik RD, Wu YR, Zimmern PE. Definition of recurrent urinary tract infections in women: Which one to adopt? *Female Pelvic Med Reconst Surg* 2018;24(6):424–429.

83. Katsumi HK, Kalisvaart JF, Ronningen LD, et al. Urethral versus suprapubic catheter: Choosing the best bladder management for male spinal cord injury patients with indwelling catheters. *Spinal Cord* 2010;48(4):325–329.

84. Bayrak Ö, Dmochowski RR. Undeactive bladder: A review of the current treatment concepts. *Turk J Urol* 2019;45(6):401–409.

85. Sugaya K, Kadekawa K, Onaga T, et al. Effect of distigmine at 5 mg daily in patients with detrusor underactivity. *Nihon Hinyokika Gakkai Zasshi* 2014;105(1):10–16.

86. deGroat WC, Vizzard MA, Araki I, et al. Spinal interneurons and preganglionic neurons in sacral autonomic reflex pathways. *Prog Brain Res* 1996;107:97–111.

87. Dasgupta R, Fowler CJ. The management of female voiding dysfunction: Fowler's syndrome—a contemporary update. *Curr Opin Urol* 2003;13(4):293–299.

88. Dasgupta R, Wiseman OJ, Kitchen N, et al. Long-term results of sacral neuromodulation for women with urinary retention. *BJU Int* 2004;94(3):335–337.

89. Dasgupta R, Critchley HD, Dolan RJ, et al. Changes in brain activity following sacral neuromodulation for urinary retention. *J Urol* 2005;174(6):2268–2272.

90. Scheepens WA, de Bie RA, Weil EH, et al. Unilateral versus bilateral sacral neuromodulation in patients with chronic voiding dysfunction. *J Urol* 2002;168(5):2046–2050.

91. Turner LC, Kantartzis K, Shepherd JP. Predictors of postoperative acute urinary retention in women undergoing minimally invasive sacral colpopexy. *Female Pelvic Med Reconstr Surg* 2015;21(1):39–42.

92. Book NM, Novi B, Novi JM, et al. Postoperative voiding dysfunction following posterior colporrhaphy. *Female Pelvic Med Reconstr Surg* 2012;18(1):32–34.

93. Yune JJ, Cheng JW, Wagner H, et al. Postoperative urinary retention after pelvic organ prolapse repair: Vaginal versus robotic transabdominal approach. *Neurourol Urodyn* 2018;37(5):1794–1800.

94. Balai M, Gupta LK, Kumari A. Urethral caruncle in a perimenopausal female: Dramatic response to topical estrogen cream. *Indian J Urol* 2018;34(4):308–309.

95. Lane GI, Smith AL, Stambakio H, et al. Treatment of urethral stricture disease in women: A multi-institutional collaborative project from the SUFU research network. *Neurourol Urodyn* 2020;39(8):2433–2441.

96. Kim-Fine S, El-Nashar SA, Linder BJ, et al. Patient satisfaction after sling revision for voiding dysfunction after sling placement. *Female Pelvic Med Reconstr Surg* 2016;22(3):140–145.

97. Klutke C, Siegel S, Carlin B, et al. Urinary retention after tension-free vaginal tape procedure: Incidence and treatment. *Urology* 2001;58(5):697–701.

98. Rardin CR, Rosenblatt PL, Kohli N, et al. Release of tension-free vaginal tape for the treatment of refractory postoperative voiding dysfunction. *Obstet Gynecol* 2002;100(5 Pt 1):898–902.

99. Costantini E, Lazzeri M, Bini V, et al. Open-label, longitudinal study of tamsulosin for functional bladder outlet obstruction in women. *Urol Int* 2009;83(3):311–315.

100. Sussman RD, Drain A, Brucker BM. Primary bladder neck obstruction. *Rev Urol* 2019;21(2–3):53–62.

101. Zhang P, Wu Z-J, Xu L, et al. Bladder neck incision for female bladder neck obstruction: Long-term outcomes. *Urology* 2014;83(4):762–767.

102. McKenna PH, Herndon CD, Connery S, et al. Pelvic floor muscle retraining for pediatric voiding dysfunction using interactive computer games. *J Urol* 1999;162(3 Pt 2):1056–1063.

103. Pannek J, Einig E-M, Einig W. Clinical management of bladder dysfunction caused by sexual abuse. *Urol Int* 2009;82(4):420–425.

104. Franco I, Landau-Dyer L, Isom-Batz G, et al. The use of botulinum toxin A injection for the management of external sphincter dyssynergia in neurologically normal children. *J Urol* 2007;178(4 Pt 2):1775–1780.

105. Tarcan T, von Gontard A, Apostolidis A, et al. Can we improve our management of dysfunctional voiding in children and adults: International Consultation on Incontinence Research Society; ICI-RS2018? *Neurourol Urodyn* 2019;38(Suppl 5):S82–S89.

106. De Ridder D, Ost D, Bruyninckx F. The presence of Fowler's syndrome predicts successful long-term outcome of sacral nerve stimulation in women with urinary retention. *Eur Urol* 2007;51(1):229–234.

107. Swinn MJ, Kitchen ND, Goodwin RJ, et al. Sacral neuromodulation for women with Fowler's syndrome. *Eur Urol* 2000;38(4):439–443.

108. Datta SN, Chaliha C, Singh A, et al. Sacral neurostimulation for urinary retention: 10-Year experience from one UK centre. *BJU Int* 2008;101(2):192–196.

109. Jiang YH, Chen SF, Jhang JF, et al. Therapeutic effect of urethral sphincter onabotulinumtoxinA injection for urethral sphincter hyperactivity. *Neurourol Urodyn* 2018;37(8):2651–2657.

110. Chancellor MB, Yoshimura N, Pruchnic R, et al. Gene therapy strategies for urological dysfunction. *Trends Molec Med* 2001;7(7):301–306.

111. Goins WF, Yoshimura N, Phelan MW, et al. Herpes simplex virus mediated nerve growth factor expression in bladder and afferent neurons: Potential treatment for diabetic bladder dysfunction. *J Urol* 2001;165(5):1748–1754.

112. Huard J, Yokoyama T, Pruchnic R, et al. Muscle derived cell-mediated ex vivo gene therapy for urological dysfunction. *Gene Ther* 2002;9(23):1617–1626.

113. Kwon D, Minnery B, Kim Y, et al. Neurologic recovery and improved detrusor contractility using muscle-derived cells in rat model of unilateral pelvic nerve transection. *Urology* 2005;65(6):1249–1253.

114. Lee JY, Cannon TW, Pruchnic R, et al. The effects of periurethral muscle-derived stem cell injection on leak point pressure in a rat model of stress urinary incontinence. *Int Urogynecol J Pelvic Floor Dysfunct* 2003;14(1):31–37.

115. Yokoyama T, Huard J, Pruchnic R, et al. Muscle-derived cell transplantation and differentiation into lower urinary tract smooth muscle. *Urology* 2001;57(4):826–831.

CHAPTER 27

LOWER URINARY TRACT DYSFUNCTION DUE TO NEUROLOGIC DISEASE

Brendan Thomas Frainey • Howard B. Goldman

Introduction

Neurogenic lower urinary tract dysfunction (NLUTD), or "neurogenic bladder" as it is commonly referred to, describes dysfunction of the bladder and urethra due to a clinically confirmed neurologic disorder.[1,2] NLUTD is not a single entity but a variety of clinical signs and symptoms resulting in abnormal urinary storage and/or micturition.[1] Similarly, NLUTD is due to a heterogenous group of neurologic diseases, which can be congenital (i.e., spina bifida [SB]) or acquired (i.e., stroke and spinal cord injury [SCI]) in nature and affect either the central (i.e., multiple sclerosis [MS]) and/or peripheral nervous system (i.e., pelvic plexus injury). As a result, NLUTD is quite common, with 40% to 90% of patients with MS, 37% to 72% with Parkinson disease (PD), 70% to 84% with spinal cord injuries, and 15% with stroke estimated to have some element of NLUTD.[3,4] NLUTD can present in a variety of ways, but patients commonly note a change in baseline voiding function, reporting symptoms such as urinary urgency, frequency, incontinence, slow urinary stream, incomplete emptying, and recurrent urinary tract infection.

Although the clinical presentations and associated disease processes are diverse, the overarching goals of management for these patients are not. The main principles include protection of the upper urinary tract, prevention of urinary tract infections and sepsis, and maintenance of social continence and quality of life. To effectively do this, it is essential for the practicing urogynecologist to have a baseline understanding of normal micturition, the appropriate evaluation of patients with presumed NLUTD, and the main neurologic disease processes that can result in NLUTD so that these patients can be managed competently. In this chapter, we cover each of these topics and also provide a basic framework for categorizing patterns of NLUTD so that general treatment principles can be applied.

NEUROPHYSIOLOGY OF MICTURITION

In order to understand how pathology in the nervous system may affect the lower urinary tract, it is critical to first understand normal micturition. At the most basic level, normal micturition involves a storage phase and emptying phase. Passive, low-pressure urinary storage requires relaxation of the smooth muscle within the bladder and an appropriate resting tone of both the internal urethral sphincter (IUS) and external urethral sphincter (EUS) to prevent incontinence. Emptying, or voiding, requires an adequate detrusor contraction coordinated with relaxation of the pelvic musculature and IUS and EUS.[3,5-7]

The neural control governing micturition requires synchronized input from the central nervous system (CNS), autonomic nervous system (both parasympathetic and sympathetic), and somatic nervous system.[3,6] During bladder filling (storage phase), sympathetic and pudendal (somatic) nerves mediate tonic contraction of the IUS and EUS, respectively, via the sacral spinal cord and Onuf nucleus, creating a "guarding reflex" while the compliant bladder wall relaxes due to sympathetic inhibition of the detrusor muscle via the thoracolumbar spinal cord, preventing involuntary contractions during filling.[5,7,8]

Once the bladder reaches a critical volume (approximately 400 to 500 mL), stretch receptors within the detrusor illicit a spinal reflex, the "voiding reflex," mediated by the pontine micturition center (PMC), or Barrington nucleus, within the brainstem.[8,9] However, normal voiding is not initiated by a spinal reflex but is a voluntary decision primarily under cortical control. During bladder filling, the PMC is tonically inhibited, via the prefrontal cortex and periaqueductal gray in the midbrain. When it is socially acceptable to void, suppression of the voiding reflex ceases and micturition can occur.[5,8,10] Voiding (emptying phase) is then primarily driven by parasympathetic stimulation of the detrusor muscle via the sacral spinal cord, resulting in a bladder contraction, but also relaxation of the pelvic musculature, bladder neck, and EUS, creating an open, unobstructed urinary channel.[5,9]

Therefore, for successful micturition to occur, there must be intact neural signaling between the cerebral cortex, brainstem, spinal cord, and peripheral nerves,

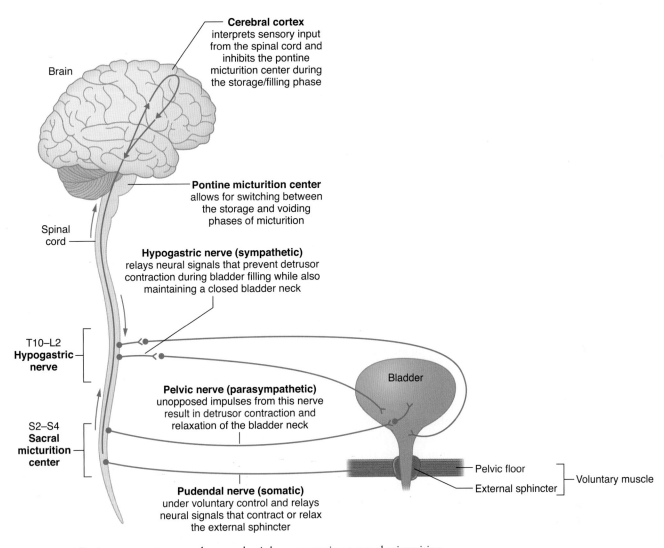

Cerebral cortex
interprets sensory input
from the spinal cord and
inhibits the pontine
micturition center during
the storage/filling phase

Brain

Pontine micturition center
allows for switching between
the storage and voiding
phases of micturition

Spinal
cord

Hypogastric nerve (sympathetic)
relays neural signals that prevent detrusor
contraction during bladder filling while also
maintaining a closed bladder neck

T10–L2
**Hypogastric
nerve**

Bladder

Pelvic nerve (parasympathetic)
unopposed impulses from this nerve
result in detrusor contraction and
relaxation of the bladder neck

S2–S4
**Sacral
micturition
center**

Pelvic floor

External sphincter

Voluntary muscle

Pudendal nerve (somatic)
under voluntary control and relays
neural signals that contract or relax
the external sphincter

FIGURE 27.1 Basic neuroanatomy and neurophysiology governing normal micturition.

which is demonstrated in Figure 27.1. When diseases or injury to the nervous system occur, it can lead to differing forms of lower urinary tract dysfunction (LUTD), which is described later.

EVALUATION

As with the assessment of any urogynecologic patient, evaluation of a patient with NLUTD requires a detailed history, physical examination, and appropriate laboratory and diagnostic studies. In this section, we review each of the major components of the history and physical, highlighting the unique aspects for patients with NLUTD.

History

The key components of the history include discussion of current symptoms (history of present illness) and

characterization of the neurologic disease process while placing these items in the context of the patient's overall lower urinary tract function. Other essential elements include assessment of bowel habits, sexual function, urinary tract infection and stone history, gynecologic history (if applicable), past medical and surgical history, current medications, family history, social history, functional status, and prior diagnostic studies performed (if applicable).[2,3,11,12]

Assessment of lower urinary tract function should involve questions regarding both storage and emptying symptoms. Storage symptoms include urinary urgency, frequency, nocturia, and urgency incontinence, whereas emptying symptoms include hesitancy, straining, intermittency, and reduced force of the urinary stream. The clinician should inquire if the patient self-catheterizes to empty the bladder. If so, document the frequency of catheterization, the type of catheter used, and if the patient is incontinent between catheterizations. A 2- to 3-day voiding diary is also recommended and can provide objective data regarding voiding habits and urine volumes to support the reported history.[12–14] Additionally, the frequency of symptomatic, culture-proven urinary tract infections must be evaluated because repeated infection can lead to long-term renal dysfunction.

When characterizing the neurologic disease or injury, several key components must be addressed[2]:

1. The location of the neurologic insult or "level of the lesion"—this aids the clinician in thinking about how normal micturition might be affected and predict patterns of LUTD (See "Classification" section for more details.)
2. The timing or onset of neurologic dysfunction—*is the condition congenital or acquired? What is the time course from neurologic insult/disease to urologic symptomatology? Has there been a significant change from baseline?*
3. The extent of the loss in function and the likelihood for progression—this will help determine appropriate management strategies and possible limitations for certain therapeutic options (i.e., manual dexterity and ability to self-catheterize)

The last several fundamental aspects of the history include assessment of bowel habits, presence of autonomic dysreflexia (AD), and functional status. Key questions regarding bowel function include *Does the patient sense passage of flatus or stool? How frequently do they have a bowel movement? Are they on a bowel regimen, and what does this entail (laxatives, enemas, digital stimulation)? Are they incontinent of stool?* These questions are critical as significant constipation can contribute to voiding dysfunction and must be managed aggressively. AD is a life-threatening clinical syndrome that can occur in patients with history of SCI. SCI patients, particularly those with lesions at thoracic level T6 or above, must be asked about a history of AD and associated signs and symptoms, which typically include severe hypertension, reflex bradycardia, sweating, flushing, and headache. Finally, the clinician must assess the patient's functional status including mobility, dexterity, occupation, and support system at home because these will all impact management strategies.

Physical Exam

Essential elements of a focused neurourologic exam include assessment of gross motor function, abdominal exam, a brief skin exam, and genitourinary (GU) exam, including digital rectal exam, pelvic exam, reflex testing, and sacral sensitivity testing.[13]

When assessing gross motor function, the clinician is able gain most of the relevant information just on initial inspection. *Does the patient use assistive devices or a wheelchair? Are the patient's extremities contracted? Do they have manual dexterity?* If the patient is able to stand or sit up, examine their back to assess for scoliosis, surgical scars, costovertebral angle tenderness, or lesions along the lower back such as a sacral dimple or hair tuft. If able to ambulate, assess the patient's gait.

Next, the abdominal exam consists of inspection for surgical scars, hernias, stomas, or catheterizable channels. The abdomen can be palpated to assess for suprapubic discomfort or abdominal distention secondary to an overdistended bladder or severe constipation if there is concern for bowel dysfunction. A brief examination of the skin to assess for ulceration in dependent areas such as the sacrum, hips, and lower extremities is critical in patients who use a wheelchair or orthotics for ambulation.

The last major component consists of the GU exam, including a pelvic exam in females. Assess for traumatic hypospadias if the patient has a history of chronic indwelling catheter. The clinician can next proceed to sacral sensitivity and reflex testing. Sacral sensitivity testing consists of light touch, pinprick, and proprioceptive maneuvers to determine if there is decreased sensitivity in any of the sacral dermatomes.[13] Abnormal findings can suggest lesions of the lumbosacral cord and their associated peripheral nerves. Reflex testing includes the bulbocavernosus reflex and anal reflex. The bulbocavernosus reflex is elicited by pinching the glans or applying pressure to the clitoris with a cotton swab while simultaneously assessing for anal sphincter contraction. In the female, one can often feel the bulbocavernosus contraction when two fingers are placed in the vagina. The anal reflex is performed by stroking the skin lateral to the anus and observing for anal contraction. For both, an absent reflex typically indicates a defect with the sacral reflex arc.[12,13,15,16] However, in neurologically intact females, the bulbocavernosus reflex can be absent in 30% of women and is not considered pathologic.[17] Finally, digital rectal exam should be performed to assess for prostatic enlargement in males and to assess for sphincter tone and fecal impaction in both males and females.

Laboratory and Diagnostic Studies

Relevant laboratory studies include urinalysis as well as urine culture if appropriate. Measurement of a postvoid residual urine volume (PVR), either via a portable bladder ultrasound device or straight catheterization, is also an essential component of the initial evaluation and provides important data regarding the patient's ability to effectively empty their bladder.[9,12,18,19] Although elevated residual volumes indicate voiding dysfunction, they unfortunately do not identify the etiology of incomplete emptying which can be secondary to poor detrusor function or an obstructed outlet.[9] Renal function panel and renal bladder ultrasound (RBUS) should also be considered, especially in patients with a history of chronic kidney disease or with elevated risk for upper tract deterioration.[9,12,20] European Association of Urology guidelines recommend RBUS be performed every 6 months.[12]

Urodynamic testing is a cornerstone in the assessment of NLUTD. Per the International Continence Society, urodynamics (UDS) are recommended for the "initial and long-term surveillance" of NLUTD.[21] However, it should always be used with a specific question in mind to help guide management.[2] Patient presentation may also determine need for UDS. For example, all would agree that a recent SCI patient should have baseline UDS; yet, many would not require UDS for a very functional patient with MS who has overactive bladder symptoms but empties easily without a significant PVR.

Multichannel urodynamics consists of a filling cytometry phase and a voiding pressure flow study and provides the most objective assessment of the lower urinary tract. The addition of electromyography (EMG) provides a gross estimation of pelvic floor and EUS function. The use of fluoroscopy during urodynamics, or videourodynamics (VUDS), provides real-time assessment of anatomic and functional information during bladder filling and emptying.

UDS provides a great deal of clinical information on lower urinary tract mechanics. Specifically, during filling, it allows for determination of detrusor overactivity, compliance, bladder capacity, and incontinence. The pressure-flow portion provides information regarding voiding pressures, sphincter coordination, and the ability to empty effectively. As seen in Table 27.1, poor compliance, elevated detrusor leak point pressures (DLPP; >40 cm H_2O), vesicoureteral reflux (VUR), and detrusor external sphincter dyssynergia (DESD) are key findings on VUDS suggestive of NLUTD and place the patient at risk for upper tract deterioration.[1,22,23]

TABLE 27.1

High-Risk Features Seen on Videourodynamics (VUDS)*

HIGH-RISK FEATURES SEEN ON VUDS
Poor compliance (<12 mL/cm H_2O)
Elevated DLPP (>40 cm H_2O)
DESD
VUR

*Presence of any of these high-risk features which can be seen on VUDS can place a patient at risk for upper tract deterioration.

CLASSIFICATION

Because of the heterogeneity in both clinical presentation and neurologic disease processes that can result in NLUTD, the authors believe that creating a classification system is useful to assist clinicians in predicting expected lower urinary tract symptoms (LUTS) and urodynamic findings. Although not absolute, we believe that categorization based on the location of the neurologic pathology or "level of the lesion" is the most intuitive way to recognize patterns of presentation for these patients, which is depicted in Figure 27.2 and Table 27.2.

Another method of characterizing patients with NLUTD uses a more functional classification system with urodynamic findings as an objective adjunct. With this system, the type of NLUTD can be categorized as a "failure to store" versus a "failure to empty" where either the bladder, the outlet (urinary sphincters), or both may be effected. The authors believe that this type of categorization may better assist clinicians in developing appropriate treatment and management strategies for these patients.

GENERAL TREATMENT PRINCIPLES

The principles of management for patients with NLUTD include protection of the upper urinary tract, prevention of urinary tract infections, and maintenance of social continence and quality of life.[9,12] All treatment considerations should take into account the patient's functional capability, level of social support, and goals of care. Urogynecologists should use a multidisciplinary approach with neurologists, physical medicine and rehabilitation specialists, and primary care physicians in order to provide this group of patients with appropriate, coordinated care.

Our method for determining the appropriate management strategy involves (1) identifying the location of the neurologic insult/lesion and (2) defining its effects on storage, emptying, or both. Treatment decisions should typically be based on objective urodynamic findings, but occasionally, therapies can be started prior to UDS if LUTS are straightforward and there is low risk for upper tract deterioration. Urodynamics can not only define whether there is a storage or emptying issue but also if it is a detrusor or outlet issue. Once these elements have been defined, the clinician can more easily determine the appropriate treatment approach. The various treatment approached based on functional assessment can be seen in Table 27.3. If the patient has abnormalities with both storage and emptying or both detrusor and outlet, the clinician should prioritize treatment of any high-risk features that place the patient at risk for upper tract deterioration and then consider level of symptomatic bother.

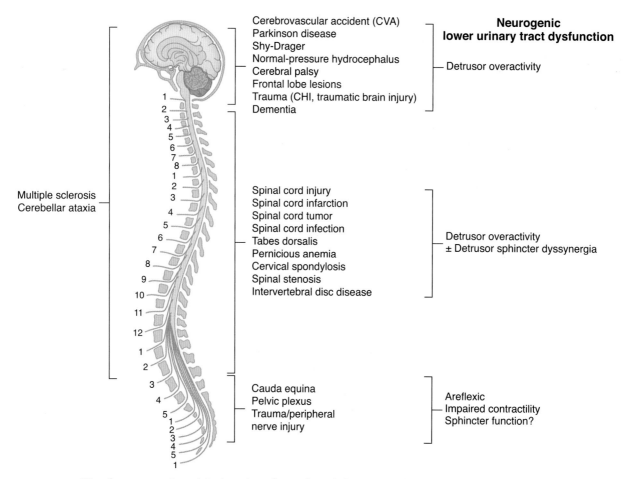

FIGURE 27.2 Visual representation of the location of neural insult for various disease states and their expected effects on lower urinary function. CHI, closed head injury.

TABLE 27.2

Classification of Expected NLUTD Based on the Location of the Neural Insult/Lesion

LEVEL OF LESION	BASIC PATHOPHYSIOLOGY	UDS FINDINGS	EXAMPLES
Suprapontine	Loss of tonic inhibition of the PMC leading to uninhibited voiding reflex	Detrusor overactivity	CVA Parkinson MS CP
Suprasacral spinal cord (pons to S2)	Development of new spinal afferent nerves during recovery which are more sensitive to low bladder volumes leading to reflexive detrusor contractions in an uncoordinated fashion with the external sphincter	All lesions: Detrusor overactivity DESD Lesions above T6: AD	SCI MS SB CP
Sacral spinal cord (S2–S4)	Parasympathetic nervous system dysfunction	Detrusor areflexia Onuf nucleus involved: Yes—flaccid sphincter No—functional sphincter	SCI SB
Peripheral nerves	Variable depending on location of injury—typically parasympathetic dysfunction	Detrusor underactivity Tonic sphincter	Pelvic plexus injury Disc disease

TABLE 27.3

Treatment Options Based on a Functional Classification System for Lower Urinary Tract Dysfunction

	FAILURE TO STORE	FAILURE TO EMPTY
Detrusor	Behavioral modification	CIC
	Anticholinergics/β_3-agonists	SNM
	Intravesical Botox	
	SNM	
	PTNS	
	Augmentation cystoplasty $+/-$	
	Continent catheterizable channel	
	Urinary diversion	
Outlet	Timed voiding	CIC
	External urinary collection device	Sphincteric Botox
		Sphincterotomy
	Bulking agent	Urinary diversion
	Urethral sling	
	Artificial urinary sphincter	
	Bladder neck/urethral closure	

Storage Dysfunction: Detrusor

This is the most commonly encountered problem because many neurologic injuries lead to detrusor overactivity and occasionally poor compliance and decreased bladder capacity. First-line therapies include behavioral modifications such as bladder training, timed voiding, fluid management, and pelvic floor rehabilitation.[2,9,24-28] Additional first-line therapy includes the use of anticholinergic agents such as oxybutynin, tolterodine, and trospium.[12] However, adverse effects, specifically on cognition, must be factored, and if the risks outweigh the benefits, use of β_3-agonists, mirabegron, or vibegron should be considered.

If these more conservative first-line options are unsuccessful, surgical options should be discussed. The intervention with the best evidence for neurogenic detrusor overactivity (NDO) is intravesical injection of botulinum toxin A (Botox).[12,29-35] Of note, 200 units is the recommended dose for NDO as compared to 100 units in the nonneurogenic setting. Long-term data has demonstrated the efficacy of repeat injections and it can be done in the office without anesthesia.[36,37] The most frequent complications include urinary tract infection and urinary retention, so the potential need for clean intermittent self-catheterization (CIC) in the postinjection period must be discussed with the patient.

Aside from Botox, other more minimally invasive surgical options include neuromodulation, specifically percutaneous tibial nerve stimulation (PTNS) and sacral neuromodulation (SNM). Although PTNS has shown some promise in MS and PD patients, it is limited by the fact that it requires frequent in-office treatments which may be difficult for this patient population.[38,39] Implantable tibial nerve stimulation devices are currently being studied and may be of benefit to these patients in the future. SNM has also been studied in MS patients but overall has been limited by concerns over the need for regular magnetic resonance imaging (MRI) studies in this cohort and the progressive nature of many neurologic diseases.[40] However, the concerns over MRI compatibility have now been obviated by the newest generation of MRI conditional SNM devices.[41]

More invasive surgical options include augmentation cystoplasty with or without concomitant continent catheterizable channel creation and urinary diversion. These options are only to be considered in appropriately selected patients where all other options have been exhausted. Augmentation cystoplasty incorporates an intestinal segment into the bladder to increase bladder capacity and lower storage pressures. Continent urinary diversions should be preferentially performed over incontinent diversions if feasible.[12]

Storage Dysfunction: Outlet

For patients with neurogenic stress urinary incontinence (SUI) due to an incompetent outlet and intrinsic sphincteric deficiency, surgical management provides the best outcomes. However, with any surgical procedure to correct SUI, there is a risk of creating obstruction. These risks and benefits must be weighed, especially in a neurogenic cohort. If the SUI is minor or the patient is a poor surgical candidate, conservative measures such as timed voiding, incontinence pessary, or use of external urinary collection devices can be considered. Conversely, if the SUI is severe, resulting in skin breakdown or significant decrement in patient quality of life, then surgical options should be discussed. Patients undergoing these procedures must be counseled on the risk for retention and possible need for CIC.

Urethral bulking agents are the least invasive option and can provide improvement in women. Urethral slings can be placed in both men and women but require different approaches. In females, slings are typically placed via a pubovaginal approach and can use mesh or autologous graft material such as rectus fascia or fascia lata. In males, slings can be placed either at the bladder neck via an abdominal approach or at the bulbar urethra via a perineal approach. Artificial urinary sphincters (AUS) can also be placed for severe incontinence but are typically only performed in males with NLUTD in the United States. In males, the cuff can be placed at either the bladder neck or the bulbar urethra with the pump located in the scrotum. An important consideration for AUS candidates is that they must have the manual dexterity to operate the pump. Finally, bladder neck closure is a "last resort" option for the end-stage outlet and should be performed concomitantly with suprapubic tube (SPT) placement and/or some form of catheterizable channel.[2,12,42]

Emptying Dysfunction: Detrusor

CIC is the first-line treatment for patients who are unable to adequately empty their bladder.[2,12] Occasionally, patients will require assistance from a caregiver or guardian if the patient does not have the manual dexterity or capability to perform CIC. The frequency of CIC is determined by urodynamic findings but is typically performed four to six times per day. Education of the patient and caregivers is essential for success.[43] Silicone catheters are typically preferred because they are less susceptible to encrustation and many NLUTD patients are latex allergic.

SNM has been U.S. Food and Drug Administration approved for the treatment of nonobstructive urinary retention since 1999.[44] It is thought to modulate the guarding reflex, facilitating voiding. However, currently, there is a dearth of evidence using SNM in patients with NLUTD.[45]

Emptying Dysfunction: Outlet

Emptying dysfunction due to the outlet in typically due to DESD. DESD refers to a detrusor contraction occurring concurrently with an involuntary contraction of the EUS and indicates inappropriate communication between the PMC and sacral spinal cord.[1] This can be identified on fluoroscopy during VUDS or on a multichannel UDS tracing as depicted in Figure 27.3A,B. As earlier, CIC is the mainstay of treatment for patients who are unable to adequately empty their bladder, whether from an underactive detrusor or obstructed outlet. However, there are several additional therapeutic options that have been well studied in this realm and may be indicated if necessary to protect the upper tracts. First, botulinum toxin A injection into the EUS has been shown to lower detrusor pressures and improve voided volumes in patients with detrusor sphincter dyssynergia but requires repeated injections.[46,47] Other endoscopic options include transurethral laser sphincterotomy which can be staged and repeated as needed so as not to totally lose sphincteric function.[47–49] Finally, urinary diversion can be considered as a last option when the bladder and sphincter are too hostile and place the upper tracts at risk.

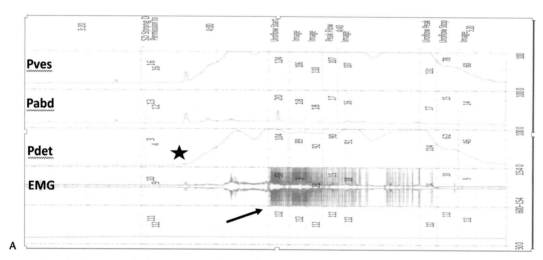

A

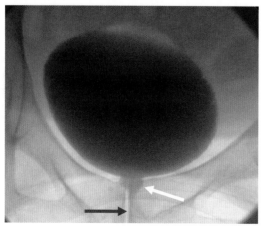

B

FIGURE 27.3 Videourodynamic findings of DESD. Fluoroscopic images obtained during videourodynamics on the right at corresponding points during urodynamic tracing on the left. **A:** Black star indicating the onset of a detrusor contraction noted by the rise in detrusor pressure (Pdet) and intravesical pressure (Pves). *Black arrow* demonstrating active contraction of the external urinary sphincter during detrusor contraction. **B:** *White arrow* indicated an open bladder neck and proximal urethra. *Red arrow* demonstrating a contracted/closed EUS not allowing passage of contrast. DESD, detrusor external sphincter dyssynergia; EUS, external urethral sphincter; Pabd, abdominal pressure.

SPECIFIC DISORDERS

In this section, we address some of the most commonly seen neurologic disorders associated with NLUTD and briefly discuss prevalence, clinical presentation, urodynamic findings, and general treatment principles for each. Although this is not exhaustive, we encourage you to use our framework for categorizing various diseases and predicting the associated clinical presentation based on the location of neurologic insult.

Multiple Sclerosis

MS is an autoimmune demyelinating disorder of the CNS and is the most common nontraumatic disabling neurologic disease in young adults.[50,51] The prevalence within the United States has been estimated at 150 per 100,000 individuals (~400,000 individuals in the United States), with females 3 times as likely as males to develop MS.[52] Demyelinating lesions can involve the cerebral cortex, spinal cord, and optic nerves, leading to a host of clinical manifestations.

LUTD is incredibly common in MS, with a reported 80% to 96% of patients pursuing urologic care.[51,53] The incidence of NLUTD appears to increase with disease duration, with most MS patients having some element of LUTD within 6 to 10 years of diagnosis.[9,54–56] Urinary urgency and frequency are the most commonly reported symptoms and are noted in 37% to 99% of MS patients. Obstructive symptoms such as incomplete emptying, hesitancy, and urinary retention are also common, occurring in 34% to 79% of patients. Urge incontinence has been reported in 19% to 80% of patients based on current series.[51,55,57,58] Importantly, about 10% of patients will have LUTD as part of their initial presentation prior to a diagnosis of MS.[53,59,60] Therefore, urogynecologist must have a high index of suspicion and refer to neurology if other findings of MS are noted on review of systems.

There are no standardized recommendations for the use of UDS in patients with MS. However, urodynamic abnormalities are abundant in MS patients and can be seen in 90% of individuals. The most common finding is detrusor overactivity (34% to 99%, mean occurrence 65%) followed by DESD (3% to 83%, mean 35%), detrusor underactivity (0% to 40%, mean 25%), and poor compliance (2% to 10%).[51,55,61] UDS findings commonly do not correlate with clinical symptoms, with one study revealing 52% of patients without LUTS had "silent" UDS abnormalities.[62] Despite this, the risk for upper tract deterioration in patients with MS is quite low, even in the presence of bladder outlet obstruction from DESD.[63–66] Therefore, the universal use of UDS in patients with MS has come into question.[53] However, UDS can be critical in determining the etiology of incomplete emptying in this group

(hypocontractile detrusor vs. bladder outlet obstruction) so that the proper management strategies can be employed. Additionally, some studies have shown that neurologic symptom severity, defined by the Expanded Disability Status Scale (EDSS), positively correlates with pathologic UDS findings.[53,67,68] Therefore, the authors believe that UDS are warranted in patients with severe neurologic symptoms or those with poor compliance or DESD on initial UDS because these patients may have higher risk for upper tract deterioration.[66,69]

Appropriate and timely treatment of NLUTD in MS patients is essential because LUTD has been shown to significantly decrease quality of life in this patient population.[70] The choice of management strategy is guided by the urodynamic findings. In patients with pure detrusor overactivity, initial therapies should include behavioral modification, pelvic floor rehabilitation, and/or pharmacologic therapy (antimuscarinics or β_3-agonist) to reduce symptom burden, improve bladder capacity, and reduce the frequency of involuntary detrusor contractions.[28,71,72] If these conservative approaches fail, intravesical botulinum toxin injection or neuromodulation (SNM, PTNS) can be considered because both have demonstrated efficacy in patients with MS.[32,33,40,72,73] Until recently, the use of SNM had been limited in this patient population due to the requirement of regular MRIs and device incompatibility. However, this limitation is being overcome by newer device generations that are now MRI compatible.[41] If there is any element of incomplete emptying, either due to detrusor overactivity with DESD or a hypocontractile detrusor, clean intermittent catheterization is an essential element of management in order to maintain a low-pressure system.[7] However, clinicians must ensure that the patient's manual dexterity and functional capabilities would allow for this. In the era of botulinum toxin and neuromodulation, major surgical interventions such as augmentation cystoplasty with catheterizable channel creation or urinary diversion are performed less commonly and must also take into consideration functional status, quality of life, and life expectancy.

Suprasacral Spinal Cord Injury

According to the National Spinal Cord Injury Database, in 2019, there were an estimated 17,810 new SCI cases per year in the United States, with a prevalence of about 294,000 individuals living with SCI. Mean age at time of injury has been steadily increasing and is currently 43 years of age. SCI has a male predominance, with 78% of new SCI cases being men.[74]

When evaluating patients with SCI, it is critical to determine the level of the injury and whether the injury is complete or incomplete in order to accurately determine the type of NLUTD expected and the extent of neurologic recovery. An intact spinal cord is required for communication between the pontine micturition central and sacral spinal cord to occur so that the bladder can appropriately transition between the storage and emptying phases of micturition. The majority of SCI are incomplete lesions and occur above the T12 vertebral level.[75,76]

Initially after SCI, there is a period of spinal shock defined by decreased excitability of spinal cord segments below the level of the injury, which clinically manifests as flaccid muscular paralysis and urinary retention secondary to an areflexic, acontractile bladder and closed EUS.[75,77] Depending on the severity of the injury, this phase can last days to weeks but is typically between 6 and 12 weeks.[78,79] During this time, the patient should be managed with CIC or an indwelling catheter. CIC is preferred because urinary incontinence between catheterizations may often be the first sign of lower urinary tract recovery.

Urologic evaluation is typically performed 3 to 6 months following the injury, with urodynamics, specifically VUDS, providing the most objective assessment of the lower urinary tract.[78–81] Eighty-one percent of all SCI patients report some form of LUTD at 1 year following injury, although symptoms often do not correlate with UDS findings.[82,83] As a result of the recovery process following neurologic insult, new afferent pathways within the spinal tract develop, resulting in reflexive detrusor contractions in response to low filling volumes which manifest as NDO on UDS or as urinary leakage or incontinence clinically.[5,76] DESD is another urodynamic hallmark of suprasacral SCI, which, in combination with NDO, can lead to elevated intravesical pressures, VUR, incomplete emptying, and ultimately upper tract deterioration.[84–86] There are no consensus guidelines as to timing for repeat urodynamics, but most agree that at minimum, yearly urologic evaluation is warranted with the frequency of UDS determined by the presence of high-risk features such as poor compliance, DESD, or DLPP >40 cm H_2O.[80] In addition to UDS, upper tract imaging, such as RBUS, should also be performed annually, given the elevated risk for upper tract deterioration as compared to other disease states associated with NLUTD.[64,81,84]

In SCI patients with lesions at or above T6, AD may occur in response to noxious stimuli below the level of the lesion. This potentially life-threatening clinical syndrome is defined by severe hypertension but can also present with headache, flushing, sweating, bradycardia, and piloerection. Common etiologies for AD including bladder overdistention or fecal impaction. Management includes removal of the noxious stimuli (i.e., drain the bladder), placing the patient in the upright position, closely monitoring vitals, and administering pharmacologic agents such as nitrates or calcium channel blockers if needed.[81,87]

The primary goals of long-term management for SCI patients are to preserve renal function and maintain quality of life by preventing incontinence and complications.[2,12,79,88] Treatment strategies should be tailored to the specific urodynamic findings but also must consider the patient's goals and functional status.[89] Although SCI patients may develop a wide variety of pathophysiology affecting either the bladder, outlet, or both during either storage or emptying phases of micturition, we will focus on the typical patient with NDO and DESD. Conservative therapies are the preferred initial management strategy with implementation of CIC being the most critical management option for patients with unsafe storage or emptying.[81,89–91] NDO should initially be managed with the addition of antimuscarinic therapy.[12,89] Alternatively, intravesical botulinum A toxin injection has also been well studied in SCI patients with NDO.[30,34,35,89,90] Transurethral botulinum A toxin injection to the EUS as well as transurethral sphincterotomy have been also been described in the setting of significant DESD but are not first-line management options.[47,49] Major surgical procedures such as augmentation cystoplasty, sacral rhizotomy, or urinary diversion should only be considered in well-selected patients where all other conservative or minimally invasive options have failed.

Parkinson Disease (PD) and Multiple Systems Atrophy

PD is a neurodegenerative disorder primarily affecting the dopaminergic neurons within the substantia nigra but also involving a heterogenous group of other neurons within the CNS. It is diagnosed clinically with defining features including bradykinesia, resting tremor, rigidity, and postural instability.[92,93] The incidence of PD significantly increases with age, with an estimated incidence of 8 to 18 per 100,000 person years. The prevalence is estimated to be 0.3% of the general population in industrialized countries, equating to about 985,000 individuals in the United States. Mean age at diagnosis is 60 years, and there is a male predominance, with males being affected 1.5 to 2 times as often as females.[92,93]

Depending on the definition used, the incidence of LUTD in patients with PD varies between 27% and 80%.[75,94–97] The onset of LUTD typically occurs an average of 6 years from PD diagnosis.[98] Additionally, the severity of LUTD appears to correlate with the degree of neuromotor disability, suggesting an association between dopaminergic neurodegeneration and LUTD.[9,76,94,99,100] When LUTD does occur, the primary symptoms are storage related (urgency, frequency, nocturia, urge incontinence), occurring in 50% to 75% of patients.[75,101,102] Nocturia is the most commonly reported symptom (~70%) and has a considerable impact on quality of life.[97] Voiding symptoms are less commonly reported, occurring in 17% to 27% of patients.[96]

The most common urodynamics finding in PD is NDO, which occurs in 45% to 93% of patients.[96,98,101,103,104] The proposed pathophysiology of NDO in PD is that the basal ganglia have an inhibitory effect on the voiding reflex via dopaminergic neurons which ceases with loss of these cells in the substantia nigra.[100,105,106] However, the neurodegeneration of higher voiding centers which regulate cortical control of voiding is also thought to contribute as well.[103,107] Other key urodynamic features include detrusor hypocontractility and pseudodyssynergia secondary to bradykinesia of the EUS, but typically, these findings do not result in urethral obstruction or elevated PVRs.[97,103–105,108]

Management of PD must factor in symptom severity and quality of life because storage symptoms may impact quality of life more substantially in patients with bradykinesia and motor dysfunction. If postvoid residuals are low (<100 mL), behavioral modifications and anticholinergic medications provide the mainstay of symptom management, although no randomized clinical trials have been performed in this group.[109] If there is concern for cognitive impairment, which is common in PD patients, consideration for β$_3$-agonists such as mirabegron or vibegron may be a more appropriate pharmacologic agent given its reduced side effect profile.[97] Intravesical botulinum toxin A injection is an option for refractory neurogenic urgency incontinence and has demonstrated efficacy in several small series of PD patients.[29,110] SNM has been studied in this patient population as well but with mixed results.[111–113] In the setting of an elevated PVR, urodynamic findings should guide management. If detrusor hypocontractility is present, initiation of CIC may be all that is necessary if the patient has the dexterity necessary to perform it. Deep brain stimulation of the subthalamic nucleus is a promising option for PD patients because it has not only been proved to ameliorate motor symptoms but can also improve both LUTS and UDS parameters.[97,114–116]

Multiple systems atrophy (MSA) is another progressive neurodegenerative disorder with parkinsonian features in addition to cerebellar and autonomic symptoms.[75,109] It is often misdiagnosed as PD early on in the disease course. However, unlike with PD, up to 60% of patients with MSA have urologic symptoms that precede parkinsonian symptoms.[109,117,118] Other key features that favor MSA over PD are elevated PVRs, open bladder neck on VUDS, and striated sphincter denervation on EMG.[119] Historically, transurethral procedures for treatment of benign prostatic hypertrophy were contraindicated in men with PD due to increased risk for postoperative incontinence. However, when patients with MSA were excluded, more recent studies have demonstrated improvement in lower urinary tract function following transurethral procedures in men with PD. Therefore, transurethral

procedures in men with PD can be performed as long as a diagnosis of MSA is excluded first.[75]

Cerebrovascular Accident

An estimated 795,000 people suffer a cerebrovascular accident (CVA), or stroke, each year.[120] Although stroke is the fifth leading cause of mortality in the United States, 75% of CVA victims ultimately survive, resulting in significant morbidity and disability.[120,121] In 2008, there were an estimated 5.8 million stroke survivors.[122] Eighty-seven percent of strokes are ischemic in nature with the remaining 13% hemorrhagic.[120] Although strokes typically occur in the elderly, 34% of stroke victims in 2009 were younger than 65 years old.[123]

Both ischemic and hemorrhagic CVA ultimately lead to areas of infarction within the brain, some of which may negatively impact cortical control of voiding via inhibition of the micturition reflex.[75] The acute phase after stroke presents similar to spinal shock, with urinary retention reported in 50% of patients within 3 days following CVA due to detrusor areflexia.[124] However, urinary incontinence is also noted in 32% to 79% of CVA victims on admission and can persist in 12% to 19% at about 6 months.[125,126]

Following the acute phase, up to 80% of patients may report LUTD, with nocturia (70%), incontinence (~35%), and frequency (18%) being the most commonly reported symptoms.[127] Similarly, the most common urodynamic finding following CVA is detrusor overactivity.[128,129] Because the lesion is above the PMC, DESD is typically not present and both sphincters are coordinated.[125,129] The second most common urodynamic finding is detrusor underactivity with elevated PVR, which is present in about one-third of patients following CVA.[124] Studies have suggested that hemorrhagic strokes may be more likely to present with detrusor underactivity than ischemic strokes.[124,130]

Treatment of CVA is similar to that of PD because both are suprapontine lesions with NDO and an intact EUS as their predominant finding. Initial management should include behavioral modifications such as timed voiding, fluid management and urge suppression, pelvic floor physical therapy, and judicious use of anticholinergics or β$_3$-agonists if PVRs are low.[131] If detrusor underactivity and elevated PVRs are seen on UDS, CIC should be introduced if dexterity allows. Botulinum toxin A has not been well studied in patients with CVA but has shown efficacy in several small studies and could be considered in appropriately selected patients where the need to perform CIC is not an issue.[31,131,132] Data on PTNS is limited but has shown promise as a minimally invasive third-line option.[133] Surgical therapies on the prostate should be avoided for at least 6 to 12 months following CVA because LUTS and UDS findings may evolve during this time period.

Spina Bifida

SB, or myelodysplasia, is a congenital condition that arises due to the incomplete closure of the vertebral column with or without associated malformation of the neural tube. SB entails a wide spectrum of malformations which range in severity from a fatty filum terminale (least severe) to myelomeningocele (most severe). The incidence of SB in the United States is 1 to 2 cases per 1,000 population, with about 1,500 infants born with myelomeningocele each year. The estimated prevalence is 166,000 individuals living with SB in the United States.[134] The overall incidence has been decreasing in large part due to folate supplementation.

LUTD is determined by the level of neural tube defect with 2% of myelomeningocele with a cervical level, 5% thoracic, 26% lumbar, 47% lumbosacral, and 20% sacral.[75] Most studies suggest LUTD in 90% of patients, with incontinence being a key finding. In one study analyzing the National Spina Bifida Patient Registry, 34% of patients remained incontinent over the study period.[135] Symptoms typically begin in infancy/childhood but can recur or worsen later in life, which should raise concern for retethering of the spinal cord.

UDSs are an essential component of evaluation in SB patients because history and neurourologic exam often do no correlate with UDS findings. Detrusor overactivity with DESD is the most common urodynamic pattern seen because the majority of the lesions are suprasacral. However, any combination of detrusor and sphincteric findings can be seen.[136] Additionally, many patients with SB can have poorly compliant bladders.[137,138] Therefore, VUDS are often preferred over standard UDS to assess for VUR, bladder neck and sphincteric competence/synergy, bladder trabeculations, and other high-risk features.

Although survival has improved drastically, protection of the upper tracts remains the priority for management in patients with SB given their elevated risk for renal deterioration.[22,64,139-141] The second major component of management is promoting urinary continence. To accomplish these goals, all patients and parents are educated on CIC at an early age and started on anticholinergic medications. Reconstructive procedures such as augmentation cystoplasty, creation of a continent catheterizable channel, and bladder neck procedures should be reserved for patients refractory to conservative therapies and require extensive preoperative discussion with patients and guardians.

Pelvic Plexus Injury

The pelvic plexus, or inferior hypogastric plexus, is a paired autonomic nerve plexus which runs alongside the anterolateral rectum and lateral vagina in females, innervating the viscera of the pelvic cavity. The pelvic plexus is composed of both sympathetic fibers from the hypogastric nerve and parasympathetic nerves from the pelvic nerve.[75,142] Injury to this plexus can occur commonly during radical pelvic surgery leading to LUTD. Incidence of pelvic plexus injury is estimated at 20% to 68% for abdominoperineal resection, 16% to 80% for radical hysterectomy, 20% to 25% for low anterior resection, and 10% to 20% for proctocolectomy.[75] However, these rates are likely overestimates given the development of nerve-sparing techniques.[143-145]

Approximately one-third of patients report some element of LUTD, with common complaints being poor emptying, urgency, frequency, and incontinence. The type of LUTD depends on the specific nerves injured and the extent of injury. However, the most common initial presentation is difficulty emptying and urinary retention. Key urodynamic features include impaired detrusor contractility, decreased compliance, open bladder neck, and fixed EUS.[146-149] Management should be directed at maintaining low-pressure storage and protecting the upper urinary tracts with CIC. The majority of patients will have resolution of voiding dysfunction by 6 to 12 months, but 15% to 20% may have permanent LUTD. Therefore, more invasive therapies should be avoided early on and the patient should be monitored clinically for improvement.[75]

Cerebral Palsy

Cerebral palsy (CP) is a heterogenous disorder of movement and posture resulting from an insult to the immature brain.[150] CP often presents within the first 3 years of life and is defined by the nonprogressive nature of the neurologic deficit and wide variation in motor impairment.[75,151] The etiology of CP is unknown in up to 80% of cases but is often attributed to perinatal hypoxia or infection. The incidence varies between 2 and 2.5 per 1,000 live births with a prevalence of approximately 400,000 individuals living in the United States with CP at any given time.[151,152] In addition to motor impairment, CP is often associated with disturbances of sensation, cognitive deficits, communication issues, and epilepsy.

Studies indicate LUTD is present in 55% of individuals with CP. The most commonly reported symptoms include urinary incontinence (20% to 94%), urgency (38.5%), and frequency (22.5%). Voiding symptoms are less prevalent, with hesitancy noted in 2% to 51.5% of patients.[153] Urodynamic abnormalities are discovered in 85% of patients, with NDO being the most common finding with an average prevalence of 59%. Other UDS features include decreased bladder capacity (73.5%) and less commonly DESD (11%).[153-158] Importantly, several studies have found that patients with UDS abnormalities did not endorse any LUTS prior to UDS, highlighting the need for objective monitoring of lower urinary tract with UDS.[154,155] Patients with more severe significant spasticity, functional impairment, and cognitive deficits seem to be at higher risk for LUTD and UDS abnormalities.[153] Adult patients with CP and LUTD require close surveillance with UDS because they have been shown to have higher rates of poor compliance and elevated DLPP, placing them at higher risk for upper tract deterioration.[156]

Management of NLUTD in CP should begin with conservative measures, which include development of a toileting plan, a strict bowel regimen, perineal skin care, and anticholinergic medications if storage symptoms or NDO predominate.[159-161] Some experts believe CIC should be reserved for patients with recurrent urinary retention or high-risk features for upper tract deterioration, given the difficulty with CIC in this group due to fine motor impairment, contractures, and pelvic/EUS spasticity.[161] If conservative measures fail, endoscopic options (intravesical botulinum toxin A) and surgical options such as SNM or augmentation cystoplasty with or without catheterizable channel can be considered. SPT placement should be the last resort for patients unable to be successfully managed with conservative measures and poor surgical candidates.

Lumbar Disk Disease and Cauda Equina

Lumbar disc disease refers to herniation of the nucleus pulposus from the intervertebral disc space resulting in compression of the associated sacral spinal roots, most commonly at the L4/L5 and L5/S1 vertebral spaces.[162-164] Lumbar disc disease is one of the most common causes of low back pain, with an incidence of 5 to 20 cases per 1,000 adults annually. It most commonly occurs in the third to fifth decade of life and has a male predominance of 2 to 1.[163,164]

LUTD has been reported in 27% to 92% of individuals with lumbar disc disease.[162,165,166] Compression of the sacral spinal roots often leads to disruption of both the parasympathetic and somatic nervous system. Therefore, common symptoms include difficulty emptying, straining to void, or urinary retention. Urodynamics are normal in about three quarters of cases and demonstrate detrusor areflexia in the remaining quarter.[166] These patients also typically have delayed sensation but have good compliance and are at low risk for upper tract deterioration. Treatment of LUTD aims to correct the underlying cause, specifically via laminectomy. However, laminectomy may not improve lower urinary tract function in many cases.[167]

Cauda equina syndrome refers the symptoms of perineal sensory loss in addition to diminution of both anal and urinary sphincter function due to significant compression of the sacral nerve roots. Cauda equina syndrome occurs in 1% to 5% of herniated lumbar discs cases but can be a result of other etiologies as well.

Unlike with standard lumbar disc disease, cauda equina syndrome requires acute surgical decompression. Studies have shown that early decompression within 48 hours have much higher rates of resolution of their LUTD.[168]

CONCLUSION

NLUTD is quite common and is associated with a wide variety of neurologic disorders, demonstrating the importance of neural control over lower urinary tract function. Principles of management include protection of the upper urinary tract, prevention of urinary tract infections, and maintenance of social continence and quality of life.

In addition to a focused history and physical, urinalysis, PVR, and UDS form the basis of NLUTD evaluation. Typically, objective urodynamic data rather than LUTS inform management decisions for these patients, but in certain instances, UDS may not be necessary. Identification of high-risk UDS features such as poor compliance, increased DLPP, VUR, or DESD helps stratify which patients may be at increased risk for upper tract deterioration and require closer surveillance.

Knowledge of the basic NLUTD patterns and major neurologic disease states associated with NLUTD will allow clinicians to more effectively manage these patients. All management decisions should take into account the patient's functional capability, level of social support, and personal goals of care. Patients with NLUTD require multidisciplinary care and the urogynecologist can play a critical role in their health.

References

1. Gajewski JB, Drake MJ. Neurological lower urinary tract dysfunction essential terminology. *Neurourol Urodyn* 2018;37(S6): S25–S31.
2. Drake MJ, Apostolidis A, Cocci A, et al. Neurogenic lower urinary tract dysfunction: Clinical management recommendations of the Neurologic Incontinence Committee of the fifth International Consultation on Incontinence 2013. *Neurourol Urodyn* 2016;35(6):657–665.
3. Dorsher PT, McIntosh PM. Neurogenic bladder. *Adv Urol* 2012;2012:816274.
4. Ginsberg D. The epidemiology and pathophysiology of neurogenic bladder. *Am J Manag Care* 2013;19(Suppl 10):s191–s196. Accessed September 15, 2020. https://www.ajmc.com/view/ace012_jul13_ngb_ginsberg1_s191
5. Fowler CJ, Griffiths D, de Groat WC. The neural control of micturition. *Nat Rev Neurosci* 2008;9(6):453–466.
6. Brown E, Wein A, Dmochowski R. Pathophysiology and classification of lower urinary tract dysfunction: Overview. In: Partin AW, Dmochowski RR, Kavoussi LR, et al, eds. *Campbell-Walsh-Wein urology*. 12th ed. Philadelphia: Elsevier, 2020:2514–2524.
7. Chancellor MB, Yoshimura N. Neurophysiology of stress urinary incontinence. *Rev Urol* 2004;6(Suppl 3):S19–S28.

Accessed September 23, 2020. http://www.ncbi.nlm.nih.gov/pubmed/16985861

8. Drake MJ, Fowler CJ, Griffiths D, et al. Neural control of the lower urinary and gastrointestinal tracts: Supraspinal CNS mechanisms. *Neurourol Urodyn* 2010;29(1):119–127.

9. Panicker JN, Fowler CJ, Kessler TM. Lower urinary tract dysfunction in the neurological patient: Clinical assessment and management. *Lancet Neurol* 2015;14(7):720–732.

10. Griffiths D. Neural control of micturition in humans: A working model. *Nat Rev Urol* 2015;12(12):695–705.

11. Bors E, Turner RD. History and physical examination in neurological urology. *J Urol* 1960;83:759–767.

12. Groen J, Pannek J, Diaz DC, et al. Summary of European Association of Urology (EAU) guidelines on neuro-urology. *Eur Urol* 2016;69(2):324–333.

13. Giusto LL, Zahner PM, Goldman HB. Considerations for the focused neuro-urologic history and physical exam. In: Corcos J, Karsenty G, Thomas K, et al, eds. *Essentials of the adult neurogenic bladder.* Florida: CRC Press, 2020:135–144.

14. Cameron AP, Wiseman JB, Smith AR, et al. Are three-day voiding diaries feasible and reliable? Results from the Symptoms of Lower Urinary Tract Dysfunction Research Network (LURN) cohort. *Neurourol Urodyn* 2019;38(8):2185–2193.

15. Wyndaele JJ, De Sy WA. Correlation between the findings of a clinical neurological examination and the urodynamic dysfunction in children with myelodysplasia. *J Urol* 1985;133(4):638–639.

16. Schurch B, Schmid DM, Kaegi K. Value of sensory examination in predicting bladder function in patients with T12-L1 fractures and spinal cord injury. *Arch Phys Med Rehabil* 2003;84(1):83–89.

17. Lucioni A, Kobashi K. Evaluation and management of women with urinary incontinence and pelvic prolapse. In: Partin AW, Dmochowski RR, Kavoussi LR, et al, eds. *Campbell-Walsh-Wein urology.* 12th ed. Philadelphia: Elsevier, 2020:2525–2538.

18. Merritt JL. Residual urine volume: Correlate of urinary tract infection in patients with spinal cord injury. *Arch Phys Med Rehabil* 1981;62(11):558–561. Accessed September 24, 2020. https://pubmed.ncbi.nlm.nih.gov/7316711/

19. Alnaif B, Drutz HP. The accuracy of portable abdominal ultrasound equipment in measuring postvoid residual volume. *Int Urogynecol J Pelvic Floor Dysfunct* 1999;10(4):215–218.

20. Satar N, Bauer SB, Shefner J, et al. The effects of delayed diagnosis and treatment in patients with an occult spinal dysraphism. *J Urol* 1995;154(2):754–758.

21. Abrams P, Andersson KE, Birder L, et al. Fourth international consultation on incontinence recommendations of the International Scientific Committee: Evaluation and treatment of urinary incontinence, pelvic organ prolapse, and fecal incontinence. *Neurourol Urodyn* 2010;29(1):213–240.

22. McGuire EJ, Woodside JR, Borden TA. Upper urinary tract deterioration in patients with myelodysplasia and detrusor hypertonia: A followup study. *J Urol* 1983;129(4):823–826.

23. McGuire EJ. Urodynamics of the neurogenic bladder. *Urol Clin North Am* 2010;37(4):507–516.

24. Ostaszkiewicz J, Johnston L, Roe B. Timed voiding for the management of urinary incontinence in adults. *Cochrane Database Syst Rev* 2004;(1):CD002802.

25. Eustice S, Roe B, Paterson J. Prompted voiding for the management of urinary incontinence in adults. *Cochrane Database Syst Rev* 2000;(2):CD002113.

26. Gormley A, Lightner DJ, Burgio KL, et al. Diagnosis and treatment of overactive bladder (non-neurogenic) in adults: AUA/SUFU guideline. Accessed September 29, 2020. https://sufuorg.com/resources/guidelines.aspx

27. Wallace SA, Roe B, Williams K, et al. Bladder training for urinary incontinence in adults. *Cochrane Database Syst Rev* 2004;(1):CD001308.

28. De Ridder D, Vermeulen C, Ketelaer P, et al. Pelvic floor rehabilitation in multiple sclerosis. *Acta Neurol Belg* 1999;99(1):61–64. Accessed September 27, 2020. https://pubmed.ncbi.nlm.nih.gov/10218095/

29. Giannantoni A, Conte A, Proietti S, et al. Botulinum toxin type A in patients with Parkinson's disease and refractory overactive bladder. *J Urol* 2011;186(3):960–964.

30. Schurch B, Stöhrer M, Kramer G, et al. Botulinum-A toxin for treating detrusor hyperreflexia in spinal cord injured patients: A new alternative to anticholinergic drugs? Preliminary results. *J Urol* 2000;164(3, Pt 1):692–697.

31. Kuo H-C. Therapeutic effects of suburothelial injection of botulinum A toxin for neurogenic detrusor overactivity due to chronic cerebrovascular accident and spinal cord lesions. *Urology* 2006;67(2):232–236.

32. Schulte-Baukloh H, Schobert J, Stolze T, et al. Efficacy of botulinum-A toxin bladder injections for the treatment of neurogenic detrusor overactivity in multiple sclerosis patients: An objective and subjective analysis. *Neurourol Urodyn* 2006;25(2):110–115.

33. Schurch B, de Sèze M, Denys P, et al. Botulinum toxin type A is a safe and effective treatment for neurogenic urinary incontinence: Results of a single treatment, randomized, placebo controlled 6-month study. *J Urol* 2005;174(1):196–200.

34. Cruz F, Herschorn S, Aliotta P, et al. Efficacy and safety of onabotulinumtoxinA in patients with urinary incontinence due to neurogenic detrusor overactivity: A randomised, double-blind, placebo-controlled trial. *Eur Urol* 2011;60(4):742–750.

35. Ginsberg D, Gousse A, Keppenne V, et al. Phase 3 efficacy and tolerability study of onabotulinumtoxinA for urinary incontinence from neurogenic detrusor overactivity. *J Urol* 2012;187(6):2131–2139.

36. Kennelly M, Dmochowski R, Schulte-Baukloh H, et al. Efficacy and safety of onabotulinumtoxinA therapy are sustained over 4 years of treatment in patients with neurogenic detrusor overactivity: Final results of a long-term extension study. *Neurourol Urodyn* 2017;36(2):368–375.

37. Giannantoni A, Mearini E, Del Zingaro M, et al. Six-year follow-up of botulinum toxin A intradetrusorial injections in patients with refractory neurogenic detrusor overactivity: Clinical and urodynamic results. *Eur Urol* 2009;55(3):705–712.

38. Kabay SC, Kabay S, Mestan E, et al. Long term sustained therapeutic effects of percutaneous posterior tibial nerve stimulation treatment of neurogenic overactive bladder in multiple sclerosis patients: 12-Months results. *Neurourol Urodyn* 2017;36(1):104–110.

39. Kabay S, Kabay SC, Centiner M, et al. The clinical and urodynamic results of percutaneous posterior tibial nerve stimulation on neurogenic detrusor overactivity in patients with Parkinson's disease. *Urology* 2016;87:76–81.

40. Engeler DS, Meyer D, Abt D, et al. Sacral neuromodulation for the treatment of neurogenic lower urinary tract dysfunction caused by multiple sclerosis: A single-centre prospective series. *BMC Urol* 2015;15(1):105.

41. Blok B, Van Kerrebroeck P, de Wachter S, et al. A prospective, multicenter study of a novel, miniaturized rechargeable sacral neuromodulation system: 12-Month results from the RELAX-OAB study. *Neurourol Urodyn* 2019;38(2):689–695.

42. Athanasopoulos A, Gyftopoulos K, McGuire EJ. Treating stress urinary incontinence in female patients with neuropathic bladder: The value of the autologous fascia rectus sling. *Int Urol Nephrol* 2012;44(5):1363–1367.

43. Seth JH, Haslam C, Panicker JN. Ensuring patient adherence to clean intermittent self-catheterization. *Patient Prefer Adherence* 2014;8:191–198.

44. Gani J, Hennessey D. The underactive bladder: Diagnosis and surgical treatment options. *Transl Androl Urol* 2017;6(Suppl 2): S186–S195.

45. Lombardi G, Musco S, Celso M, et al. Intravesical electrostimulation versus sacral neuromodulation for incomplete spinal cord patients suffering from neurogenic non-obstructive urinary retention. *Spinal Cord* 2013;51(7):571–578.

46. Chancellor MB, Elovic E, Esquenazi A, et al. Evidence-based review and assessment of botulinum neurotoxin for the treatment of urologic conditions. *Toxicon* 2013;67:129–140.

47. Utomo E, Groen J, Blok BF. Surgical management of functional bladder outlet obstruction in adults with neurogenic bladder dysfunction. *Cochrane Database Syst Rev* 2014;(5): CD004927.

48. Perkash I. Use of contact laser crystal tip firing Nd:YAG to relieve urinary outflow obstruction in male neurogenic bladder patients. *J Clin Laser Med Surg* 1998;16(1):33–38.

49. Noll F, Sauerwein D, Stöhrer M. Transurethral sphincterotomy in quadriplegic patients: Long-term-follow-up. *Neurourol Urodyn* 1995;14(4):351–358.

50. Dobson R, Giovannoni G. Multiple sclerosis—a review. *Eur J Neurol* 2019;26(1):27–40.

51. Litwiller SE, Frohman EM, Zimmern PE. Multiple sclerosis and the urologist. *J Urol* 1999;161(3):743–757.

52. Dilokthornsakul P, Valuck RJ, Nair KV, et al. Multiple sclerosis prevalence in the United States commercially insured population. *Neurology* 2016;86(11):1014–1021.

53. Dillon DE, Lemack GE. Urodynamics in the evaluation of the patient with multiple sclerosis: When are they helpful and how do we use them? *Urol Clin North Am* 2014;41(3):439–444.

54. Nortvedt MW, Riise T, Frugård J, et al. Prevalence of bladder, bowel and sexual problems among multiple sclerosis patients two to five years after diagnosis. *Mult Scler* 2007;13(1): 106–112.

55. de Sèze M, Ruffion A, Denys P, et al. The neurogenic bladder in multiple sclerosis: Review of the literature and proposal of management guidelines. *Mult Scler* 2007;13(7):915–928.

56. del Popolo G, Panariello G, Corso F, et al. Diagnosis and therapy for neurogenic bladder dysfunctions in multiple sclerosis patients. *Neurol Sci* 2008;29(Suppl 4):S352–S355.

57. Hennessey A, Robertson NP, Swingler R, et al. Urinary, faecal and sexual dysfunction in patients with multiple sclerosis. *J Neurol* 1999;246(11):1027–1032.

58. Fernández O. Mechanisms and current treatments of urogenital dysfunction in multiple sclerosis. *J Neurol* 2002;249(1):1–8.

59. Mayo ME, Chetner MP. Lower urinary tract dysfunction in multiple sclerosis. *Urology* 1992;39(1):67–70.

60. Phé V, Chartier-Kastler E, Panicker JN. Management of neurogenic bladder in patients with multiple sclerosis. *Nat Rev Urol* 2016;13(5):275–288.

61. Stoffel JT. Chronic urinary retention in multiple sclerosis patients: Physiology, systematic review of urodynamic data, and recommendations for care. *Urol Clin North Am* 2017;44(3): 429–439.

62. Bemelmans BL, Hommes OR, van Kerrebroeck PEV, et al. Evidence for early lower urinary tract dysfunction in clinically silent multiple sclerosis. *J Urol* 1991;145(6):1219–1224.

63. Lemack GE, Frohman E, Ramnarayan P. Women with voiding dysfunction secondary to bladder outlet dyssynergia in the setting of multiple sclerosis do not demonstrate significantly elevated intravesical pressures. *Urology* 2007;69(5): 893–897.

64. Lawrenson R, Wyndaele JJ, Vlachonikolis I, et al. Renal failure in patients with neurogenic lower urinary tract dysfunction. *Neuroepidemiology* 2001;20(2):138–143.

65. Koldewijn EL, Hommes OR, Lemmens WA, et al. Relationship between lower urinary tract abnormalities and disease-related parameters in multiple sclerosis. *J Urol* 1995;154(1):169–173.

66. Fletcher SG. Renal deterioration in multiple sclerosis patients with neurovesical dysfunction. *Mult Scler* 2013;19(9): 1169–1174.

67. Giannantoni A, Scivoletto G, Di Stasi SM, et al. Lower urinary tract dysfunction and disability status in patients with multiple sclerosis. *Arch Phys Med Rehabil* 1999;80(4):437–441.

68. Wiedemann A, Kaeder M, Greulich W, et al. Which clinical risk factors determine a pathological urodynamic evaluation in patients with multiple sclerosis? An analysis of 100 prospective cases. *World J Urol* 2013;31(1):229–233.

69. Ineichen BV, Schneider MP, Hlavica M, et al. High EDSS can predict risk for upper urinary tract damage in patients with multiple sclerosis. *Mult Scler* 2018;24(4):529–534.

70. Nortvedt MW, Riise T, Myhr K-M, et al. Reduced quality of life among multiple sclerosis patients with sexual disturbance and bladder dysfunction. *Mult Scler* 2001;7(4):231–235.

71. De Ridder D, Ost D, Van der Aa F, et al. Conservative bladder management in advanced multiple sclerosis. *Mult Scler* 2005;11(6):694–699.

72. Fascelli M, Goldman H. Demyelinating neuropathies. In: Corcos J, Karsenty G, Thomas K, et al, eds. *Essentials of the adult neurogenic bladder*. Florida: CRC Press, 2020:83–94.

73. Puccini F, Bhide A, Elneil S, et al. Sacral neuromodulation: An effective treatment for lower urinary tract symptoms in multiple sclerosis. *Int Urogynecol J* 2016;27(3):347–354.

74. Model Systems Knowledge Translation Center. Spinal cord injury facts and figures at a glance. 2020 SCI data sheet. Accessed September 27, 2020. https://www.nscisc.uab.edu/Public /Facts%20and%20Figures%202020.pdf

75. Kowalik CG, Wein AJ, Dmochowski RR. Neuromuscular dysfunction of the lower urinary tract. In: Partin A, Dmochowski RR, Kavoussi L, et al, eds. *Campbell-Walsh urology*, 12th ed. Philadelphia: Elsevier, 2021:2600–2636.

76. Panicker J, DasGupta R, Batla A. Neurourology. In: Daroff RB, Jankovic J, Maziotta JC, et al, eds. *Bradley's neurology in clinical practice*, 7th ed. Philadelphia: Elsevier, 2016:605–621.

77. Ditunno JF, Little JW, Tessler A, et al. Spinal shock revisited: A four-phase model. *Spinal Cord* 2004;42(7):383–395.

78. Samson G, Cardenas DD. Neurogenic bladder in spinal cord injury. *Phys Med Rehabil Clin N Am* 2007;18(2):255–274.

79. Jeong SJ, Cho SY, Oh S-J. Spinal cord/brain injury and the neurogenic bladder. *Urol Clin North Am* 2010;37(4):537–546.

80. Schurch B, Iacovelli V, Averbeck MA, et al. Urodynamics in patients with spinal cord injury: A clinical review and best practice paper by a working group of The International Continence Society Urodynamics Committee. *Neurourol Urodyn* 2018;37(2):581–591.

81. Consortium for Spinal Cord Medicine. Bladder management for adults with spinal cord injury: A clinical practice guideline for health-care providers. *J Spinal Cord Med* 2006;29(5):527–573. Accessed September 27, 2020.https://www.ncbi.nlm.nih.gov/pmc/articles/PMC1949036/

82. Stover S, DeLisa J, Whiteneck G. *Spinal cord injury: Clinical outcomes from the model systems.* Maryland: Aspen, 1995.

83. Ku JH. The management of neurogenic bladder and quality of life in spinal cord injury. *BJU Int* 2006;98(4):739–745.

84. Weld KJ, Dmochowski RR. Association of level of injury and bladder behavior in patients with post-traumatic spinal cord injury. *Urology* 2000;55(4):490–494.

85. Kaplan SA, Chancellor MB, Blaivas JG. Bladder and sphincter behavior in patients with spinal cord lesions. *J Urol* 1991;146(1):113–117.

86. Gerridzen RG, Thijssen AM, Dehoux E. Risk factors for upper tract deterioration in chronic spinal cord injury patients. *J Urol* 1992;147(2):416–418.

87. Eldahan KC, Rabchevsky AG. Autonomic dysreflexia after spinal cord injury: Systemic pathophysiology and methods of management. *Auton Neurosci* 2018;209:59–70.

88. Abrams P, Agarwal M, Drake M, et al. A proposed guideline for the urological management of patients with spinal cord injury. *BJU Int* 2008;101(8):989–994.

89. Wyndaele JJ. The management of neurogenic lower urinary tract dysfunction after spinal cord injury. *Nat Rev Urol* 2016;13(12):705–714.

90. Burns AS, Rivas DA, Ditunno JF. The management of neurogenic bladder and sexual dysfunction after spinal cord injury. *Spine* 2001;26(24 Suppl):S129–S136.

91. Wyndaele JJ, Madersbacher H, Kovindha A. Conservative treatment of the neuropathic bladder in spinal cord injured patients. *Spinal Cord* 2001;39(6):294–300.

92. Lang AE, Lozano AM. Parkinson's disease: First of two parts. *N Engl J Med* 1998;339(15):1044–1053.

93. Lee A, Gilbert RM. Epidemiology of Parkinson disease. *Neurol Clin* 2016;34(4):955–965.

94. Uchiyama T, Sakakibara R, Yamamoto T, et al. Urinary dysfunction in early and untreated Parkinson's disease. *J Neurol Neurosurg Psychiatry* 2011;82(12):1382–1386.

95. Barone P, Antonini A, Colosimo C, et al. The PRIAMO study: A multicenter assessment of nonmotor symptoms and their impact on quality of life in Parkinson's disease. *Mov Disord* 2009;24(11):1641–1649.

96. Yeo L, Singh R, Gundeti M, et al. Urinary tract dysfunction in Parkinson's disease: A review. *Int Urol Nephrol* 2012;44(2):415–424.

97. Sakakibara R, Panicker J, Finazzi-Agro E, et al. A guideline for the management of bladder dysfunction in Parkinson's disease and other gait disorders. *Neurourol Urodyn* 2016;35(5):551–563.

98. Bonnet AM, Pichon J, Vidailhet M, et al. Urinary disturbances in striatonigral degeneration and Parkinson's disease: Clinical and urodynamic aspects. *Mov Disord* 1997;12(4):509–513.

99. Sakakibara R, Shinotoh H, Uchiyama T, et al. SPECT imaging of the dopamine transporter with [^{123}I]-β-CIT reveals marked decline of nigrostriatal dopaminergic function in Parkinson's disease with urinary dysfunction. *J Neurol Sci* 2001;187(1–2):55–59.

100. Hashimoto K, Oyama T, Sugiyama T, et al. Neuronal excitation in the ventral tegmental area modulates the micturition reflex mediated via the dopamine D_1 and D_2 receptors in rats. *J Pharmacol Sci* 2003;92(2):143–148.

101. Araki I, Kitahara M, Oida T, et al. Voiding dysfunction and Parkinson's disease: Urodynamic abnormalities and urinary symptoms. *J Urol* 2000;164(5):1640–1643.

102. Campos-Sousa RN, Quagliato E, da Silva BB, et al. Urinary symptoms in Parkinson's disease: Prevalence and associated factors. *Arq Neuropsiquiatr* 2003;61(2):359–363.

103. Stocchi F, Carbone A, Inghilleri M, et al. Urodynamic and neurophysiological evaluation in Parkinson's disease and multiple system atrophy. *J Neurol Neurosurg Psychiatry* 1997;62(5):507–511.

104. Fitzmaurice H, Fowler J, Rickards D, et al. Micturition disturbance in Parkinson's disease. *Br J Urol* 1985;57(6):652–656.

105. Blackett H, Walker R, Wood B. Urinary dysfunction in Parkinson's disease: A review. *Parkinsonism Relat Disord* 2009;15(2):81–87.

106. Sakakibara R, Tateno F, Kishi M, et al. Pathophysiology of bladder dysfunction in Parkinson's disease. *Neurobiol Dis* 2012;46(3):565–571.

107. Kitta T, Kakizaki H, Furuno T, et al. Brain activation during detrusor overactivity in patients with Parkinson's disease: A positron emission tomography study. *J Urol* 2006;175(3):994–998.

108. Pavlakis AJ, Siroky MB, Goldstein I, et al. Neurourologic findings in Parkinson's disease. *J Urol* 1983;129(1):80–83.

109. Winge K, Fowler CJ. Bladder dysfunction in Parkinsonism: Mechanism, prevalence, symptoms, and management. *Mov Disord* 2006;21(6):737–745.

110. Anderson RU, Orenberg EK, Glowe P. OnabotulinumtoxinA office treatment for neurogenic bladder incontinence in Parkinson's disease. *Urology* 2014;83(1):22–27.

111. Wallace PA, Lane FL, Noblett KL. Sacral nerve neuromodulation in patients with underlying neurologic disease. *Am J Obstet Gynecol* 2007;197(1):96.e1–96.e5.

112. Kessler TM, La Framboise D, Trelle S, et al. Sacral neuromodulation for neurogenic lower urinary tract dysfunction: Systematic review and meta-analysis. *Eur Urol* 2010;58(6):865–874.

113. Peters KM, Kandagatla P, Killinger KA, et al. Clinical outcomes of sacral neuromodulation in patients with neurologic conditions. *Urology* 2013;81(4):738–744.

114. Finazzi-Agrò E, Peppe A, D'Amico A, et al. Effects of subthalamic nucleus stimulation on urodynamic findings in patients with Parkinson's disease. *J Urol* 2003;169(4):1388–1391.

115. Seif C, Herzog J, van der Horst C, et al. Effect of subthalamic deep brain stimulation on the function of the urinary bladder. *Ann Neurol* 2004;55(1):118–120.

116. Zong H, Meng F, Zhang Y, et al. Clinical study of the effects of deep brain stimulation on urinary dysfunctions in patients with Parkinson's disease. *Clin Interv Aging* 2019;14:1159–1166.

117. Sakakibara R, Hattori T, Uchiyama T, et al. Urinary dysfunction and orthostatic hypotension in multiple system atrophy: Which is the more common and earlier manifestation? *J Neurol Neurosurg Psychiatry* 2000;68(1):65–69.

118. Beck RO, Betts CD, Fowler CJ. Genitourinary dysfunction in multiple system atrophy: Clinical features and treatment in 62 cases. *J Urol* 1994;151(5):1336–1341.

119. Fowler CJ. Urinary disorders in Parkinson's disease and multiple system atrophy. *Funct Neurol* 2001;16(3):277–282. Accessed October 1, 2020. https://pubmed.ncbi.nlm.nih.gov/11769873/

120. Mozaffarian D, Benjamin EJ, Go AS, et al. Heart disease and stroke statistics—2016 update: A report from the American Heart Association. *Circulation* 2016;133(4):38–e48.

121. Addo J, Ayerbe L, Mohan KM, et al. Socioeconomic status and stroke: An updated review. *Stroke* 2012;43(4):1186–1191.
122. Grysiewicz RA, Thomas K, Pandey DK. Epidemiology of ischemic and hemorrhagic stroke: Incidence, prevalence, mortality, and risk factors. *Neurol Clin* 2008;26(4):871–895.
123. Hall MJ, Levant S, Defrances CJ. Hospitalization for stroke in U.S. hospitals, 1989–2009. *NCHS Data Brief* 2012;(95):1–8.
124. Burney TL, Senapati M, Desai S, et al. Acute cerebrovascular accident and lower urinary tract dysfunction: A prospective correlation of the site of brain injury with urodynamic findings. *J Urol* 1996;156(5):1748–1750.
125. Kolominsky-Rabas PL, Hilz MJ, Neundoerfer B, et al. Impact of urinary incontinence after stroke: Results from a prospective population-based stroke register. *Neurourol Urodyn* 2003;22(4):322–327.
126. Brittain KR, Peet SM, Castleden CM. Stroke and incontinence. *Stroke* 1998;29(2):524–528.
127. Williams MP, Srikanth V, Bird M, et al. Urinary symptoms and natural history of urinary continence after first-ever stroke—a longitudinal population-based study. *Age Ageing* 2012;41(3):371–376.
128. Gupta A, Taly A, Srivastava A, et al. Urodynamics post stroke in patients with urinary incontinence: Is there correlation between bladder type and site of lesion? *Ann Indian Acad Neurol* 2009;12(2):104–107.
129. Tsuchida S, Noto H, Yamaguchi O, et al. Urodynamic studies on hemiplegic patients after cerebrovascular accident. *Urology* 1983;21(3):315–318.
130. Han KS, Heo SH, Lee SJ, et al. Comparison of urodynamics between ischemic and hemorrhagic stroke patients; can we suggest the category of urinary dysfunction in patients with cerebrovascular accident according to type of stroke? *Neurourol Urodyn* 2010;29(3):387–390.
131. Panfili Z, Metcalf M, Griebling TL. Contemporary evaluation and treatment of poststroke lower urinary tract dysfunction. *Urol Clin North Am* 2017;44(3):403–414.
132. Jiang Y-H, Liao C-H, Tang D-L, et al. Efficacy and safety of intravesical onabotulinumtoxinA injection on elderly patients with chronic central nervous system lesions and overactive bladder. *PLoS One* 2014;9(8):e105989.
133. Monteiro ÉS, de Carvalho LBC, Fukujima MM, et al. Electrical stimulation of the posterior tibialis nerve improves symptoms of poststroke neurogenic overactive bladder in men: A randomized controlled trial. *Urology* 2014;84(3):509–514.
134. National Institute of Neurological Disorders and Stroke. Spina bifida fact sheet. Accessed September 29, 2020. https://www.ninds.nih.gov/Disorders/Patient-Caregiver-Education/Fact-Sheets/Spina-Bifida-Fact-Sheet
135. Liu T, Ouyang L, Thibadeau J, et al. Longitudinal study of bladder continence in patients with spina bifida in the National Spina Bifida Patient Registry. *J Urol* 2018;199(3):837–843.
136. van Gool JD, Dik P, de Jong TP. Bladder-sphincter dysfunction in myelomeningocele. *Eur J Pediatr* 2001;160(7):414–420.
137. Webster GD, el-Mahrouky A, Stone AR, et al. The urological evaluation and management of patients with myelodysplasia. *Br J Urol* 1986;58(3):261–265.
138. Sakakibara R, Hattori T, Uchiyama T, et al. Uroneurological assessment of spina bifida cystica and occulta. *Neurourol Urodyn* 2003;22(4):328–334.
139. Singhal B, Mathew KM. Factors affecting mortality and morbidity in adult spina bifida. *Eur J Pediatr Surg* 1999;9(Suppl 1):31–32.
140. Dik P, Klijn AJ, van Gool JD, et al. Early start to therapy preserves kidney function in spina bifida patients. *Eur Urol* 2006;49(5):908–913.
141. Mourtzinos A, Stoffel JT. Management goals for the spina bifida neurogenic bladder: A review from infancy to adulthood. *Urol Clin North Am* 2010;37(4):527–535.
142. Aoun F, van Velthoven R. Lower urinary tract dysfunction after nerve-sparing radical hysterectomy. *Int Urogynecol J* 2015;26(7):947–957.
143. Zhou M-W, Huang X-Y, Chen Z-Y, et al. Intraoperative monitoring of pelvic autonomic nerves during laparoscopic low anterior resection of rectal cancer. *Cancer Manag Res* 2018;11:411–417.
144. Wu J, Liu X, Hua K, et al. Effect of nerve-sparing radical hysterectomy on bladder function recovery and quality of life in patients with cervical carcinoma. *Int J Gynecol Cancer* 2010;20(5):905–909.
145. Chen C, Li W, Li F, et al. Classical and nerve-sparing radical hysterectomy: An evaluation of the nerve trauma in cardinal ligament. *Gynecol Oncol* 2012;125(1):245–251.
146. Aagaard J, Gerstenberg TC, Knudsen JJ. Urodynamic investigation predicts bladder dysfunction at an early stage after abdominoperineal resection of the rectum for cancer. *Surgery* 1986;99(5):564–568.
147. Hamada K, Kihana T, Kataoka M, et al. Urinary disturbance after therapy for cervical cancer: Urodynamic evaluation and β_2-agonist medication. *Int Urogynecol J Pelvic Floor Dysfunct* 1999;10(6):365–370.
148. Benedetti-Panici P, Zullo MA, Plotti F, et al. Long-term bladder function in patients with locally advanced cervical carcinoma treated with neoadjuvant chemotherapy and type 3-4 radical hysterectomy. *Cancer* 2004;100(10):2110–2117.
149. Axelsen SM, Petersen LK. Urogynaecological dysfunction after radical hysterectomy. *Eur J Surg Oncol* 2006;32(4):445–449.
150. Bax MC. Terminology and classification of cerebral palsy. *Dev Med Child Neurol* 1964;6(3):295–297.
151. Sawyer J, Spence D. Cerebral palsy. In: Azar FM, Canale ST, Beaty JH, eds. *Campbell's operative orthopaedics*. 13th ed. Philadelphia: Elsevier, 2020:1249–1303.
152. Reddihough DS, Collins KJ. The epidemiology and causes of cerebral palsy. *Aust J Physiother* 2003;49(1):7–12.
153. Samijn B, Van Laecke E, Renson C, et al. Lower urinary tract symptoms and urodynamic findings in children and adults with cerebral palsy: A systematic review. *Neurourol Urodyn* 2017;36(3):541–549.
154. Houle AM, Vernet O, Jednak R, et al. Bladder function before and after selective dorsal rhizotomy in children with cerebral palsy. *J Urol* 1998;160(3, Pt 2):1088–1091.
155. Chiu PK-F, Yam K-Y, Lam T-Y, et al. Does selective dorsal rhizotomy improve bladder function in children with cerebral palsy? *Int Urol Nephrol* 2014;46(10):1929–1933.
156. Cotter KJ, Levy ME, Goldfarb RA, et al. Urodynamic findings in adults with moderate to severe cerebral palsy. *Urology* 2016;95:216–221.
157. Mayo ME. Lower urinary tract dysfunction in cerebral palsy. *J Urol* 1992;147(2):419–420.
158. Karaman M, Kaya C, Caskurlu T, et al. Urodynamic findings in children with cerebral palsy. *Int J Urol* 2005;12(8):717–720.
159. Murphy KP, Boutin SA, Ide KR. Cerebral palsy, neurogenic bladder, and outcomes of lifetime care. *Dev Med Child Neurol* 2012;54(10):945–950.
160. Reid CJD, Borzyskowski M. Lower urinary tract dysfunction in cerebral palsy. *Arch Dis Child* 1993;68(6):739–742.

161. Goldfarb RA, Pisansky A, Fleck J, et al. Neurogenic lower urinary tract dysfunction in adults with cerebral palsy: Outcomes following a conservative management approach. *J Urol* 2016;195(4):1009–1013.

162. Goldman HB, Appell RA. Voiding dysfunction in women with lumbar disc prolapse. *Int Urogynecol J Pelvic Floor Dysfunct* 1999;10(2):134–138.

163. Dydyk AM, Massa RN, Mesfin FB. *Disc herniation.* Florida: StatPearls Publishing, 2018.

164. Willems P. Decision making in surgical treatment of chronic low back pain: The performance of prognostic tests to select patients for lumbar spinal fusion. *Acta Orthop Suppl* 2013;84(349):1–37.

165. Rosomoff HL, Johnston JD, Gallo AE, et al. Cystometry in the evaluation of nerve root compression in the lumbar spine. *Surg Gynecol Obstet* 1963;117:263–270. Accessed October 1, 2020. https://pubmed.ncbi.nlm.nih.gov/14080336/

166. Bartolin Z, Gilja I, Bedalov G, et al. Bladder function in patients with lumbar intervertebral disk protrusion. *J Urol* 1998;159(3): 969–971.

167. O'Flynn KJ, Murphy R, Thomas DG. Neurogenic bladder dysfunction in lumbar intervertebral disc prolapse. *Br J Urol* 1992;69(1):38–40.

168. Ahn UM, Ahn NU, Buchowski JM, et al. Cauda equina syndrome secondary to lumbar disc herniation. *Spine* 2000;25(12): 1515–1522.

CHAPTER 28

AVOIDANCE AND MANAGEMENT OF GENITOURINARY COMPLICATIONS

Javier F. Magrina

Introduction

If you operate long enough, you will have complications. Because the ureters and the bladder are very close neighbors to the uterus and adnexa, they are at risk for injury ANYTIME you operate in the pelvis.

INCIDENCE

Take home message: Genitourinary injuries remain at about the same incidence for the past 20 years. Bladder injuries are more common than ureteral injuries.

Bladder and ureteral injuries remain a common problem. Although their mortality is very low, they are a frequent cause of litigation when diagnosed postoperatively and specially when associated with complications deriving from their repair. The overall incidence of urinary injuries associated with laparoscopic gynecologic surgery has remained stable during the past 20 years ranging from 0.02% to 1.7%,[1,2] with bladder injuries being more common than ureteral injuries. When considering only laparoscopic hysterectomy, the overall urinary tract injury is 0.7%, with injury rates of 0.02% to 0.4% for ureters and 0.05% to 0.7% for bladder.[3] In a more recent review considering open, vaginal, and laparoscopic hysterectomy in 296,130 patients, ureteral injuries were diagnosed in 1% and bladder injuries in 0.7%.[4] The open hysterectomy had a higher risk for urinary injury than vaginal and laparoscopic.

DELAYED INJURIES

Take home message: Most ureteral injuries remain unrecognized during surgery.

Unrecognized ureteral injuries are more common than bladder injuries, and symptoms may be delayed for up to 6 weeks or longer. Ureteral entrapments can be permanently silent. In a more recent review of 45,139 open, vaginal, and laparoscopic hysterectomies, during the period of 2014 to 2016, the incidence of delayed injuries during the first 30 days was 0.2%, including ureteral obstruction in 0.1% of patients, ureteral fistula in 0.07%, and bladder fistula in 0.06%.[4]

INTRAOPERATIVE VERSUS POSTOPERATIVE DIAGNOSIS (RECOGNIZED VS. UNRECOGNIZED)

Take home message: Bladder injuries are more commonly diagnosed intraoperatively, whereas ureteral injuries are more commonly diagnosed postoperatively. Performing a cystoscopy will diagnose unrecognized intraoperative injuries but not all types of injuries and not in all patients.

There is no doubt intraoperative recognition is favorable for the patient and the surgeon. In a series of 223,872 patients undergoing hysterectomy, ureteral injuries occurred in 0.7% of them, and it was unrecognized in 62.4% of them.[5] In a systematic review of benign laparoscopic surgery, 60% of ureteral injuries were recognized postoperatively.[6]

Unrecognized ureteral injuries increase the risk of readmission, sepsis, urinary fistula, renal insufficiency, and death as compared to recognized injuries.[5]

Intraoperative diagnosis of a ureteral injury required surgical repair in only 9% of patients (most were corrected by cutting a suture or placing a stent), whereas postoperative diagnosis required a surgical repair in 61% of patients.[3]

Intravenous indigo carmine is helpful to diagnose an intraoperative ureteral leak. Bladder distension with methylene blue will diagnose a leak or a near full-thickness injury.

Cystoscopy is a friendly tool which identifies most, but not all, injuries. You will not regret performing a negative cystoscopy, but you will if an injury is diagnosed after the patient is discharged and you did not perform a cystoscopy. Routine cystoscopy decreased postoperative ureteral injuries from 0.16% to 0.07%. Delayed bladder injuries were diagnosed in 0.08% and 0.1% without and with cystoscopy, respectively.[2]

Ureteral obstruction (suture or sealing) or transection is revealed by lack of a ureteral jet. Full-thickness or near full-thickness thermal bladder injuries are identified by blanching of the vesical urothelium.

Incomplete thermal injuries of the ureter or sutures involving near fullness of the bladder wall in the cuff closure will not be diagnosed by cystoscopy.

AVOIDANCE OF BLADDER INJURY

Preparation for Dissecting the Vesicovaginal Space

For a safe dissection, you need to place the anterior vaginal fornix and the bladder wall under stretch and sometimes distend the bladder with 300 mL of water.

- A vaginal probe, a cervical cup, or a uterine manipulator is necessary for a safe bladder dissection and identification of the cervicovaginal junction.
- A distended bladder is useful to identify its margins if unclear. We use a three-way Foley catheter in all patients to distend the bladder with water whenever necessary during the operation or to visualize its integrity at the end. There should never be a bladder injury with normal anatomy.

Bladder Dissection

Take home message: In the absence of adhesions, start the dissection of the vesicovaginal space in the midline. There are no vessels in the vesicovaginal space, so if you encounter bleeding, you are in the wrong plane of dissection.

In the absence of obliteration of the vesicovaginal space (i.e., no adhesions), always start the dissection in the midline to avoid bleeding from the lateral vesicouterine ligaments (bladder pillars).

There are no vessels in the vesicovaginal space; therefore, if you encounter bleeding, you are either in the cervix, the vagina, or the detrusor muscle, and you are not in the vesicovaginal space.

Stop, distend the bladder with 300 mL of water, clearly visualize its contour, and find the correct space.

How far to dissect the vesicovaginal space?

Continue the dissection in the midline past 2 cm from the cervicovaginal junction and then widen the space laterally.

Why 2 cm?

Simply because the vaginal wall is stretched from the manipulator and once it is removed with the uterus, the vaginal wall will retract and the distance from the vaginal cuff to the bladder will be reduced to 1 cm or less.

This distance is adequate to take 5-mm bites away from the cut adventitial edge of the vagina without risk of including the bladder wall.

Bladder Adhesions and/or Obliteration of the Vesicovaginal Space

Take home message: Distend the bladder with 300 mL of water and start the dissection of the vesicovaginal space lateral to the adhesions such as from a cesarean scar.

The most common cause of midline adhesions is a previous cesarean section (Fig. 28.1A). In that case, the dissection always starts lateral to the cesarean scar.

The vesicovaginal space is not usually obliterated from a cesarean because the myotomy is in the lower uterine segment and not in the lower part of the cervix or vagina. Therefore, once you are past the cesarean scar, the rest of the dissection is in virginal territory.

Distend the bladder with 300 mL of water at the start of the dissection, which will delineate the area of bladder–uterus attachment. ALWAYS start the dissection of the vesicovaginal space lateral to the scar, right or left. Continue the dissection until you identify the vesicovaginal space free of adhesions (Fig. 28.1B,C). This outlines the cesarean scar, superiorly and inferiorly, which then can be safely divided (maintaining a full bladder), starting on the right or left and proceeding to the contralateral side (Fig. 28.1D,E). If you have any doubts about the plane of dissection, dissect deeper on the uterus instead than on the bladder.

You will end up with the cesarean scar left in the bladder wall which does not need to be removed (unless it has myometrium or the patient had bladder symptoms).

If the adhesions are from infiltrating endometriosis, proceed as if a cesarean, but you will need to resect a portion of the bladder wall to obtain clearance of the lesion.

Checking for Bladder Integrity

Distend the bladder with 300 mL of water or diluted methylene blue and observe for a leak or bulging blue urothelium, indicating near full bladder wall damage. A cystoscopy is another option.

AVOIDANCE OF URETERAL INJURY

Take home message: The only reliable method to prevent ureteral injury is to identify the ureters in all patients. Ureteral stents do not reduce ureteral injuries.

There is no other proven method for avoidance of ureteral injury than ureteral identification in every pelvic operation, even in patients with normal anatomy. If they are not identified, there is a high risk (88% to 97%)[3] of unrecognized injury.

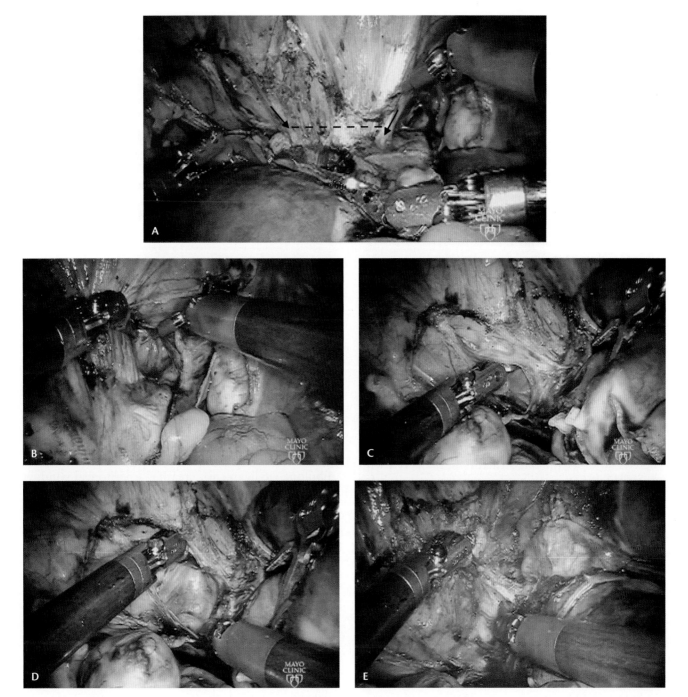

FIGURE 28.1 Bladder dissection in the presence of a cesarean scar. **A:** The bladder is distended with 300 mL of water and the cesarean scar clearly delineated by a *broken line* between the *two arrows*. **B:** The dissection starts lateral to the scar; in this case, on the right side until the free vesicovaginal space is identified. **C:** The same dissection is performed on the opposite left side, creating a tunnel underneath the cesarean scar. **D:** The cesarean scar is partially divided, being safe from the bladder wall. **E:** The cesarean scar is almost completely divided.

FIGURE 28.2 A peritoneal window has been created to prevent ureteral injury when sealing the right ovarian vessels. The right ureter is below and lateral to the window.

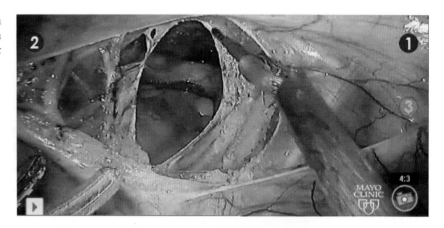

Why Do You Need to Identify the Ureters in All Patients?

The ureters are never in the exact location in all patients, and in a given patient, they may not be in the same location on each side of the pelvis.

What is the Single Feature the Ureters Have that When Identified it Guarantees is a Ureter?

Peristalsis

There is no other tubular structure in the pelvis with peristalsis. If you are a patient surgeon and wait for peristalsis before sealing a tubular structure, you will avoid more than one ureteral injury.

How frequent is peristalsis?

The frequency of peristalsis is directly related to the hydration level of the patient. If you are operating on a dehydrated patient, you have to wait much longer for peristalsis than on a well-hydrated one. In case of doubt, 5 mg of intravenous furosemide will produce active peristalsis within 8 minutes. Waiting 8 minutes can save you 60 minutes of repairing a ureter.

How Good Is Cystoscopy to Diagnose Ureteral Injury?

No ureteral jet is a fast diagnosis of ureteral obstruction or transection. It does not diagnose ureteral thermal injuries. Rare causes of absence of ureteral jet are unilateral renal agenesis or nonfunctioning kidney.

Do Ureteral Stents Prevent Ureteral Injuries?

As a general rule, no. A prospective randomized trial showed the same incidence of ureteral injuries with and without ureteral stents.

Are there Exceptions to the Rule?

Yes. In some instances, stents will help you to identify the location of a ureter immersed in fibrosis or in an unusual position. Palpating a rigid tube inside a tubular structure with minimal or no peristalsis due to fixation from fibrosis will help to identify it as a ureter. There is no doubt that cutting a ureter, partial or complete, with a stent inside will allow you to recognize the injury very easily.

Is it possible to prevent all ureteral injuries at endoscopic hysterectomy and adnexectomy with normal pelvic anatomy?

Yes. At the level of the ovarian vessels (i.e., infundibulopelvic ligament), creating a peritoneal window between the vessels superiorly and the ureter inferiorly will guarantee ureteral safety when sealing the ovarian vessels (Fig. 28.2).

At the level of the cardinal ligaments, 1 out of 8 patients have at least one ureter within 5 mm from the lateral cervical wall as measured by computed tomography scan.[7]

The uterine manipulator is probably helpful to increase the distance of the ureter to the uterine artery or lateral cervical wall in some patients but not in all.

Transection of the uterine artery at the crossing with the ureter allows lateral displacement of the ureter and safe sealing of the uterine vessels. This is the only option for ureters adjacent to the cervix.

At the end of every operation, visually inspect bladder and ureters (also bowel) for any apparent injuries and dictate the findings in the operative report. Intraoperative recognition and repair is more favorable for a good outcome than a delayed diagnosis in a patient medically compromised due to the injury.

MANAGEMENT OF BLADDER INJURIES

The most common location of bladder injury during a hysterectomy is immediately posterior to the interureteric ridge. Depending on the proximity to the

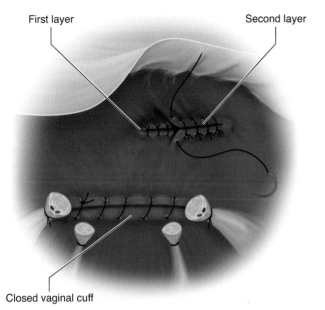

First layer   Second layer

Closed vaginal cuff

FIGURE 28.3 Cystotomy repair. The opening has been closed in two layers with 4-0 DAS, the second layer imbricating the first layer. If there is redundancy of the peritoneum, a flap is created and interposed between the vaginal cuff and the cystotomy repair to prevent fistula formation, which is unlikely with a good closure and in the absence of infection.

intramural portion of the ureter, stent placement may be necessary. Complete your operation and then proceed to repair the injury.

The edges of the injury must be sharp, fresh, clean of burned tissue, and easily identifiable.

The defect is closed in whichever direction the edges can be approximated without tension, vertically or transversely. The first layer consists of a continuous suture of 4-0 delayed absorbable suture (DAS) including full thickness or near full thickness of the bladder wall. A second continuous imbricating layer including near full thickness of the bladder wall and using the same suture material is used to reduce

tension, bring additional blood supply, and reinforce the closure (Fig. 28.3).

A Foley catheter is left for 7 days. A cystogram is then performed, and if negative, the catheter is removed. The surgeon may consider the use of antibiotics until the catheter is removed.

MANAGEMENT OF URETERAL INJURIES

Adventitia

Small adventitial defects do not require suturing. Large defects may devascularize a segment of the ureter and result in stricture. If approximation of the adventitia is performed, it must be in a transverse fashion to avoid stenosis using a few interrupted 5-0 DAS.

If no closure is performed due to a lengthy longitudinal adventitial defect, an omental J flap is superimposed over the devascularized area to bring blood supply.

Thermal Injury

Thermal injuries can be direct or indirect. Direct injuries caused by direct application of an electrocautery instrument are easily noted because of the char on the ureteral wall (Fig. 28.4). In that case, the charred area is superficially excised with cold scissors to determine depth and extension. If small, an omental J flap is superimposed to bring blood supply. If large, it is treated as an indirect thermal injury.

Indirect thermal injuries are caused by increased temperature of the ureter due to the application of an electrocautery device in its immediate vicinity and have no charring. They are diagnosed intraoperatively when a blanching area devoted to blood supply is noted. The injured area must be fully resected until there is bleeding at each cut end of the ureter. The cut ends

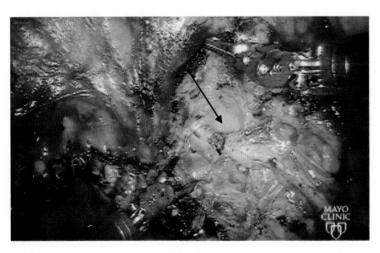

FIGURE 28.4 Direct right ureteral thermal injury near the vaginal cuff. The charred area is clearly noted on the right ureter at the tip of the *arrow*. The charred tissue was removed, and an omental J flap was placed over it without a stent. There were no subsequent complications.

are spatulated and an end-to-end anastomosis or reimplantation is performed (see following discussion), depending on vascularization of the remaining ureter and distance to the bladder. In case of doubt, reimplantation is preferable because the bladder wall has superior blood supply than the ureter.

URETEROTOMIES

Incomplete

Incomplete ureter transections are repaired in a transverse fashion with a few interrupted sutures of 5-0 DAS including full thickness of the ureteral walls. A closed suction drain is left for 24 to 48 hours.

Complete

Complete transections require a spatulated end-to-end anastomosis or spatulated reimplantation depending on the degree of vascularization and level of the injury. As stated before, reimplantation is preferable because the bladder wall has good blood supply and is less likely to result in stricture. Reimplantation can be achieved even in the upper third of the pelvis with mobilization of the bladder from the space of Retzius, unilateral or bilateral division of its peritoneal attachments, and suturing the bladder to the psoas tendon (psoas hitch) with permanent sutures. Transections within 2 cm of the intramural portion of the ureter are best repaired by reimplantation. Rarely, a Boari flap (a transverse incision of the bladder sutured longitudinally in which proximal end the ureter is anastomosed) is needed.

End-to-End Anastomosis

All end-to-end anastomoses are performed with spatulated ends of each ureter to create a larger inner diameter at the anastomotic site because the resulting fibrosis from healing will produce a constriction (Fig. 28.5). They require good blood supply to each ureteral ends and approximation without tension.

A 5-mm linear incision is made at the 6 o'clock of the proximal ureteral end and at the 12 o'clock of the distal end. The first suture, using 5-0 DAS, includes the V end of the distal incision and the 6 o'clock of the proximal end. It is tied and cut long to be used later to rotate the ureter to facilitate suturing in the opposite, lower aspect of the anastomosis.

Next, the two tips of the resulting V incision from spatulation are sutured to each other with 5-0 DAS including full thickness to full thickness of each ureteral wall. The remaining of the anastomosis is completed with a few interrupted sutures of the same material.

A second imbricating layer should be attempted if possible, suturing the proximal with the distal periureteral tissue to reduce tension and improve blood supply.

Anastomosis of one ureter to the contralateral ureter is not recommended because stricture at the anastomotic site may result in bilateral ureteral obstruction.

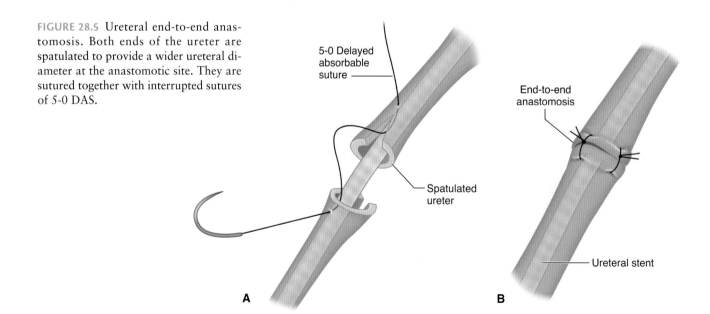

FIGURE 28.5 Ureteral end-to-end anastomosis. Both ends of the ureter are spatulated to provide a wider ureteral diameter at the anastomotic site. They are sutured together with interrupted sutures of 5-0 DAS.

5-0 Delayed absorbable suture

Spatulated ureter

End-to-end anastomosis

Ureteral stent

A   B

Reimplantation

The following is performed in all or near all instances of reimplantation.

1. The bladder is mobilized from the space of Retzius with 300 mL of water. The lateral peritoneal attachments of the bladder are transected unilaterally or bilaterally depending if additional mobilization is required. The bladder wall is then sutured near full thickness to the ipsilateral psoas tendon with 0 DAS.
2. The ureteral end is spatulated, a 5-mm incision is made at the 6 o'clock of the ureter, and a 4-0 DAS is passed through the base of the resulting V incision to retrieve the ureter into the bladder.
3. A drain is used for 24 to 48 hours because a urine leak is highly irritating to peritoneal surfaces.
4. A Foley catheter is left for 7 to 10 days and a double-J ureteral stent for 6 weeks at which time a retrograde ureterogram is performed. It is repeated at 3 months to ensure there is no stricture. Antibiotics are used until the Foley is removed.

Transvesical Technique

A small vertical bladder incision is made in the extraperitoneal superior portion of the bladder, which will be closed transversely in two layers (Fig. 28.6). A curved grasper is used to outdent the bladder wall from the inside to the outside at the selected site of anastomosis, and a full-thickness nick is made by avulsion of its arms or with the help of scissors. The ureter is brought into the bladder by grasping the previously placed suture. It is anastomosed with a few interrupted 5-0 DAS incorporating full thickness of the ureteral wall to near full thickness of the bladder wall including the mucosa.

A second layer of interrupted 5-0 DAS is placed extravesically around the site of entrance of the ureter into the bladder, incorporating near full thickness of the bladder wall and the periureteral tissue which has intentionally been preserved for this layer. This has four functions: removes tension from the anastomosis, reduces bladder leaks, improves blood supply, and creates a tunnel-shaped anastomosis.

Extravesical

The extravesical technique is more commonly used for the correction of vesicoureteral reflux (Fig. 28.7). In this approach, there is no bladder incision other than a small cystotomy for the ureterovesical anastomosis. A vertical linear incision, about 4 times as long as the ureter's width, is created in the distended bladder wall

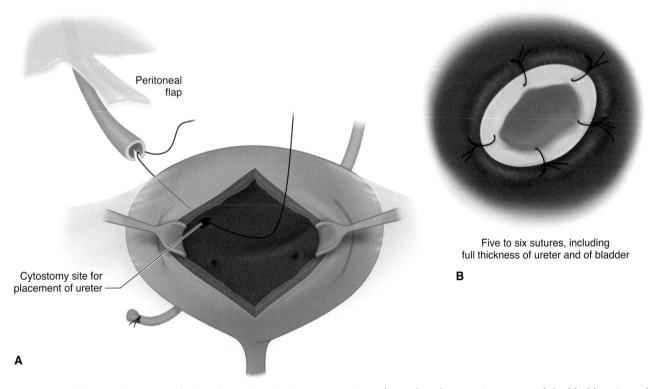

Peritoneal flap

Cytostomy site for placement of ureter

Five to six sutures, including full thickness of ureter and of bladder

A

B

FIGURE 28.6 Transvesical ureteral reimplantation. **A:** A cystotomy is performed in the superior aspect of the bladder. A small opening is made in a selected site for the reimplantation, usually superior and medial to the original ureteral meatus. **B:** The ureter is anastomosed to the bladder wall with full-thickness bites on the ureter and near full-thickness bites on the bladder wall using 5-0 DAS. (Redrawn with permission from Mayo Foundation for Medical Education and Research. All rights reserved.)

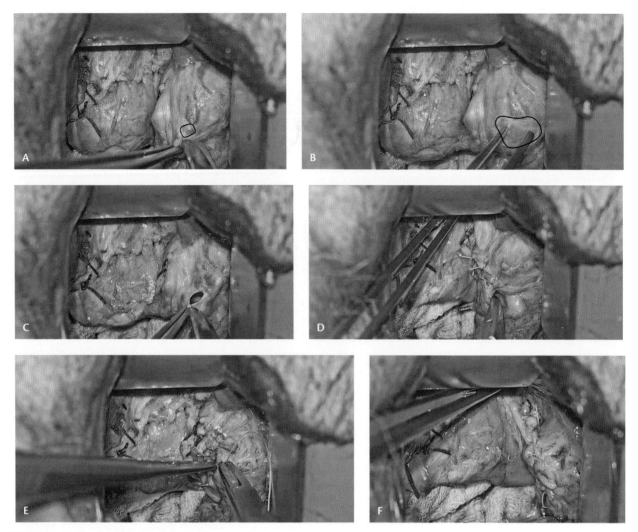

FIGURE 28.7 Extravesical left ureteral reimplantation in a cadaver performed through a vaginal approach. **A:** A small detrusor incision *(small circle)* has been made down to the bladder mucosa, which is elongated and widened (**B**) to create a trough where the ureter will be placed *(large circle)*. **C:** A small mucosal opening is made for the ureteral anastomosis. **D:** The ureter has been anastomosed with full ureteral bites and near full-thickness bladder wall bites using 5-0 DAS. **E:** The ureteral trough is closed with imbricating near full bladder thickness interrupted sutures of 5-0 DAS over the ureter. **F:** The left ureter lays in the created detrusor tunnel.

without opening the mucosa. The bladder is drained, and a small opening is made in the mucosa at the superior end of the incision. The spatulated end of the ureter is sutured with a few interrupted sutures of 5-0 DAS including full thickness of the ureteral wall to near full thickness of the bladder wall. The sutures are tied once they are all placed. The detrusor trough created is then closed with imbricating interrupted sutures of 5-0 DAS including near full thickness of the bladder wall without including the ureter. This creates a tunnel which removes tension, brings blood supply, and prevents vesicoureteral reflux.

RESULTS OF INTRAOPERATIVE REPAIR

Intraoperative identification of a ureteral injury is favorable for the patient and the surgeon; however, it does not guarantee a successful outcome, even when properly performed. This information is valuable to share with the patient and family. In a series of 296,130 hysterectomies (open, vaginal, and laparoscopic), there were 1% of ureteral and 0.7% of bladder injuries repaired during the hysterectomy. Postoperatively, urinary fistula developed in 0.3% of the patients.[4]

Ureteral strictures are a potential late complication occurring in about 10% of end-to-end anastomosis for the repair of ureteral injury.[8] They are uncommon with ureteral reimplantation due to improved blood supply from the detrusor muscle.

Ureteral reflux is expected in patients in whom an antirefluxing type of reimplantation is not performed. In the adult, reflux generally does not lead to long-term problems with infection or pyelonephritis, and renal deterioration is uncommon.

Fistula formation is very uncommon (<1% of repairs)[8] especially if the repair is stented and drained. Ureteric fistulas are typically caused by distal obstruction.

References

1. Magrina JF. Complications of laparoscopic surgery. *Clin Obstet Gynecol* 2002;45(2):469–480.

2. Teeluckdharry B, Gilmour D, Flowerdew G. Urinary tract injury at benign gynecologic surgery and the role of cystoscopy: A systematic review and meta-analysis. *Obstet Gynecol* 2015;126(6):1161–1169.

3. Adelman MR, Bardsley TR, Sharp HT. Urinary tract injuries in laparoscopic hysterectomy: A systematic review. *J Minim Invasive Gynecol* 2014;21(4):558–566.

4. Bretschneider CE, Casas-Puig V, Sheyn D, et al. Delayed recognition of lower urinary tract injuries following hysterectomy for benign indications: A NSQIP-based study. *Am J Obstet Gynecol* 2019;221(2):132.e1–132.e13.

5. Blackwell RH, Kirshenbaum EJ, Shah AS, et al. Complications of recognized and unrecognized iatrogenic ureteral injury at time of hysterectomy: A population based analysis. *J Urol* 2018;199(6):1540–1545.

6. Wong JMK, Bortoletto P, Tolentino J, et al. Urinary tract injury in gynecologic laparoscopy for benign indication: A systematic review. *Obstet Gynecol* 2018;131(1):100–108.

7. Hurd WW, Chee SS, Gallagher KL, et al. Location of the ureters in relation to the uterine cervix by computed tomography. *Am J Obstet Gynecol* 2001;184(3):336–339.

8. Santucci RA, Doumanian LR. Section IX. Upper urinary tract obstruction and trauma. Upper urinary tract trauma. In: McDougal WS, Wein AJ, Kavoussi LR, eds. *Campbell-Walsh urology*, 10th ed. Philadelphia: Elsevier, 2012: 1169–1189.

CHAPTER 29

MIDURETHRAL SLINGS

Emily L. Whitcomb • Emily Helena Frisch

TENSION-FREE VAGINAL TAPE

Since its introduction in 1996 by Ulmsten et al., the tension-free vaginal tape (TVT) has become the most commonly performed and "gold standard" surgery for stress urinary incontinence (SUI).[1] The TVT gained popularity due to its minimally invasive approach without the voiding dysfunction, de novo urgency urinary incontinence, and longer recovery seen in other procedures. Cure rates for the TVT are higher than those of the Burch colposuspension and at least equivalent to traditional sling procedures.[2–5] Although based on the traditional sling technique, TVT has several characteristics that distinguish it, including placement of the sling at the midurethra, sling arms that are "self-fixing" and do not require suturing to the rectus fascia, the use of trocars that pass the sling from the urethra to the abdomen ("bottom-up" trocar passage), the use of loosely knitted polypropylene mesh for the sling material, and "tension-free" placement (Table 29.1). TVT is indicated for the primary treatment of SUI, or stress-predominant mixed urinary incontinence (MUI), with urethral hypermobility and is also commonly used with modified success in women with intrinsic sphincter deficiency (ISD).[6] In addition, it has a role as a salvage operation in subjects who have failed previous SUI surgery.[7]

Mechanism

Petros and Ulmsten developed the TVT based on the integral theory wherein SUI results from impairment in the pubourethral ligaments that connect the anterior wall of the bladder and the proximal urethra to the posterior surface of the pubic bone.[8–10] The proposed goal of the TVT was to correct "inadequate urethral support from the pubourethral vesical ligaments."[9,11] As such, the TVT is placed under the midurethra where, based on urethral pressure profilometry, the pubourethral ligaments were assumed to have their functional attachment.

Although the most important anatomic landmark of the integral theory, the role of the pubourethral ligaments in maintaining continence has been called into question by some anatomic and radiologic studies.

An anatomic study by Fritsch et al.[12] concluded that the female urethra has no direct ligamentous fixation to the pubic bone. They identified "delicate cords" of smooth muscle running form the pubic bone to the bladder neck, which they proposed should be called the "pubovesical muscles" rather than pubourethral ligaments. They concluded that because of the low content of connective tissue and small dimensions of these structures, they cannot be considered a supportive structure of the urethra.[12] In contrast, anatomic and histologic study by Petros[13] found the pubourethral ligaments to be "strong finite structures" consisting of smooth muscle, elastin, collagen, nerves, and blood vessels. Magnetic resonance imaging and sonographic data also demonstrate the urethra is a mobile structure that moves up and down and is not fixed to the pubic bone.[14,15] These findings suggest the integral theory may not provide the best explanation for the effectiveness of the TVT.

A more plausible mechanism of action for the TVT is that of transient urethral kinking during stress.[16,17] Unlike traditional sling procedures or retropubic colposuspensions, the effectiveness of the TVT does not appear to be related to correction of urethral hypermobility. Most patients with urethral hypermobility preoperatively continue to have urethral hypermobility postoperatively while still achieving high cure rates.[18] Ultrasound studies demonstrate that during Valsalva or a cough, dynamic urethral kinking occurs in the presence of the TVT, with the suburethral portion of the sling serving as the fulcrum.[19,20] At rest, there is no compression or kinking of the urethra. This suggests that urethral mobility may be important in the mechanism of action of the TVT.

There is debate regarding the appropriate position of the urethral tape along the urethra. Urodynamic studies demonstrate an increase in pressure transmission ratios after a TVT with no change in maximum urethral closure pressure.[21] Although midurethral placement is often emphasized, postoperative ultrasonography demonstrates marked variation of sling placement relative to the urethra, with little apparent effect on symptoms or continence rates.[22,23] In contrast, other studies have shown a greater risk of treatment failure when the tape was located under the

TABLE 29.1

Comparison of the Tension-Free Vaginal Tape to Traditional Sling Procedures

	TRADITIONAL SLING	TENSION-FREE VAGINAL TAPE
Sling placement (urethra)	Bladder neck	Midurethra
Sling arms	Fixed to rectus fascia or pubic bone	Self-fixing
Sling material	Variable	1 × 40 cm polypropylene mesh
Instrument passage through retropubic space	Abdomen to vagina ("top down") with guidance from the surgeon's fingers	Vagina to abdomen ("bottom-up"); passed blindly
Sling tension	Variable	Tension-free
Mechanism of cure:		
Repositions bladder neck?	Yes	No
Urethral compression?	Variable	No
Urethral kinking with stress?	?	Yes

proximal urethra.[24,25] In a prospective study investigating whether the location of the tape may influence outside-in transobturator sling outcome, the highest failure rate was associated with the tape under the proximal third of the urethra.[26] As such, the authors concluded that both the middle and distal sections of the urethra may be regarded as targets for transobturator tape (TOT) placement.[23] Proximal midurethral sling (MUS) placement has also been shown to have a weak association with irritative voiding symptoms.[22]

Technique

Although in their original description of the TVT technique, Ulmsten et al.[11] used local anesthesia with intravenous sedation, general or regional anesthesia is also acceptable. The patient is placed in the dorsal lithotomy position in high stirrups and the vagina and lower abdomen are prepped and draped. A Foley catheter is placed to dependent drainage. Using a pen, the suprapubic sites for the two stab incisions are marked just superior to the pubic symphysis 2 fingerbreadths (2 cm) lateral to the midline on each side. Local anesthetic such as 1% lidocaine is often injected at the two suprapubic sites, 10 mL on each side. Using a spinal needle, the injection is carried down behind the pubic bone and should include the rectus muscle, fascia, and skin. In a randomized, double-blind trial of 42 women undergoing MUS, retropubic injection of 0.125% bupivacaine decreased short-term postoperative pain as measured by VAS scores up to 24 hours compared to no injection.[27]

Attention is turned to the vagina, where a weighted speculum is placed for exposure. The midurethra is identified with traction on the Foley catheter, allowing identification of the urethrovesical junction and

the distal urethra. The vaginal epithelium at this level is often grasped with Allis clamps. Local anesthetic (10 mL) with dilute epinephrine or vasopressin is infiltrated in the anterior vaginal wall at the location of the midurethra and laterally to the inferior pubic rami for hydrodissection and hemostasis. A 1.5-cm midurethral incision is made vertically at least 1 cm from the external urethral meatus and the dissection is carried laterally with Metzenbaum scissors to create a tunnel to the inferior pubic ramus bilaterally. The TVT kit (Gynecare Worldwide, a division of Ethicon, Somerville, New Jersey) includes two curved stainless-steel trocars connected by a 1 cm × 40 cm piece of polypropylene mesh encased in a plastic sheath and a nondisposable handle that attaches to the trocars. The plastic sheath covering the mesh consists of two pieces that overlap in the midline, allowing for easy removal after the sling is placed. A hemostat placed in the middle of the sling in the area of overlap can be useful for marking the midline and preventing sheath slippage during placement. One of the two trocars is attached to the trocar handle. Prior to each trocar passage, the bladder is drained, and a rigid catheter guide is placed in the Foley catheter and directed to the ipsilateral side of trocar placement to displace the urethrovesical junction away from the path of the trocar. Of note, in two retrospective cohort studies, Foley catheter guide use did not decrease the risk of lower urinary tract injury during retropubic MUS placement.[28,29]

The trocar handle is held in the hand contralateral to the side of trocar placement while the thumb of the ipsilateral hand stabilizes the trocar as it curves into the vagina and the index finger maintains proper alignment of the tip. The tip of the trocar is placed in the periurethral tunnel and directed toward the patient's ipsilateral shoulder and the marked suprapubic exit site. The endopelvic fascia is perforated and the trocar is directed along the back of the pubic symphysis—with great care to hug the posterior aspect of the bone—to exit at the previously marked abdominal incisions. In a modification of the TVT using a top-to-bottom approach, the two needle trocars are inserted through the suprapubic incisions, passed through the retropubic space behind the pubic bone on top of the operator's finger and exit through a vaginal incision.

After each trocar placement—although it can be performed after passage of both trocars—the Foley catheter is removed, and the bladder is inspected with a 70-degree cystoscope. It is important that the bladder is filled to capacity during cystoscopy so that a bladder perforation is not missed behind a mucosal fold. The area at highest risk for bladder perforation is the anterolateral portion of the bladder dome.

After bladder integrity is confirmed, the handle is detached from the trocar and the trocar is pulled through the abdominal incision. The encased mesh is clamped just below the trocar and cut so that the trocar can be removed from the operative field. The second trocar is then placed on the opposite side using the same technique. Should bladder perforation occur, the trocar is withdrawn, the bladder is drained, the appropriate landmarks are reviewed, and a second attempt at trocar placement is made, taking care to stay as close as possible to the posterior surface of the pubic bone. As the typical TVT bladder injury is small (less than 1 cm), extraperitoneal, and in the bladder dome, it is usually unnecessary to perform any type of repair. Although some surgeons prefer short-term catheterization after such an injury, findings from a retrospective case series found the majority of subjects experiencing a cystotomy during MUS were successfully discharged home the day of surgery without catheter drainage.[30]

The tension of the TVT sling is adjusted to allow for dynamic urethral kinking while avoiding compression of the urethra at rest. The original technique specified the sling to be "loosely placed—without elevation—around the urethra" and it was intended for an intraoperative cough stress testing to determine the tension.[17] If the procedure is performed using local anesthesia as initially described, the patient may be asked to cough repeatedly with a bladder volume of 250 to 300 mL. The sling is tightened so that a few drops of urine are present at the external meatus during coughing. This ensures that the sling is not too tight and minimizes the risk of urinary retention. If general anesthesia is used, the sling is tightened empirically without the benefit of the cough test. Some surgeons use a spacer between the urethra and the sling such as a blunt scissor, Hegar dilator, or Babcock clamp to ensure a tension-free application.[31–33] Others use a Credé maneuver with a full bladder to simulate a Valsalva.[34] In patients who receive regional anesthesia, any of the above

techniques may be used, depending on the patient's level of consciousness and ability to perform forceful cough or Valsalva. The use of the cough test to guide TVT tensioning was originally thought to be an important component of the TVT procedure; however, numerous authors have reported high cure rates with a low incidence of voiding dysfunction in patients who received general anesthesia or when the cough test was otherwise omitted.[35–40] Some authors have found that when compared with general anesthesia, the use of local anesthesia with a cough test improved continence rates, whereas others have found no relationship between anesthesia type and TVT efficacy.[41,42] Adamiak et al. randomized 103 women with SUI to undergo a TVT with either local anesthetic or spinal anesthesia and found no difference in efficacy or safety between the two types of anesthesia.[37] One randomized, double-blind, multicenter trial compared tensioning with scissors or Babcock clamp and found high rates of objective and subjective cure in both groups; however, women in the Babcock group experienced higher vaginal mesh erosion rates (5.3% vs. 0.7%) and women in the scissor group were more likely to have uroflowmetry suggestive of urinary obstruction (26% vs. 15%).[33]

Once the desired tension is achieved, the sheath encasing the sling is removed while stabilizing the sling below the urethra. The abdominal ends of the sling are cut below the skin surface and the incisions are closed with absorbable suture, Steri-strips, or skin adhesive. The vaginal incision is closed with 2-0 or 3-0 absorbable suture in a running fashion. A voiding trial is typically performed in the recovery room. A commonly described technique is the backfill-assisted voiding trial wherein the bladder is retrograde filled with 300 mL of sterile fluid, the catheter removed, and the patient allowed to void. If the patient voids at least two-thirds of the instilled volume, she is discharged without a catheter. This technique has been found to be more efficient than a simple voiding trial wherein the catheter is removed and a postvoid residual measured after spontaneous void.[43] In a randomized, double-blinded trial of backfill standard voiding trial compared to patients' subjective evaluation based on the assessment of force of stream after MUS, there were no differences in rates of catheterization up to 6 weeks postoperatively.[44]

TRANSOBTURATOR SLINGS

In 2001, Delorme[45] described the transobturator suburethral sling. Similar to the TVT, this is a minimally invasive synthetic MUS; however, it is placed using a transobturator rather than retropubic approach. Transobturator slings are positioned under the midurethra and brought laterally through the obturator membrane in either an inside-out or outside-in approach. The inside-out technique involves the blind passage of a curved trocar from the periurethral incision through the obturator internus muscle, obturator membrane, and obturator externus muscle to an incision in the groin.[46] The outside-in approach involves the reverse blind passage of the trocar from the groin incision around the ischiopubic ramus and out the vaginal incision at the level of the midurethra.[45,47] The anatomic approach of the TOT differs from other sling procedures because the retropubic space is not entered. Additionally, the relationship between the sling and the urethra is different for the TOT than for other slings. In other sling techniques, including the TVT, the sling axis is roughly vertical, or U-shape, in relation to the urethral axis.[47] In contrast, the axis of the TOT is more horizontal in relation to the urethral axis. As such, the TOT potentially provides less circumferential compression of the urethra than do traditional or retropubic slings.

Obturator Anatomy

Because of the popularity of the TOT technique, pelvic surgeons should have an intimate knowledge of

obturator compartment and medial thigh anatomy in order to properly perform this procedure and manage its complications (Fig. 29.1). The obturator membrane is a fibrous sheath that spans the obturator foramen, through which the obturator neurovascular bundle penetrates via the obturator canal. The obturator internus muscle lies on the superior (intrapelvic) side of the obturator membrane. The obturator internus origin is on the inferior margin of the superior pubic ramus and the pelvic surface of the obturator membrane. Its tendon passes through the lesser sciatic foramen to insert onto the greater trochanter of the femur to externally rotate the thigh. The obturator artery and vein originate as branches of the internal iliac vessels. As they emerge from the cranial side of the obturator membrane via the obturator canal and enter the obturator space, they divide into many small branches supplying the muscles of the adductor compartment of the thigh (Fig. 29.2). Cadaveric study by Whiteside and Walters[47] has contradicted previous reports of the obturator vessels bifurcating into medial and lateral branches. Rather, the vessels are predominantly small

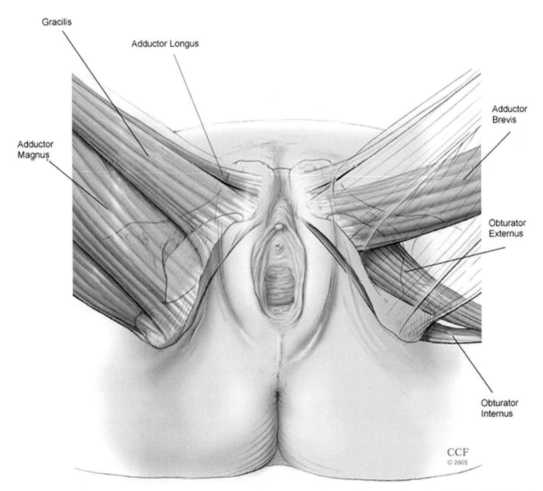

FIGURE 29.1 Muscles of the obturator compartment. The superficial muscles are illustrated on the **left**. On the **right**, the superficial muscles have been made transparent to illustrate the deeper muscles. (Reprinted with permission, Cleveland Clinic Foundation © 2022. All rights reserved.)

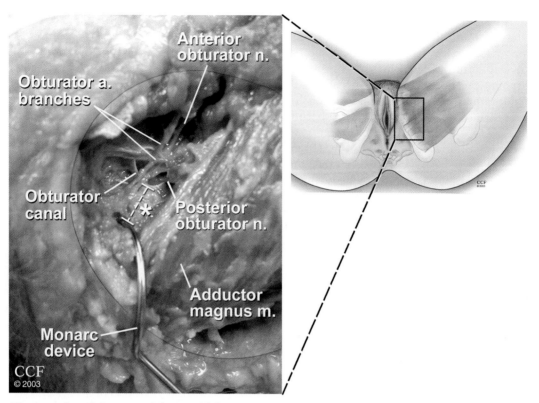

FIGURE 29.2 Photograph and drawing of dissected left external obturator region. Margins of the obturator foramen are highlighted in the photograph. Displayed are the anterior and posterior obturator nerves (n) as they emerge from the obturator canal (ghosted). Multiple obturator artery (a) branches are displayed after emergence from the canal along with adductor magnus muscle (m). The TOT device is shown passing around the left ischiopubic ramus. The distance from the device to the canal *(asterisk)* is on average 2.3 cm. (Reprinted by permission from Springer: Whiteside JL, Walters MD. Anatomy of the obturator region: Relations to a trans-obturator sling. *Int Urogynecol J Pelvic Floor Dysfunct* 2004;15[4]:223–226.)

(less than 5 mm in diameter) and splinter into variable courses. The muscles of the medial thigh and adductor compartment are, from superficial to deep, the gracilis, adductors longus, adductors brevis, adductors magnus, and obturator externus muscles.

In contrast to the vessels, the obturator nerve emerges from the obturator canal and bifurcates into anterior and posterior divisions traveling distally down the thigh to supply the adductor muscles.[47] In a recent cadaveric study by Shah et al.,[48] the anterior nerve divided into smaller branches that perforated the adductor brevis and adductor longus muscles. The posterior nerve divided into smaller branches that perforated the gracilis, adductor brevis, adductor magnus, and obturator externus muscles.[48] With the patient in the dorsal lithotomy position, the nerves and vessels follow the thigh and course laterally away from the ischiopubic ramus.

Technique

The TOT may be performed under general, regional, or local anesthesia with sedation. The peatient is placed in dorsal lithotomy position in high stirrups. The vagina,

lower abdomen, and inner thighs are prepped and draped, and a Foley catheter is placed to dependent drainage. Important landmarks in the obturator compartment are identified, including the ischiopubic ramus and the adductor longus tendon. When using an outside-in approach, the location of the inner thigh incisions is identified by palpating the notch below the adductor longus tendon just lateral to the labia majora. A pen is used to mark the location of the incisions on each side within this notch at the level of the clitoris. The location of these incision sites is approximately 2.5 cm medial to the obturator neurovascular bundle as it exits the obturator canal.[47] If the procedure is being performed using local anesthetic, 10 to 60 mL of local anesthetic with dilute epinephrine is injected into the incision site and carried down through underlying muscle to the level of the obturator membrane just lateral to the ischiopubic ramus on each side. A 1-cm stab incision is made at the marked sites.

A weighted speculum is placed in the vagina for exposure. Using the marking pen, the site for the 2-cm midurethral incision is marked vertically beginning at least 1 cm from the external urethral meatus. Local anesthetic with dilute epinephrine or vasopressin is infiltrated in the anterior vaginal wall at the location of the urethral incision site and laterally to the inferior pubic rami for hydrodissection and hemostasis. The vaginal epithelium at the midurethra is incised, and the dissection is carried laterally with Metzenbaum scissors to create a tunnel, large enough to allow an index finger, to the inferior pubic ramus on each side of the urethra.

Several different transobturator slings have been marketed, with some using helical trocars and others using curved trocars. The surgeon should follow the manufacturer's recommendations for each sling. The angle of trocar passage from the thigh incision to the periurethral incision is approximately 30 to 40 degrees. The trocar is oriented appropriately and held with the ipsilateral hand. The surgeon's contralateral index finger is inserted into the periurethral tunnel to the medial edge of the ramus. The trocar passes through the following layers as it is passed around the ischiopubic ramus: skin, subcutaneous fat, gracilis muscle, adductor brevis, obturator externus muscle, obturator membrane, obturator internus muscle, and periurethral endopelvic fascia (Fig. 29.3).[47] If passed properly, the trocar tip will meet the surgeon's finger as it passes around the ramus so that it can be guided out the periurethral tunnel lateral to the urethra. The sling is connected to the trocar and pulled through the periurethral tunnel, around the ischiopubic ramus and out the inner thigh incision (Fig. 29.4). The sling is

clamped and cut just below the trocar, and the trocar is removed from the operative field. This procedure is repeated on the opposite side (Fig. 29.5). Although some have suggested that intraoperative cystoscopy may be unnecessary with the TOT, bladder injuries have been reported.[49,50] Routine cystoscopy is recommended because of the significant adverse consequences that can occur with an unrecognized bladder injury involving an exposed foreign body within the bladder.

The sling is adjusted in a tension-free application beneath the midurethra. Tensioning techniques are similar to those described for the TVT. Some authors have suggested that TOT slings should be tensioned somewhat tighter than a TVT; however, there are no randomized trials evaluating different TOT tensioning techniques. Once the desired tension is achieved, the sheath encasing the sling is removed while stabilizing the sling below the urethra. The outer ends of the sling are cut below the skin surface and the incisions are closed with 4-0 absorbable suture or skin adhesive. The vaginal incision is closed with 2-0 or 3-0 absorbable suture in a running fashion. A voiding trial is typically performed in the recovery room.

Unlike other TOT kits, the TVT Obturator (TVT-O) system (Ethicon, Somerville, New Jersey) uses an inside-out approach. Like the TOT procedure, a 2-cm midurethral incision is made, and the periurethral tunnels are developed bilaterally. Unlike the TOT,

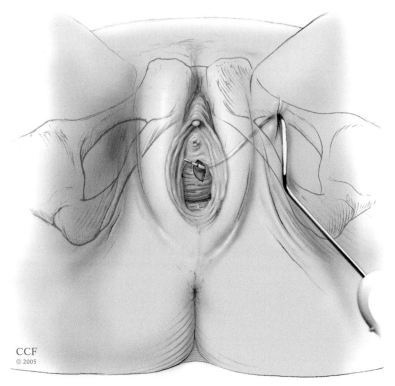

FIGURE 29.3 Transobturator sling placed using outside-in technique. (Reprinted with permission, Cleveland Clinic Foundation © 2022. All rights reserved.)

CCF
© 2005

FIGURE 29.4 Transobturator sling is connected to the trocar and pulled through the periurethral tunnel, around the ischiopubic ramus and out the inner thigh incision. (Reprinted with permission, Cleveland Clinic Foundation © 2022. All rights reserved.)

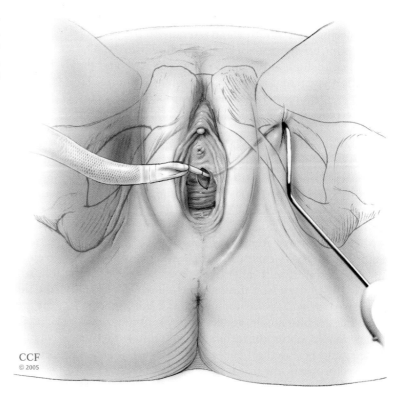

FIGURE 29.5 Transobturator sling. (Reprinted with permission, Cleveland Clinic Foundation © 2022. All rights reserved.)

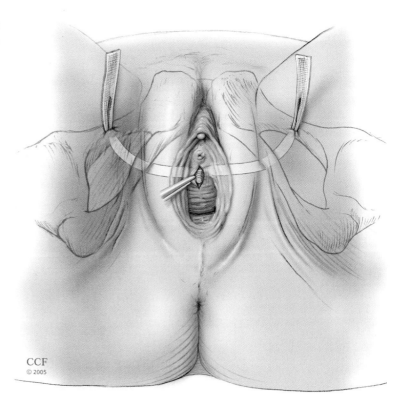

where the dissection stops at the ischiopubic ramus, the obturator membrane is perforated with the tip of the scissors in this approach. Included within the TVT-O kit is a winged metal trocar guide whose purpose is to help guide the helical TVT-O trocars around the ischiopubic ramus. The winged guide is inserted into the periurethral tunnels, and the tip is pushed just beyond the perforated obturator membrane. The tip of the helical trocar is passed into the periurethral tunnel just inside the metal guide (Fig. 29.6). The trocar is then rotated around the ischiopubic ramus to exit the skin through stab incisions (Fig. 29.7). The groin incisions of the TVT-O are somewhat lateral to those of the outside-in technique, located 2 cm above a horizontal line at the level of the urethral meatus and 2 cm outside the thigh folds. The sling is then pulled through the thigh incision and held. The same procedure is repeated on the opposite side. The sling is tensioned and the procedure completed similar to technique described earlier.

Retropubic Midurethral Sling Complications

One of the aspects of the TVT procedure that differentiates it from more traditional continence procedures is the blind trocar passage through the retropubic space.

This blind trocar passage has been the source of some concern, particularly regarding perioperative complications. Generally, the complication rate with the TVT procedure is low; however, in meta-analysis of comparative data, bladder perforations were more common after MUS compared to Burch colposuspensions, and lower urinary tract symptoms and reoperation were more common after traditional sling procedures.[3,51,52] Long-term outcomes following surgical treatment for SUI have been evaluated in several population-based datasets. Muller et al.[53] used National Health Service administrative data to compare the risk of reoperation up to 10 years after retropubic colposuspension, mesh sling insertion, and autologous sling in 96,020 women. They found retropubic colposuspension was associated with a higher risk of reoperation in the first 10 years after SUI surgery compared with mesh sling insertion or autologous sling procedures (21.3% compared to 10.9% and 12%, respectively).[53]

The complication rates noted in early nationwide registries from Finland and Austria are shown in Table 29.2. The one complication that occurs more frequently with TVT than with other procedures is bladder injury, ranging from 2.9% to 9% in the literature.[54–57] Fortunately, the long-term sequelae from these bladder perforations appear to be minimal, assuming

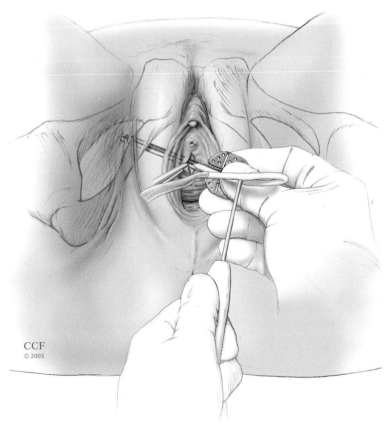

FIGURE 29.6 The trocar of the TVT-O procedure is passed using an inside-out technique. The tip of the helical trocar is passed into the periurethral tunnel just inside the winged metal guide. (Reprinted with permission, Cleveland Clinic Foundation © 2022. All rights reserved.)

FIGURE 29.7 TVT-O trocar rotating around the ischiopubic ramus to exit out the skin through stab incisions on inner thigh. (Reprinted with permission, Cleveland Clinic Foundation © 2022. All rights reserved.)

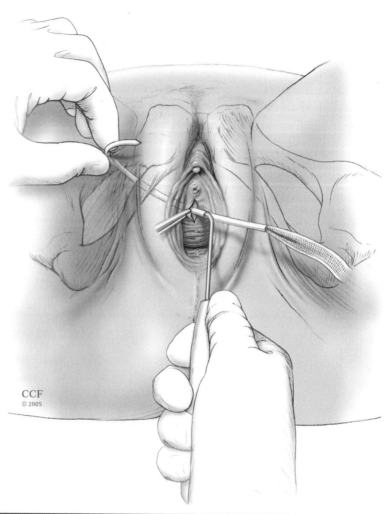

CCF
© 2005

TABLE 29.2		
Complications of the Tension-Free Vaginal Tape Procedure (TVT) in Two Nationwide Registries		
COMPLICATIONS	**AUSTRIAN TVT REGISTRY**[54]	**FINNISH NATIONWIDE TVT STUDY**[55]
n	5,578	1,455
Bladder perforation	2.7%	3.8%
Urethral injury	0%	0.1%
Bowel perforation	0.02%	0%
Increased blood loss	1.9%	1.9%
Retropubic hematoma	1.1%	1.9%
Reoperation for hematoma	0.8%	0.5%
Blood transfusion	0.3%	0.3%
Mesh erosion	0.7%	0.1%
Reoperation for voiding dysfunction	1.3%	2.3%
Urinary tract infection	4.1%	17%
Vesicovaginal fistula	0%	0.1%

they are identified intraoperatively. Trocar injuries to the bladder are typically small and extraperitoneal, requiring no intervention other than replacement of the trocar in the proper location. Trocar injuries of the bowel and major blood vessels have been reported but are exceedingly rare.[54,55,57]

On average, the intraoperative blood loss from a TVT is less than that from an open or laparoscopic Burch colposuspension[35,56]; however, the rate of postoperative bleeding and retropubic hematomas is higher with the TVT.[56] Postoperative hematomas develop in up to 4.1% of patients; however, the majority can be managed expectantly.[58,59] The rate of blood transfusion after TVT ranges from 0.3% to 0.6% in a large series.[58] Correct orientation of the TVT trocar during placement is critical for avoiding a cystotomy and damage to major blood vessels. The orientation of the trocar and handle is best kept slightly lateral to the midline sagittal plane and directed to the ipsilateral shoulder during retropubic passage.[60] Care must be taken to minimize external or internal rotation of the device, as the average distance to major vascular structures ranges from 3.2 to 4.9 cm away from the proper trocar path (Fig. 29.8).[60]

Generally, return to normal voiding occurs more quickly with the TVT than with traditional continence procedures.[56,61] Short-term voiding dysfunction has been estimated to be as high as 24%.[62,63] However, over 80% of women with short-term voiding dysfunction will have resolution of their symptoms by 6 weeks after surgery.[64] In a 2016 study, Ripperda et al.[62] found that of the almost 22% of MUS patients who failed the initial voiding trial, 90% and 38.5% succeeded at the second and third trials respectively.

In a subanalysis of the Trial of Midurethral Slings (TOMUS), a randomized controlled trial comparing retropubic and transobturator slings, only 38 of 586 (6%) reported any catheter use at 2 weeks, and only 9 of 587 (2%) reported any catheter use by 6 weeks.[65] Women with incomplete bladder emptying at discharge were more likely to have had a retropubic MUS and to report preoperative voiding symptoms such as straining to void.

Urinary retention requiring transection of the tape occurs in 1% to 5% of subjects.[54,55,64,66] The risk of urinary retention is greater in women who have had a previous incontinence procedure (odds ratio [OR] 2.9) compared to women treated for primary SUI.[64] In women with prolonged urinary retention, vaginal transection of the TVT tape almost universally resolves the voiding dysfunction, with only a small proportion developing recurrent SUI.[67] De novo urinary urgency after TVT has been reported at rates similar to or lower than that of other continence operations.[56,68,69]

The rate of vaginal mesh exposure after TVT is 1% or less.[54,55,70] This rate is lower than that typically reported for traditional slings using synthetic materials and is likely the result of a combination of factors, including the use of monofilament, loosely knitted polypropylene mesh and a small vaginal incision with minimal dissection. In patients who are asymptomatic and have small (less than 1 cm) exposures, topical estrogen therapy and observation may result in reepithelialization. In symptomatic patients and those with larger exposures, reoperation to excise the exposed mesh and reapproximate the vaginal epithelium is required. Excision of a larger portion of the mesh or the entire sling is necessary only in cases of severe infection or

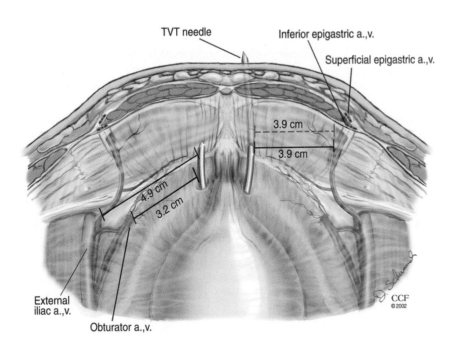

FIGURE 29.8 The relationship of the TVT needle to the vascular anatomy of the anterior abdominal wall and retropubic space. Numbers represent the mean distance from the lateral aspect of the TVT needle to the medial edge of the vessels. a, artery; v, vein. (From Muir TW, Tulikangas PK, Fidela Paraiso M, et al. The relationship of tension-free vaginal tape insertion and the vascular anatomy. *Obstet Gynecol* 2003;101[5 Pt 1]:933–936.)

intractable pain. Mesh exposures into the bladder and urethra have occurred but are very rare. The presence of the TVT mesh in the bladder or urethra in the postoperative period is more likely the result of intraoperative perforation that was missed during cystoscopy than a postoperative exposure.

Transobturator Midurethral Sling: Comparative Complications

TOT has been advocated because it avoids the retropubic space and, as such, has been shown to have lower morbidity—including decreased risk of bladder, bowel, and iliac vessel injury—and more favorable operating time, blood loss, and length of hospital stay compared to the retropubic approach.[2,57,65,71-73] Comparative studies have confirmed a lower rate of bladder injury for TOT than TVT.[57,74-76] Some authors have suggested that the rate of bladder injury with TOT is low enough that routine cystoscopy is not necessary.[45,76] However, although uncommon, lower urinary tract injuries can occur with TOT, with bladder injuries reported in up to 0.5% of cases, and urethral injuries occur in up to 1.1% of cases.[45,49,50] Minaglia et al.[50] reported 3 bladder injuries in their first 61 cases of TOT, 2 of which would not have been identified without routine intraoperative cystoscopy.[50] Given the adverse consequences of an unrecognized bladder injury, intraoperative cystoscopy is recommended.

The novel anatomic approach of the TOT, while avoiding the space of Retzius and thereby reducing the risk of bladder injury, does allow the potential for other complications, including obturator neurovascular injury and lower extremity complications not seen with other approaches. Hematomas and abscesses of the obturator compartment have been reported. Although early studies of TOT showed either absent or low rates of obturator nerve injuries, thigh hematomas, infections, and low rates of postoperative leg pain (0.5%),[73] subsequent randomized or quasi-randomized controlled trials have consistently demonstrated higher rates of groin pain in women undergoing transobturator compared to retropubic MUS (relative risk [RR] 4.12, 95% confidence interval [CI] 2.71 to 6.27).[57]

The less compressive nature of the TOT sling translates into a lower rate of voiding dysfunction and irritative bladder symptoms than the TVT. In a retrospective comparison of the TOT to TVT, Barber et al.[74] found subjects who received TVT were more likely to require urethrolysis for voiding dysfunction or urinary urgency (OR 3.2, 95% CI 1.2 to 10.1) and more likely to use anticholinergic medications postoperatively (OR 2.1, 95% CI 1.02 to 4.70) than those who received TOT. Similarly, in the 2017 Cochrane review evaluating 6,200 participants across 37 trials, lower rates of postoperative voiding dysfunction

were demonstrated in the transobturator compared to retropubic groups (RR 0.53, 95% CI 0.43 to 0.65).[57] Voiding dysfunction was also more frequent, and vaginal perforation less frequent, in the inside-out compared to outside-in route.[57]

In a systematic review of English-language randomized controlled trials through 2013 performed by the Society of Gynecologic Surgeons (SGS) Systematic Review Group, retropubic slings had lower rates of sling exposure, reoperation for sling erosion, nerve injury, ureteral injury, groin or leg pain, and vaginal perforation. Obturator slings had shorter operative time, lower blood loss, fewer bladder and urethral perforations, less perioperative pain, fewer urinary tract infections, and fewer overactive bladder symptoms.[72]

In a meta-analysis of retropubic and transobturator slings, bladder perforations and bleeding were more common with retropubic MUS, whereas vaginal perforations and neurologic symptoms were more common with transobturator MUS. Operative time was significantly longer for retropubic MUS than transobturator MUS. There were no differences in mesh exposure, urinary retention, infection, lower urinary tract symptoms, and length of hospital stay.[73]

In a more recent retrospective cohort study of 1,881 women at a single institution with median follow-up of almost 5 years, women undergoing a transobturator sling had an increased risk of reoperation for recurrent SUI compared to women undergoing a retropubic sling.[77] Women in the retropubic group had a higher rate of intraoperative complications compared with those in the transobturator group, the majority of which were bladder perforations, and a higher risk of sling revision for urinary retention (hazard ratio 8.11, 95% CI 1.08 to 61.17).

In a retrospective cohort study of over 17,000 patients undergoing primary MUS—including retropubic (63%), transobturator (27%) and single incision (10%)—within a large health maintenance organization, the reoperation rate for mesh revision or removal was 0.7% at 1 year, 1.0% at 5 years, and 1.1% at 9 years. Reoperation for recurrent SUI was 1.6% at 1 year, 3.9% at 5 years, and 5.2% at 9 years.[78] Low rates of readmission and reoperation were similarly described in an American College of Surgeons National Surgical Quality Improvement Program database study of 9,910 patients undergoing isolated MUS.[79] They found 58 (0.59%) patients were readmitted (urinary retention [27.6%], non–surgical site-related infection [15.5%], and medical related issues [15.5%]) and 81 (0.82%) had reoperation. Most recently, using a population-based cohort of 334,601 commercially insured women, Dejene et al.[80] found that the 10- and 15-year cumulative risks of midurethral sling revision were 6.9% and 7.9%, respectively. Nearly half of the sling revisions were due to mesh exposure. The 10- and

15-year risks of repeat SUI surgery were 14.5% and 17.9%, respectively.[80]

Although the overall risk of adverse events after both retropubic and transobturator MUS is low, they do vary by approach; as such, surgeons should engage patients in a shared decision-making process that includes discussion of these unique risks.

OUTCOMES

MUS have been the most extensively studied surgical treatment for female SUI.[57] Randomized controlled clinical trials have repeatedly demonstrated the efficacy of synthetic polypropylene mesh slings at 15 to 17 years (Table 29.3).[51,57] The first randomized controlled equivalence trial comparing retropubic and transobturator slings was the TOMUS.[71] This multicenter study enrolled 597 women and reported on 1-, 2-, and 5-year outcomes. The primary outcome was treatment success defined by objective (negative stress test, negative pad test, and no retreatment) and subjective (self-reported absence of symptoms, no leakage episodes on voiding diary, and no retreatment) criteria at 12 months. At 1 year, the retropubic and transobturator slings were objectively

---

TABLE 29.3

Summary of Comparative Trials: Retropubic versus Transobturator

COMPARISON	IMPORTANT STUDIES	SUMMARY
Retropubic vs. transobturator	Cochrane review (Ogah et al., 2009)[3]	Slightly higher objective cure with retropubic slings but no difference in subjective cure; higher blood loss, bladder perforations, and voiding dysfunction with retropubic vs. transobturator slings
	Trial of Midurethral Slings (TOMUS) RCT (Richter et al., 2010)[71]	Similar subjective and objective success rates; higher voiding dysfunction with retropubic and higher neurologic symptoms with transobturator slings
	TOMUS 5-year follow-up (Kenton et al., 2015)[81]	Treatment success decreased at 5 years for retropubic and transobturator slings; high satisfaction in both groups; more sustained improvement in urinary symptoms and sexual function with transobturator slings; similar low rates of new mesh erosions in both groups
	Society of Gynecologic Surgeons (SGS) review (Schimpf et al., 2014)[72]	Similar efficacy and satisfaction; higher bladder perforations, pain, urinary tract infections, and overactive bladder with retropubic and higher erosion, groin pain, and vaginal perforation with transobturator slings
	RCT, 5-year (Laurikainen et al., 2014)[82]	No difference in cure rate between retropubic and transobturator slings; high patient satisfaction in both groups
	Meta-analysis (Seklehner et al., 2015)[83]	Higher objective and subjective cure rates with retropubic slings; higher rates of bladder perforation and bleeding with retropubic slings; higher rates of neurologic symptoms and vaginal perforation with transobturator slings
	Meta-analysis (Maggiore et al., 2017)[84]	Similar long-term effectiveness and safety, objective and subjective cure rates and complications, regardless of specific approach
Retropubic top-down vs. bottom-up	SGS review (Schimpf et al., 2014)[72]	Insufficient evidence
	Cochrane review (Ford et al., 2017)[57]	Bottom-up was more effective for subjective cure and had less voiding dysfunction, fewer bladder perforations and mesh erosions
Transobturator inside-out vs. outside-in	SGS review (Schimpf et al., 2014)[72]	Insufficient evidence
	Cochrane review (Ford et al., 2017)[57]	No differences in short- and medium-term subjective cure rates
Single Incision vs. full length	Review (Mostafa et al., 2013)[85]	No difference in cure rates when excluding TVT-Secur
	SGS review (Schimpf et al., 2014)[72]	Improved cure rates with full-length slings
	Cochrane review (Ford et al., 2017)[57]	Higher rates of persistent SUI after single-incision slings when including TVT-Secur
	Meta-analysis (Kim et al., 2019)[86]	Higher objective cure after long-term follow-up, with more favorable immediate postoperative pain, intraoperative blood loss, and postoperative voiding dysfunction in mini-sling group

RCT, randomized controlled trial; SUI, stress urinary incontinence; TVT, tension-free vaginal tape.

equivalent, with 80.8% of the retropubic and 77.7% of the obturator groups demonstrating treatment success. The rates of subjective treatment success were slightly higher in retropubic compared to transobturator slings (62.2% and 55.8%, respectively); however, this did not meet the prespecified criteria for equivalence. There were no significant differences in urgency urinary incontinence, satisfaction with the procedure, or quality of life measures. Voiding dysfunction requiring surgery was significantly higher in the retropubic slings (2.7% vs. 0%), and neurologic symptoms were higher in the transobturator slings (9.4% vs. 4.0%). A post hoc comparison of the TOMUS showed no significant differences in success between the inside-out and outside-in approaches.[71] The use of a composite outcome and the inclusion of both objective and subjective outcomes are thought to account for the lower rates of treatment success compared to commonly reported rates in the literature.

In a 5-year longitudinal follow-up of 404 of the 597 (68%) of the original cohort, surgical success—defined as no retreatment or self-reported stress incontinence symptoms—was slightly higher in the retropubic compared to the transobturator slings (51.3% vs. 43.4%); however, this did not meet criteria for equivalence.[81] Although overall urinary and sexual function were improved after surgery, sexual function, urgency urinary incontinence and quality of life measures demonstrated greater improvement in the transobturator group. Overall satisfaction decreased at 5 years; however, satisfaction remained high in both groups (94% to 79% TVT, 92% to 85% TOT).

Another multicenter randomized clinical trial of retropubic compared to transobturator MUS in Finland of 95% of the 268 enrolled women reported 5-year outcomes. Objective treatment success was similarly defined by a negative stress test, negative 24-hour pad test, and no retreatment for stress incontinence. Condition-specific quality of life questionnaires assessed patient satisfaction.[82] Objective cure rate (84.7% in the retropubic and 86.2% in the transobturator group), subjective satisfaction (94.2% in the retropubic and 91.7% in the transobturator groups), and complications were similar between groups.

Meta-analyses of retropubic and transobturator midurethal slings have either favored[71] or demonstrated significant improvements in objective cure and subjective cure with the retropubic approach.[73] Authors of one of those meta-analyses found in a separate study that the transobturator approach was more cost-effective than the retropubic approach[83]; this supports the brief economic commentary from the Cochrane review also favoring the transobturator over the retropubic approach.[57]

A Cochrane Collaboration review (2017) of MUS operations identified 81 randomized trials evaluating 12,113 women with SUI, urodynamic SUI, or mixed urinary incontinence (MUI).[57] In this review of mostly moderate-quality evidence comparing retropubic and transobturator routes, including 8,652 women in 55 trials, short-term (up to 1 year) rates of subjective cure ranged from 62% to 98% in the transobturator group and from 71% to 97% in the retropubic group; objective cure was similar in both groups. In the more limited review of medium- and long-term data, subjective cure was similar between the groups, with long-term rates ranging from 43% to 92% in the transobturator group and from 51% to 88% in the retropubic group. A European systematic review similarly found similar long-term objective and subjective cure rates, and complication rates, for retropubic and transobturator techniques regardless of the specific approach.[84]

Moderate-quality evidence in this review indicated the retropubic bottom-to-top route was more effective than top-to-bottom route for subjective cure and was associated with less voiding dysfunction, fewer bladder perforations, and vaginal tape exposures. There were no differences in short- and medium-term subjective cure rates between transobturator slings passed using an inside-out compared to an outside-in approach.

In summary, strong level evidence supports the short and medium term—with accruing evidence in the longer term—efficacy and safety of MUS. The various approaches do differ in their complications, and discussion of these should be incorporated into a shared surgical decision-making process with the individual patient.

Modifying Factors

Although weight loss should be considered first-line therapy for the treatment of SUI, MUS are safe and effective in obese women. TOT and TVT MUS procedures are associated with significant improvement in obese women with SUI, although patient-reported outcome measures for SUI are inversely correlated with body mass index.[87] The reason for the higher failure rate in obese patients is a subject of debate,[88] with some postulating the increasing intra-abdominal pressure during daily activity[89] and others suggesting sling malposition.[90] Rafii et al.[91] prospectively compared the success of TVT in 149 normal and overweight women to 30 obese women and found that obese women had a higher rate of postoperative urgency urinary incontinence (18% vs. 5%, $P = .02$), with no effect on objective or subjective cure of SUI. In contrast, retrospective studies have demonstrated satisfactory efficacy for TVT in obese women comparable to nonobese women.[92] A meta-analysis including 28 studies comparing TVT versus TOT MUS procedures found superior objective and subjective cure rates in obese patients undergoing TVT compared to TOT MUS (94.9% vs. 82% success rate).[93]

The postoperative complication rate also varies between obese and nonobese women. In a systematic review of 13 studies, there were no significant differences in postoperative urinary retention or rates of sling excision between obese and nonobese women.[88,94] However, in an analysis of 11,859 women over 9 years, higher rates of worsening overactive bladder symptoms were found as body mass index increased. This study also showed higher rates of perforation at the low and high extremes of body mass index.[87] Given the diverse outcomes and complications in this patient population, patients should be thoroughly counseled regarding the realistic benefits and risk of MUS.[95]

Mixed Urinary Incontinence

Historically, caution against surgical intervention for MUI has been advised because there is potential to worsen the urgency component. In addition, because there is no objective criterion for measuring MUI, the literature contains a wide range of success rates, with most relying on patient reported outcomes.

Davis et al.[96] evaluated predictors of patient satisfaction after TVT in a prospective cohort of 97 women. They found that the only preoperative predictors of decreased satisfaction 1 year after surgery were symptoms of overactive bladder or voiding difficulty before surgery, corroborating the findings of others that preexisting detrusor overactivity increased the risk of de novo urgency and urgency urinary incontinence.[97] Although several early studies demonstrated similar cure rates in women with preoperative MUI symptoms and those with pure stress incontinence symptoms,[82,97,98] subsequent studies suggest that those with mixed incontinence symptoms have higher long-term failure.[99,100]

A systematic review including six randomized trials and seven prospective studies (average to good-quality data) assessed the effectiveness of MUS in women with symptomatic ± urodynamic MUI who underwent TVT or TOT.[101] The overall subjective cure from the seven prospective studies was 56.4% at 35-month follow-up. The overall cure of urgency and urgency urinary incontinence component was 30% to 85% at a follow-up of few months to 5 years, with most studies demonstrating that this cure did not persist over time. The cure rate of SUI varied from 85% to 97%. On meta-analysis of five randomized controlled trials, which included women with MUI symptoms, the odds of overall subjective cure with TVT versus TOT were similar at 6 to 33 months follow-up. This finding persisted in a subgroup analysis of women with MUI who did not have detrusor overactivity on urodynamics.

In a clinical review of MUI, a MEDLINE search resulted in 785 articles of which a total of 73 articles were included.[102] Although high-quality evidence for treating either SUI or UUI existed, direct high-quality evidence for the diagnosis and treatment of women with MUI was lacking. As such, convention typically has been to treat MUI with management emphasizing the most bothersome or predominant symptom first; this has been supported by data demonstrating good concordance between the dominant type of incontinence and urodynamic findings.[103]

Gleason et al.[104] undertook a retrospective cohort study of women with SUI only versus women with MUI who underwent primary MUS surgery for SUI. MUI was defined as at least "moderately" bothersome urgency and SUI on the Urinary Distress Inventory (UDI-6) subscale of the Pelvic Floor Distress Inventory-20 (PFDI-20). They found women in the MUI group not only had an increased risk of SUI failure but also experienced greater improvements in urinary symptoms and symptom impact on quality of life compared to women with SUI only.

In summary, MUS are generally indicated for women with stress-predominant MUI or in the carefully evaluated and counseled women with equal stress and urgency urinary incontinence.[105] Although the cure of SUI is consistently good with patients with MUI, urgency outcomes are more variable and not as durable.[101] As such, personalized approaches to the treatment of MUI are recommended, and patients should be explicitly counseled regarding the possibility of persistent overactive bladder symptoms and urgency urinary incontinence requiring additional treatment.[105]

Intrinsic Sphincter Deficiency

Although preoperative urethral immobility (urethral straining angle less than 30 degrees) was traditionally considered a contraindication to MUS due to overall lower success rates compared to women without ISD, more recent evidence suggests MUS are effective in treating women with ISD.[6,16,18,74] Unfortunately, the lack of a standardized definition of ISD has limited comparisons in the literature. Although originally described as severe form of SUI with an immobile urethra, it is now commonly accepted to be maximal urethral closure pressure <20 cm H_2O or Valsalva leak point pressure (VLPP) of <60 cm H_2O.

Some studies have found similar cure rates in women with low compared to normal urethral closure pressures,[106,107] whereas others have found low maximum urethral closure pressures to be an independent risk factor for treatment failure.[108] In an analysis of a randomized controlled trial of retropubic and transobturator MUS, when patients were stratified for preoperative VLPP ($\leq$ or $>$ of 60 cm H_2O), preoperative VLPP was not linked to outcome after TVT or TOT procedures.[109] In the TOMUS, women with a VLPP or maximum urethral closure pressure in the lowest quartile were nearly twofold more likely to experience SUI 1 year after transobturator or retropubic MUS.[110] The differences in these studies is likely due to differences in the definitions of ISD and the difficulties in standardizing measurements of urethral insufficiency. Highlighting the lack of a universal definition of ISD—and the significant role urethral hypermobility plays in SUI—are the findings of Haliloglu et al.[111] who found in a cohort of 65 women undergoing TOT, women with ISD with a fixed urethra had the poorest outcome compared to women who had ISD with a hypermobile urethra at 2-year follow-up.

In a systematic review and meta-analysis of 12 randomized controlled trials that reported on data specifically for women with ISD, the retropubic approach resulted in higher subjective cure rates in the short and medium term compared with the transobturator approach.[6] The were no significant differences in objective cure, postoperative voiding dysfunction, or urgency urinary incontinence in the two groups; however, repeat incontinence surgery in the long-term was higher in the transobturator route. In the SGS systematic review referenced above, there were too few studies that specifically examined those with ISD to allow meta-analysis.[72]

Salvage Surgery

Several studies suggest that TVT is effective as a salvage surgery in women who have failed previous surgical treatment with something other than an MUS. A retrospective multicenter study of 245 consecutive women with urodynamic SUI treated with TVT demonstrated cure rates in women with recurrent SUI were similar to those with primary SUI (85% vs. 87%) at a mean follow-up of 38 weeks.[112] Similarly, two prospective studies of women with recurrent SUI treated with TVT with a mean follow-up over 4 years found success rates of 82% and 84.7%, respectively.[106,113]

In a recent systematic review of the evidence on the effectiveness of MUS for recurrent SUI, the pooled objective cure rates across 24 studies, including a total of 858 cases, was 68.5%. Success rates for repeat MUS as a salvage surgery for those who failed a previous MUS varied from 40% to 100% according to study sample sizes, definitions of success, types of MUS used and length of follow-up.[7] The transobturator approach had lower success rates compared to the retropubic approach in repeat MUS surgery, with 72.8% of patients cured with TVT compared to 55.4% of patients cured with TOT as a secondary procedure.[7] In a more recent and more rigorous Cochrane review (2019) of interventions for the treatment of recurrent SUI after failed minimally invasive synthetic MUS, there was insufficient data—and no published papers reporting exclusively on women with a history of MUS—to assess the effects of treatment for recurrent SUI after failed MUS.[114]

Concomitant Pelvic Organ Prolapse Repair

Because women undergoing pelvic organ prolapse (POP) repair are at risk for developing SUI, the use of an MUS—much like that of the Burch colposuspension at time of sacrocolpopexy—to decrease the risk of postoperative SUI has been examined.[115] In a multicenter trial involving 327 women without symptoms of SUI and at least stage 2 anterior vaginal wall prolapse planning vaginal prolapse surgery, women were randomly assigned to undergo either an MUS or a sham surgical incisions. At 12 months, urinary incontinence was present in 27.3% and 43.0% of patients in the MUS and sham groups, respectively ($P = .002$). Bladder perforations, urinary tract infection, major bleeding complications, and incomplete bladder emptying were higher in the MUS group compared to the sham group (6.7% vs. 0%).[116] The number needed to treat in order to prevent one case of SUI was 6.[116]

In a 2018 Cochrane review aimed to determine the impact on postoperative bladder function of surgery for symptomatic POP with or without concomitant continence procedures to treat or prevent SUI, low to moderate data from 19 randomized controlled trials including 2,717 women was reviewed.[117] In women with SUI undergoing vaginal prolapse repair, concomitant MUS improved postoperative rates of subjective SUI (RR 0.30, 95% CI 0.19 to 0.48) and decreased the need for further incontinence surgery (RR 0.04, 95% CI 0.00 to 0.74). In those undergoing vaginal repair with concomitant compared to delayed MUS, there was little or no difference in postoperative SUI. In women with occult SUI undergoing vaginal prolapse repair, MUS improved rates of subjective postoperative SUI (RR 0.38, 95% CI 0.26 to 0.55). In continent women undergoing vaginal prolapse repair with or without MUS, there was no conclusive evidence of a difference in rates of subjective postoperative SUI (RR 0.69, 95% CI 0.47 to 1.00). The authors concluded in women with POP and either symptomatic or occult SUI, "a concurrent MUS probably reduces postoperative SUI and should be discussed in counselling."

Mini-Slings

The single-incision sling, or mini-sling, was developed in 2006 as an alternative to the transobturator approach in order to reduce complications because it does not pass through the retropubic space or obturator membrane.[118] As such, the advantages include less tissue disruption, lower rates of urinary retention, and less risk of visceral injury. Mini-slings are shorter than standard-length retropubic and transobturator slings, and no suprapubic or groin incisions are required.[85] Also made of the same type 1 wide pore monofilament polypropylene mesh, they are inserted through a vaginal incision and fixed in a U-shaped position connecting tissue of the urogenital diaphragm or in a hammock position into the obturator internus muscle. Mini-slings may be placed in an outpatient surgery center under local anesthesia, and they allow for a 1-week return to activity.[118]

Two meta-analyses of randomized controlled trials have demonstrated that MUS are significantly more successful than mini-slings. A 2017 Cochrane Review comparing the mini-sling to the MUS found that women were more likely to experience persistent SUI after mini-slings compared to retropubic slings (41% vs. 26%) and inside-out transobturator slings (30% vs. 11%).[119] It is important to note that many of the comparative studies included the TVT-Secur which was removed from the market in 2013 for commercial reasons. The adverse event profile of mini-slings was significantly worse, including higher risks of vaginal mesh exposure, bladder or urethral exposure, and operative blood loss. Postoperative pain, however, was less common following single-incision slings.

In a 2019 meta-analysis, long-term efficacy of mini-slings, excluding TVT-Secur, was compared to MUS.[86] MUS demonstrated superior objective cure after long-term follow-up, however, mini-slings had more favorable immediate postoperative pain, intraoperative blood loss, and postoperative voiding dysfunction. They found no significant differences in the length of hospital stay, bladder injury, postoperative sexual function, urinary tract infection, urinary retention, de novo urgency, mesh extrusion, vaginal erosion, tape release, or reoperation rate between the mini-sling and MUS.[86]

Thus, the risk–benefit profile for each procedure, along with the patient's goals and expectations, should be considered in determining the preferred sling type for each individual. Mini-slings may be considered in patients in whom surgical complications must be kept to a minimum.

Vaginal Mesh Controversy

In 2011, the U.S. Food and Drug Administration[120] (FDA) released a safety communication on transvaginal mesh placement for POP in response to growing safety concerns. In their database review of reports that included injury, death, and malfunctions, the FDA stated that serious adverse events were not rare and that transvaginally placed mesh for POP repair did not conclusively improve clinical outcomes over traditional nonmesh repair. The FDA ultimately banned the production and sale of transvaginal mesh for POP repair in April 2019. Although the FDA warning specifically excluded surgical mesh for SUI, the resultant mass litigation—and class action lawsuits—included both transvaginal mesh for POP and SUI.[121] In 2012, MUS were specifically excluded from the call for postmarket surveillance studies. In 2013, the FDA released their statement saying, "The safety and effectiveness of multi-incision slings is well-established in clinical trials that followed patients for up to one-year."[120] In 2016, the FDA upclassified transvaginal mesh for POP from class 2 to 3; however, they explicitly excluded mesh for SUI in this reclassification.[121]

Nevertheless, relevant organizations and medical societies were called on to examine implantable mesh for both POP and SUI.[122] The Scientific Committee on Emerging and Newly Identified Health Risks has advised that mesh implanted for SUI—with far fewer mesh-related complications—be viewed differently than mesh for POP. They have recommended "synthetic sling SUI surgery is an accepted procedure with proven efficacy and safety in the majority of patients with moderate to severe SUI when used by an experienced and appropriately trained surgeon."[123] Since then, most major relevant national and international societies have supported the placement of mesh slings for SUI by rigorously trained surgeons in carefully selected and counseled patients. These include the International Urogynecological Association, the American Urogynecologic Society, the American Urologic Association, the Society of Urodynamics, Female Pelvic Medicine & Urogenital Reconstruction, the Royal Australian and New Zealand College of Obstetricians and Gynaecologists, the European Association of Urology, and the American College of Obstetrics and Gynecology.

CONCLUSION

MUS are the most studied surgical treatment for SUI and are accruing strong level data to suggest they are the most effective and durable procedures currently available for the surgical management of SUI. As such, they should be considered the "gold standard" to which newer operations are compared. Because they can be performed in an ambulatory setting and are associated with less pain, quicker recovery, and quicker return to normal voiding, MUS are the optimal choice for the management of isolated primary SUI. They have demonstrated success in the treatment of obese women; those undergoing concomitant POP repair; and women with MUI, ISD, and recurrent SUI. Although meta-analyses favor full-length over mini-slings, mini-slings have a role in patients in whom complications must be minimized.

ACKNOWLEDGMENT

The authors of this chapter would like to acknowledge Dr. Matthew Barber, who contributed to the last edition of this chapter.

References

1. Nager CW. Long-term data support slings as the best surgical procedures for stress urinary incontinence. *Am J Obstet Gynecol* 2021;225(6):591–592.
2. Fusco F, Abdel-Fattah M, Chapple CR, et al. Updated systematic review and meta-analysis of the comparative data on colposuspensions, pubovaginal slings, and midurethral tapes in the surgical treatment of female stress urinary incontinence. *Eur Urol* 2017;72(4):567–591.

3. Ogah J, Cody JD, Rogerson L. Minimally invasive synthetic suburethral sling operations for stress urinary incontinence in women. *Cochrane Database Syst Rev* 2009;(4):CD006375.

4. Wang AC, Chen M-C. Comparison of tension-free vaginal taping versus modified Burch colposuspension on urethral obstruction: A randomized controlled trial. *Neurourol Urodyn* 2003;22(3):185–190.

5. Imamura M, Hudson J, Wallace SA, et al. Surgical interventions for women with stress urinary incontinence: Systematic review and network meta-analysis of randomised controlled trials. *BMJ* 2019;365:l1842.

6. Ford AA, Ogah JA. Retropubic or transobturator mid-urethral slings for intrinsic sphincter deficiency-related stress urinary incontinence in women: A systematic review and meta-analysis. *Int Urogynecol J* 2016;27(1):19–28.

7. Nikolopoulos KI, Betschart C, Doumouchtsis SK. The surgical management of recurrent stress urinary incontinence: A systematic review. *Acta Obstet Gynecol Scand* 2015;94(6):568–576.

8. Petros P, Abendstein B. Knowledge of urethral closure mechanics helps to optimize surgical methodology of the midurethral sling operation. *Cent European J Urol* 2018;71(3):334–337.

9. Petros PE, Ulmsten UI. An integral theory of female urinary incontinence. Experimental and clinical considerations. *Acta Obstet Gynecol Scand Suppl* 1990;153:7–31.

10. Nikolopoulos KI, Chrysanthopoulou E, Pergialiotis V, et al. An animal experimental study on pubourethral ligament restoration with platelet rich plasma for the treatment of stress urinary incontinence. *Cent European J Urol* 2019;72(2):134–141.

11. Ulmsten U, Henriksson L, Johnson P, et al. An ambulatory surgical procedure under local anesthesia for treatment of female urinary incontinence. *Int Urogynecol J Pelvic Floor Dysfunct* 1996;7(2):81–86.

12. Fritsch H, Pinggera GM, Lienemann A, et al. What are the supportive structures of the female urethra? *Neurourol Urodyn* 2006;25(2):128–134.

13. Petros PE. The pubourethral ligaments—An anatomical and histological study in the live patient. *Int Urogynecol J Pelvic Floor Dysfunct* 1998;9(3):154–157.

14. Brandt FT, Albuquerque CD, Lorenzato FR, et al. Perineal assessment of urethrovesical junction mobility in young continent females. *Int Urogynecol J Pelvic Floor Dysfunct* 2000;11(1):18–22.

15. Fielding JR, Griffiths DJ, Versi E, et al. MR imaging of pelvic floor continence mechanisms in the supine and sitting positions. *AJR Am J Roentgenol* 1998;171(6):1607–1610.

16. Lo K, Marcoux V, Grossman S, et al. Cost comparison of the laparoscopic burch colposuspension, laparoscopic two-team sling procedure, and the transobturator tape procedure for the treatment of stress urinary incontinence. *J Obstet Gynaecol Can* 2013;35(3):252–257.

17. Lo T-S, Wang AC, Horng S-G, et al. Ultrasonographic and urodynamic evaluation after tension free vagina tape procedure (TVT). *Acta Obstet Gynecol Scand* 2001;80(1):65–70.

18. Klutke JJ, Carlin BI, Klutke CG. The tension-free vaginal tape procedure: Correction of stress incontinence with minimal alteration in proximal urethral mobility. *Urology* 2000;55(4):512–514.

19. Lo T-S, Horng S-G, Liang C-C, et al. Ultrasound assessment of mid-urethra tape at three-year follow-up after tension-free vaginal tape procedure. *Urology* 2004;63(4):671–675.

20. Sarlos D, Kuronen M, Schaer GN. How does tension-free vaginal tape correct stress incontinence? Investigation by perineal ultrasound. *Int Urogynecol J Pelvic Floor Dysfunct* 2003;14(6):395–398.

21. Mutone N, Mastropietro M, Brizendine E, et al. Effect of tension-free vaginal tape procedure on urodynamic continence indices. *Obstet Gynecol* 2001;98(4):638–645.

22. Dietz HP, Mouritsen L, Ellis G, et al. How important is TVT location? *Acta Obstet Gynecol Scand* 2004;83(10):904–908.

23. Ng CCM, Lee LC, Han WHC. Use of three-dimensional ultrasound scan to assess the clinical importance of midurethral placement of the tension-free vaginal tape (TVT) for treatment of incontinence. *Int Urogynecol J Pelvic Floor Dysfunct* 2005;16(3):220–225.

24. Jiang Y-H, Wang C-C, Chuang F-C, et al. Positioning of a suburethral sling at the bladder neck is associated with a higher recurrence rate of stress urinary incontinence. *J Ultrasound Med* 2013;32(2):239–245.

25. Kociszewski J, Rautenberg O, Perucchini D, et al. Tape functionality: Sonographic tape characteristics and outcome after TVT incontinence surgery. *Neurourol Urodyn* 2008;27(6):485–490.

26. Bogusiewicz M, Monist M, Gałczyński K, et al. Both the middle and distal sections of the urethra may be regarded as optimal targets for "outside-in" transobturator tape placement. *World J Urol* 2014;32(6):1605–1611.

27. Dunivan GC, Parnell BA, Connolly A, et al. Bupivacaine injection during midurethral sling and postoperative pain: A randomized controlled trial. *Int Urogynecol J* 2011;22(4):433–438.

28. Miranne JM, Dominguez A, Sokol AI, et al. Foley catheter guide use during midurethral slings: Does it make a difference? *Can J Urol* 2015;22(3):7811–7816.

29. Tavakoli A, Nasiri A, Lane F. The impact of the rigid catheter guide on trocar injury during mid-urethral sling placement. *Int Arch Urol Complic* 2019;5(1):057. https://clinmedjournals.org/articles/iauc/international-archives-of-urology-and-complications-iauc-5-057.php?jid=iauc

30. Crosby EC, Vilasagar S, Duecy EE, et al. Expectant management of cystotomy at the time of midurethral sling placement: A retrospective case series. *Int Urogynecol J* 2013;24(9):1543–1546.

31. Cundiff GW, Azziz R, Bristow RE. *Te Linde's atlas of gynecologic surgery*. Philadelphia: Lippincott Williams & Wilkins; 2013:382.

32. Mishra VC, Mishra N, Karim OMA, et al. Voiding dysfunction after tension-free vaginal tape: A conservative approach is often successful. *Int Urogynecol J Pelvic Floor Dysfunct* 2005;16(3):210–214.

33. Brennand EA, Wu G, Houlihan S, et al. Two intraoperative techniques for midurethral sling tensioning: A randomized controlled trial. *Obstet Gynecol* 2020;136(3):471–481.

34. Partoll LM. Efficacy of tension-free vaginal tape with other pelvic reconstructive surgery. *Am J Obstet Gynecol* 2002;186(6):1292–1298.

35. Paraiso MF, Falcone T, Walters MD. Laparoscopic surgery for genuine stress incontinence. *Int Urogynecol J Pelvic Floor Dysfunct* 1999;10(4):237–247.

36. Abdel-Fattah M, Barrington JW, Arunkalaivanan AS. Pelvicol pubovaginal sling versus tension-free vaginal tape for treatment of urodynamic stress incontinence: A prospective randomized three-year follow-up study. *Eur Urol* 2004;46(5):629–635.

37. Adamiak A, Milart P, Skorupski P, et al. The efficacy and safety of the tension-free vaginal tape procedure do not depend on the method of analgesia. *Eur Urol* 2002;42(1):29–33.

38. El-Barky E, El-Shazly A, El-Wahab OA, et al. Tension free vaginal tape versus Burch colposuspension for treatment of female stress urinary incontinence. *Int Urol Nephrol* 2005;37(2):277–281.

39. Lim YN, Muller R, Corstiaans A, et al. Suburethral sling-plasty evaluation study in North Queensland, Australia: The SUSPEND trial. *Aust N Z J Obstet Gynaecol* 2005;45(1):52–59.

40. Moore KH, Shahab RB, Walsh CA, et al. Randomized controlled trial of cough test versus no cough test in the tension-free vaginal tape procedure: Effect upon voiding dysfunction and 12-month efficacy. *Int Urogynecol J* 2012;23(4):435–441.

41. Ghezzi F, Cromi A, Raio L, et al. Influence of the type of anesthesia and hydrodissection on the complication rate after tension-free vaginal tape procedure. *Eur J Obstet Gynecol Reprod Biol* 2005;118(1):96–100.

42. Murphy M, Culligan PJ, Arce CM, et al. Is the cough-stress test necessary when placing the tension-free vaginal tape? *Obstet Gynecol* 2005;105(2):319–324.

43. Foster RT, Borawski KM, South MM, et al. A randomized, controlled trial evaluating 2 techniques of postoperative bladder testing after transvaginal surgery. *Am J Obstet Gynecol* 2007;197(6):627.e1–627.e4.

44. Tunitsky-Bitton E, Murphy A, Barber MD, et al. Assessment of voiding after sling: A randomized trial of 2 methods of postoperative catheter management after midurethral sling surgery for stress urinary incontinence in women. *Am J Obstet Gynecol* 2015;212(5):597.e1–597.e9.

45. Delorme E. Transobturator urethral suspension: Mini-invasive procedure in the treatment of stress urinary incontinence in women. *Prog Urol* 2001;11(6):1306–1313.

46. de Leval J. Novel surgical technique for the treatment of female stress urinary incontinence: Transobturator vaginal tape inside-out. *Eur Urol* 2003;44(6):724–730.

47. Whiteside JL, Walters MD. Anatomy of the obturator region: Relations to a trans-obturator sling. *Int Urogynecol J Pelvic Floor Dysfunct* 2004;15(4):223–226.

48. Shah NM, Jackson LA, Phelan JN, et al. Medial thigh anatomy in female cadavers: Clinical applications to the transobturator midurethral sling. *Female Pelvic Med Reconstr Surg* 2020;26(9):531–535.

49. Mellier G, Benayed B, Bretones S, et al. Suburethral tape via the obturator route: Is the TOT a simplification of the TVT? *Int Urogynecol J Pelvic Floor Dysfunct* 2004;15(4):227–232.

50. Minaglia S, Ozel B, Klutke C, et al. Bladder injury during transobturator sling. *Urology* 2004;64(2):376–377.

51. Novara G, Artibani W, Barber MD, et al. Updated systematic review and meta-analysis of the comparative data on colposuspensions, pubovaginal slings, and midurethral tapes in the surgical treatment of female stress urinary incontinence. *Eur Urol* 2010;58(2):218–238.

52. Jones R, Abrams P, Hilton P, et al. Risk of tape-related complications after TVT is at least 4%. *Neurourol Urodyn* 2010;29(1):40–41.

53. Muller P, Gurol-Urganci I, van der Meulen J, et al. Risk of reoperation 10 years after surgical treatment for stress urinary incontinence: a national population-based cohort study. *Am J Obstet Gynecol* 2021;225(6):645.e1–645.e14. doi:10.1016/j.ajog.2021.08.059

54. Tamussino K, Hanzal E, Kölle D, et al; for the Austrian Urogynecology Working Group. The Austrian tension-free vaginal tape registry. *Int Urogynecol J Pelvic Floor Dysfunct* 2001;12(Suppl 2):S28–S29.

55. Kuuva N, Nilsson CG. A nationwide analysis of complications associated with the tension-free vaginal tape (TVT) procedure. *Acta Obstet Gynecol Scand* 2002;81(1):72–77.

56. Ward K, Hilton P; for the United Kingdom and Ireland Tension-Free Vaginal Tape Trial Group. Prospective multicentre randomised trial of tension-free vaginal tape and colposuspension as primary treatment for stress incontinence. *BMJ* 2002;325(7355):67.

57. Ford AA, Rogerson L, Cody JD, et al. Mid-urethral sling operations for stress urinary incontinence in women. *Cochrane Database Syst Rev* 2017;(7):CD006375.

58. Kölle D, Tamussino K, Hanzal E, et al. Bleeding complications with the tension-free vaginal tape operation. *Am J Obstet Gynecol* 2005;193(6):2045–2049.

59. Flock F, Reich A, Muche R, et al. Hemorrhagic complications associated with tension-free vaginal tape procedure. *Obstet Gynecol* 2004;104(5 Pt 1):989–994.

60. Muir TW, Tulikangas PK, Fidela Paraiso M, et al. The relationship of tension-free vaginal tape insertion and the vascular anatomy. *Obstet Gynecol* 2003;101(5 Pt 1):933–936.

61. Geynisman-Tan J, Dave-Heliker B, Bochenska K, et al. Duration of catheterization after retropubic midurethral sling. *Female Pelvic Med Reconstr Surg* 2019;25(5):369–371.

62. Ripperda CM, Kowalski JT, Chaudhry ZQ, et al. Predictors of early postoperative voiding dysfunction and other complications following a midurethral sling. *Am J Obstet Gynecol* 2016;215(5):656.e1–656.e6.

63. Norton PA, Nager CW, Chai TC, et al. Risk factors for incomplete bladder emptying after midurethral sling. *Urology* 2013;82(5):1038–1041.

64. Sokol AI, Jelovsek JE, Walters MD, et al. Incidence and predictors of prolonged urinary retention after TVT with and without concurrent prolapse surgery. *Am J Obstet Gynecol* 2005;192(5):1537–1543.

65. Brubaker L, Norton PA, Albo ME, et al. Adverse events over two years after retropubic or transobturator midurethral sling surgery: Findings from the Trial of Midurethral Slings (TOMUS) study. *Am J Obstet Gynecol* 2011;205(5):498.e1–498.e6.

66. Meschia M, Pifarotti P, Bernasconi F, et al. Tension-free vaginal tape: Analysis of outcomes and complications in 404 stress incontinent women. *Int Urogynecol J Pelvic Floor Dysfunct* 2001;12(Suppl 2):S24–S27.

67. Shaw J, Wohlrab K, Rardin C. Recurrence of stress urinary incontinence after midurethral sling revision: A retrospective cohort study. *Female Pelvic Med Reconstr Surg* 2017;23(3):184–187.

68. Lee JK-S, Dwyer PL, Rosamilia A, et al. Which women develop urgency or urgency urinary incontinence following midurethral slings? *Int Urogynecol J* 2013;24(1):47–54.

69. Smith A. A prospective randomised controlled trial of open and laparoscopic colposuspension. Paper presented at the 35th meeting of International Continence Society, Montreal, Canada, 2005. Accessed March 10, 2022. https://www.cochranelibrary.com/central/doi/10.1002/central/CN-00549494/full

70. Ward KL, Hilton P; and the United Kingdom and Ireland Tension-Free Vaginal Tape Trial Group. A prospective multicenter randomized trial of tension-free vaginal tape and colposuspension for primary urodynamic stress incontinence: Two-year follow-up. *Am J Obstet Gynecol* 2004;190(2):324–331.

71. Richter HE, Albo ME, Zyczynski HM, et al. Retropubic versus transobturator midurethral slings for stress incontinence. *N Engl J Med* 2010;362(22):2066–2076.

72. Schimpf MO, Rahn DD, Wheeler TL, et al. Sling surgery for stress urinary incontinence in women: A systematic review and metaanalysis. *Am J Obstet Gynecol* 2014;211(1):71.e1–71.e27.

73. Seklehner S, Laudano MA, Xie D, et al. A meta-analysis of the performance of retropubic mid urethral slings versus transobturator mid urethral slings. *J Urol* 2015;193(3):909–915.

74. Barber MD, Gustilo-Ashby AM, Chen CCG, et al. Perioperative complications and adverse events of the MONARC transobturator tape, compared with the tension-free vaginal tape. *Am J Obstet Gynecol* 2006;195(6):1820–1825.

75. David-Montefiore E, Frobert J-L, Grisard-Anaf M, et al. Perioperative complications and pain after the suburethral sling procedure for urinary stress incontinence: A French prospective randomised multicentre study comparing the retropubic and transobturator routes. *Eur Urol* 2006;49(1):133–138.

76. Fischer A, Fink T, Zachmann S, et al. Comparison of retropubic and outside-in transoburator sling systems for the cure of female genuine stress urinary incontinence. *Eur Urol* 2005;48(5):799–804.

77. Trabuco EC, Carranza D, El Nashar SA, et al. Reoperation for urinary incontinence after retropubic and transobturator sling procedures. *Obstet Gynecol* 2019;134(2):333–342.

78. Berger AA, Tan-Kim J, Menefee SA. Long-term risk of reoperation after synthetic mesh midurethral sling surgery for stress urinary incontinence. *Obstet Gynecol* 2019;134(5):1047–1055.

79. Hokenstad ED, Glasgow AE, Habermann EB, et al. Readmission and reoperation after midurethral sling. *Int Urogynecol J* 2018;29(9):1367–1370.

80. Dejene SZ, Funk MJ, Pate V, et al. Long-term outcomes after midurethral mesh sling surgery for stress urinary incontinence. *Female Pelvic Med Reconstr Surg* 2021 [Epub ahead of print]. doi:10.1097/SPV.0000000000001094

81. Kenton K, Stoddard AM, Zyczynski H, et al. 5-Year longitudinal followup after retropubic and transobturator mid urethral slings. *J Urol* 2015;193(1):203–210.

82. Laurikainen E, Valpas A, Aukee P, et al. Five-year results of a randomized trial comparing retropubic and transobturator midurethral slings for stress incontinence. *Eur Urol* 2014;65(6):1109–1114.

83. Seklehner S, Laudano MA, Te AE, et al. A cost-effectiveness analysis of retropubic midurethral sling versus transobturator midurethral sling for female stress urinary incontinence. *Neurourol Urodyn* 2014;33(8):1186–1192.

84. Maggiore ULR, Agrò EF, Soligo M, et al. Long-term outcomes of TOT and TVT procedures for the treatment of female stress urinary incontinence: A systematic review and meta-analysis. *Int Urogynecol J* 2017;28(8):1119–1130.

85. Mostafa A, Agur W, Abdel-All M, et al. Multicenter prospective randomized study of single-incision mini-sling vs tension-free vaginal tape-obturator in management of female stress urinary incontinence: A minimum of 1-year follow-up. *Urology* 2013;82(3):552–559.

86. Kim A, Kim MS, Park Y-J, et al. Clinical outcome of single-incision slings, excluding TVT-Secur, vs standard slings in the surgical management of stress incontinence: An updated systematic review and meta-analysis. *BJU Int* 2019;123(4):566–584.

87. Bach F, Hill S, Toozs-Hobson P. The effect of body mass index on retropubic midurethral slings. *Am J Obstet Gynecol* 2019;220(4):371.e1–371.e9.

88. Fuselier A, Hanberry J, Margaret Lovin J, et al. Obesity and stress urinary incontinence: impact on pathophysiology and treatment. *Curr Urol Rep* 2018;19(1):10.

89. Haverkorn RM, Williams BJ, Kubricht WS III, et al. Is obesity a risk factor for failure and complications after surgery for incontinence and prolapse in women? *J Urol* 2011;185(3):987–992.

90. Majkusiak W, Pomian A, Tomasik P, et al. Does the suburethral sling change its location? *Int J Urol* 2017;24(12):848–853.

91. Rafii A, Daraï E, Haab F, et al. Body mass index and outcome of tension-free vaginal tape. *Eur Urol* 2003;43(3):288–292.

92. Mukherjee K, Constantine G. Urinary stress incontinence in obese women: Tension-free vaginal tape is the answer. *BJU Int* 2001;88(9):881–883.

93. Kim DR, Wang E, McGeehan B, et al. Randomized controlled trial of transcranial magnetic stimulation in pregnant women with major depressive disorder. *Brain Stimul* 2019;12(1):96–102.

94. Weltz V, Guldberg R, Lose G. Efficacy and perioperative safety of synthetic mid-urethral slings in obese women with stress urinary incontinence. *Int Urogynecol J* 2015;26(5):641–648.

95. Mamza JB, Geary R, El-Hamamsy D, et al. Variation in surgical treatment advice for women with stress urinary incontinence: A study using clinical case vignettes. *Int Urogynecol J* 2020;31(6):1153–1161.

96. Davis TL, Lukacz ES, Luber KM, et al. Determinants of patient satisfaction after the tension-free vaginal tape procedure. *Am J Obstet Gynecol* 2004;191(1):176–181.

97. Debodinance P, Delporte P, Engrand JB, et al. Tension-free vaginal tape (TVT) in the treatment of urinary stress incontinence: 3 Years experience involving 256 operations. *Eur J Obstet Gynecol Reprod Biol* 2002;105(1):49–58.

98. Rezapour M, Ulmsten U. Tension-free vaginal tape (TVT) in women with mixed urinary incontinence—A long-term follow-up. *Int Urogynecol J Pelvic Floor Dysfunct* 2001;12(Suppl 2):S15–S18.

99. Holmgren C, Nilsson S, Lanner L, et al. Long-term results with tension-free vaginal tape on mixed and stress urinary incontinence. *Obstet Gynecol* 2005;106(1):38–43.

100. Ankardal M, Heiwall B, Lausten-Thomsen N, et al. Short- and long-term results of the tension-free vaginal tape procedure in the treatment of female urinary incontinence. *Acta Obstet Gynecol Scand* 2006;85(8):986–992.

101. Jain P, Jirschele K, Botros SM, et al. Effectiveness of midurethral slings in mixed urinary incontinence: A systematic review and meta-analysis. *Int Urogynecol J* 2011;22(8):923–932.

102. Myers DL. Female mixed urinary incontinence: A clinical review. *JAMA* 2014;311(19):2007–2014.

103. Digesu GA, Salvatore S, Fernando R, et al. Mixed urinary symptoms: What are the urodynamic findings? *Neurourol Urodyn* 2008;27(5):372–375.

104. Gleason JL, Parden AM, Jauk V, et al. Outcomes of midurethral sling procedures in women with mixed urinary incontinence. *Int Urogynecol J* 2015;26(5):715–720.

105. Welk B, Baverstock RJ. The management of mixed urinary incontinence in women. *Can Urol Assoc J* 2017;11(6 Suppl 2):S121–S124.

106. Rezapour M, Falconer C, Ulmsten U. Tension-free vaginal tape (TVT) in stress incontinent women with intrinsic sphincter deficiency (ISD)—A long-term follow-up. *Int Urogynecol J Pelvic Floor Dysfunct* 2001;12(Suppl 2):S12–S14.

107. Meschia M, Pifarotti P, Buonaguidi A, et al. Tension-free vaginal tape (TVT) for treatment of stress urinary incontinence in women with low-pressure urethra. *Eur J Obstet Gynecol Reprod Biol* 2005;122(1):118–121.

108. Paick J-S, Ku JH, Shin JW, et al. Tension-free vaginal tape procedure for urinary incontinence with low Valsalva leak point pressure. *J Urol* 2004;172(4 Pt 1):1370–1373.

109. Costantini E, Lazzeri M, Giannantoni A, et al. Preoperative MUCP and VLPP did not predict long-term (4-year) outcome after transobturator mid-urethral sling. *Urol Int* 2009;83(4):392–398.

110. Nager CW, Sirls L, Litman HJ, et al. Baseline urodynamic predictors of treatment failure 1 year after mid urethral sling surgery. *J Urol* 2011;186(2):597–603.

111. Haliloglu B, Karateke A, Coksuer H, et al. The role of urethral hypermobility and intrinsic sphincteric deficiency on the outcome of transobturator tape procedure: A prospective study with 2-year follow-up. *Int Urogynecol J* 2010;21(2):173–178.

112. Rardin CR, Kohli N, Rosenblatt PL, et al. Tension-free vaginal tape: Outcomes among women with primary versus recurrent stress urinary incontinence. *Obstet Gynecol* 2002;100(5 Pt 1): 893–897.

113. Nilsson CG, Kuuva N, Falconer C, et al. Long-term results of the tension-free vaginal tape (TVT) procedure for surgical treatment of female stress urinary incontinence. *Int Urogynecol J Pelvic Floor Dysfunct* 2001;12(Suppl 2):S5–S8.

114. Bakali E, Johnson E, Buckley BS, et al. Interventions for treating recurrent stress urinary incontinence after failed minimally invasive synthetic midurethral tape surgery in women. *Cochrane Database Syst Rev* 2019;(9):CD009407.

115. Wei JT, Nygaard I, Richter HE, et al. A midurethral sling to reduce incontinence after vaginal prolapse repair. *N Engl J Med* 2012;366(25):2358–2367.

116. van der Ploeg JM, van der Steen A, Zwolsman S, et al. Prolapse surgery with or without incontinence procedure: A systematic review and meta-analysis. *BJOG* 2018;125(3):289–297.

117. Baessler K, Christmann-Schmid C, Maher C, et al. Surgery for women with pelvic organ prolapse with or without stress urinary incontinence. *Cochrane Database Syst Rev* 2018;(8):CD013108.

118. Gon LM, Riccetto CLZ, de Campos CCC, et al. Mini-sling ophira at 8 years follow-up: Does it sustain results? *Urol Int* 2019;102(3):326–330.

119. Nambiar A, Cody JD, Jeffery ST, et al. Single-incision sling operations for urinary incontinence in women. *Cochrane Database Syst Rev* 2017;(7):CD008709.

120. U.S. Food and Drug Administration. Urogynecologic surgical mesh implants. Accessed March 10, 2022. https://www.fda.gov/medical-devices/implants-and-prosthetics/urogynecologic-surgical-mesh-implants

121. Nager CW. Midurethral slings: Evidence-based medicine vs the medicolegal system. *Am J Obstet Gynecol* 2016;214(6): 708.e1–708.e5.

122. Ford AA, Taylor V, Ogah J, et al. Midurethral slings for treatment of stress urinary incontinence review. *Neurourol Urodyn* 2019;38(Suppl 4):S70–S75.

123. Scientific Committee on Emerging and Newly Identified Health Risks. *Opinion on the safety of surgical meshes used in urogynecological surgery*. Luxembourg: European Union, 2015.

CHAPTER 30

AUTOLOGOUS PUBOVAGINAL SLING PLACEMENT

Brian J. Linder

Introduction

Female stress urinary incontinence is a highly prevalent and bothersome condition that can have a large impact on quality of life. In fact, in the United States, it is estimated that by age 80 years, roughly 13% of women will undergo an anti-incontinence surgery.[1] Of the available surgeries (i.e., urethral slings with various materials and approaches, periurethral bulking agents, retropubic urethropexy) the risks, benefits, and durability of each procedure is variable and shared decision-making with patients regarding treatment selection is crucial.[2] This chapter reviews the history, indications, surgical techniques, outcomes, and postoperative management strategies for autologous pubovaginal sling placement.

BRIEF HISTORY OF URETHRAL SLING DEVELOPMENT AND TECHNIQUES

The use of autologous material for urethral sling placement was initially described in 1907 with utilization of a sling based on the gracilis muscle.[3] Over the ensuing decades, numerous modifications to the procedure have been described.[4,5] In 1978, McGuire and Lytton[6] described the use of a rectus fascial urethral sling, where the sling was left attached on one side and then tunneled through the rectus muscle, under the urethra, and reattached to the other side of the rectus fascia. Further modification of this technique, to the more contemporary version, was reported in 1988 by Blaivas and Olsson[7] who described fully detaching the strip of rectus fascia and then perforating the endopelvic fascia for sling placement. Additional modifications regarding intraoperative (e.g., sling tensioning) and postoperative management continue to evolve.[8,9]

Further developments for urethral sling placement continued to occur in the late 1990s and beyond. These modifications included use of synthetic materials instead of harvesting autologous tissue and development of the transobturator approach.[10,11] The use of synthetic material avoided morbidity from tissue harvest (e.g., wound infection, hernia), although added the risk of mesh-related complications (e.g., vaginal mesh exposure, dyspareunia, mesh erosion).[12,13] Likewise, the risk of postoperative dysfunctional voiding or urinary retention is lower following synthetic midurethral sling placement than with pubovaginal slings. In part for these reasons, synthetic sling placement has supplanted pubovaginal slings as the most commonly performed anti-incontinence procedure among gynecologists and urologists alike.[14,15]

Although midurethral slings are commonly performed, they have been subject to increased scrutiny by patients, surgeons, and the legal community following U.S. Food and Drug Administration (FDA) notifications regarding the use of transvaginal mesh for managing pelvic organ prolapse.[16] Indeed, in a review of 1% of a legal database for cases related to mesh placement, 63% of cases involved slings for urinary incontinence, 13% mesh for prolapse, and 23% involved both.[17] For a variety of reasons, around the time of the FDA notifications, while synthetic slings remained the most common procedures performed, at some academic centers an increase in autologous sling placements was identified.[18]

INDICATIONS FOR PUBOVAGINAL SLING PLACEMENT

Autologous pubovaginal sling placement can be considered in the setting of either primary or reoperative anti-incontinence surgery. Patient-specific comorbidities or preferences may necessitate avoidance of polypropylene mesh sling materials in some cases.

One of the notable uses of autologous slings is in the setting of concomitant urethral reconstructive procedures, where use of polypropylene mesh may impact wound healing and lead to mesh-related complications. For instance, if placing a sling at the time of urethrovaginal fistula repair, urethral diverticulectomy, or excision of a urethral mesh erosion, fascial slings are the mainstay of anti-incontinence therapy. Although not uniformly necessary during urethral diverticulectomy, concomitant placement of a fascial sling may be useful in some cases. Potential scenarios to consider placement of an autologous sling during diverticulectomy include patients with preoperative stress incontinence, larger diverticulum sizes, and those in a proximal urethral location.[19,20] However, it is worth noting that baseline stress incontinence may resolve in many patients undergoing diverticulectomy and one can consider delayed sling placement as needed.[21–23]

An additional clinical scenario where the 2017 American Urological Association (AUA)/Society of Urodynamics, Female Pelvic Medicine & Urogenital Reconstruction (SUFU) guideline on female stress urinary incontinence suggests considering alternatives to synthetic mesh use is in patients at risk for poor wound healing.[2] Although there is limited direct evidence on predictors of urethral erosion, those with compromised tissue may be at increased risk. Clinical comorbidities that may impact wound healing in this setting include prior pelvic radiation treatment, long-term steroid use, immunosuppression, and significant scarring from prior vaginal surgeries.[2]

An additional role for pubovaginal sling placement is when urethral obstruction is intended, for instance for a patient with a neurogenic bladder with both urinary retention (necessitating self-catheterization) and outlet incompetence (resulting in stress incontinence). In this setting, a fascial sling can be placed with more tension than a mesh sling, where urethral erosion over time would be a larger concern.

SURGICAL TECHNIQUE FOR PUBOVAGINAL SLING PLACEMENT

An overview of the procedure is shown in Figure 30.1 and a demonstration is available in the accompanying Video 30.1. The patient is typically placed in the dorsolithotomy position with movable stirrups to allow for changes in position during the abdominal (rectus fascial harvest) and vaginal dissections. The abdomen and vagina are prepared and draped to create the sterile field and perioperative antibiotics are given. Unless there is a concomitant urethral reconstruction to be performed or it is uncertain if a sling will be needed, the procedure starts with the graft harvest. This is to prevent ongoing bleeding from the vaginal dissection during the time of graft harvest.

Rectus Fascia Harvest

In most cases, we use rectus fascia as the sling material. For graft harvest a 7- to 8-cm Pfannenstiel incision is made roughly two fingerbreadths above the pubic bone.

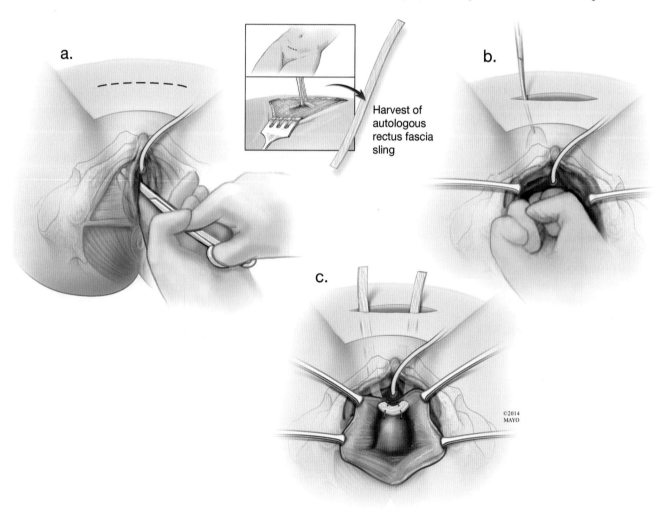

a.

Harvest of autologous rectus fascia sling

b.

c.

©2014 MAYO

FIGURE 30.1 Procedural overview for pubovaginal sling placement with rectus fascia harvest. (Used with permission of Mayo Foundation for Medical Education and Research. All rights reserved.)

The dissection continues with electrocautery through the subcutaneous tissues to the level of the rectus fascia. Once an area of the fascia has been cleared of adipose, two parallel incisions are made in the rectus fascia approximately 2 cm apart. This will correspond to the width of the sling. The underlying muscle is then separated from the fascia. The surgeon places the index finger of their nondominant hand through the two incisions and underneath the fascial strip which allows for countertraction to aid the dissection (Fig. 30.2). The incisions are then carried laterally with slight upward curve toward the anterior superior iliac spine, to avoid the ilioinguinal and iliohypogastric nerves. Care is taken to maintain the 2 cm width of the sling throughout its entire course. The dissection is carried approximately 5 cm laterally to each side, so the final fascial sling is roughly 10 cm in total length.

Prior to transecting the lateral edges of the fascia, a monofilament permanent suture is secured to the fascial fibers (Fig. 30.3). The tail of this suture is left as long as possible and tagged because it will be used later in the procedure to pass the sling from the vaginal dissection to the abdominal dissection. Leaving the fascia attached laterally facilitates placement of these sutures given fixation of the tissue, as opposed to trying to place these on a back table. Likewise, if exposure of the corner of the fascial defect is difficult, a stay suture for fascial closure can be placed prior to freeing the lateral attachments of the sling. Following this, the lateral edge of the sling is transected, and the fascial strip is freed from any remaining attachments to the underlying muscle. This is repeated on the contralateral side. Typically, the midline portion of the sling is freed last because this is where more scar may be encountered in those with prior surgeries, and this is the portion that will rest underneath the urethra. With the fascial strip completely detached, excess subcutaneous adipose tissue is removed from the graft. Following this, it is stored in normal saline until it is ready for placement.

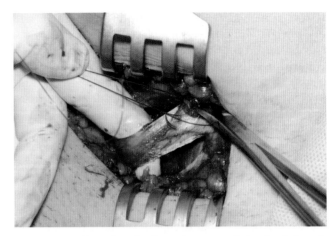

FIGURE 30.3 Securing the lateral aspect of the fascial graft with a permanent suture while the graft remains in situ.

The rectus fascial edges are then mobilized slightly from the muscle underneath, if needed, to allow for a tension-free closure. The fascial incision is closed with a running delayed absorbable suture. Of note, for the lateral aspects of the fascial closure, it is important to include all layers of the fascia because they may have separated in the lateral portion of the incision. A local anesthetic is injected to aid in postoperative analgesia. Typically, we use a long-acting liposomal formulation for this. The subcutaneous tissue and skin are left open at this point to allow a space for trocar passage and tensioning the sling later in the procedure.

In patients with significant retropubic scarring, prior to fascial closure, the rectus muscle can be separated in the midline and an extraperitoneal dissection of the retropubic space performed under direct visualization. Here, staying in the space of Retzius, the intended area for sling passage can be cleared sharply. The fascia can be left open until the sutures have been passed from the vagina to the abdomen. Although this is not routinely necessary, this technique can be useful when significant retropubic scarring is anticipated.

Fascia Lata Harvest

The use of fascia lata for the sling material, rather than rectus fascia, may be considered secondary to patient comorbidities, patient or surgeon preference. For instance, in those with multiple prior abdominal surgeries, ventral hernias repairs (especially with mesh use in the abdominal wall), or morbid obesity, this approach may be preferable.

For the graft harvest, the patient is placed in the lateral position, with the leg intended for graft harvest rotated internally at the hip. The anterior and lateral thigh are prepared and draped from the knee to the anterior superior iliac spine. A 3-cm longitudinal incision is made several centimeters above the patella and superior to the iliotibial tract. The incision is made in

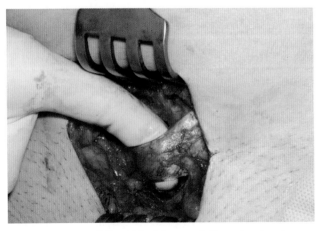

FIGURE 30.2 Initial fascial incisions and dissection for the rectus fascia harvest. The incisions are parallel and 2 cm apart.

the direction of the greater trochanter and dissection carried down to the fascia lata. Once identified, two parallel longitudinal incisions are made 2 cm apart, in the direction of the fascial fibers. A permanent monofilament suture is placed through the end of the fascial strip, similar to what is described above for a rectus fascial harvest. The two parallel incisions are connected to create a free end, and a thin malleable retractor is used to dissect it from the subcutaneous above and muscle below. A fascial stripper then used to extend the fascial incision and divide the fascia proximally to allow for removal. An additional permanent monofilament suture is used to secure the other end of the graft. The wound is then inspected for hemostasis, closed in multiple layers, and a compressive wrapped dressing is placed.[24,25]

Vaginal Dissection and Sling Placement

In preparation for the vaginal portion of the surgery, a Foley catheter is placed, the bladder drained, and a weighted speculum placed in the posterior vagina. With palpation of the Foley balloon, the bladder neck is identified and marked. A wide Allis clamp is placed immediately inferior to the urethral meatus for traction. Hydrodissection is performed with injectable normal saline at the midurethral, bladder neck, and periurethral tissues.

We typically prefer an inverted U-shaped incision because it gives superior visualization and access to the endopelvic fascia. The incision starts roughly 2 cm below the meatus and is then extended as it progresses laterally to the level of the bladder neck (Fig. 30.4). A wide base to the incision is needed to avoid flap devitalization. Notably, a midline incision could be used either for surgeon preference or patient factors, such as a narrow vaginal introitus. A wide Allis clamp is placed on the cut edge of the inverted U-incision to provide counter traction for the dissection. The surgeon then uses the index finger of their nondominant hand for

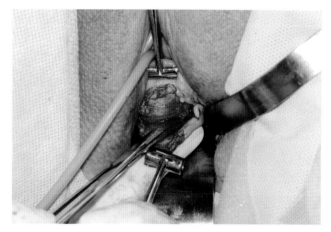

FIGURE 30.5 Anterior vaginal wall dissection.

tension, and the anterior vaginal wall dissection is carried out superficial to the periurethral and pubocervical fascia (Fig. 30.5). Palpation of the Foley balloon confirms the extent of the proximal dissection. The dissection is then carried posterolaterally until the underside of the pubic bone can be palpated. Care is taken to avoid urethral or bladder neck injury during the dissection. This forms the lateral channel along which the sling will lay. Following this dissection, an index finger can be used to palpate the underside of the bone and endopelvic fascia.

Next, the bladder is drained, the patient placed in a slight Trendelenburg position, and the endopelvic fascia is perforated. In general, the scissors are rotated away from the midline in the direction of the ipsilateral shoulder, with tips oriented laterally, and at a steep upward angle, so it is travelling along the posterior aspect of the pubic bone. Once perforated, the scissors are spread and removed with the blades open to create a 2 cm wide opening (Fig. 30.6). An index finger is used to bluntly develop the space of Retzius up to the level of the rectus muscle belly. Care is taken to clear connective tissue, sweeping lateral to medial to avoid the

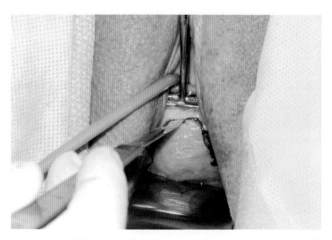

FIGURE 30.4 The inverted U incision in the anterior vaginal wall.

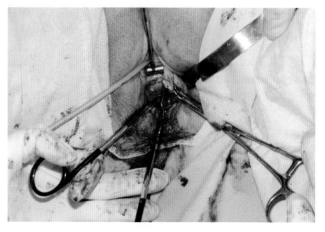

FIGURE 30.6 Perforation of the endopelvic fascia.

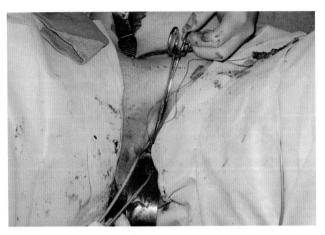

FIGURE 30.7 Trocar passage for transferring the permanent sutures on the sling from the vaginal incision to the abdominal incision.

bladder and bladder neck tissues. This process is then repeated on the contralateral side.

With the vaginal dissection completed, attention is turned to trocar passage for placing the sling. An index finger is placed through the vaginal dissection and a Pereyra needle passer inserted through the abdominal incision which was previously left open. The needle passer is placed immediately above the edge of the pubic bone and advanced to the index finger that has been inserted from below in to the space of Retzius. The trocar is then advanced through to the vaginal incision. The tagged ends of the permanent suture on the previously harvested fascial sling are then placed through the eyelets of the needle passer (Fig. 30.7). The permanent suture is retracted up to the abdominal incision and the tags transferred to secure the sutures. This is repeated on the contralateral side. The sling is then palpated throughout its length to ensure it is not rolling at the level of the endopelvic fascia.

Rigid cystoscopy with a 70° lens is performed to evaluate for bladder or ureteral injury. Additionally, evaluation with a 0° lens is used to confirm there is no urethral injury and that the sling is located at the bladder neck as urethral coaptation is seen when tension is added to the sling. The vaginal dissection is evaluated to ensure the sling is symmetric, with the urethra at the midpoint when it is placed (Fig. 30.8). The sling is then secured to the periurethral tissue with a rapid absorbable suture in four quadrants at the level of the urethrovesical junction, immediately distal to the bladder neck. The securing sutures are placed at the proximal and distal aspect of the sling on each side (Fig. 30.9). The vaginal incision is then closed with interrupted 2-0 absorbable polyglactin sutures.

The sling is then tensioned via the abdominal incision. Here, the cystoscope sheath is left in place and while applying downward traction in the urethra, the sutures are tied across the midline. Care is taken

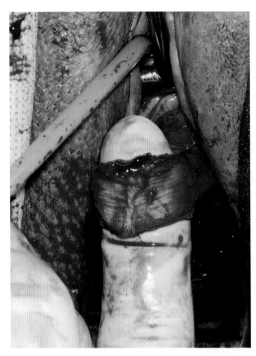

FIGURE 30.8 Ensuring the sling lays flat with the midportion of the sling centered on the urethra.

to leave at least two to three fingerbreadths of space between the tied sutures and the level of the fascia to avoid overcorrection. Interestingly, a recent study noted that a lax sling height of less than 4 cm above the fascia was associated with a higher risk of urinary retention, need for self-catheterization, and urethrolysis.[9]

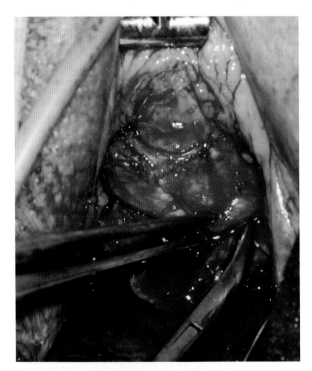

FIGURE 30.9 Securing the sling to the periurethral tissues in four quadrants so it remains flat and centered.

The cystoscope sheath is then removed, a Foley catheter inserted, and a vaginal packing is placed. The packing is removed prior to the patient's voiding trial, and self-catheterization is used as needed. In patients that are unable or unwilling to perform self-catheterization if needed, a suprapubic tube could be placed at the time of surgery. This performed under direct cystoscopic visualization.

Of note, if a fascial sling is being performed with a concomitant urethral reconstruction, the sling can be harvested and placed prior to closing the urethral defect. The sling is then left loose and tucked away during the urethral reconstruction. After completion of the reconstruction the sling is tensioned. Using this sequence decreases the need for additional tissue mobilization and repeat cystoscopy after completion of the urethral reconstruction.

PUBOVAGINAL SLING OUTCOMES

Multiple studies, across several clinical scenarios, demonstrate that autologous sling placement is an effective and durable treatment for female stress urinary incontinence. In the early reports on pubovaginal sling outcomes, high success rates, with variable definitions of success, were noted. For instance, in their 1978 report, McGuire and Lytton[6] noted a satisfactory result with good urinary control in 50 of 52 women treated. Similar success was identified by Blaivas and Jacobs[26] in their review of 67 patients with a mean follow-up of 3.5 years. Here, 82% of patients were dry, with only two women having persistent stress incontinence.

In more contemporary studies, success rates have varied from 75% to 92%, with 3- to 10-year follow-up.[13,27–30] In a randomized study with 10-year follow-up, 75% of women available for follow-up (n = 61) were significantly improved, and 51% were completely continent.[28] In addition to the subjective and objective incontinence outcomes, pubovaginal sling placement has also been associated with high patient satisfaction rates (82% to 92%).[27,29,31]

Several randomized studies have compared outcomes between a pubovaginal sling and retropubic urethropexy.[32] For instance, the Stress Incontinence Surgical Treatment Efficacy Trial (SISTEr) randomized women with stress urinary incontinence to undergo pubovaginal sling or Burch urethropexy.[33] Here, success rates at 24 months were greater in the pubovaginal sling group for overall continence (47% vs. 38%; P = .01) and stress-specific continence (66% vs. 49%; P < .001).[33] Those undergoing sling placement were also more likely to have urinary tract infections, difficulty voiding, and postoperative urge incontinence.[33] Sustained improvements, with success rates continuing to favor pubovaginal sling placement were reported in the 5-year follow-up study, although continence rates in both groups decreased over time (31% vs. 24%).[34]

Satisfaction at 5 years was related to continence status and was higher in women undergoing a pubovaginal sling (83% vs. 73%; P = .04).[34] Similar findings have been reported in a recent Cochrane Review of the available randomized trials, with women being less likely to need repeat continence surgery after pubovaginal sling placement than retropubic urethropexy (relative risk [RR] 0.15, 95% confidence interval [CI] 0.05 to 0.42).[32]

When compared to midurethral slings, similar continence success rates for pubovaginal slings have been identified at medium term (1- to 5-year) follow-up (67% vs. 74% odds ratio [OR] 0.67, 95% CI 0.44 to 1.02).[32,35] Data regarding longer term outcomes is limited. In one randomized study comparing pubovaginal sling and retropubic synthetic midurethral sling placement (median follow-up 10 years), pubovaginal sling placement was associated with superior complete continence rates (51% vs. 32%; P = .04) and similar success rates (75% vs. 73%).[28] Of note, in terms of clinical success, these continence rates would need to be contextualized regarding the different morbidity and risk profiles of the various slings available.

An additional clinical role for the pubovaginal sling is in the setting of recurrent stress incontinence after a prior synthetic midurethral sling. Here, smaller single institution studies have demonstrated adequate success rates, ranging from 52% to 85% depending on the criteria applied.[27,36,37] In a series of 66 women with a mean follow-up of 14.5 months, a stress incontinence cure rate of 70% was identified, including 38% of women who were completely dry.[36] In a smaller series with longer follow-up (n = 21, median 74 months), 52% of women were dry or had slight incontinence, and 86% would recommend the procedure.[37]

PUBOVAGINAL SLING COMPLICATIONS AND MANAGEMENT

Voiding Dysfunction/Urinary Retention

One of the issues regarding pubovaginal sling placement is the risk of postoperative voiding dysfunction or urinary retention. Overall, it is estimated that in roughly 8% to 14% of cases, there is a need for ongoing self-catheterization or sling incision/urethrolysis.[33,38] Of note, there may be a greater risk of this in patients with preoperative storage urinary symptoms, detrusor underactivity, or in those who void via Valsalva mechanism.[39,40] However, these associations have not been consistent across studies.[41,42] For instance, in a secondary analysis of the SISTEr data (Burch vs. pubovaginal sling), no preoperative factors, including noninvasive testing and multichannel urodynamic testing, were associated with the risk of voiding dysfunction.[41]

Early in the postoperative course, it is not uncommon for patients to need self-catheterization. Many of these patients will resume voiding within 4 to 6 weeks following the procedure. As such, early in the postoperative course, conservative management is typically used. For those who would be unwilling or unable to perform self-catheterization, a suprapubic tube can be placed at the time of the sling. This can remain in until the patient can adequately void to a low postvoid residual.

For those with persistent significant voiding dysfunction or complete retention, early management (roughly 6 weeks) can include an attempt at sling loosening or sling incision/urethrolysis. Sling loosening is accomplished in the operating room by applying inferior pressure to the urethra with a cystoscope. Farther out in the postoperative course, this is unlikely to be successful given the degree of periurethral scarring. When sling incision is to be performed, it is important to discuss with patients the risk of recurrent stress urinary incontinence or persistent obstruction following this procedure.[43] The risk of recurrent incontinence increases with additional urethrolysis, and as such, we typically attempt to relieve the obstruction with sling lysis first.[44,45] Across several series, sling incision is successful in relieving the obstruction in 84% to 100% of cases.[44–47] The risk of recurrent stress incontinence in most series is 9% to 21%, with retreatment in 7% to 14%.[43–45,48] In those where initial sling incision is not successful at relieving the obstruction, additional more aggressive urethrolysis can be undertaken.[49]

Of note, overactive bladder symptoms may persist or develop following sling release. This may be related preoperative overactive bladder symptoms or the duration of outlet obstruction prior to intervention.[48,50–52] For those with de novo overactive bladder or persistent residual symptoms following relief of outlet obstruction, management typically proceeds in a stepwise fashion with treatments following the current guidelines for overactive bladder care.[53]

Wound Infection

Given the added incision and dissection for graft harvest, placement of a pubovaginal sling carries with it the risk of wound infection, seroma, hematoma, or incisional hernia. In the randomized SISTEr study (pubovaginal sling vs. Burch), the rate of wound complications necessitating a surgical procedure in the sling group was 3.3%, and an additional 11.6% had minor abdominal wound complications.[33] In a meta-analysis from a prior version of the AUA guideline on female stress urinary incontinence, the risk of wound-related complications following pubovaginal sling placement was estimated to be 8%.[54] Lower rates, roughly 1%, have been noted in a two large single-institution series.[29,30] In a recent retrospective series, the harvest of fascia lata was associated with a nonsignificant trend toward lower wound infection rates than rectus fascia (0% vs. 14%; $P = .12$).[55]

CONCLUSION

Autologous pubovaginal sling placement is a durable and efficacious treatment in both the primary and reoperative setting. As such, it is a vital tool in the armamentarium of pelvic floor surgeons and should be discussed with patients considering anti-incontinence surgery. This chapter reviews technical considerations for intraoperative and postoperative management of autologous pubovaginal slings.

References

1. Wu JM, Matthews CA, Conover MM, et al. Lifetime risk of stress urinary incontinence or pelvic organ prolapse surgery. *Obstet Gynecol* 2014;123(6):1201–1206.
2. Kobashi KC, Albo ME, Dmochowski RR, et al. Surgical treatment of female stress urinary incontinence: AUA/SUFU guideline. *J Urol* 2017;198(4):875–883.
3. Giordano D. Guérison par autoplastie musculo–nerveuse d'une incontinence vésicale, suite de 'befida spina.' *Cong Franc de Chir* 1907;20:506.
4. Aldridge A. Transplantation of fascia for the relief of urinary stress incontinence. *Am J Obstet Gynecol* 1942;44(3):398–411.
5. Frangenheim P. Zur operative behaundlung der inkontinenz der mannlichen harnohre. *Verh Dtsch Ges Chir* 1914;43:149–158.
6. McGuire EJ, Lytton B. Pubovaginal sling procedure for stress incontinence. *J Urol* 1978;119(1):82–84.
7. Blaivas JG, Olsson CA. Stress incontinence: Classification and surgical approach. *J Urol* 1988;139(4):727–731.
8. Blaivas JG, Simma-Chiang V, Gul Z, et al. Surgery for stress urinary incontinence: Autologous fascial sling. *Urol Clin North Am* 2019;46(1):41–52.
9. Preece PD, Chan G, O'Connell HE, et al. Optimising the tension of an autologous fascia pubovaginal sling to minimize retentive complications. *Neurourol Urodyn* 2019;38(5):1409–1416.
10. Ulmsten U, Petros P. Intravaginal slingplasty (IVS): An ambulatory surgical procedure for treatment of female urinary incontinence. *Scand J Urol Nephrol* 1995;29(1):75–82.
11. Delorme E. Transobturator urethral suspension: Mini-invasive procedure in the treatment of stress urinary incontinence in women. *Prog Urol* 2001;11(6):1306–1313.
12. Linder BJ, Elliott DS. Synthetic midurethral slings: Roles, outcomes, and complications. *Urol Clin North Am* 2019;46(1):17–30.
13. Blaivas JG, Purohit RS, Benedon MS, et al. Safety considerations for synthetic sling surgery. *Nat Rev Urol* 2015;12(9):481–509.
14. Chughtai BI, Elterman DS, Vertosick E, et al. Midurethral sling is the dominant procedure for female stress urinary incontinence: Analysis of case logs from certifying American Urologists. *Urology* 2013;82(6):1267–1271.
15. Palmerola R, Peyronnet B, Rebolos M, et al. Trends in stress urinary incontinence surgery at a tertiary center: Midurethral sling use following the AUGS/SUFU position statement. *Urology* 2019;131:71–76.
16. Chapple CR, Raz S, Brubaker L, et al. Mesh sling in an era of uncertainty: Lessons learned and the way forward. *Eur Urol* 2013;64(4):525–529.
17. Souders CP, Eilber KS, McClelland L, et al. The truth behind transvaginal mesh litigation: Devices, timelines, and provider characteristics. *Female Pelvic Med Reconstr Surg* 2018;24(1):21–25.

18. Rac G, Younger A, Clemens JQ, et al. Stress urinary incontinence surgery trends in academic female pelvic medicine and reconstructive surgery urology practice in the setting of the Food and Drug Administration public health notifications. *Neurourol Urodyn* 2017;36(4):1155–1160.

19. Stav K, Dwyer PL, Rosamilia A, et al. Urinary symptoms before and after female urethral diverticulectomy—Can we predict de novo stress urinary incontinence? *J Urol* 2008;180(5): 2088–2090.

20. Seth JH, Naaseri S, Solomon E, et al. Correlation of MRI features of urethral diverticulum and pre- and post-operative stress urinary incontinence. *Neurourol Urodyn* 2019;38(1):180–186.

21. Barratt R, Malde S, Pakzad M, et al. The incidence and outcomes of urodynamic stress urinary incontinence in female patients with urethral diverticulum. *Neurourol Urodyn* 2019;38(7): 1889–1900.

22. Bradley SE, Leach DA, Panza J, et al. A multicenter retrospective cohort study comparing urethral diverticulectomy with and without pubovaginal sling. *Am J Obstet Gynecol* 2020;223(2):273.e1–273.e9.

23. Reeves FA, Inman RD, Chapple CR. Management of symptomatic urethral diverticula in women: A single-centre experience. *Eur Urol* 2014;66(1):164–172.

24. Gomelsky A, Dmochowski RR. Slings: Autologous, biologic, synthetic, and mid-urethral. In: Partin AW, Peters CA, Kavoussi LR, et al. *Campbell-Walsh-Wein urology*, 12th ed. Philadelphia: Elsevier, 2021:2830–2876.

25. Walter AJ, Hentz JG, Magrina JF, et al. Harvesting autologous fascia lata for pelvic reconstructive surgery: Techniques and morbidity. *Am J Obstet Gynecol* 2001;185(6):1354–1359.

26. Blaivas JG, Jacobs BZ. Pubovaginal fascial sling for the treatment of complicated stress urinary incontinence. *J Urol* 1991;145(6):1214–1218.

27. Athanasopoulos A, Gyftopoulos K, McGuire EJ. Efficacy and preoperative prognostic factors of autologous fascia rectus sling for treatment of female stress urinary incontinence. *Urology* 2011;78(5):1034–1038.

28. Khan ZA, Nambiar A, Morley R, et al. Long-term follow-up of a multicentre randomised controlled trial comparing tension-free vaginal tape, xenograft and autologous fascial slings for the treatment of stress urinary incontinence in women. *BJU Int* 2015;115(6):968–977.

29. Morgan TO Jr, Westney OL, McGuire EJ. Pubovaginal sling: 4-YEAR outcome analysis and quality of life assessment. *J Urol* 2000;163(6):1845–1848.

30. Chaikin DC, Rosenthal J, Blaivas JG. Pubovaginal fascial sling for all types of stress urinary incontinence: Long-term analysis. *J Urol* 1998;160(4):1312–1316.

31. Richter HE, Varner RE, Sanders E, et al. Effects of pubovaginal sling procedure on patients with urethral hypermobility and intrinsic sphincteric deficiency: Would they do it again? *Am J Obstet Gynecol* 2001;184(2):14–19.

32. Saraswat L, Rehman H, Omar MI, et al. Traditional suburethral sling operations for urinary incontinence in women. *Cochrane Database Syst Rev* 2020;1(1):CD001754.

33. Albo ME, Richter HE, Brubaker L, et al. Burch colposuspension versus fascial sling to reduce urinary stress incontinence. *N Engl J Med* 2007;356(21):2143–2155.

34. Brubaker L, Richter HE, Norton PA, et al. 5-year continence rates, satisfaction and adverse events of burch urethropexy and fascial sling surgery for urinary incontinence. *J Urol* 2012;187(4):1324–1330.

35. Fusco F, Abdel-Fattah M, Chapple CR, et al. Updated systematic review and meta-analysis of the comparative data on colposuspensions, pubovaginal slings, and midurethral tapes in the surgical treatment of female stress urinary incontinence. *Eur Urol* 2017;72(4):567–591.

36. Milose JC, Sharp KM, He C, et al. Success of autologous pubovaginal sling after failed synthetic mid urethral sling. *J Urol* 2015;193(3):916–920.

37. Petrou SP, Davidiuk AJ, Rawal B, et al. Salvage autologous fascial sling after failed synthetic midurethral sling: Greater than 3-year outcomes. *Int J Urol* 2016;23(2):178–181.

38. Leach GE, Dmochowski RR, Appell RA, et al. Female Stress Urinary Incontinence Clinical Guidelines Panel summary report on surgical management of female stress urinary incontinence. The American Urological Association. *J Urol* 1997;158(3 Pt 1): 875–880.

39. Bhatia NN, Bergman A. Urodynamic predictability of voiding following incontinence surgery. *Obstet Gynecol* 1984;63(1):85–91.

40. Iglesia CB, Shott S, Fenner DE, et al. Effect of preoperative voiding mechanism on success rate of autologous rectus fascia suburethral sling procedure. *Obstet Gynecol* 1998;91(4): 577–581.

41. Lemack GE, Krauss S, Litman H, et al. Normal preoperative urodynamic testing does not predict voiding dysfunction after Burch colposuspension versus pubovaginal sling. *J Urol* 2008;180(5):2076–2080.

42. Miller EA, Amundsen CL, Toh KL, et al. Preoperative urodynamic evaluation may predict voiding dysfunction in women undergoing pubovaginal sling. *J Urol* 2003;169(6): 2234–2237.

43. Clifton MM, Linder BJ, Lightner DJ, et al. Risk of repeat anti-incontinence surgery following sling release: A review of 93 cases. *J Urol* 2014;191(3):710–714.

44. Goldman HB. Simple sling incision for the treatment of iatrogenic urethral obstruction. *Urology* 2003;62(4):714–718.

45. Nitti VW, Carlson KV, Blaivas JG, et al. Early results of pubovaginal sling lysis by midline sling incision. *Urology* 2002;59(1):47–52.

46. Carr LK, Webster GD. Voiding dysfunction following incontinence surgery: Diagnosis and treatment with retropubic or vaginal urethrolysis. *J Urol* 1997;157(3):821–823.

47. Thiel DD, Pettit PD, McClellan WT, et al. Long-term urinary continence rates after simple sling incision for relief of urinary retention following fascia lata pubovaginal slings. *J Urol* 2005;174(5):1878–1881.

48. South MM, Wu JM, Webster GD, et al. Early vs late midline sling lysis results in greater improvement in lower urinary tract symptoms. *Am J Obstet Gynecol* 2009;200(5):564.e1–564.e5.

49. Scarpero HM, Dmochowski RR, Nitti VW. Repeat urethrolysis after failed urethrolysis for iatrogenic obstruction. *J Urol* 2003;169(3):1013–1016.

50. Leng WW, Davies BJ, Tarin T, et al. Delayed treatment of bladder outlet obstruction after sling surgery: Association with irreversible bladder dysfunction. *J Urol* 2004;172(4 Pt 1):1379–1381.

51. Metcalfe PD, Wang J, Jiao H, et al. Bladder outlet obstruction: Progression from inflammation to fibrosis. *BJU Int* 2010;106(11):1686–1694.

52. Van den Broeck T, De Ridder D, Van der Aa F. The value of surgical release after obstructive anti-incontinence surgery: An aid for clinical decision making. *Neurourol Urodyn* 2015;34(8):736–740.

53. Lightner DJ, Gomelsky A, Souter L, et al. Diagnosis and treatment of overactive bladder (non-neurogenic) in adults: AUA/SUFU guideline amendment. *J Urol* 2019;202(3):558–563.

54. Dmochowski RR, Blaivas JM, Gormley EA, et al. Update of AUA guideline on the surgical management of female stress urinary incontinence. *J Urol* 2010;183(5):1906–1914.

55. Peng M, Sussman RD, Escobar C, et al. Rectus fascia versus fascia lata for autologous fascial pubovaginal sling: A single-center comparison of perioperative and functional outcomes. *Female Pelvic Med Reconstr Surg* 2020;26(8):493–497.

CHAPTER 31

BURCH COLPOSUSPENSION

Ankita Gupta • Sean L. Francis

Introduction

The International Continence Society defines stress urinary incontinence (SUI) as involuntary leakage on effort, exertion, sneezing, or coughing.[1] SUI can be treated by surgical options including Burch colposuspension; pubovaginal slings; urethral bulking; and retropubic, transobturator, or single-incision midurethral slings (MUS).[2] Although synthetic MUS have been the procedure of choice for several years,[3] the use of surgical mesh has become a public health problem and, as of writing this chapter, its use has been suspended in the United Kingdom.[3,4] Therefore, the well-trained pelvic floor surgeon should be comfortable offering nonmesh options for SUI including retropubic colposuspensions.

HISTORICAL PERSPECTIVE

Described in 1949, the Marshall-Marchetti-Krantz was the first retropubic procedure for SUI and involved placement of interrupted sutures into the periosteum of the pubic symphysis.[5] This procedure was modified by John Burch in 1961. Dr. Burch described the bilateral placement of three interrupted sutures between the periurethral tissue and the iliopectineal (Cooper) ligament which is the thick band of fibrous tissue found on the superior surface of the superior ramus of the pubic bone.[5,6] Most surgeons will recognize the Tanagho modification, first described in 1976, that involves bilateral placement of two sutures in the anterior vaginal wall, one in the midurethra and the second at the level of bladder neck, avoiding the urethral sphincter complex (Figs. 31.1 and 31.2).[5,7] Since these early descriptions, the Burch colposuspension has waxed and waned in popularity.[3] The open Burch colposuspension was long considered the gold standard of treatment for SUI, although its popularity decreased after the widespread adoption of MUS.[2,8–11] The advent of minimally invasive surgery and the scrutiny around the use of mesh has led to an increase in safe and effective use of minimally invasive techniques for Burch colposuspension.[8,12] The landmark articles for the Burch colposuspension have been listed in Table 31.1.

INDICATIONS

The choice of surgical treatment for SUI varies based on clinical scenario, coexisting conditions, and specialty or preference of the surgeon.[8,9] Although Burch colposuspension may be offered to any patient, the ideal clinical scenario is a mesh-averse patient, a history of mesh infection, or previous mesh complication. The surgery may also be appropriate for women with stress incontinence and a hypermobile urethra undergoing abdominal surgery for other indications.[9] The addition of Burch colposuspension at the time of abdominal sacral colpopexy in continent women should be individualized.[13,14] This decision is more challenging in patients with intrinsic sphincter deficiency (ISD) where surgical outcomes data is conflicting.[15–17] In the surgical treatment of ISD, experts recommend MUS or pubovaginal sling over Burch colposuspension.[16]

MECHANISM OF ACTION

To maintain continence, the urethral closure pressure must exceed the pressure within the bladder. A common theory postulates that the transmission of intra-abdominal pressure to the bladder, and bladder neck can only be maintained when the urethra remains above the pelvic floor.[18] Displacement of the urethra outside the abdomen may occur secondary to changes around the bladder neck due to pelvic organ prolapse or tissue damage.[11,19] By resuspending the anterior vaginal wall, the Burch colposuspension is thought to restore the hypermobile urethra to its normal anatomy.[20] This has been corroborated by imaging studies where shorter distance between the bladder neck and levator ani muscles was associated with surgical success.[21] An additional mechanism is the mechanical compression provided to the urethra by a stable anterior vaginal wall and the pubic symphysis. Older studies have suggested that the Burch procedure may affect urethral resistance or increase obstruction as a mechanism for stress continence.[22,23] In a large multicenter study, Kraus et al.[24,25] demonstrated increased urethral resistance and obstructive changes on urodynamics 2 years after a Burch procedure.

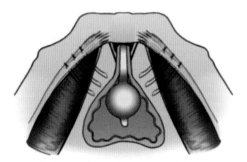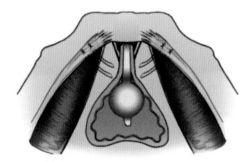

FIGURE 31.1 **Left:** Suture placement for the original Burch colposuspension. **Right:** Suture placement for the Tanagho-modified Burch urethropexy.

RETROPUBIC ANATOMY

The retropubic space is an extraperitoneal, avascular, potential space commonly encountered during anti-incontinence surgery. It is also known as the "space of Retzius" and lies between the pubic symphysis and the bladder, behind the transversalis muscle but in front of the peritoneum.[11] It is bound laterally by the pubic bone and obturator internus muscle, whereas the arcus tendinous fascia pelvis (ATFP) forms the posterolateral boundaries, and the floor is formed by the anterior vagina and its endopelvic attachments, inserting in to the ATFP.[11,26] Specific to the Burch procedure, the points of interest include the midurethra, the urethrovesical junction, and the Cooper or iliopectineal ligament which can be found lateral to the pubic tubercle beneath the superior margin of the pubic ramus (Fig. 31.3; Video 31.1). Vascular landmarks in this space include the external iliac vessels which are approximately 2.9 cm from the lateral Cooper ligament and the obturator neurovascular bundle which lies 2.6 cm away.[27] The obturator neurovascular bundle exits the pelvis at the level of the obturator foramen and can contribute to the "corona mortis" which is an anastomosis between the obturator and inferior epigastric vessels and can be a source of bleeding during retropubic surgery.[11] The anterior vaginal wall is composed of fibroadipose tissue, nerves, and blood vessels which can also bleed while placing sutures through the vaginal fibromuscular layer as recommended by Tanagho.[7,26]

SURGICAL TECHNIQUE

As previously described, the original technique involved placement of three sutures via laparotomy and was modified by Tanagho[7] to two sutures placed on each side. With the advent of laparoscopic colposuspension in 1991, modifications to this technique were described using some combination of suture, staples, or mesh to compensate for the steep learning curve associated with laparoscopic suturing.[10,28,29] However, the use of these modifications, including placement of clips, surgical mesh, and one suture instead of two, have all demonstrated inferior outcomes to the original modification described by Tanagho.[7,10,30–34]

FIGURE 31.2 Permanent sutures on either side of the bladder neck for the Burch urethropexy. The more proximal pair of sutures are lateral to the bladder neck, and the more distal pair of sutures are at the level of the midurethra. The proximal sutures are placed through the more lateral aspect of Cooper ligament with the distal sutures placed more medially. (Adapted from Tanagho EA. Colpocystourethropexy: The way we do it. *J Urol* 1976;116[6]:751–753. Copyright © 1976 Wolters Kluwer. With permission.)

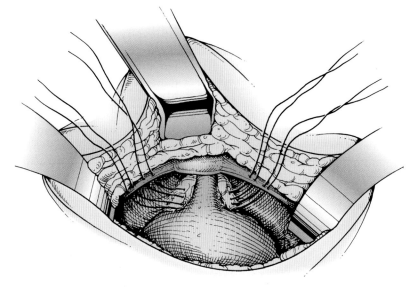

TABLE 31.1

Landmark Articles for Burch Colposuspension

FIRST AUTHOR	TITLE	JOURNAL	YEAR OF PUBLICATION	STUDY TYPE	NUMBER OF SUBJECTS	FOLLOW-UP TIME	CONCLUSION
John C. Burch[6,20]	"Urethrovaginal Fixation to Cooper's Ligament for Correction of Stress Incontinence, Cystocele, and Prolapse"	*American Journal of Obstetrics & Gynecology*	1961	Observational	53	2–17 mo	Initial description of Burch colposuspension; experience with Cooper ligament urethrovaginal suspension indicated that it is a superior operation for urinary stress incontinence.
Emil A. Tanagho[7]	"Colpocystourethropexy: The Way We Do It"	*Journal of Urology*	1976	Observational	NA	NA	Description of Tanagho modification for Burch colposuspension
Kimberly Kenton[43]	"Open Burch Urethropexy Has a Low Rate of Perioperative Complications"	*American Journal of Obstetrics & Gynecology*	2002	Retrospective	151	3 mo	Open Burch urethropexy has a low rate of perioperative complications in a tertiary teaching hospital.
Marie Fidela Paraiso[58]	"Laparoscopic Burch Colposuspension versus Tension-Free Vaginal Tape: A Randomized Trial"	*Obstetrics and Gynecology*	2004	Interventional	72	20.6 ± 8 mo (range 12–43)	Retropubic sling results in greater objective and subjective cure rates for UDSI than does laparoscopic Burch colposuspension.
Linda Brubaker[14]	"Abdominal Sacrocolpopexy with Burch Colposuspension to Reduce Urinary Stress Incontinence"	*The New England Journal of Medicine*	2006	Interventional	322	3 mo	In women without stress incontinence undergoing abdominal sacrocolpopexy For prolapse, Burch colposuspension significantly reduced postoperative symptoms of stress incontinence without increasing other lower urinary tract symptoms.
Michael E. Albo[44]	"Burch Colposuspension versus Fascial Sling to Reduce Urinary Stress Incontinence"	*The New England Journal of Medicine*	2007	Interventional	520	24 mo	The autologous fascial sling results in a higher rate of successful treatment of stress incontinence but also greater morbidity than the Burch colposuspension.

NA, not applicable; UDSI, urodynamic stress incontinence.

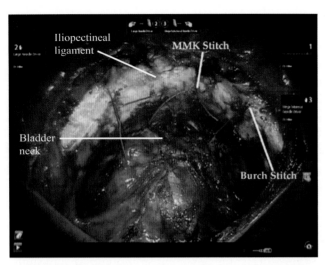

FIGURE 31.3 Retropubic anatomy. MMK, Marshall-Marchetti-Krantz. (Reprinted from Jones HW, Rock JA. *Te Linde's operative gynecology*, 11th ed. Philadelphia: Wolters Kluwer, 2015.)

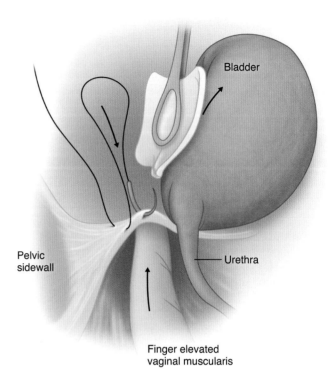

FIGURE 31.4 Use of vaginal finger for assistance with dissection and placement of Burch colposuspension sutures with medial displacement of bladder.

At this time, Burch colposuspension can be offered via open, minilaparotomy, laparoscopic, or robotic routes. Preoperative antibiotics are administered as recommended for clean-contaminated procedures.[35]

Open Burch

In this technique, the patient is placed in a low lithotomy position with feet in adjustable stirrups, allowing access to both the abdomen and vagina. A Foley catheter is placed, and the bladder may be drained or left half full to allow demarcation of bladder borders. A larger catheter with a 30-mL balloon can also be used to facilitate visualization of the urethra and urethrovaginal junction from above. The abdomen may be entered through a transverse or longitudinal incision, and the dissection in to the retropubic space can be intraperitoneal or extraperitoneal. Intraperitoneal access will allow for concomitant hysterectomy or other prolapse procedures, whereas extraperitoneal entry may be adequate if Burch colposuspension is the only procedure planned. Using blunt dissection, the rectus abdominis muscles are separated, and the transversalis fascia is separated from the pubic symphysis. The surgeon places their nondominant hand in the vagina to assist with dissection and allow better identification of paravaginal tissue and urethrovesical junction (Fig. 31.4). Bleeding from vaginal vessels can be encountered during dissection or placement of sutures, and upward pressure with the vaginal hand can be employed to compress the vaginal vasculature until sutures are placed. Gentle traction on the Foley balloon can also assist with dissection and hemostasis. The obturator vessels and ATFP are identified laterally and form the outer most limits of dissection. Dissection should be avoided directly over the urethra or at the urethrovesical junction to prevent surgical trauma to the urethra.[36] Permanent suture is used to place the proximal suture through the vaginal muscularis at the level of the bladder neck, 2 cm lateral to the urethra to avoid placement in the ATFP laterally and urethra or bladder medially.[26,27] The midurethral suture is placed about 1 cm distal to the bladder neck and 1 to 1.5 cm lateral to the urethra in the vaginal muscularis. Each suture is passed through the vaginal muscularis twice and then passed through the Cooper ligament on the same side, such that the knot can be tied above the ligament without tension. A suture bridge is desired, and two fingers should easily pass between the pubic symphysis and urethra. A cystoscopy is performed to rule out any injuries to the bladder or urethra.

Laparoscopic or Robotic Burch

Both laparoscopic and robotic techniques for Burch colposuspension have been well described.[12,37,38] Minimally invasive techniques allow faster recovery and return to activity with shorter length of hospital stay.[8,39–41] These techniques also allow for additional prolapse surgeries at the time of incontinence procedure as indicated. Disadvantages of these techniques can include steeper learning curve and higher cost of equipment. Data continues to support the use of two sutures bilaterally at the time of surgery, similar to the open technique, and the use of staples, bone tacks, or mesh is not recommended.

The patient is placed in low lithotomy position to allow access to both, the abdomen and vagina. When performed laparoscopically, three trocars are placed including the umbilical laparoscopic trocar and two lower quadrant trocars to facilitate dissection and suturing. An additional suprapubic trocar can be placed as needed, with at least one trocar large enough to allow passage of the needle. When performed robotically, we dock on the right side with two robotic arms on the right and one robotic arm and assistant port on the left. The bladder is identified by backfilling with a three-way Foley. In order to maintain sterility, the three-way Foley is connected to a fluid bag using sterile cystoscopy tubing. The monopolar scissors are used to incise the peritoneum 1 to 2 cm above the bladder dome between the medial umbilical ligaments that act as the lateral most dissection points. The retropubic space is entered using a combination of blunt and sharp dissection and is carried down to the level of the pubic symphysis. The landmarks are identified as described in the open dissection earlier. Adipose tissue is cleared from the vaginal walls and Cooper ligament to facilitate future fibrosis and scarring of opposed tissues, as described by Tanagho.[7] Vaginal retraction is facilitated by a Lucite rod or fingers placed in the vagina by the assistant or surgeon during laparoscopic surgery. As described earlier, two sutures are placed using permanent suture on each side and allowing for a suture bridge. We prefer to use nonbraided permanent suture due to high risk of suture-related complications with braided permanent suture including vaginal bleeding and granulation tissue formation, which can be challenging to manage.[42] The second bite through the vaginal muscularis typically assists with hemostasis. Tensioning of the sutures is determined by visual or tactile inspection ensuring that the urethral angle is at approximately 0°. A cystoscopy is performed to confirm urethral patency and bladder integrity. The peritoneum is closed using an absorbable suture (Video 31.2).

Although uncommon, extraperitoneal approach to laparoscopic colposuspension may be preferred by some surgeons and involves entry into the preperitoneal incision through the infraumbilical incision. This dissection is carried to the retropubic space, and the retropubic space is insufflated with carbon dioxide to create a "pneumoretzius." Historically, special trocars were available with expandable balloons which would create and maintain a retropubic operative space; however, the widespread availability of these trocars is uncertain (Fig. 31.5). Additional trocars are placed, and the remainder of the surgery is similar to the intraperitoneal approach.[5]

COMPLICATIONS

In general, the rate of complications after Burch colposuspension is low. In a study of open Burch colposuspension, Kenton et al.[43] demonstrated less than 1% of lower urinary tract injury and 3.5% incision cellulitis. Albo reported similar rates (3.9%) of wound complications requiring surgical intervention, and 10% of patients developed cystitis by 6 weeks after surgery, which was significantly lower than the 24% in the pubovaginal sling group.[44,45] Demirci and Petri[46] also described low rates of complications and an additional 0.7% to 2.3% risk of blood transfusion, discussing the possibility of injuring the external iliac or accessory obturator artery and vein while placing the lateral suture on Cooper ligament. A systematic review reported that rates of complications were similar between open Burch colposuspension and other open surgeries.[47] There were significantly fewer perioperative complications in the laparoscopic colposuspension group when compared to open procedure (relative risk [RR] 0.67, 95% confidence interval [CI] 0.47 to 0.94, low-quality evidence) but similar or higher rates of bladder perforations (RR 1.72, 95% CI 0.90 to 3.29).[48] Two studies reported cases of laceration to the obturator vein during laparoscopic colposuspension.[39]

The most common long-term complication after Burch colposuspension is de novo overactive bladder. Ciećwież et al.[49] reported a rate of 14% de novo overactive bladder at 3 months and 17% at 6 months compared to 5% and 7% in the transobturator tape group. However, on comparison with tension-free vaginal tape (TVT) and traditional fascial slings, Burch colposuspension had similar rates of de novo urgency.[24,25,47,49,50] The laparoscopic Burch colposuspension had similar rates of de novo detrusor overactivity when compared with the open approach up to 5 years (1.22, 95% CI 0.4 to 3.75).[39] Transient voiding dysfunction occurs in 6% to 37% of patients after Burch, based on its definition, but persistent voiding dysfunction is uncommon.[5] Voiding dysfunction is significantly more common after a pubovaginal sling when compared with Burch colposuspension.[44]

OUTCOMES

The outcomes of Burch colposuspension have been differentiated by route of surgery.[39,47] The open Burch colposuspension was traditionally considered the "gold standard" for management of SUI. A systematic review found that for women with clinically identified

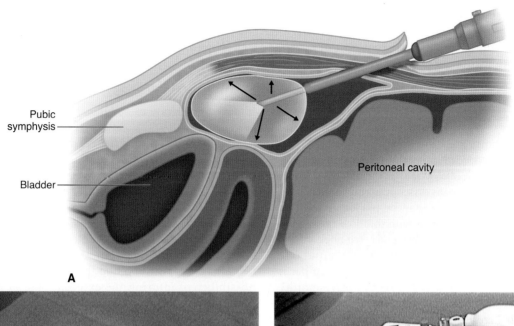

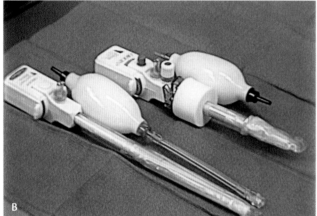

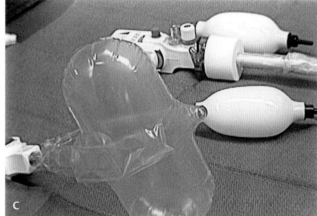

FIGURE 31.5 **A–C:** Extraperitoneal trocars for retropubic dissection. *Arrows* demonstrate direction of insufflation within the extraperitoneal trocar expanding the retropubic space (**A**).

or urodynamic stress incontinence (UDSI), overall continence rates were 85% to 90% within the first year and up to 80% by 5 years after open Burch surgery.[47] Albo et al.[44] found that fascial slings had better success (66% vs. 49% in Burch) at 2 years at the expense of more voiding dysfunction, but comparative data on the newer, minimally invasive slings is limited and shows similar continence rates at 5 years.[51-53] Although there was no evidence of greater morbidity after open colposuspension, there was a greater risk of postoperative pelvic organ prolapse, especially vault and posterior wall prolapse, when compared with isolated anterior repair or slings for SUI.[47,53-55] Open Burch colposuspension had better cure rates when compared to conservative management, anterior colporrhaphy, or Pereyra needle suspension.[56] In patients without SUI undergoing surgery for pelvic organ prolapse, Brubaker and colleagues[14] found a significant improvement in postoperative SUI with the addition of Burch colposuspension as compared to abdominal sacral colpopexy alone. However, a systematic review

found inadequate evidence to support this claim (RR 1.31, 95% CI 0.19 to 9.01).[13]

Unsurprisingly, laparoscopic Burch colposuspension is associated with less postoperative pain, less blood loss, shorter hospital stay and quicker return to activities when compared with the open Burch procedures.[39,57] At 18 months, subjective cure rates after laparoscopic Burch were similar to the open procedure (62% to 100% vs. 58% to 96% in open) and objective cure rates were similar up to 5 years (RR 1.01, 95% CI 0.88 to 1.16).[39] There were similar rates of de novo detrusor overactivity (RR 1.29, 95% CI 0.72 to 2.30) and voiding dysfunction (RR 0.81, 95% CI 0.50 to 1.31) between the groups.[48] When comparing laparoscopic Burch to TVT, Paraiso et al.[58] found significantly longer operating time in Burch (132 vs. 79 minutes) and higher rates of UDSI at 1 year (19% vs. 3% in TVT group). This was similar to Trabuco et al.[59] who found higher stress-specific continence at both 1 and 2 years after sacral colpopexy with retropubic MUS when compared with Burch procedure (70% sling vs. 45% Burch at 2 years). All five systematic reviews conducted on this comparison agree that there was no difference in subjective cure at 18 months after laparoscopic Burch when compared with slings, but objective cure may favor slings.[2,39,48,50,60] In addition, TVT has been noted to be quicker to perform and has a shorter length of hospital stay.[50] Based on current cost and efficacy data, it has also been suggested that the TVT is more cost-effective than Burch colposuspension, but laparoscopic Burch colposuspension is slightly more cost-effective than the open procedure at 24 months.[39,47,61–63]

Sexual function has been investigated after surgery for SUI with mixed results. Although Cayan et al.[64] reported a decrease in sexual arousal, desire, orgasm, and lubrication scores after Burch procedure, Ward and Hilton[53] noted an improvement in sexual function, pain, and incontinence during intercourse after Burch procedure.[64,65] Brubaker et al.[66] also reported an improvement in sexual function after surgery for SUI, with no difference between Burch colposuspension and sling groups. At this time, there is not enough data to make conclusions regarding the impact of Burch colposuspension on sexual function.[67]

CONCLUSION

Open Burch colposuspension remained the procedure of choice for several years until the widespread acceptance of the synthetic MUS. With the advent of laparoscopic and robotic techniques and increased public and government pressure against mesh, this procedure has seen a resurgence. Although surgeons have not reported it as their procedure of choice,[68] it should be considered in certain patients. It can be offered concurrently at the time of other procedures or as the primary procedure in patients who are mesh averse or suffered a mesh complication. It has similar cure rates and adverse event profile and less voiding dysfunction when compared with fascial slings. Burch colposuspension therefore holds an important place and should be offered to patients and taught to trainees worldwide.

References

1. Abrams P, Cardozo L, Fall M, et al. The standardisation of terminology of lower urinary tract function: Report from the standardisation sub-committee of the International Continence Society. *Neurourol Urodyn* 2002;21(2):167–178.
2. Oliveira LM, Dias MM, Martins SB, et al. Surgical treatment for stress urinary incontinence in women: A systematic review and meta-analysis. *Rev Bras Ginecol Obstet* 2018;40(8):477–490.
3. Zacche MM, Mukhopadhyay S, Giarenis I. Changing surgical trends for female stress urinary incontinence in England. *Int Urogynecol J* 2019;30(2):203–209.
4. Mangir N, Roman S, Chapple CR, et al. Complications related to use of mesh implants in surgical treatment of stress urinary incontinence and pelvic organ prolapse: Infection or inflammation? *World J Urol* 2020;38(1):73–80.
5. Barber MD. Surgical treatment of stress urinary incontinence. In: Bent AE, Cundiff GW, Swift SE, eds. *Ostergard's urogynecology and pelvic floor dysfunction*, 6th ed. Philadelphia: Lippincott Williams & Wilkins, 2007:225–262.
6. Burch JC. Urethrovaginal fixation to Cooper's ligament for correction of stress incontinence, cystocele, and prolapse. *Am J Obstet Gynecol* 1961;81:281–290.
7. Tanagho EA. Colpocystourethropexy: The way we do it. *J Urol* 1976;116(6):751–753.
8. Dean NM, Ellis G, Wilson PD, et al. Laparoscopic colposuspension for urinary incontinence in women. *Cochrane Database Syst Rev* 2006;(3):CD002239.
9. Dwyer PL, Karmakar D. Surgical management of urinary stress incontinence—Where are we now? *Best Pract Res Clin Obstet Gynaecol* 2019;54:31–40.
10. Sohlberg EM, Elliott CS. Burch colposuspension. *Urol Clin North Am* 2019;46(1):53–59.
11. Veit-Rubin N, Dubuisson J, Ford A, et al. Burch colposuspension. *Neurourol Urodyn* 2019;38(2):553–562.
12. Francis SL, Agrawal A, Azadi A, et al. Robotic Burch colposuspension: A surgical case and instructional video. *Int Urogynecol J* 2015;26(1):147–148.
13. Baessler K, Christmann-Schmid C, Maher C, et al. Surgery for women with pelvic organ prolapse with or without stress urinary incontinence. *Cochrane Database Syst Rev* 2018;(8):CD013108.
14. Brubaker L, Cundiff GW, Fine P, et al. Abdominal sacrocolpopexy with Burch colposuspension to reduce urinary stress incontinence. *N Engl J Med* 2006;354(15):1557–1566.
15. Ford AA, Ogah JA. Retropubic or transobturator mid-urethral slings for intrinsic sphincter deficiency-related stress urinary incontinence in women: A systematic review and meta-analysis. *Int Urogynecol J* 2016;27(1):19–28.
16. Medina CA, Costantini E, Petri E, et al. Evaluation and surgery for stress urinary incontinence: A FIGO working group report. *Neurourol Urodyn* 2017;36(2):518–528.
17. Hsieh GC, Klutke JJ, Kobak WH. Low Valsalva leak-point pressure and success of retropubic urethropexy. *Int Urogynecol J Pelvic Floor Dysfunct* 2001;12(1):46–50.
18. Enhorning G. Simultaneous recording of intravesical and intraurethral pressure. A study on urethral closure in normal and stress incontinent women. *Acta Chir Scand Suppl* 1961;Suppl 276:1–68.
19. Cundiff GW. The pathophysiology of stress urinary incontinence: A historical perspective. *Rev Urol* 2004;6(Suppl 3): S10–S18.
20. Burch JC. Cooper's ligament urethrovesical suspension for stress incontinence. Nine years' experience—Results, complications, technique. *Am J Obstet Gynecol* 1968;100(6):764–774.
21. Digesu GA, Bombieri L, Hutchings A, et al. Effects of Burch colposuspension on the relative positions of the bladder neck to the levator ani muscle: An observational study that used magnetic resonance imaging. *Am J Obstet Gynecol* 2004;190(3):614–619.
22. Bélair G, Tessier J, Bertrand PE, et al. Retropubic cystourethropexy: Is it an obstructive procedure? *J Urol* 1997;158(2): 533–538.
23. Klutke JJ, Klutke CG, Bergman J, et al. Urodynamics changes in voiding after anti-incontinence surgery: An insight into the mechanism of cure. *Urology* 1999;54(6):1003–1007.
24. Kraus SR, Lemack GE, Richter HE, et al. Changes in urodynamic measures two years after Burch colposuspension or autologous sling surgery. *Urology* 2011;78(6):1263–1268.

25. Kraus SR, Lemack GE, Sirls LT, et al. Urodynamic changes associated with successful stress urinary incontinence surgery: Is a little tension a good thing? *Urology* 2011;78(6):1257–1262.

26. Hamner JJ, Carrick KS, Ramirez DMO, et al. Gross and histologic relationships of the retropubic urethra to lateral pelvic sidewall and anterior vaginal wall in female cadavers: Clinical applications to retropubic surgery. *Am J Obstet Gynecol* 2018;219(6):597.e1–597.e8.

27. Kinman CL, Agrawal A, Deveneau NE, et al. Anatomical relationships of Burch colposuspension sutures. *Female Pelvic Med Reconstr Surg* 2017;23(2):72–74.

28. Liu CY. Laparoscopic retropubic colposuspension (Burch procedure). A review of 58 cases. *J Reprod Med* 1993;38(7):526–530.

29. Vancaillie TG, Schuessler W. Laparoscopic bladderneck suspension. *J Laparoendosc Surg* 1991;1(3):169–173.

30. Ankardal M, Ekerydh A, Crafoord K, et al. A randomised trial comparing open Burch colposuspension using sutures with laparoscopic colposuspension using mesh and staples in women with stress urinary incontinence. *BJOG* 2004;111(9):974–981.

31. Persson J, Wølner-Hanssen P. Laparoscopic Burch colposuspension for stress urinary incontinence: A randomized comparison of one or two sutures on each side of the urethra. *Obstet Gynecol* 2000;95(1):151–155.

32. Ross J. Two techniques of laparoscopic Burch repair for stress incontinence: A prospective, randomized study. *J Am Assoc Gynecol Laparosc* 1996;3(3):351–357.

33. Zullo F, Morelli M, Russo T, et al. Two techniques of laparoscopic retropubic urethropexy. *J Am Assoc Gynecol Laparosc* 2002;9(2):178–181.

34. Souza RJ, Resende JAD Jr, Miglio CG, et al. Can reducing the number of stitches compromise the outcome of laparoscopic Burch surgery in the treatment of stress urinary incontinence? Systematic review and meta-analysis. *Rev Col Bras Cir* 2017;44(6):649–654.

35. American College of Obstetricians and Gynecologists Committee on Practice Bulletins—Gynecology. ACOG Practice Bulletin No. 195: Prevention of infection after gynecologic procedures. *Obstet Gynecol* 2018;131(6):e172–e189.

36. Walters MD. Retropubic operations for stress urinary incontinence. In: Walters MD, Karram MM. *Urogynecology and reconstructive pelvic surgery*, 4th ed. Pennsylvania: Elsevier: 253–261.

37. Hill AJ, Jallad K, Walters MD. Laparoscopic Burch colposuspension using a 3-trocar system: Tips and tricks. *J Minim Invasive Gynecol* 2017;24(3):344.

38. Bora GS, Gupta VG, Mavuduru RS, et al. Robotic Burch colposuspension—Modified technique. *J Robot Surg* 2017;11(3):381–382.

39. Dean N, Ellis G, Herbison GP, et al. Laparoscopic colposuspension for urinary incontinence in women. *Cochrane Database Syst Rev* 2017;7(7):CD002239.

40. Miannay E, Cosson M, Lanvin D, et al. Comparison of open retropubic and laparoscopic colposuspension for treatment of stress urinary incontinence. *Eur J Obstet Gynecol Reprod Biol* 1998;79(2):159–166.

41. Tan E, Tekkis PP, Cornish J, et al. Laparoscopic versus open colposuspension for urodynamic stress incontinence. *Neurourol Urodyn* 2007;26(2):158–169.

42. Toglia MR, Fagan MJ. Suture erosion rates and long-term surgical outcomes in patients undergoing sacrospinous ligament suspension with braided polyester suture. *Am J Obstet Gynecol* 2008;198(5):600.e1–600.e4.

43. Kenton K, Oldham L, Brubaker L. Open Burch urethropexy has a low rate of perioperative complications. *Am J Obstet Gynecol* 2002;187(1):107–110.

44. Albo ME, Richter HE, Brubaker L, et al. Burch colposuspension versus fascial sling to reduce urinary stress incontinence. *N Engl J Med* 2007;356(21):2143–2155.

45. Chai TC, Albo ME, Richter HE, et al. Complications in women undergoing Burch colposuspension versus autologous rectus fascial sling for stress urinary incontinence. *J Urol* 2009;181(5):2192–2197.

46. Demirci F, Petri E. Perioperative complications of Burch colposuspension. *Int Urogynecol J Pelvic Floor Dysfunct* 2000;11(3):170–175.

47. Lapitan MCM, Cody JD, Mashayekhi A. Open retropubic colposuspension for urinary incontinence in women. *Cochrane Database Syst Rev* 2017;7(7):CD002912.

48. Freites J, Stewart F, Omar MI, et al. Laparoscopic colposuspension for urinary incontinence in women. *Cochrane Database Syst Rev* 2019;12(12):CD002239.

49. Ciećwież S, Chełstowski K, Brodowska A, et al. Association between the urinary bladder volume and the incidence of "de novo" overactive bladder in patients with stress urinary incontinence subjected to sling surgeries or Burch procedure. *Biomed Res Int* 2019(2019):9515242.

50. Dean N, Herbison P, Ellis G, et al. Laparoscopic colposuspension and tension-free vaginal tape: A systematic review. *BJOG* 2006;113(12):1345–1353.

51. Ward K, Hilton P. Prospective multicentre randomised trial of tension-free vaginal tape and colposuspension as primary treatment for stress incontinence. *BMJ* 2002;325(7355):67.

52. Ward KL, Hilton P. A prospective multicenter randomized trial of tension-free vaginal tape and colposuspension for primary urodynamic stress incontinence: Two-year follow-up. *Am J Obstet Gynecol* 2004;190(2):324–331.

53. Ward KL, Hilton P. Tension-free vaginal tape versus colposuspension for primary urodynamic stress incontinence: 5-year follow up. *BJOG* 2008;115(2):226–233.

54. Asicioglu O, Gungorduk K, Besimoglu B, et al. A 5-year follow-up study comparing Burch colposuspension and transobturator tape for the surgical treatment of stress urinary incontinence. *Int J Gynaecol Obstet* 2014;125(1):73–77.

55. Holdø B, Verelst M, Svenningsen R, et al. Long-term clinical outcomes with the retropubic tension-free vaginal tape (TVT) procedure compared to Burch colposuspension for correcting stress urinary incontinence (SUI). *Int Urogynecol J* 2017;28(11):1739–1746.

56. Colombo M, Vitobello D, Proietti F, et al. Randomised comparison of Burch colposuspension versus anterior colporrhaphy in women with stress urinary incontinence and anterior vaginal wall prolapse. *BJOG* 2000;107(4):544–551.

57. Carey MP, Goh JT, Rosamilia A, et al. Laparoscopic versus open Burch colposuspension: A randomised controlled trial. *BJOG* 2006;113(9):999–1006.

58. Paraiso MF, Walters MD, Karram MM, et al. Laparoscopic Burch colposuspension versus tension-free vaginal tape: A randomized trial. *Obstet Gynecol* 2004;104(6):1249–1258.

59. Trabuco EC, Linder BJ, Klingele CJ, et al. Two-year results of Burch compared with midurethral sling with sacrocolpopexy: A randomized controlled trial. *Obstet Gynecol* 2018;131(1):31–38.

60. Fusco F, Abdel-Fattah M, Chapple CR, et al. Updated systematic review and meta-analysis of the comparative data on colposuspensions, pubovaginal slings, and midurethral tapes in the surgical treatment of female stress urinary incontinence. *Eur Urol* 2017;72(4):567–591.

61. Laudano MA, Seklehner S, Chughtai B, et al. Cost-effectiveness analysis of tension-free vaginal tape vs Burch colposuspension for female stress urinary incontinence in the USA. *BJU Int* 2013;112(2):E151–E158.

62. Rawlings T, Zimmern PE. Economic analyses of stress urinary incontinence surgical procedures in women. *Neurourol Urodyn* 2016;35(8):1040–1045.

63. Wu JM, Visco AG, Weidner AC, et al. Is Burch colposuspension ever cost-effective compared with tension-free vaginal tape for stress incontinence? *Am J Obstet Gynecol* 2007;197(1):62.e1–62.e5.

64. Cayan F, Dilek S, Akbay E, et al. Sexual function after surgery for stress urinary incontinence: vaginal sling versus Burch colposuspension. *Arch Gynecol Obstet* 2008;277(1):31–36.

65. Thiagamoorthy G, Srikrishna S, Cardozo L. Sexual function after urinary incontinence surgery. *Maturitas* 2015;81(2):243–247.

66. Brubaker L, Chiang S, Zyczynski H, et al. The impact of stress incontinence surgery on female sexual function. *Am J Obstet Gynecol* 2009;200(5):562.e1–562.e7.

67. Bicudo-Fürst MC, Borba Leite PH, Araújo Glina FP, et al. Female sexual function following surgical treatment of stress urinary incontinence: Systematic review and meta-analysis. *Sex Med Rev* 2018;6(2):224–233.

68. Giarenis I, Thiagamoorthy G, Zacchè M, et al. Management of recurrent stress urinary incontinence after failed midurethral sling: A survey of members of the International Urogynecological Association (IUGA). *Int Urogynecol J* 2015;26(9):1285–1291.

CHAPTER 32

PERIURETHRAL AND TRANSURETHRAL BULKING AGENTS

Christopher E. Wolter

Introduction

Stress urinary incontinence (SUI) has been and will continue to be a significant problem for women worldwide. It can affect women of a variety of ages and activity levels through several etiologies. Peak prevalence rates for any SUI are seen in women between ages 40 and 59 years according to the International Consultation on Incontinence (ICI), indicating that this is not only a problem for the frail or elderly.[1] There is a significant economic impact as well from direct treatment costs within the health care system as well as indirect costs borne by individual women. There can also be significant emotional and social effects seen in women as SUI can frequently alter normal activity and interactions.[2]

After failed conservative management, patients frequently desire more definitive procedural therapy. Surgical treatment options vary widely for this condition and can range from invasive (pubovaginal slings and colposuspensions), to minimally invasive (midurethral slings [MUS] and bulking agent injections), of which MUS are now the most commonly performed surgical procedures.[3] Bulking agents are attractive for women because of their low risk, endoscopic, minimally invasive nature. Given ongoing apprehension regarding the use of polypropylene mesh, they appeal even further.[4,5] This is especially true for those who do not desire to undergo more invasive surgery.

BULKING AGENTS

Bulking agents for SUI are space-occupying injectable substances that can be performed in the office or operating room setting. They are made of a variety of substances, both biologic and synthetic, particulate and nonparticulate.[4] The goal of bulking agent injection therapy is to increase urethral resistance and the overall inherent seal effect of the urethra through submucosal deposition of these substances in the proximal urethra by likely increasing the functional length of the continence mechanism.[6] The end result should allow for increased intraurethral pressure and urethral coaptation

at rest and during Valsalva maneuvers, yet still allow for flow through the urethra at the time of voiding.[5,7]

The ideal bulking agent should have the following properties: biocompatibility, nonantigenicity, cause minimal reaction, encapsulation, or inflammation. Additionally, there should be minimal degradation or migration.[7] There should also be a prolonged duration of treatment effect. There has not been an ideal agent produced yet. That being said, there are several agents available for use that combine one or more, but not all, of these ideal properties. There does not appear to be an obvious advantage to any one of the bulking agents currently commercially available over another.[8]

PATIENT SELECTION

The ideal patient candidate for bulking agent injection should be one who is willing to accept lower success rates in exchange for ease of application. Patients declining pelvic floor physical therapy, incontinence pessary, and those with a fixed urethra due to prior surgery or radiation are also candidates. Urethral mobility in women does not appear to influence the success of bulking agents.[9] However, some suggest hypermobility may influence relative success with these agents, or infer other suspension therapies would be superior in those otherwise not well supported.[5,10] In these patients, ideally, they would be treatment failures with sling or suspension surgery but who have a well-supported urethra with continued intrinsic sphincter deficiency (ISD).[11,12] Additional considerations for treatment with bulking agents include those who cannot discontinue anticoagulant medications, women of childbearing age who desire more children in the future, those who are poor candidates for other surgical therapies, and those who are at high risk for urinary retention.[5]

Patients undergoing urethral bulking injections need to be counseled about several things. First, they should be told that this treatment is likely not as effective as sling surgery in overall efficacy in treating their SUI. They should also be told that they likely will need more than one treatment to either achieve or maintain optimum results and that they may not be able to achieve complete continence with this therapy. Overall, long-term data regarding this therapy is lacking. Patients should be counseled that regarding the specific agents available, there is no data to necessarily support the use of one agent over another, as few head to head studies have been performed. Management of patient expectations should incorporate all these points.[5,7,8,10] Finally, patients should be counseled that while uncommon, complications can occur with bulking agent injections, although most are minor and self-limited. However, serious complications have been reported over the years, requiring more invasive surgical interventions for management.[13]

Conventional teaching warns against the use of injectable agents in patients with a history or previous radiation therapy (RT) for pelvic cancers, but there is evidence to refute this. Patients with a history of previous pelvic RT are considered poor bulking candidates due to poor tissue quality and stiffness of the urethral layers, making coaptation of the urethra difficult as a result.[7] However, in a review by Dobberfuhl,[14] bulking agents were described as the only incontinence treatment studied in a prospective fashion specifically in radiated women, and although not randomized, had the highest level of evidence. In one trial, Krhut et al.[15] compared two groups treated with polyacrylamide hydrogel, with one group having previous RT, and the other was radiation naïve. Although the RT patients did not have quite as good of an outcome as the nonradiated group, the differences were nonsignificant for several parameters and they concluded that bulking therapy is valuable for radiated patients.

INJECTION PROCEDURE

Patient Preparation

General considerations apply to all periurethral injection procedures. Patient counseling should be done as outlined in the previous section. The setting of expectations cannot be minimized given the repetitive nature of these treatments, and if patients want something more definitive, they should seek another therapy. They should be counseled regarding the possibility of urinary retention and its management. They should also be told it is normal to have dysuria, hematuria, urgency, and frequency after the procedure and that there is a possibility for infection afterward. A preprocedure urine culture should be obtained and treated and repeated as appropriate. If a patient has a history of hypersensitivity or allergy to any of the injectable components, that particular agent is contraindicated. One of the most commonly used agents before it was discontinued, Contigen (glutaraldehyde cross-linked bovine collagen), actually required a skin test 30 days prior to treatment to rule out allergy to this xenographic agent. This point is largely historical at this time, however.[7,10]

Injection Techniques

Urethral bulking agents can be administered by either a transurethral or periurethral injection technique. For either procedure, they can be done under local anesthesia or under general anesthesia/sedation per the preference of the surgeon and patient. Both techniques use cystoscopic guidance in order to visually confirm the correct location of injection of the agent in use. The main difference lies with where the needle is inserted, and there can be advantages to both techniques. The transurethral technique is purported to allow for better visualization of the injection site, thus allowing for more precise placement of the agent, whereas the periurethral route is less likely to result in extravasation of the material due because there is no puncture of the urethral lumen in this case. Ultrasound guided techniques have also been described.[4,5,7,10]

Transurethral injection technique

The patient is placed in the dorsal lithotomy position and should be prepped and draped using sterile technique. Local anesthesia in the form of lidocaine jelly given intraurethrally should be administered next, if the patient is awake, and given proper dwell time for effect. Optionally, a periurethral block can be used here as well (Fig. 32.1). Using a rigid cystoscope, it should first be advanced into the bladder and the bladder should be drained completely. With a 30° lens, the injection needle should then be advanced into view and then the scope is then withdrawn into the urethra and the location of the midproximal urethra should be noted. The needle is deflected 30° to 45° and starting at the lateral position (3 or 9 o'clock), is placed against the mucosa until it indents slightly. The scope and needle are then advanced

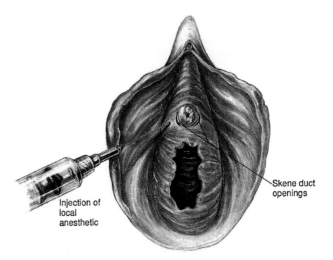

FIGURE 32.1 Periurethral bulking technique with periurethral block. Injection of local anesthetic lateral to Skene duct openings. (Reprinted from Bent AE. Periurethral collagen injections. *Oper Tech Gynecol Surg* 1997;2:52. Copyright © 1997, with permission from Elsevier.)

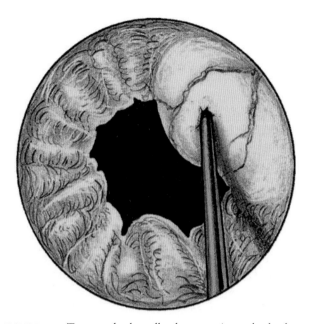

FIGURE 32.2 Transurethral needle placement in urethral submucosa. (Reprinted from Bent AE. Periurethral collagen injections. *Oper Tech Gynecol Surg* 1997;2:54. Copyright © 1997, with permission from Elsevier.)

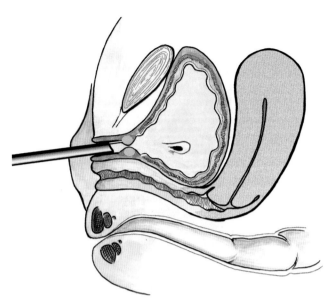

FIGURE 32.3 Under cystoscopic visualization, a transurethral needle injects a bulking agent into multiple submucosal sites in the proximal urethra to increase urethral resistance. (Illustration by J. Tan-Kim, MD.)

until the needle pierces the mucosa and advances a slight amount in the submucosal space. Care should be taken that the needle insertion site is not too proximal on the urethra so that when it is advanced it does not continue into the lumen of the bladder.[5,7,10]

Without moving the position of the needle, the bulking agent can then slowly be injected in an amount sufficient to cause a mass effect akin to coaptation (Fig. 32.2). This process is then repeated on the opposite side and when injecting the agent, the end result should show good urethral coaptation in the proximal portion of the urethra (Fig. 32.3). Advancing the scope back into the bladder should be avoided so as to not crush, distort, or cause extravasation of the injectable agent that has just been administered.[7,10]

Periurethral injection technique

The patient is placed in the dorsal lithotomy position and should be prepped and draped using sterile technique. If the patient is awake, local anesthesia in the form of lidocaine jelly given intraurethral should be administered next and given proper dwell time for effect. In this case, a periurethral block *should* be used here as described before (see Fig. 32.1), especially in an awake patient as the injection needle is usually large and will be inserted in this location. Next, a rigid cystoscope sheath should be inserted to drain the bladder. A 30° lens should then be used, and the scope is withdrawn into the urethra, visualizing the anticipated site of injection. The bulking agent injection needle is then inserted at the lateral aspect of the meatus and advanced through

the submucosa. The cystoscope is there to visualize its position throughout the process. Care should be taken to ensure that the mucosa is not violated. If this occurs, the needle should be withdrawn and advanced in a new, similar location to avoid extravasation. The needle can be carefully rocked side to side in order to confirm its location.[7,10]

When the needle is positioned correctly, the bulking agent can then slowly be injected. The process is then repeated for the other side of the urethra. The goal is similar to the other technique, with the end result being enough agent used to achieve good urethral coaptation in the proximal region of the urethra (Fig. 32.4). Similar to the transurethral technique, the cystoscope should not be advanced further through the area of injection to avoid disrupting the agent.[10] Also, regardless of technique, if extravasation of the injectable agent is seen, the process should be repeated in another location, usually in a more anterior orientation. This should be avoided as much as possible because the first try is usually the most ideal in terms of conditions and visualization.

Postprocedure Care

After the procedure is completed and the patient is well on their way to recovery, they need to be able to demonstrate they can void on their own sufficiently before discharge. If they are in urinary retention, in-and-out straight catheterization can be performed once with a small catheter (12 French or less). If they ultimately still cannot void, they can be sent home with a small indwelling catheter and voiding can be attempted in the

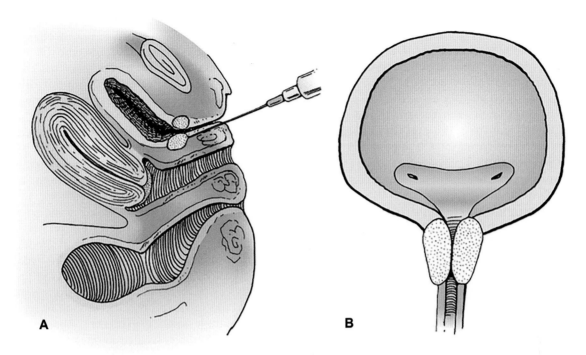

FIGURE 32.4 **A:** Periurethral injection at the bladder neck. **B:** Bulking of bladder neck and proximal urethra. (Reprinted from Handa L, Van Le V. *Te Linde's operative gynecology*, 12th ed. Philadelphia: Wolters Kluwer, 2019.)

clinic 1 to 2 days later. If prolonged retention occurs, the patient can be taught intermittent self-catheterization or a suprapubic catheter can be placed until they can void on their own. Repeated or indwelling catheterization should be avoided overall to prevent the injectable agent from being mechanically dissipated.[7,10]

AVAILABLE AND HISTORICAL INJECTABLE AGENTS

There have been numerous injectable agents developed and used over the last few decades. Again, no ideal agent has quite met all the criteria mentioned earlier. When considering these options, it should be noted again that data does not exist to recommend the use of one injectable agent over another unless serious safety issues have been uncovered leading to market withdrawal. Although not all inclusive of everything historically tried, the following sections summarize representative agents used over the years.

Available Agents (Listed Alphabetically)

Bulkamid (polyacrylamide hydrogel, Contura International, Soeborg, Denmark): This agent is the most recently approved in the United States for use in female stress incontinence (January 2020). The unique

feature when compared to other agents is that this is nonparticulate which in theory alleviates the risk of particle migration seen with particulate agents. Bulkamid is nonresorbable, biocompatible, nonbiodegradable, and is composed of water and cross-linked polyacrylamide suspended as a hydrophilic gel.[16] It comes in 1-mL prefilled syringes and is injected through a 23G 12-cm needle. The product is available with an 11 cm, 0° scope, and needle guide intended for transurethral use.

Overall, clinical trials with Bulkamid have shown good efficacy and durability of the treatment response. In one multicenter trial of 135 patients with stress incontinence or stress predominant mixed urinary incontinence. Toozs-Hobson et al.[17] reported 67% and 64% success at 12 and 24 months, respectively with minimal safety issues. In another randomized, prospective trial, 345 patients were treated with Bulkamid versus collagen. Subjects could receive up to 3 injections at 1-month intervals and were assessed at 3, 6, 9, and 12 months after last injection. Bulkamid was found to be noninferior to collagen in terms of both efficacy and safety in this analysis.[18] Collagen (covered later) has long been considered the "gold standard" of treatments but is no longer available after being withdrawn from the market in 2009. Yet another noninferiority trial with Bulkamid compared it to MUS placement in 224 women (111 transvaginal tape [TVT], 113 Bulkamid). In this case, Bulkamid was found to be inferior to

TVT at 1 year, with roughly 95% of patients achieving success with the TVT group, whereas the Bulkamid cohort was about 60% successful.[19] Long-term data on Bulkamid also appears to be favorable. Brosche et al.[20] looked at long-term follow-up with 7-year outcomes from a single institution. Efficacy and safety were both found to be durable in their review of 388 patients treated with Bulkamid as either a primary or secondary procedure (cure/improved 67.1% and 61.5% respectively, 65.2% overall).

Coaptite (calcium hydroxyapatite, Boston Scientific, Natick, MA): Coaptite was U.S. Food and Drug Administration (FDA) approved in 2005. This agent is composed of an injectable, sterile, nonpyrogenic implant composed of spherical particles of calcium hydroxylapatite (CaHA) 75 to 125 μm in diameter, suspended in an aqueous-based gel carrier. The gel carrier is composed of sodium carboxymethylcellulose, sterile water for injection, and glycerin. The gel carrier suspends the CaHA particles, allowing their delivery through injection needles, and is dissipated in vivo, whereas the CaHA particles remain at the injection sites to provide soft tissue augmentation. The carrier degrades over time leaving the CaHA particles in place to facilitate tissue in-growth.[5,21] A unique characteristic is that this agent is radiopaque, allowing it to be visualized on standard x-ray or computed tomography imaging.[7] It is administered through a standard cystoscopic technique through a 21 gauge needle end- or side-firing needle. No special storage is required and it comes in 1-mL prefilled syringes. The material is fairly viscous and becomes more so once injection starts, so moving expediently through the procedure is advised.

Efficacy with Coaptite has been well studied over the years. In the initial randomized, multicenter trial of this agent in 296 patients, Mayer and colleagues[22] found that it had similar efficacy to collagen (63% vs. 57%, P = nonsignificant) at 12 months. One factor favoring Coaptite was that fewer patients in that group required fewer treatments and an overall lower volume of material injected compared to the subjects receiving collagen (4.0 vs. 6.6 mL, respectively, P < .0001). Adverse events were rare, but in the patients treated with Coaptite, vaginal erosion of the agent, subtrigonal migration, granuloma formation, and urethral prolapse after treatment have been reported.[7]

Durasphere (carbon-coated zirconium beads, Coloplast, Minneapolis, MN): Durasphere was FDA approved in 1999. It is composed of pyrolytic carbon-coated zirconium beads in a water-based carrier gel containing beta-glucan.[23] It was initially formulated with a large particle size to avoid concerns with migration, although asymptomatic occurrences of this have been reported. However, the initial formulation was difficult to inject, so smaller particles were formulated

(still >80 μm to prevent migration) and introduced by Durasphere EXP.[7] It is injected through either the transurethral or periurethral route, and the beads themselves are nondegradable and permanent. The supplied injection needle is specifically made for this product and comes in either 18 or 20G size and comes in 1- and 3-mL prefilled syringes.

Success of this agent when compared to collagen injection has also been reported. In the initial multicenter, randomized controlled trial of 355 women with ISD, Durasphere was shown to be noninferior at 12 months when compared to collagen in improvement in continence grade (80.3% vs. 69.1%, P = nonsignificant). Similarly, to other agents tested versus collagen, Durasphere also required less material injected, and complications were similar between the two groups.[24] Complications in other case reports and series were infrequent overall. Notable complications reported are urethral prolapse, carbon beads found in regional and distant lymph nodes, periurethral abscess formation in 4 of 135 patients studied in one series, and pseudoabscess formation in one other case report after the patient had undergone sling placement.[7]

Macroplastique (polydimethylsiloxane [silicone], Cogentix Medical, United Kingdom): Macroplastique was FDA approved for use in 2006. It is composed of nonpyrogenic, injectable bulking agent composed of polydimethylsiloxane (silicone elastomer) particles suspended in a polyvinylpyrrolidone carrier gel.[25] Once implanted, the elastomer is encapsulated and remains, whereas the carrier is absorbed. It is variable in particle size from 50 to 400 μm which could cause concern for particle migration, although the encapsulation is thought to prevent any migration.[26] It is highly viscous, so injection requires the use of a specialized injector gun. It can be injected through a transurethral route, either endoscopically or with a nonendoscopic transurethral injection device. Like the other agents, it does not require specific storage or handling and comes in 2.5-mL preloaded syringes.

In a large, randomized, multicenter study by Ghoniem et al.[26] of 247 women with ISD, subjects were randomized to either Macroplastique or collagen injection. In this case, Macroplastique was actually shown to be statistically more effective than collagen. This was actually for two outcomes, with 61.5% versus 48% of patients attaining improvement of at least one continence grade, and 36.9% versus 24.8% achieving cure/dry status, both favoring the Macroplastique group. Maher et al.[27] also directly compared Macroplastique to pubovaginal sling in a prospective, randomized controlled trial. Here, they found that although subjective cure rates were similar, the objective success rate clearly favored the pubovaginal sling, and long-term data favored the sling group overall (continence 69% vs. 21%, satisfaction 69% vs 29%, P = .057).[27]

Historical Agents

In addition to the currently available bulking agents, there have been numerous others used in the past that are no longer available for various reasons. Collagen deserves special mention for its significance. As mentioned before, collagen, or glutaraldehyde cross-linked bovine collagen (Contigen, Allergan, Inc, Irvine, CA), had been considered the "gold standard" of bulking agent injection therapy. It was initially approved for use in 1993 and had a long track record of use and success and was often the direct comparator to the newer agents seeking approval. It did require frequent reinjections due to degradation and reabsorption of this agent and was seldom satisfactory for patients over the long term.[5,7] Contigen was ultimately removed from the market in 2010 voluntarily after hyaluronic acid emerged as an alternative cosmetic filler and production was discontinued.[7]

Other previously used agents were removed from the market or were shown to be inferior as well. Historical attempts to use autologous fat were unsuccessful, and there were important safety concerns with migration and embolism reported.[5] Teflon (PTFE/polytetrafluoroethylene) was another agent used that had significant migration concerns and was ultimately never approved for use in the United States for safety reasons.[5] One agent that did go through clinical trials and that had FDA approval was Tegress (ethylene vinyl alcohol, CR Bard, Covington, GA). It was shown to be equivalent in efficacy to collagen in clinical trials. Postmarket follow-up, however, revealed an unacceptable urethral erosion rate of 37% of subjects, and it was subsequently voluntarily removed from the market.[28] Finally, Dextranomer/hyaluronic acid (Zuidex/Deflux, Q-Med, Uppsala, Sweden) was another such agent that underwent the rigors of a clinical trial in the United States and did not ultimately gain approval. Initially marketed as Deflux and used extensively in children with vesicoureteral reflux, this agent was quite familiar to many urologists. In a 2:1 randomized study, it failed to reach equivalency with endoscopically injected collagen.[29] Additionally, there was concern for noninfectious pseudoabscess formation in up to 16% of patients, and ultimately, the agent was deemed neither safe nor efficacious.[30]

CELL THERAPY

A more recent development in the treatment of SUI is the advent of cell-based therapy (see Chapter 22) in the form of autologous muscle–derived cell injection. Clinical trials are ongoing with this therapy, and as of the time of this writing, there has not been approval of this therapy. The American Urological Association guidelines specifically point out that cell therapy should not be offered outside the setting of a clinical trial at this time.[8] Cell therapy is promising because of the potential to restore striated and smooth muscle lost to the various pathologies that cause SUI. Theoretical restoration or improvement of endothelial and nerve/neuromuscular synapse function has also been proposed but has not been the subject or outcome in trials looking at cell therapy for SUI as of yet.[31]

Striated muscle has been the subject of cell therapy research data for SUI to date. The theory is that lost or damaged could be restored or replaced using autologous skeletal muscle cells, muscle cell progenitor cells, or stem cells themselves. Use of the muscle-derived cells, specifically the satellite cells derived from muscle biopsy, has proven to be the most feasible and the urethral rhabdosphincter may prove to be a very favorable target for repair due to the relatively small size of it. This latter point is important as the overall amount of tissue required to transfer is relatively small, thus allowing for easier harvest, culture growth, and ultimately, uptake, especially as ex vivo expansion of satellite cells is not easy.[31,32]

In a pilot study, Carr et al.[33] looked at eight patients who were treated with autologous-derived muscle cells (ADMCs) over 12 months of therapy. Patients underwent urethral injection of cells derived from a quadriceps biopsy. A beneficial effect was seen in five of the eight patients, with a sustained benefit seen at median follow-up of 10 months.[7,33] Building off this, they then looked at 38 patients in a dose ranging study to evaluate the effect of increasingly larger numbers of ADMCs administered to the area of the rhabdosphincter. The low-dose injection groups were given 1, 2, 4, 8, or 16×10^6 ADMCs, whereas the high-dose group was injected with 32, 64, or 128×10^6 ADMCs derived from the quadriceps femoris. The muscle biopsy was sent to a cell processing facility at Cook Myosite Incorporated (Pittsburg, PA) and underwent a proprietary processing method to extract and expand the ADMCs used. The results favored the higher dosage group, with a higher percentage of those patients achieving 50% or greater reduction in pad usage (88.9% vs. 61.5%), 50% or greater reduction in voiding diary reported stress leaks (77.8% vs. 53.3%), and 0 to 1 leaks during a 3-day period (88.9% vs. 33.3%).[34] Overall, safety was good, and complications were infrequent and minor.

Building off this, a study looking at pooled data from two open-label phase I/II trials was reported by Peters et al.[35] where again increasingly escalated doses (10, 50, 100, or 200×10^6 ADMCs) were used on 80 patients. Similarly, their results favored the higher dosage groups in terms of achieving success defined by at least 50% reduction in stress leaks and pad weight improvement at 12 months. All groups actually achieved significant improvement in Urogenital Distress Inventory, Short Form (UDI-6) and Incontinence Impact Questionnaire, Short Form (IIQ-7) scores as well when compared to baseline values. Overall safety was good as well with no reported adverse events due to the ADMCs and minor biopsy-related complications only reported.[35] Phase III trials of this therapy are ongoing.

Although cell therapy is extremely promising, there are some challenges inherent to this therapy. Obtaining the ADMC product is challenging and infrastructure heavy. Cells need to undergo very specific handling and processing under sometimes extreme refrigeration; therefore, there is risk in the handling of the specimen that could lead to contamination or nonviability. There is also an issue with variability in cell growth across samples, thus there is a risk that certain threshold cell numbers may not be met without rebiopsy of these patients.[35] Overall, despite the challenges, the prospect of this therapy is extremely appealing and further study and adoption will be exciting to see in the future.

CONCLUSION

Urethral bulking agent therapy is clearly established and should be in the armamentarium of physicians treating SUI. Available treatments have been shown to be safe and well tolerated with reasonable efficacy. Careful patient selection and education can lead to satisfactory outcomes for both physician and patient alike. Although the ideal injectable agent has not been discovered, ongoing research into injectable cell therapy holds much promise for upcoming research and clinical applications.

References

1. Buckley BS, Lapitan MC. Prevalence of urinary incontinence in men, women, and children—Current evidence: Findings of the fourth International Consultation on Incontinence. *Urology* 2010;76(2):265–270.
2. Kirchin V, Page T, Keegan PE, et al. Urethral injection therapy for urinary incontinence in women. *Cochrane Database Syst Rev* 2017;(7):CD003881.
3. Fusco F, Abdel-Fattah M, Chapple CR, et al. Updated systematic review and meta-analysis of the comparative data on colposuspensions, pubovaginal slings, and midurethral tapes in the surgical treatment of female stress urinary incontinence. *Eur Urol* 2017;72(4):567–591.
4. Chapple C, Dmochowski R. Particulate versus non-particulate bulking agents in the treatment of stress urinary incontinence. *Res Rep Urol* 2019;11:299–310.
5. Reynolds WS, Dmochowski RR. Urethral bulking: A urology perspective. *Urol Clin North Am* 2012;39(3):279–287.
6. Wasenda EJ, Kirby AC, Lukacz ES, et al. The female continence mechanism measured by high resolution manometry: Urethral bulking versus midurethral sling. *Neurourol Urodyn* 2018;37(5):1809–1814.
7. Boone TB, Stewart JN, Martinez LM. Additional therapies for storage and emptying failure. In: Partin AW, Peters CA, Kavoussi LR, et al, eds. *Campbell-Walsh-Wein urology*. Philadelphia: Elsevier, 2021:2889–2904.e4.
8. Kobashi KC, Albo ME, Dmochowski RR, et al. Surgical treatment of female stress urinary incontinence: AUA/SUFU guideline. *J Urol* 2017;198(4):875–883.
9. ter Meulen PH, Berghmans LC, Nieman FH, et al. Effects of Macroplastique implantation system for stress urinary incontinence and urethral hypermobility in women. *Int Urogynecol J Pelvic Floor Dysfunct* 2009;20(2):177–183.
10. Brown ET, Cohn JA, Kaufman MR, et al. Bulking agents for incontinence. In: *Hinman's atlas of urologic surgery*. Philadelphia: Elsevier, 2018:764–765.
11. Daly CME, Mathew J, Aloyscious J, et al. Urethral bulking agents: A retrospective review of primary versus salvage procedure outcomes. *World J Urol* 2021;39(6):2107–2112.
12. Gomelsky A, Athanasiou S, Choo MS, et al. Surgery for urinary incontinence in women: Report from the 6th International Consultation on Incontinence. *Neurourol Urodyn* 2019;38(2):825–837.
13. de Vries AM, Wadhwa H, Huang J, et al. Complications of urethral bulking agents for stress urinary incontinence: An extensive review including case reports. *Female Pelvic Med Reconstr Surg* 2018;24(6):392–398.
14. Dobberfuhl AD. Evaluation and treatment of female stress urinary incontinence after pelvic radiotherapy. *Neurourol Urodyn* 2019;38(Suppl 4):S59–S69.
15. Krhut J, Martan A, Jurakova M, et al. Treatment of stress urinary incontinence using polyacrylamide hydrogel in women after radiotherapy: 1-Year follow-up. *Int Urogynecol J* 2016;27(2):301–305.
16. U.S. Food and Drug Administration. Bulkamid® urethral bulking system: Instructions for use. Accessed January 2020. https://www.accessdata.fda.gov/cdrh_docs/pdf17/P170023D.pdf
17. Toozs-Hobson P, Al-Singary W, Fynes M, et al. Two-year follow-up of an open-label multicenter study of polyacrylamide hydrogel (Bulkamid®) for female stress and stress-predominant mixed incontinence. *Int Urogynecol J* 2012;23(10):1373–1378.
18. Sokol ER, Karram MM, Dmochowski R. Efficacy and safety of polyacrylamide hydrogel for the treatment of female stress incontinence: A randomized, prospective, multicenter North American study. *J Urol* 2014;192(3):843–849.
19. Itkonen Freitas AM, Mentula M, Rahkola-Soisalo P, et al. Tension-free vaginal tape surgery versus polyacrylamide hydrogel injection for primary stress urinary incontinence: A randomized clinical trial. *J Urol* 2020;203(2):372–378.
20. Brosche T, Kuhn A, Lobodasch K, et al. Seven-year efficacy and safety outcomes of Bulkamid for the treatment of stress urinary incontinence. *Neurourol Urodyn* 2021;40(1):502–508.
21. U.S. Food and Drug Administration. Summary of safety and effectiveness data: Coaptite® injectable implant for soft tissue augmentation. Accessed November 2005. https://www.accessdata.fda.gov/cdrh_docs/pdf4/P040047b.pdf
22. Mayer RD, Dmochowski RR, Appell RA, et al. Multicenter prospective randomized 52-week trial of calcium hydroxylapatite versus bovine dermal collagen for treatment of stress urinary incontinence. *Urology* 2007;69(5):876–880.
23. U.S. Food and Drug Administration. Summary of safety and effectiveness data: Durasphere™ injectable bulking agent. Accessed September 1999. https://www.accessdata.fda.gov/cdrh_docs/pdf/P980053b.pdf
24. Lightner D, Calvosa C, Andersen R, et al. A new injectable bulking agent for treatment of stress urinary incontinence: Results of a multicenter, randomized, controlled, double-blind study of Durasphere. *Urology* 2001;58(1):12–15.

25. U.S. Food and Drug Administration. Summary of safety and effectiveness data: Macroplastique® implants injectable urethral bulking agent. Accessed October 2006. https://www.accessdata.fda.gov/cdrh_docs/pdf4/p040050b.pdf

26. Ghoniem G, Corcos J, Comiter C, et al. Cross-linked polydimethylsiloxane injection for female stress urinary incontinence: Results of a multicenter, randomized, controlled, single-blind study. *J Urol* 2009;181(1):204–210.

27. Maher CF, O'Reilly BA, Dwyer PL, et al. Pubovaginal sling versus transurethral Macroplastique for stress urinary incontinence and intrinsic sphincter deficiency: A prospective randomised controlled trial. *BJOG* 2005;112(6):797–801.

28. Hurtado E, McCrery R, Appell R. The safety and efficacy of ethylene vinyl alcohol copolymer as an intra-urethral bulking agent in women with intrinsic urethral deficiency. *Int Urogynecol J Pelvic Floor Dysfunct* 2007;18(8):869–873.

29. Lightner D, Rovner E, Corcos J, et al; for Zuidex Study Group. Randomized controlled multisite trial of injected bulking agents for women with intrinsic sphincter deficiency: Mid-urethral injection of Zuidex via the Implacer versus proximal urethral injection of Contigen cystoscopically. *Urology* 2009;74(4):771–775.

30. Lightner DJ, Fox J, Klingele C. Cystoscopic injections of dextranomer hyaluronic acid into proximal urethra for urethral incompetence: Efficacy and adverse outcomes. *Urology* 2010;75(6):1310–1314.

31. Hart ML, Izeta A, Herrera-Imbroda B, et al. Cell therapy for stress urinary incontinence. *Tissue Eng Part B Rev* 2015;21(4):365–376.

32. Maclean S, Khan WS, Malik AA, et al. The potential of stem cells in the treatment of skeletal muscle injury and disease. *Stem Cells Int* 2012;2012:282348.

33. Carr LK, Steele D, Steele S, et al. 1-year follow-up of autologous muscle-derived stem cell injection pilot study to treat stress urinary incontinence. *Int Urogynecol J Pelvic Floor Dysfunct* 2008;19(6):881–883.

34. Carr LK, Robert M, Kultgen PL, et al. Autologous muscle derived cell therapy for stress urinary incontinence: A prospective, dose ranging study. *J Urol* 2013;189(2):595–601.

35. Peters KM, Dmochowski RR, Carr LK, et al. Autologous muscle derived cells for treatment of stress urinary incontinence in women. *J Urol* 2014;192(2):469–476.

CHAPTER 33

BOTULINUM TOXIN THERAPY FOR URINARY INCONTINENCE

Christopher John Chermansky • Linda Burkett

HISTORY

Botulinum as a disease was first described by Kerner in 1822,[1] and the toxin was first isolated for medical treatment in 1857 by van Ermengem.[2] Schurch et al.[3] first used onabotulinumtoxinA (onaBoNT-A) within urology for detrusor sphincter dyssynergia in 2000, and then onaBoNT-A was widely adopted for neurogenic detrusor overactivity (NDO) in 2011 after publication of phase 3 trials and U.S. Food and Drug Administration (FDA) approval.[4,5] In 2013, intradetrusor onaBoNT-A was approved by the FDA for use in patients with overactive bladder (OAB) refractory to oral medications after publication of phase 3 OAB trials.[6,7]

Idiopathic overactive bladder (iOAB) is defined by the International Continence Society and the International Urogynecological Association as urinary urgency, usually accompanied by urinary frequency and nocturia, with or without urgency urinary incontinence (UUI), in the absence of urinary tract infection (UTI) or other obvious pathology.[8] The American Urological Association (AUA) and the Society of Urodynamics, Female Pelvic Medicine and Urogenital Reconstruction (SUFU) have published guidelines for the treatment of iOAB in adults.[9] Intradetrusor onaBoNT-A injection is considered third-line treatment for iOAB patients who have failed to improve with behavioral modifications and oral agents such as antimuscarinics and/or beta-adrenoceptor agonists.

MECHANISM OF ACTION AND FORMULATIONS

Botulinum toxin is derived from the bacteria *Clostridium botulinum*.[10] There are seven serotypes, and serotype A is used most commonly in clinical applications including intradetrusor injection for iOAB. Serotype B is also available for clinical use, but it has decreased potency and duration of action compared to serotype A. The different formulations of serotype A botulinum toxin include onaBoNT-A (Botox), abobotulinumtoxinA (Dysport), and incobotulinumtoxinA (Xeomin). Currently, the most studied and only FDA-approved formulation is onaBoNT-A.[6,7] A small number of studies have been published on the use of intradetrusor abobotulinumtoxinA for iOAB; however, larger multicenter clinical trials are needed to confirm safety and efficacy.[11–13] It should be noted the dosages differ between formulations, and the conversion of onaBoNT-A to abobotulinumtoxinA is 1:2.5. Botulinum toxin is usually labeled by dosage in units (U), and this describes its potency.

The mechanism of action of botulinum toxin is by cleaving the synaptosome-associated protein 25 kDa within presynaptic neurons, thereby preventing the release of acetylcholine at the neuromuscular junction. By inactivating cholinergic transmission, botulinum toxin results in temporary muscle paralysis.[10] Furthermore, botulinum toxin affects afferent transmission within the bladder by inhibiting the release of adenosine triphosphate and substance P with a reduction in axonal expression of purinergic and vanilloid receptors.[14] The duration of blockade differs by neuron type, lasting 3 to 6 months within skeletal muscle and up to 12 months within smooth muscle.[10] There has been limited research evaluating presence of antibodies to onaBoNT-A after intradetrusor injection and its impact in decreasing therapeutic efficacy.[15] No patients developed antibodies to onaBoNT-A in the two phase 3 randomized controlled trials (RCTs) studying the 100-U dose for iOAB.[6,7]

TECHNIQUES OF DELIVERY

General Technique

Patients choosing intradetrusor onaBoNT-A should be counseled regarding risk of transient urinary retention seen in 6% of patients given 100 U in the FDA qualifying trials and 8% given 200 U in the 6-month Refractory Overactive Bladder: Sacral Neuromodulation vs. Botulinum Toxin Assessment (ROSETTA) trial.[6,7,16] Despite these low risks of urinary retention, it is recommended that patients learn clean intermittent catheterization (CIC) prior to the procedure to be prepared in case it is needed. Urinalysis is performed on the day of injection to rule out UTI. To avoid canceling injection on the date scheduled because of symptomatic UTI, it is recommended that the patient submit a urine culture at least 1 week prior to allow time to result and treat with antibiotics. Any anticoagulation must be held prior to the injection to decrease problematic hematuria that could necessitate a trip to the operating room (OR) for fulguration and clot evacuation.

Antibiotics are typically given prior to injection of intradetrusor onaBoNT-A. In the phase 3 RCTs for iOAB evaluating the 100-U dose of onaBoNT-A versus placebo, the incidence of UTIs was reported to be 25.5% in those treated with onaBoNT-A ($n = 557$) compared to 9.6% in those treated with placebo ($n = 548$), $P < .001$.[6,7] In a retrospective study of 284 patients who received either one dose of ceftriaxone intramuscularly ($n = 236$) or a 3-day course of oral fluoroquinolone starting the day prior to onaBoNT-A administration ($n = 48$), Houman et al.[17] found that the UTI rate was 20.8% for those receiving the fluoroquinolone versus 36% in the ceftriaxone group, $P = .04$.

Intradetrusor onaBoNT-A injection can be performed either in the office using local anesthesia or in the OR under sedation. Intravesical instillation of 60 mL of 1% lidocaine for 20 to 30 minutes prior to injection is commonly used for office injection. The onaBoNT-A is injected into the bladder wall using direct cystoscopic visualization. An injection needle (27G) is introduced into the bladder lumen under direct visualization, and the needle is placed between 2 and 4 mm into the bladder wall for multiple injections. Each 100 U of onaBoNT-A is gently mixed with 0.9% injectable saline in a 10-mL syringe. Twenty injections (each 0.5 mL) are placed into the extratrigonal bladder walls.[18] The injections should be limited to the bottom half of the bladder.

After completion of all injections, full visualization of the bladder should be performed to confirm hemostasis at all sites. Bleeding at any injection site can be treated with either pressure for 1 to 2 minutes using the cystoscope tip or with cautery using a Bugbee electrode. Because cautery may be needed in rare cases, it is recommended to use sterile water as the cystoscopic fluid. All patients should follow-up in 2 to 3 weeks after injection to assess efficacy and to check postvoid residual (PVR) volume for urinary retention that may require temporary CIC.

Dosages

Varying injection techniques and dosages of onaBoNT-A have been described for the treatment of OAB. We will review the literature supporting current recommendations by the AUA/SUFU for the FDA-approved dosage of 100 U of onaBoNT-A for the treatment of iOAB refractory to first and second line OAB treatments.[9] The risk of side effects increase with doses more than 100 U, and these include urinary retention and UTI. Temporary retention necessitating CIC was seen in 6% of OAB patients given 100 U ($n = 1,105$) in the FDA qualifying trials[6,7] and in 8% of the OAB patients given 200 U ($n = 192$) in the 6-month ROSETTA trial.[16] The risks of UTIs, all uncomplicated with no upper tract involvement, was 25.5% for the OAB patients given 100 U in the FDA qualifying trials[6,7] and 35% for the OAB patients given 200 U in the 6-month ROSETTA trial[16] and 24% during longer follow-up in the 2-year ROSETTA trial.[19]

Several RCTs have focused on establishing the dose response by varying doses of botulinum A compared to placebo. Dmochowski et al.[20] performed a randomized dose-ranging trial of onaBoNT-A in OAB patients with eight or more episodes of UUI per week, and they demonstrated that onaBoNT-A 100 U maximized symptom improvement while minimizing urinary retention for which CIC was initiated. Fowler et al.[21] compared different doses of onaBoNT-A to placebo in OAB patients, and they found improvement from baseline in Incontinence Quality of Life (I-QOL) at 36 weeks in groups given more than 100 U, $P < .05$. Rovner et al.[22] compared onaBoNT-A doses for OAB ranging from 50 to 300 U, and after 12 weeks, the number of patients with more than 75% improvement in urgency and UUI episodes (UUIEs) was 6% for patients given 50 U compared to 42% for both 100 and 150 U groups. Denys et at.[23] performed a double-blinded, placebo-controlled, multicenter RCT comparing onaBoNT-A 50 U, 100 U, 150 U, and placebo, and after 5 months, dry rates were 15.8%, 45%, 45.8%, and 7.1%, $P < .009$. For patients given 50 U, there was no significant symptomatic improvement above placebo at any time point. Likewise, Cohen et al.[24] found no difference in urinary frequency or urodynamics measures with either the 100- or 150-U doses after 3 months; however, there was a trend toward improved dry rates in patients receiving 150 U.

For dosages of abobotulinumtoxinA, de Sá Dantas Bezerra et al.[25] compared 300 U versus 500 U in a prospective, randomized study of 21 women with OAB, and they found at 12 weeks, there were similar dry rates of 91% and similar increases of 86 mL (300 U) and 71 mL (500 U) in maximum cytometric capacity, $P = .27$; however, by 24 weeks, 50% of patients given 300 U saw incontinence return compared to 0% given 500 U group. A similar trend in both groups at 24 weeks was seen in the Patient Global Impression of Improvement (PGI-I) scores. Because there was no significant difference in PVR at 4 weeks between 300 U (71.7 mL) and 500 U (96.5 mL) and no difference in UTI rates, these authors concluded that the 500-U dose was superior with a longer duration of effect and no increase in adverse events (AEs).

Injection Techniques

Various techniques for the delivery of intradetrusor ona-BoNT-A have been studied to evaluate efficacy and AEs. These techniques compare supratrigonal-only versus inclusion of trigonal injections, and they evaluate different depths of injection. Earlier studies, including the FDA qualifying studies, advocated for supratrigonal injection to minimize the potential development of vesicoureteral reflux (VUR) from injections placed too close to the ureteral orifices.[6,7] Kuo[26] compared delivering onaBoNT-A 100 U into either only the bladder body ($n = 37$), 75 U into the bladder body and 25 U into the trigone ($n = 35$), or 50 U into the bladder base and 50 U into the trigone ($n = 33$). The study enrolled 105 patients, including 57 women and 48 men, and all patients completed the injection and at least two follow-up visits. Success was defined as moderate or marked improvement in the patient's perception of bladder condition. Kuo[26] found no significant differences between treatment success (72%) or dry rates (also 72%) among the groups at 3 months. Acute urinary retention was 6% overall with no difference between groups ($P = .127$), but the bladder base and trigone injection group had no retention and no patient with trigone injection developed VUR at 3 months. More recently, Jo et al.[27] performed a meta-analysis of eight studies (419 subjects), including the Kuo study, evaluating the effect of intradetrusor onaBoNT-A according to injection site. Compared to trigone sparing techniques, injecting onaBoNT-A into the trigone demonstrated significant symptom score (I-QOL and Overactive Bladder Symptom Score [OABSS]) improvement ($P = .04$), higher dryness rates ($P = .002$), and fewer UUIEs ($P = .02$). When comparing intradetrusor to suburothelial injection, there were no differences in the incidence of VUR, PVR, or UTIs. Jo et al.[27] concluded that injecting onaBoNT-A into the trigone was more efficacious that supratrigonal-only injections, and the risks of AEs was similar between techniques. Also, the depth of onaBoNT-A injection did not change either efficacy or safety.

Manecksha et al.[28] compared trigone-sparing versus trigone-including injection techniques of 500 U abobotulinumtoxinA in 22 OAB patients, and the primary outcome was the OABSS measured at 6 weeks. The mean total OABSS improved from 22.4 at baseline to 8.7 at 6 weeks ($P < .001$) in the trigone-including group compared with an OABSS improvement from 22.7 to 13.4 ($P < .03$) in the trigone-sparing group, a difference of 4.4 points in favor of the trigone-including group ($P = .03$). PVRs were similar between the groups, and no trigone-injecting patient developed VUR. Thus, they concluded that trigone-including injections are superior, and this technique did not result in VUR.

The number of injections and different injection volumes have both been investigated. The original FDA qualifying studies evaluating onaBoNT-A 100 U for OAB used 20 supratrigonal injections, each 0.5 mL.[6,7] It has been postulated that fewer injections with larger dilution volumes could result in greater suburothelial diffusion to allow for toxin action on a larger muscle surface area.[29] Yet, larger injection volumes could increase serosal extravasations, thereby decreasing efficacy. Liao et al.[30] compared 10, 20, or 40 injections of suburothelial onaBoNT-A 100 U in 10 mL given under intravenous sedation with a prospective randomized study of 67 refractory OAB patients. The OABSS and patient perception of bladder condition scores were comparable between the groups at 3 and 6 months, and there was no difference in AEs between groups. The authors concluded that decreasing the number of intravesical injections while maintaining the same dose of onaBoNT-A and injection volume resulted in equal efficacy. Finally, MacDiarmid et al.[31] conducted an Allergan-sponsored, multicenter RCT of 120 refractory OAB patients (115 women and 5 men) receiving either placebo ($n = 40$) or onaBoNT-A 100 U ($n = 80$) mixed with 5 mL of injectable saline and administered as eight peritrigonal and two trigonal injections (each 0.5 mL). Of the patients receiving onaBoNT-A using this alternative injection paradigm (Fig. 33.1), 51.4% achieved a ≥50% reduction in urinary incontinence episodes per day at week 12 (similar to the FDA qualifying studies), and CIC was not required in any of the women injected.

EFFICACY AND ADVERSE EVENTS WITH INTRADETRUSOR BOTOX FOR OVERACTIVE BLADDER

FDA Qualifying Phase 3 Randomized Controlled Trials and Extension Study of OnabotulinumtoxinA

Allergan sponsored two multicenter, placebo-controlled, phase 3 RCTs studying the efficacy and tolerability of onaBoNT-A 100 U in the treatment of OAB that led to FDA approval.[6,7] Sievert et al.[18] pooled these two studies and summarized the data. To qualify for these studies, the 1,105 OAB patients recruited had three or more urge urinary incontinence episodes (UUIEs) over 3 days and eight or more voids per day. All patients were refractory to anticholinergic drugs either due to inadequate efficacy or intolerable side effects. Patients had a baseline PVR less than 100 mL, and they all had to be willing to initiate CIC if necessary. Patients were randomized 1:1 to receive either placebo using normal saline ($n = 548$) or onaBoNT-A 100 U ($n = 557$). Independent onaBoNT-A reconstitution was used to maintain the blind, and 20 injections (each 0.5 mL) were placed into the supratrigonal bladder wall using a cystoscope. The coprimary end points measured at week 12 were the change from baseline in the number

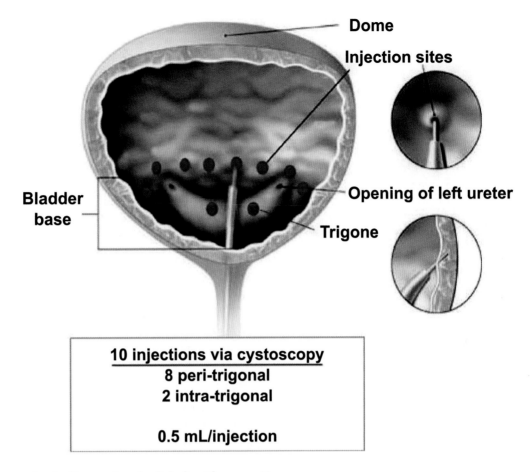

Alternative onabotulinumtoxinA injection pattern

FIGURE 33.1 Alternative onaBoNT-A injection pattern. (Reprinted from MacDiarmid S, Glazier D, Shapiro A, et al. Treatment of overactive bladder with a peritrigonal injection paradigm of onabotulinumtoxinA is associated with a low incidence of clean intermittent catheterization. Paper presented at: ICS 2019 Gothenburg Scientific Programme; September 4, 2019; Gothenburg, Sweden. https://www.ics.org/2019/abstract/186.)

of UUIEs per day and the proportion of patients reporting a positive response on the Treatment Benefit Scale (TBS). Secondary end points included measuring changes from baseline in urgency and micturition episodes per day, I-QOL, King's Health Questionnaire (KHQ), and the proportion of patients achieving a ≥50% or a 100% reduction in UUIEs.

The results of the pooled data showed a mean decrease of 2.80 UUIEs per day at week 12 in the onaBoNT-A group compared to a decrease of 0.95 UUIEs per day in the placebo group, $P < .001$. Also, 27.1% of the onaBoNT-A patients became dry at week 12 compared to 8.4% of the patients given placebo, $P < .001$. In addition, 60.5% of the patients treated with onaBoNT-A demonstrated a ≥50% reduction from baseline in UUIEs per day compared to 31% in the placebo group, $P < .001$. Subgroup analyses of the pooled data were performed looking at the number of prior anticholinergics and at the reasons for inadequate anticholinergic therapy. Neither the number of prior anticholinergics nor the reason(s) why anticholinergics

were stopped influenced the decreases in UUIEs seen with onaBoNT-A. In addition, urinary urgency episodes per day decreased from baseline by 3.30 and 1.23 in the onaBoNT-A and placebo groups, respectively, $P < .001$. Also, micturition episodes per day decreased from baseline by 2.35 and 0.87 in the onaBoNT-A and placebo groups, respectively, $P < .001$.

As for the other primary end point, 61.8% of the patients treated with onaBoNT-A were greatly improved or improved on the TBS compared to 28.0% in the placebo group, $P < .001$. Also, neither the number of prior anticholinergics nor the reason(s) why anticholinergics were stopped impacted the TBS responses seen with onaBoNT-A. Furthermore, changes from baseline in I-QOL and the KHQ were studied in both of the phase 3 RCTs. At baseline, all patients had poor QOL as seen by low I-QOL scores and high KHQ scores. Nitti et al.[6] showed that the I-QOL score increased by 21.9 with onaBoNT-A versus 6.8 with placebo, $P < .001$. Similarly, Chapple et al.[7] showed that the I-QOL score increased by 23.1 with onaBoNT-A versus

6.3 with placebo, $P < .001$. Likewise, improvements from baseline in all seven domains of the KHQ in both studies were noted after onaBoNT-A versus placebo, $P < .001$, for each domain.

Subjects in both phase 3 RCTs investigating onaBoNT-A for OAB were invited to participate in a long-term extension study.[32] Of the 839 patients that entered the extension study, 430 of 839 (51.3%) completed the 3.5-year study period. After 3.5 years or six treatment cycles, the reductions in mean UUIEs per day as measured at 12 weeks after each onaBoNT-A injection were between 2.9–4.5 in all subgroups.

The proportion of patients reporting high satisfaction as measured by the TBS was 70% to 90%. The rate of discontinuation due to lack of efficacy was 5.7% (47 of 839 patients). The majority of patients discontinued due to either personal reasons, loss to follow-up, or study burden and other–treatment-related reasons.

Predictors of Response to OnabotulinumtoxinA for Overactive Bladder

To evaluate potential predictors of nonresponse to treatment with onaBoNT-A in women with refractory detrusor overactivity (DO), Owen et al.[33] performed a secondary analysis of baseline and 6-week follow-up data of their initial randomized trial of onaBoNT-A versus placebo in women with refractory DO.[34] Univariate and multivariate logistic regression were used to assess demographic factors and baseline clinical parameters on nonresponse to treatment defined as 20% or less improvement in urinary urgency and leakage episodes, 10% or less in voiding frequency, not achieving continence, and "no change" or worse on PGI-I score at 6 weeks. At the 10% significance threshold, age, baseline voiding frequency, and I-QOL scores were potential predictors of nonresponse in voiding frequency. Age and body mass index (BMI) were associated with nonresponse on the PGI-I scale. Having accounted for all associated factors in the multivariate analysis, only increasing age and BMI showed a marginal association with nonresponse on the PGI-I scale.

Liao and Kuo[35] assessed outcomes in the frail older adults (age older than 65 years and unintentional weight loss, self-reported exhaustion, weakness, slow walking speed, and/or low physical activity), the older adults (age older than 65 years without frailty), and patients younger than 65 years of age. The frail older adults were more likely to have a large PVR, develop urinary retention, need longer period of recovery, and have lower success than the other groups. Wang et al.[36] compared patients with idiopathic DO that had diabetes mellitus (DM) to those without DM, and they found no difference in either OAB symptoms or urodynamic

parameters 3 months following onaBoNT-A; however, those with DM were more likely to have PVR ≥ 150 mL and general weakness post treatment.

As to the predictive benefit of urodynamics prior to onaBoNT-A injection, Sahai et al.[37] sought to determine if urodynamic parameters predict outcomes in OAB patients undergoing onaBoNT-A injections. They found that a high maximum detrusor pressure of more than 110 cm H_2O was found to be predictive of poor response to onaBoNT-A. In contrast, Rovner et al.[22] found that OAB symptom improvement after onaBoNT-A was independent of the urodynamic presence of DO.

ROSETTA predictors was a planned secondary analysis of the National Institutes of Health (NIH) Pelvic Floor Disorders Network (PFDN) ROSETTA study performed to identify baseline clinical and demographic factors associated with treatment response and satisfaction in women participating in ROSETTA.[38] The variables examined included age, race, BMI, functional comorbidity index (FCI), UUIEs per day, urodynamic variables (maximum bladder capacity, presence of DO), and health-related QoL on the Health Utility Index-3 (HUI-3). For women receiving onaBoNT-A 200 U, a greater reduction in mean daily UUIEs was seen in when DO was present. Also, those with higher HUI-3 scores had greater reductions in daily UUIE, and greater patient age was associated with less UUIEs per day reduction, both $P < .001$. Finally, a higher FCI score was associated with a decreased odds of achieving a 50% or greater reduction in UUIEs. In summary, older women with multiple comorbidities and decreased functional and health-related QOL had reduced treatment response and satisfaction with onaBoNT-A 200 U.

Duration of OnabotulinumtoxinA Therapy for Overactive Bladder

The pooled analysis for both FDA qualifying phase 3 studies showed that the median time to request retreatment was 9 months following onaBoNT-A 100 U treatment.[6,7] In the 3.5-year long-term extension study of onaBoNT-A for OAB, the median duration of effect was 7.6 months.[32] Dowson et al.[39] reported on a prospective single-center study of 100 patients who received at least one onaBoNT-A 200 U injection for refractory iOAB, and the median interval between injections was 10.7 months. For the ROSETTA 2-year outcomes paper which compared onaBoNT-A 200 U ($n = 192$) to sacral neuromodulation ($n = 184$), the median interval between the first and second onaBoNT-A injections was 350 days, interquartile range (IQR) = 242 to 465.[19] In addition, the median interval between the second and third onaBoNT-A injections was 273 days, IQR = 224 to 350. Thus, the duration of onaBoNT-A therapy for OAB clearly increases by several months with the higher 200-U dose.

Adverse Events with OnabotulinumtoxinA Therapy for Overactive Bladder

UTIs and urinary retention were the most common AEs found in the phase 3 RCTs studying onaBoNT-A for OAB.[6,7] The incidence of UTIs was reported in 25.5% of those treated with onaBoNT-A compared to 9.6% of those treated with placebo, $P < .001$. Urinary retention requiring CIC was found in 5.8% of the patients given onaBoNT-A versus 0.4% of the patients given placebo. CIC was initiated if the PVR greater than 350 mL regardless of symptoms or if the PVR was ≥200 mL and less than 350 mL with symptoms of difficult voiding or constant bladder fullness. In the 3.5-year long-term extension study of onaBoNT-A 100 U, the most common AE was UTI.[32] The rate of de novo catheterization after the first treatment was 4.0%, and it ranged from 0.6% to 1.7% after subsequent treatments. The rate of onaBoNT-A discontinuation due to AEs was 5.1% (42 of 839). In the Dowson study evaluating onaBoNT-A 200 U for OAB, the need to start CIC was seen in 35% of patients, and UTIs were seen in 21% of patients.[39] Finally, for the ROSETTA 2-year outcomes paper, 24% of the patients receiving onaBoNT-A 200 U developed recurrent UTIs, and 6% required CIC postsecond injection.[19]

Efficacy and Adverse Events with AbobotulinumtoxinA for Overactive Bladder

Craciun and Irwin[40] reported on 170 patients treated with abobotulinumintoxinA 250 U at a single center over a 10-year period, and they showed that 26% achieved dryness, and urinary incontinence severity was reduced by 44%. Furthermore, OABSS improved by a mean of 35% ($P < .001$), with the OABSS improving by 2 or more points in 65% of cases. The mean interval between repeat abobotulinumtoxinA injection treatments was 21.3 months, and de novo self-catheterization was required in 18.2% of cases.

Ravindra et al.[12] prospectively compared onaBoNT-A 200 U ($n = 101$) and abobotulinumtoxinA 500 U ($n = 106$) in patients with iOAB (80% women).[12] All patients were routinely reviewed at 2 weeks to assess for symptomatic urinary retention and then at 3 months to assess response. Similar reductions in daytime urinary frequency, nocturia, and incontinence episodes were observed after treatment. Also, there is no difference in duration of effect between those receiving onaBoNT-A (10.65 months) and abobotulinumtoxinA (10.87 months), $P = .83$. Yet, urinary retention requiring CIC was seen in 42% of patients receiving abobotulinumtoxinA compared to 23% of patients receiving onaBoNT-A, $P = .009$.

COMPARISONS TO OTHER OVERACTIVE BLADDER TREATMENTS

OnabotulinumtoxinA versus Oral Overactive Bladder Drugs (Anticholinergics and Mirabegron)

The NIH PFDN Anticholinergic versus Botulinum Toxin Comparison (ABC) trial by Visco et al.[41] was a double-blind, double-placebo–controlled, RCT of women with idiopathic UUI who received either daily oral anticholinergic medication (solifenacin, 5 mg initially, with possible escalation to 10 mg and, if necessary, subsequent switch to trospium XR, 60 mg) or onaBoNT-A 100 U. The primary outcome was the reduction from baseline in mean UUIEs per day over the 6-month period, and the mean reduction was 3.4 in the anticholinergic group ($n = 118$) and 3.3 in the onaBoNT-A group ($n = 113$), $P = .81$. Yet, 27% of patients receiving onaBoNT-A achieved dryness compared to 13% of patients receiving anticholinergic group, $P = .003$. As stated by the authors, the rate of reduction of UUIEs per day with anticholinergics in this study was twice that seen in a Cochrane review of anticholinergics for OAB (0.6 to 1.7 UUIEs per day).[42] It is likely that the baseline education about lifestyle modifications and/or the frequent study phone calls and visits improved patient compliance with anticholinergics, thereby impacting the decrease seen in UUIEs per day.

In a meta-analysis of 56 RCTs, Drake et al.[43] compared the efficacy of onaBoNT-A 100 U and oral OAB drugs (anticholinergics and mirabegron) for the treatment of OAB. The comparative analysis found that after 12 weeks of treatment, patients receiving onaBoNT-A 100 U, compared to placebo, had the greatest reductions in UUIEs per day, urgency episodes, and voids compared to oral OAB drugs: reductions of 1.55 UUIEs more per day (credible interval or CrI of 1.10 to 2.01), 2.01 urgency episodes more per day (CrI of 1.48 to 2.54), and 1.37 voids more per day (CrI of 1.03 to 1.70). In addition, onaBoNT-A therapy had higher odds of achieving complete dryness and seeing a ≥50% decrease in UUIEs per day compared to other treatment options. The authors concluded the need for more well-designed head-to-head trials that assess therapy adherence and persistence. Although Allergan was involved at the protocol stage of the review, it was not involved in either data collection or analysis.

OnabotulinumtoxinA versus Sacral Neuromodulation

ROSETTA was an open-label, multicenter, randomized trial of 364 women with idiopathic refractory UUI randomized to either onaBoNT-A 200 U ($n = 190$) or staged sacral neuromodulation with the Medtronic

InterStim ($n = 174$).[16] The primary outcome of ROSETTA was the change from baseline in mean UUIEs per day averaged over 6 months, as recorded for 3 consecutive days in monthly bladder diaries. The authors found that onaBoNT-A had a greater mean daily UUIEs per day reduction over 6 months than did the sacral neuromodulation group, -3.9 versus -3.3 episodes per day, $P = .01$. Also, women treated with onaBoNT-A showed greater improvement in the Overactive Bladder Questionnaire Short Form (OAB-q-SF) for symptom bother compared to treatment with sacral neuromodulation, -46.7 versus -38.6; $P = .002$. Although statistically significant, onaBoNT-A resulted in greater reduction of UUIE, but this was limited by the small magnitude of the difference (less than one episode per day). Furthermore, 83% of patients receiving onaBoNT-A were considered clinical responders (more than 50% decrease in UUIEs per day at 1 month) compared to 84% of patients receiving first-stage sacral neuromodulation lead (more than 50% decrease in UUIEs per day during the 7- to 14-day testing phase).

The same authors performed an extension trial of ROSETTA comparing the efficacy and safety of onaBoNT-A 200 U with sacral neuromodulation over a 2-year period.[19] The primary objective was the change from baseline in mean number of daily UUIE over 2 years. Outcome data were available for 87% of the clinical responders from the original 6-month study. Both treatments had sustained improvements in the daily reduction of UUIE, and there was no difference between the two treatments at 24 months: decrease of 3.9 UUIEs per day for those receiving repeat onaBoNT-A versus a decrease of 3.5 UUIEs per day for those continuing with sacral neuromodulation, $P = .15$. Yet, patients receiving onaBoNT-A maintained higher treatment satisfaction and treatment endorsement across 24 months compared to those receiving sacral neuromodulation, $P < .001$. Other QOL measures (OAB-q-SF, Urogenital Distress Inventory short form, Incontinence Impact Questionnaire, and Sandvik Incontinence Severity Index) showed no difference between the treatments.

Harvie et al. conducted a secondary analysis of ROSETTA to assess the cost-effectiveness of staged sacral neuromodulation versus onaBoNT-A 200 U for the treatment of UUI in women with OAB.[44] The analysis was from the health care system perspective with primary within-trial analysis for 2 years and secondary 5-year decision analysis. Effectiveness was measured in quality-adjusted life-years (QALYs) and reductions in UUIEs per day. Two-year costs were higher for sacral neuromodulation than for onaBoNT-A 200 U ($35,680 vs. $7,460, $P < .01$), and this persisted through 5 years ($36,550 vs. $12,020, $P < .01$). The authors found no significant differences in effectiveness between the two therapies across multiple effectiveness measures including QALYs, UUIEs per day, and condition-specific symptom and health-related QOL outcomes. The probability that sacral neuromodulation is cost-effective relative to onaBoNT-A is $<.025$ for all willingness to pay values below $580,000 per QALY at 2 years and $204,000 per QALY at 5 years. The authors concluded that although both treatments were effective, the high cost of sacral neuromodulation was not a good value for treating UUI compared to onaBoNT-A 200 U.

OnabotulinumtoxinA versus Posterior Tibial Nerve Stimulation

In an RCT comparing percutaneous tibial nerve stimulation (PTNS) with Urgent PC to onaBoNT-A 100 U in 60 patients (85% female), Sherif et al.[45] found statistically significant improvements in overall OAB symptom score and urgency scores in both groups at 6 months. Yet, in the PTNS group the improvements were not significant at 9 months. The authors concluded that onaBoNT-A was more durable than PTNS; however, the authors did not report doing maintenance (monthly) PTNS after patients completed the initial 12-week therapy.

OPTIMIZING INTRADETRUSOR ONABOTULINUMTOXINA

Methods that could potentially improve delivery of intradetrusor onaBoNT-A and/or reduce AEs include different injection protocols (volume/dilution, number of injections) and enhanced drug delivery modalities that seek to deliver the Botox to the bladder wall without injections, thereby reducing the risk of bleeding and giving patients who cannot come off blood thinners access to bladder onaBoNT-A. Different injection protocols were discussed earlier in this chapter.

Liposomes and hydrogel, both embedded with onaBoNT-A, have been investigated as intravesical, injection-free treatments for patients with OAB. Chuang et al.[46] published a double-blind RCT performed at two sites whereby 62 OAB patients were randomized to either lipotoxin (liposomes containing onaBoNT-A 200 U) or saline. One month after treatment, urinary frequency decreased by 4.6 voids over 3 days in the lipotoxin group versus 0.19 voids over 3 days in the placebo group, $P = .025$. Also, Lipotoxin resulted in a decrease in urgency severity scores compared to placebo, $P = .018$. Furthermore, PVRs did not increase, and there was no increased risk of UTIs. TheraCoat (TC-3) is an inert, heat-sensitive hydrogel which when placed into the bladder solidifies and provides a slow release of embedded drug.[47] Krhut et al.[47] randomized 39 women with OAB into four groups receiving 50 mL of an intravesical instillation of either placebo (0.9% sodium chloride), TC-3 gel embedded with onaBoNT-A 200 U, TC-3 gel embedded with onaBoNT-A 200 U and dimethyl sulfoxide (DMSO), and DMSO.

OAB parameters (UUIEs per day and urgency episodes per day) and questionnaires (OABSS and Patient Perception of Bladder Condition) were compared before and 1 month after instillation, and the group receiving TC-3 embedded with onaBoNT-A group was found to be superior. Allergan has recently completed a phase 2, multicenter, randomized, double-blind, placebo-controlled, single-treatment, two-stage, dose-finding study evaluating onaBoNT-A admixed with the TC-3 hydrogel (NCT03320850). The onaBoNT-A doses evaluated are 100 U, 300 U, 400 U, and 500 U. The primary outcome measurement is the change from baseline at week 12 in the average number of UUIEs per day as measures in a 3-day bladder diary. The results of this trial are forthcoming.

FUTURE RESEARCH AND CONCLUSION

The use of intradetrusor onaBoNT-A has expanded greatly in clinical practice; however, larger, multicenter trials would continue to improve our understanding and likely be more representative of the general population. Furthermore, more direct head-to-head comparisons would greatly improve our understanding of advanced OAB therapies like intradetrusor onaBoNT-A. In addition, better standardizing the definition of PVR that necessitates the initiation of CIC would allow better comparisons between studies. Furthermore, there is a need to develop alternative methods for delivering onaBoNT-A. As clinical use and understanding expands, the hope would be to change payer limitations requiring diagnosis of refractory OAB (failed first- and second-line treatments) to access onaBoNT-A, thereby allowing faster access to benefitting populations.

References

1. Santos-Silva A, da Silva CM, Cruz F. Botulinum toxin treatment for bladder dysfunction. *Int J Urol* 2013;20:956–962.
2. van Ermengem E. A new anaerobic bacillus and its relation to botulism. *Rev Infect Dis* 1979;1(4):701–719.
3. Schurch B, Schmid D, Stohrer M, et al. Treatment of neurogenic incontinence with botulinum toxin. *N Engl J Med* 2000;342(9):665.
4. Ginsberg D, Gousse A, Keppenne V, et al. Phase 3 efficacy and tolerability study of onabotulinumtoxinA for urinary incontinence from neurogenic detrusor overactivity. *J Urol* 2012;187(6):2131–2139.
5. Cruz F, Herschorn S, Aliotta P, et al. Efficacy and safety of onabotulinumtoxinA in patients with urinary incontinence due to neurogenic detrusor overactivity: A randomized, double-blind, placebo controlled trial. *Eur Urol* 2011;60(4):742–750.
6. Nitti VW, Dmochowski R, Herschorn S, et al. OnabotulinumtoxinA for the treatment of patients with overactive bladder and urinary incontinence: Results of a phase 3, randomized, placebo controlled trial. *J Urol* 2013;189(6):2186–2193.
7. Chapple C, Sievert K-D, MacDiarmid S, et al. OnabotulinumtoxinA 100 U significantly improves all idiopathic overactive bladder symptoms and quality of life in patients with overactive bladder and urinary incontinence: A randomized, double-blind, placebo-controlled trial. *Eur Urol* 2013;64(2):249–256.
8. Haylen BT, De Ridder D, Freeman RM, et al. An International Urogynecological Association (IUGA)/International Continence Society (ICS) joint report on the terminology for female pelvic floor dysfunction. *Neurourol Urodyn* 2010;29(1):4–20.
9. Gormley EA, Lightner DJ, Burgio KL, et al. Diagnosis and treatment of overactive bladder (non-neurogenic) in adults: AUA/SUFU guideline. *J Urol* 2012;188(6 Suppl):2455–2463.
10. Chancellor MB, Fowler CJ, Apostolidis A, et al. Drug insight: Biological effects of botulinum toxin A in the lower urinary tract. *Nat Clin Pract Urol* 2008;5:319–328.
11. Abeywickrama L, Arunkalaivanan A, Quinlan M. Repeated botulinum toxin type A (Dysport®) injections for women with intractable detrusor overactivity: A prospective outcome study. *Int Urogynecol J Pelvic Floor Dysfunct* 2014;25(5):601–605.
12. Ravindra P, Jackson BL, Parkinson RJ. Botulinum toxin type A for the treatment of non-neurogenic overactive bladder: Does using onabotulinumtoxinA (Botox®) or abobotulinumtoxinA (Dysport®) make a difference? *BJU Int* 2013;112(1):94–99.
13. Flint R, Rantell A, Cardozo L. AbobotulinumtoxinA for the treatment of overactive bladder. *Expert Opin Biol Ther* 2018;18(10):1005–1013.
14. Apostolidis A, Dasgupta P, Fowler CJ. Proposed mechanism for the efficacy of injected botulinum toxin in the treatment of human detrusor overactivity. *Eur Urol* 2006;49(4):644–650.
15. Hegele A, Frohme C, Varga Z, et al. Antibodies after botulinum toxin A injection into musculus detrusor vesicae: Incidence and clinical relevance. *Urol Int* 2011;87(4):439–444.
16. Amundsen CL, Richter HE, Menefee SA, et al; for the Pelvic Floor Disorders Network. OnabotulinumtoxinA vs sacral neuromodulation on refractory urgency urinary incontinence in women. A randomized clinical trial. *JAMA* 2016;316(13):1366–1374.
17. Houman J, Moradzadeh A, Patel DN, et al. What is the ideal antibiotic prophylaxis for intravesically administered Botox injection? A comparison of two different regimens. *Int Urogynecol J* 2019;30(5):701–704.
18. Sievert KD, Chapple C, Herschorn S, et al. OnabotulinumtoxinA 100U provides significant improvements in overactive bladder symptoms in patients with urinary incontinence regardless of the number of anticholinergic therapies used or reason for inadequate management of overactive bladder. *Int J Clin Pract* 2014;68(10):1246–1256.
19. Amundsen CL, Komesu YM, Chermansky C, et al; for the Pelvic Floor Disorders Network. Two-year outcomes of sacral neuromodulation versus onabotulinumtoxinA for refractory urgency urinary incontinence: A randomized trial. *Eur Urol* 2018;74(1):66–73.
20. Dmochowski R, Chapple C, Nitti VW, et al. Efficacy and safety of onabotulinumtoxinA for idiopathic overactive bladder: A double-blind, placebo controlled, randomized, dose ranging trial. *J Urol* 2010;184(6):2416–2422.
21. Fowler CJ, Auerbach S, Ginsberg D, et al. OnabotulinumtoxinA improves health-related quality of life in patients with urinary incontinence due to idiopathic overactive bladder: A 36-week, double-blind, placebo-controlled, randomized, dose-ranging trial. *Eur Urol* 2012;62(1):148–157.
22. Rovner E, Kennelly M, Schulte-Baukloh H, et al. Urodynamic results and clinical outcomes with intradetrusor injections of onabotulinumtoxinA in a randomized, placebo-controlled dose-finding study in idiopathic overactive bladder. *Neurourol Urodyn* 2011;30(4):556–562.

23. Denys P, Le Normand L, Ghout I, et al. Efficacy and safety of low doses of onabotulinumtoxinA for the treatment of refractory idiopathic overactive bladder: A multicentre, double-blind, randomised, placebo-controlled dose-ranging study. *Eur Urol* 2012;61(3):520–529.

24. Cohen BL, Barboglio P, Rodriguez D, et al. Preliminary results of a dose-finding study for botulinum toxin-A in patients with idiopathic overactive bladder: 100 versus 150 units. *Neurourol Urodyn* 2009;28(3):205–208.

25. de Sá Dantas Bezerra D, de Toledo LGM, da Silva Carramão S, et al. A prospective randomized clinical trial comparing two doses of abobotulinumtoxinA for idiopathic overactive bladder. *Neurourol Urodyn* 2019;38(2):660–667.

26. Kuo H-C. Bladder base/trigone injection is safe and as effective as bladder body injection of onabotulinumtoxinA for idiopathic detrusor overactivity refractory to antimuscarinics. *Neurourol Urodyn* 2011;30(7):1242–1248.

27. Jo JK, Kim KN, Kim DW, et al. The effect of onabotulinumtoxinA according to site of injection in patients with overactive bladder: A systematic review and meta-analysis. *World J Urol* 2018;36(2):305–317.

28. Manecksha RP, Cullen IM, Ahmad S, et al. Prospective randomised controlled trial comparing trigone-sparing versus trigone-including intradetrusor injection of abobotulinumtoxinA for refractory idiopathic detrusor overactivity. *Eur Urol* 2012;61(5):928–935.

29. Rapp DE, Lucioni A, Bales GT. Botulinum toxin injection: A review of injection principles and protocols. *Int Braz J Urol* 2007;33(2):132–141.

30. Liao C-H, Chen S-F, Kuo H-C. Different number of intravesical onabotulinumtoxinA injections for patients with refractory detrusor overactivity do not affect treatment outcome: A prospective randomized comparative study. *Neurourol Urodyn* 2016;35(6):717–723.

31. MacDiarmid S, Glazier D, Shapiro A, et al. Treatment of overactive bladder with a peritrigonal injection paradigm of onabotulinumtoxinA is associated with a low incidence of clean intermittent catheterization. *Neurourol Urodyn* 2019;38(Suppl 3):S123–S124.

32. Nitti VW, Ginsberg D, Sievert K-D, et al; for the 191622-096 Investigators. Durable efficacy and safety of long-term onabotulinumtoxinA treatment in patients with overactive bladder syndrome: Final results of a 3.5-year study. *J Urol* 2016;196(3):791–800.

33. Owen RK, Abrams KR, Mayne C, et al. Patient factors associated with onabotulinum toxin A treatment outcome in women with detrusor overactivity. *Neurourol Urodyn* 2017;36(2):426–431.

34. Tincello DG, Kenyon S, Abrams KR, et al. Botulinum toxin a versus placebo for refractory detrusor overactivity in women: A randomised blinded placebo-controlled trial of 240 women (the RELAX study). *Eur Urol* 2012;62(3):507–514.

35. Liao C-H, Kuo H-C. Increased risk of large post-void residual urine and decreased long-term success rate after intravesical onabotulinumtoxinA injection for refractory idiopathic detrusor overactivity. *J Urol* 2013;189(5):1804–1810.

36. Wang C-C, Liao C-H, Kuo H-C. Diabetes mellitus does not affect the efficacy and safety of intravesical onabotulinumtoxinA injection in patients with refractory detrusor overactivity. *Neurourol Urodyn* 2014;33(8):1235–1239.

37. Sahai A, Khan MS, Le Gall N, et al. Urodynamic assessment of poor responders after botulinum toxin-A treatment for overactive bladder. *Urology* 2008;71(3):455–459.

38. Richter HE, Amundsen CL, Erickson SW, et al. Characteristics associated with treatment response and satisfaction in women undergoing onabotulinumtoxinA and sacral neuromodulation for refractory urgency urinary incontinence. *J Urol* 2017;198(4):890–896.

39. Dowson C, Watkins J, Khan MS, et al. Repeated botulinum toxin type A injections for refractory overactive bladder: Medium-term outcomes, safety profile, and discontinuation rates. *Eur Urol* 2012;61(4):834–839.

40. Craciun M, Irwin PP. Outcomes for intravesical abobotulinumtoxin A (Dysport) treatment in the active management of overactive bladder symptoms—A prospective study. *Urology* 2019;130(4):54–58.

41. Visco AG, Brubaker L, Richter HE, et al; for the Pelvic Floor Disorders Network. Anticholinergic therapy vs. onabotulinumtoxinA for urgency urinary incontinence. *N Engl J Med* 2012;367(19):1803–1813.

42. Nabi G, Cody JD, Ellis G, et al. Anticholinergic drugs versus placebo for overactive bladder syndrome in adults. *Cochrane Database Syst Rev* 2006;(4):CD003781.

43. Drake MJ, Nitti VW, Ginsberg DA, et al. Comparative assessment of the efficacy of onabotulinumtoxinA and oral therapies (anticholinergics and mirabegron) for overactive bladder: A systematic review and network meta-analysis. *BJU Int* 2017;120(5):611–622.

44. Harvie HS, Amundsen CL, Neuwahl SJ, et al. Cost-effectiveness of sacral neuromodulation versus onabotulinumtoxinA for refractory urgency urinary incontinence: Results of the ROSETTA randomized trial. *J Urol* 2020;203(5):969–977.

45. Sherif H, Khalil M, Omar R. Management of refractory idiopathic overactive bladder: Intradetrusor injection of botulinum toxin type A versus posterior tibial nerve stimulation. *Can J Urol* 2017;24(3):8838–8846.

46. Chuang YC, Kaufmann JH, Chancellor DD, et al. Bladder instillation of liposome encapsulated onabotulinumtoxinA improves overactive bladder symptoms: A prospective, multicenter, double-blind, randomized trial. *J Urol* 2014;192(6):1743–1749.

47. Krhut J, Navratilova M, Sykora R, et al. Intravesical instillation of onabotulinum toxin A embedded in inert hydrogel in the treatment of idiopathic overactive bladder: A double-blind randomized pilot study. *Scand J Urol* 2016;50(3):200–205.

CHAPTER 34

RECOGNITION AND MANAGEMENT OF GENITOURINARY FISTULA

Jeffrey L. Cornella

Introduction

This chapter discusses recognition and management of postsurgical fistulas in the developed world. Genitourinary fistulas in the developed world are primarily postsurgical, although the tenets of repair are also applicable for operative obstetrical injury. There is a separate chapter in this textbook which addresses extensive field-effect fistula secondary to prolonged obstructed obstetrical labor.

ANATOMIC CONSIDERATIONS

It is imperative that surgeons have a thorough understanding and appreciation of pelvic anatomy in order to reduce genitourinary injury. Anatomic relationships of the ureter, bladder, and urethra have been further elucidated in recent studies.[1,2] Avoidance of fistulas following gynecologic surgery requires strict attention to tissue planes, hemostasis, tissue vascularization, and appropriate use of instruments.

RISK FACTORS AND RECOGNITION

The risks for genitourinary fistula are affected by the radicality and route of surgery. Hilton and Cromwell[3] reported on the risks of vesicovaginal fistula following hysterectomy in a National Health Service cohort study. The highest rate occurred in patients undergoing surgery for cervical cancer, and the lowest incidence was found in patients undergoing vaginal prolapse surgery. In 286,053 women undergoing benign hysterectomy, 339 fistulas were later identified (0.12%). The risk for vesicovaginal fistula following vaginal prolapse surgery was estimated to be 1 in 3,861 (0.02%).

A 2019 California population-based cohort study assessing fistula after hysterectomy for benign indications reviewed 296,130 patients.[4] A total of 5,455 (1.80%) patients experienced at least one genitourinary injury. There were 2,817 (1.0%) ureteral injuries, 2,058 (0.7%) bladder injuries, and 834 (0.3%) patients developed subsequent genitourinary fistulas. The number of genitourinary injuries recognized during surgery was 4,701 (86.2%), and the number of unrecognized injuries was 754 (13.8%). In the injury cohort, 174 women (3.2%) sustained a complex injury involving both the bladder and ureter. These combined injuries had a rate of fistula formation which was 2 times higher compared to single-site injury patients, even with immediate identification. The risk of fistula occurrence was 9 times higher if recognition of complex injury was not immediate (2.7% vs. 25.0%). The overall risk for developing a fistula in the total injury cohort despite immediate recognition and repair was 9.5%.

Repairing a recognized ureteral injury or cystotomy must be done in a way to optimize healing and reduce the risk of a subsequent fistula. Principles of assuring adequate blood supply, suture lines without tension, catheter drainage, and tissue interposition are important in minimizing the risk of fistula. In a study of recognized incidental cystotomy at the time of benign hysterectomy, 11.7% developed a subsequent fistula.[5]

There is a significant difference in morbidity when comparing recognized and unrecognized genitourinary injuries at the time of surgery. A National Surgical Quality Improvement Program (NSQIP)-based study reviewed the incidence and risk factors for genitourinary injury recognized in the postoperative period following hysterectomy for benign indications.[6] The study assessed 45,139 patients undergoing benign hysterectomy with an incidence of lower urinary tract complication at 0.2%. The unrecognized ureteral obstruction rate was 0.1% with 0.07% of patients developing a ureteral fistula and 0.6% experiencing a bladder fistula. Unrecognized ureteral obstruction has significant morbidity and requirements for additional hospitalization and surgery. A review of patients with recognized and unrecognized ureteral injury was reported in a study using a California inpatient database reviewing patients with ureteral injuries following hysterectomy.[7] The study identified 1,753 ureteral injuries in 223,872 patients following hysterectomy, with a delayed recognition rate of 62.4% (1,094 patients). The unrecognized injuries increased the risk of acute renal insufficiency (aOR 23.8, 95% confidence interval [CI] 20.1 to 28.2) and death (a1.4, 95% CI 1.03 to 1.9, $P = .0032$).

Unrecognized bladder injury during hysterectomy frequently occurs during the dissection of the bladder base from the underlying vagina and cervix. This dissection should always be done sharply, with attention paid to the lateral bladder pillars and fine-tissue visual characteristics. Several centimeters of endopelvic fascial dissection prior to vaginal incision allow separation of tissue planes for subsequent cuff closure. If bladder wall thinning is observed, it should be reinforced by fine-gauge, delayed absorbable interrupted sutures with attention to any vascular compromise. A three-way Foley catheter can allow bladder filling during surgical dissection to assist in recognition of boundaries.

The ureters should be identified throughout their course during abdominal and laparoscopic surgery and assessed during vaginal surgery. It is incumbent on the surgeon to carefully examine all tissues and structures at the termination of the procedure to rule out any unrecognized injury. This would include use of cystoscopy to assess bladder integrity and bilateral efflux of urine at the termination of the procedure.[8]

Additional detail on avoidance of injury at pelvic surgery can be found in Chapter 28 of this textbook.

CLINICAL RECOGNITION (VIDEOS 34.1 TO 34.3)

A high index of suspicion is required for recognition of delayed bladder and ureteral injuries. The postoperative patient who presents with fluid leaking per vagina warrants careful clinical assessment. This includes a thorough history and physical examination. A fistula may present days or weeks following a pelvic surgery. Late presentations are often related to delayed necrosis of tissues.

Patients with urinary incontinence have episodes of leakage between longer dry periods. Patients who have a fistula may experience almost constant drips of urine depending on body position. The vast majority of postsurgical fistulas are supratrigonal in location. The cuff should carefully be examined to rule out fluid coming from the peritoneum or bladder. Simple filling of the bladder in the office with repeat inspection of the vagina may show influx of fluid into the vagina along the cuff. The tampon test of Moir can often identify small pinpoint fistulas after placement of dye within the bladder fluid. Three gauze pledgets are placed into the vagina with subsequent placement of dyed saline into the bladder. The patient is asked to stand, cough, walk, and void prior to pledget removal. The pledget closest to the introitus will be stained from voiding. If the upper portion of the second pledget or the third pledget is stained, a fistula should be suspected. A ureterovaginal fistula will not show coloration unless dye was given intravenously or if the patient had previously received oral phenazopyridine. A computed tomography (CT) urogram or other imaging is mandatory to rule out ureteral or complex fistula (concomitant ureteral and bladder fistulas) in all patients requiring repair. A concomitant ureteral injury may be present in up to 12% of cases of vesicovaginal fistula.[9] If a ureteral fistula is suspected, a retrograde pyelogram is beneficial for localization.

Some patients with vesicovaginal fistulas may have a negative CT urogram in the supine position but immediately leak urine via the fistula when standing. Cystoscopies can also fail to show an overt fistula if scarring and/or inflammation is present. This further illustrates the importance of a detailed history and high index of suspicion, as some patients have received unnecessary incontinence operations in the presence of an occult fistula.

MANAGEMENT PRINCIPLES

The most important features of fistula management involve careful evaluation and assessment of the entire clinical picture prior to surgery. This includes careful assessment of tissue integrity, status of the ureters, bladder characteristics, and urethral sphincteric function. History should include past issues relative to the bladder and social considerations. The surgeon should be cognizant of overall bladder capacity, vaginal limitations, tissue inflammation, sphincteric function, presence of multiple fistulae, and ureteral integrity prior to planning the operative approach. The surgeon can then make thoughtful decisions regarding timing and route of surgery.

There is an ongoing debate regarding the timing of fistula repair following surgical injury. This is reflective of the body's tendency to create deleterious inflammation following surgery. Early recognition of injury allows early repair (either at the time of surgery or within several days following operation). Patients who present greater than 10 days following injury should have assessment of the fistula by cystoscopy to determine the size and degree of reactive inflammation, swelling, and absence of infection. Historically, if significant inflammation is noted, recommendations have been to delay surgery for a period of 2 to 3 months from the original operative insult in order to allow resolution of inflammation and improve healing of suture lines. There are articles in the literature advocating early repair of posthysterectomy fistulas no matter the time of discovery. The vast majority of these articles employ an abdominal or transvesical approach with larger excision of surrounding tissue.[9] Those who advocate early repair of post-obstetrical fistulas in the developing world use a vaginal approach.[10]

The surgical goal is healing of the fistula with optimal subsequent bladder function. In order to reduce the risk of persistent fistula, surgical principles of precise sharp tissue dissection, observation of vascularity, avoidance of tension along suture lines, watertight closure, placement of an interposition flap, and postoperative drainage are followed.

The length of postoperative bladder drainage may depend on characteristics of the fistula and surrounding tissue. A suprapubic catheter placed for duration of 2 weeks, followed by a cystogram prior to removal, is a reasonable clinical approach. There are ongoing studies assessing optimal length of postoperative bladder drainage in large obstetrical fistulas secondary to tissue necrosis.[11]

Studies assessing use of interposition flaps have shown mixed results depending on the type of fistula and causation. It is clinically recommended to protect suture lines with an interposition flap because it is not time-consuming relative to the patient's bother and may decrease the risk of persistent fistula. It should always be recognized that an interposition flap will not compensate for an inadequate bladder closure. Omental and Martius flaps can be useful when increased blood supply is beneficial for tissue healing.[12]

A systematic review and meta-analysis in the management of the vesicovaginal fistulas following benign gynecologic surgery was reported in 2017.[13] Following review, 124 articles were included for assessment involving 1,379 patients. The fistula closure rate in this group was 97.98%. The transvaginal approach was performed in the majority of patients (39%), followed by the transabdominal/transvesical route (36%), and a laparoscopic/robotic approach (15%). Prolonged catheter drainage was initially used in 239 patients, with 19 (8%) achieving success without surgery. The remainder of patients not responding to conservative catheter drainage underwent surgical repair.

An analysis of fistula characteristics, treatments, and complications of surgical repair were reported using the American College of Surgeons (ACS) NSQIP database. Two hundred patients were reported of which 65% were repaired vaginally. Compared to the vaginal approach, the abdominal approach had higher overall morbidity (22% vs. 7%, $P = .017$); longer hospital stay; and were more likely to be associated with sepsis, blood transfusion, and readmission.[14] This difference in morbidity may be reduced in the future secondary to minimally invasive surgery and limitations of dissection, including unnecessary bivalving of the bladder.

OPERATIVE APPROACHES

Cystotomy Repair

The first tenet of repairing an incidental cystotomy at the time of surgery is recognition of the injury. Therefore, the bladder should be carefully examined at the termination of surgery including by cystoscopy. The majority of incidental cystotomies are in a supratrigonal location. A recognized cystotomy has a risk of future fistula development and must be carefully repaired at the time of surgery, including placement of a peritoneal or other tissue graft for interposition. In a multicenter study of 5,698 hysterectomies performed for benign disease, 102 (1.8%) patients sustained cystotomies with 6 (5.9%) developing a vesicovaginal fistula.[15] A cystotomy which involves the urethra is at a greater risk for development of subsequent fistula and requires special considerations and a longer term of catheter drainage.[5] The risks of urethral injury are further illustrated by acute trauma patients with bladder outlet injury.[16] These injuries have increased risks of bladder-related complications despite immediate repair. The surgeon must perform careful closure with the consideration of providing increased blood supply with a concomitant Martius flap. An intraoperative consultation with a urologist for shared management should be considered.

Cystotomies in a dependent location of the bladder or at an intraperitoneal location require a double- or triple-layer closure with interrupted fine-gauge, delayed absorbable sutures (Figs. 34.1 and 34.2). A watertight closure is confirmed by filling the bladder and observing for any loss of fluid. This is followed by an interposition flap. A cystoscopy at the termination of the procedure confirms bilateral efflux of urine and allows visualization of the suture line prior to catheter drainage. A follow-up cystogram at the time of catheter removal is recommended.

Vaginal Approach to Fistula Repair

The majority of fistulas can be repaired vaginally. This has been demonstrated both in developed and nondeveloped countries.[17] It has been demonstrated over a range of fistula severity. The benefits include a high fistula closure rate and lower rates of complications compared with traditional abdominal approaches.

Adequate vaginal retraction and visualization is highly important and can be achieved with modern lighting sources and self-retaining retractors (e.g., the Magrina-Bookwalter vaginal retractor). Cystoscopy precedes incision with placement of a #8 French Foley catheter from the vagina through the fistula into the bladder. The distances to the course of the ureters are assessed. Stents are usually not required in the absence of ureteral involvement.

FIGURE 34.1 A cystotomy is created in the muscularis of the bladder during hysterectomy. Sharp dissection in the proper plane reduces the incidence of such injury. (Reprinted from Lee RA. *Atlas of gynecologic surgery*. Philadelphia: W.B. Saunders, 1992. Copyright © 1992, with permission from Elsevier.)

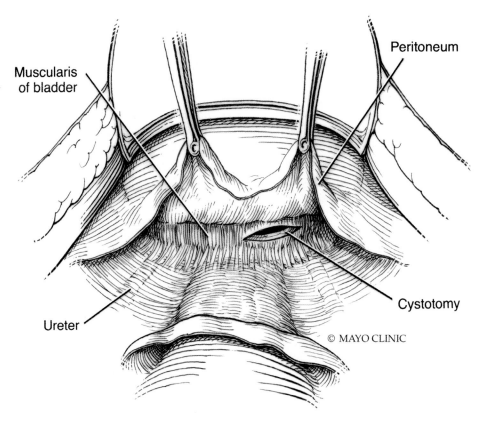

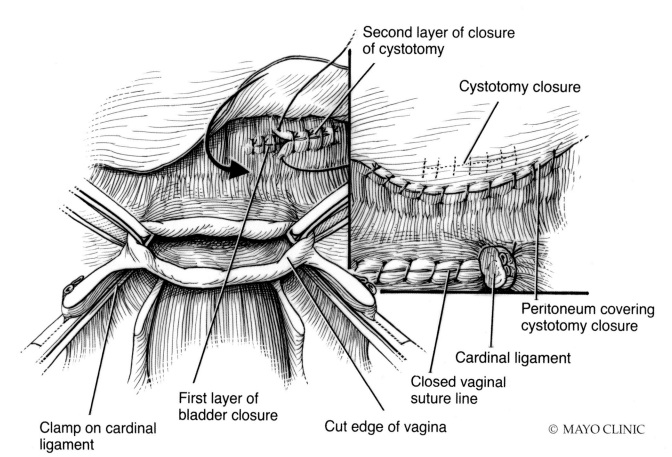

FIGURE 34.2 A peritoneal interposition flap is used over a double-layer closure of the bladder muscularis. (Reprinted from Lee RA. *Atlas of gynecologic surgery*. Philadelphia: W.B. Saunders, 1992. Copyright © 1992, with permission from Elsevier.)

The standard flap-splitting repair of the supratrigonal fistula involves making a circular incision around the fistula tract (Fig. 34.3). This is extended to a transverse vaginal incision with separation of the bladder from the vagina (Fig. 34.4). The small catheter facilitates subsequent dissection of tissue planes and eventual removal of any scar tissue surrounding the fistula. Tissue planes are developed allowing sufficient mobility for subsequent tension-free closure of the bladder and vagina. Following complete hemostasis, a circular incision is made around the fistula scar which is removed along with the #8 French Foley catheter (Fig. 34.5). The initial

suture line consists of 3-0 delayed absorbable suture placed in an extramucosal fashion and extending beyond the opening by 3 to 4 mm (Fig. 34.6). A secondary interrupted suture line is placed in a similar fashion involving the bladder muscularis (Fig. 34.7). A 2-0 delayed absorbable suture is used for this imbricating layer. The bladder is filled with sterile milk or saline dyed with methylene blue and tested for watertight status. An interposition flap is then placed using either peritoneum or a Martius flap (Fig. 34.8). The vagina is then closed in a transverse fashion followed by bladder catheter drainage (Fig. 34.9).

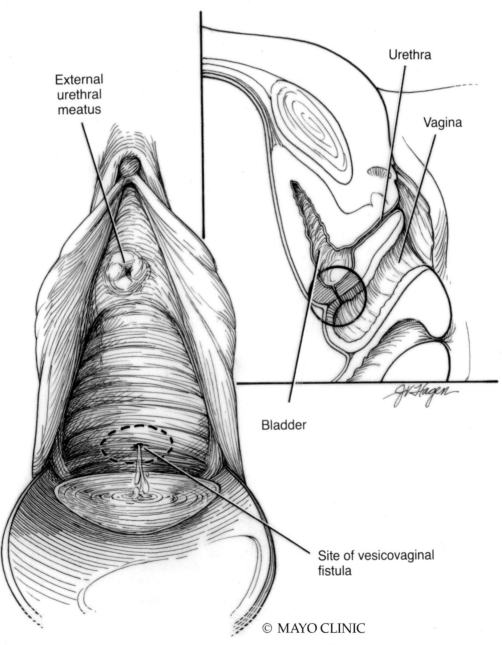

External urethral meatus

Urethra

Vagina

Bladder

Site of vesicovaginal fistula

© MAYO CLINIC

FIGURE 34.3 Fistulas occurring after hysterectomy are usually in a supratrigonal location along the vaginal cuff. A small Foley catheter placed through the fistula can facilitate dissection. (Reprinted from Lee RA. *Atlas of gynecologic surgery.* Philadelphia: W.B. Saunders, 1992. Copyright © 1992, with permission from Elsevier.)

FIGURE 34.4 A flap-splitting dissection results in mobilization of tissues and decreased tension on subsequent suture lines. (Reprinted from Lee RA. *Atlas of gynecologic surgery*. Philadelphia: W.B. Saunders, 1992. Copyright © 1992, with permission from Elsevier.)

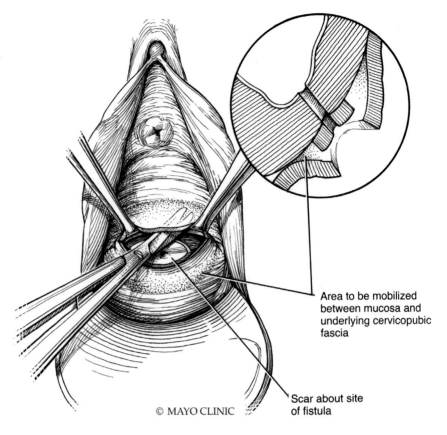

Area to be mobilized between mucosa and underlying cervicopubic fascia

Scar about site of fistula

© MAYO CLINIC

FIGURE 34.5 Following complete dissection of tissue planes, a sharp incision is made around the fistula scar with its subsequent removal. (Reprinted from Lee RA. *Atlas of gynecologic surgery*. Philadelphia: W.B. Saunders, 1992. Copyright © 1992, with permission from Elsevier.)

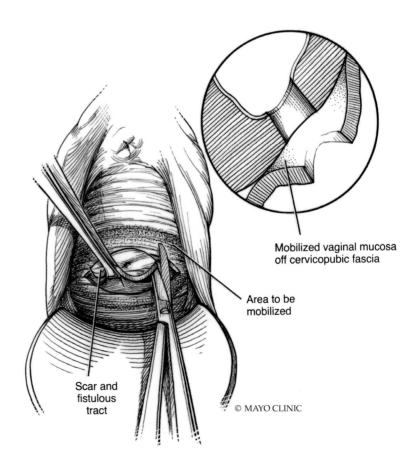

Mobilized vaginal mucosa off cervicopubic fascia

Area to be mobilized

Scar and fistulous tract

© MAYO CLINIC

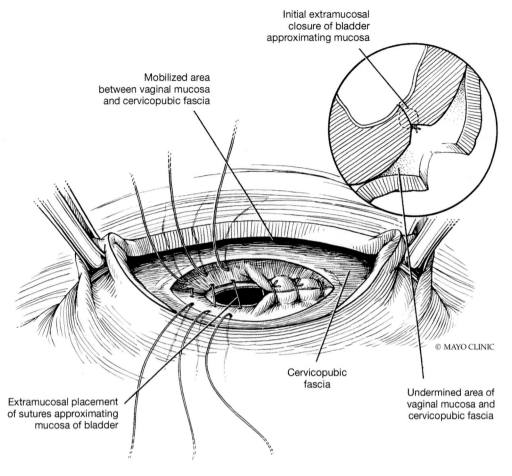

Initial extramucosal
closure of bladder
approximating mucosa

Mobilized area
between vaginal mucosa
and cervicopubic fascia

Cervicopubic
fascia

Undermined area of
vaginal mucosa and
cervicopubic fascia

Extramucosal placement
of sutures approximating
mucosa of bladder

© MAYO CLINIC

FIGURE 34.6 The initial suture line consists of interrupted, 3-0 delayed absorbable suture placed in an extramucosal fashion. (Reprinted from Lee RA. *Atlas of gynecologic surgery*. Philadelphia: W.B. Saunders, 1992. Copyright © 1992, with permission from Elsevier.)

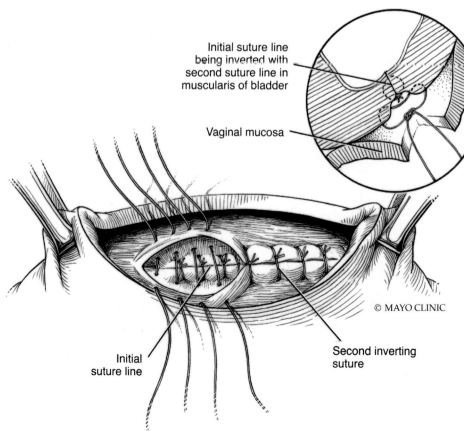

Initial suture line
being inverted with
second suture line in
muscularis of bladder

Vaginal mucosa

Initial
suture line

Second inverting
suture

© MAYO CLINIC

FIGURE 34.7 A second suture line of interrupted, 2-0 delayed absorbable suture imbricates the first suture line completing a watertight closure. (Reprinted from Lee RA. *Atlas of gynecologic surgery*. Philadelphia: W.B. Saunders, 1992. Copyright © 1992, with permission from Elsevier.)

FIGURE 34.8 An interposition flap is placed after testing for watertight closure. This usually consists of peritoneum, although other types of interposition flaps may be used. (Reprinted from Lee RA. *Atlas of gynecologic surgery.* Philadelphia: W.B. Saunders, 1992. Copyright © 1992, with permission from Elsevier.)

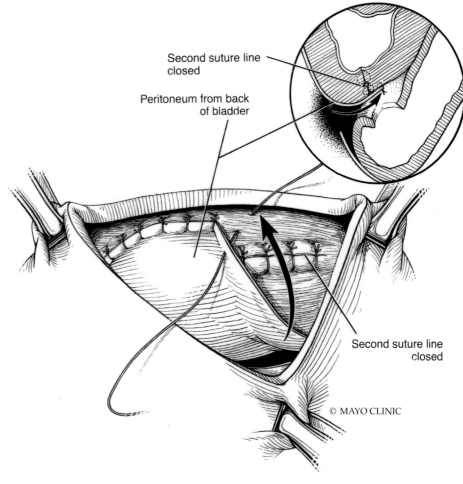

FIGURE 34.9 The vagina is closed in a transverse fashion. A catheter is then placed for sustained drainage. (Reprinted from Lee RA. *Atlas of gynecologic surgery.* Philadelphia: W.B. Saunders, 1992. Copyright © 1992, with permission from Elsevier.)

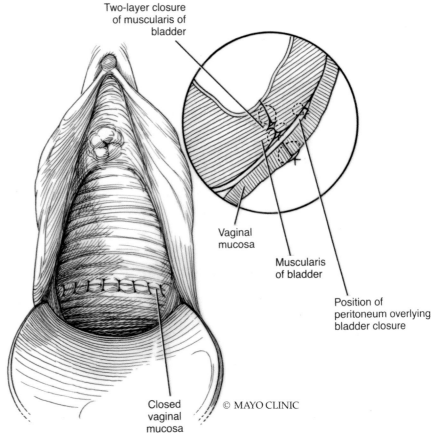

Abdominal Approach to Fistula Repair

Historically, the vaginal approach to fistula repair was joined by abdominal routes of surgery as the sciences of anesthesia and germ theory were developed. The techniques developed in the 19th century continued into the 21st century. It is only in the first two decades of the 21st century that minimally invasive surgery allowed modification of these techniques to decrease morbidity.

It benefits any fistula surgeon to review the historical development of fistula repair by surgeons such as Dittel, Forgue, Legueu, Mackenrodt, Lambelle, Trendelenburg, Roonhuysen, and others. Suffice it to say, the classic abdominal approach used in the United States for decades was developed in Europe. O'Conor and Sokol[18] popularized techniques already described as the Dittel-Forgue-Legueu operation which involved bivalving the bladder, separating the vagina from bladder, removal of the fistula, closure of the vagina, placement of an interposition flap, and closure of the bladder. It has been demonstrated over time that bivalving the bladder significantly increases morbidity.

The abdominal route of surgery was often chosen by surgeons unfamiliar with vaginal techniques and approaches. Reasons for an abdominal approach to fistula repair may include vaginal scarification, complex fistulas involving the ureter, history of irradiation, the multiple-operated fistula, the presence of persistent bladder inflammation, or other factors prohibiting a vaginal approach.

The classic abdominal technique opens the dome of the bladder and the incision is extended in the midline to the fistula (Fig. 34.10). Ureteral stents may be placed through the incision. The bladder is dissected from the vagina surrounding the fistula and scar tissue is removed. The vagina is then closed with 0-gauge delayed absorbable suture (Fig. 34.11). The bladder is then closed in an extramucosal fashion using an initial air of 3-0 gauge delayed absorbable suture. This is followed by a secondary imbricating layer of interrupted 2-0 gauge delayed absorbable suture (Fig. 34.12). The peritoneum or omentum is used as an interposition flap (Fig. 34.13). A suprapubic Foley catheter may be placed.

Laparoscopic and Robotic Approaches to Fistula Repair (Videos 34.4 and 34.5)

Morbidity related to the classic abdominal approach can be reduced with technique modifications and minimally invasive surgery.[19] The primary difference in

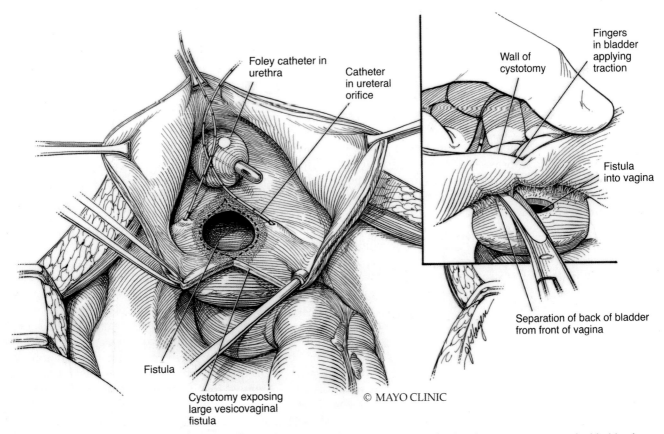

Foley catheter in urethra

Catheter in ureteral orifice

Wall of cystotomy

Fingers in bladder applying traction

Fistula into vagina

Separation of back of bladder from front of vagina

Fistula

Cystotomy exposing large vesicovaginal fistula

© MAYO CLINIC

FIGURE 34.10 A bladder incision exposes the fistula. The fistula scar is removed, and further dissection separates the bladder from the vagina allowing the establishment of wide tissue planes. (Reprinted from Lee RA. *Atlas of gynecologic surgery.* Philadelphia: W.B. Saunders, 1992. Copyright © 1992, with permission from Elsevier.)

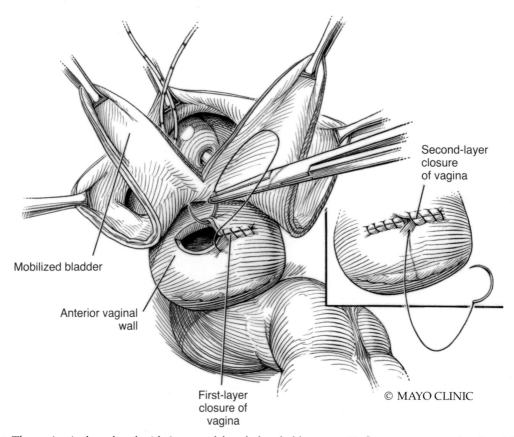

Second-layer
closure
of vagina

Mobilized bladder

Anterior vaginal
wall

First-layer
closure of
vagina

© MAYO CLINIC

FIGURE 34.11 The vagina is then closed with 0-gauge delayed absorbable suture. Tacking sutures may be placed for subsequent connection to an interposition flap. (Reprinted from Lee RA. *Atlas of gynecologic surgery*. Philadelphia: W.B. Saunders, 1992. Copyright © 1992, with permission from Elsevier.)

technique is to avoid bivalving the bladder and simply separate the bladder and vagina along a broad tissue plane with identification of the openings into the bladder and vagina.[20] The bladder opening may have its edges freshened to improve healing, but the overall size of the opening is not extended. Cystoscopy and examination of the bladder interior via the laparoscope allows continued identification of the ureters. A systematic review comparing classic abdominal fistula repair to minimally invasive repair showed similar cure rates.[21]

The technique of laparoscopic or robotic vesicovaginal fistula repair begins with cystoscopy and vaginal examination. A #8 French Foley catheter is placed from the vagina into the bladder via the fistula. A suprapubic catheter is placed into the dome of the bladder under direct cystoscopic vision and is plugged. A three-way Foley catheter is placed within the bladder to allow bladder filling at the time of abdominal surgery to assist with initial identification of bladder and vaginal tissue planes. The distance between the fistula and the ureters is observed, and ureteral stenting may be considered in a low percentage of cases.

Following establishment of pneumoperitoneum, the courses of the ureters are examined. A Lucite rod or vaginal probe is placed into the vagina, and bladder filling may be considered with the three-way Foley catheter. Fistulas following hysterectomy may have resulted in effects on cuff healing secondary to constant drainage and inflammation. The cuff may easily separate, and this facilitates further dissection of the vagina from the bladder. If the cuff remains closed, the surgeon dissects the bladder from the vagina in a wide plane until the fistula and small catheter are encountered. Further dissection of the bladder from the vagina follows to allow optimal subsequent closure of each of the two structures. During dissection, the small Foley catheter may be removed from the bladder and any scar surrounding the fistula resected. A balloon may be placed in the vagina to maintain pneumoperitoneum. The inside of the bladder and ureteral orifices can be examined through the small opening by gentle traction on the opening. The vagina is closed with delayed absorbable suture in a longitudinal direction. The bladder is then closed transversely in two layers. A 3-0 Vicryl may be used in interrupted fashion on the first

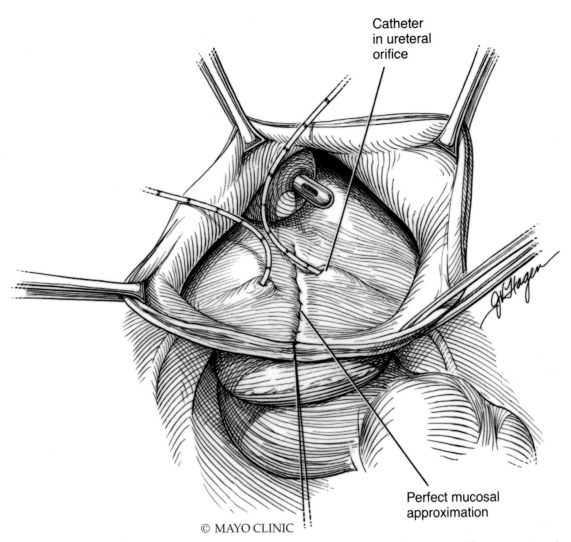

Catheter
in ureteral
orifice

Perfect mucosal
approximation

© MAYO CLINIC

FIGURE 34.12 The bladder is closed in an extramucosal fashion and the stents removed. (Reprinted from Lee RA. *Atlas of gynecologic surgery*. Philadelphia: W.B. Saunders, 1992. Copyright © 1992, with permission from Elsevier.)

layer followed by an imbricating layer of interrupted 2-0 Vicryl. The bladder is then filled with the three-way Foley catheter to assess for a watertight closure. A cystoscopy is performed to examine internal suture lines and to confirm bilateral efflux of urine following bladder closure. An interposition flap is then placed either consisting of peritoneum, omentum, or less commonly sigmoid epiploica. An omental flap may be facilitated at the time of trocar entry by assessing or creating the required tissue length for later placement.

Future primary vesicovaginal fistula repairs in developed countries will most likely be accomplished by either a vaginal or a laparoscopic/robotic approach. The former classic method of abdominal fistula repair through an open incision should be limited, unless extenuating factors are present. This will decrease the morbidity of surgical fistula repair. If a complex fistula involving a ureter is present, this can also be

accomplished robotically. This may include robotic ureteroneocystostomy with a psoas hitch depending on the extent and location of the ureteral injury.[22]

Intravesical Vesicovaginal Fistula Repair

A laparoscopic approach via the dome of the bladder with carbon dioxide bladder distension has been reported in the literature by case reports.[23] The technique is feasible but may not reduce morbidity in comparison to robotic approaches, especially when an interposition flap is desired.[24]

Transvaginal Repair of Vesicovaginal Fistula by Latzko Technique

The procedure known as the Latzko repair also has a long history going back to the work of Gustav Simon in 1854, followed by Sir Henry Collis describing a

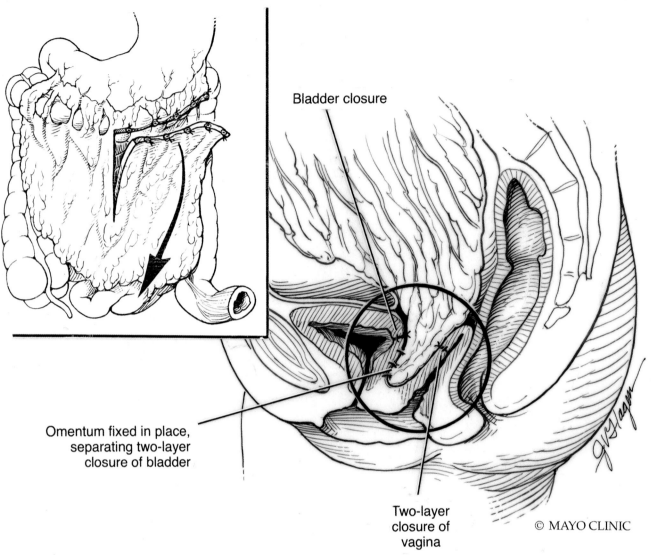

FIGURE 34.13 Omentum is interposed between the bladder and vagina protecting the suture lines and increasing blood supply. (Reprinted from Lee RA. *Atlas of gynecologic surgery*. Philadelphia: W.B. Saunders, 1992. Copyright © 1992, with permission from Elsevier.)

layered closure technique in 1861. This procedure involves a limited colpocleisis by denuding the vaginal mucosa surrounding the fistula. The endopelvic fascia (vaginal wall minus mucosa) and mucosa are closed in separate layers. This results in some shortening of the vagina in comparison to the flap-splitting technique. The technique is often used in small noncomplicated fistulas. Fewer papers have been written on this technique following the year 2006, although it continues to be taught and used by some institutions.[25]

Ureterovaginal Fistula

The etiology of ureterovaginal fistula is most commonly related to gynecologic or urologic surgery in developed countries. This differs from developing countries where causation more commonly relates to cesarean

procedures, including cesarean hysterectomy. A 2012 cohort of 17 cases of ureterovaginal fistula in Pakistan reported 10 (58.8%) following hysterectomy and 7 (41.1%) following cesarean section.[26]

Current management of isolated ureterovaginal fistulas involves stenting and endourology, which is preferred over reimplantation.[27] This may include ureteroscopic stenting which may be successful in a majority of patients. The ureteroscope overcomes inherent angulation and allows passage of a guidewire for subsequent stent placement. Unsuccessful stenting may relate to severe angulation of the ureter relative to the bladder and may require antegrade techniques.

A study from Loyola University in Chicago described the experience of 18 patients with posthysterectomy ureterovaginal fistula.[28] An additional patient experienced the ureterovaginal fistula following a cesarean section. Ureteral stenting was successful in 11 (92%) of 12 patients. Reimplantation was required in 6 cases with 1 additional patient experiencing spontaneous resolution. Conservative management was successful in 10 (83%) of 12 cases.

Patients with concomitant vesicovaginal and ureterovaginal fistula will require repair of the bladder. A retrograde urogram should be accomplished early for ureteral stenting and planning for subsequent surgery. Healing of the ureterovaginal component may occur, and if a ureteral stricture is absent, it may be possible to repair the vesicovaginal fistula separately without ureteral reimplantation.

In a London database review of 116 patients referred for management of vesicovaginal fistula, 4 (3.4%) had associated ureteric injury.[29] The patients were managed by concomitant ureteral reimplantation at the time of vesicovaginal fistula repair.

Vesicouterine Fistula

Vesicouterine fistula is fairly rare and requires a high index of suspicion, as there may be a delayed diagnosis. The majority of vesicouterine fistulas relate to cesarean section (83% to 93%).[30] The tract runs between the posterior bladder and cesarean section scar and may be lined by endometrial cells.[31] Less common causes include obstructed labor, vaginal birth after cesarean, endometriosis, foreign devices, uterine artery embolization, and injury from operative delivery.[32] Symptoms may include menouria, urinary incontinence, cyclic hematuria, and possibly amenorrhea. A constellation of these symptoms including apparent amenorrhea is known as Youssef syndrome.

The diagnosis may be made by hysterosalpingogram, magnetic resonance imaging, cystogram, or intravesical contrast-enhanced ultrasound.[33] A Scandinavian cohort was reported with 22 cases, all of which followed cesarean section.[30] Total incontinence was noted in 7 women, 15 patients had occasional leakage, and cyclic hematuria was noted in 17. The operative approach included a circumferential incision around the fistula with excision of the tract and separate closure of the bladder and uterus. The omentum was used for interposition. Only 1 patient required hysterectomy which was for dysfunctional uterine bleeding. The authors stated that the fistula repairs were successful in all patients.

The vesicouterine fistula is best repaired using a minimally invasive approach via laparoscopy or robotics.[32]

PREDICTORS OF RECURRENCE

A multicountry prospective cohort study assessing factors related to fistula outcome showed that prognosis for fistula closure is related to preoperative bladder size,

previous unsuccessful repair, vaginal scarring, and urethral involvement.[17] Surgical outcomes in developing countries relate to multiple factors including fistula location, degree of scarification, presence of a circumferential fistula, overall bladder capacity, prior attempt at fistula repair, and urethral damage.[34] In general, greater tissue damage and complexity trend toward persistent morbidities and mixed outcomes. Further studies are needed assessing these factors for persistent fistula risk in developed countries.[35]

There have been several classification systems for genitourinary fistula.[36] The purpose is to identify patients who are at a risk for persistent vesicovaginal fistula and allow academic comparison of surgical outcomes. The classification systems have been used primarily in developing countries which relates to the prevalence of large fistulas with surrounding tissue damage seen in prolonged obstructed delivery. Factors which affect the risk of persistent fistula include the number of fistulas present, the involved anatomic structures, the presence of inflammation, size of the fistula, amount of scarring or tissue deficit, relationship to the ureters, and any field-effect damage. The prognostic values of existing classification systems have been limited.[37] There is currently no accepted standardized classification for fistula in the developing world.[38]

CONCLUSION

It is incumbent on the gynecologic surgeon to have an extensive knowledge of anatomy, surgical principles, and techniques which reduce the risk of genitourinary injury. Vital structures should be identified and mobilized away from the area of extirpative dissection. If injuries occur, they should be recognized at the time of surgery to reduce morbidity and mortality. Surgical repair of fistula should consider the entire patient, including social considerations, nutrition, and factors which increase successful healing and outcomes. A minimally invasive approach to fistula following established tenets of repair including tension-free suture lines, hemostasis, and interposition placement can be successfully accomplished, decreasing morbidity.

References

1. Jackson LA, Ramirez DMO, Carrick KS, et al. Gross and histologic anatomy of the pelvic ureter: Clinical applications to pelvic surgery. *Obstet Gynecol* 2019;133(5):896–904.
2. Rahn DD, Bleich AT, Wai CY, et al. Anatomic relationships of the distal third of the pelvic ureter, trigone, and urethra in unembalmed female cadavers. *Am J Obstet Gynecol* 2007;197(6):668.e1–668.e4.
3. Hilton P, Cromwell DA. The risk of vesicovaginal and urethrovaginal fistula after hysterectomy performed in the English National Health Service—a retrospective cohort study examining patterns of care between 2000 and 2008. *BJOG* 2012;119(12):1447–1454.

4. Dallas KB, Rogo-Gupta L, Elliott CS. Urologic injury and fistula after hysterectomy for benign indications. *Obstet Gynecol* 2019;134(2):241–249.

5. Duong TH, Gellasch TL, Adam RA. Risk factors for the development of vesicovaginal fistula after incidental cystotomy at the time of a benign hysterectomy. *Am J Obstet Gynecol* 2009;201(5):512.e1–512.e4.

6. Bretschneider CE, Casas-Puig V, Sheyn D, et al. Delayed recognition of lower urinary tract injuries following hysterectomy for benign indications: A NSQIP-based study. *Am J Obstet Gynecol* 2019;221(2):132.e1–132.e13.

7. Blackwell RH, Kirshenbaum EJ, Shah AS, et al. Complications of recognized and unrecognized iatrogenic ureteral injury at time of hysterectomy: A population based analysis. *J Urol* 2018;199(6):1540–1545.

8. Ibeanu OA, Chesson RR, Echols KT, et al. Urinary tract injury during hysterectomy based on universal cystoscopy. *Obstet Gynecol* 2009;113(1):6–10.

9. Moses RA, Gormley EA. State of the art for treatment of vesicovaginal fistula. *Curr Urol Rep* 2017;18(8):60.

10. Pope R, Beddow M. A review of surgical procedures to repair obstetric fistula. *Int J Gynaecol Obstet* 2020;148(Suppl 1):22–26.

11. Barone MA, Widmer M, Arrowsmith S, et al. Breakdown of simple female genital fistula repair after 7 day versus 14 day postoperative bladder catheterisation: A randomised, controlled, open-label, non-inferiority trial. *Lancet* 2015;386(9988):56–62.

12. Malde S, Spilotros M, Wilson A, et al. The uses and outcomes of the Martius fat pad in female urology. *World J Urol* 2017;35(3):473–478.

13. Bodner-Adler B, Hanzal E, Pablik E, et al. Management of vesicovaginal fistulas (VVFs) in women following benign gynaecologic surgery: A systematic review and meta-analysis. *PLoS One* 2017;12(2):e0171554.

14. Theofanides MC, Sui W, Sebesta EM, et al. Vesicovaginal fistulas in the developed world: An analysis of disease characteristics, treatments, and complications of surgical repair using the ACS-NSQIP database. *Neurourol Urodyn* 2017;36(6):1622–1628.

15. Duong TH, Taylor DP, Meeks GR. A multicenter study of vesicovaginal fistula following incidental cystotomy during benign hysterectomies. *Int Urogynecol J* 2011;22(8):975–979.

16. Anderson RE, Keihani S, Moses RA, et al. Current management of extraperitoneal bladder injuries: Results from the Multi-Institutional Genito-Urinary Trauma Study (MiGUTS). *J Urol* 2020;204(3):538–544.

17. Barone MA, Frajzyngier V, Ruminjo J, et al. Determinants of postoperative outcomes of female genital fistula repair surgery. *Obstet Gynecol* 2012;120(3):524–531.

18. O'Conor VJ, Sokol JK. Vesicovaginal fistula from the standpoint of the urologist. *J Urol* 1951;66(4):579–585.

19. Agrawal V, Kucherov V, Bendana E, et al. Robot-assisted laparoscopic repair of vesicovaginal fistula: A single-center experience. *Urology* 2015;86(2):276–281.

20. Schimpf MO, Morgenstern JH, Tulikangas PK, et al. Vesicovaginal fistula repair without intentional cystotomy using the laparoscopic robotic approach: A case report. *JSLS* 2007;11(3):378–380.

21. Miklos JR, Moore RD, Chinthakanan O. Laparoscopic and robotic-assisted vesicovaginal fistula repair: A systematic review of the literature. *J Minim Invasive Gynecol* 2015;22(5):727–736.

22. Laungani R, Patil N, Krane LS, et al. Robotic-assisted ureterovaginal fistula repair: Report of efficacy and feasibility. *J Laparoendosc Adv Surg Tech A* 2008;18(5):731–734.

23. Liu S, Ye H, Li Q, et al. Intravesical laparoscopic repair of vesicovaginal fistula. *Beijing da Xue Xue Bao Yi Xue Ban* 2010;42(4):458–460.

24. Grange P, Shakir F, Thiagamoorthy G, et al. Combined laparoscopic, vesicoscopic, and vaginal repair of a vesicovaginal fistula. *J Minim Invasive Gynecol* 2016;23(6):859–860.

25. Ansquer Y, Mellier G, Santulli P, et al. Latzko operation for vault vesicovaginal fistula. *Acta Obstet Gynecol Scand* 2006;85(10):1248–1251.

26. Murtaza B, Mahmood A, Niaz WA, et al. Ureterovaginal fistula—etiological factors and outcome. *J Pak Med Assoc* 2012;62(10):999–1003.

27. Rajamaheswari N, Chhikara AB, Seethalakshmi K. Management of ureterovaginal fistulae: An audit. *Int Urogynecol J* 2013;24(6):959–962.

28. Chen Y, Wolff BJ, Kenton KS, et al. Approach to ureterovaginal fistula: Examining 13 years of experience. *Female Pelvic Med Reconstr Surg* 2019;25(2):e7–e11.

29. Seth J, Kiosoglous A, Pakzad M, et al. Incidence, type and management of ureteric injury associated with vesicovaginal fistulas: Report of a series from a specialized center. *Int J Urol* 2019;26(7):717–723.

30. Ali-El-Dein B, El-Tabey N, El-Hefnawy A, et al. Diagnosis, treatment and need for hysterectomy in management of postcaesarean section vesicouterine fistula. *Scand J Urol* 2014;48(5):460–465.

31. Jóźwik M, Jóźwik M, Kozłowski R, et al. Structural arrangement of vesicouterine fistula revisited: An immunohistochemical study documenting the presence of the endometrium. *J Obstet Gynaecol Res* 2018;44(2):341–346.

32. Perveen K, Gupta R, Al-Badr A, et al. Robot-assisted laparoscopic repair of rare post-cesarean section vesicocervical and vesicouterine fistula: A case series of a novel technique. *Urology* 2012;80(2):477–482.

33. Sun F, Cui L, Zhang L, et al. Intravesical contrast-enhanced ultrasound (CEUS) for the diagnosis of vesicouterine fistula (VUF): A case report. *Medicine (Baltimore)* 2018;97(17):e0478.

34. Arrowsmith SD, Barone MA, Ruminjo J. Outcomes in obstetric fistula care: A literature review. *Curr Opin Obstet Gynecol* 2013;25(5):399–403.

35. Beardmore-Gray A, Pakzad M, Hamid R, et al. Does the Goh classification predict the outcome of vesico-vaginal fistula repair in the developed world? *Int Urogynecol J* 2017;28(6):937–940.

36. Lee D, Zimmern P. Vaginal approach to vesicovaginal fistula. *Urol Clin North Am* 2019;46(1):123–133.

37. Frajzyngier V, Li G, Larson E, et al. Development and comparison of prognostic scoring systems for surgical closure of genitourinary fistula. *Am J Obstet Gynecol* 2013;208(2):112.e1–112.e11.

38. Pope R. Research in obstetric fistula: Addressing gaps and unmet needs. *Obstet Gynecol* 2018;131(5):863–870.

CHAPTER 35

COMPLEX OBSTETRICAL FISTULA

Steven D. Arrowsmith

Introduction

In the realm of pelvic reconstructive surgery, perhaps the most daunting challenge could be that of the obstetric fistula. In its full-blown form, this entity has virtually and thankfully disappeared from wealthy nations. However, because fistulas do occur from after a variety of injuries (trauma, surgical misadventure, and radiation) in developed countries,[1] it is useful to consider principles developed to deal with obstetric fistula, which can still be seen in high volume in endemic areas, and apply the lessons learned to injuries that might be less complex. The subject matter deserves an entire textbook of its own, and so this, overview can only hope to outline some of the challenges complex fistula presents.

One of the unfortunate realities of fistula care has been, because the vast majority of complex fistula care has been delivered in some of the most resource-challenged areas on earth, quality clinical data collection is one victim of the impoverished context. Many of the assertions presented here would be widely agreed on within the fistula community, but a robust evidence base, although finally starting to accrue, is still essentially lacking.

Fistulas seen in wealthy nations tend to be iatrogenic, resulting from the unintentional, direct cutting of pelvic structures, or devascularization of pelvic structures via ischemia resulting from ligature, indiscrete clamping, or overexuberant cautery. In nonobstetric fistula, these insults are generally limited to an area a few millimeters in size. With untreated obstructed labor, wide areas of pelvic tissue are subject to unrelenting pressure from the presenting fetal part, resulting in the compromise of arterial inflow and finally the ischemic loss of regions, and not small foci, of pelvic tissue. The only equivalent in Western medicine may be fistulas resulting from radiation therapy, especially early in the development in this technology, which caused vascular compromise to wide areas in the pelvis. It is the etiology of obstetric fistula that renders these injuries so severe and so varied. In obstetric fistula, much of the bladder, all of the urethra, the anterior rectum, the cervix, and much of the vagina may simply be lost.

Thankfully, large strides have been made in the prevention of obstetric fistula through the push toward improved access to emergency obstetric services addressed by strategies like the Millennium Development Goals and Sustainable Development Goals.[2] These efforts have significantly impacted rates of maternal mortality and morbidity, and after many millennia of despair, the number of obstetric fistula cases may finally be trending downward.

DEFINITION

Surgeons attempting fistula repair often refer to "simple," "moderate," and "complex" fistulas. Although there seems to be an unspoken understanding of what roughly comprises each category, there has never been an accepted definition to exactly delineate the boundaries between these categories. For example, some would argue that the size of the defect is an important distinctive of complex fistulas; yet, there are many difficult small fistulas and simple large ones. In 2013 to 2014, a large multicenter prospective clinical trial was organized to study the need for long-duration catheterization after fistula repair.[3] It was agreed that, for the sake of consistency of data, the study would be limited to women with simple fistula. Several group exercises were carried out in which a range of fistula surgeons were presented with a series of drawings depicting a wide range of fistula cases and then surveyed as to the consistency that the labels of "simple," "moderate," and "complex" agreed across the group. It was apparent that although there was good agreement on the characteristics of a simple fistula, there was far less consistency reporting of injuries felt to be moderate versus complex.

The "classic" simple fistula is a case where the defect is small, the location of the fistula and caliber of the vagina are such that the defect can be easily approached during repair, and vital structures like the urethra and it's continence mechanism or ureters are not involved. Conversely, a complex fistula might be associated with a scarred vagina making surgical exposure challenging. Involvement of the bladder neck and urethra make the functional repair of the damage far more challenging. In the most severe cases, enough bladder can be lost to require augmentation or urinary diversion. The concomitant presence of rectovaginal fistula from ischemia directed posteriorly threatens successful repair because of the constant contamination with fecal flora. Involvement of the ureters might require an abdominal approach and formal ureteral reimplantation. The sad fact is that, in obstetric fistula at least, if the ischemia has been widespread enough in the pelvis to produce any one of the injuries, then some or all of the others may occur as well. So perhaps the most significant distinctive of complex fistula repair is the tendency of never-ending combinations of injury to present all at once.[4] Complex cases may require a staged approach or multiple attempts at repair, and some would argue that a history of previous repair would move an individual case into a complex category.

HISTORY

Fistula can be documented back to more than 4,000 years ago, as an Egyptian mummy, thought to possibly be that of a wife of a Pharaoh, was noted to have a complex fistula.[5] The basic techniques of fistula repair began to be published in the mid-1800s, and from beginning, it was necessary to address approaches to complex injuries. Indeed, a surgical text in 1846 describes the use of an island flap in fistula repair,[6] perhaps one of the earliest examples of the use of this tool from the armamentarium of plastic surgery. Therefore, complex fistula might rightfully be thought of as a major driving force in modern surgical innovation.

PRESENTATION

In terms of the symptoms a patient may describe, vesicovaginal fistula presents with total urinary incontinence. Generally, there is no difference in the degree of urinary leakage between women with simple fistulas and those whose injuries are more complex. It is astounding to see that a tiny pinhole fistula can destroy quality of life just as effectively as a massive complex fistula.

Women with complex fistula are more likely to present with symptoms and quality of life impacts arising from the presence of comorbidities that are not so commonly seen in association with a simple fistula.[4] In addition to urinary incontinence, women suffering complex fistula may present with fecal incontinence from concomitant rectovaginal fistula, impairment of sexual function because of vaginal stenosis, and foot drop resulting from peripheral nerve damage during prolonged labor. Other issues related to severe, complex fistula may not appear until after an initial procedure to close the fistula. Once the defect has been dealt with and continuity of the urinary tract restored, it is only then that the woman may display post-repair incontinence because of damage to the continence mechanism

and urethra or debilitating urinary frequency from loss of bladder tissue resulting in reduced bladder capacity. The cause for these ongoing symptoms is present at presentation but not expressed until the patient resumes function of the lower urinary tract.

EVALUATION

The initial physical examination in women with fistula should be focused on delineating as completely as possible the extent of injury, all with the intent of planning the best approach to repair.

Factors to be evaluated include the following:

- **The condition of the vagina:** Is there any compromise in vaginal depth or caliber from ischemic injury? In complex fistula, dense bands of scar may traverse the vagina, especially posteriorly at the junction of the proximal one-third and distal two-thirds of the vagina.
- **The status of the urethra.** Has it been spared injury? Partially damaged? Completely destroyed? The urethral length should be measured. This is most easily accomplished by inserting a bladder catheter and noting the distance between the inflated balloon and the urethral meatus. Is the urethra scarred and stiff? In complex fistula, it is not unusual to encounter urethral stricture while attempting passage of the catheter.
- **Status of the bladder:** Does there appear to be significant loss of bladder storage capacity? By definition, the bladder is unable to store urine with a fistula present, so it is not possible to determine bladder capacity with bedside or formal urodynamic studies. Likewise, a cystoscopy is generally unfeasible as the bladder cannot retain any irrigating fluid.
  - In very large fistulas, it is not unusual for prolapse of the dome of the bladder to occur. This is not to be confused with classic prolapse of the bladder, where the anterior vaginal wall loses support and the bladder base and vesicourethral junction descend. Instead, the bladder can simply evert via the fistula defect. While distressing in appearance, this finding is generally associated with an abundance of bladder tissue which has survived the initial trauma.
  - It may be possible to easily note and record the location of the ureteral orifices as urine "jets" into the bladder. The more complex the fistula, the more derangement of local anatomy occurs, and the possibility of injuring the distal ureters increases.
- **Status of the upper urinary tract:** In high-resource settings, it is preferable to image the kidneys and ureters with ultrasound. This may reveal hydronephrosis from a ureteric injury or compromise of

renal cortical thickness from renal failure in long-term fistula patients. In poor nations, imaging may be entirely unavailable, and ureteric injury can only be implied when a dye test shows that the bladder can retain saline tinged with a vital dye and, with the bladder filled, the leakage into the vagina is clear.

- **Overall medical status of the patient:** Complex fistulas tend to occur after complex trauma. Especially with women in the developing world with complex fistula, it is very common for nutritional compromise, anemia, varying degrees of renal failure, and other challenges to her general health. Because fistula repair is elective surgery, these issues must be identified and corrected as far as possible before repair is attempted.

MANAGEMENT

Cancer care over just the past few decades has seen a rapid recognition and implementation of a team approach to each individual patient so that anyone presenting for care might benefit from surgery, medical therapies, radiation treatments, newer immunotherapies, and now even gene therapy. It is recognized that no individual provider can possibly master all of these needed skill sets. In the same way a women suffering from complex fistula injuries might require surgeons with training and experience in plastic techniques such as complex skin flaps and grafts, urologic interventions for postrepair incontinence, complete urethral reconstruction, bladder augmentation, or urinary diversion; colorectal expertise for complicated rectovaginal fistula; or general surgery experience that might lead to skill in replacing an injured or destroyed vagina with a segment of bowel. Gynecologists offer the most expert insight into how these interventions can be fashioned in a way to preserve or restore sexual and reproductive function. It is only through high-volume exposure and years of experience that individual surgeons can begin to straddle the boundaries between these surgical disciplines and offer the range of skill sets that complex fistulas demand. If we continue to make strides in reducing the incidence of fistula as we strive toward eradication, we may become increasingly forced into a team paradigm for dealing with complex fistula.

Fistula Closure

For all vesicovaginal fistula repairs, the overall approach for many decades has been to employ aggressive dissection to separate bladder and vaginal tissue planes so that the tissue edges can be reapproximated with no tension. Generally speaking, this is also true in the repair of complex injuries. However, in complex fistula, the dissection often must be done either via a scarred and narrowed vagina, or by an abdominal approach, or even both. If performed vaginally, complex repairs can require relaxing incisions to allow access. Because these incisions are tailored to cut where the scar is the densest and most limiting, it is probably not appropriate to employ the term *episiotomy* in this particular setting. During dissection, normal tissue planes may be obliterated and anatomy, such as the location of the distal ureters, can be quite distorted. The tissue about the circumference of the defect may have lost pliability and vascular supply and therefore may have questionable viability as they are mobilized to span a fistula defect.

Because the most severe cases of fistula tend to occur in the world's poorest countries, technology such as laparoscopy equipment is very rarely available. And so, it is probably too soon for there to be a sufficient volume of accumulated clinical experience to assess whether or not a laparoscopic approach to truly complex fistula repair is useful when access vaginally is compromised.

Although far too early to assess on the grounds of large clinical studies, there is exciting hope that new science in tissue engineering[7] may provide a more robust menu of options with the degree of loss of bladder and vaginal tissue is severe.

Special Cases

One common variant of a complex vesicovaginal fistula is known as the "circumferential defect." For these unfortunate women, the ischemia of prolonged labor seems to be directed unrelentingly at the area of the vesicourethral junction. Continuity between the bladder and urethra is totally lost, and there may be a gap of several centimeters between the stump of the urethra and the remnant of the bladder base. Technically, a relatively new approach has gained wide acceptance among surgeons providing complex fistula care in which these fistula repairs are approached not as the closure of a discrete defect in the bladder but rather of the reanastomosis of the bladder to the urethra. Both the distal extent of the remaining tissue of the bladder base and the proximal urethra are mobilized until a full-circumference closure like that seen in repair of a ureteral defect or a small bowel closure. The reason that circumferential fistulas are dreaded is that it is easy to conceptualize that an injury of this extent in this anatomic location is bound to compromise the function of the "closing mechanism" responsible for urinary continence.

Ureteral Issues

In complex fistula, it is not at all uncommon to find the orifice of one or both ureters either within the edge of the fistula or retracted back away from the defect. There is not a large body of literature to direct a best approach to repair in these cases. Although some ureteral surgery for distal stone retrieval was performed via a vaginal approach in the pre-ureteroscopy era, formal reimplantation of the ureter into the bladder has been thought of as an abdominal surgery. Especially in the context of the scarring produced during the global ischemia of obstructed labor, mobilizing a ureter for a length sufficient to allow reimplantation is very difficult in complex fistula repair.

Incontinence after Repair

One extremely frustrating outcome of complex fistula repair, both for surgeon and patient, is the significant chance of urinary incontinence that becomes apparent once a fistula is closed and the lower urinary tract begins to function again. The reported incidence of post-repair incontinence in highly complex fistula varies widely in the available literature, but has been reported as potentially approaching 100%.[8]

As a urologist, the author would contend that fistula victims may have the most vexing and varied issues with urinary incontinence of any single group of patients. This issue has for decades been grossly mislabeled as "stress incontinence." This label has led to the treatment of women with interventions designed for stress urinary incontinence, which, in its pure form, only represents a small percentage of women who remain wet after fistula closure. Conceptually, women who have had untreated obstructed labor have pathophysiologic justification for nearly any type of incontinence. The fistula defect often incorporates the region of the bladder (the base, between the ureteral orifices) know to be the anatomic site of entry for some of the most important innervation to the bladder and to have the highest concentration of neuroreceptors. It is as if an attack had been made on the local "command center" for voiding and continence. Therefore, some women present with total incontinence from a wildly overactive bladder, whereas others present with overflow incontinence from bladder atony. Some have debilitating frequency and urgency because they have been left with a tiny storage capacity due to tremendous loss of bladder tissue. Some develop an overdistended bladder because they lose sensation telling them when to void. Some have total loss, either anatomically, physiologically, or both, of the contribution of the bladder neck and urethra to continence. Although a few exhibit the hypermobility of the bladder neck that is associated with standout stress urinary incontinence, complex fistula victims more generally have a lower urinary tract that is entombed in dense scar, leading not to hypermobility but rather to "hyperimmobility," preventing the normal pattern of bladder closure. Worst of all, any individual item on this "menu" of injury generally presents in combination with others, with endless variations and bizarre combinations of lower urinary tract dysfunction.

The result of this panoply of possibly pathologies means that fistula surgeons, working within the most resource-challenged facilities on earth, probably need full capability for urodynamic studies to sort out this diagnostic mess. Junior gynecologists with little or no exposure to complex continence care find themselves up against a scenario demanding skills in the most complex set of urologic skills. These patients may require familiarity with techniques of bowel-segment bladder augmentation, may need a full range of medications for continence, may benefit from state-of-the-art capability in physical therapy for continence care, and may be required to attempt suspension procedures like the pubovaginal sling in the presence of a pelvis frozen in scar. The dismal rates of the achievement of long-term continence in this group starkly outline the harm of the blanket diagnosis of "stress" and the mismatch between diagnosis and treatment that ensues.

Urethral Involvement

The group of women with direct injury to the urethra often find themselves in the "post-repair incontinence" group discussed earlier. Loss of the female urethra is an exceedingly unusual injury in Western practice, but may account for 5%[4] of women with complex fistula. Some women present with a flat plate of tissue where the urethra formerly resided, tissue that does not appear to be vaginal wall or scar, but rather pink-colored urethral epithelium. This appearance suggests that urethral tissue has been lost in the posterior midline, allowing the tubular urethra to splay itself open in to a two-dimensional flat structure. For this subgroup, it is possible to carefully dissect and mobilize the full thickness of this plate around a small catheter and reform a urethral tube, one that presumably contains the normal urethral urothelium and muscular layers. This maneuver is relatively quick and easy to accomplish and can result in a continent patient.

Far more difficult are the cases where the urethra is totally absent, leaving behind a layer of vaginal epithelium over the bony public arch. Obviously, this scenario calls for more advanced and complete reconstruction. Simply rolling vaginal epithelial tissue into a tube does not result in a functional urethra. One common choice here is the use of an anterior bladder wall flap popularized by fistula pioneer Dr. Tom Elkins (Fig. 35.1).[8] However, Dr. Elkins himself recommended that this procedure be combined with a pubovaginal sling, pointing to a high level of residual incontinence even when the neourethra is built of bladder musculature and lined with urothelium.

The Incurable Fistula

Herein lies yet another issue in basic nomenclature, as the inevitable question, in the absence of formal consensus on the definition of this term,[9] is "incurable for

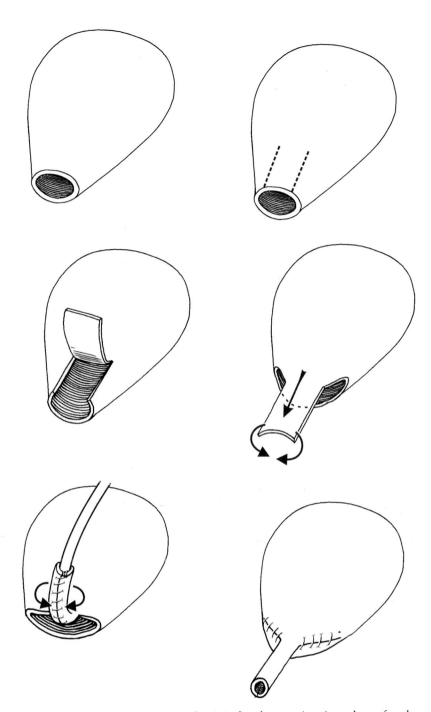

FIGURE 35.1 The Elkins neourethral reconstruction. In obstetric fistula, massive tissue loss often leaves the patient with no native tissue to repair. This technique takes a strip of anterior bladder wall tissue and rolls into a tube to act as the neourethra. The advantages over older approaches using skin flaps include the presence of transitional epithelium, similar muscular anatomy, and at least the possibility of some function for continence.

whom, where, and when?" Is the surgeon in possession of all of the clinical skills currently known for complex repair? Does the facility offer a full range of specialty care, physiotherapy, and necessary continence-related medications? Are there plans for an expert to visit in the near future? Complex fistula injuries, occurring in combination as they so often do, can easily sum up to a scenario where there is simply no reasonable hope of

restoring normal continence of urine and stool; normal sexual function; or the ability of the woman to become pregnant, carry a pregnancy to term, and deliver vaginally. A practical definition of the spectrum of injuries that lead to such a "hopeless" clinical state is critically important. Women with complex fistula are often desperate for help, often disempowered to challenge the suggestion of a zealous surgeon, and often ill-informed of reasonable expectations of a positive outcome. So, many with the most severe injuries wander over large geographic space seeking help. The author has seen a woman present for evaluation after 13 prior and failed attempts at repair. Not only do the chances of a positive outcome fall with each subsequent attempt, but also the odds of surgical harm accrue. Therefore, it is contingent on any provider dealing with complex fistula to have a full set of skills offered in a fully capable institution and to be willing, for the sake of the patient, to be honest and realistic in counseling women with injuries not amenable to surgery to say "no." In these cases, a full range of social interventions is needed to encourage and assist the woman with living and supporting herself in spite of her incontinence.

The line of last resort in surgical interventions in complex fistula is urinary diversion. This field has exploded over the past few decades from a place where originally the only option might have been ureterosigmoidostomy, a procedure with potentially life-threatening metabolic consequences, to a panoply of reconstructive options falling under the heading of "continent urinary diversion." There is an ever-growing experience[10–12] in the use of diversion in complex fistula. However, it can be difficult to choose appropriate candidates when one considers the life-long need for follow-up medical and surgical care after these procedures.[13,14]

FUTURE

There is an alarming trend that is changing the face of fistula care. Even in areas traditionally enduring a large incidence of obstetric fistula, there is a steep upward trend in the area of iatrogenic fistula. Although formal data are just beginning to be reported, fistula as a complication of pelvic surgery now makes up upward of 70% to 80% of incoming new cases in certain geographic areas. When technically compared with obstetric fistula, iatrogenic fistulas tend to be less demanding simply because most involve a discrete focal area of injury instead of a swatch of ischemic mayhem. However, iatrogenic injuries, most often associated with hysterectomy, tend to be "high" or at the proximal extent of the vagina, where visualization of the injury area can be difficult and surgical access awkward.

References

1. Hillary CJ, Osman NI, Hilton P, et al. The aetiology, treatment, and outcome of urogenital fistulae managed in well- and low-resourced countries: A systematic review. *Eur Urol* 2016;70(3):478–492.
2. United Nations General Assembly. Intensifying efforts to end obstetric fistula within a generation: Report of the Secretary-General. Published July 31, 2018. Accessed March 8, 2022. https://undocs.org/A/73/285.
3. Barone MA, Widmer M, Arrowsmith S, et al. Breakdown of simple female genital fistula repair after 7 day versus 14 day postoperative bladder catheterisation: A randomised, controlled, open-label, non-inferiority trial. *Lancet* 2015;386(9988):56–62.
4. Arrowsmith S, Hamlin EC, Wall L. Obstructed labor injury complex: Obstetric fistula formation and the multifaceted morbidity of maternal birth trauma in the developing world. *Obstet Gynecol Surv* 1996;51(9):568–574.
5. Zacharin RF. *Obstetric fistula*. New York: Springer Publishing, 1998.
6. Pancoast J. *A treatise operative surgery: Comprising a description of the various processes of the art, including all the new operations; exhibiting the state of surgical science in its present advanced condition.* Philadelphia: Carey and Hart, 1846.
7. Pope R, Wilkinson J. Surgical innovation for obstetric fistula patients. *BJOG* 2018;125(6):750.
8. Browning A. Prevention of residual urinary incontinence following successful repair of obstetric vesico-vaginal fistula using a fibro-muscular sling. *BJOG* 2004;111(4):357–361.
9. Elkins TE, Ghosh TS, Tagoe GA, et al. Transvaginal mobilization and utilization of the anterior bladder wall to repair vesicovaginal fistulas involving the urethra. *Obstet Gynecol* 1992;79(3):455–460.
10. Fistula Care, Harvard Humanitarian Initiative. *Meeting the needs of women with fistula deemed incurable: Creating a culture of possibility—Report of a consultative meeting, Harvard club, Boston: September 19–20, 2011.* New York: Fistula Care, 2012.
11. Kirschner CV, Lengmang S, Zhou Y, et al. Urinary diversion for patients with inoperable obstetric vesicovaginal fistula: The Jos, Nigeria experience. *Int Urogynecol J* 2016;27(6):865–870.
12. Morgan MA, Polan ML, Melecot HH, et al. Experience with a low-pressure colonic pouch (Mainz II) urinary diversion for irreparable vesicovaginal fistula and bladder extrophy in East Africa. *Int Urogynecol J Pelvic Floor Dysfunct* 2009;20(10):1163–1168.
13. Alemu MH. Mainz II pouch: Continent urinary diversion, for bladder extrophy epispadia complex and irreparable VVF: A 5 year comprehensive retrospective analysis. *Ethiop Med J* 2010;48(1):57–62.
14. Arrowsmith S. Urinary diversion in the vesico-vaginal fistula patient: General considerations regarding feasibility, safety, and follow-up. *Int J Gynaecol Obstet* 2007;99(Suppl 1):S65–S68.

CHAPTER 36

URETHRAL DIVERTICULUM

Nicola Dykes • Peter L. Dwyer

Introduction

Female urethral diverticulum (UD) was originally described more than 200 years ago by Hey.[1] It is a relatively uncommon condition with an estimated incidence of between 0.02% and 4.7%[2,3] and is thought to account for up to 1.4% of women presenting to urology services with incontinence.[2] This figure could be an underestimate due to the nonspecific plethora of symptoms that this condition may present with, the difficulties and delays in making a diagnosis due to a lack of awareness of the condition, and the potential for the condition to remain asymptomatic. A prevalence rate of 3% in an asymptomatic population was reported based on positive pressure urethrography in women being investigated for cervical cancer.[4] The median age at time of diagnosis or treatment is between 36 and 46 years.[5-9] A trend has been noted toward an increased rate of diagnosis over the last few decades,[3] presumably due to increased awareness and diagnosis of this condition rather than an increasing prevalence.

ANATOMY AND PATHOPHYSIOLOGY

The female urethra is a 4-cm-long tubular structure originating at the bladder neck and extending to the external urethral meatus. There are three distinct layers: the mucosal epithelium, the submucosal layer of elastic tissue which includes an extensive vascular network, and an outer muscular layer. The proximal third is lined by transitional epithelium and the distal two-thirds by stratified squamous epithelium (Fig. 36.1).[10,11] The anatomy of the paraurethral ducts has been described by Huffman[12] in detail, with variable numbers of paraurethral ducts terminating in tubular glands (Fig. 36.2), which exist over the entire length of the urethra posterolaterally and secrete mucous material that provide urethral lubrication. They are most prominent over the distal two-thirds, with the majority of the glands draining into the distal third of the urethra.[13]

A UD is commonly described as a benign, sac-like protrusion from the urethra with a surface lining that is continuous with the epithelial lumen of the urethra.[14,15]

However, there has been considerable variability of definitions used in the literature given the pathologic terms "diverticulum," which implies the presence of all layers of the urethra including muscle, and "pseudodiverticulum," which denotes the absence of at least one layer.[16] This latter term more closely approximates the true histology of UD, with muscle tissue not being identified as a component of the diverticular wall on histopathology.[16] Histologic examination of the epithelium of UD has identified the same findings as those seen in paraurethral cysts, with predominant cell types of squamous (42%), columnar (32%), combined squamous and columnar, and cuboidal.[16]

Given the indistinguishable histology of UD and paraurethral cysts,[16] and with the dorsolateral anatomical position of the paraurethral glands in relation to the urethra also correlating with the location of two-thirds of UD,[17] a common origin is implicated and is in keeping with the most widely accepted hypothesis for UD development which is that of an acquired condition. The most common cause for UD is thought to be from infection of the periurethral glands, which can lead to obstruction and subsequent abscess formation as first described by Routh[18] in 1890. When the abscess ruptures into the urethral lumen, it creates a fistulous connection with subsequent epithelialization of the tract. However, the causation of UD can be multifactorial with the final position and appearance of the diverticulum varying with its etiology. The urethral orifice may be midline or mediolateral and vary in size and position (Fig. 36.3), entering the proximal, mid, or distal urethra which can influence symptoms. Purulent material may be expressed on urethral compression (Fig. 36.4).

Alongside infection, other causes of acquired UD have been described, including trauma due to urethral surgery such as urethrovaginal fistula repair (Fig. 36.5), these UD are usually open and shallow as a result of a muscular defect in the posterior urethral wall. Other causes such as vaginal birth, urethral catheterization, urethral dilatation, and urethrotomy[14,19] have also been reported. Previous synthetic midurethral sling has also been described as a possible aetiologic factor.[19,20] More recently, another etiology has been proposed for

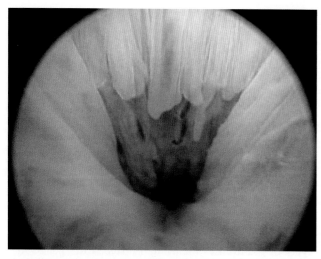

FIGURE 36.1 Urethroscopy of keratinized stratified squamous epithelium changing to nonkeratinized stratified squamous and then transitional epithelium in the urethra. (Reproduced from Dwyer PL, ed. *Atlas of urogynecological endoscopy.* London: Informa, 2007. © Informa UK, 2007, reproduced by arrangement with Taylor & Francis Group.)

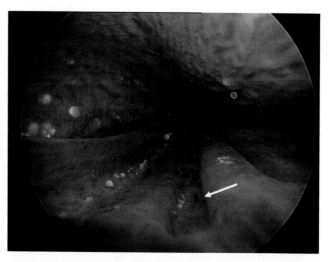

FIGURE 36.3 Small midline posterior UD orifice. (Reproduced from Dwyer PL, ed. *Atlas of urogynecological endoscopy.* London: Informa, 2007. © Informa UK, 2007, reproduced by arrangement with Taylor & Francis Group.)

development of proximal to midurethral UD, that of high pressure within the proximal urethra during voiding due to a high-tone nonrelaxing sphincter.[21]

Congenital UD has been described but is rare[22]; however, it is important as can often be associated with other congenital urogenital abnormalities including persistence of Gartner duct with ectopic ureters (Figs. 36.6, 36.7, and 36.8).[23] Possible etiologies proposed

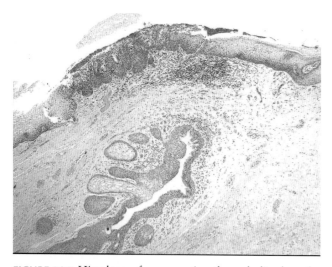

FIGURE 36.2 Histology of cross-section through distal uretha showing mucinous paraurethral glands that open into the urethra. The keratinized stratified squamous epithelium of the distal urethra changes to nonkeratinized stratified squamous epithelium seen above these glands more proximally. (Reproduced from Dwyer PL, ed. *Atlas of urogynecological endoscopy.* London: Informa, 2007. © Informa UK, 2007, reproduced by arrangement with Taylor & Francis Group.)

are congenital dilatations of the paraurethral cysts or glands, faulty union of urogenital sinus folds, cloacogenic rests during development, or Mullerian duct cysts.[14,17]

A cyst or abscess of Skene gland and duct will also present as a paraurethral mass of the distal urethra with discharge and can be easily confused with UD. Although initially described by Skene[24] in 1880, their function is still not well understood. Wernert et al.[25] described the Skene gland as a group of glands arranged in long distal structures situated in the caudal two-thirds of the urethra, mainly in the dorsal and lateral mucosal stroma but extending in some cases to the smooth musculature of the septum urethrovaginale. They are tubuloalveolar formations on long ductal structures and resemble male prostate glands prior to puberty and androgenic stimulation and contain prostate-specific antigen and prostatic acid phosphatase on immunostaining. Controversy exists regarding the function of these glands: whether simply an embryologic remnant in the female or whether they have a role in sexual arousal and the ejaculation of lubricating fluid with orgasm[26] similar to the male prostate gland. Moalem and Reidenberg[27] have suggested that gland secretions may have antimicrobial qualities and protect from urinary tract infections.

Skene cysts of the gland or duct are found lateral to the distal urethra and external urethral meatus and when infection occurs can cause pain, dysuria, vaginal discharge, and dyspareunia. On examination, a palpable painful mass is present and purulent material can be expressed from the ductal orifice (Figs. 36.9 and 36.10A,B). The difference between a UD and a Skene cyst is the duct of the Skene cyst exits laterally and inferiorly

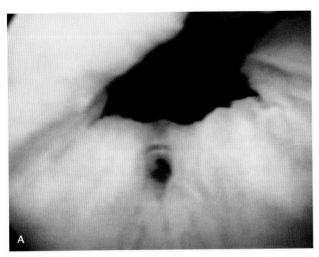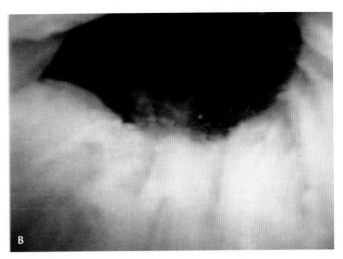

FIGURE 36.4 **A,B:** Purulent material expressed from the UD orifice on urethral compression. (Reproduced from Dwyer PL, ed. *Atlas of urogynecological endoscopy.* London: Informa, 2007. © Informa UK, 2007, reproduced by arrangement with Taylor & Francis Group.)

to the external urethral meatus and does not communicate with the urethra. When symptomatic, treatment is surgical drainage and complete cyst excision, as recurrent cyst and abscess formation is not uncommon (Fig. 36.10C,D). Histopathology of the cyst wall is always appropriate. As there is no communication with the urethra, the risk of fistula formation is less, although urethral injury is possible.

Although UD is commonly seen as a benign condition, stones or malignancy may develop within the diverticulum which can be easily missed, as seen on a magnetic resonance imaging (MRI) showing an intradiverticular filling defect which was a urethral

adenocarcinoma (Fig. 36.11). This was missed by the other imaging modalities of ultrasound (USS) and computed tomography (CT) scanning.[28] Leiomyomas within UD have also been reported.[29] Stones are diagnosed with urethroscopy (Fig. 36.12) or radiology imaging and arise due to urinary stasis and cellular debris within the UD (Fig. 36.13). Malignancy has been reported in up to 6% of cases when examined histologically, with up to 10% of histology overall showing atypical glandular findings.[6] Two-thirds of malignancies arising within UD are adenocarcinomas,[30] with transitional cell carcinomas exceedingly rare.[31] Squamous cell cancer can also occur as in this woman who presented with a painless urethral mass (Fig. 36.14). Another study found the risk of unexpected tumors at surgery to be 2%[32]; however, a high index of suspicion is needed for cancer with histologic review of all diverticulum pathology is essential. If the UD is small and asymptomatic, a conservative approach with regular imaging seems appropriate.

UD are commonly described as simple (20% to 40%), horseshoe or U-shaped (24% to 57%), or circumferential (23% to 37%) based on MRI findings.[19,33,34] In 1993, Leach et al.[35] outlined a classification system for UD, called L/N/S/C3, with L relating to location within the urethra; N, number; S, size expressed in centimeters; and C3 standing for configuration, communication, and continence configuration. C1 identifies whether the UD is single, multiloculated, or saddle shaped; C2 identifies the site of communication with the urethral lumen, that is, whether it is distal, mid, or proximal; and C3 indicates the presence of stress urinary incontinence (SUI).[35] This classification does not appear to have been widely adopted, with only 10% of studies published after the classification was created using this system when analyzed in a 2016 systematic review.[36]

FIGURE 36.5 Large open UD which developed following successful urethrovaginal fistula repair.

FIGURE 36.6 Woman with UD caused by persistence of a Gartner duct cyst. Other congenital abnormalities were a right ectopic ureter, absent right kidney, and uterus didelphys shown in Figures 36.6 and 36.7. (Reprinted from Dwyer PL, Rosamilia A. Congenital urogenital anomalies that are associated with the persistence of Gartner's duct: A review. *Am J Obstet Gynecol* 2006;195[2]:354–359. Copyright © 2006, with permission from Elsevier.)

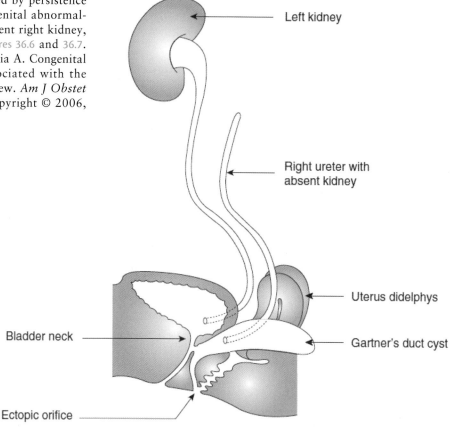

FIGURE 36.7 Ostium of ectopic ureter inferolateral to external urethral meatus, with indwelling Foley catheter. (Reprinted from Dwyer PL, Rosamilia A. Congenital urogenital anomalies that are associated with the persistence of Gartner's duct: A review. *Am J Obstet Gynecol* 2006;195[2]:354–359. Copyright © 2006, with permission from Elsevier.)

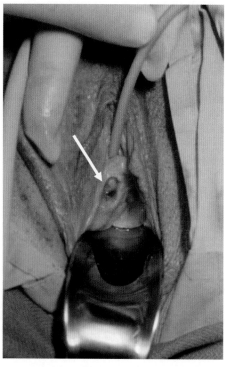

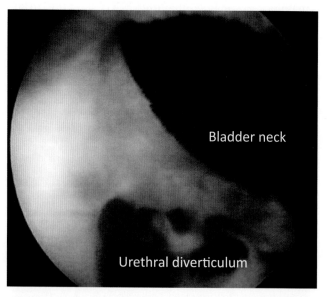

FIGURE 36.8 Urethroscopic photograph of bladder neck and large posterior UD and Gartner duct cyst with the surrounding urethral wall transparently thin. (Reprinted from Dwyer PL, Rosamilia A. Congenital urogenital anomalies that are associated with the persistence of Gartner's duct: A review. *Am J Obstet Gynecol* 2006;195[2]:354–359. Copyright © 2006, with permission from Elsevier.)

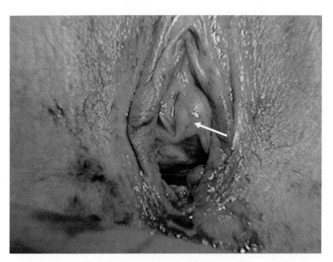

FIGURE 36.9 An infected Skene cyst with duct orifice at 5 o'clock relative to the meatus. (Reprinted by permission from Dwyer PL. Skene's gland revisited: Function, dysfunction and the G spot. *Int Urogynecol J* 2012;23[2]:135–137. Copyright 2012.)

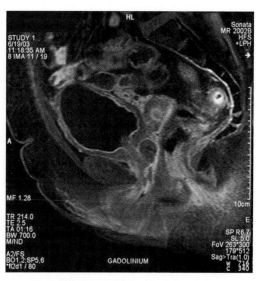

FIGURE 36.11 MRI showing an intradiverticular filling defect which was a urethral adenocarcinoma. This was missed by the other imaging modalities of ultrasound and CT scanning. (Reprinted by permission from Foster RT, Amundsen CL, Webster GD. The utility of magnetic resonance imaging for diagnosis and surgical planning before transvaginal periurethral diverticulectomy in women. *Int Urogynecol J Pelvic Floor Dysfunct* 2007;18[3]:315–319. Copyright 2007.)

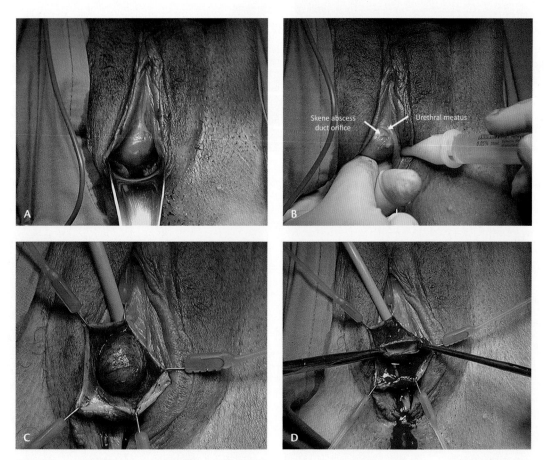

FIGURE 36.10 **A:** Woman with a Skene abscess on speculum examination. **B:** Expressed purulent material on compression of Skene abscess. **C:** Vaginal dissection of Skene abscess. **D:** Drainage of Skene abscess prior to excision.

FIGURE 36.12 Multiple intradiverticular calculi seen on urethroscopy. (Reproduced from Dwyer PL, ed. *Atlas of urogynecological endoscopy*. London: Informa, 2007. © Informa UK, 2007, reproduced by arrangement with Taylor & Francis Group.)

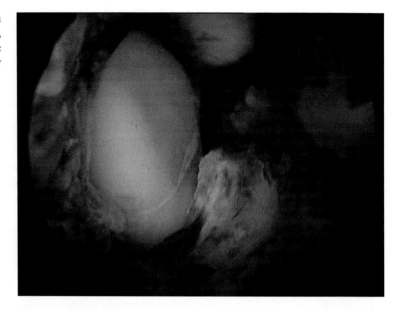

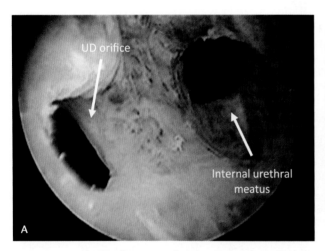

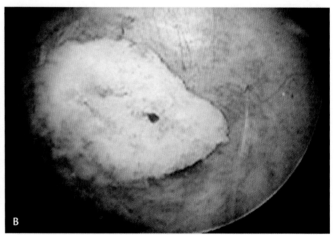

FIGURE 36.13 **A:** Urethroscopy showing internal urethral meatus above and right lateral UD orifice. **B:** Inside the UD is cellular debris. (Reproduced from Dwyer PL, ed. *Atlas of urogynecological endoscopy*. London: Informa, 2007. © Informa UK, 2007, reproduced by arrangement with Taylor & Francis Group.)

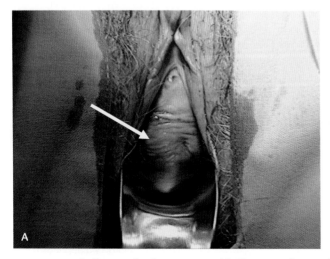

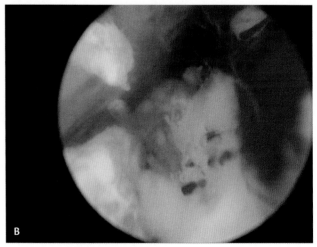

FIGURE 36.14 **A.** Paraurethral mass seen with Sims speculum and **B.** On urethroscopy and biopsy was an invasive squamous cell carcinoma.

CLINICAL PRESENTATION

There is significant discrepancy in the reported symptoms of UD due to the challenges in awareness and hence delay or difficulties in diagnosing this condition. Given the heterogeneity of symptoms that women can present with, often the diagnosis of UD can be significantly delayed and misdiagnosis is common. Historically, the presentation of UD has been described as the "three D's": dysuria, dyspareunia, and postmicturition dribbling, although with larger case series of women, it has become apparent that using this triad of symptoms for diagnosis would only identify 5% to 20% of cases[15,37] with up to 27% of women having none of these symptoms.[37] UD have been found in up to 3% of asymptomatic women.[4] In our own series, the most common presenting symptoms were urinary urgency and frequency (60%), and dyspareunia (56%) with 88% having a tender anterior vaginal wall mass and 40% a urethral discharge.[38]

Commonly, women may present with nonspecific irritative symptoms of the lower urinary tract such as urinary frequency and urgency, alongside SUI, recurrent urinary tract infections, and pain. The most common presenting symptoms are outlined in Table 36.1.[5,9,13,19,32–34,37,39–41]

On physical examination, a tender palpable mass can be identified in 34% to 88% of cases (Fig. 36.15A).[5,9,37,38] Compression of the mass may result in purulent discharge being expressed per the urethral meatus in 40% to 66%[38,40] of cases; this clinical finding has been reported to have a sensitivity of 66% and a specificity of 95%.[40]

Given the varied clinical presentation, there are several differential diagnoses that need to be considered (Table 36.2).[15,42–44] Other presenting complaints may be overactive bladder, SUI, and bladder pain syndrome.

TABLE 36.1

Common Presenting Symptoms of Urethral Diverticulum

SYMPTOM	FREQUENCY (%)
Pain	21–61
Urinary incontinence	22–62
SUI	36–50
Dyspareunia	10–60
Frequency/urgency	22–100
Vaginal lump	21–82
Recurrent UTIs	7–70
Dysuria	22–73
Postvoid dribble	5–48
Urinary retention	4

UTIs, urinary tract infections.

TABLE 36.2

Differential Diagnosis of Periurethral and Anterior Vaginal Wall Masses

UD
Simple vaginal cysts
Embryologic cystic remnants of Gartner duct
Skene gland cysts or abscess
Leiomyoma
Ectopic urethrocele
Vaginal wall inclusion cyst
Müllerian cyst (Gartner cyst)
Urothelial cyst
Periurethral injections for stress incontinence
Endometriosis
Vaginal wall abscess (e.g., infected urethral sling)
Nephrogenic adenoma
Benign and malignant conditions, including carcinoma and sarcoma of the urogenital tracts
Cystocele

Reproduced from Dwyer PL, ed. *Atlas of urogynecological endoscopy.* London: Informa, 2007. © Informa UK, 2007, reproduced by arrangement with Taylor & Francis Group.

INVESTIGATIONS

As with any patient presenting with lower urinary tract symptoms, a midstream urine sample should be obtained to exclude a urinary tract infection.

Over time, the preferred modality of imaging has changed, from voiding urethrocystography being the initial preferred investigation (Fig. 36.16) to now more commonly an MRI (see Fig. 36.11), CT, or USS.[5,8]

Cystourethroscopy

Cystourethroscopy with a 0° scope and Sachse sheath is often advocated in the initial investigation of UD, including by the authors.[45] Distension of the urethra with irrigation fluid facilitates the identification of the UD ostium and intradiverticular examination (see Fig. 36.13). Although evidence of a diverticular ostium is highly specific for the diagnosis of UD (100%), this investigative tool has been reported to have a low sensitivity of 39% in one study, which is thought to be due to the operator-dependent nature of the procedure. Visualization of the ostium may be facilitated by digital compression of the suspected diverticulum vaginally in order to milk purulent discharge into the urethral lumen (see Fig. 36.4).[15] This is a low-cost

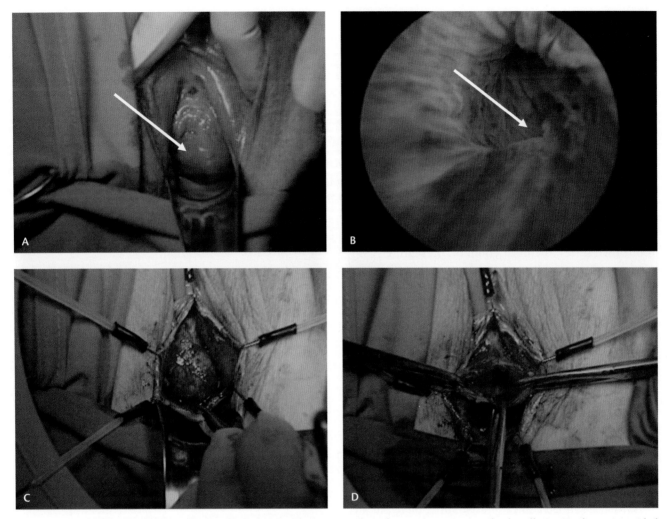

FIGURE 36.15 **A:** Woman with a UD on speculum examination. **B:** UD orifice on posterior urethral wall. **C:** UD dissection aided by a Brantley Scott retractor. **D:** UD opened revealing urethral orifice and ready for excision.

and readily accessible investigation which can be performed in the outpatient setting using a rigid or flexible urethroscope.

Voiding Cystourethrography

This was the traditional technique used for UD diagnosis historically, with a reported accuracy of UD identification of between 24% and 95%.[41,46] After filling the bladder with contrast agent, images are obtained during filling, voiding, and after voiding in order to identify filling of a UD cavity. Limitations of this technique include the inability to define the orifice of the UD with accuracy as well as only being able to identify the orifice when it is patent.[47]

Positive Pressure Urethrography

This technique uses catheters with either a second balloon or a retention plug proximal to the balloon at the catheter tip in order to use positive pressure to force contrast agent into the UD (Figs. 36.16 and 36.17). Although earlier studies identified a much greater

sensitivity of diagnosing UD with a double-balloon urethrography relative to a voiding cystourethrogram,[48,49] there are several disadvantages including the requirement of experienced radiologists, use of radiation and specialized equipment, and the propensity to cause patient discomfort and infection.[47]

Ultrasound

In more recent years, the use of USS has become more common due to the perceived benefits of being non-invasive, no requirement for ionizing radiation, wide availability, appropriateness for pregnant patients, and good discrimination in differentiating solid from cystic lesions. Disadvantages include interoperator variability and technical difficulty.[47] USS has also been used intra-operatively to assist with demonstrating the neck of the UD.[50] Transvaginal contrast-enhanced sonourethrography has been reported as a useful tool in the assistance of identifying UD, with findings correlating well with the surgical findings of size, location, configuration and opening of the UD.[51]

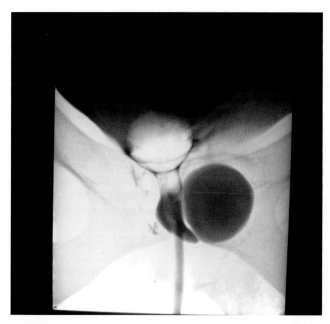

FIGURE 36.16 UD with Trattner catheter and voiding urethrography. (Reproduced from Dwyer PL, ed. *Atlas of urogynecological endoscopy*. London: Informa, 2007. © Informa UK, 2007, reproduced by arrangement with Taylor & Francis Group.)

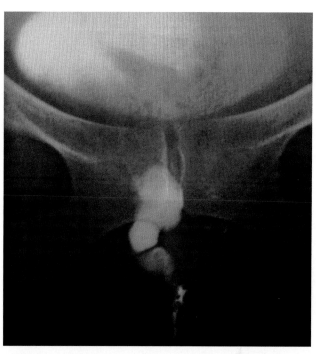

FIGURE 36.17 Trattner catheter and multiple diverticula.

Translabial USS may provide a minimally invasive and reproducible method of diagnosing UD, providing information on size, complexity, and presence/location of diverticular neck as well as content of the UD.[52] A recent paper looking at translabial USS for the detection of UD found a cystic structure crossing the urethral sphincter had a high predictive value for urethroscopic diagnosis of UD and reported this to be a valid, noninvasive method for diagnosis.[53] In a study of 42 women with a paraurethral cyst, three-dimensional pelvic floor USS correlated with surgical findings of either a UD or a Gartner duct cyst in 95%.[54] As this technique becomes more widely used, it may contribute to the more accurate diagnosis of UD.

Computed Tomography Voiding Urethrography

During the CT, the bladder and urethra are scanned with the patient voiding contrast material, which provides an accurate measurement of diverticulum size and location. Use of radiation and technical difficulty for the patients are disadvantages.

Magnetic Resonance Imaging

MRI is rapidly becoming the investigation of choice for UD, with a reported 83% specificity and 100% sensitivity for the diagnosis of UD.[40] Although MRI is minimally invasive and avoids the use of ionizing radiation, it is also an expensive diagnostic test which is not available in all institutions. It is an excellent modality for examining periurethral anatomy due to multiplanar capabilities and soft tissue contrast[55] and has proven to be beneficial for complex UD localization, orifice detection, and in providing accurate estimates of size and complexity (see Fig. 36.11). T2-weighted imaging (highlighting differences on the T2 relaxation time of tissues) is preferred for the detection of hyperintense fluid within a UD as the increased water content creates a bright signal, whereas intravenous gadolinium-based contrast aids in the detection of inflammation and adenocarcinoma.[47]

Urodynamic Studies

Urinary symptoms are the most common presentation in women with a UD; therefore, urodynamics should be performed to assess lower urinary tract function in order to assist with adequate preoperative counseling. Postoperative incontinence, voiding dysfunction, and urethrovaginal fistulas are common complications following UD repair with possible legal consequences. Video urodynamics can be useful for the ability to provide additional information[33] on establishing the underlying cause for incontinence, either true SUI as opposed to "paradoxical" incontinence with leakage from the UD with stress maneuvers.[35] It is thought that urodynamic studies (UDS) may identify abnormal findings in 62% including SUI in 48%.[41] One large series performed baseline UDS in all patients referred for refractory urinary symptoms and identified to have a UD, and identified urodynamic SUI in 27%, detrusor overactivity in 23%, and bladder outlet obstruction in 43%.[19] The pathophysiology of SUI with UD may be either as a result of damage to the urethral sphincteric musculature by the diverticular mass or inflammation[38] but is typically not the usual cause of SUI being a poorly supported urethra, although this can coexist. For this reason, SUI requiring surgical repair is uncommon following good excision and tension-free repair.[38] Postmicturition dribble is a symptom typical of UD and is caused by urine filling the UD and not then being controlled by the normal urethral sphincter mechanism.

MANAGEMENT

Although surgery is the mainstay of treatment for symptomatic UD, conservative management may be appropriate for women who are asymptomatic and with no signs suspicious for malignancy or calculus on imaging.[36] It may also be considered in women who decline surgical intervention due to medical comorbidities or pregnancy. The risk of underlying malignancy or progression to malignancy must be discussed in order for the patient to make an informed decision.

UD diagnosed during pregnancy are best treated conservatively with antibiotics and symptom relief. Vaginal delivery is appropriate in most cases, and the diverticular mass can be aspirated or drained if obstructing labor.[56] Surgical excision and repair of symptomatic UD can be performed at an appropriate time following pregnancy.

Multiple surgical procedures have been described for UD including transurethral deroofing, marsupialization of distal UD, and transvaginal diverticulectomy. To date, no studies have been performed comparing the different surgical procedures.

Transvaginal Resection with Urethral Reconstruction

The most common and effective procedure performed is a transvaginal resection with urethral reconstruction, otherwise referred to as a diverticulectomy, which was performed in 84% of patients examined in a large systematic review of surgical treatments.[36] This procedure involves a midline or inverted U incision on the anterior vaginal wall, with excision of the UD and a multilayer tension-free watertight closure. The suture lines are traditionally nonoverlapping to reduce the risk of fistula formation, and absorbable suture material is used. This procedure aims to identify and completely excise the UD sac with identification and closure of the ostia[45] with preservation of the periurethral fascia and rhabdosphincter in order to preserve continence.

Operative technique of transvaginal resection with urethral reconstruction is described below.[45]

1. A diagnostic cystourethroscopy is performed with a 0° scope and Sachse sheath.
2. A midline incision is made in the vaginal mucosa with wide lateral dissection and into the retropubic space if necessary to enable tissue mobilization and tension-free urethral closure. The surgical approach is the same whether the UD is small, bulbous, and ventral, or a much larger horseshoe-shaped UD extending into the retropubic space. For the larger diverticulum, the dissection is more extensive and the bladder and urethra frequently need to be completely mobilized off the vagina and pelvic sidewall prior to UD excision. Popat and Zimmern[57] reported good long-term outcomes with the surgical treatment of horseshoe UD, and our study confirms this.[38] However, UD larger than 30 mm and proximal urethral location were significant factors for the development of de novo SUI postsurgery.[38]
3. A Brantley Scott retractor (Lone Star Surgical) provides excellent surgical visualization and access (see Fig. 36.15C,D).
4. The diverticular sac is opened usually at the thinnest point, and the full extent of the diverticulum and the urethral orifice is assessed (see Fig. 36.15D).
5. A probe is used to identify the opening from the diverticulum into the urethra; there may be multiple openings and diverticula.
6. The diverticular mucosa is excised and sent for histology. The urethral mucosa is closed with 4.0 Vicryl in a continuous fashion avoiding excessive mucosa excision or stricture. The top and bottom sutures are tagged to mark the boundaries of the incision.
7. A second layer closure is performed and a tension-free closure is ensured.
8. A further two or three layers of closure of 2.0 or 3.0 delayed absorbable sutures are performed using the diverticular muscle wall and periurethral fascia to provide additional support to the repair.
9. A 0° urethroscope with Sachse sheath or flexible scope is performed to ensure watertight urethral closure.
10. A Martius labial fat pad if necessary can be placed over the entire length of the repair and sutured into position. Martius grafts are generally not needed except where the urethral defect is extensive or for recurrent cases.
11. The vaginal wall is closed with interrupted sutures with 2.0 Vicryl sutures.

Other Surgical Options

In 1970, Spence and Duckett[58] described a procedure of vaginal marsupialization for distal urethral diverticula, where the UD is opened from the vaginal aspect into the urethra, commonly referred to as a Spence procedure. This procedure creates a shorter urethral length and a more patulous urethral meatus.[36] Although this procedure may be used for small distal UD, excessive proximal incision could result in urethral sphincteric injury, and there is a risk of urethrovaginal fistulas development. This procedure has been reported in small case series only, limiting the evaluation of success and complications for this procedure.

Transurethral excision of the urethral floor using a knife electrode has also been described as an option for distal UD, converting a narrow opening into a wider diverticulum opening and thereby allowing drainage.[59] Due to the nature of the procedure, this has in the past not been recommended for more proximal UD due to the risk of iatrogenic injury to the urethral sphincter and only reported in small case series. However, in a recent larger case series of 22 women, Wu et al.[60] used transurethral endoscopic incision of the roof of complex proximal UD to open the UD widely and allow drainage of pus and infection. They reported a high long-term symptom resolution rate of 81.8% and a low de novo SUI rate of 13.6%.[60] The authors suggest that as complex UD have a higher recurrence rate than simple UD when treated via transvaginal diverticulectomy, transurethral endoscopic excision may prove to be a beneficial and less invasive treatment option for less experienced vaginal surgeons. Comparative studies are needed to determine the functional results of recurrence, complications, and SUI following both procedures, but the endoscopic approach does avoid the need for difficult vaginal surgery in complex UD.

There are case reports of the abdominal approach to treat UD.[61] With the increasing popularity of laparoscopic and robotic surgery, and lack of experience of urologists in vaginal surgery, this will only increase. However, with the excellent surgical exposure and low morbidity of the vaginal approach, and the need for accurate watertight tension-free urethral closure of the diverticulum orifice, when the UD is positioned posteriorly or posterolaterally, this makes the use of the abdominal retropubic approach alone problematic. A combined abdominal vaginal approach may occasionally be necessary for large UD extending into the retropubic space. Recently, our unit was referred a woman who had a UD excision and repair with Burch colposuspension performed robotically and subsequently developed a urethrovaginal fistula. Fistula repair was attempted unsuccessfully from above using a robotic approach; the permanent colposuspension sutures were found to be intravesical and were removed (Fig. 36.18). This case demonstrates the dangers of using the abdominal approach alone to surgically treat UD and the difficulty of closing posterior urethral defects retropubically.

POSTOPERATIVE CARE

At the completion of surgery, a vaginal pack may be placed for 1 day to assist with hemostasis, and an indwelling catheter or a suprapubic catheter is sited. Similar to urinary fistula repair, the duration of catheterization will depend on surgeon preference and complexity of the procedure; we usually remove the catheter after only 1 to 2 days. Some centers advocate

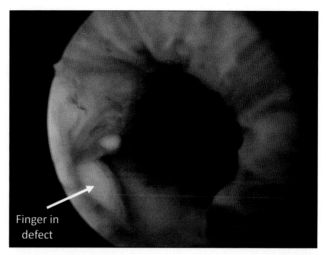

Finger in defect

FIGURE 36.18 A 30-year-old nulliparous woman with UD and urinary incontinence had a robotic laparoscopic excision of the UD and a Burch colposuspension with Ethibond sutures which resulted in urethrovaginal fistula. Repair was attempted unsuccessfully robotically with removal of the intravesical Ethibond sutures and calculus and attempted closure of the fistula from above. On urethroscopy postoperatively there was a 1-cm urethrovaginal fistula at 7 o'clock with an examining finger pushing through the defect from the vagina. The fistula was successfully closed transvaginally with a layered closure and a Martius graft.

longer catheterization and a voiding cystourethrogram at time of catheter removal[15,57] to ensure healing is confirmed; this is not our routine practice. Broad-spectrum antibiotics are commonly prescribed for 24 to 48 hours postoperatively followed by prophylactic oral antibiotics until catheter removal.

COMPLICATIONS OF SURGERY

Potential complications of surgery may include recurrent diverticula, urethrovaginal fistula, urethral strictures, pain and dyspareunia, and de novo SUI,[36] which have been reported at various frequencies in the literature due to variable lengths of follow-up (Table 36.3).[5,8,19,32,34,36,57]

TABLE 36.3	
Complications of Surgery	
COMPLICATION	**FREQUENCY (%)**
De novo SUI	0–16
Urethrovaginal fistula	0–8
Urethral strictures	0–5
Recurrent UTIs	7–31
Recurrent diverticula	3–23

UTI, urinary tract infection.

ADDITIONAL SURGICAL CONSIDERATIONS

Martius Graft

The use of a Martius labial fat pad interposition (MLFP) has been used in an attempt to prevent fistula formation and reduce the risk of recurrent UD, especially in cases of secondary repair where tissue quality and vascularity may be suboptimal (Video 36.1).[45] Although historically used in cases where poor quality or insufficient periurethral fascia was available, or a large urethral defect was evident after UD removal,[8,32] Malde et al.[19] in a retrospective series of 70 cases with routine use of MLFP alongside urethral diverticulectomy achieved high success rates of almost 99% at medium-term follow-up with low complication rates as well as identifying a low morbidity rate from the MLFP harvest at 4%. This study found this approach also led to 41% of women having complete resolution of preoperative SUI, thereby potentially preventing the need for further surgical intervention. It should however be noted that high rates of SUI resolution have also been reported in cases managed without an MLFP.[38] The placement of an MLFP has also been thought to prevent scarring so that future autologous fascial slings may be placed without significant difficulty if required.[32] It has been argued that given a high rate of success can be achieved with simple diverticulectomy in cases of simple and U-shaped UDs, that placement of an MLFP is not required in all patients,[34] although is likely to be of greater benefit when performed as an adjunct to repair of circumferential or recurrent UDs.

Stress Urinary Incontinence Surgery

SUI surgery can be performed as a combined procedure in women with coexistent SUI or as a prophylactic measure. The risk of SUI requiring surgical treatment after primary surgery for a UD is low despite the relatively high rates of SUI that are diagnosed on preoperative urodynamics, and it is estimated that 40% to 60% of preoperative SUI may resolve with diverticulectomy alone, with or without an MLFP.[19,32] Rates of de novo SUI postoperatively have been reported as between 0% and 16% (see Table 36.3) with between 3% and 16% of patients overall requiring incontinence surgery at a later date.[32,34,38,57] A large retrospective cohort study of 485 cases by Bradley et al.[62] demonstrated that the addition of a pubovaginal sling at the time of a urethral diverticulectomy led to a greater resolution of SUI; however, there was an increased risk of postoperative urinary retention and recurrent urinary tract infections in the sling group. A large systematic review by Bodner-Adler et al.[36] has concluded there is currently insufficient data to recommend a concomitant incontinence procedure at time of diverticulectomy. The risk

of postoperative stress incontinence requiring surgery is low at less than 5% in our experience,[38] and with pubovaginal slings having a significant incidence of short- and long-term voiding problems, the benefit of reduced SUI may be outweighed by voiding difficulties and recurrent urinary tract infection. First, do no harm.

Predictive factors for the development of de novo SUI postoperatively have been identified as a UD larger than 30 mm and proximal urethral location,[38] suggesting that patients with these elements identified preoperatively could be considered for concomitant incontinence surgery. If concomitant SUI surgery is to be performed at the time of UD repair, traditionally, it has been recommended that the treatment of choice is a fascial sling in order to prevent implant complications from a synthetic sling or injectable agents.[63]

OUTCOMES

Reported success rates for diverticulectomy range from 77% to 98%,[2,5,19,34,64] when success is defined as the absence of recurrence on follow-up. This figure may vary according to the method used for defining recurrence, as some studies define recurrence as the need for reoperation and others on the evidence of recurrent UD on MRI scans. Several features have been identified as risk factors for failure/recurrence and include multiple diverticula, proximal diverticula, U-shaped or circumferential UD, and those with previous urethral surgery.[34,45,55,64] A reoperation rate for recurrent UD of up to 17% has been reported at 5 years from the original procedure.[5] Up to 81% of women have reported long-term improvement in symptoms,[8] with a large systematic review identifying a complete resolution of presenting symptoms in 69% of a cohort of 1,044 patients.[36] Sexual function can also improve for women after UD repair, with an improvement in female sexual function index in women treated for UD.[65]

MANAGEMENT OF RECURRENT URETHRAL DIVERTICULUM

Outcomes for recurrent UD repair have been reported to have success rates of up to 75%,[34] with potentially a higher cure rate with the use of an MLFP compared to those performed without (83% vs. 69%, not significant). The authors have previously published a video detailing the management of a recurrent UD with mobilization and repositioning of a previously placed MLFP with a good outcome (see Video 36.1).[45] Due to the technically challenging nature of repairing a recurrent UD due to scarring and loss of surgical planes, this procedure should only be performed by surgeons with experience in complex repairs in order to optimize the surgical outcome.

CONCLUSION

Female UD is a relatively uncommon condition but may present to gynecologists and urologists with irritable bladder symptoms and incontinence, vaginal mass, and dyspareunia. Etiology is multifactorial with infection of paraurethral glands the most common cause. Diagnostic assessment with urethroscopy and imaging with USS, CT, or MRI are the primary investigations. Transvaginal diverticular mucosal excision and urethral reconstruction for symptomatic UD is the treatment of choice. The use of a Martius graft or pubovaginal slings will be useful at times, but the evidence does not support their routine use.

References

1. Hey W. *Practical observations in surgery*. Philadelphia: James Humphreys Publishers, 1805.
2. Crescenze IM, Goldman HB. Female urethral diverticulum: Current diagnosis and management. *Curr Urol Rep* 2015;16(10):71.
3. El-Nashar SA, Bacon MM, Kim-Fine S, et al. Incidence of female urethral diverticulum: A population-based analysis and literature review. *Int Urogynecol J* 2014;25(1):73–79.
4. Andersen MJ. The incidence of diverticula in the female urethra. *J Urol* 1967;98(1):96–98.
5. El-Nashar SA, Singh R, Bacon MM, et al. Female urethral diverticulum: Presentation, diagnosis, and predictors of outcomes after surgery. *Female Pelvic Med Reconstr Surg* 2016;22(6):447–452.
6. Thomas AA, Rackley RR, Lee U, et al. Urethral diverticula in 90 female patients: A study with emphasis on neoplastic alterations. *J Urol* 2008;180(6):2463–2467.
7. Rufford J, Cardozo L. Urethral diverticula: A diagnostic dilemma. *BJU Int* 2004;94(7):1044–1047.
8. Ljungqvist L, Peeker R, Fall M. Female urethral diverticulum: 26-Year followup of a large series. *J Urol* 2007;177(1):219–224.
9. Romanzi LJ, Groutz A, Blaivas JG. Urethral diverticulum in women: Diverse presentations resulting in diagnostic delay and mismanagement. *J Urol* 2000;164(2):428–433.
10. Surabhi VR, Menias CO, George V, et al. Magnetic resonance imaging of female urethral and periurethral disorders. *Radiol Clin North Am* 2013;51(6):941–953.
11. Gosling JA, Dixon JS, Humpherson JR. *Functional anatomy of the urinary tract. An integrated text and colour atlas*. London: Gower Medical, 1983.
12. Huffman JW. The detailed anatomy of the para-urethral ducts in the adult human female. *Am J Obstet Gynecol* 1948;55(1):86–101.
13. Rovner ES. Urethral diverticula: A review and an update. *Neurourol Urodyn* 2007;26(7):972–977.
14. Lee JW, Fynes MM. Female urethral diverticula. *Best Pract Res Clin Obstet Gynaecol* 2005;19(6):875–893.
15. Greenwell TJ, Spilotros M. Urethral diverticula in women. *Nat Rev Urol* 2015;12(12):671–680.
16. Tsivian M, Tsivian A, Shreiber L, et al. Female urethral diverticulum: A pathological insight. *Int Urogynecol J Pelvic Floor Dysfunct* 2009;20(8):957–960.
17. Bennett SJ. Urethral diverticula. *Eur J Obstet Gynecol Reprod Biol* 2000;89(2):135–139.
18. Routh A. Urethral diverticula. *Br Med J* 1890;1:361.
19. Malde S, Sihra N, Naaseri S, et al. Urethral diverticulectomy with Martius labial fat pad interposition improves symptom resolution and reduces recurrence. *BJU Int* 2017;119(1):158–163.
20. Hammad FT. TVT can also cause urethral diverticulum. *Int Urogynecol J Pelvic Floor Dysfunct* 2007;18(4):467–469.
21. Mukhtar BMB, Solomon E, Naaseri S, et al. Urethral diverticula in women are associated with increased urethra-sphincter complex volumes: A potential role for high-tone nonrelaxing sphincter in their etiology? *Neurourol Urodyn* 2019;38(7):1859–1865.
22. Glassman TA, Weinerth JL, Glenn JF. Neonatal female urethral diverticulum. *Urology* 1975;5(2):249–251.
23. Dwyer PL, Rosamilia A. Congenital urogenital anomalies that are associated with the persistence of Gartner's duct: A review. *Am J Obstet Gynecol* 2006;195(2):354–359.
24. Skene A. The anatomy and pathology of two important glands of the female urethra. *Am J Obs Dis Women Child* 1880;13:265–270.
25. Wernert N, Albrech M, Sesterhenn I, et al. The 'female prostate': Location, morphology, immunohistochemical characteristics and significance. *Eur Urol* 1992;22(1):64–69.
26. Dwyer PL. Skene's gland revisited: Function, dysfunction and the G spot. *Int Urogynecol J* 2012;23(2):135–137.
27. Moalem S, Reidenberg JS. Does female ejaculation serve an antimicrobial purpose? *Med Hypotheses* 2009;73(6):1069–1071.
28. Foster RT, Amundsen CL, Webster GD. The utility of magnetic resonance imaging for diagnosis and surgical planning before transvaginal periurethral diverticulectomy in women. *Int Urogynecol J Pelvic Floor Dysfunct* 2007;18(3):315–319.
29. Karadag D, Caglar O, Haliloglu AH, et al. Leiomyoma in a female urethral diverticulum. *Jpn J Radiol* 2010;28(5):369–371.
30. Oluyadi F, Ramachandran P, Gotlieb V. A rare case of advanced urethral diverticular adenocarcinoma and a review of treatment modalities. *J Investig Med High Impact Case Rep* 2019;7:2324709619828408.
31. Manning J. Case report: Transitional cell carcinoma in situ within a urethral diverticulum. *Int Urogynecol J* 2012;23(12):1801–1803.
32. Reeves FA, Inman RD, Chapple CR. Management of symptomatic urethral diverticula in women: A single-centre experience. *Eur Urol* 2014;66(1):164–172.
33. Barratt R, Malde S, Pakzad M, et al. The incidence and outcomes of urodynamic stress urinary incontinence in female patients with urethral diverticulum. *Neurourol Urodyn* 2019;38(7):1889–1900.
34. Ko KJ, Suh YS, Kim TH, et al. Surgical outcomes of primary and recurrent female urethral diverticula. *Urology* 2017;105:181–185.
35. Leach GE, Sirls LT, Ganabathi K, et al. L N S C3: A proposed classification system for female urethral diverticula. *Neurourol Urodyn* 1993;12(6):523–531.
36. Bodner-Adler B, Halpern K, Hanzal E. Surgical management of urethral diverticula in women: A systematic review. *Int Urogynecol J* 2016;27(7):993–1001.
37. Baradaran N, Chiles LR, Freilich DA, et al. Female urethral diverticula in the contemporary era: Is the classic triad of the "3Ds" still relevant? *Urology* 2016;94:53–56.
38. Stav K, Dwyer PL, Rosamilia A, et al. Urinary symptoms before and after female urethral diverticulectomy—can we predict de novo stress urinary incontinence? *J Urol* 2008;180(5):2088–2090.
39. Patel AK, Chapple CR. Female urethral diverticula. *Curr Opin Urol* 2006;16(4):248–254.

40. Pathi SD, Rahn DD, Sailors JL, et al. Utility of clinical parameters, cystourethroscopy, and magnetic resonance imaging in the preoperative diagnosis of urethral diverticula. *Int Urogynecol J* 2013;24(2):319–323.

41. Ganabathi K, Leach GE, Zimmern PE, et al. Experience with the management of urethral diverticulum in 63 women. *J Urol* 1994;152(5, Pt 1):1445–1452.

42. Fletcher SG, Lemack GE. Benign masses of the female periurethral tissues and anterior vaginal wall. *Curr Urol Rep* 2008;9(5):389–396.

43. Blaivas JG, Flisser AJ, Bleustein CB, et al. Periurethral masses: Etiology and diagnosis in a large series of women. *Obstet Gynecol* 2004;103(5, Pt 1):842–847.

44. Dwyer P, ed. Urethral and periurethral conditions. In: *Atlas of urogynecological endoscopy*. London: Informa, 2007:51–72.

45. Dykes N, Dwyer P, Rosamilia A, et al. Video and review of the surgical management of recurrent urethral diverticulum. *Int Urogynecol J* 2020;31(12):2679–2681.

46. Arunkalaivanan AS, Baptiste M, Sami T. Urethral diverticulum in women: Retrospective case series. *J Obstet Gynaecol India* 2016;66(1):47–51.

47. Chou CP, Levenson RB, Elsayes KM, et al. Imaging of female urethral diverticulum: An update. *Radiographics* 2008;28(7):1917–1930.

48. Jacoby K, Rowbotham RK. Double balloon positive pressure urethrography is a more sensitive test than voiding cystourethrography for diagnosing urethral diverticulum in women. *J Urol* 1999;162(6):2066–2069.

49. Golomb J, Leibovitch I, Mor Y, et al. Comparison of voiding cystourethrography and double-balloon urethrography in the diagnosis of complex female urethral diverticula. *Eur Radiol* 2003;13(3):536–542.

50. El-Zein C, Khoury N, El-Zein Y, et al. Intraoperative translabial ultrasound for urethral diverticula: A road map for surgeons. *Eur J Radiol* 2009;70(1):133–137.

51. Dai Y, Wang J, Shen H, et al. Diagnosis of female urethral diverticulum using transvaginal contrast-enhanced sonourethrography. *Int Urogynecol J* 2013;24(9):1467–1471.

52. Gugliotta G, Calagna G, Adile G, et al. Use of trans-labial ultrasound in the diagnosis of female urethral diverticula: A diagnostic option to be strongly considered. *J Obstet Gynaecol Res* 2015;41(7):1108–1114.

53. Gillor M, Dietz HP. Translabial ultrasound imaging of urethral diverticula. *Ultrasound Obstet Gynecol* 2019;54(4):552–556.

54. Liu D, Qing Z, Wen L. The use of tomographic ultrasound imaging on three-dimensional translabial ultrasound: A diagnostic sign for urethral diverticulum. *Int Urogynecol J* 2020;31(7):1451–1456.

55. Han DH, Jeong YS, Choo MS, et al. Outcomes of surgery of female urethral diverticula classified using magnetic resonance imaging. *Eur Urol* 2007;51(6):1664–1670.

56. Moran PA, Carey MP, Dwyer PL. Urethral diverticula in pregnancy. *Aust N Z J Obstet Gynaecol* 1998;38(1):102–106.

57. Popat S, Zimmern PE. Long-term outcomes after the excision of horseshoe urethral diverticulum. *Int Urogynecol J* 2016;27(3):439–444.

58. Spence HM, Duckett JW Jr. Diverticulum of the female urethra: Clinical aspects and presentation of a simple operative technique for cure. *J Urol* 1970;104(3):432–437.

59. Lapides J. Transurethral treatment of urethral diverticula in women. *J Urol* 1979;121(6):736–738.

60. Wu B, Bai S, Yao Z, et al. Transurethral endoscopic extensive incision of complex urethral diverticula in symptomatic women: Case series in a single center experience with long-term follow-up. *Int Urol Nephrol* 2021;53(7):1279–1287.

61. Sivarajan G, Glickman L, Faber K, et al. Transabdominal robot-assisted laparoscopic urethral diverticulectomy of a complex anterior horseshoe diverticulum of the proximal urethra. *J Endourol Case Rep* 2015;1(1):33–35.

62. Bradley SE, Leach DA, Panza J, et al. A multicenter retrospective cohort study comparing urethral diverticulectomy with and without pubovaginal sling. *Am J Obstet Gynecol* 2020;223(2):273.e271–273.e279.

63. Kobashi KC, Albo ME, Dmochowski RR, et al. Surgical treatment of female stress urinary incontinence: AUA/SUFU guideline. *J Urol* 2017;198(4):875–883.

64. Zhou L, Luo DY, Feng SJ, et al. Risk factors for recurrence in female urethral diverticulectomy: A retrospective study of 66 patients. *World J Urol* 2017;35(1):139–144.

65. Sun Y, Tang C, Li N, et al. Risk factors of postoperative sexual function in patients with urethral diverticulum and their partners: A cohort study of 83 women. *Int Braz J Urol* 2019;45(6):1216–1226.

CHAPTER 37

LOWER URINARY TRACT INFECTION

Sarah E.S. Jeney • Yuko M. Komesu

Introduction

Urinary tract infections (UTIs) are common and are most common in women.[1] Approximately 50% to 80% of women will have at least one UTI in their lifetime, and 30% to 44% with an initial UTI will experience an additional UTI within 3 months.[2] In women with two UTIs, half will experience another recurrence.[2] UTIs ultimately cost the United States over 2 to 3 billion dollars yearly and are one of the most common indications for outpatient antibiotics, contributing to an epidemic of multidrug resistance.[1,3,4] These issues heighten concerns regarding UTIs, their treatment, and appropriate antibiotic stewardship.[5]

URINARY TRACT INFECTION DEFINITIONS

Although definitions vary,[1,6,7] UTI classifications include uncomplicated acute lower UTI (acute cystitis), uncomplicated recurrent UTI (rUTI), complicated UTI, and asymptomatic bacteriuria. This chapter focuses on uncomplicated acute UTI, rUTI, and asymptomatic bacteriuria.

Acute uncomplicated lower UTI: a single symptomatic infection confined to the bladder without fever, systemic symptoms, or upper tract involvement.[7] Some require an anatomically normal urinary tract without prior instrumentation to qualify for this definition.[1,6]

Complicated UTI: UTI with involvement beyond the bladder (pyelonephritis or systemic symptoms).[8] Some also include presence of functional/structural urinary tract abnormalities, history of urinary instrumentation, renal transplantation, or insufficiency or underlying immunodeficiency in this definition.[1,6]

Uncomplicated rUTI: a symptomatic lower UTI occurring twice in 6 months or three times in 1 year in those without anatomic abnormalities or pyelonephritis.[2,6,9,10]

Asymptomatic bacteriuria: bacteria present in the bladder without attendant urinary symptoms (e.g., dysuria, increased urgency/frequency or incontinence, suprapubic tenderness, hematuria, fever, costovertebral angle tenderness).[11]

CURRENT UNDERSTANDING OF URINARY TRACT INFECTION PATHOPHYSIOLOGY

Studies of UTI pathophysiology were originally based on bacterial culture data. Recent advent of culture-independent methods expanded understanding of the relationship between bacteria and humans. The science advanced following initiation of the Human Microbiome Project (HMP), established in 2008 by the National Institutes of Health.[12] Using bacterial gene sequencing, the HMP sought to characterize bacterial communities in various human sites, collectively known as the human microbiome.

The HMP characterized bacteria inhabiting anatomic niches, offering the ability to view individual bacteria and bacterial communities within the ecologic background of their host. Human microbiome findings present a framework to evaluate specific bacteria, their metabolic profiles, and their interactions within differing environments, allowing improved understanding of bacteria, hosts, and habitats. Although knowledge about UTI pathophysiology is incomplete, this framework also applies to the study of UTI.

Bacterial Gene Sequencing

Bacteria have their own characteristic genetic profiles. Culture-independent sequencing of bacterial DNA allows characterization of the many bacteria residing in humans. The technology identifies individual bacteria by either sequencing entire bacterial genomes using whole-genome shotgun sequencing (shotgun metagenomics) or by targeting a specific genetic region for sequencing.[13] The latter typically uses the 16S ribosomal RNA bacterial gene to identify bacteria. The 16S gene has highly conserved regions that are identical in all bacteria as well as variable regions that serve as genetic signatures identifying bacteria to the genus or, in some cases, to the species level.[13] Both methods have advantages and disadvantages. Shotgun metagenomics may be more costly but may offer greater taxonomic and functional resolution, whereas 16S is less costly and may be used to analyze large numbers of samples.[14]

Notably, both methods involve lysis of human cells and neither can distinguish between live and dead bacteria in samples.[13]

The HMP found that the humans harbor bacteria that are characteristic for specific niches.[15,16] The original HMP did not evaluate the lower urinary tract because urine was believed to be sterile. Sequencing technology has since discovered that although urinary bacterial biomass is relatively sparse, urinary bacterial communities do exist.[13,16–18] Traditionally, cultures were developed to identify *Escherichia coli*, the most common uropathogen. Recognition of the existence of the urinary microbiome led to development of nontraditional culture techniques identifying a wider range of bacteria, complementing sequence findings. The expanded quantitative urine culture (EQUC) technique cultivates bacteria under aerobic and/or anaerobic conditions with longer incubation, better identifying fastidious organisms.[17,18] In contrast to gene sequencing, EQUC identifies live bacteria verifying that bacteria found with 16S methods can represent live bacteria in urine, an environment previously considered sterile.[17,18] EQUC, following bacterial identification with genetic sequencing, better quantifies bacteria in samples and may better identify them to the species level.[17] EQUC disadvantages include an inability to identify all bacteria in samples[13] and because eukaryotic cells are not lysed during EQUC, intracellular bacterial communities (see following discussion) may remain unrecognized. Nonetheless, nontraditional culturing, genomics, and metabolomics (study of bacterial metabolic products) work in tandem to increase understanding of UTI.

Vaginal microbiome studies illustrate how genomics and metabolomics have altered interpretation of bacterial associations with health and disease. Vaginal *Lactobacillus* has historically been equated with health, dating back to Döderlein's 1892 report of a lactic acid producing bacillus (later identified as *Lactobacillus*) inhibiting pathogen growth.[19] This resulted in the prevalent, although perhaps simplistic view, that *Lactobacillus* ensures health.[19] Microbiome studies have since found that *Lactobacillus* dominates vaginal communities in many but not all women and that *Lactobacillus* nondominant communities can also provide a healthy, acidic environment.[20] Understanding differences in the relative abundance and characteristics of *Lactobacilli* to the *Lactobacillus* species level provides further insight into their interactions with pathogens. *Lactobacillus crispatus*, *Lactobacillus iners*, *Lactobacillus gasseri*, and *Lactobacillus jensenii* are the most common vaginal *Lactobacillus* species.[16,20,21] Their relative abundance in women differs with age, ethnicity/race, and behaviors (e.g., contraceptive, antibiotic, and hormonal use and sexual activity).[16,22] *Lactobacillus* species metabolomes also vary. *L. iners* cannot synthesize D-lactic acid, which is more protective against dysbiosis than the L-lactic acid produced by

L. iners.[22] *L. iners* has been associated with vaginal dysbiosis and greater susceptibility to HIV and Chlamydia infections.[22] This contrasts with *L. crispatus*, which synthesizes both D- and L-lactic acid and has been reported to be associated with vaginal stability and health.[22] *Lactobacilli* are also relevant to the urinary microbiome. Presence of *Lactobacillus* species in the vagina correlates highly with their presence in urine, as demonstrated in a comparative study of 197 paired vaginal and urine samples.[23] Furthermore, in a phase 2 randomized controlled trial of reproductive-aged women with rUTI, *L. crispatus* provided as a vaginal supplement resulted in decreased rUTI in those who achieved high-level colonization of *L. crispatus*.[24]

Bacterial Virulence and Survival Factors

Lactobacilli developed survival mechanisms beneficial to both host and bacteria, or homeostatic mutualism. In contrast, pathogenic bacteria developed mechanisms detrimental to the host, or bacterial virulence. The most common bacteria responsible for UTI are uropathogenic *E. coli* (UPEC) followed by *Klebsiella pneumoniae*, *Enterococcus faecalis*, *Proteus mirabilis*, group B *Streptococcus*, *Pseudomonas aeruginosa*, *Staphylococcus* species, and *Candida* species.[10,25]

UTI often occurs when bacteria from nearby niches migrate to the urinary tract, adhere to, and then colonize or destroy host cells.[10,16,25] Murine and UPEC models have enhanced understanding of bacterial factors associated with human UTI (Fig. 37.1).[10,16,25] Bacterial pili, commonly found on UPEC, *Klebsiella*, *Proteus*, and *Enterococcus* species, facilitate bacterial migration and mediate adherence to host cells.[10,25] UPEC also invade superficial umbrella cells of mice, forming intracellular bacterial communities.[10,25] Although intracellular communities (in humans and mice) develop acutely, some persist chronically, allowing bacteria to multiply, avoid host surveillance, and serve as bacterial reservoirs in rUTI or asymptomatic bacteriuria.[10,26,27] Bacteria also form biofilms; the adhesive proteins (adhesins) produced by pili form a scaffold for bacterial adherence, acting as an extracellular matrix barrier to the host and antibiotics. UPEC, *Proteus*, *Klebsiella*, *Enterococcus*, and *Staphylococcus* are all capable of biofilm production enhanced in the presence of foreign bodies, such as urinary catheters.[10,25] A final example of bacterial virulence is production of enzymes (e.g., proteases, urease) and toxins (e.g., cytotoxic necrotizing factor in UPEC, hemolysin in UPEC, *Proteus* species) that lyse host cells, releasing nutrients in the nutrient-poor bladder, enhancing bacterial survival.[10] These capabilities are not limited to pathogens. *Lactobacilli* are also capable of cell adherence; biofilm formation; and hydrogen peroxide, lactic acid, and bacteriocin production, capabilities that are antagonistic to other bacteria and beneficial to the host.[28–31]

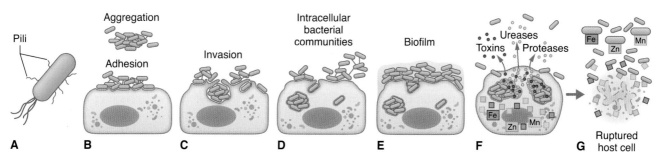

FIGURE 37.1 Bacterial survival and virulence factors. Bacterial virulence factors include the presence of bacterial pili or production of adhesins (**A**) allowing attachment to host uroepithelium (**B**) and/or host cell invasion (**C**). Successful reproduction and survival of intracellular bacteria can result in intracellular bacterial communities (IBCs) that can either remain quiescent, evading host surveillance and serving as bacterial reservoirs, or result in bacterial dispersal, repeating the reproduction of new IBCs (**D**). Some bacteria are capable of forming biofilms, a scaffold of extracellular matrices surrounding bacterial communities, which also subvert host detection and destruction (**E**). Other bacteria produce substances that lyse cells (e.g., toxins, proteases, urease), releasing much-needed nutrients into the nutrient-poor urinary environment, enhancing bacterial survival (**F**). An example of bacterial production of substances competing with the host for nutrients, include siderophore production that improves scavenging of iron (**G**).

Host Factors

Host mechanisms preventing UTI include urinary turbulence accompanying voiding (impeding bacterial passage to the bladder), presence of bladder umbrella cells (mucosal barriers to bacterial invasion), and host immune responses aiding bacterial destruction.[26] UTI occurs when host defenses are breached. Epidemiologic studies indicate that host susceptibility to rUTI increases with a family history of UTI, age, menopause, spermicide use, and sexual activity.[3,25] Urinary microbiome studies in older women have increased understanding of genetic influences in rUTI. A microbiome study in twins found that almost one-third of the bacteria present in twin urinary microbiomes were attributable to genetic predisposition.[32] *Escherichia* and certain *Lactobacillus* species exhibited particularly high heritability in these subjects. Increased heritability of specific bacteria suggests

human genetics influence the urinary microbiome, predisposing women to rUTI.[32]

Last, host immunity affects rUTI. Murine models offer insight into the molecular basis of this susceptibility. Transurethral inoculation of UPEC in susceptible mice results either in spontaneous resolution within 2 weeks or development of chronic cystitis. Mice that more commonly develop rUTI more commonly express cyclooxygenase 2, suggesting that specific immunologic reactions affect UTI recurrence.[25] Chronic cystitis is also associated with prolonged tumor necrosis factor signaling, suggesting that prior UTI may increase host susceptibility to future infection.[25] On a cellular level, chronic cystitis likely occurs by infection-induced monocyte recruitment, followed by exfoliation of superficial bladder umbrella cells (Fig. 37.2). This initially decreases bacterial load but exposes underlying transitional epithelium

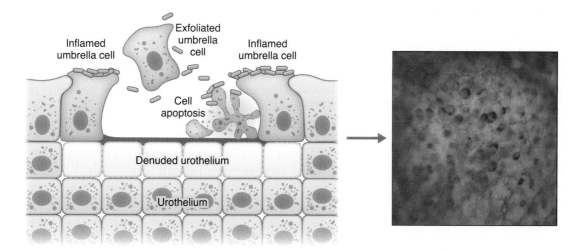

FIGURE 37.2 Host inflammatory factors. Host inflammatory response to bacteria can result in the host's umbrella cell apoptosis or exfoliation which may decrease bacterial load but also exposes the underlying transitional epithelium to continued inflammation and potential bacterial invasion.

to bacterial invasion and development of intracellular bacterial communities.[25] Although these mechanisms have yet to be fully validated in humans, women with UPEC rUTI exhibit increased inflammatory biomarkers and bladder histology similar to that of mice with chronic cystitis, suggesting that maladaptive inflammatory reactions contribute to rUTI in humans.[25] Interplay between bacteria, their communities, surrounding niches, and the host result in UTI resistance or susceptibility.[16,25] Future studies will likely continue to explore the yet-to-be-identified "core" urinary, vaginal, and gut microbiomes; the interactions between these neighboring microbiomes; and their metabolic profiles.

EVALUATION AND DIAGNOSIS: ASYMPTOMATIC BACTERIURIA, ACUTE URINARY TRACT INFECTION, AND RECURRENT URINARY TRACT INFECTION

Patient Presentation

Asymptomatic bacteriuria

Consider asymptomatic bacteriuria as the diagnosis when patients lack typical UTI symptoms as all bacteriuria may not be associated with UTI.

Uncomplicated acute lower urinary tract infection

Acute-onset dysuria is the most specific symptom of UTI. Other symptoms include new or worsening urinary frequency, urgency, or urinary incontinence; suprapubic pain; or hematuria.[3,9,33] Fever and/or flank pain differentiate acute complicated UTI involving the upper UTI (pyelonephritis) from acute uncomplicated lower UTI (cystitis).

Although UTI symptoms may be more subtle in older women, genitourinary symptoms remain specific for UTI with acute-onset dysuria or new or acutely worsening incontinence.[6,34,35] When the diagnosis is unclear, the 2019 American Urological Association (AUA)/Canadian Urological Association (CUA)/Society of Urodynamics, Female Pelvic Medicine & Urogenital Reconstruction (SUFU) guideline emphasizes the importance of chronicity in assessing UTI symptoms.[3] Worsening chronic incontinence is not reliably associated with UTI; urine testing in this setting may lead to unnecessary antibiotics.[6]

Uncomplicated recurrent lower urinary tract infection

Acute change in genitourinary symptoms suggests an acute UTI in women with rUTI. Obtain a detailed history in women presenting with rUTI, including past medical, surgical, gynecologic, and obstetric history, symptoms associated with prior UTI, related events (such as intercourse), and prior treatment (prescribed and homeopathic regimens). History should also include sequelae of treatment including antibiotic allergies, side effects, deleterious effects on the microbiome including diarrhea, *Clostridium difficile* or *Candida* infection, colonization by multidrug-resistant organisms (MDRO), and review of modifiable factors such as spermicide use and fluid intake.[1,3,9]

Laboratory Evaluation

Asymptomatic bacteriuria

AUA guidelines indicate that asymptomatic bacteriuria of any magnitude fits this definition with no upper limit of colony forming units (CFUs).[3]

Uncomplicated acute lower urinary tract infection

Empiric treatment with antibiotics based on symptoms alone has become acceptable in primary care settings based in part on cost-effectiveness analyses of UTI treatment in young women from the 1990s and early 2000s.[36,37] Neither of these models included the cost of increasing antibiotic resistance.

Society recommendations regarding empiric treatment for acute UTI differ. The American College of Obstetricians and Gynecologists (ACOG) Practice Bulletin for UTI treatment recommends urine testing, including urinalysis and/or urine culture to diagnose UTI.[1] ACOG states that women with a prior culture-proven UTI may be empirically treated without testing based on presence of symptoms similar to prior UTIs.[1] The 2018 American Urogynecologic Society (AUGS) Best-Practice Statement allows infrequent UTI to be assessed with "less rigor and treated empirically" than UTI in women with rUTI.[9] Empiric treatment is reasonable in young women with classic acute-onset dysuria without concomitant vaginal symptoms, as the probability of UTI is 90%.[33] Urine dipstick testing for leukocyte esterase or nitrites may be used as a screening test to rule out UTI in low-risk women, with a sensitivity of 75% and specificity of 82% for bacteriuria.[7] This should be followed by confirmatory urine culture in women at risk for development of MDRO, including a history in the last 3 months of prior MDRO; travel to high MDRO regions; admission to a health care facility; or treatment with fluroquinolones, trimethoprim-sulfamethoxazole (TMP-SMX), or broad-spectrum beta lactams.[7] Urinalysis demonstrating pyuria (more than 10 white blood cells per high-power field) may be clinically useful in women with symptoms less typical for UTI.[7]

Urine culture is useful in women with persistent or recurrent urinary symptoms after treatment. Clinical microbiology laboratories may offer expanded culture techniques to evaluate non–*E. coli* uropathogens.[17] Non-UTI pathology may present with dysuria. *Neisseria gonorrhoeae, Chlamydia trachomatis, Ureaplasma, Candida, Trichomonas vaginalis*, bacterial vaginosis, or human simplex virus infections may cause dysuria and should be excluded if dysuria persists after empiric antibiotics. Genitourinary syndrome of menopause, bladder pain syndrome/interstitial cystitis, and pelvic floor myalgia also cause symptoms inadvertently attributed to UTI.

Acute urinary tract infection in women with recurrent lower urinary tract infection

Extending the treatment pathway in women with a single, acute UTI to women with rUTI is not appropriate antibiotic stewardship. Urine dipstick testing is not recommended in women with rUTI as these women should have pretreatment urine culture and sensitivity testing.[3,9] To be considered a UTI requiring treatment, UTI symptoms should occur in conjunction with urinary isolation of a uropathogen, usually *E. coli* (75% to 95%). Other uropathogens include *Enterobacteriaceae, P. mirabilis, K. pneumoniae*, and *Staphylococcus saprophyticus*.[3] Surveillance testing in asymptomatic women with rUTI should not be performed; this can detect clinically insignificant bacteriuria leading to unnecessary antibiotics.[9] Young women treated with antibiotics for asymptomatic bacteriuria are more likely to develop subsequent infections and to develop antibiotic resistance than those who are untreated.[9,38]

Definitions of a positive urine culture in acute and recurrent urinary tract infection

Traditionally, bacteriuria of 10^5 CFUs/mL on clean catch voided samples defined clinically significant bacteriuria.[39] One hundred thousand CFUs per milliliter in a clean catch urine specimen was the threshold where bacteriuria on voided samples correlated with bacteriuria on catheterized samples in asymptomatic women. In women with UTI symptoms, lower colony counts on voided samples may still define a UTI. Colony counts of 10^2 CFUs/mL on voided samples have high positive predictive values for bacteriuria on catheterized samples.[40] AUA guidelines propose that >10^2 CFUs/mL may be a reasonable cutoff for bacteriuria in carefully selected (i.e., those with acute change in genitourinary symptoms) women with pyuria. The Society of Obstetricians and Gynecologists of Canada

recommends cutoffs of 10^2 CFUs/mL in symptomatic patients,[41] and European Association of Urology recommends 10^3 CFUs/mL in symptomatic patients.[42] The 2018 AUGS Best-Practice Statement notes that because microbiology laboratories may report growth less than 10^4 CFUs/mL as "no growth," it is important to know local laboratory policies. If laboratories reports urine cultures as "contaminated" in symptomatic patients, consider repeat testing with catheterized samples.[3]

Physical Examination and Imaging

Uncomplicated acute lower urinary tract infection

A physical examination or additional diagnostic testing is not necessary in women with acute uncomplicated UTI.

Uncomplicated recurrent urinary tract infection or refractory urinary tract infection

Abdominopelvic examination including postvoid residual is recommended in women with rUTI or persistent symptoms after antibiotic treatment.[3,9] There are no specific guidelines for imaging in women with rUTI. AUA/CUA/SUFU guidelines do not recommend imaging in patients initially presenting with rUTI. A meta-analysis of the utility of cystoscopy and imaging in women with uncomplicated rUTI found that cystoscopy and upper tract imaging were not useful.[43] Another study found that only 3.8% of patients with rUTI had specific findings on cystoscopy.[44] Cystourethroscopy and upper urinary tract imaging is appropriate in a woman with prior pelvic surgery, a clinical history concerning for fistula, or with clinical worsening. AUA/CUA/SUFU guidelines suggests imaging in patients with complicated UTI or prior pelvic surgery[3]; ACOG recommends imaging women who do not respond to appropriate antibiotic treatment for UTI[1]; and AUGS recommends imaging women with worsening clinical status, rapid recurrence after treatment, suspected stones or obstruction, and in those with anatomic abnormalities or history of genitourinary surgery.[9]

A renal ultrasound is recommended as first-line imaging to evaluate renal obstruction and does not expose the patient to radiation. CT urogram may also be used to evaluate the genitourinary system for possible abscess or stones,[1] although a simple X-ray may identify stones. A CT urogram is the preferred modality to evaluate pyelonephritis or perinephric abscess in nonpregnant women for whom imaging will alter clinical care.

Future diagnostic tools

Molecular diagnostic and next-generation testing

Novel urine diagnostics are gaining in popularity but present a clinical challenge because these are relatively new tools. The promise of these tests lies in their potential to rapidly detect uropathogens and confirm antibiotic sensitivity. Next-generation sequencing detects nucleic material consistent with the signatures of particular uropathogens. In contrast to next-generation sequencing, molecular sensing mechanisms detect living microbes using machine learning to conduct rapid antibiotic sensitivity testing. These new diagnostic methods may allow identification of antimicrobial susceptibility within hours in contrast to traditional culture and sensitivity testing. Currently, there are insufficient data to interpret these tests or guide treatment based on their results.

TREATMENT: ASYMPTOMATIC BACTERIURIA, ACUTE UNCOMPLICATED URINARY TRACT INFECTION, RECURRENT URINARY TRACT INFECTION

The Infectious Diseases Society of America (IDSA) describes appropriate UTI treatment as that providing "the shortest effective course."[45] Antibiotic stewardship is critical to combat antibiotic resistance and its threat to public health. Antibiotic resistance increases in a dose-dependent manner with antibiotic exposure. The incidence of extended spectrum beta lactamase producing *Enterobacteriaceae* in urine of kidney transplant recipients rose from 13% to 45% from the first to third UTI episode.[46] Understanding antibiotics' deleterious effects on microbial ecology and on overall antibiotic resistance currently guides UTI treatment.

Treatment of Asymptomatic Bacteriuria

Treatment of asymptomatic bacteriuria is recommended in specific populations and clinical circumstances. See Table 37.1 for IDSA guidance on screening and treatment in special populations.[45] The IDSA recommends screening and treatment of asymptomatic bacteriuria in early pregnancy to reduce pyelonephritis and potentially low birth weight and premature labor. A 2019 Cochrane review of 15 randomized controlled trials found treatment decreased pyelonephritis risk, although data regarding preterm delivery and low birth weight reduction were less robust.[47] Clinicians also often screen and treat elderly women with altered mental status or functional decline for bacteriuria. The IDSA reviewed available observational data and issued a "strong recommendation" not to treat bacteriuria in older adults with decreased functional or cognitive status *without* the presence of genitourinary symptoms.[45] Although earlier observational studies found increased prevalence of bacteriuria in patients with delirium, these studies inadequately controlled for confounders (age, comorbidities, reduced mobility). Subsequent studies adjusting for these factors did not show higher prevalence of bacteriuria in delirium patients nor did antibiotic treatment

TABLE 37.1

Guidance on Screening for Asymptomatic Bacteriuria in Special Populations

POPULATION	IDSA (2019) RECOMMENDATIONS
Pregnancy	Screen and treat once. Insufficient data guiding retest or retreatment
Older, functionally or cognitively impaired	Do not screen or treat.
Diabetics	Do not screen or treat.
Patients with an indwelling bladder catheter (<30 d)	Do not screen or treat. Insufficient data guiding screening or treating at the time of catheter removal
Patients with an indwelling bladder catheter (>30 d)	Do not screen or treat.
Patients undergoing nonurologic surgery	Do not screen or treat.
Patients undergoing endourologic surgery (associated with mucosal trauma)	Screen and treat preoperatively to reduce sepsis. A short course (1–2 doses) is recommended rather than prolonged.

From Nicolle LE, Gupta K, Bradley SF, et al. Clinical practice guideline for management of asymptomatic bacteriuria: 2019 Update by the Infectious Diseases Society of America. *Clin Infect Dis* 2019;68(10):e83–e110 and Owens DK, Davidson KW, Krist AH, et al; and the U.S. Preventive Task Force. Screening for asymptomatic bacteriuria in adults: US Preventive Services Task Force recommendation statement. *JAMA* 2019;322(12):1188–1194.

increase their survival; the studies did show increased morbidity from adverse drug reactions and antimicrobial resistance.[34,45,48–50]

Treatment of Acute Uncomplicated Urinary Tract Infection

Antibiotics are usually prescribed for acute, uncomplicated UTI. The 2018 AUGS Best-Practice Statement for rUTI states that nonantimicrobial, symptomatic (or "conditional") treatment, including nonsteroidal anti-inflammatory use, may treat UTI symptoms in young, healthy women, followed by antibiotics if symptoms persist or progress.[9] Conditional treatment results in

UTI resolution in 47% to 54% of women, although the risk of pyelonephritis (2% to 5%) is higher than in those treated with nonsteroidals compared to antibiotics.[51,52] Despite usual treatment of acute cystitis with antimicrobials, the low risk of progression to upper tract infection offers reassurance that awaiting urine cultures prior to prescribing antibiotics is safe.

IDSA Guidelines for uncomplicated, acute UTI treatment recommends that antimicrobials chosen for first-line therapy maximize clinical efficacy and minimize risk of collateral microbial ecologic harm.[53] These antibiotics, their bacterial coverage, and dosages are in Table 37.2. First-line treatment includes nitrofurantoin monohydrate macrocrystals, TMP-SMX, or fosfomycin

TABLE 37.2

Recommended Oral Antibiotic Regimens for Acute Uncomplicated Lower Urinary Tract Infection

ANTIMICROBIAL	DOSING	UROPATHOGEN COVERAGE	SERIOUS ADVERSE EFFECTS
Nitrofurantoin Monohydrate/Macrocrystals			
	100 mg twice daily for 5 d	Relatively narrow uropathogen coverage; *Escherichia coli, Enterococcus faecalis, Klebsiella pneumoniae, Staphylococcus saprophyticus*, including beta lactamase producing	Pulmonary fibrosis (with prolonged use), peripheral neuropathy Decreased efficacy in reduced renal function (CrCl <30 mL/min)
TMP-SMX			
	160/800 mg (1 double-strength tablet) twice daily for 3 d	Broad gram-negative bacilli coverage, *Staphylococcus aureus* (including MRSA)	Toxic epidermal necrolysis, neurologic effects (tremor, gait changes), blood dyscrasia, hemolysis (G6PD deficiency), P450 enzyme inhibition
Fosfomycin Trometamol			
	3 g once	*E. coli, E. faecalis, K. pneumoniae*, including beta lactamase producing	
Beta Lactam Agents (Amoxicillin-Clavulanate, Cefdinir, Cefaclor, Cefalexin, Cefpodoxime-Proxetil)			
	3–7 d	Non–beta lactamase-producing gram-negative bacilli (including *E. coli, K. pneumoniae*)	Relatively high rate of collateral ecologic damage (selection for MDRO, *Clostridium difficile* colitis)
Fluoroquinolones			
	Twice daily for 3 d	Broad gram-negative bacilli coverage including beta lactamase producing	QT prolongation, tendonitis, peripheral neuropathy, aortic dissection, aortic aneurysm rupture
Fluconazole			
	200 mg daily for 2 wk	*Candida albicans*; less activity against *Candida glabrata* and *Candida krusei*	P450 enzyme inhibition

CrCl, creatinine clearance; MRSA, methicillin-resistant *Staphylococcus aureus*; G6PD, glucose-6-phosphate dehydrogenase.

From Kronenberg A, Bütikofer L, Odutayo A, et al. Symptomatic treatment of uncomplicated lower urinary tract infections in the ambulatory setting: Randomised, double blind trial. *BMJ* 2017;359:j4784.

Adapted from information in Gupta K, Hooton TM, Naber KG, et al. International clinical practice guidelines for the treatment of acute uncomplicated cystitis and pyelonephritis in women: A 2010 update by the Infectious Diseases Society of America and the European Society for Microbiology and Infectious Diseases. *Clin Infect Dis* 2011;52(5):e103–e120 and Pappas PG, Kauffman CA, Andes DR, et al. Clinical practice guideline for the management of candidiasis: 2016 Update by the Infectious Diseases Society of America. *Clin Infect Dis* 2016;62(4):e1–e50.

(pivmecillinam, unavailable in North America, is excluded from Table 37.2). In the event of allergy or documented microbial resistance, fluoroquinolones or beta lactams (avoiding ampicillin or amoxicillin alone) may be used. True allergy, compared to antibiotic intolerance, should be based on patient history. Allergy testing is beneficial in women with rUTI and childhood or unclear penicillin allergy.

Nitrofurantoin, TMP-SMX, and fosfomycin have clinical cure rates of 88% to 100% with minimal collateral damage to the gut and vaginal microbiomes. Nitrofurantoin's renal excretion and urinary concentration decreases its efficacy in patients with decreased creatinine clearance (see Table 37.2). As nitrofurantoin is bacteriostatic and not bactericidal, it should not be used in suspected pyelonephritis. Prolonged nitrofurantoin use has been reported (rarely) to be associated with pulmonary fibrosis due to buildup of metabolites.[9] TMP-SMX covers a broad treatment spectrum. Due to growing bacterial resistance to TMP-SMX, clinicians should limit its use if local resistance is >20%.[3] Fosfomycin tromethamine benefits include its relatively low levels of antimicrobial resistance as well as its single dosing regimen, attributable to its persistence in urine for 30 to 40 hours.[5,54,55]

When antibiotic resistance or patient allergies/intolerance limit first-line therapies, clinicians may initiate second-line regimens. These do have limitations. Beta lactams (cefpodoxime, cefixime, cefalexin) can be used but have lower cure rates than TMP-SMX and fluoroquinolones.[20,39] Amoxicillin and ampicillin are not concentrated in urine and have poor efficacy. Their rare use should be guided by antibiotic sensitivity testing.[32,39] Due to increasing resistance and adverse events, fluoroquinolones are not first-line treatments.[45,53]

Treatment of Uncomplicated Recurrent Urinary Tract Infection

Because of increased antibiotic resistance in women with rUTI, clinicians should await sensitivity results prior to prescribing antibiotics. If waiting is not clinically feasible, patient history and local antibiogram sensitivities should guide antibiotic choice. Antimicrobial therapy guidelines for rUTI are similar to guidelines for acute UTI. Duration of treatment for acute UTI in women with rUTI is unknown but recommended to be no longer than 7 days and individualized as clinically appropriate.[3,9] Evidence favors shorter compared to longer (5- to 7-day) treatment for acute and rUTI due to similar effectiveness in symptom relief, improved compliance, decreased costs, and lower rates of adverse reaction.[53,56,57] Because of high rates of bacteriuria, UTI symptoms should drive urine culture testing. Clinicians should not perform a posttreatment "test of cure" in asymptomatic patients but should use urine cultures to guide further treatment in women with persistent symptoms.[3]

The 2018 AUGS Best-Practice Statement and AUA/CUA/SUFU 2019 guidelines confirm that clinicians may offer self-start treatment in carefully selected patients unable to submit urine specimens prior to therapy. Appropriate patients for self-start antibiotics are those who clearly recognize UTI symptoms, are inappropriate for long-term prophylaxis, or do not wish to take daily antibiotics.[3,9] These patients should seek care if symptoms do not improve in a short time frame (AUGS recommends 48 hours). In acute cystitis resistant to all oral antibiotics, parental antibiotics can be used for as short a duration as necessary and for no longer than 7 days.[3]

Patients with rUTI are at risk for developing candiduria due to deleterious effects of repeated antimicrobial use on the normal genitourinary microbiome. In 2016, the IDSA issued Practice Guidelines for candidiasis management, including candiduria.[58] The IDSA did not recommend treating asymptomatic candiduria unless the patient was at high risk for disseminated candidemia (neutropenic patients or those undergoing urologic manipulation). Like asymptomatic bacteriuria, asymptomatic candiduria rarely leads to systemic infection.[59,60]

Candida albicans is the most common cause of symptomatic candida cystitis. Recommended treatment for *C. albicans* cystitis is fluconazole 200 mg daily for 2 weeks.[61] Fluconazole is renally excreted, reaching urinary concentrations 10 to 20 times that of serum.[62] Organisms resistant to fluconazole, such as *Candida glabrata*, are treated with amphotericin B deoxycholate, 0.3 to 0.6 mg/kg daily × 1 to 7 days or oral flucytosine, 25 mg/kg four times daily.[61] *Candida krusei* is treated with amphotericin B deoxycholate, 0.3 to 0.6 mg/kg daily × 1 to 7 days. Alternatively, amphotericin B deoxycholate bladder irrigation (50 mg/L sterile water daily × 5 days) decreases toxicity.[58]

PREVENTION OF RECURRENT URINARY TRACT INFECTION

Preventive strategies of varying efficacy may reduce rUTI in women. These include diluting or acidifying urine, decreasing bacterial load, preventing bacterial adhesion, or outcompeting uropathogenic bacteria by restoring a normal local microbiome. Risk–benefit discussions are essential to set expectations and foster shared decision-making.

Vaginal estrogen and prophylactic antibiotics are the best-studied preventive treatments. In postmenopausal women with rUTI, vaginal estrogen has the best efficacy to side effect profile for UTI prevention.

Low-dose vaginal estrogen is available in cream, suppository, or ring formulations. Vaginal estrogen restores abundance of hydrogen peroxide-producing *Lactobacillus* in the vaginal microbiome, decreasing vaginal pH and *Enterobacteriaceae*.[9] Vaginal estrogen also improves genitourinary syndrome of menopause symptoms, including voiding discomfort that may be confused with UTI.[63] AUGS Guidelines reviewed two seminal randomized controlled trials regarding vaginal estrogen in postmenopausal women with rUTI: (1) a comparison of vaginal estriol cream versus placebo reported fewer UTI episodes in the estriol group (0.5 vs. 5.9 UTI episodes per patient-year, $P < .001$) with greater likelihood of being UTI-free at 4 months (0.95 [95% CI 0.88 to 1] vs. 0.30 [95% CI 0.16 to 0.46]) and (2) a comparison of estradiol vaginal ring versus no treatment found that at 9 months the likelihood of remaining UTI free in the estradiol group was approximately 45% versus 20% in controls ($P = .008$).[9] Although data suggest low systemic absorption of low-dose vaginal estrogen and no increased morbidity or mortality from estrogen-mediated disease,[64–66] women may be reluctant to use exogenous estrogen. This is especially true in those with a history of estrogen-dependent cancer or antiestrogen therapy following cancer treatment. Collaboration with oncology may be useful when treating these women.

Oral antibiotic prophylaxis can be offered postcoitally or daily in appropriate women to reduce rUTI. The 2019 AUA/CUA/SUFU guideline, reporting pooled results of prophylactic antibiotics compared to placebo or no antibiotic, found antibiotics decreased likelihood of UTI recurrence (RR 0.26, 95% CI 0.18 to 0.37).[3] Continuous therapy consists of a daily low dose antibiotic. AUGS recommends a negative urine culture prior to initiating therapy, reviewing efficacy of continuous prophylaxis after 3 months of treatment, typically continuing no longer than 6 months.[9] A postcoital antibiotic taken immediately after intercourse is appropriate for UTI temporally associated with sexual activity. This therapy is as effective as daily therapy.[67]

Intravesical drug administration for rUTI prophylaxis offers targeted therapy with reduced side effects. Case series using gentamicin irrigation in patients with complicated rUTI suggest that it is safe, effective, and is an option for treatment of MDRO.[68,69] This offers targeted delivery into the bladder without the potentially deleterious effects of systemic administration. Intravesical, nonantibiotic instillations of chondroitin sulfate, heparin, and hyaluronic acid may also reduce rUTI via urothelial glycosaminoglycan restoration.[70–72]

Evidence is conflicting regarding efficacy of existing rUTI products that interfere with bacterial adhesion. Mechanistically, cranberry supplement's proanthocynidin compounds (PAC) inhibit *E. coli* binding to the urothelium. PAC concentrations differ between cranberry formulations (juice, cocktail, tablet), making it difficult to pool study findings. National societies disagree on the utility of cranberry supplements for rUTI prevention. A 2012 Cochrane review concluded that evidence was insufficient to recommend cranberry supplementation for rUTI.[73] A synopsis by the same authors noted that the volume of cranberry juice consumption required for prophylaxis resulted in poor adherence and that the active ingredient was only available for 10 to 12 hours, likely limiting its efficacy. The authors recommended that future trials require therapeutic amounts of PACs, 36 mg per day.[74] The AUA/CUA/SUFU 2019 systematic review pooled five studies of cranberry versus placebo and concluded that cranberry was associated with decreased risk of rUTI (RR 0.67 [95% CI 0.54 to 0.83]).[3] After reviewing the limits and heterogeneity of the available studies, the AUA/CUA/SUFU guideline stated that clinicians could offer cranberry prophylaxis for rUTI (grade C evidence). In contrast, the AUGS 2018 Best-Practice Statement concludes that cranberry supplementation is ineffective for UTI prevention. Overall, cranberry supplementation seems to be low risk, although juice formulations may contribute to hyperglycemia in sensitive populations. D-mannose is a sugar that, like cranberry, prevents bacterial adhesion to the urothelium. A recent meta-analysis concluded that D-mannose appeared well tolerated and was protective for rUTI versus placebo (RR 0.23, 95% CI 0.14 to 0.37) with possible similar effectiveness as antibiotics (RR 0.39, 95% CI 0.12 to 1.25).[75]

Methenamine salts have also been reported to decrease rUTI. Methenamine converts to formaldehyde and ammonia in the urine, creating a bacteriostatic environment with 1 g twice daily being the smallest dose studied. A 2012 Cochrane review concluded methenamine studies were limited by heterogeneity in outcome definitions and study populations.[76] The review did conclude that short-term methenamine treatment (≤1 week) might be effective in those with an anatomically normal urinary tract.

Oral hydration in premenopausal women represents a low-risk strategy to decrease rUTI. In a single study of younger women with rUTI, hydration of ≥1.5 L per day modestly decreased acute cystitis episodes over 12 months; mean UTI episodes 1.7 (95% CI 1.5 to 1.8) hydration group versus 3.2 (95% CI 3.0 to 3.4) controls.[77] In summary, multiple UTI preventive therapies are currently used or are under investigation (Table 37.3).[25,29,78–90] Although we currently lack definitive human trials validating these potential interventions, therapeutic options are expanding.

TABLE 37.3

Possible Future Urinary Tract Infection Treatments

CATEGORY	POTENTIAL INTERVENTION	MECHANISM	EVIDENCE FOR POTENTIAL TREATMENTS AND NOTES
Alter Bacterial Adhesion			
Interfere with bacterial pili	Mannosides	Bind UPEC type 1 pili, decreasing ability to bind with host cell[25]	Based on murine models
	Galactosides	Bind with pili inhibiting adhesion to host cell[25]	Based on chronic UTI murine models
	Vaccines	Thus far, have targeted UPEC (1) type 1 pili, (2) *Staphylococcus* species, or (3) *Enterococcus* species[25]	(1) and (2) completed phase 1 clinical trials. (3) is based on murine bladder and catheter adherence.[25]
Other	Lactoferrin	Decreases UPEC adhesion to bladder epithelium and might have immune modulatory effect[25]	Intravesical human lactoferrin ↓ UPEC burden in mice and human cell adherence in vitro[25]
Alter Cell Invasion			
	Alter immune modulation to ↓ cell invasion	Use of hypoxia-inducible factor 1α to decrease UPEC cell adhesion and invasion[25,78]	In vitro and in murine models[25,78]
Alter Biofilm Formation			
	Vaccine targeting/blocking pili adhesins	Block *Enterococcus* species adhesins that bind to catheter-associated fibrinogen, decreasing biofilm production[25]	*Enterococcus* catheter–associated UTIs in mice[25]
	Target bacterial quorum sensing	Interferes with bacterial quorum sensing autoinducers responsible for intra-/interbacterial signaling, decreasing bacterial aggregation, multiplication, biofilm production[79,80]	rUTIs (e.g., UPEC), catheter/stone-associated pathogens (e.g., *Proteus*)[80]
Alter Ability to Compete for Nutrients			
	Vaccine targeting siderophores	UPEC: potentially develop vaccines targeting outer membrane UPEC siderophores/metal binding sites to ameliorate bacterial virulence[25]	UPEC rUTI in mice[25]
Increase Competition for Niches			
	Probiotics	UPEC and other pathogens Theory—increase *Lactobacillus* species to compete with pathogenic bacteria[25,29]	Variable results in vivo human UTI prophylaxis studies[3]
	Other non-UPEC *Escherichia coli*	Nonpathogenic *E. coli* may compete successfully with UPEC.[25]	Effective in some human studies[25]
	Fecal transplants	Fecal transplants treating *C. difficile* might ↓ pathogens with loss of antibiotic resistance genes.[81]	Case reports of ↓ rUTI with fecal transplants[82–85,90]
Bacterial Destruction			
	Bacteriophage therapy	Use viruses (phages) that invade and lyse uropathogenic bacteria.[86] Phage therapy might also have immune modulatory effect.[80,86,87]	United States and Western Europe use waned and stopped following ↑ antibiotics use. Available for human use in Russia/Eastern Europe.[86]

TABLE 37.3 *(Continued)*			
Possible Future Urinary Tract Infection Treatments			
CATEGORY	**POTENTIAL INTERVENTION**	**MECHANISM**	**EVIDENCE FOR POTENTIAL TREATMENTS AND NOTES**
Modify Host Immune Response			
	NSAIDs	UPEC: inhibit host inflammatory response (e.g., COX1, COX2 production) to UPEC, decrease umbrella cell sloughing[25]	Human trials demonstrate some efficacy in UTI symptom resolution.[25]
	Vaccine OM-89	*E. coli* lysate immune stimulant tested in humans.[88,89] Murine models suggested may also decrease bladder inflammation.[89]	rUTI prophylaxis: European Association of Urology[88,89] Unavailable in United States
	Other immune modulators	Stabilization of other immune modulators (e.g., HIF-1α above) ↓ host inflammatory response[25]	Murine models[25]

NSAIDs, nonsteroidal anti-inflammatory drugs; COX1, cyclooxygenase 1; COX2, cyclooxygenase 2; OM-89, Uro-Vaxom; HIF-1α, hypoxia-inducible factor 1α.

CONCLUSION

UTIs are a common and costly problem with evolving paradigms for diagnosis and treatment of acute uncomplicated UTI (acute cystitis), rUTI, and asymptomatic bacteriuria. Recent developments, including increased antibiotic resistance and advances in basic science research, have modified our understanding and treatment of UTIs. Genetic sequencing of genitourinary microbiota associated with health and disease provide insight into UTI pathophysiology, illustrating the complex interplay between the environment, host, and microbiota. The discovery that urine is not sterile informs interpretation of urine tests; clinical presentation drives treatment rather than absolute urine colony counts. The worldwide increase in antibiotic resistance highlights the need for judicious antibiotic use. Although empiric antibiotic treatment for acute cystitis may be appropriate in certain situations, when the diagnosis is uncertain, it is also reasonable to await urine culture results prior to antibiotic treatment, as progression to upper tract or systemic infection is unlikely. Acute UTI symptoms in women with rUTI also warrants, if possible, UTI confirmation with urine culture and antimicrobial sensitivity testing prior to appropriate treatment. The IDSA recommends avoidance of antibiotics for asymptomatic bacteriuria in nonpregnant women due to adverse drug reactions and worsening antibiotic resistance. Future diagnostic and therapeutic advances will continue to improve the understanding, diagnosis, and treatment of UTIs, a condition present throughout the ages. For now, the critically important tenet of antibiotic stewardship underlies culture-based treatment strategies.

References

1. American College of Obstetricians and Gynecologists. Treatment of urinary tract infections in non-pregnant women. ACOG Practice Bulletin No. 91. *Obstet Gynecol* 2008;111(3): 785–794.
2. Gupta K, Trautner BW. Diagnosis and management of recurrent urinary tract infections in non-pregnant women. *BMJ* 2013;346:f3140.
3. Anger JL, Lee U, Ackerman AL, et al. Recurrent uncomplicated urinary tract infections in women: AUA/CUA/SUFU guideline. *J Urol* 2019;202(2):282–289.
4. Shapiro DJ, Hicks LA, Pavia AT, et al. Antibiotic prescribing for adults in ambulatory care in the USA, 2007-09. *J Antimicrob Chemother* 2014;69(1):234–240.
5. Walker E, Lyman A, Gupta K, et al. Clinical management of an increasing threat: Outpatient urinary tract infections due to multidrug-resistant uropathogens. *Clin Infect Dis* 2016;63(7):960–965.
6. Mody L, Juthani-Mehta M. Urinary tract infections in older women: A clinical review. *JAMA* 2014;311(8):844–854.
7. Hooton TM, Gupta K. Acute simple cystitis in women. Published 2020. Accessed September 6, 2020. http://www.uptodate.com/contents/acute-simple-cystitis-in-women
8. Hooton TM, Gupta K. Acute complicated urinary tract infection (including pyelonephritis) in adults. Published 2020. Accessed September 6, 2020. http://www.uptodate.com/contents/acute-complicated-urinary-tract-infection-including-pyelonephritis-in-adults
9. Brubaker L, Carberry C, Nardos R, et al. American Urogynecologic Society best-practice statement: Recurrent urinary tract infection in adult women. *Female Pelvic Med Reconstr Surg* 2018;24(5):321–335.
10. Flores-Mireles AL, Walker JN, Caparon M, et al. Urinary tract infections: Epidemiology, mechanisms of infection and treatment options. *Nat Rev Microbiol* 2015;13(5):269–284.
11. Owens DK, Davidson KW, Krist AH, et al; and the U.S. Preventive Task Force. Screening for asymptomatic bacteriuria

in adults: US Preventive Services Task Force recommendation statement. *JAMA* 2019;322(12):1188–1194.

12. Institute for Genome Sciences, University of Maryland School of Medicine. NIH human microbiome project. Accessed September 8, 2020. https://www.hmpdacc.org

13. Karstens L, Asquith M, Caruso V, et al. Community profiling of the urinary microbiota: Considerations for low-biomass samples. *Nat Rev Urol* 2018;15(12):735–749.

14. Jovel J, Patterson J, Wang W, et al. Characterization of the gut microbiome using 16S or shotgun metagenomics. *Front Microbiol* 2016;7:459.

15. Human Microbiome Project Consortium. Structure, function and diversity of the healthy human microbiome. *Nature* 2012;486(7402):207–214.

16. Neugent ML, Hulyalkar NV, Nguyen VH, et al. Advances in understanding the human urinary microbiome and its potential role in urinary tract infection. *mBio* 2020;11(2):e00218–e00220.

17. Hilt EE, McKinley K, Pearce MM, et al. Urine is not sterile: Use of enhanced urine culture techniques to detect resident bacterial flora in the adult female bladder. *J Clin Microbiol* 2014;52(3):871–876.

18. Price TK, Dune T, Hilt EE, et al. The clinical urine culture: Enhanced techniques improve detection of clinically relevant microorganisms. *J Clin Microbiol* 2016;54(5):1216–1222.

19. Hickey RJ, Zhou X, Pierson JD, et al. Understanding vaginal microbiome complexity from an ecological perspective. *Transl Res* 2012;160(4):267–282.

20. Ravel J, Gajer P, Abdo Z, et al. Vaginal microbiome of reproductive-age women. *Proc Natl Acad Sci U S A* 2011;108(Suppl 1): 4680–4687.

21. Brotman RM, Shardell MD, Gajer P, et al. Association between the vaginal microbiota, menopause status, and signs of vulvovaginal atrophy. *Menopause* 2014;21(5):450–458.

22. Amabebe E, Anumba DOC. The vaginal microenvironment: The physiologic role of *Lactobacilli*. *Front Med (Lausanne)* 2018;5:181.

23. Komesu YM, Dinwiddie DL, Richter HE, et al. Defining the relationship between vaginal and urinary microbiomes. *Am J Obstet Gynecol* 2020;222(2):154.e1–154.e10.

24. Stapleton AE, Au-Yeung M, Hooton TM, et al. Randomized, placebo-controlled phase 2 trial of a Lactobacillus crispatus probiotic given intravaginally for prevention of recurrent urinary tract infection. *Clin Infect Dis* 2011;52(10):1212–1217.

25. Klein RD, Hultgren SJ. Urinary tract infections: Microbial pathogenesis, host-pathogen interactions and new treatment strategies. *Nat Rev Microbiol* 2020;18(4):211–226.

26. Hannan TJ, Totsika M, Mansfield KJ, et al. Host-pathogen checkpoints and population bottlenecks in persistent and intracellular uropathogenic *Escherichia coli* bladder infection. *FEMS Microbiol Rev* 2012;36(3):616–648.

27. Duraiswamy S, Chee JLY, Chen S, et al. Purification of intracellular bacterial communities during experimental urinary tract infection reveals an abundant and viable bacterial reservoir. *Infect Immun* 2018;86(4):e00740-17.

28. Younes JA, van der Mei HC, van den Heuvel E, et al. Adhesion forces and coaggregation between vaginal staphylococci and lactobacilli. *PLoS One* 2012;7(5):e36917.

29. Salas-Jara MJ, Ilabaca A, Vega M, et al. Biofilm forming *Lactobacillus*: New challenges for the development of probiotics. *Microorganisms* 2016;4(3):35.

30. Ventolini G, Mitchell E, Salazar M. Biofilm formation by vaginal *Lactobacillus* in vivo. *Med Hypotheses* 2015;84(5):417–420.

31. Martinez S, Garcia JG, Williams R, et al. *Lactobacilli spp.*: Real-time evaluation of biofilm growth. *BMC Microbiol* 2020;20(1):64.

32. Adebayo AS, Ackermann G, Bowyer RCE, et al. The urinary tract microbiome in older women exhibits host genetic and environmental influences. *Cell Host Microbe* 2020;28(2):298–305.

33. Hooton T. Uncomplicated urinary tract infection. *N Engl J Med* 2012;366(11):1028–1037.

34. Juthani-Mehta M, Quagliarello V, Perrelli E, et al. Clinical features to identify urinary tract infection in nursing home residents: A cohort study. *J Am Geriatr Soc* 2009;57(6):963–970.

35. Medina-Bombardo D, Segui-Diaz M, Roca-Fusalba C, et al. What is the predictive value of urinary symptoms for diagnosing urinary tract infection in women? *Fam Pract* 2003;20(2):103–107.

36. Barry HC, Ebell MH, Hickner J. Evaluation of suspected urinary tract infection in ambulatory women: A cost-utility analysis of office-based strategies. *J Fam Pract* 1997;44(1):49–60.

37. Fenwick EA, Briggs AH, Hawke CI. Management of urinary tract infection in general practice: A cost-effectiveness analysis. *Br J Gen Pract* 2000;50(457):635–639.

38. Cai T, Nesi G, Mazzoli S, et al. Asymptomatic bacteriuria treatment is associated with a higher prevalence of antibiotic resistant strains in women with urinary tract infections. *Clin Infect Dis* 2015;61(11):1655–1661.

39. Platt R. Quantitative definition of bacteriuria. *Am J Med* 1983;75(1B):44–52.

40. Giesen LG, Cousins G, Dimitrov BD, et al. Predicting acute uncomplicated urinary tract infection in women: A systematic review of the diagnostic accuracy of symptoms and signs. *BMC Fam Pract* 2010;11:78.

41. Epp A, Larochelle A. No. 250—Recurrent urinary tract infection. *J Obstet Gynaecol Can* 2017;39(10):e422–e431.

42. Grabe M, Bartoletti R, Bjerklund Johansen TE, et al. Guidelines on urological infections. Accessed September 30, 2020. https://uroweb.org/wp-content/uploads/18-Urological-Infections_LR.pdf

43. Santoni N, Ng A, Skews R, et al. Recurrent urinary tract infections in women: What is the evidence for investigating with flexible cystoscopy, imaging and urodynamics? *Urol Int* 2018;101(4):373–381.

44. Pagano MJ, Barbalat Y, Theofanides MC, et al. Diagnostic yield of cystoscopy in the evaluation of recurrent urinary tract infection in women. *Neurourol Urodyn* 2017;36(3):692–696.

45. Nicolle LE, Gupta K, Bradley SF, et al. Clinical practice guideline for the management of asymptomatic bacteriuria: 2019 Update by the Infectious Diseases Society of America. *Clin Infect Dis* 2019;68(10):e83–e110.

46. Pinheiro HS, Mituiassu AM, Carminatti M, et al. Urinary tract infection caused by extended-spectrum beta-lactamase-producing bacteria in kidney transplant patients. *Transplant Proc* 2010;42(2):486–487.

47. Smaill FM, Vazquez JC. Antibiotics for asymptomatic bacteriuria in pregnancy. *Cochrane Database Syst Rev* 2019;(11):CD000490.

48. Petty LA, Vaughn VM, Flanders SA, et al. Risk factors and outcomes associated with treatment of asymptomatic bacteriuria in hospitalized patients. *JAMA Intern Med* 2019;179(11):1519–1527.

49. Balogun SA, Philbrick JT. Delirium, a symptom of UTI in the elderly: Fact or fable? A systematic review. *Can Geriatr J* 2014;17(1):22–26.

50. Das R, Towle V, Van Ness PH, et al. Adverse outcomes in nursing home residents with increased episodes of observed bacteriuria. *Infect Control Hosp Epidemiol* 2011;32(1):84–86.

51. Gagyor I, Bleidorn J, Kocen M, et al. Ibuprofen versus fosfomycin for uncomplicated urinary tract infection in women: Randomised controlled trial. *BMJ* 2015;351:h6544.

52. Kronenberg A, Bütikofer L, Odutayo A, et al. Symptomatic treatment of uncomplicated lower urinary tract infections in the ambulatory setting: Randomised, double blind trial. *BMJ* 2017;359:j4784.

53. Gupta K, Hooton TM, Naber KG, et al. International clinical practice guidelines for the treatment of acute uncomplicated cystitis and pyelonephritis in women: A 2010 update by the Infectious Diseases Society of America and the European Society for Microbiology and Infectious Diseases. *Clin Infect Dis* 2011;52(5):e103–e120.

54. Seroy JT, Grim SA, Reid GE, et al. Treatment of MDR urinary tract infections with oral fosfomycin: A retrospective analysis. *J Antimicrob Chemother* 2016;71(9):2563–2568.

55. Michalopoulos AS, Livaditis IG, Gougoutas V. The revival of fosfomycin. *Int J Infect Dis* 2011;15(11):e732–e739.

56. Hooton T. Recurrent urinary tract infection in women. *Int J Antimicrob Agents* 2001;17:259–268.

57. Milo G, Katchman E, Paul M, et al. Duration of antibacterial treatment for uncomplicated urinary tract infection in women. *Cochrane Database Syst Rev* 2005;(2):CD004682.

58. Pappas PG, Kauffman CA, Andes DR, et al. Clinical practice guideline for the management of candidiasis: 2016 Update by the Infectious Diseases Society of America. *Clin Infect Dis* 2016;62(4):e1–e50.

59. Kauffman C, Vazquez J, Sobel J, et al. Prospective multicenter surveillance study of funguria in hospitalized patients. *Clin Infect Dis* 2000;30(1):14–18.

60. Paul N, Mathai E, Abraham O, et al. Factors associated with candiduria and related mortality. *J Infect* 2007;55(5):450–455.

61. Fisher JF, Sobel JD, Kauffman CA, et al. Candida urinary tract infections—treatment. *Clin Infect Dis* 2011;52(Suppl 6):S457–S466.

62. Ashley ESD, Lewis R, Lewis JS, et al. Pharmacology of systemic antifungal agents. *Clin Infect Dis* 2006;43(Suppl 1):S28–S39.

63. Rahn DD, Carberry C, Sanses TV, et al. Vaginal estrogen for genitourinary syndrome of menopause: A systematic review. *Obstet Gynecol* 2014;124(6):1147–1156.

64. Sánchez-Rovira P, Hirschberg A, Gil-Gil M, et al. A phase II prospective, randomized, double-blind, placebo-controlled and multicenter clinical trial to assess the safety of 0.005% estriol vaginal gel in hormone receptor-positive postmenopausal women with early stage breast cancer in treatment with aromatase inhibitor in the adjuvant setting. *Oncologist* 2020;25(12):e1846–e1854.

65. Chambers LM, Herrmann A, Michener CM, et al. Vaginal estrogen use for genitourinary symptoms in women with a history of uterine, cervical, or ovarian carcinoma. *Int J Gynecol Cancer* 2020;30(4):515–524.

66. Streff A, Chu-Pilli M, Stopeck A, et al. Changes in serum estradiol levels with Estring in postmenopausal women with breast cancer treated with aromatase inhibitors. *Support Care Cancer* 2021;29(1):187–191.

67. Stapleton A, Latham R, Johnson C, et al. Postcoital antimicrobial prophylaxis for recurrent urinary tract infection. *JAMA* 1990;264(6):703–706.

68. Stalenhoef JE, Nieuwkoop Cv, Menken PH, et al. Intravesical gentamicin treatment for recurrent urinary tract infections caused by multidrug resistant bacteria. *J Urol* 2019;201(3):549–555.

69. van Nieuwkoop C, den Exter PL, Elzevier HW, et al. Intravesical gentamicin for recurrent urinary tract infection in patients with intermittent bladder catheterisation. *Int J Antimicrob Agents* 2010;36(6):485–490.

70. Damiano R, Quarto G, Bava I, et al. Prevention of recurrent urinary tract infections by intravesical administration of hyaluronic acid and chondroitin sulphate: A placebo-controlled randomised trial. *Eur Urol* 2011;59(4):645–651.

71. Dutta S, Lane F. Intravesical instillations for the treatment of refractory recurrent urinary tract infections. *Ther Adv Urol* 2018;10(5):157–163.

72. De Vita D, Giordano S. Effectiveness of intravesical hyaluronic acid/chondroitin sulfate in recurrent bacterial cystitis: A randomized study. *Int Urogynecol J* 2012;23(12):1707–1713.

73. Jepson R, Williams G, Craig JC. Cranberries for preventing urinary tract infections. *Cochrane Database Syst Rev* 2012;(10):CD001321.

74. Jepson R, Craig JC, Williams G. Cranberry products and prevention of urinary tract infections. *JAMA* 2013;310(13):1395–1396.

75. Lenger S, Bradley M, Thomas D, et al. D-mannose vs other agents for recurrent urinary tract infection prevention in adult women: A systematic review and meta-analysis. *Am J Obstet Gynecol* 2020;223(2):265.e1–265.e3.

76. Lee BS, Bhuta T, Simpson JM, et al. Methenamine hippurate for preventing urinary tract infections. *Cochrane Database Syst Rev* 2012;(10):CD003265.

77. Hooton TM, Vecchio M, Iroz A, et al. Effect of increased daily water intake in premenopausal women with recurrent urinary tract infections: A randomized clinical trial. *JAMA Intern Med* 2018;178(11):1509–1515.

78. Liu AE, Beasley FC, Olson J, et al. Role of hypoxia inducible factor-1alpha (HIF-1alpha) in innate defense against uropathogenic *Escherichia coli* infection. *PLoS Pathog* 2015;11(4):e1004818.

79. Dickey SW, Cheung GYC, Otto M. Different drugs for bad bugs: Antivirulence strategies in the age of antibiotic resistance. *Nat Rev Drug Discov* 2017;16(7):457–471.

80. Delcaru C, Alexandru I, Podgoreanu P, et al. Microbial biofilms in urinary tract infections and prostatitis: Etiology, pathogenicity, and combating strategies. *Pathogens* 2016;5(4):65.

81. Allegretti JR, Kassam Z, Mullish BH, et al. Effects of fecal microbiota transplantation with oral capsules in obese patients. *Clin Gastroenterol Hepatol* 2020;18(4):855–863.e2.

82. Tariq R, Pardi DS, Tosh PK, et al. Fecal microbiota transplantation for recurrent *Clostridium difficile* infection reduces recurrent urinary tract infection frequency. *Clin Infect Dis* 2017;65(10):1745–1747.

83. Biehl LM, Cruz Aguilar R, Farowski F, et al. Fecal microbiota transplantation in a kidney transplant recipient with recurrent urinary tract infection. *Infection* 2018;46(6):871–874.

84. Hocquart M, Pham T, Kuete E, et al. Successful fecal microbiota transplantation in a patient suffering from irritable bowel syndrome and recurrent urinary tract infections. *Open Forum Infect Dis* 2019;6(10):ofz398.

85. Wang T, Kraft CS, Woodworth MH, et al. Fecal microbiota transplant for refractory *Clostridium difficile* infection interrupts 25-year history of recurrent urinary tract infections. *Open Forum Infect Dis* 2018;5(2):ofy016.

86. Garretto A, Miller-Ensminger T, Wolfe AJ, et al. Bacteriophages of the lower urinary tract. *Nat Rev Urol* 2019;16(7):422–432.

87. de Miguel T, Rama JLR, Sieiro C, et al. Bacteriophages and lysins as possible alternatives to treat antibiotic-resistant urinary tract infections. *Antibiotics (Basel)* 2020;9(8):466.

88. Bankat G, Bartoletti R, Bruyère F, et al. EAU guidelines on urological infections. Accessed Oct 20, 2020. https://uroweb.org/guideline/urological-infections/

89. Haddad JM, Ubertazzi E, Cabrera OS, et al. Latin American consensus on uncomplicated recurrent urinary tract infection—2018. *Int Urogynecol J* 2020;31(1):35–44.

90. Jeney SES, Lane F, Oliver A, et al. Fecal microbiota transplantation for the treatment of refractory recurrent urinary tract infection. *Obstet Gynecol* 2020;136(4):771–773.

CHAPTER 38

Painful Conditions of the Lower Urinary Tract and Bladder

Kristina Cvach • Anna Rosamilia

Introduction

Painful conditions of the bladder and urethra fall under chronic pelvic pain syndrome (CPPS) as outlined in the International Association for the Study of Pain taxonomy document.[1] In general, these conditions present with persistent or recurrent pain that the patient attributes to the bladder or urethra with no identifiable local pathology as the causative agent. Although peripheral mechanisms exist, central nervous system neuromodulation may be more important and systemic disorders such as fibromyalgia, irritable bowel syndrome, or chronic fatigue syndrome may also be present.[2] As in most chronic pain states, there is an association with emotional, behavioral, and sexual dysfunction.

Although diagnosis and management of CPPS is challenging, much can be achieved by employing the primary principles of pain management: education; psychological support; and physical, medical, and complementary and alternative medical (CAM) therapies. Using multiple strategies and working across craft groups, to provide multimodal and multidisciplinary management, provides optimal care of the patient with chronic pain.

BLADDER PAIN SYNDROME

Bladder pain syndrome (BPS) is a condition characterized by pain attributable to the bladder. Although at least one other bladder-related symptom (urinary frequency/nocturia and/or urgency) is required to define the syndrome, pain perception is always the primary complaint. The use of the word *syndrome* connotes that pain is the disease process where the role of the nervous system in generating the sensations is pivotal. Patients may have difficulty describing their symptoms and not always report the presence of pain. The use of the word *pain* has many cultural overtones; for instance, in Japan women would rarely volunteer the symptom of pain.[3] Other descriptors used may be pressure, discomfort, burning, or a constant awareness of the bladder. The urinary frequency is driven by fear of pain or discomfort,

not of incontinence; this is a key difference with overactive bladder syndrome. Patients often describe increasing pain/pressure with bladder filling and relief, albeit temporary, with voiding; however, many patients will also describe dysuria or increasing pain after voiding.

It is important to exclude other conditions with overlapping symptomatology such as urinary tract infection, overactive bladder syndrome, urethral diverticulum, or underlying bladder pathology such as malignancy. The duration of symptoms needed to be classified as BPS varies according to different guidelines. The American Urological Association (AUA) only requires 6 weeks of symptoms in an effort to institute treatment in a timely fashion.[4] The European Association of Urology (EAU) and the European Society for the Study of Bladder Pain Syndrome/Interstitial Cystitis (ESSIC) define the condition if there has been persistent or recurrent pain over 6 months, in an effort to capture those patients with fluctuating symptoms.[5,6] However, there is an absence of evidence to support either definition of BPS based on duration of symptoms. This has prompted the most recent publication from the International Consultation on Incontinence (ICI) Committee to suggest that the duration of symptoms required to diagnose the chronic condition be up to the discretion of the clinician and patient.[7]

Interstitial cystitis (IC) was first described by Skene[8] as an inflammatory condition destroying the mucous membrane of the bladder, but over the last two decades, the nomenclature has changed to reflect a broader symptom complex defined as BPS which is not necessarily associated with histologic changes. A full description of the historical changes in terminology is beyond the scope of this chapter but can be found in the ICI BPS document.[7] In 1915, Hunner described a bladder ulcer, now termed *Hunner lesion* (HL), identified at time of cystoscopy in patients with frequency and bladder pain. HL, although initially thought to have a prevalence rate of 5% to 10% of BPS patients, has also been reported with prevalence rates of up to 57%.[9,10] The appearance is of patches of red mucosa and small vessels radiating to a central pale scar, which

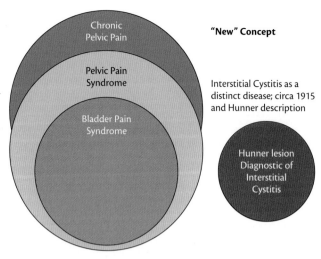

FIGURE 38.1 International Consultation conception of bladder pain syndrome and interstitial cystitis. (From Abrams P, Cardozo L, Wagg A, Wein A. *Incontinence*, 6th ed. Bristol: International Consultation on Incontinence, 2017.)

ruptures following bladder distension. Ronstrom and Lai[11] have recently published an atlas of HL which is useful in identifying the variations in appearance of HL. Fall et al.[12] described BPS as a heterogenous syndrome comprising two main categories: ulcerative and nonulcerative. The term *interstitial cystitis* is now reserved for those patients who have mucosal (HLs) and histologic (evidence of inflammatory infiltrate on biopsy) changes at cystoscopy and hydrodistension and are thought to represent a distinct phenotype of BPS (Fig. 38.1).[13]

Epidemiology

Clear and accurate estimates of the prevalence of BPS are difficult to ascertain due to changing definitions of the condition, different populations studied, and the methodology used to collect the data. Acknowledging these difficulties in producing prevalence data, a United States-based study found prevalence rates of 2.7% to 6.5%.[14] BPS is 2 to 5 times more common in females than males.[15–17]

Etiology

Although there is no unifying model or definitive evidence for the pathogenesis of BPS, a number of *theories* have been proposed to be involved in the initiation and maintenance of the disease process that then results in the clinical condition of BPS.

Urothelial dysfunction/increased bladder permeability

The urothelium is a highly specialized transitional epithelium lining the upper and lower urinary tracts (Fig. 38.2). It consists of three layers of cells. The basal layer is responsible for all cell division; the partially differentiated intermediate layer is responsible for rapid differentiation to replace lost apical/umbrella cells; and the apical layer provides the main protective barrier through tight intercellular junctions, plaques of uroplakins (cell membrane proteins), and the glycosaminoglycan (GAG) layer.[18] The urothelium provides

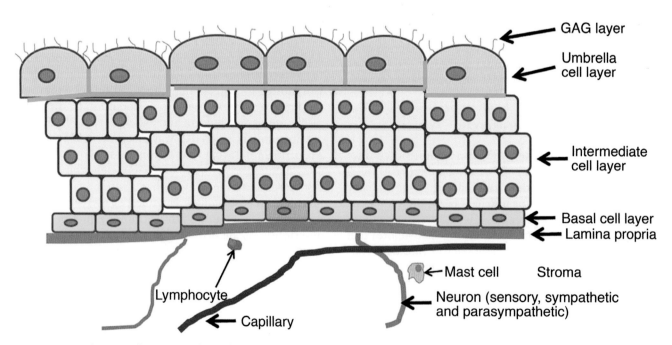

FIGURE 38.2 Schematic illustration of bladder anatomy. (Republished with permission of AME Publishing Company, from Hurst RE, Greenwood-Van Meerveld B, Wisniewski AB, et al. Increased bladder permeability in interstitial cystitis/painful bladder syndrome. *Transl Androl Urol* 2015;4[5]:563–571, permission conveyed through Copyright Clearance Center, Inc.)

the interface between the bladder lumen and the interstitium which collectively contains the connective and muscular tissue, the vasculature and neural networks. It prevents urinary solutes, toxins, and bacteria from penetrating into the interstitium. It is postulated that dysfunction of the tight intercellular junctions allows these noxious agents to permeate into the interstitium, setting up the inflammatory and neural pathways that are proposed to drive the disease process.[19,20]

A defect in the protective GAG layer of the urothelium may also play a role in the increased permeability of the urothelium seen in patients with BPS. The GAG layer is composed of hyaluronic acid, chondroitin sulphate, heparin sulphate, dermatan sulphate, and keratin sulphate.[21] This GAG layer also provides protection against absorption of urine constituents into the interstitium. Parsons et al.[22] noted the increased uptake of urea in patients with BPS compared with normal controls (25% vs. 4.5%, $P < .005$) and that patients with HLs had higher absorption than those BPS patients without HLs (34.5% vs. 22.8%, $P = .002$). Hauser et al.[23] also showed GAG layer abnormalities with a change in the distribution of the proteoglycans in controls versus BPS. Control bladder biopsies showed a greater expression of the proteoglycans in the luminal layer of the urothelium with decreased expression down through to the basal layers, whereas biopsies from patients with BPS showed uniform expression throughout the urothelium with absent strong luminal staining.[23]

Impairment of cell proliferation

Defects in the GAG layer may result in an alteration in the actions of cytokines which then result in increased urothelial permeability due to failure of the urothelium to differentiate properly in patients with BPS. This has been postulated to occur through a number of mechanisms. Hauser et al.[23] suggested that GAGs are able to bind a number of cytokines such as tissue growth factor-beta, platelet-derived growth factor and vascular endothelial growth factor thereby regulating the availability of each ligand. A deficiency in GAGs could then potentially alter the growth and differentiation of urothelial cells from the basal and intermediate layers and result in deficient replacement of the apical cells.[23]

Inflammation

The role of the immune system in the inflammatory response seen in patients with BPS, and particularly in those with HLs, has been widely studied. Mast cells, which are highly specialized immune cells involved in autoimmune and neurogenic immune responses, can be activated by the damaged or dysfunctional urothelium seen in BPS. They secrete several biologically active molecules, including histamine, serotonins, leukotrienes, and cytokines. These proinflammatory mediators are capable of inducing the inflammation, vasodilation and angiogenesis, fibrosis, and smooth muscle contraction associated with BPS.[24]

In support of the role of mast cell activation in BPS, several studies have identified increased concentrations of histamine and its metabolites in the urine of patients with BPS, higher eosinophil density and prostaglandin E2 (also known as dinoprostone) excretion, and high mast cell density particularly in the detrusor muscle.[25] Although detrusor mastocytosis has been proposed as a biomarker for BPS with density cutoffs of greater than 20 microcoulomb/mm² to greater than 32 microcoulomb/mm², the sensitivity and positive predictive values are variable.[26-28]

Neural upregulation

The neural control of bladder function is a complex interplay between the peripheral and central nervous system, with ultimate conscious control of voiding by the prefrontal cortex. Sensory signals originating from the bladder arise from afferents embedded within the detrusor muscle and urothelium. They are sensitive to mechanical distension as well as transmitting sensory stimuli resulting from bladder infection, urothelial inflammation, and barrier breakdown[29] and are therefore responsible for inducing sensations ranging from fullness to pain.[30]

Proinflammatory mediators are known to directly sensitize the bladder afferent nerve terminals,[31] leading to the peripheral sensitization that is an essential mechanism for the induction of normal wound healing.[32] During prolonged or severe inflammation, chronic sensitization of the afferents can occur, reducing the pain threshold and amplifying the responsiveness of nociceptors. This process drives the allodynia and hyperalgesia to bladder distension that is observed in patients with BPS. Both animal and human studies have shown a role for upregulation of receptors and channels associated with nociception (predominantly driven by C fibers, which respond to chemical, mechanical and thermal stimuli) in BPS as well as increased levels of serum and urinary nerve growth factor with resultant increase in afferent nerve density.[33-35]

Central sensitization with changes within the spinal cord and brain can occur following persistent activation of dorsal horn neurons. These changes can then result in the mediation of pain even after resolution of inflammation or other pelvic insult. Central sensitization is a common feature of chronic pain conditions, and functional brain imaging has enhanced knowledge of central nervous system control of the bladder and other pelvic organs. For instance, increased functional brain activation in regions known to be involved in sensory perception and pain has been shown in BPS patients with a full bladder. White matter changes have also been noted in women with BPS compared to controls and correlated with bladder pain and urinary symptoms.[36]

The peripheral and central sensitization occurring in BPS may also explain the high prevalence of vulvodynia of 50% to 85% observed in women with BPS.[37,38] Patients with vulvodynia have been found to have increased nociceptors (specialized sensory neurons that respond to noxious or injurious stimuli), with enhanced pain signaling, compared to normal controls.[39]

Pelvic organ cross talk

Shared sensory pathways involving the dorsal root ganglia, the spinal cord, and the brain exist between the colon, bladder, and reproductive organs. These pathways are necessary for the mediation of normal pelvic organ function; however, this also provides a pathway for dysfunction of one pelvic organ leading to functional changes in another.[40]

Animal and clinical studies have shown that diseases of the colon (irritable bowel syndrome, inflammatory bowel disease) can induce pathology in the bladder. In a mouse model of colitis, changes in bladder voiding parameters that replicate urgency/frequency, increased bladder permeability, as well as increased bladder afferent sensitivity to bladder distension have been observed.[41–43] Conversely, induced bladder inflammation has resulted in colonic changes with lower thresholds for sensation of distension and increased colonic permeability in the absence of inflammatory changes.

Pelvic organ cross talk may also be responsible for the observation that women with endometriosis develop or have coexisting BPS. Prevalence studies have identified that, of women presenting with CPPS with a diagnosis of endometriosis, up to 60% will have BPS.[44,45] A recent population-based study assessing the incidence of BPS in women with endometriosis has shown a hazard ratio for BPS among these women of 3.74 compared to that of controls.[46]

Urinary microbiome

Although once considered sterile, it is now known that urine contains extensive numbers of bacteria in the healthy individual, much like the vagina and gastrointestinal tract. This population of bacteria is referred to as the urinary microbiome and has been shown to be altered in a number of pathologic states. The role of the urinary microbiome in BPS is unclear with conflicting study results. Abernethy et al.[47] studied the urinary microbiome in 40 women with and without BPS and found women with BPS had a less diverse microbiome, with fewer *Lactobacillus* species and higher levels of proinflammatory cytokines. Meriwether et al.,[48] in a study of 41 women with and without BPS, did not find a significant difference in either urinary or vaginal microbiomes.

Cortical regulation: stress, anxiety, depression

There is mounting evidence that chronic stress can result in changes in the balance of autonomic function with a shift to sympathetic nervous system predominance. This then can lead to an exacerbation of sympathetic-mediated pain sensation. This may be one mechanism by which psychological stress increases the severity and duration of pain symptoms in BPS.[49,50]

Diagnosis and Assessment

The diagnosis of BPS is largely based on the clinical criteria of bladder "pain," urinary frequency/nocturia, and/or urgency. As previously discussed, it is a diagnosis of exclusion and duration of symptoms required to make the diagnosis is also variable. The National Institute of Diabetes and Digestive and Kidney Diseases proposed a definition of IC with very strict inclusion and exclusion criteria.[51] This definition was devised in order to homogenize patients participating in IC research studies and not to serve as a diagnostic tool. It has subsequently been shown to be too restrictive, but the list of conditions under exclusion criteria still holds and is mirrored by the ESSIC list of confusable diseases (Table 38.1) and must be assessed for in the workup of any patients presenting with irritative voiding symptoms. These are broadly urogenital malignancy and infection, cystitis (radiation, chemotherapy, immunotherapy, anti-inflammatory), urethral diverticulum, bladder outlet obstruction (BOO)/urinary retention, and urinary tract stone disease. It is important, however, to understand that patients may have a confusable disease *and* BPS.

History

Patients may have difficulty in describing the pain component of BPS and often have trouble localizing or describing their sensations. The pain may be referred to other areas of the pelvis. Besides the typical pain over the suprapubic area, which may be relieved by voiding, BPS patients may complain of referred urethral pain, such as dysuria, strangury, or constant burning. They may also complain of low back pain, vulval pain, rectal pain, and dyspareunia. Quantitation of the severity of pain is quite difficult because of the waxing–waning presentation of symptoms, and there are no formal quantitative objective measures of bladder or pelvic pain.

Urinary urgency is another symptomatic component of BPS that can be difficult to separate from pain in some patients. BPS patients may describe a constant strong urge to void, despite low bladder volumes, that

TABLE 38.1

ESSIC Confusable Diseases (Excluding Male Pathology)

CONFUSABLE DISEASES	EXCLUDED OR DIAGNOSED BY
Carcinoma and carcinoma in situ	Cystoscopy and biopsy
Infection with	
Common intestinal bacteria	Routine bacterial culture
C. trachomatis, U. urealyticum	Special cultures
Mycoplasma hominis, Mycoplasma genitalium	
Corynebacterium urealyticum, Candida sp	
Mycobacterium tuberculosis	Dipstick; if "sterile" pyuria, culture for Mycobacterium tuberculosis
Herpes simplex, human papillomavirus	Physical examination
Radiation	Medical history
Chemotherapy, including immunotherapy	Medical history
Anti-inflammatory therapy	Medical history
Bladder neck obstruction, neurogenic outlet obstruction	Uroflowmetry, ultrasound
Bladder stone	Imaging or cystoscopy
Lower ureteric stone	Medical history and/or hematuria; upper urinary tract imaging CT IVP
Urethral diverticulum	Medical history and physical examination
Urogenital prolapse	Medical history and physical examination
Endometriosis	Medical history and physical examination
Vaginal candidiasis	Medical history and physical examination
Cervical, uterine, ovarian cancer	Physical examination
Incomplete bladder emptying (retention)	Postvoid residual urine volume
Overactive bladder	Medical history and urodynamics
Pudendal nerve entrapment	Medical history, physical examination, nerve block may prove diagnostic
Pelvic floor muscle–related pain	Medical history, physical examination

CT IVP, computed tomography intravenous pyelogram.

when severe is described as pain. Urinary frequency is a manifestation of the actual act of voiding, but BPS patients have been known not to void because they realize that frequent voiding does not necessarily lead to relief of pain and urge sensations. From the standpoint of quantification of BPS symptoms, measurement of voiding frequency may be the best objective parameter.

Other points on history:

- History of previous urinary tract infections
- Urologic/pelvic surgery
- Triggers
  - Diet: Although no research links BPS symptoms to certain foods or drinks, some patients may notice worsening symptoms with ingestion of caffeinated beverages, carbonated drinks, alcohol, tomatoes, hot and spicy foods, chocolate, citrus juices and drinks, monosodium glutamate, and high-acid foods.
  - Hormonal: Some women note perimenstrual flares in BPS symptoms.[52]
- Evidence of pelvic organ cross talk or systemic disease clusters: endometriosis, bowel symptoms (irritable bowel syndrome, inflammatory bowel disease), fibromyalgia, chronic fatigue syndrome, migraine, autoimmune diseases (Sjögren disease)
- Psychological conditions: anxiety, depression

Examination

General physical examination is important but focused on the abdomen and pelvis. Pain mapping should be performed.

- Suprapubic tenderness
- Vulva—exclude vulval/vestibular disease, cotton swab test to assess and score sites of tenderness
- Vagina—evidence of vaginismus, tenderness on palpation of the urethra or anterior vaginal wall/bladder base, evidence of levator ani spasm/trigger points suggestive of pelvic floor hypertonicity; exclude urethral diverticulum (suburethral mass)

Symptom questionnaires

Although not diagnostic, symptom questionnaires can help in tracking response to treatment, with lower scores generally indicating less severe symptoms. Questionnaires also provide objective assessment of treatment effect in research studies with a number of validated questionnaires available.

One questionnaire instrument was developed by O'Leary et al.[53] in 1997 specifically to assess BPS patients. The questionnaire has two subscales to quantify symptoms and their impact on quality of life: the Interstitial Cystitis Symptom Index (ICSI) and Interstitial Cystitis Problem Index (ICPI). A second symptom measurement instrument, the University of Wisconsin IC Scale (UW-ICS), has also been developed and validated.[54] The UW-ICS is a 7-point, 0-to-6 rating scale with each item anchored between the extremes of 0 (not at all) and 6 (a lot). Parsons et al.[55] developed the Pelvic Pain and Urgency/Frequency (PUF) questionnaire to capture symptoms of pelvic pain and dyspareunia in patients with BPS, assessing both symptom severity and impact on quality of life. Any of these validated instruments should be administered to the patient with BPS to quantitate symptoms during the course of evaluation and treatment. It is important to use these standardized instruments so that changes in a patient's symptoms and quality of life can be followed as objectively as possible.

Specific assessment of pain can be achieved on a visual analog scale, a validated subjective measure for acute and chronic pain. Scores are recorded by making a handwritten mark on a 10-cm line that represents a continuum between "no pain" and "worst pain" (Table 38.2).

Bladder diary

A bladder diary provides a very useful insight into the patient's bladder function over 1 to 3 days. This typically shows increased urinary frequency during the day and overnight, with small voided volumes and low maximal functional bladder capacity. It also allows assessment of fluid intake which may require adjustment as patients often limit their fluid intake to minimize voiding frequency, not understanding that severe fluid restriction leading to concentrated urine may exacerbate their symptoms. Changes in voiding parameters can be objectively monitored as treatment progresses, hopefully providing independent positive feedback to the patient or highlighting that current management is not working and prompting change in treatment strategies. In mild BPS without significant pain, bladder retraining using repeat bladder diaries can be a useful therapeutic strategy.

Investigations

Urine microscopy and culture must be performed to exclude intercurrent urinary tract infection. It also allows assessment of microscopic hematuria or sterile pyuria to direct further investigations, that is, urine cytology/cystoscopy/renal imaging to exclude renal tract malignancy or stone disease and urine culture for tuberculosis. There is more emphasis on the possibility of low-grade intracellular infection with elevated urinary leucocyte count causing lower urinary tract symptoms (LUTS) which in some units are being treated with prolonged low-dose antibiotics with some success and controversy.[56]

Screening for voiding dysfunction to exclude it as a cause of urinary frequency/urgency/bladder pressure should be performed. This can be done by catheter or preferably by bedside bladder scan or formal renal tract imaging. If screening is positive, then urodynamic testing should be carried out. Otherwise, the use of urodynamics in the assessment of patients with BPS is not recommended and is usually extremely uncomfortable. If performed, the findings would include voiding dysfunction, a low-capacity bladder, or poor compliance. The Interstitial Cystitis Database Study Group analyzed urodynamic data and compared them to data collected from voiding diaries.[57] It showed that urodynamic data closely correlated with the findings of the voiding diaries, and therefore, it has been suggested that urodynamics are unnecessary in the evaluation of BPS because the voiding diary, which is noninvasive, captures the necessary information.

Cystoscopy without anesthesia can be used to exclude confusable bladder pathology such as malignancy or bladder stone disease and on inspection can reveal HLs on filling but does not allow for sufficient hydrodistension of the bladder and assessment for the presence of glomerulations (pinpoint petechial hemorrhages), cascade bleeding, maximum bladder capacity, or therapeutic interventions. Although there are technical variations in how hydrodistention is performed, Nordling et al.[58] outlined a detailed description. It is performed with the patient under general or regional anesthesia with a full cystoscopic examination of the bladder performed first. Cystoscopic irrigant (water, saline, or glycine) is then

TABLE 38.2	
Interstitial Cystitis Symptoms Quantitation	
IC SYMPTOM INDEX (ICSI)	**IC PROBLEM INDEX (ICPI)**

IC SYMPTOM INDEX (ICSI)

1. During the past month, how often have you felt the strong urge to urinate with little or no warning?
   - 0_____not at all
   - 1_____less than 1 time in 5
   - 2_____less than half the time
   - 3_____about half the time
   - 4_____more than half the time
   - 5_____almost always
2. During the past month, have you had to urinate less than 2 hours after you finished urinating?
   - 0_____not at all
   - 1_____less than 1 time in 5
   - 2_____less than half the time
   - 3_____about half the time
   - 4_____more than half the time
   - 5_____almost always
3. During the past month, how often did you most typically get up at night to urinate?
   - 0_____not at all
   - 1_____less than 1 time in 5
   - 2_____less than half the time
   - 3_____about half the time
   - 4_____more than half the time
   - 5_____almost always
4. During the past month, have you experienced pain or burning in your bladder?
   - 0_____not at all
   - 1_____less than 1 time in 5
   - 2_____less than half the time
   - 3_____about half the time
   - 4_____more than half the time
   - 5_____almost always

IC PROBLEM INDEX (ICPI)

During the past month, how much has each of the following been a problem for you?

1. Frequent urination during the day
   - 0_____no problem
   - 1_____very small problem
   - 2_____small problem
   - 3_____medium problem
   - 4_____big problem
2. Getting up at night to urinate
   - 0_____no problem
   - 1_____very small problem
   - 2_____small problem
   - 3_____medium problem
   - 4_____big problem
3. Need to urinate with little warning
   - 0_____no problem
   - 1_____very small problem
   - 2_____small problem
   - 3_____medium problem
   - 4_____big problem
4. Burning pain, discomfort, or pressure in your bladder
   - 0_____no problem
   - 1_____very small problem
   - 2_____small problem
   - 3_____medium problem
   - 4_____big problem

infused at a pressure of 80 to 100 cm H_2O (this distance above the bladder, i.e., gravity fill) into the bladder until filling into the drip chamber stops; this may require urethral occlusion as water may bypass the cystoscope around the urethra. During filling, the anesthetist may note patient tachycardia or increased respiratory rate indicative of pain. The bladder is distended for 2 to 5 minutes before all the irrigant is released from the bladder under direct vision. The volume of instilled fluid is measured and noted as the patient's anesthetic bladder capacity. Glomerulations may be noted as petechial hemorrhages during bladder emptying and should be quantified as to the number of bladder quadrants in which they are observed (Fig. 38.3). The bladder is then refilled to 20% to 50% of bladder capacity to allow visualization of HLs (Fig. 38.4), appearing as fissures or cracks in the epithelium (these findings are often seen on first fill), and biopsies (both superficial and deep including detrusor muscle) taken if required. Although HLs are considered pathognomic of IC, the presence of

glomerulations is not, occurring in up to 45% of normal subjects without symptoms of BPS at volumes higher than their usual functional bladder capacity. For example, 9 out of 20 asymptomatic women had glomerulations when having tubal ligation and cystoscopy with bladder fill volume of 950 mL.[59] Conversely, glomerulations are often not found in subjects with symptomatic BPS, and therefore, absence of identifiable epithelial changes at cystoscopy does not exclude BPS.

The role of histology in BPS is predominantly to exclude other diseases, particularly malignancy. A variety of histologic appearances have been documented on biopsies in BPS and IC patients. Rosamilia et al.[60] reported 55% of biopsies in BPS patients were indistinguishable from normal controls; however, only those patients with BPS were found to have denuded epithelium, and this was more common in those with severe disease. Other histologic features more commonly found in BPS patients were submucosal edema, congestion, ectasia, as well as inflammatory infiltrate.[60]

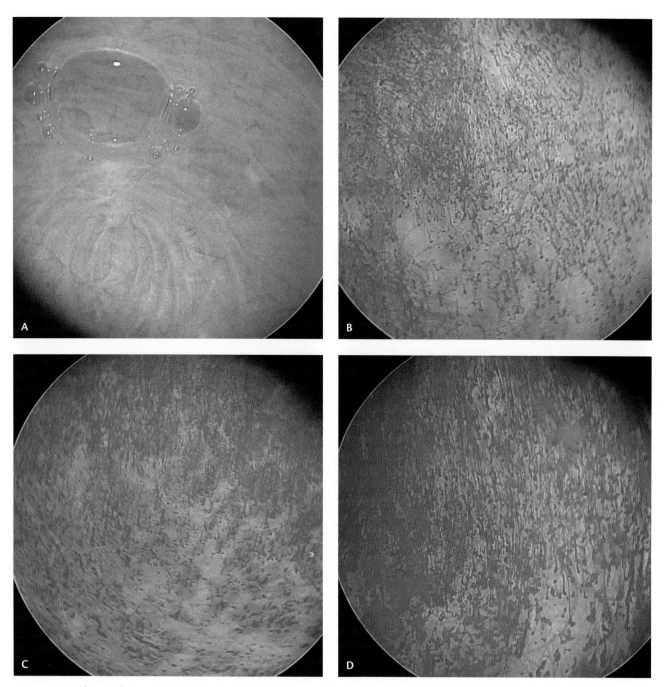

FIGURE 38.3 Glomerulations. **A:** A 66-year-old female presented with a 3-month history of bladder pain, frequency, and urgency. On filling, the bladder mucosa had a normal appearance but anesthetic capacity of 500 mL. (Image courtesy of Kristina Cvach.) **B–D:** On emptying the bladder, extensive glomerulations (pinpoint petechial hemorrhages) with cascade bleeding were noted in all four bladder quadrants. Bladder biopsy was reported as normal. (Image courtesy of Kristina Cvach.)

The role of phenotyping of bladder pain syndrome

The role and timing of cystoscopy and hydrodistension in the diagnosis of BPS varies according to different guidelines. The AUA guidelines[4] suggest its use in "complicated disease" with concurrent incontinence, urinary tract infection, hematuria, and gynecologic symptoms/signs. ESSIC and the EAU place greater emphasis on the role of cystoscopy and bladder biopsy in the diagnosis and classification of BPS,[6] with the ultimate aim being identification of the two main phenotypes of BPS, namely, HL (IC) and non-HL (BPS).

IC and BPS patients have been shown to differ in terms of demographic profile, cystoscopic and histologic findings, as well as the response to all forms of treatment. In the recent ICI BPS document, a new paradigm was suggested, excluding IC completely from BPS, recognizing it

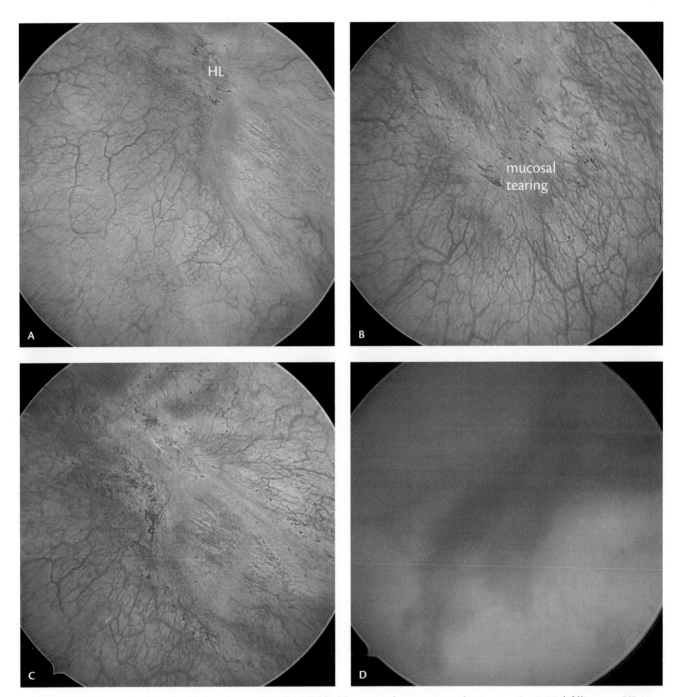

FIGURE 38.4 HL. **A:** A 63-year-old female presented with bladder pain, frequency, and urgency. On initial filling, an HL was noted at the left dome. (Image courtesy of Kristina Cvach.) **B–D:** With filling, the mucosa around the HL became more erythematous with subsequent mucosal tearing and petechial hemorrhages. The anesthetic capacity was 450 mL. On emptying, four quadrant glomerulations were noted. On relook cystoscopy, clot was noted on the HL and the view was obscured by blood. Biopsy of the HL showed ulcerated mucosa, overlying fibrin, stromal inflammatory infiltrate, and vascular congestion, with no malignant features. (Image courtesy of Kristina Cvach.)

as a distinct disease.[7] Patients with IC have been shown to be older with more severe bladder-centric symptoms and lower anesthetic bladder capacity than patients with BPS.[9,61] Schachar et al.[62] studied anesthetic bladder capacity of less than 400 mL as a marker of bladder-centric disease. Patients with lower bladder capacity had higher validated questionnaire scores (signifying more severe symptoms and greater impact on quality of life), higher incidence of HLs (47% vs. 5%), higher levels of acute and chronic inflammation, and erosion on microscopy. These patients were also noted to have a different bladder biopsy gene expression profile characterized by a downregulation of urothelial adhesion molecules and an upregulation of inflammatory markers.

Biomarkers

The ideal biomarker would detect the presence of a disease at early stage, differentiate the disease from other similar symptom complexes, and provide information about the severity of the disease process. BPS is an ideal candidate for establishment of a biomarker or a biomarker cluster due to the absence of a gold standard diagnostic procedure and poor correlation of a patient's clinical condition with findings at cystoscopy/hydrodistension and on histology.

A unique antiproliferative factor (APF) has been found only in the urine of BPS patients. It is capable of inhibiting bladder urothelial cell proliferation and repair processes primarily through its effect on reducing thymidine incorporation into bladder epithelial cells and is highly sensitive (94%) and specific (95%) for BPS.[63] The concentrations of urine epithelial cell growth factors have been shown to be altered in BPS patients compared to controls. Heparin-binding epidermal growth factor (HB-EGF) is significantly decreased, and epidermal growth factor (EGF) is increased in BPS patients.[19] APF has been shown to inhibit HB-EGF production in urothelial cells of BPS patients, and APF activity was inhibited by recombinant human HB-EGF, suggesting the urothelial abnormalities in BPS patients are caused by a negative autocrine growth factor that inhibits cell proliferation by downregulating HB-EGF production.[64]

Although the use of urinary biomarkers is promising, the studies to date have used complicated techniques of detecting APF activity from cultured bladder urothelial cells, therefore limiting clinical use. Most studies were also published over a decade ago suggesting biomarkers in BPS patients and controls, and therefore, further research comparing BPS, IC, and overactive bladder patients will provide further evidence to support the validity of using APF, HB-EGF, and/or EGF as diagnostic biomarkers.

In summary, the clinical presentation of BPS is characterized by chronic urinary frequency, urgency, and pelvic pain in the absence of precise identifiable etiologic features. These symptoms do not necessarily follow a set pattern and may be quite different from one patient to another. BPS patients may have one symptomatic component that predominates over the others. Finally, BPS symptoms typically wax and wane, which further complicates the evaluation and treatment of this condition. The key is to rule out identifiable and potentially reversible causes of the bladder symptoms.

Management

The management of patients with BPS is often empiric as there is no clear underlying pathologic mechanism to treat. It is worthwhile adhering to the principles of management of any chronic pain condition, employing a multimodal and multidisciplinary team approach to optimize care and outcomes for these patients.

Education

A diagnosis of BPS can be a relief for patients, many of whom have suffered for years without a clear understanding of the cause of their recurrent symptoms. However, it also comes with the knowledge that it is a chronic, often debilitating condition without a cure. Therefore, it is important to provide education about the condition and management through a variety of mediums. Written information that the patient can take home to read following the consultation can be very helpful in reinforcing the information initially given. There are a number of organizations that provide detailed condition-specific information on their websites (see list at end of chapter) which the patient can be referred to as well as BPS support groups that provide a forum for patients to share their experiences.

Fluid management is an important first step in management of BPS. Ensuring adequate, and not excessive, fluid intake of 1.5 to 2 L over 24 hours is advised. Many patients reduce their fluid intake in an effort to reduce their urinary frequency. Completion of a bladder diary can help with assessment of intake and guidance on any changes required. Timed voiding and bladder training for women with milder symptoms may help reduce urinary frequency and gradually increase voiding intervals.

Complementary and alternative medicine

Although the evidence for many complementary and alternative medicines (CAMs) used by patients to manage BPS symptoms is lacking, there is no doubt that conservative management selectively incorporating a number of CAMs can be beneficial. A survey published in 2013 of patients' ratings of CAM therapies identified a number of them to be considered helpful, especially diet and pain management adjuncts, such as physical therapy, heat and cold, meditation and relaxation, acupuncture, stress reduction, exercise, and sleep hygiene.[65] The AUA BPS management guidelines incorporate diet and physical therapy into first-line management.

Dietary modification

Although limited, there is some evidence to suggest that certain foods/fluids can exacerbate the symptoms of BPS.[66,67] The most common triggers are caffeinated, alcoholic, or carbonated beverages and acidic (tomatoes, citrus) and spicy foods. Patients should be advised of these dietary triggers and consider an elimination diet. The involvement of a dietitian/nutritionist may be beneficial for women with food triggers to ensure as least restrictive a diet as possible. Ingestion of calcium glycerophosphate (Prelief) appears to reduce symptoms of BPS in those patients with identified food triggers.[68]

Physical therapy

Pelvic floor hypertonicity is a common finding in women with BPS, and this can contribute to overall pelvic pain as well as dyspareunia. Other muscles of the pelvic/hip girdle, low back and abdominals may also be overactive, leading to low back pain and gait disturbance. Involvement of pelvic physiotherapists is therefore recommended in those women with evidence of muscle overactivity. A small case series of direct myofascial release of pelvic floor trigger points has shown reduction in urinary frequency and suprapubic pain, improvement in OLS scores, and reduction in dyspaurenia.[69] A randomized controlled trial (RCT) of myofascial physical therapy (MPT: targeted internal and external tissue manipulation focusing on the pelvic floor, hip girdle, and abdomen) and global therapeutic massage (a traditional full-body Western massage program, focusing on generalised relaxation and relief of muscle tension through massage) in newly diagnosed women with BPS showed significantly greater improvement based on global response assessment in those undergoing MPT (59% vs. 26%, $P = .0012$).[70] Both groups showed similar improvements in pain, urgency, frequency, and quality-of-life outcomes.

The goal of physical therapy is to lengthen the contracted muscles by decreasing tension, releasing trigger points in the levator muscles, reeducating the muscles to a normal range of motion, and improving patient awareness. Other than physiotherapist-guided activities, yoga and Pilates with their focus on stretching and flexibility may also provide relief of symptoms related to hip girdle, lower back, and abdominal muscle overactivity.

Stress reduction

As previously discussed, chronic stress leads to sympathetic overactivity with modulation of pain response. Patients with BPS have been shown to experience intensified pain due to stress and experience higher levels of psychological stress than those without BPS.[71,72] Although there is no evidence to support stress reduction and relaxation, given what is known about stress and its impact on pain experience, it makes sense to advise BPS patients to try to minimize the stressful components of their lives if possible. Psychological support and counselling may also be helpful.

Medical management

Assessment and management of pain should occur at every level along the treatment algorithm. Analgesia requirements will differ for each patient as the experience of pain varies. Simple analgesics such as paracetamol and anti-inflammatories should always be tried first. The use of heat and cold (hot and cold packs) can also be beneficial. Escalation to opioid medication should be avoided but, if required, then referral to a pain physician/chronic pain team is preferable to manage this on a continuing basis.

Oral neuromodulatory agents have been used in the management of chronic neuropathic pain to modulate the central sensitization. These agents are also used in BPS patients with varying success. Amitriptyline is a tricyclic antidepressant with multiple sites of action; among others, it stabilizes mast cells and inhibits painful nociception from the bladder at the level of the central nervous system, and urine storage may be facilitated by its beta-adrenergic receptor stimulation. Sedation is often a beneficial side effect, providing some respite from nocturia. However, this is one of the main reasons for cessation; therefore, slow dose escalation from 10 mg is recommended, aiming for 50 to 75 mg. An RCT comparing amitriptyline to placebo in patients undergoing a standardized education and behavioral modification program showed that, although amitriptyline overall resulted in a nonsignificant improvement based on global response assessment compared to placebo (55% vs. 45%, $P = .12$), 66% of those patients able to achieve at least a 50-mg dosing of amitriptyline had improvement compared to 47% in the placebo arm ($P = .01$).[73] Patients are often reluctant to take an antidepressant so should be provided with a clear explanation of the rationale for using amitriptyline. Gabapentin and pregabalin are antiepileptic agents also used for neuropathic pain. Evidence for their use in BPS is limited but promising.

Pentosan polysulfate sodium (PPS) is the only U.S. Food and Drug Administration–approved oral agent for BPS. It is a synthetic polysaccharide postulated to repair the disrupted GAG layer. Initial trials provided evidence of efficacy with improvement in symptoms of greater than 25% in 28% of PPS treated patients compared to 13% in the placebo group ($P = .03$).[74] A more recent RCT of 368 patients evaluating efficacy of PPS 100 mg three times a day versus PPS 100 mg daily versus placebo did not show a significant difference in the primary outcome of 30% reduction from baseline of ICSI total score (42.6% vs. 39.8% vs. 40.7%, respectively).[75] The current recommended dose is 100 mg three times a day. Oral therapy results in low urine concentrations of the drug, and therefore, there may be a lag time of up to 6 months before clinical improvement is achieved. With the more recent publication of studies showing an association between use of PPS and progressive maculopathy, the Food and Drug Administration in the US have issued a black box warning for PPS.[76]

Antihistamines have been studied in BPS due to the mastocytosis evident in the bladder wall of BPS patients, in particular those with HL. The use of antihistamines may theoretically reduce the activation of mast cells and therefore help reduce frequency and urgency symptoms. In a single RCT of 36 patients, cimetidine 400 twice a day over 3 months resulted in significant reductions in symptom scores, suprapubic pain, and nocturia compared to placebo.[77]

Other medical management

Cyclosporin A (CyA) is an immunosuppressant used in transplant medicine. It is currently suggested as fifth-line therapy in the AUA treatment guidelines. Due to concerns around toxicity and renal impairment, it is seldom used in the BPS patient population; however, the lower doses required to treat BPS may mean these complications are less likely. A number of small nonblinded/randomized studies have shown efficacy for CyA, particularly in patients with HL. Forrest et al.[78] conducted a retrospective review of 44 patients from three tertiary centers, 34 of which had HL. Response to treatment was defined as marked improvement on Global Response Assessment (GRA) or a greater than 50% reduction in ICSI score. Sixty-eight percent of patients with HL had improvement compared with 30% of those without HL. For all responders, improvement occurred within 4 months of commencing treatment.[78] Crescenze et al.[79] conducted an open-label study of CyA in 26 patients who had failed two prior treatments. At 3 months, 31% were considered improved on GRA, with 15% and 19% improved on ICSI and ICPI. The presence of HL predicted improvement in ICSI (odds ratio [OR] 15.4, $P = .01$); however, numbers were small.[79] During therapy, monitoring of blood pressure, renal function, and drug levels is mandatory.

A number of novel therapies have undergone assessment in small trials but require further investigation in larger RCTs. The oral SHIP 1 (SH2-containing inositol-5'-phospatase 1) activator compound AQX-1125 modulates immune/inflammatory regulation and showed promise in a small phase II trial.[80] However, the larger phase III trial assessing AQX-1125 versus placebo in 298 patients showed no significant difference in pain, frequency, GRA, or questionnaire scores at 3 months.[81]

Women who experience perimenstrual flares in their BPS symptoms may benefit from hormonal modulation through the combined oral contraceptive pill (COCP). A trial of COCP with continuous hormonal use (skipping periods by taking only the hormone tablets) is appropriate in these women and may significantly reduce the number and severity of BPS flares.

Intravesical therapy

Intravesical therapy can be considered for second-line treatment of BPS if patients have not had response to behavioral and medical management. Intravesical treatment provides localized therapy to the bladder, delivering high concentrations of the agent and minimizing systemic side effects. It is however important to continue with the behavioral and lifestyle changes including bladder training as well as focus on pain control as management of BPS is often achieved through the incremental benefits of multiple treatment strategies.

There are a number of agents that are currently available, and these are summarized in Table 38.3.

The evidence for these agents varies from small case series to RCTs, and it is important to note that efficacy rates are modest for all of the treatments, in the order of 60% to 70%. Most intravesical therapies require instillation of the solution via a catheter with the patient awake and may result in a flare in pain following treatment and increases the risk of urinary tract infection. Most treatments are administered over a period of weeks to months with responses often not seen until a number of treatments have been given.

Cystoscopy/hydrodistension

Cystoscopy and hydrodistension has been shown to provide short-term relief of BPS symptoms, although the mechanism by which this occurs is unknown. A small cohort study showed hydrodistension resulted in 56% of patients having improvement in symptoms but with a mean duration of effect of only 2 months.[82]

Cystoscopic treatment of Hunner lesions

Given the evidence that patients with HL have poorer responses to oral and intravesical therapies, the EAU and ESSIC have advocated for earlier use of diagnostic cystoscopy to identify those patients with HL who would benefit from earlier detection and specific treatment of the HL. Prior to treatment, biopsy of the lesion should be performed to exclude malignancy.

Triamcinolone is a long-acting synthetic steroid which can be directly injected into the center and periphery of the HL at the time of cystoscopy, with concentrations of 12 to 40 mg/mL diluted in normal saline or bupivacaine/lidocaine. Funaro et al.[83] used a lower concentration of triamcinolone and reported on significant reductions in pain (Visual Analogue Scale [VAS] pain score pretest 8.3 vs. posttest 3.8, $P < .001$) and nocturia bother with median interval between injections of 10 months (313 days, range 77 to 717).[83] Crescenze et al.[84] used the higher concentration and found 85% of patients had symptomatic improvement, with significant improvements in AUA symptom scores and quality of life. Median time between injections was 8 months (range 4 to 13).[84]

Alternatively, HL can be treated by transurethral coagulation/fulguration (TUC) or transurethral resection (TUR) of the lesion. An RCT of 126 patients with HL underwent TUC or TUR. The primary outcome was recurrence-free time, and this did not significantly differ between the two groups (TUC 11.5 months vs. TUR 12.2 months, $P = .735$). Response rates based on questionnaire scores (O'Leary Sant Symptom Index, O'Leary Sant Problem Index, PUF) also did not differ between groups and at 3 months posttreatment were 65% for TUC and 69% for TUR. Bladder perforations occurred in 2 patients in the TUC group (3.4%) and 5 patients in the TUR group (7.9%).[85]

TABLE 38.3				
Intravesical Therapy				
AGENT	**MECHANISM OF ACTION**	**TREATMENT PROTOCOL**	**EVIDENCE**	**TREATMENT RESPONSE**
Dimethyl sulfoxide (DMSO)	Anti-inflammatory	Often administered as a cocktail with steroid/alkalinized lidocaine/heparin sulphate	RCT DMSO vs. placebo; response based on urodynamics and symptoms[110]	Objective 93% vs. 35%; subjective 53% vs. 18%
	Analgesic	Twice weekly for 4 wk, weekly for 4 wk (total 12 instillations)	Long-term follow-up to 4 y[111]	Improvement in ICSI/ICPI and VAS pain score 23% to 47%; lower response with anesthetic bladder capacity <500 mL
	Smooth muscle relaxation	Repeat or maintenance therapy for recurrent/persistent symptoms		
Heparin	Replenishment of GAG layer	Both agents can be administered individually but more commonly in combination.	Case series 12 weekly instillations of heparin 20,000 U/5 mL, 4% lidocaine/25 mL, 7% sodium bicarbonate[112]	GRA response 76% at 12 wk, reduction to 16% at 6 mo posttreatment
Lidocaine	Topical anesthetic			
Intravesical PPS	Replenishment of GAG layer	Twice-weekly instillations for 3 mo	RCT intravesical PPS (30 mg in 50 mL normal saline) vs. placebo[113]	Subjective improvement 40% PPS vs. 20% placebo
	Inhibits histamine release from mast cells			
Sodium hyaluronate (HA)	Replenishment of GAG layer	Both agents can be administered individually but more commonly in combination (iAluRil: 1.6% HA and 2% CS).	RCT HA/CS vs. DMSO; 13 weekly instillations	Pain reduction significant in both groups; >50% reduction in pain scores at 3 mo 70% HA/CS vs. 55% DMSO
Chondroitin sulphate (CS)	Replenishment of GAG layer			
Botulinum toxin A	Inhibits release of acetylcholine from afferent and efferent nerve endings	Use is off-label for BPS	Systematic review of 5 studies (282 patients) Botox vs. placebo[114]	Significant improvements in VAS pain, OLSI/OLPI Botox vs. placebo
	Inhibits ATP release from urothelium	Suburothelial injections of Botulinum toxin A 100 U under anesthetic		
Oxychlorosene sodium (Clorpactin)	Degranulation of bladder nociceptive nerve endings; anti-inflammatory	0.4% solution (2 g in 500 mL normal saline) instilled into bladder under anesthetic; option for retreatment	RCT Clorpactin vs hydrodistension[115]	GRA improvement at 3 mo Clorpactin 56% vs. hydrodistension 4.5%

ATP, adenosine triphosphate; OLSI, O'Leary Sant Symptom Index; OLPI, O'Leary Sant Problem Index; PPS, pentosan polysulfate sodium.

Sacral neuromodulation

Implantable neuromodulator devices are used in chronic pain conditions and are thought to suppress pain via the gate-control theory, whereby non-noxious input closes the "gates" to painful input. Sacral neuromodulation with lead placement at S3 is approved for use in overactive bladder, nonobstructive voiding dysfunction, and fecal incontinence but is not currently approved for use in BPS. Its efficacy in BPS has been assessed in only a small number of clinical trials. Most published studies show reductions in VAS pain scores of 40% to 63% with explantation rates of 0% to 50%.[86–88]

Bladder augmentation/cystectomy

Patients with refractory BPS/IC with severely fibrosed, contracted small capacity bladders may consider more invasive surgical management although this is considered a last resort. A recent review of surgical management of refractory BPS/IC found that of 448 patients undergoing surgery (a combination of subtotal cystectomy with cystoplasty, cystectomy and orthotopic neobladder or cystectomy and ileal conduit), 77% had symptom improvement. Complications occurred in 27% with overall mortality 1.3%. However, the authors noted the findings should be interpreted with caution given small patient numbers, multiple centres involved and the use of variable outcome measures.[89]

PAINFUL CONDITIONS OF THE URETHRA

Urethral Caruncle

A urethral caruncle is the most common female urethral lesion and is due to eversion of the distal portion of the posterior urethral meatus. It is usually small, soft, smooth or friable, bright pink to dark, and usually single but can be pedunculated up to 1 to 2 cm long. It most commonly occurs in postmenopausal women but can occur in premenopausal and prepubertal girls.[90] It is assumed that estrogen deficiency leads to urothelial atrophy and retraction of the vagina. Histologically, a caruncle contains blood vessels and loose connective tissue covered by urothelium and squamous epithelium.

Most women are asymptomatic, and caruncles are often an incidental finding on pelvic examination. A study looked at the effects of asymptomatic caruncles on micturition and found that 6% (50 out of 850) of women who presented with urinary incontinence were noted to have caruncles; this suggests no association. There was no effect on micturition, and all caruncles were less than 1 cm.[91] Symptoms can include postmenopausal bleeding, a palpable lump, dysuria, and pain. Voiding dysfunction has also been reported.[92] Biopsy is not necessary unless the appearance is atypical and diagnosis uncertain or if there is a suspicion of malignancy.[93]

There are no large studies or RCTs evaluating various treatment strategies. Asymptomatic women do not require treatment; observation could be offered or advice on the use of topical estrogen in order to prevent future symptoms. Women who are symptomatic should be treated with topical estrogen cream, and this may require indefinite, twice-weekly, or intermittent treatment. Self-inspection could guide this. Referral to a urogynecologist, gynecologist, or urologist should be considered in cases of large persistent lesions. If initial therapy with topical estrogen fails, surgical treatment can be considered. Excision with suturing can be performed under local or general anesthesia, with the specimen sent for histopathology. Diathermy or cryosurgery should be avoided as this precludes histologic assessment. Risks include bleeding or rarely external urethral meatal stenosis.

Urethral Prolapse

Female urethral prolapse is uncommon and defined as eversion of the urethral mucosa circumferentially through the distal urethra. It is usually seen in prepubertal or postmenopausal women. Pathogenesis of urethral prolapse may be due to separation of the two muscular layers of the urethra, which can be congenital or acquired,[91] or, similar to that of urethral caruncle, a lack of estrogen leading to urothelial atrophy and retraction of the vaginal epithelium.[94]

Prepubertal girls are usually asymptomatic; the diagnosis is often made as an incidental finding during examination. The most common symptom is vaginal bleeding along with a urethral mass.[95] In contrast, postmenopausal women are often symptomatic with vaginal bleeding and discomfort. Voiding symptoms are common. Urethral prolapse can also be seen in association with severe stage pelvic organ prolapse or uncommonly after prolapse correction.

Diagnosis is by physical examination. Urethral prolapse presents as a circumferential, small doughnut-shaped mass protruding from the anterior vaginal wall; the external urethral meatus is in the middle (Fig. 38.5). It can be erythematous, congested, infected, or even ulcerated. There are some case series of differential diagnosis of urethral malignancy. Postmenopausal

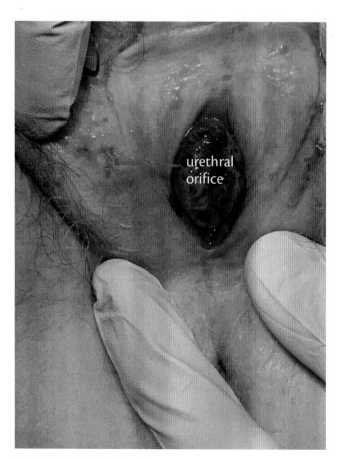

FIGURE 38.5 Urethral prolapse.

asymptomatic women generally with milder degrees of urethral prolapse are usually initially treated with topical estrogen therapy. In symptomatic or more severe degrees of urethral prolapse, excisional biopsy with suturing of epithelial edges with a short period of urethral catheterization is the usual management. There are some instances of urinary incontinence following urethral prolapse excision and repair.

Urethritis

Urethritis is inflammation of the urethra and most commonly associated with sexually transmitted infection (STI). *Neisseria gonorrhoeae* and *Chlamydia trachomatis* are the most common causes and coinfection can occur. Other possible causative organisms include *Mycoplasma genitalium*, *Trichomonas vaginalis*, herpes simplex virus, and, uncommonly, *Treponema pallidum*, *Haemophilus influenzae*, *Neisseria meningitidis*, *Ureaplasma urealyticum*, and *Candida* species.

Noninfectious etiologies include trauma following catheterization or instrumentation or foreign-body reaction. Friction or irritation to the vulva and external urethra may be associated with urethritis due to rubbing from tight clothing or sex; bicycle riding; and irritants including soaps, body powders, and spermicides.

Urethritis is commonly asymptomatic, but symptoms may include dysuria, pruritus, burning, and discharge at the urethral meatus. Gonorrhea presents most commonly with frank purulent discharge, whereas chlamydia often presents with dysuria alone. Dysuria with the development of painful genital ulcers is most likely herpes simplex virus.

Urethritis is clinically suspected when any sexually active patient presents with symptoms consistent with urethritis including pruritus, discharge, or dysuria. It is mostly a clinical diagnosis based on history and physical examination.

Microbiologic diagnosis depends on the availability of point-of-care testing. The Gram stain test has been traditionally the gold standard for the diagnosis of urethritis. *N. gonorrhoeae* is diagnosed initially with nucleic acid amplification testing with first-catch urine or urethral swab. A urethral culture provides information regarding antibiotic resistance.

C. trachomatis is diagnosable in females based on urinalysis revealing pyuria with no organisms reported on Gram stain or culture. The laboratory test of choice is the nucleic acid amplification test with a first-void urine.

The recommended treatment of choice for gonococcal urethritis is a single dose of ceftriaxone 250-mg intramuscular injection and a single dose of oral 1 g of azithromycin to cover for coinfection with chlamydia. The alternative for chlamydia would be doxycycline 100 mg twice a day for 7 days. Azithromycin is the recommended treatment for pregnant women. Patient education and partner treatment should occur. All patients need repeat testing 3 months after treatment, and reinfection should receive therapy with azithromycin.

For *M. genitalium*, the recommended antibiotic of choice is also azithromycin 1 g orally as a single dose. *T. vaginalis* urethritis, including in pregnant patients, should be treated with 7 days of metronidazole 500 mg orally twice a day.

Genitourinary Syndrome of Menopause

This is a collection of symptoms and signs caused by hypoestrogenic changes to the labia majora/minora, clitoris, vestibule/introitus, vagina, urethra, and bladder that occur in postmenopausal women. This term was introduced in 2014 and replaced the term *urogenital atrophy* or *atrophic vaginitis*. The syndrome may include, but is not limited to, genital symptoms of dryness, burning, and irritation; sexual symptoms of lack of lubrication, discomfort or pain, and impaired function; and urinary symptoms of urgency, dysuria, and recurrent urinary tract infections. Some or all of the signs and symptoms may be present.

In premenopausal women, a hypoestrogenic state may occur during the postpartum period or lactation, hypothalamic amenorrhea, or due to antiestrogenic drugs.

Urinary tract structures are derived from the same embryologic origin as the genital tract and also contain estrogen receptors. Thus, the bladder, urethra, pelvic floor musculature, and endopelvic fascia are affected by a hypoestrogenic state. Examination findings include labia minora resorption or fusion; tissue fragility/fissures/petechiae; introital retraction; loss of hymenal remnants; prominence of the urethral meatus; urethral eversion or prolapse; vulvovaginal pallor/erythema, loss of vaginal rugae; and decreased vulvovaginal secretions, lubrication, and elasticity.

Topical estrogen is the most common treatment for symptoms attributable to a low estrogen state. These preparations include estradiol, estriol, and conjugated equine estrogen in the form of creams or pessaries. Choice of preparation is largely related to personal choice, although there is evidence to suggest that estriol preparations have less systemic absorption. Women are advised to commence night time application for 2 weeks to provide a loading dose and then reduce to weekly or twice-weekly application for maintenance. Some women do describe increased vaginal burning or irritation as well as increased episodes of candidal infection resulting in cessation of treatment. In some cases, the author would commence and retain treatment at twice-weekly dosing which may be associated with less side effects. Women should be advised that vaginal estrogen is a hormonal product but with minimal risk regarding breast/uterine/ovarian cancer risk due to its minimal absorption; however, if the woman has a personal history of estrogen-sensitive malignancy, a discussion with her surgeon or oncologist is warranted to determine the safety of its use.

Female Urethral Stricture

Urethral strictures in females are considered rare. Bladder outlet obstruction (BOO) is a relatively uncommon cause of LUTS in women. It has been estimated that BOO accounts for between 3% to 8% of women with LUTS.[96] In those women with known BOO, female urethral stricture (FUS) account for between 4% and 18% of these cases so in total 0.3% to 1% of all women with LUTS.[97] Symptoms of FUS may be variable but often include hesitancy, poor flow, dribbling, frequency, urgency, urethral pain, and dysuria and may lead to recurrent urinary tract infection and overt urinary retention.

The causes of FUS may include trauma, iatrogenic injury, infection, malignancy, and radiation. The differential diagnosis may include functional BOO that is more common, urethral diverticulum, or, even rarely, urethral malignancy. Uroflowmetry with measurement of the postvoid residual represents the first level of investigation, whereas urethroscopy and videourodynamics are performed to confirm the presence of a urethral stricture and its location and to exclude concomitant conditions of the lower urinary tract. Magnetic resonance imaging (MRI) of the pelvis may also be performed to assess for anatomical abnormalities of urethral or periurethral tissues or features suggestive of malignancy.[98]

Initial surgical management is usually urethral dilatation; this has been associated with a greater than 50% success rate when combined with intermittent self-dilatation.[99] Endoscopic management with cold knife or laser incision of midurethral stricture has been suggested, typically incising at the 3 and 9 o'clock positions. Urethral reconstruction techniques depend on the location of the stricture. Meatotomy or meatoplasty involve circumferential excision of the meatal stenosis, followed by reapproximation of the urethral lumen to the vaginal epithelium performed over a Foley catheter; this would be appropriate for stenosis involving the distal 1 cm of the urethra.[96]

Vaginal flap urethroplasty using a dorsal or ventral approach has been described in addition to vaginal graft urethroplasty which can also be dorsal or ventral; an example of the latter is the ventral inlay labial graft urethroplasty.[100] Several published series have described good outcomes after urethroplasty for FUS using buccal or lingual mucosa in a dorsal onlay technique and small series using a ventral onlay technique.[101]

Urethral Pain Syndrome

The EUA CPP document describes urethral pain syndrome (UPS) as the occurrence of chronic or recurrent episodic pain perceived in the urethra, in the absence of proven infection or other obvious local pathology. It is often associated with negative cognitive, behavioral, sexual, or emotional consequences as well as with symptoms suggestive of lower urinary tract, sexual, bowel, or gynecologic dysfunction.[102]

The International Continence Society terminology document of CPPS in 2016 describes the patient assessment requiring a thorough history of the patient's perception of pain or discomfort: duration (at least 6 months), perception (identify inciting event and/or triggers), and modality (persistent/recurrent).[103] The document states that the terms *chronic urethritis* and *urethral syndrome* are no longer recommended.

Urethral pain is perceived to be in the urethra, usually when voiding, with increased day- and nighttime frequency. It may be combined with a feeling of dull pressure and sometimes radiates toward the groin, sacrum, and perineum. Features include the persistence or recurrence of pain with no history of current infection or other obvious pathology and that it may occur subsequent to a previous urinary tract infection or urethral instrumentation.

The typical patient is of reproductive age with urethral pain and has often seen multiple clinicians. Pain episodes may be intermittent, and there may be identifiable triggers. As with BPS/IC, many patients have other disorders such as fibromyalgia, vulvodynia, irritable bowel syndrome, chronic fatigue syndrome, or allergies. They may have been diagnosed with urethritis, treated with multiple courses of antibiotics and undergone extensive gynecologic or urologic workups including urethral dilations.[104] These patients have been identified as more likely to contact providers; have more office visits, procedures, and medication changes; report more pain; have higher depression scores; and have more "health care–seeking behaviors."[105]

The diagnosis of urethral pain syndrome is one of exclusion; for instance, urinary tract, vaginal, and STIs; local causes such as genitourinary syndrome of menopause; Bartholin gland cysts or infections; or urethral diverticulum. Conditions such as BOO, urethral stenosis, stone disease, tumors, endometriosis, and constipation should be ruled out. A thorough history including past medical, surgical, family, and social histories including gynecologic and sexual history.[104] This includes a screening assessment of the gastrointestinal, neurologic, and musculoskeletal systems.

The examination includes palpation of the lower abdomen for bladder fullness and tenderness and a complete pelvic examination including the external genitalia. This would include the vulva, urethra, and vagina, assessing for the presence of atrophy, stage 2 or more pelvic organ prolapse, or pelvic masses. Cotton swab mapping of the suprapubic, pubic, labial, perineal, and introital areas with a VAS (0 to 10 out of 10 in terms of pain) can be helpful. This scale can also be used to score tenderness to digital palpation of the suburethral area, anterior and posterior vaginal walls, uterus or apex, and pelvic floor muscles. The latter can be checked at rest and while performing a pelvic floor muscle contraction, and those sites could be described as tender points. Specific to the lower urinary tract, the examination should check for suburethral mass or discharge or any ectopic or unusual anatomy.

The investigations include urinalysis and culture; STI, vaginal, *Ureaplasma*, and *Mycoplasma* cultures should be sent if appropriate. A bladder diary is a useful baseline investigation. Imaging such as renal and bladder ultrasound will screen for calculi and check postvoid residual; translabial/transvaginal ultrasound is a very useful bedside investigation to screen for urethral diverticulum and anterior vaginal wall cysts, to identify transvaginal mesh, and to estimate postvoid residual volume. Other investigations which can be used selectively include MRI to exclude urethral diverticulum (beware prior bulking agent injection as this will often be reported as diverticulum), uroflowmetry/urodynamic testing to assess bladder capacity and function, and cystourethroscopy with or without bladder biopsy.

Some of the possible etiologies for urethral pain syndrome share many features with BPS with processes such as neuropathic hypersensitivity and pelvic floor dysfunction thought to be contributory. Other possible etiologies included psychogenic factors, diet, BOO, and infectious causes including fastidious organisms of the paraurethral glands, although this is not proven.[104] Indeed, lower rates of *Mycoplasma* and *Ureaplasma* in women with UPS have been identified compared with controls.[106] Hypoestrogenism is another etiologic process put forward; however, this does not fit with peak prevalence in women of reproductive age.

The EAU CPP states that treatment for urethral pain syndrome must be multidisciplinary and take a "trial-and-error" approach. Finally, the therapeutic guidelines for UPS should mirror the guidelines for BPS/IC as recommended by the AUA: Conservative therapy should be initiated first, gradually followed by more invasive interventions. Many proposed interventions have not been tested against placebo which is associated with up to a 30% improvement in chronic pain conditions.

A recent Swedish study surveyed gynecology, urology, and venereology services for their treatment practices for urethral pain syndrome; 70% used local steroid instillation, 67% local estrogen, 50% urethral dilatation, 36% local anesthetic, and 25% used local or oral antibiotics. There were lower rates of other options such as alpha-blockers, mucosal protecting agents, acupuncture, antidepressants, bladder training, and physical therapy. This was similar to findings from their 2006 survey. RCT evidence is lacking.[107]

The rationale for anti-inflammatories is that histology of urethral biopsies from women with UPS show inflammatory changes in the mucosa and the paraurethral glands. A retrospective pilot study of 30 patients underwent an average of five instillations of 2-mL 0.05% clobetasol cream + 2-mL lidocaine gel (unknown strength) intraurethrally. There was a 60% rate of relief reported by the patients in the study, and at 6 months, 57% were symptom free. Of the surveyed group of clinicians, 93%

would consider clobetasol + lidocaine for retreatment in the event of a relapse.[108]

A large study of 500 female patients with UPS was conducted over a 2-year period and found that two-thirds had improvement of symptoms with urethral dilation to 26 to 28 French. However, the study concluded "there currently exists no justification" for use of urethral dilation as a treatment modality. Common complications of urethral dilation include infection, urethral perforation, bleeding, and pain. Women who undergo repetitive urethral dilation may suffer from more significant complications like the development of FUS disease.[109] Anecdotally, these patients tend to obtain relief immediately after dilation; this may be due to a response similar to the concept of hydrodistention in BPS/IC. However, symptoms recur with time. Thus, with other treatment options available, the risks of repetitive urethral dilation outweigh the benefits.

Some patients may have overlapping symptoms with BPS/IC and treatments with dimethyl sulfoxide, other instillations, hydrodistention, neuromodulation, and intradetrusor Botox injections may be helpful. In a similar manner to the treatment approach for BPS/IC, the management algorithm begins with patient counseling, education, behavioral modification with stress reduction and dietary modifications; pelvic floor muscle trigger point therapy; topical estrogen therapy for postmenopausal women; and urethral instillations. Other medications which have been trialed depending on symptoms include alpha-blockers, beta3-agonists, anticholinergics and antidepressants, psychological counseling, and support for anxiety symptoms.

Urethral pain syndrome is a diagnosis of exclusion and requires individualized, multimodal therapy in similar fashion to BPS/IC and other chronic pain conditions.

References

1. Kennedy R, Abd-Elsayed A. The International Association for the Study of Pain (IASP) Classification of Chronic Pain Syndromes. In: Abd-Elsayed, ed. *Pain.* Switzerland: Springer, 2019:1101–1103.
2. Rodríguez MÁB, Afari N, Buchwald DS, et al; and the National Institute of Diabetes and Digestive and Kidney Diseases Working Group on Urological Chronic Pelvic Pain. Evidence for overlap between urological and nonurological unexplained clinical conditions. *J Urol* 2013;189(1 Suppl):S66–S74.
3. Ueda T. The legendary beginning of the International Consultation on Interstitial Cystitis. *Int J Urol* 2003;10(Suppl 1):S1–S2.
4. Hanno P, Erickson D, Moldwin R, et al. Diagnosis and treatment of interstitial cystitis/bladder pain syndrome: AUA guideline amendment. *J Urol* 2015;193:1545.
5. Engeler D, Baranowski AP, Berghmans B, et al. Chronic pelvic pain. European Association of Urology. Accessed November 25, 2021. https://uroweb.org/guideline/chronic-pelvic-pain/
6. van de Merwe JP, Nordling J, Bouchelouche P, et al. Diagnostic criteria, classification, and nomenclature for painful bladder syndrome/interstitial cystitis: An ESSIC proposal. *Eur Urol* 2008;53(1):60–67.

7. Hanno P, Cervigni M, Dinis P, et al. Bladder pain syndrome. In: Abrams P, Cardozo L, Wagg A, et al, eds. *Incontinence*, 6th ed. United Kingdom: ICI-ICS International Continence Society, 2017:2203–2301.

8. Skene AJC. *Diseases of the bladder and urethra*. New York: William Wood and Company, 1878.

9. Logadottir Y, Fall M, Kabjorn-Gustafsson C, et al. Clinical characteristics differ considerably between phenotypes of bladder pain syndrome/interstitial cystitis. *Scand J Urol Nephrol* 2012;46(5):365–370.

10. Rais-Bahrami S, Friedlander JI, Herati AS, et al. Symptom profile variability of interstitial cystitis/painful bladder syndrome by age. *BJU Int* 2012;109(9):1356–1359.

11. Ronstrom C, Lai HH. Presenting an atlas of Hunner lesions in interstitial cystitis which can be identified with office cystoscopy. *Neurourol Urodyn* 2020;39(8):2394–2400.

12. Fall M, Johansson SL, Aldenborg F. Chronic interstitial cystitis: A heterogeneous syndrome. *J Urol* 1987;137(1):35–38.

13. Whitmore KE, Fall M, Sengiku A, et al. Hunner lesion versus non-Hunner lesion interstitial cystitis/bladder pain syndrome. *Int J Urol* 2019;26:26–34.

14. Konkle KS, Berry SH, Elliott MN, et al. Comparison of an interstitial cystitis/bladder pain syndrome clinical cohort with symptomatic community women from the RAND Interstitial Cystitis Epidemiology study. *J Urol* 2012;187(2):508–512.

15. Clemens JQ, Meenan RT, O'Keeffe MC, et al. Prevalence of interstitial cystitis symptoms in a managed care population. *J Urol* 2005;174(2):576–580.

16. Clemens JQ, Link CL, Eggers PW, et al. Prevalence of painful bladder symptoms and effect on quality of life in black, Hispanic and white men and women. *J Urol* 2007;177(4):1390–1394.

17. Berry SH, Stoto MA, Elliott M, et al. Prevalence of interstitial cystitis/painful bladder syndrome in the United States. *J Urol* 2009;181(4S):20–21.

18. Khandelwal P, Abraham SN, Apodaca G. Cell biology and physiology of the uroepithelium. *Am J Physiol Renal Physiol* 2009;297(6):F1477–F1501.

19. Zhang C-O, Wang J-Y, Koch KR, et al. Regulation of tight junction proteins and bladder epithelial paracellular permeability by an antiproliferative factor from patients with interstitial cystitis. *J Urol* 2005;174(6):2382–2387.

20. Shie J-H, Kuo H-C. Higher levels of cell apoptosis and abnormal E-cadherin expression in the urothelium are associated with inflammation in patients with interstitial cystitis/painful bladder syndrome. *BJU Int* 2011;108(2 Pt 2):E136–E141.

21. Hurst RE, Moldwin RM, Mulholland SG. Bladder defense molecules, urothelial differentiation, urinary biomarkers, and interstitial cystitis. *Urology* 2007;69(4 Suppl):17–23.

22. Parsons CL, Lilly JD, Stein P. Epithelial dysfunction in nonbacterial cystitis (interstitial cystitis). *J Urol* 1991;145(4):732–735.

23. Hauser PJ, Dozmorov MG, Bane BL, et al. Abnormal expression of differentiation related proteins and proteoglycan core proteins in the urothelium of patients with interstitial cystitis. *J Urol* 2008;179(2):764–769.

24. Furuta A, Suzuki Y, Igarashi T, et al. Angiogenesis in bladder tissues is strongly correlated with urinary frequency and bladder pain in patients with interstitial cystitis/bladder pain syndrome. *Int J Urol* 2019;26(Suppl 1):35–40.

25. Sant GR, Kempuraj D, Marchand JE, et al. The mast cell in interstitial cystitis: Role in pathophysiology and pathogenesis. *Urology* 2007;69(4 Suppl):34–40.

26. Gamper M, Regauer S, Welter J, et al. Are mast cells still good biomarkers for bladder pain syndrome/interstitial cystitis? *J Urol* 2015;193(6):1994–2000.

27. Malik ST, Birch BR, Voegeli D, et al. Distribution of mast cell subtypes in interstitial cystitis: Implications for novel diagnostic and therapeutic strategies? *J Clin Pathol* 2018;71(9):840–844.

28. Kim A, Han J-Y, Ryu C-M, et al. Histopathological characteristics of interstitial cystitis/bladder pain syndrome without Hunner lesion. *Histopathology* 2017;71(3):415–424.

29. Spencer NJ, Greenheigh S, Kyloh M, et al. Identifying unique subtypes of spinal afferent nerve endings within the urinary bladder of mice. *J Comp Neurol* 2018;526(4):707–720.

30. Fowler CJ, Griffiths D, de Groat WC. The neural control of micturition. *Nat Rev Neurosci* 2008;9(6):453–466.

31. Davidson S, Copits BA, Zhang J, et al. Human sensory neurons: Membrane properties and sensitization by inflammatory mediators. *Pain* 2014;155(9):1861–1870.

32. Abraham SN, Miao Y. The nature of immune responses to urinary tract infections. *Nat Rev Immunol* 2015;15(10):655–663.

33. Grundy L, Erickson A, Caldwell A, et al. Tetrodotoxin-sensitive voltage-gated sodium channels regulate bladder afferent responses to distension. *Pain* 2018;159(12):2573–2584.

34. Chen W, Ye D-Y, Han D-J, et al. Elevated level of nerve growth factor in the bladder pain syndrome/interstitial cystitis: A meta-analysis. *Springerplus* 2016;5(1):1072.

35. Regauer S, Gamper M, Fehr MK, et al. Sensory hyperinnervation distinguishes bladder pain syndrome/interstitial cystitis from overactive bladder syndrome. *J Urol* 2017;197(1):159–166.

36. Farmer MA, Huang L, Martucci K, et al; for the MAPP Research Network. Brain white matter abnormalities in female interstitial cystitis/bladder pain syndrome: A MAPP Network neuroimaging study. *J Urol* 2015;194(1):118–126.

37. Gardella B, Porru D, Ferdeghini F, et al. Insight into urogynecologic features of women with interstitial cystitis/painful bladder syndrome. *Eur Urol* 2008;54(5):1145–1151.

38. Peters K, Girdler B, Carrico D, et al. Painful bladder syndrome/interstitial cystitis and vulvodynia: A clinical correlation. *Int Urogynecol J* 2008;19(5):665–669.

39. Goetsch MF, Morgan TK, Korcheva VB, et al. Histologic and receptor analysis of primary and secondary vestibulodynia and controls: A prospective study. *Am J Obstet Gynecol* 2010;202(6):614.e1–614.e8.

40. Malykhina AP. Neural mechanisms of pelvic organ cross-sensitization. *Neuroscience* 2007;149(3):660–672.

41. Yoshikawa S, Kawamorita N, Oguchi T, et al. Pelvic organ cross-sensitization to enhance bladder and urethral pain behaviors in rats with experimental colitis. *Neuroscience* 2015;284:422–429.

42. Greenwood-Van Meerveld B, Mohammadi E, Tyler K, et al. Mechanisms of visceral organ crosstalk: Importance of alterations in permeability in rodent models. *J Urol* 2015;194(3):804–811.

43. Towner RA, Smith N, Saunders D, et al. Assessment of colon and bladder crosstalk in an experimental colitis model using contrast-enhanced magnetic resonance imaging. *Neurogastroenterol Motil* 2015;27(11):1571–1579.

44. Cheng C, Rosamilia A, Healey M. Diagnosis of interstitial cystitis/bladder pain syndrome in women with chronic pelvic pain: A prospective observational study. *Int Urogynecol J* 2012;23(10):1361–1366.

45. Tirlapur SA, Kuhrt K, Chaliha C, et al. The 'evil twin syndrome' in chronic pelvic pain: A systematic review of prevalence

studies of bladder pain syndrome and endometriosis. *Int J Surg* 2013;11(3):233–237.

46. Wu C-C, Chung S-D, Lin HC. Endometriosis increased the risk of bladder pain syndrome/interstitial cystitis: A population-based study. *Neurourol Urodyn* 2018;37(4):1413–1418.

47. Abernethy MG, Rosenfeld A, White JR, et al. Urinary microbiome and cytokine levels in women with interstitial cystitis. *Obstet Gynecol* 2017;129(3):500–506.

48. Meriwether KV, Lei Z, Singh R, et al. The vaginal and urinary microbiomes in premenopausal women with interstitial cystitis/bladder pain syndrome as compared to unaffected controls: A pilot cross-sectional study. *Front Cell Infect Microbiol* 2019;9:92.

49. Gil D, Wang J, Gu C, et al. Role of sympathetic nervous system in rat model of chronic visceral pain. *Neurogastroenterol Motil* 2016;28(3):423–431.

50. Charrua A, Pinto R, Taylor A, et al. Can the adrenergic system be implicated in the pathophysiology of bladder pain syndrome/interstitial cystitis? A clinical and experimental study. *Neurourol Urodyn* 2015;34(5):489–496.

51. Gillenwater JY, Wein AJ. Summary of the National Institute of Arthritis, Diabetes, Digestive and Kidney Diseases Workshop on Interstitial Cystitis, National Institutes of Health, Bethesda, Maryland, August 28–29, 1987. *J Urol* 1988;140(1):203–206.

52. Powell-Boone T, Ness TJ, Cannon R, et al. Menstrual cycle affects bladder pain sensation in subjects with interstitial cystitis. *J Urol* 2005;174(5):1832–1836.

53. O'Leary MP SG, Fowler FJ Jr, et al. The interstitial cystitis symptom index and problem index. *Urology* 1997;49(5):58–63.

54. Goin JE, Olaleye D, Peters KM, et al. Psychometric analysis of the University of Wisconsin Interstitial Cystitis Scale: Implications for use in randomized clinical trials. *J Urol* 1998;159(3):1085–1090.

55. Parsons CL, Dell J, Stanford EJ, et al. Increased prevalence of interstitial cystitis: Previously unrecognized urologic and gynecologic cases identified using a new symptom questionnaire and intravesical potassium sensitivity. *Urology* 2002;60(4):573–578.

56. Swamy S, Barcella W, De Iorio M, et al. Recalcitrant chronic bladder pain and recurrent cystitis but negative urinalysis: What should we do? *Int Urogynecol J* 2018;29(7):1035–1043.

57. Teichman JM, Nielsen-Omeis BJ, McIver BD. Modified urodynamics for interstitial cystitis. *Tech Urol* 1997;3(2):65–68.

58. Nordling J, Anjum FH, Bade JJ, et al. Primary evaluation of patients suspected of having interstitial cystitis (IC). *Eur Urol* 2004;45(5):662–669.

59. Waxman JA, Sulak PJ, Kuehl TJ. Cystoscopic findings consistent with interstitial cystitis in normal women undergoing tubal ligation. *J Urol* 1998;160(5):1663–1667.

60. Rosamilia A, Igawa Y, Higashi S. Pathology of interstitial cystitis. *Int J Urol* 2003;10(Suppl):S11–S15.

61. Doiron RC, Tolls V, Irvine-Bird K, et al. Clinical phenotyping does not differentiate Hunner lesion subtype of interstitial cystitis/bladder pain syndrome: A relook at the role of cystoscopy. *J Urol* 2016;196(4):1136–1140.

62. Schachar JS, Evans RJ, Parks GE, et al. Histological evidence supports low anesthetic bladder capacity as a marker of a bladder-centric disease subtype in interstitial cystitis/bladder pain syndrome. *Int Urogynecol J* 2019;30(11):1863–1870.

63. Keay SK, Zhang CO, Shoenfelt J, et al. Sensitivity and specificity of antiproliferative factor, heparin-binding epidermal growth factor–like growth factor, and epidermal growth factor as urine markers for interstitial cystitis. *Urology* 2001;57(6):9–14.

64. Keay S, Kleinberg M, Zhang CO, et al. Bladder epithelial cells from patients with interstitial cystitis produce an inhibitor of heparin-binding epidermal growth factor-like growth factor production. *J Urol* 2000;164(6):2112–2118.

65. O'Hare PG, Hoffmann AR, Allen P, et al. Interstitial cystitis patients' use and rating of complementary and alternative medicine therapies. *Int Urogynecol J* 2013;24(6):977–982.

66. Shorter B, Lesser M, Moldwin RM, et al. Effect of comestibles on symptoms of interstitial cystitis. *J Urol* 2007;178(1):145–152.

67. Bassaly R, Downes K, Hart S. Dietary consumption triggers in interstitial cystitis/bladder pain syndrome patients. *Female Pelvic Med Reconstr Surg* 2011;17(1):36–39.

68. Bologna RA, Gomelsky A, Lukban JC, et al. The efficacy of calcium glycerophosphate in the prevention of food-related flares in interstitial cystitis. *Urology* 2001;57(6 Suppl 1):119–120.

69. Lukban J, Whitmore K, Kellogg-Spadt S, et al. The effect of manual physical therapy in patients diagnosed with interstitial cystitis, high-tone pelvic floor dysfunction, and sacroiliac dysfunction. *Urology* 2001;57(6 Suppl 1):121–122.

70. FitzGerald MP, Payne CK, Lukacz ES, et al. Randomized multicenter clinical trial of myofascial physical therapy in women with interstitial cystitis/painful bladder syndrome and pelvic floor tenderness. *J Urol* 2012;187(6):2113–2118.

71. Nickel JC, Tripp DA, Pontari M, et al. Psychosocial phenotyping in women with interstitial cystitis/painful bladder syndrome: A case control study. *J Urol* 2010;183(1):167–172.

72. Lai H, Gardner V, Vetter J, et al. Correlation between psychological stress levels and the severity of overactive bladder symptoms. *BMC Urol* 2015;15(1):14.

73. Foster HE Jr, Hanno PM, Nickel JC, et al. Effect of amitriptyline on symptoms in treatment naïve patients with interstitial cystitis/painful bladder syndrome. *J Urol* 2010;183(5):1853–1858.

74. Mulholland SG, Hanno P, Parsons CL, et al. Pentosan polysulfate sodium for therapy of interstitial cystitis. A double-blind placebo-controlled clinical study. *Urology* 1990;35(6):552–558.

75. Nickel JC, Herschorn S, Whitmore KE, et al. Pentosan polysulfate sodium for treatment of interstitial cystitis/bladder pain syndrome: Insights from a randomized, double-blind, placebo controlled study. *J Urol* 2015;193(3):857–862.

76. Lyons RJ, Ahmad S, Ansari S, et al. Pentosan polysulfate-associated macular disease in patients with interstitial cystitis. *Obstet Gynecol* 2020;135(5):1091–1094.

77. Thilagarajah R, Witherow RO, Walker MM. Oral cimetidine gives effective symptom relief in painful bladder disease: A prospective, randomized, double-blind placebo-controlled trial. *BJU Int* 2001;87(3):207–212.

78. Forrest JB, Payne CK, Erickson DR. Cyclosporine A for refractory interstitial cystitis/bladder pain syndrome: Experience of 3 tertiary centers. *J Urol* 2012;188(4):1186–1191.

79. Crescenze IM, Tucky B, Li J, et al. Efficacy, side effects, and monitoring of oral cyclosporine in interstitial cystitis-bladder pain syndrome. *Urology* 2017;107:49–54.

80. Nickel JC, Egerdie B, Davis E, et al. A phase II study of the efficacy and safety of the novel oral SHIP1 activator AQX-1125 in subjects with moderate to severe interstitial cystitis/bladder pain syndrome. *J Urol* 2016;196(3):747–754.

81. Nickel JC, Moldwin R, Hanno P, et al. Targeting the SHIP1 pathway fails to show treatment benefit in interstitial cystitis/bladder pain syndrome: Lessons learned from evaluating potentially effective therapies in this enigmatic syndrome. *J Urol* 2019;202(2):301–308.

82. Ottem DP, Teichman JMH. What is the value of cystoscopy with hydrodistension for interstitial cystitis? *Urology* 2005;66(3):494–499.

83. Funaro MG, King AN, Stern JNH, et al. Endoscopic injection of low dose triamcinolone: A simple, minimally invasive, and effective therapy for interstitial cystitis with Hunner lesions. *Urology* 2018;118:25–29.

84. Crescenze IM, Gupta P, Adams G, et al. Advanced management of patients with ulcerative interstitial cystitis/bladder pain syndrome. *Urology* 2019;133:78–83.

85. Ko KJ, Cho WJ, Lee Y-S, et al. Comparison of the efficacy between transurethral coagulation and transurethral resection of Hunner lesion in interstitial cystitis/bladder pain syndrome patients: A prospective randomized controlled trial. *Eur Urol* 2020;77(5):644–651.

86. Peters KM, Feber KM, Bennett RC. A prospective, single-blind, randomized crossover trial of sacral vs pudendal nerve stimulation for interstitial cystitis. *BJU Int* 2007;100(4):835–839.

87. Gajewski JB, Al-Zahrani AA. The long-term efficacy of sacral neuromodulation in the management of intractable cases of bladder pain syndrome: 14 years of experience in one centre. *BJU Int* 2011;107(8):1258–1264.

88. Marinkovic SP, Gillen LM, Marinkovic CM. Minimum 6-year outcomes for interstitial cystitis treated with sacral neuromodulation. *Int Urogynecol J* 2011;22(4):407–412.

89. Osman N, Braff DG, Downey AP, et al. A systematic review of surgical interventions for the treatment of bladder pain syndrome/interstitial cystitis. *Eur Urol Focus* 2021;7(4):877–885.

90. Kim KK, Sin DY, Park HW. Urethral caruncle occurring in a young girl—A case report. *J Korean Med Sci* 1993;8(2):160–161.

91. Ozkurkcugil C, Ozkan L, Tarcan T. The effect of asymptomatic urethral caruncle on micturition in women with urinary incontinence. *Korean J Urol* 2010;51(4):257–259.

92. Çoban S, Bıyık I. Urethral caruncle: Case report of a rare acute urinary retension cause. *Can Urol Assoc J* 2014;8(3–4):E270–E272.

93. Dolan MS, Hill C, Valea FA. Benign gynecologic lesions. In: Lobo RA, Gerhenson DM, Lentz GM, et al, eds. *Comprehensive gynecology*, 7th ed. Philadelphia: Elsevier; 2017:370–422.

94. Lowe FC, Hill GS, Jeffs RD, et al. Urethral prolapse in children: Insights into etiology and management. *J Urol* 1986;135(1):100–103.

95. Anveden-Hertzberg L, Gauderer M, Elder JS. Urethral prolapse: An often misdiagnosed cause of urogenital bleeding in girls. *Pediatr Emerg Care* 1995;11(4):212–214.

96. Rosenblum N, Nitti VW. Female urethral reconstruction. *Urol Clin North Am* 2011;38(1):55–64.

97. Groutz A, Blaivas JG, Chaikin DC. Bladder outlet obstruction in women: Definition and characteristics. *Neurourol Urodyn* 2000;19(3):213–220.

98. Santucci R, Chen M. Evaluation and treatment of female urethral stricture disease. *Curr Bladder Dysfunct Rep* 2013;8:123–127.

99. Romman AN, Alhalabi F, Zimmern PE. Distal intramural urethral pathology in women. *J Urol* 2012;188(4):1218–1223.

100. Hoag N, Chee J. Surgical management of female urethral strictures. *Transl Androl Urol* 2017;6(Suppl 2):S76–S80.

101. Osman NI, Chapple CR. Contemporary surgical management of female urethral stricture disease. *Curr Opin Urol* 2015;25(4):341–345.

102. Fall M, Baranowski AP, Elneil S, et al. EAU guidelines on chronic pelvic pain. *Eur Urol* 2010;57(1):35–48.

103. Doggweiler R, Whitmore KE, Meijlink JM, et al. A standard for terminology in chronic pelvic pain syndromes: A report from the chronic pelvic pain working group of the International Continence Society. *Neurourol Urodyn* 2017;36(4):984–1008.

104. Chowdhury ML, Javaid N, Ghoniem GM. Urethral pain syndrome: A systematic review. *Curr Bladder Dysfunct Rep* 2019;14(2):75–82.

105. Clemens JQ, Stephens-Shields A, Naliboff BD, et al; for the MAPP Research Network. Correlates of health care seeking activities in patients with urological chronic pelvic pain syndromes: Findings from the MAPP cohort. *J Urol* 2018;200(1):136–140.

106. Kyndel A, Elmér C, Källman O, et al. Mycoplasmataceae colonizations in women with urethral pain syndrome: A case-control study. *J Low Genit Tract Dis* 2016;20(3):272–274.

107. Ivarsson LB, Lindström BE, Olovsson M, et al. Treatment of urethral pain syndrome (UPS) in Sweden. *PloS One* 2019;14(11):e0225404.

108. Lindström BE, Hellberg D, Lindström AK. Urethral instillations of clobetasol propionate and lidocaine: A promising treatment of urethral pain syndrome. *Clin Exp Obstet Gynecol* 2016;43(6):803–807.

109. Bazi T, Abou-Ghannam G, Khauli R. Female urethral dilation. *Int Urogynecol J* 2013;24(9):1435–1444.

110. Perez-Marrero R, Emerson LE, Feltis JT. A controlled study of dimethyl sulfoxide in interstitial cystitis. *J Urol* 1988;140(1):36–39.

111. Lim YN, Karmakar D, Murray C, et al. A long term study of intravesical dimethyl sulfoxide (DMSO)/heparin/hydrocortisone/bupivacaine therapy for interstitial cystitis/bladder pain syndrome (BPS). *Int Urogynecol J* 2015;26(Suppl 1):S127–S128.

112. Nomiya A, Naruse T, Niimi A, et al. On- and post-treatment symptom relief by repeated instillations of heparin and alkalized lidocaine in interstitial cystitis. *Int J Urol* 2013;20(11):1118–1122.

113. Bade JJ, Laseur M, Nieuwenburg A, et al. A placebo-controlled study of intravesical pentosanpolysulphate for the treatment of interstitial cystitis. *Br J Urol* 1997;79(2):168–171.

114. Shim SR, Cho YJ, Shin I-S, et al. Efficacy and safety of botulinum toxin injection for interstitial cystitis/bladder pain syndrome: A systematic review and meta-analysis. *Int Urol Nephrol* 2016;48(8):1215–1227.

115. Cvach K, Rosamilia A, Dwyer P, et al. Efficacy of Clorpactin in refractory bladder pain syndrome/interstitial cystitis: A randomized controlled trial. *Int Urogynecol J* 2021;32(5):1177–1183.

Associations with Useful Information Regarding Bladder Pain Syndrome/Interstitial Cystitis

International Urogynecological Association (IUGA)
  http://www.yourpelvicfloor.org
American Urological Association (AUA)
  http://www.auanet.org
International Society for the Study of Bladder Pain Syndrome (ESSIC)
  http://www.essic.org
Interstitial Cystitis Association
  https://www.ichelp.org
International Continence Society
  http://www.ics.org
International Painful Bladder Foundation
  http://www.painful-bladder.org
Interstitial Cystitis Network
  http://www.ic-network.com

CHAPTER 39

EVALUATION AND MANAGEMENT OF MICROSCOPIC HEMATURIA

Ellen O'Connor • Aoife McVey • Nathan Lawrentschuk

Introduction

Microscopic hematuria (MH) is a common incidental finding present in up to 1 in 5 women.[1] MH may indicate presence of underlying pathology such as urothelial cancer, urolithiasis, or infection; however, only 30% of patients presenting with MH are found to have an identifiable cause.[1,2] Many existing guideline recommendations for evaluation of MH reflect male urologic malignancy risk despite known gender disparities in urologic cancer.[3] In the female patient demographic, unconstrained investigation of patients with MH may lead to individual and public health implications associated with adverse clinical and economic effects.[4,5] Despite this, bladder cancer remains to account for 125,000 cancer diagnoses in women worldwide annually; therefore, a risk-stratified approach to evaluation and management of MH is essential.[6]

DEFINITION AND ETIOLOGY

Terminology and definitions used for MH can vary; the terms "microscopic hematuria," "microhematuria," "nonvisible hematuria," and "dipstick hematuria" are all commonly and interchangeably used. The definition of MH varies according to guidelines; however, majority require microscopic evaluation for diagnosis with a threshold ranging from 2 to 25 red blood cells per high-power field (RBCs/HPF).[7-9] An appropriately collected urine sample for interpretation requires a freshly voided, clean-catch, midstream specimen.[7,9] Dipstick hematuria is a common incidental finding because it is a universally used screening tool for a variety of indications. It is important to note, however, that urine dipstick analysis can be prone to false positives due to myoglobinuria, dehydration, and menstrual blood among other factors.[10] It is for this reason that most guidelines suggest that dipstick hematuria be further investigated with formal urine microscopy for diagnosis of MH to be confirmed.[7] A single finding of MH on urine microscopy is sufficient to warrant further investigation due to the known transient nature of MH present in even malignant conditions.

Causes of MH can be classified according to anatomical site of origin (kidney, ureter, bladder, urethra) or etiology (malignant, obstructive, infectious/inflammatory, nephrogenic, transient) (Table 39.1). Transient and benign causes for MH, such as urinary tract infection, trauma, viral illness, vigorous exercise, and recent urologic instrumentation, should be considered prior to commencing initial evaluation for underlying pathology.[11] Additionally, female-specific conditions such as urogenital tract atrophy, pelvic organ prolapse, and menstruation can lead to urinary contamination resulting in false-positive findings of MH.[9,12,13] In these patients, a clean-catch specimen may be obtained using in-and-out catheterization to avoid introital contamination.

Hematuria is an established clinical indicator for bladder cancer, a disease that results in 200,000 deaths worldwide annually and attributable to 3% of new cancer diagnoses.[14] Although the incidence of bladder cancer is higher in men than in women (3.1:1 ratio), women disproportionally present with more advanced disease and have a high mortality rate compared to their male counterparts.[15,16] Studies looking at women evaluated within dedicated urogynecology clinics for MH, with and without symptoms, identified a 0.4% to 1.7% incidence rate of urologic malignancy.[17-20] Despite the low prevalence of bladder cancer in women with MH, risk-stratified referral for investigation is widely recommended.[21] Women are more likely to experience delay in time to evaluation and time to diagnosis of bladder cancer.[15,22] Although the precise reasons for this remain unknown, this delay may be attributed to repeated testing, initial management of presumed infection, and hesitancy to overinvestigate.[23] Furthermore, some studies report nonadherence to guideline recommendations for cystoscopy and upper tract imaging in up to 20% of female patients.[20]

TABLE 39.1

Causes of Microscopic Hematuria

ETIOLOGY	CAUSE	ORIGIN
Transient	Exercise induced	Bladder
	Trauma	Urethra
	Sexual intercourse	
Malignant	Urothelial cancer	Bladder/ureter/ renal pelvis
	Renal cell carcinoma	Kidney
Infectious/ inflammatory	Lower urinary tract infection	Bladder
	Radiation cystitis	
	Foreign body	
Renal medical disease	IgA nephropathy	Kidney
	Thin basement membrane disease	
	Hereditary nephritis	
Obstructive	Urolithiasis	Kidney/ureter

IgA, immunoglobulin A.

EVALUATION

Initial evaluation for MH should incorporate careful history and physical examination. Presence of lower urinary tract symptoms, such as urinary frequency, dysuria, and urgency may reflect urinary tract infection. Obstructive pathology may be indicated with hesitancy, incomplete emptying, and reduced urinary flow. Flank or abdominal pain favors potential urolithiasis, trauma, or pyelonephritis. History of risk factors for urologic malignancy should be carefully considered, with smoking history and increased age as the greatest risk factors (Table 39.2). Use of anticoagulation or antiplatelet agents does not exclude a patient from requiring further evaluation.

Physical examination should include abdominal and urogenital examination as well as blood pressure assessment. Speculum examination can be used to rule out vaginal, cervical, and uterine sources of MH. Laboratory investigations include serum creatinine, urea and glomerular filtration rate, and urinalysis to assess for potential renal parenchymal disease. Evaluation of urinary cytology has a high sensitivity in patients with high-grade urothelial cancer and may be used as an adjunct to cystoscopy and radiologic evaluation. Negative cytology, however, does not exclude the possibility of malignancy due to low sensitivity in detection of low-grade tumors.[25] Furthermore, cytologic evaluation can be impaired in the presence of urinary tract infection

TABLE 39.2

Risk Factors for Urinary Tract Malignancy in Patients with Microscopic Hematuria

RISK FACTORS[3,7,20,24]

Age

History of gross hematuria

Irritative lower urinary tract symptoms

Smoking (current or past history)

Occupational exposure (dyes, benzenes, aromatic amines)

Cyclophosphamide exposure

History of chronic urinary tract infection

History of pelvic irradiation

and urolithiasis. Full diagnostic workup for MH should include radiologic and cystoscopic assessment of both the upper and lower urinary tract, respectively, with referral to urologic services.

Selection of women who require further investigation for MH can be a contentious issue as there are many transient and benign causes that may not require a full diagnostic workup. A suggested algorithm for MH evaluation is depicted in Figure 39.1. Patients suspected of having urinary tract infection should undergo urine culture and be treated with antibiotics, if indicated, followed by repeat urinalysis to ensure resolution of MH.[26] Women with other suspected transient and benign causes should have repeat urine microscopy following resolution of the suspected cause. If MH persists, then further evaluation is warranted. Several medical organizations offer guidelines regarding selection and methods of evaluation for patients with MH (Table 39.3). The American Urological Association 2020 guideline for MH recommends investigation of patients who present with a single sample of ≥3 RBCs/HPF based on a risk-stratified approach following initial evaluation.[7] Women younger than the age of 50 years with no risk factors and 3 to 10 RBCs/HPF should have a discussion regarding cystoscopic and ultrasound evaluation, with the alternative option for repeat urinalysis within 6 months. Intermediate and high-risk women are determined based on degree of MH, significance of risk factors, and prior history of hematuria, with a preference for axial imaging over ultrasonography in the high-risk group.

Although the European Association of Urology has not released a dedicated guideline regarding the diagnosis and evaluation of hematuria, rather detailing recommendations based on disease status, they do recommend either renal ultrasound or computed tomography (CT) urography together with cystoscopy

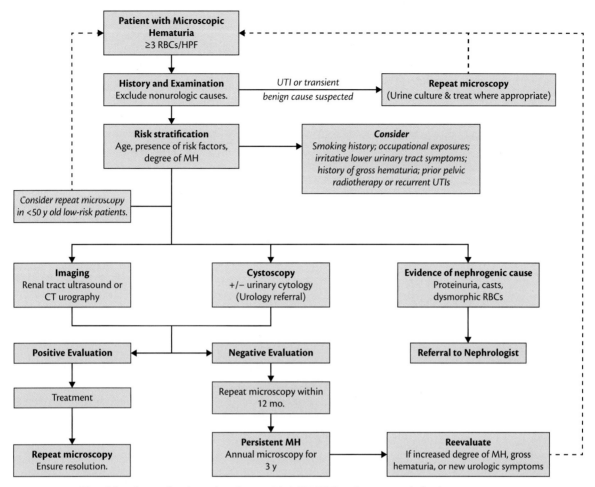

FIGURE 39.1 Algorithm for evaluation of patients with MH. UTI, urinary tract infection.

for investigation of hematuria.[31] In a recent systematic review and meta-analysis on the subject, Jubber et al.[32] recommends evaluation using cystoscopy and upper tract imaging (either ultrasound or CT urography) in patients with dipstick positive hematuria, older than the age of 40 years, following exclusion of potential precipitating factors. With regard to female-specific patient groups, a joint statement by the American College of Obstetricians and Gynecologists and American Urogynecologic Society acknowledges the gender disparities in incidence of urologic malignancy.[9] As such, they recommend evaluation for low-risk, asymptomatic women aged 35 to 50 years only if greater than 25 RBCs/HPF are identified on microscopy.

Choice of imaging modality to investigate MH, as with any investigation, should be performed using the least invasive option where clinically appropriate. Multiphase CT urography (Fig. 39.2) has the highest sensitivity and specificity for identifying upper tract pathology; however, it is associated with increased cost as well as radiation and intravenous contrast exposure.[33,34] Renal ultrasound is a relatively cheaper mode of investigation and obtains reasonable assessment for renal

cortical lesions; however, it is less accurate in detection of urolithiasis and urothelial lesions.[34] A risk-stratified approach may be employed in this setting whereby patients deemed low- or intermediate-risk undergo renal tract ultrasound, and high-risk patients be investigated using multiphase CT urography.[7] Where there are contraindications to CT urography, alternative imaging modalities including magnetic resonance (MR) urography, noncontrast CT, or retrograde pyelogram should be considered.

Cystoscopy is the accepted gold standard for evaluation of the bladder in patients with MH. Although CT urography also has a high sensitivity for detection of bladder tumors (0.95 compared to 0.98 for cystoscopy), it may be unable to detect flat lesions such as small nonmuscle invasive tumors or carcinoma in situ (Fig. 39.3). In additional, cystoscopy may be able to identify alternative causes of MH such as anatomical abnormalities (urethral stricture, diverticulum), inflammatory pathology or bladder calculi. Flexible cystoscopy is the diagnostic procedure of choice; however, should the patient have an identified bladder lesion on CT or ultrasound, they should be referred directly for rigid cystoscopy in the first instance.

TABLE 39.3

Guideline Recommendations for Evaluation of Microscopic Hematuria

GUIDELINE	DEFINITION	CRITERIA FOR INVESTIGATION	IMAGING	CYSTOSCOPY	FOLLOW-UP
AUA/SUFU (2020)[7]	≥3 RBCs/HPF on single microscopy	*Low*[a]: age <50 y, never or <10 pack-year smoker, 3–10 RBCs/HPF, no risk factors *Intermediate*[b]: age 50–59 y, 10–30 pack-year smoker, 11–25 RBCs/HPF, single risk factor *High*[b]: age >60 y, >30 pack-year smoker, >25 RBCs/HPF, history gross hematuria	*Low*: repeat UA with 6 mo or renal ultrasound *Intermediate*: renal ultrasound *High*: multiphase CT urography	*Low*: repeat UA within 6 mo or cystoscopy *Intermediate*: cystoscopy *High*: cystoscopy	Repeat UA within 12 mo for those with negative evaluation Shared decision-making if persistent MH Reevaluate if new risk factors.
ACOG/AUGS (2017)[9]	≥25 RBCs/HPF on single microscopy	Women aged 35–50 y, nonsmokers, absence of other risk factors	Avoid unless ≥25 RBCs/HPF (in stated population).	Avoid unless ≥25 RBCs/HPF (in stated population).	No recommendation
CUA (2009)[8]	>2 RBCs/HPF on two microscopy specimens	No recommendation	Renal ultrasound in all patients	Cystoscopy in age >40 y, risk factors or positive/atypical cytology	Repeat UA, cytology, and BP at 6, 12, 24, and 36 mo Reevaluate if new risk factors or symptoms.
Canadian consensus document (2015)[27]	≥3 RBCs/HPF on single microscopy	aMH: age ≥35 y or age <35 y with risk factors sMH: any age	Ultrasound or CT urography for aMH CT urography for sMH	Cystoscopy in all patients	Annual UA for 3 y Reevaluate if new risk factors or symptoms.
ACP (2016)[28]	≥3 RBCs/HPF on single microscopy	No recommendation	Any asymptomatic adult in absence of benign cause	Any asymptomatic adult in absence of benign cause	No recommendation
BAUS/RA (2008)[29]	Either dipstick (1+ or more) or MH	aMH: age >40 y, confirmed on two samples sMH: any age	Imaging in all patients, no further recommendation	Cystoscopy in all patients	Annual assessment as long as the MH persists Reevaluate if new risk factors or symptoms.
NICE (2015)[30]	No recommendation	Age >60 y with either dysuria of raised serum white cell count	No recommendation	No recommendation	No recommendation

[a]Meets all criteria.
[b]Meets one of the criteria.
AUA, American Urological Association; SUFU, Society of Urodynamics, Female Pelvic Medicine & Urogenital Reconstruction; UA, urinalysis; ACOG, American College of Obstetricians and Gynecologists; AUGS, American Urogynecologic Society; CUA, Canadian Urological Association; aMH, asymptomatic microscopic hematuria; sMH, symptomatic microscopic hematuria; ACP, American College of Physicians; BAUS, British Association of Urological Surgeons; BP, blood pressure; mo, months; RA, Renal Association; NICE, National Institute for Health and Care Excellence; y, year.

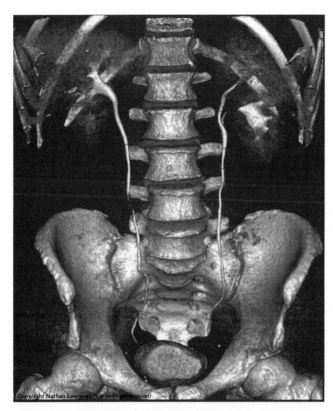

FIGURE 39.2 Three-dimensional reconstructed CT urography demonstrating normal renal collecting system and ureters. (Courtesy of Professor Nathan Lawrentschuk, Australia.)

Hematuria during Pregnancy

MH in pregnancy is not uncommon; recorded in 3% to 20% of pregnant women.[35] Anatomical changes secondary to the gravid uterus may result in idiopathic MH, with external compression elevating the trigone and increasing vascularity.[11] Although rare, urologic cancers do occur in pregnancy with renal cell carcinoma being the most common.[36] Pregnancy-specific conditions such as

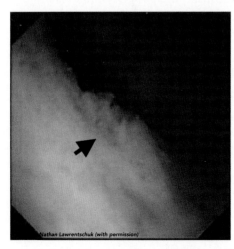

FIGURE 39.3 Endoscopic appearance of low-grade carpet urothelial cancer (arrow). (Courtesy of Professor Nathan Lawrentschuk, Australia.)

preeclampsia and placenta percreta may result in MH; however, infection, urolithiasis, and trauma remain to be the most likely identifiable causes.[11] Although no clear guidelines exist for MH in pregnancy, it is suggested that evaluation and investigation is with the same approach as nonpregnant women given etiologies are similar.

A clear barrier to investigation of MH in pregnancy is choice of imaging technique. However, it is worth noting that pregnant women are less likely to exhibit significant risk factors due to their demographics (age <60 years, <30 pack-year smoker) and therefore in the low- to intermediate-risk group with ultrasound renal tract being the most appropriate investigation of choice regardless. If pregnant women do fall into high-risk category (e.g., gross hematuria), then MR urography can be considered.[7]

MANAGEMENT

Urologic Pathology

Patients identified to have urolithiasis or potentially malignant causes for MH require urologic review for further management. Primary treatment for bladder tumor is transurethral resection of the tumor followed by either surveillance, intravesical immunotherapy, or radical surgery depending on disease stage.[31] Where cystoscopic evaluation has been performed by an experienced urogynecologist, documentation should include a detailed operative report, intraoperative photography where possible, and biopsy histology where completed. Patients with risk factors for bladder cancer, symptomatic MH, or suspicious cystoscopic findings should be referred for urologic review promptly. There is no guideline consensus regarding adequacy of urogynecologic-led cystoscopic evaluation for MH; therefore, clinicians should be cognizant of pitfalls in missing potentially significant pathology in this patient demographic. Referral to a dedicated urology service should be performed in all patients in the event of uncertainty.

Presence of nonobstructing renal calculi on upper tract imaging does not exclude other potentially malignant causes for MH, therefore, even asymptomatic patients with urolithiasis require referral to urology for discussion of results or further investigation as indicated.

Renal Pathology

MH with evidence of glomerulopathic disease on urinalysis, renal insufficiency, or hypertension in those aged younger than 40 years should be referred to a nephrologist for further investigation. Potential nephrogenic causes of MH will result in proteinuria, dysmorphic RBCs, and red cell casts on urinalysis, an indication of glomerular injury. The most common glomerular cause of MH is immunoglobulin A nephropathy, followed by thin basement membrane disease and hereditary nephritis.[37]

Percutaneous renal biopsy is considered in this populations for diagnosis of glomerular or tubulointerstitial causes of MH. Risk-based urologic referral is still indicated for patients with suspicion of medical renal disease as urologic malignancy may still occur in these populations.[7]

Management following Initial Negative Workup

Appropriate management of patients with MH following primary negative workup requires shared decision-making and a risk-stratified approach. In the first instance, in those women without potential transient causes, with normal cystoscopy and upper tract imaging, a repeat urinalysis should be performed within 12 months. Although there is no clear consensus regarding the number of negative annual urinalyses prior to safely discontinuing surveillance, one per year for 1 to 2 years is thought to be sufficient.[7,27]

Persistent MH necessitates consideration of further investigation. In women representing with new symptoms such as gross hematuria, significant increase in degree of MH, lower urinary tract symptoms, and renal impairment or pain, a complete reevaluation is essential due to uncertainty of underlying pathology.[38] Shared decision-making for low-risk women with persistent MH should involve discussion regarding repeat urinalysis versus reevaluation. In this instance, annual urinalysis for at least 3 years together with urinary cytology has been recommended. Rediscussion of repeat renal tract imaging and cystoscopy in the event of ongoing MH should be performed at this time.[27]

CONCLUSION

MH is a common finding in women and may indicate serious underlying pathology in a small proportion of individuals. Up to 70% of women with MH will have no identifiable etiology, with transient and benign causes likely. A risk-stratified approach to evaluation of MH is essential for early diagnosis and treatment of potential urologic malignancy, with prompt referral for cystoscopy and upper tract imaging especially important in women with risk factors present. Women who have no pathology identified should have repeat urinary microscopy performed within 12 months to rule out persistent MH.

References

1. Lippmann QK, Slezak JM, Menefee SA, et al. Evaluation of microscopic hematuria and risk of urologic cancer in female patients. *Am J Obstet Gynecol* 2017;216(2):146.e141–146.e147.
2. Khadra MH, Pickard RS, Charlton M, et al. A prospective analysis of 1,930 patients with hematuria to evaluate current diagnostic practice. *J Urol* 2000;163(2):524–527.
3. Jeppson PC, Jakus-Waldman S, Yazdany T, et al; for American Urogynecologic Society Systematic Review Committee. Microscopic hematuria as a screening tool for urologic malignancies in women. *Female Pelvic Med Reconstr Surg* 2021;27(1):9–15.
4. Linder BJ, Bass EJ, Mostafid H, et al. Guideline of guidelines: Asymptomatic microscopic haematuria. *BJU Int* 2018;121(2):176–183.
5. Harmanli O, Yuksel B. Asymptomatic microscopic hematuria in women requires separate guidelines. *Int Urogynecol J* 2013;24(2):203–206.
6. Bray F, Ferlay J, Soerjomataram I, et al. Global cancer statistics 2018: GLOBOCAN estimates of incidence and mortality worldwide for 36 cancers in 185 countries. *CA Cancer J Clin* 2018;68(6):394–424.
7. Barocas D, Boorjian S, Alvarez R, et al. Microhematuria: AUA/SUFU guideline. *J Urol* 2020;204(4):778–786.
8. Wollin T, Laroche B, Psooy K. Canadian guidelines for the management of asymptomatic microscopic hematuria in adults. *Can Urol Assoc J* 2009;3(1):77–80.
9. American College of Obstetricians and Gynecologists Committee on Gynecologic Practice, American Urogynecologic Society. Committee Opinion No. 703: Asymptomatic microscopic hematuria in women. *Obstet Gynecol* 2017;129(6):e168–e172.
10. Dune TJ, Kliethermes S, Mueller ER, et al. Screening for microscopic hematuria in a urogynecologic population. *Female Pelvic Med Reconstr Surg* 2020;26(6):382–386.
11. Partin AW, Peters CA, Kavoussi LR, et al. *Campbell-Walsh-Wein urology.* 12th ed. Philadelphia: Elsevier, 2021.
12. Shalom DF, Lin SN, St. Louis S, et al. The prevalence of microscopic hematuria in women with pelvic organ prolapse. *Female Pelvic Med Reconstr Surg* 2011;17(6):290–292.
13. Pillalamarri N, Shalom D, Sanidad S, et al. The prevalence of microscopic hematuria in a cohort of women with pelvic organ prolapse. *Int Urogynecol J* 2015;26(1):85–90.
14. Richters A, Aben KKH, Kiemeney LALM. The global burden of urinary bladder cancer: An update. *World J Urol* 2020;38(8):1895–1904.
15. Cohn JA, Vekhter B, Lyttle C, et al. Sex disparities in diagnosis of bladder cancer after initial presentation with hematuria: A nationwide claims-based investigation. *Cancer* 2014;120(4):555–561.
16. Garg T, Pinheiro LC, Atoria CL, et al. Gender disparities in hematuria evaluation and bladder cancer diagnosis: A population based analysis. *J Urol* 2014;192(4):1072–1077.
17. Wu JM, Williams KS, Hundley AF, et al. Microscopic hematuria as a predictive factor for detecting bladder cancer at cystoscopy in women with irritative voiding symptoms. *Am J Obstet Gynecol* 2006;194(5):1423–1426.
18. Goldberg RP, Sherman W, Sand PK. Cystoscopy for lower urinary tract symptoms in urogynecologic practice: The likelihood of finding bladder cancer. *Int Urogynecol J Pelvic Floor Dysfunct* 2008;19(7):991–994.
19. Bradley MS, Willis-Gray MG, Amundsen CL, et al. Microhematuria in postmenopausal women: Adherence to guidelines in a tertiary care setting. *J Urol* 2016;195(4, Pt 1):937–941.
20. Richter LA, Lippmann QK, Jallad K, et al. Risk factors for microscopic hematuria in women. *Female Pelvic Med Reconstr Surg* 2016;22(6):486–490.
21. Packiam VT, Barocas DA, Boorjian SA. Microscopic hematuria: Diagnosis is only half the battle. *European Urology* 2020;77(5):599–600.
22. Lyratzopoulos G, Abel GA, McPhail S, et al. Gender inequalities in the promptness of diagnosis of bladder and renal

cancer after symptomatic presentation: Evidence from secondary analysis of an English primary care audit survey. *BMJ Open* 2013;3(6):e002861.

23. Ngo B, Perera M, Papa N, et al. Factors affecting the timeliness and adequacy of haematuria assessment in bladder cancer: A systematic review. *BJU Int* 2017;119(Suppl 5):10–18.

24. Lim Joon D, Foroudi F, Wasiak J, et al. The collaborative management of late urological complications after radiation therapy. *BJU Int* 2019;123(Suppl 5):8–9.

25. Tan WS, Sarpong R, Khetrapal P, et al. Does urinary cytology have a role in haematuria investigations? *BJU Int* 2019;123(1): 74–81.

26. Lawrentschuk N, Ooi J, Pang A, et al. Cystoscopy in women with recurrent urinary tract infection. *Int J Urol* 2006;13(4):350–353.

27. Kassouf W, Aprikian A, Black P, et al. Recommendations for the improvement of bladder cancer quality of care in Canada: A consensus document reviewed and endorsed by Bladder Cancer Canada (BCC), Canadian Urologic Oncology Group (CUOG), and Canadian Urological Association (CUA), December 2015. *Can Urol Assoc J* 2016;10(1–2):E46–E80.

28. Nielsen M, Qaseem A; for High Value Care Task Force of the American College of Physicians. Hematuria as a marker of occult urinary tract cancer: Advice for high-value care from the American College of Physicians. *Ann Intern Med* 2016;164(7): 488–497.

29. Anderson J, Fawcett D, Feehally J, et al. *Joint consensus statement on the initial assessment of haematuria. Prepared on behalf of the Renal Association and British Association of Urological Surgeons.* London: British Association of Urological Surgeons, 2008.

30. National Institute for Health and Care Excellence. Suspected cancer: Recognition and referral 2015. Accessed September 16, 2020. https://www.nice.org.uk/guidance/ng12 /chapter/1-Recommendations-organised-by-site-of-cancer

31. Babjuk M, Burger M, Compérat EM, et al. *EAU guidelines on non-muscle-invasive urothelial carcinoma of the bladder.* Arnhem: European Association of Urology, 2020.

32. Jubber I, Shariat SF, Conroy S, et al. Non-visible haematuria for the detection of bladder, upper tract, and kidney cancer: An updated systematic review and meta-analysis. *Eur Urol* 2020;77(5):583–598.

33. Bagheri MH, Ahlman MA, Lindenberg L, et al. Advances in medical imaging for the diagnosis and management of common genitourinary cancers. *Urol Oncol* 2017;35(7):473–491.

34. Tan WS, Sarpong R, Khetrapal P, et al. Can renal and bladder ultrasound replace computerized tomography urogram in patients investigated for microscopic hematuria? *J Urol* 2018;200(5):973–980.

35. Shahraki AD, Bardeh ME, Najarzadegan MR. Investigation of the relationship between idiopathic microscopic hematuria (in the first and second trimesters) and major adverse outcomes of pregnancy. *Adv Biomed Res* 2016;5:186.

36. Yilmaz E, Oguz F, Tuncay G, et al. Renal cell carcinoma diagnosed during pregnancy: A case report and literature review. *J Int Med Res* 2018;46(8):3422–3426.

37. Cohen RA, Brown RS. Microscopic hematuria. *N Engl J Med* 2003;348(23):2330–2338.

38. Schmitz-Dräger BJ, Kuckuck EC, Zuiverloon TC, et al. Microhematuria assessment an IBCN consensus-based upon a critical review of current guidelines. *Urol Oncol* 2016;34(10):437–451.

CHAPTER 40

URINARY CATHETERS AND URETERAL STENTS

Mary Van Meter Baker • John A. Occhino

Introduction

Urinary catheters and ureteral stents are tools commonly used by the urogynecologist for a variety of clinical indications. Catheters are hollow tubes used throughout medicine, but in urogynecology are used to drain urine from the bladder to outside the body. Stents, which are used to maintain patency of tubular structures, are useful in the field of urogynecology for identification and maintenance of integrity of the ureters. This chapter highlights the types of urinary catheters and ureteral stents, indications for use, and general instructions and risks associated with placement. The risk of infection associated with these devices constitutes a major consideration with their use and is discussed in the following text.

URINARY CATHETERS

Background and Indications

By allowing urine to freely drain from the bladder without coordinated micturition, urinary catheters are essential tools in gynecologic surgery. In addition to their role in draining and thereby preventing distention of the bladder during prolonged surgical procedures, catheters assist in the management of postoperative voiding dysfunction associated with many common pelvic reconstructive procedures. When bladder injury occurs, whether incidentally or intentionally, they prevent bladder distension and assist in healing. Urinary catheters bypass the need for conscious voiding in cases of immobility and may be indicated for long-term use in cases of neural or muscular injury to the bladder.

Foley

Transurethral catheters with self-retaining balloons were first described by Dr. Frederick Foley[1] in 1929. The Foley catheter is a latex or silicone catheter with two channels: one for draining urine and a smaller valved channel that allows for inflation of a balloon to keep the catheter in place within the bladder. Foley catheters are sized in French units, with 3 French

equivalent to 1.0 mm in diameter. Although smaller pediatric sizes are available, common sizes range from 10 to 28 French, with 14 and 16 French most commonly used for adult women. Balloon inflation amounts vary and are generally listed on packaging inserts, with a risk of expulsion and balloon rupture with under and over inflation, respectively. Of note, larger diameter Foley catheters are also used for mechanical cervical dilation in obstetrical induction of labor.

Suprapubic

Although transurethral catheters are common and allow bladder drainage through the natural orifice of the urethra, various pathologies necessitate urinary bypass of the urethra. Suprapubic catheters (SPCs) are inserted, often under direct cystoscopic guidance, transabdominally into the dome of the bladder. A distal balloon at the catheter tip allows for self-retention, although a stitch may be placed at the skin insertion site and wrapped around the catheter for reinforcement and to decrease postoperative drainage from the incision site. Although they are the most invasive and do require surgical placement, they are advantageous in that patients may attempt voiding while the SPC is in place (see Table 40.1 for patient instructions), and they may be associated with less bacterial growth and pain.

Self-Catheters

In addition to indwelling catheters, which are held in place with balloons inflated within the bladder to prevent expulsion of the catheter tubing, transurethral catheters may be inserted and removed by the patient for the purpose of bladder emptying. In addition to increasing patient comfort, self-intermittent catheterization (SIC) has been shown to decrease rates of catheter-associated urinary tract infections (CAUTIs) when compared to indwelling uretheral catheters.[2] Therefore, SIC is an excellent option in patients experiencing postoperative voiding dysfunction. Patients do require education in order to successfully self-catheterize, but over 90% of patients can successfully learn self-catheterization expediently in a single teaching episode.[3] Suggested

TABLE 40.1
Patient Instructions for Bladder Retraining following Suprapubic Catheter Placement
1. First, begin plugging the catheter for 4 hours.
2. Attempt to void every 2 hours.
3. Check residual urine after voiding at 4 hours.
4. When residual urine is <150 mL on two consecutive occasions, increase plugging interval (intervals go from 4 to 6, 8, 12, and then 24 hours).
5. Catheter should be unclamped any time you become distressed because of distension of the bladder.
6. Once residual urine is <150 mL at 24 hours, the SPC may be removed.
7. After removal, a pressure dressing should be applied to the catheter site. Void frequently for the next 4 hours to allow the bladder to heal.

TABLE 40.2
Patient Instructions for Self-Intermittent Catheterization for Postoperative Voiding Dysfunction
1. Attempt urination when you have the urge to void or every 4 hours if you do not feel the urge to void.
2. Each time you void urine—measure the voided volume.
3. Perform self-catheterization immediately after voiding and measure the residual catheterized urine volume.
4. Record the time and both voided and catheterized volumes.
5. When your postvoid residual urine volume is <150 mL for three consecutive voids, you may stop catheterization and stop measuring urine.
6. If you ever feel the sensation that you have not completely emptied your bladder or are unable to urinate when you feel the need, we encourage you to self-catheterize and measure the residual volume of urine.

instructions for patient self-catheterization following surgery are detailed in Table 40.2.

Clinical Correlates

Patient instructions

See Tables 40.1 and 40.2.

Catheter-associated urinary tract infections avoidance and best practices

CAUTIs are the most common health care–associated infection and are the major morbidity associated with catheter usage. Risk of CAUTI increases with duration of use; therefore, catheters should be used for the minimal amount of time necessary to avoid unnecessary risk of infection. Estimated incidence is 5.3 per 100 catheterizations, with female sex as an independent factor for increased risk.[4] However, urinary tract infection (UTI) is defined differently by different organizations and even different specialties, making accurate incidence reporting difficult. The National Surgical Quality Improvement Program has specific diagnostic criteria for postoperative UTI.[5] CAUTI should be distinguished from asymptomatic bacteriuria, because most long-term indwelling catheters will result in eventual bacterial colonization, and treatment in the absence of symptoms risks development of multidrug-resistant organisms. Most experts agree that asymptomatic bacteriuria in the setting of catheters does not require antibiotic treatment.[6]

Although the Centers for Disease Control and Prevention recommends removal of indwelling catheters when clinically able, this is of limited utility given the variety of indications for urinary catheter use. The American Urological Association (AUA) suggests indwelling urethral catheters remain in place for 3 to 21 days from surgery following cystotomy repair, vesicovaginal and enterovesical fistula repair, urethral injury, or urethral diverticulum repair. Indwelling catheters may remain in place 1 to 7 days following female pelvic medicine and reconstructive surgery reconstructive procedures including pubovaginal slings, urethrolysis, anterior and apical prolapse repairs, and mesh removal.[7]

In a subset of patients, long-term indwelling catheters may be required for chronic incontinence or inability to perform intermittent catheterization. Development of CAUTI is a significant cause for morbidity in this patient population. In patients requiring chronic bladder drainage, SIC is generally preferred; however, it is not always possible based on patient body habitus, motor function, and ability. In patients not able to perform SIC, SPCs are often preferred over indwelling urethral catheters. One study showed that nursing home residents with SPCs may be less likely to have CAUTI and fewer hospitalizations and antibiotic prescriptions, than patients with indwelling urethral catheters.[8] However, SPCs are more likely to be colonized by multidrug-resistant pathogens. A Cochrane meta-analysis revealed SPCs reduce asymptomatic bacteriuria, recatheterization, and pain compared to indwelling urethral catheters. The rates of symptomatic UTI between indwelling urethral catheters and SPCs are inconclusive.[9] In these settings, utilization of silver alloyed catheters have been suggested to reduce the risk of CAUTI.[10]

STENTS

Background and Indications

Ureteral stents can be used to facilitate ureteral identification during pelvic surgery, relieve ureteral obstruction, or promote healing of the ureter following injury or surgical repair. They are commonly placed cystoscopically but may also be placed via direct cystotomy or percutaneously under fluoroscopic guidance. For the purposes of this chapter, we will not address ureteral stents for urologic indications such as obstruction due to kidney stones or urologic cancers.

Sizing

Ureteral stents vary both in width (generally 4 to 7 French with 6 French most commonly used) and in length. Choosing the correct length is important to prevent stent migration and patient discomfort.[11] Although measurements based on imaging or direct measurement with a guidewire are occasionally used, stents are commonly sized based on patient height.[12,13] Generally, 22 to 26 cm is appropriate for average-sized adults.

Types

External ureteral stents are straight and typically have blunt ends with a lateral opening (whistle tip) to allow for direct placement without the need for a guidewire. The stents are long in length and made of polyurethane or silicone. This allows for the stent to be placed so the tip is in the renal pelvis, the body traverses down the ureter, enters the bladder, and exits through the urethra. These are typically placed for ureteral identification at the time of pelvic surgery, and they can easily be removed following surgery without the need for cystoscopy. They are typically secured with a tie to the urinary catheter to prevent migration or accidental removal.

Double J (also called JJ or pigtail) ureteral stents feature a coil at both stent ends, allowing self-retention in the renal pelvis and urinary bladder with decreased risk of transposition. These are typically placed when a longer duration of use is expected, such as following ureteral injury or reimplantation. They typically remain in place following the placement for days to weeks, depending on the indication for placement. They are able to be removed in the office without the need for sedation using a cystoscope and cystoscopic graspers.

Lighted ureteral stents may be used in select cases to facilitate intraperitoneal identification of the ureter and reduce risk of injury.[14] These stents are open ended and may be passed over a guidewire, with a lighted filament passed through the open stent after placement. The illumination may be continuous or intermittent, and certain models require a dedicated light source with a green lens and light cord.[15] They are typically removed at the conclusion of surgery.

Clinical Correlates

Placement

Ureteral stents are typically marked at each centimeter with unique markings every 5 cm, although it is best to inspect any stent prior to placement to understand how each mark correlates with stent length. Stents are most commonly placed under cystoscopic guidance, with or without the use of an Albarran (deflector) bridge. Traditional external stents are inserted into the ureteral orifice and advanced until slight resistance is met or until approximately 24 cm in a standard-sized adult. Following appropriate placement, the cystoscope lens and bridge are disassembled and removed while the cystoscope sheath remains in place. The sheath is then removed, and the stent may be affixed to an indwelling catheter.

Double J stents are also typically placed under cystoscopic guidance. Best practices for double J stent placement include the use of direct fluoroscopic guidance (Video 40.1). Prior to stent placement, a guidewire (typically 0.035 mm size) is passed up the ureter and advanced under fluoroscopic guidance to the renal pelvis. The double J stent is then placed over the guidewire and advanced to the renal pelvis with the use of stent pusher (packaged with each stent). The guidewire is slowly removed and fluoroscopy is used to ensure a full 360-degree coil of the stent is seen in the renal pelvis. Confirming a full coil in the renal pelvis prevents dislodgement and decreases the incidence of stent pain.[11,16] Retrograde pyelography may be performed at the time of stent placement in order to visualize the ureter and renal pelvis and evaluate for areas of stricture, dilation, or injury.

Antibiotics and management

Urinary tract infection risk

As with any implanted device, placement of ureteral stents is associated with a risk of upper urinary tract infection. Colonization rates increase with duration of use, most commonly by *Enterococcus* or *Escherichia coli*.[17] The AUA recommends antibiotic prophylaxis for stent placement. A single dose of fluoroquinolones (500 mg oral ciprofloxacin or 400 mg intravenous ciprofloxacin) or trimethoprim-sulfamethoxazole (160/800 mg oral trimethoprim-sulfamethoxazole) is considered treatment of choice, with aminoglycosides with or without ampicillin, first- or second-generation cephalosporins, or amoxicillin/clavulanate, all considered acceptable alternatives.[18] Confirmation of a UTI warrants treatment for complicated UTI. Indwelling ureteral stents should be exchanged every 3 months to decrease the risk of infection; however, urogynecologic patients rarely require stents to be in place for that duration of time.[19,20]

Pain management

In addition to the risk of infection with an indwelling prosthetic device, indwelling ureteral stents may cause hematuria, dysuria, flank pain, and suprapubic pain. The majority of these symptoms are related to bladder irritation and may be managed with anticholinergic medications and/or α-blockers. Persistent pain warrants evaluation and verification of proper stent placement.

Removal

Stents not removed at the conclusion of surgery may be removed in the outpatient setting without return to the operating room.[21] External stents and stents with external dangles may be removed manually. Alternatively, stent removal can be accomplished with office cystoscopy and a grasper inserted through a cystoscopic channel. Patients should be counseled to expect pain during and/or following removal, which can generally be managed with nonsteroidal anti-inflammatory medications.

References

1. Foley FE. Cystoscopic prostatectomy a new procedure and instrument; Preliminary report. *J Urol* 1929;21(3):289–306.
2. Li M, Yao L, Han C, et al. The incidence of urinary tract infection of different routes of catheterization following gynecologic surgery: A systematic review and meta-analysis of randomized controlled trials. *Int Urogynecol J* 2019;30(4):523–535.
3. Bickhaus JA, Drobnis EZ, Critchlow WA, et al. The feasibility of clean intermittent self-catheterization teaching in an outpatient setting. *Female Pelvic Med Reconstr Surg* 2015;21(4):220–224.
4. Daniels KR, Lee GC, Frei CR. Trends in catheter-associated urinary tract infections among a national cohort of hospitalized adults, 2001–2010. *Am J Infect Control* 2014;42(1):17–22.
5. American College of Surgeons. Variable and definitions. In: *NSQIP operations manual*. San Diego: American College of Surgeons; 2013:107.
6. Vance J. AMDA-choosing wisely. *J Am Med Dir Assoc* 2013;14(9):639–641.
7. Averch TD, Stoffel J, Goldman HB, et al. Catheter-associated urinary tract infections: Definitions and significance in the urologic patient. Published 2014. Accessed February 3, 2022. https://www.auajournals.org/doi/10.1016/j.urpr.2015.01.005
8. Gibson KE, Neill S, Tuma E, et al. Indwelling urethral versus suprapubic catheters in nursing home residents: Determining the safest option for long-term use. *J Hosp Infect* 2019;102(2):219–225.
9. Kidd EA, Stewart F, Kassis NC, et al. Urethral (indwelling or intermittent) or suprapubic routes for short-term catheterisation in hospitalised adults. *Cochrane Database Syst Rev* 2015;(12):CD004203.
10. Schumm K, Lam TB. Types of urethral catheters for management of short-term voiding problems in hospitalized adults: A short version Cochrane review. *Neurourol Urodyn* 2008;27(8):738–746.
11. Slaton JW, Kropp KA. Proximal ureteral stent migration: An avoidable complication? *J Urol* 1996;155(1):58–61.
12. Pilcher JM, Patel U. Choosing the correct length of ureteric stent: A formula based on the patient's height compared with direct ureteric measurement. *Clin Radiol* 2002;57(1):59–62.
13. Kawahara T, Ito H, Terao H, et al. Which is the best method to estimate the actual ureteral length in patients undergoing ureteral stent placement? *Int J Urol* 2012;19(7):634–638.
14. Boyan WP Jr, Lavy D, Dinallo A, et al. Lighted ureteral stents in laparoscopic colorectal surgery; a five-year experience. *Ann Transl Med* 2017;5(3):44.
15. Pedro RN, Kishore TA, Hinck BD, et al. Comparative analysis of lighted ureteral stents: Lumination and tissue effects. *J Endourol* 2008;22(11):2555–2558.
16. Breau RH, Norman RW. Optimal prevention and management of proximal ureteral stent migration and remigration. *J Urol* 2001;166(3):890–893.
17. Paick SH, Park HK, Oh S-J, et al. Characteristics of bacterial colonization and urinary tract infection after indwelling of double-J ureteral stent. *Urology* 2003;62(2):214–217.
18. Wolf JS Jr, Bennett CJ, Dmochowski RR, et al. Best practice policy statement on urologic surgery antimicrobial prophylaxis. *J Urol* 2008;179(4):1379–1390.
19. Lam JS, Gupta M. Tips and tricks for the management of retained ureteral stents. *J Endourol* 2002;16(10):733–741.
20. el-Faqih SR, Shamsuddin AB, Chakrabarti A, et al. Polyurethane internal ureteral stents in treatment of stone patients: Morbidity related to indwelling times. *J Urol* 1991;146(6):1487–1491.
21. Loh-Doyle JC, Low RK, Monga M, et al. Patient experiences and preferences with ureteral stent removal. *J Endourol* 2015;29(1):35–40.

Evaluation and Surgical Treatment of Pelvic Organ Prolapse

CHAPTER 41

Pathophysiology of Pelvic Support Disorders

Danielle Patterson • Victoria L. Handa

Introduction

Pelvic organ prolapse is a prevalent condition, especially among older women. Despite our efforts to understand the genesis of this condition, its origins and its pathophysiology are still not known. This chapter reviews current theories regarding the etiology of pelvic support disorders.

CONNECTIVE TISSUE SUPPORT OF THE PELVIC ORGANS

The connective tissue supports of the pelvic organs are collectively referred to as the "endopelvic fascia." This fascia is a continuous, complex web of connective tissue that envelops and supports the bladder, vagina, and rectum.[1] Pelvic fascia can be divided into two types. The parietal fascia, which covers the levator ani and other skeletal muscles, is composed of a dense layer of organized collagen, mostly types I and III. In contrast, the visceral fascia, which envelops the pelvic organs, is a loose, poorly organized connective tissue layer.[2] On a histologic basis, this is a loose, areolar connective tissue layer composed of smooth muscle, collagen, and elastin fibers.[2] Much of the collagen and smooth muscle in the visceral fascia is perivascular.[3] The contrast between parietal and visceral fascia parallels the functions of these two layers: The parietal fascia provides support for the muscles of the pelvic floor and abdominal cavity, whereas the visceral fascia envelops the organs, providing autonomic innervation to these organs and allowing for dramatic changes in their volumes (e.g., bladder filling).

Within the endopelvic fascia, there are several surgically identifiable structures, such as the arcus tendineus fascia pelvis (ATFP) and the uterosacral and cardinal ligaments. However, these "ligaments" are not discrete structures but rather consist of blood and lymphatic vessels, nerves, adipose tissue, and loose areolar connective tissue. Absent from these ligaments is any dense connective tissue composed of type I collagen like that found in skeletal ligaments.[4] Nevertheless, the uterosacral and cardinal ligaments (Fig. 41.1) are thought to provide important support to the uterus and upper vagina.[5] They originate along the greater sciatic foramen and lateral sacrum and insert into the lateral aspect of the vaginal apex. On magnetic resonance imaging (MRI), the deep uterosacral ligament has a band-like appearance, whereas the cardinal ligament appears as a weblike structure following the branches of the internal iliac vessels.[6,7] In the standing position, the cardinal ligament provides vertical support for the uterus and vaginal apex[5,8] and pulls the vaginal apex and cervix toward the sacrum (Fig. 41.2), maintaining the position of these structures over the levator plate.[8] If these ligaments are deficient or lax, the vaginal apex might be positioned above the levator hiatus, thereby increasing the risk of prolapse. As these organs descend into the levator hiatus, the support of the cardinal and uterosacral ligaments becomes insufficient and fails. Norton[9] likened this to a boat in dock (Fig. 41.3). In this analogy, the uterosacral and cardinal ligaments hold the ship (uterus and vagina) in position, but they are not sufficient to support the ship if the water (levator ani) is withdrawn.

Laterally, the anterior vagina is attached to the pelvic sidewall at the ATFP or "white line."[5,10] This line is a condensation of the fascia of the obturator internus muscle. Posteriorly, there is a similar attachment of the vaginal wall to the arcus tendineus fascia rectovaginalis (ATFR), which is a condensation along the fascia of the levator ani muscle.[11] The ATFR fuses with the ATFP at a point 4 cm above the posterior fourchette.[11] Separations in the lateral attachment of the anterior vaginal wall have been observed in women with vaginal wall prolapse.[5] However, a biomechanical model developed by Chen and colleagues[12] suggests that apical support and levator ani muscle function are more important to the development of cystocele than is paravaginal support.

The composition and role of the rectovaginal (Denonvilliers) fascia and pubocervical fascia are debated.[2,13] In the distal rectovaginal septum, there is a dense connective tissue layer.[14] However, this is limited to the lower vagina, and there is no histologic evidence of a substantial fascial layer in the upper rectovaginal septum.[14,15] Histologically, there is little evidence for

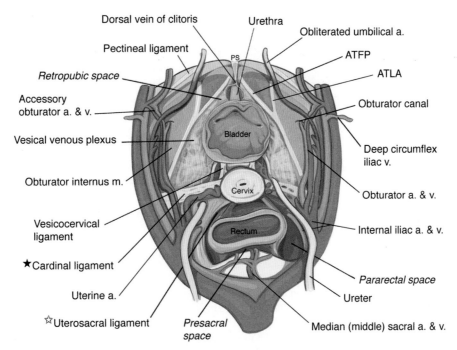

FIGURE 41.1 The cardinal ligament *(black stars)* and uterosacral ligament *(open stars)* provide support for the cervix and vaginal apex. They originate along the greater sciatic foramen and lateral sacrum. PS, pubic symphysis; ATLA, arcuate tendon levator ani; a., artery; v., vein. (Reprinted by permission from Springer: Tamakawa M, Murakami G, Takashima K, et al. Fascial structures and autonomic nerves in the female pelvis: A study using macroscopic slices and their corresponding histology. *Anat Sci Int* 2003;78[4]:228–242.)

pubocervical "fascia." Cadaveric studies of the anterior vaginal wall suggest that the visceral fascia in this location is composed of a thin areolar layer that separates the vaginal wall from the bladder.[14,16] Surgical repair of cystocele and rectocele has long relied on repair of the "endopelvic fascia," but the anatomic absence of a supportive, organized fascial layer

in this location casts doubt on this concept of surgical repair. The "fascia" (or "adventitia") used in vaginal repairs is more accurately described as "vaginal submucosa" or "vaginal muscularis,"[11,14,15] in recognition that this layer is part of the vaginal wall. However, others have suggested that defects in these layers result in cystocele and rectocele. This theory is the argument

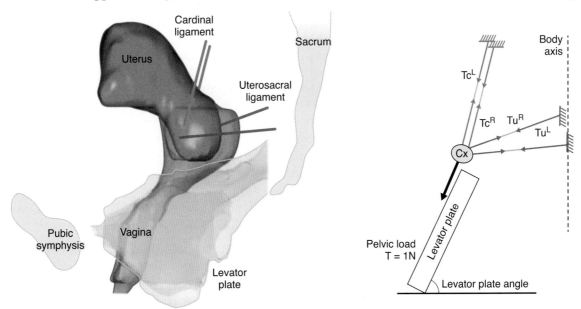

FIGURE 41.2 Three-dimensional model based on MRI. The uterus and vagina *(pink)* are positioned over the levator plate. The levator ani muscle is shown in *transparent blue*. The lines of action of the cardinal and uterosacral ligament are shown schematically. (Reprinted by permission from Springer: Chen L, Ramanah R, Hsu Y, et al. Cardinal and deep uterosacral ligament lines of action: MRI based 3D technique development and preliminary findings in normal women. *Int Urogynecol J* 2013;24[1]:37–45.)

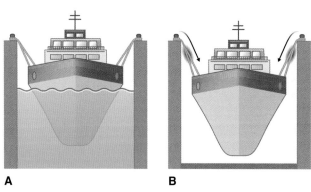

FIGURE 41.3 "Boat in dry dock" analogy for support of the cervix and vaginal apex. The water (analogous to the levator ani muscle complex) provides support for the boat. The lines (analogous to the uterosacral and cardinal ligaments) maintain the position of the boat. If the water is removed, the lines cannot support the weight of the boat. Thus, a loss of pelvic muscle function may inevitably lead to failure of the ligaments. (From Norton PA. Pelvic floor disorders: The role of fascia and ligaments. *Clin Obstet Gynecol* 1993;36[4]:926–938.)

for the "defect-directed" approach to the correction of cystocele and rectocele.[17,18] Objective defects cannot always be demonstrated, however.[2,19] Debate continues regarding the role of endopelvic connective tissue in the genesis of pelvic organ support defects and the implications for surgical repair of these defects.

There is also a role for connective tissue quality in maintaining vaginal support. Animal models show that defects in connective tissue remodeling and homeostasis contribute to prolapse. Fibulin-5 and lysyl oxidases are needed for normal elastic fiber synthesis. Mice with a genetic deficiency in fibulin-5 develop spontaneous prolapse.[20] Further work with these mice has shown that vaginal fibulin-5 during development is not only crucial for baseline pelvic organ support but is also important for protection and recovery from parturition and elastase-induced prolapse.[21] Lysyl oxidase like 1 gene (LOXL-1) knockout mice typically develop prolapse only after a traumatic event such as parturition.[22] This suggests the mechanism may be impaired recovery and repair. These murine models suggest that interventions to improve connective tissue repair, such as regenerative medicine or stem cell transplantation, may hold promise in effective repair after pregnancy and delivery.[23,24]

There is also increasing evidence for genetic variation in human women with prolapse. Variants in the expression collagen type III alpha 1 chain gene (COL3A1) and bone morphogenetic protein 1 gene (BMP1) have been associated with prolapse.[25,26]

ROLE OF THE LEVATOR ANI IN PELVIC ORGAN SUPPORT

Levator ani muscles are important structures with respect to pelvic organ function, and there is increasing

evidence of their role in pelvic organ support.[1] The levator ani muscle complex is composed of the iliococcygeus, pubococcygeus, and puborectalis muscles. The pubococcygeus, which has attachments to the vagina and anus, is sometimes called the pubovisceral muscle. The urethra, vagina, and rectum pass through the levator hiatus, the space between these paired muscles. These are unique skeletal muscles because they maintain tone in the absence of voluntary contraction.[3] The tone of the levator muscles keeps the levator hiatus closed[27] and likely prevents chronic tension on the parietal fascia. In addition to baseline tone, the normal response of the levator ani to Valsalva effort is increased tone, thereby closing the levator hiatus.[27] Laxity of the levator ani leads to a widening of the genital hiatus, and this has been suggested to be a potential initiating event for pelvic organ prolapse. We know that women with prolapse have a wider genital hiatus on MRI and three-dimensional ultrasound imaging.[28,29] Similarly, on physical examination, a wider genital hiatus is associated with the development of prolapse.[29,30] However, although these associations have been consistently demonstrated, they might not be causal.

ROLE OF THE BONY PELVIS

Preliminary research suggests an association between prolapse and the shape and size of the bony pelvis. Whereas some studies have suggested that women with prolapse have a wider pelvic diameter than women without prolapse,[31,32] other studies have been unable to confirm this association.[33,34] An "at-risk" bony pelvis could explain apparent racial differences in prolapse. Specifically, prolapse is less common in black women[35] who are more likely to have an anthropoid pelvis, with a narrow transverse inlet and wide obstetrical conjugate.[36]

There are several potential mechanisms for the role of pelvic architecture in the development of prolapse. First, certain pelvic shapes may increase the risk of obstetrical soft tissue trauma to the pelvic floor. Second, the physical support provided by the pelvic bones to the pelvic viscera may differ for different pelvic types. Finally, pelvic type may be a marker for other unmeasured factors.

PATHOPHYSIOLOGY OF PELVIC ORGAN PROLAPSE

The pathophysiology of prolapse is incompletely understood. Any framework for understanding the pathophysiology of prolapse must account for the epidemiologic risk factors, which include age, parity, obesity, and race.[35,37,38] However, these risk factors do not accurately predict who will develop prolapse. For example, although childbirth is one of the dominant risk factors for prolapse, this condition can occur in the absence of parity.[35,37] This raises the possibility of genetic or familial susceptibility factors. One paradigm for understanding the pathophysiology is to divide causal mechanisms into predisposing factors, initiating factors, and promoting factors.[39]

Predisposition might be mediated via differences in pelvic connective tissue mechanics or metabolism. Research has suggested that the ligaments of women with prolapse have decreased collagen content[40,41] or qualitative alterations in collagen composition.[42] In women with prolapse, the collagen fibrils become loose, disorderly, and discontinuous as well as stiffer than those without prolapse. Additionally, strong mechanical stress and an imbalance of tissue derived inhibitors of metalloproteinases can lead to collagen anabolism abnormalities causing changes in collagen content and structure.[43] There is also emerging evidence that elastin density, heparanase expression, and β3-adrenoreceptor activity can be implicated in development of prolapse.[44–46] There is evidence for an impact of joint hypermobility and connective tissue disorders.[47–50] However, studies to date have been limited by small size, lack of standardized measures of prolapse, and limited characterization of connective tissue biomechanics. Racial differences in connective tissue have not been investigated with respect to the apparent differences in susceptibility to prolapse. Also, it is not clear whether observed differences are a cause or result of prolapse.[51] Variations in connective tissue may explain apparent variations in susceptibility.

Given the strong association between parity and childbirth, childbirth has been viewed as an important initiating or inciting factor in the development of prolapse.[39] Investigators have postulated that acquired injury to connective tissue supports during labor and delivery is a likely mechanism for the development of prolapse.[1] Prolapse is strongly associated with vaginal versus cesarean birth, and odds of prolapse are highest for women who have had at least one operative birth.[52] They are many reasons that vaginal delivery may lead to prolapse. Levator ani strength is reduced after vaginal delivery compared to cesarean delivery and among vaginally parous women.[53] In addition, vaginal childbirth is associated with levator ani muscle avulsion, an obstetrical injury that is observed after 20% of spontaneous vaginal deliveries.[1,54] Levator ani muscle avulsion is strongly associated with poor muscle strength, as well as a wider levator hiatus, two alterations that are independently associated with prolapse.[55] Another reason may be maternal adaptation in preparation for childbirth. This is evidenced by deterioration in pelvic organ support during normal pregnancy.[56] It has been shown that mild prolapse is more common among pregnant nulliparous women compared to nonpregnant nulliparous women.[57] Additionally, inadequate pelvic floor adaptation during pregnancy could predispose a woman to levator avulsion during delivery and then lead to prolapse. In a randomized trial, a device designed to mechanically stretch the levator ani muscle during the last month of pregnancy, the Epi-No birth trainer tested this theory.[58] The trainer included progressive vaginal distension, by use of an inflated vaginal balloon device in late pregnancy. In this study, levator avulsions were observed in 12% of women assigned to the trainer and in 15% of controls ($P = 0.39$), suggesting that mechanical stretching of the levator may not be effective in preventing levator avulsions during vaginal delivery.

In addition to injuries associated with childbirth, injuries might also occur with recreational or occupational exposures to forces.[59–61] However, we do not know what activities have a significant impact. Most studies investigating the impact of strenuous exercise on pelvic organ support have failed to demonstrate a significant association between prolapse and either recreational or occupational activities.[62,63] Therefore, clinicians cannot currently provide evidence-based recommendations for primary or secondary prevention.

Disruption of pelvic muscle function is viewed as another potential initiating factor for prolapse. After a single vaginal delivery, gaps in the levator ani muscle are seen in 20% of women.[1,54] Although levator muscle avulsion has been linked to muscle weakness and widening of the levator hiatus,[55] changes in muscle function may be seen in the absence of overt muscle trauma. For example, the levator hiatus is transiently widened after childbirth[64,65] and also widened in women with prolapse.[27,66] Peripheral neuropathy has been observed after childbirth and might contribute to muscle dysfunction and atrophy. In one of the first studies of peripheral neuropathy in pelvic floor disorders, Sharf et al.[67] found electromyographic evidence of levator ani denervation in 50% of women with prolapse. Subsequent investigators have confirmed an association between denervation and pelvic floor disorders, including prolapse.[68,69] The role of pelvic muscle injury or denervation in the genesis of prolapse remains uncertain. Similarly, it is not known whether pelvic floor muscle exercises can reduce the incidence or progression of prolapse in susceptible individuals.

Environmental and lifestyle exposures may also play an important promoting role. For example, obesity has been associated with the development of prolapse as well as with the worsening of prolapse over time.[38,70,71] There is some suggestion that body morphology might be a stronger risk factor than obesity,[72] raising the possibility of metabolic as well as mechanical effects of obesity. Chronic straining and chronic increased intra-abdominal pressure may also play a role,[39] potentially as a result of the impact on connective tissue supports.

In cross-sectional studies, hysterectomy has been associated with prolapse.[70,73] Until recently, this was viewed as a likely causal association, attributed to disruption of connective tissue supports at the time of surgery. However, recent data from two large randomized trials of supracervical hysterectomy suggests that preserving the cervix does not reduce the risk of prolapse.[74,75] Thus, it is likely that the association between hysterectomy and prolapse is due either to preexisting prolapse among women undergoing hysterectomy or to other confounding factors associated with hysterectomy (e.g., parity). Indeed, the presence of prolapse at the time of hysterectomy is a strong risk factor for future prolapse.[76]

Retropubic urethropexy has also been blamed for subsequent development of prolapse.[77,78] Again, it is unclear whether this is due to undiagnosed prolapse at the time of bladder neck suspension, to the impact of confounding factors, or to a true causal association. It has been hypothesized that urethropexy deflects the vagina anteriorly, resulting in an increased mechanical load on the posterior vaginal wall. It is not known whether the long-term risk of prolapse is independently increased by urethropexy and whether this outcome can be minimized with other surgical treatments for stress incontinence, such as midurethral slings.

Finally, we cannot dismiss the important impact of aging. The prevalence of prolapse increases with age. Aging affects connective tissue properties and muscle function.[79] The hormonal changes of menopause may play a role. There is emerging evidence the estrogen therapy increases the tensile strength of healthy vaginal fibroblasts to help prevent prolapse.[80] This may support a role for estrogen therapy for postmenopausal women. It is hard to separate the impact of aging from other confounding factors, such as parity, obesity, vascular changes, and lifestyle changes.

CONCLUSION

While we are learning more about the mechanisms of normal pelvic organ support and the pathophysiology of prolapse, many questions remain unanswered. Identification of the specific anatomic causes will improve surgical treatments. Additional key questions include whether prolapse can be prevented (or its progression halted) by lifestyle modifications, whether elective cesarean could affect the incidence of prolapse, and whether susceptible individuals can be identified early in life. These questions are essential to understanding the pathophysiology of prolapse and critical to primary and secondary prevention.

References

1. Wei JT, DeLancey JO. Functional anatomy of the pelvic floor and lower urinary tract. *Clin Obstet Gynecol* 2004;47(1):3–17.
2. Tulikangas PK. Defect theory of pelvic organ prolapse. *Clin Obstet Gynecol* 2005;48(3):662–667.
3. Corton MM, DeLancey JOL. Surgical anatomy of the female pelvis. In: Handa VL, Van Le L, eds. *Telinde's operative gynecology*, 12th ed. Philadelphia: Wolters Kluwer, 2019:2–42.
4. Kieserman-Shmokler C, Swenson CW, Chen L, et al. From molecular to macro: The key role of the apical ligaments in uterovaginal support. *Am J Obstet Gynecol* 2020;222(5):427–436.

5. DeLancey JO. Anatomic aspects of vaginal eversion after hysterectomy. *Am J Obstet Gynecol* 1992;166(6 Pt 1):1717–1724.
6. Ramanah R, Berger MB, Chen L, et al. See it in 3D! Researchers examined structural links between the cardinal and uterosacral ligaments. *Am J Obstet Gynecol* 2012;207(5):437.e1–437.e7.
7. Iancu G, Doumouchtsis SK. A historical perspective and evolution of our knowledge on the cardinal ligament. *Neurourol Urodyn* 2014;33(4):380–386.
8. Chen L, Ramanah R, Hsu Y, et al. Cardinal and deep uterosacral ligament lines of action: MRI based 3D technique development and preliminary findings in normal women. *Int Urogynecol J* 2013;24(1):37–45.
9. Norton PA. Pelvic floor disorders: The role of fascia and ligaments. *Clin Obstet Gynecol* 1993;36(4):926–938.
10. DeLancey JO, Starr RA. Histology of the connection between the vagina and levator ani muscles. Implications for urinary tract function. *J Reprod Med* 1990;35(8):765–771.
11. Leffler KS, Thompson JR, Cundiff GW, et al. Attachment of the rectovaginal septum to the pelvic sidewall. *Am J Obstet Gynecol* 2001;185(1):41–43.
12. Chen L, Ashton-Miller JA, DeLancey JO. A 3D finite element model of anterior vaginal wall support to evaluate mechanisms underlying cystocele formation. *J Biomech* 2009;42(10):1371–1377.
13. Dariane C, Moszkowicz D, Peschaud F. Concepts of the rectovaginal septum: Implications for function and surgery. *Int Urogynecol J* 2016;27(6):839–848.
14. Kleeman SD, Westermann C, Karram MM. Rectoceles and the anatomy of the posterior vaginal wall: Revisited. *Am J Obstet Gynecol* 2005;193(6):2050–2055.
15. Farrell SA, Dempsey T, Geldenhuys L. Histologic examination of "fascia" used in colporrhaphy. *Obstet Gynecol* 2001;98(5 Pt 1):794–798.
16. Berglas B, Rubin IC. Histologic study of the pelvic connective tissue. *Surg Gynecol Obstet* 1953;97(3):277–289.
17. Cundiff GW, Weidner AC, Visco AG, et al. An anatomic and functional assessment of the discrete defect rectocele repair. *Am J Obstet Gynecol* 1998;179(6 Pt 1):1451–1457.
18. Kenton K, Shott S, Brubaker L. Outcome after rectovaginal fascia reattachment for rectocele repair. *Am J Obstet Gynecol* 1999;181(6):1360–1364.
19. Burrows LJ, Sewell C, Leffler KS, et al. The accuracy of clinical evaluation of posterior vaginal wall defects. *Int Urogynecol J Pelvic Floor Dysfunct* 2003;14(3):160–163.
20. Weislander CK, Acevedo JG, Drewes PG, et al. Pelvic organ prolapse severity increases with age in fibulin-5 knockout mice. *Int Urogynecol J* 2006;17:S371.
21. Chin K, Wieslander C, Shi H, et al. Pelvic organ support in animals with partial loss of fibulin-5 in the vaginal wall. *PLoS One* 2016;11(4):e0152793.
22. Borazjani A, Couri BM, Kuang M, et al. Role of lysyl oxidase like 1 in regulation of postpartum connective tissue metabolism in the mouse vagina. *Biol Reprod* 2019;101(5):916–927.
23. Pathi SD, Acevedo JF, Keller PW, et al. Recovery of the injured external anal sphincter after injection of local or intravenous mesenchymal stem cells. *Obstet Gynecol* 2012;119(1):134–144.
24. Gräs S, Tolstrup CK, Lose G. Regenerative medicine provides alternative strategies for the treatment of anal incontinence. *Int Urogynecol J* 2017;28(3):341–350.
25. Ward RM, Velez Edwards DR, Edwards T, et al. Genetic epidemiology of pelvic organ prolapse: A systematic review. *Am J Obstet Gynecol* 2014;211(4):326–335.

26. Borazjani A, Kow N, Harris S, et al. Transcriptional regulation of connective tissue metabolism genes in women with pelvic organ prolapse. *Female Pelvic Med Reconstr Surg* 2017;23(1):44–52.

27. Berglas B, Rubin IC. Study of the supportive structures of the uterus by levator myography. *Surg Gynecol Obstet* 1953;97(6):677–692.

28. Sammarco AG, Nandikanti L, Kobernik EK, et al. Interactions among pelvic organ protrusion, levator ani descent, and hiatal enlargement in women with and without prolapse. *Am J Obstet Gynecol* 2017;217(5):614.e1–614.e7.

29. Handa VL, Roem J, Blomquist JL, et al. Pelvic organ prolapse as a function of levator ani avulsion, hiatus size, and strength. *Am J Obstet Gynecol* 2019;221(1):41.e1–41.e7.

30. Handa VL, Blomquist JL, Carroll M, et al. Longitudinal changes in the genital hiatus preceding the development of pelvic organ prolapse. *Am J Epidemiol* 2019;188(12):2196–2201.

31. Handa VL, Pannu HK, Siddique S, et al. Architectural differences in the bony pelvis of women with and without pelvic floor disorders. *Obstet Gynecol* 2003;102(6):1283–1290.

32. Sze EH, Kohli N, Miklos JR, et al. Computed tomography comparison of bony pelvis dimensions between women with and without genital prolapse. *Obstet Gynecol* 1999;93(2):229–232.

33. Stein TA, Kaur G, Summers A, et al. Comparison of bony dimensions at the level of the pelvic floor in women with and without pelvic organ prolapse. *Am J Obstet Gynecol* 2009;200(3):241.e1–241.e5.

34. Li R, Song Y, Ma M. Relationship between levator ani and bony pelvis morphology and clinical grade of prolapse in women. *Clin Anat* 2015;28(6):813–819.

35. Rortveit G, Brown JS, Thom DH, et al. Symptomatic pelvic organ prolapse: Prevalence and risk factors in a population-based, racially diverse cohort. *Obstet Gynecol* 2007;109(6):1396–1403.

36. Moloy HC. *Moloy's evaluation of the pelvis in obstetrics.* Philadelphia: Saunders, 1959.

37. Nygaard I, Barber MD, Burgio KL, et al. Prevalence of symptomatic pelvic floor disorders in US women. *JAMA* 2008;300(11):1311–1316.

38. Hallock JL, Handa VL. The epidemiology of pelvic floor disorders and childbirth: An update. *Obstet Gynecol Clin North Am* 2016;43(1):1–13.

39. Weber AM, Richter HE. Pelvic organ prolapse. *Obstet Gynecol* 2005;106(3):615–634.

40. Zhu Y-P, Xie T, Guo T, et al. Evaluation of extracellular matrix protein expression and apoptosis in the uterosacral ligaments of patients with or without pelvic organ prolapse. *Int Urogynecol J* 2021;32(8):2273–2281.

41. Vulic M, Strinic T, Tomic S, et al. Difference in expression of collagen type I and matrix metalloproteinase-1 in uterosacral ligaments of women with and without pelvic organ prolapse. *Eur J Obstet Gynecol Reprod Biol* 2011;155(2):225–228.

42. Yucel N, Usta A, Guzin K, et al. Immunohistochemical analysis of connective tissue in patients with pelvic organ prolapse. *J Mol Histol* 2013;44(1):97–102.

43. Gong R, Xia Z. Collagen changes in pelvic support tissues in women with pelvic organ prolapse. *Eur J Obstet Gynecol Reprod Biol* 2019;234:185–189.

44. De Landsheere L, Brieu M, Blacher S, et al. Elastin density: Link between histological and biomechanical properties of vaginal tissue in women with pelvic organ prolapse? *Int Urogynecol J* 2016;27(4):629–635.

45. Ben-Zvi M, Ganer Herman H, Schrieber L, et al. Expression of heparanase in uterosacral ligaments of women with or without uterine prolapse. *Eur J Obstet Gynecol Reprod Biol* 2020;244:110–113.

46. Chong W, Fantl JA, Donovan M, et al. Beta-3 adrenoceptor expression in the uterosacral ligament in the postmenopausal women with pelvic organ prolapse. *Neurourol Urodyn* 2018;37(7):2135–2140.

47. Norton PA, Baker JE, Sharp HC, et al. Genitourinary prolapse and joint hypermobility in women. *Obstet Gynecol* 1995;85(2):225–228.

48. Carley ME, Schaffer J. Urinary incontinence and pelvic organ prolapse in women with Marfan or Ehlers Danlos syndrome. *Am J Obstet Gynecol* 2000;182(5):1021–1023.

49. el-Shahaly HA, el-Sherif AK. Is the benign joint hypermobility syndrome benign? *Clin Rheumatol* 1991;10(3):302–307.

50. Hansell NK, Dietz HP, Treloar SA, et al. Genetic covariation of pelvic organ and elbow mobility in twins and their sisters. *Twin Res* 2004;7(3):254–260.

51. Moalli PA, Shand SH, Zyczynski HM, et al. Remodeling of vaginal connective tissue in patients with prolapse. *Obstet Gynecol* 2005;106(5 Pt 1):953–963.

52. Handa VL, Blomquist JL, Knoepp LR, et al. Pelvic floor disorders 5-10 years after vaginal or cesarean birth. *Obstet Gynecol* 2011;118(4):777–784.

53. Friedman S, Blomquist JL, Nugent JM, et al. Pelvic muscle strength after childbirth. *Obstet Gynecol* 2012;120(5):1021–1028.

54. DeLancey JO, Kearney R, Chou Q, et al. The appearance of levator ani muscle abnormalities in magnetic resonance images after vaginal delivery. *Obstet Gynecol* 2003;101(1):46–53.

55. Handa VL, Blomquist JL, Roem J, et al. Levator morphology and strength after obstetrical avulsion of the levator ani muscle. *Female Pelvic Med Reconstr Surg* 2020;26(1):56–60.

56. Oliphant SS, Nygaard IE, Zong W, et al. Maternal adaptations in preparation for parturition predict uncomplicated spontaneous delivery outcome. *Am J Obstet Gynecol* 2014;211(6):630.e1–630.e7.

57. O'Boyle AL, Woodman PJ, O'Boyle JD, et al. Pelvic organ support in nulliparous pregnant and nonpregnant women: A case control study. *Am J Obstet Gynecol* 2002;187(1):99–102.

58. Kamisan Atan I, Shek KL, Langer S, et al. Does the Epi-No® birth trainer prevent vaginal birth-related pelvic floor trauma? A mulicentre prospective randomised controlled trial. *BJOG* 2016;123(6):995–1003.

59. Davis GD. Uterine prolapse after laparoscopic uterosacral transection in nulliparous airborne trainees. A report of three cases. *J Reprod Med* 1996;41(4):279–282.

60. Woodman PJ, Swift SE, O'Boyle AL, et al. Prevalence of severe pelvic organ prolapse in relation to job description and socioeconomic status: A multicenter cross-sectional study. *Int Urogynecol J Pelvic Floor Dysfunct* 2006;17(4):340–345.

61. Larsen WI, Yavorek TA. Pelvic organ prolapse and urinary incontinence in nulliparous women at the United States Military Academy. *Int Urogynecol J Pelvic Floor Dysfunct* 2006;17(3):208–210.

62. Nygaard IE, Shaw JM, Bardsley T, et al. Lifetime physical activity and pelvic organ prolapse in middle-aged women. *Am J Obstet Gynecol* 2014;210(5):477.e1–477.e12.

63. Nygaard IE, Shaw JM. Physical activity and the pelvic floor. *Am J Obstet Gynecol* 2016;214(2):164–171.

64. Sanozidis A, Mikos T, Assimakopoulos E, et al. Changes in levator hiatus dimensions during pregnancy and after delivery in nulliparas: A prospective cohort study using 3D transperineal

ultrasound. *J Matern Fetal Neonatal Med* 2018;31(11): 1505–1512.

65. Van de Waarsenburg MK, Verberne EA, van der Vaart CH, et al. Recovery of puborectalis muscle after vaginal delivery: An ultrasound study. *Ultrasound Obstet Gynecol* 2018;52(3):390–395.

66. Ghetti C, Gregory WT, Edwards SR, et al. Severity of pelvic organ prolapse associated with measurements of pelvic floor function. *Int Urogynecol J Pelvic Floor Dysfunct* 2005;16(6):432–436.

67. Sharf B, Zilberman A, Sharf M, et al. Electromyogram of pelvic floor muscles in genital prolapse. *Int J Gynaecol Obstet* 1976;14:2–4.

68. Smith AR, Hosker GL, Warrell DW. The role of partial denervation of the pelvic floor in the etiology of genitourinary prolapse and stress incontinence of urine. A neurophysiological study. *Br J Obstet Gynaecol* 1989;96(1):24–28.

69. Weidner AC, Barber MD, Visco AG, et al. Pelvic muscle electromyography of levator ani and external anal sphincter in nulliparous women and women with pelvic floor dysfunction. *Am J Obstet Gynecol* 2000;183(6):1390–1401.

70. Mant J, Painter R, Vessey M. Epidemiology of genital prolapse: Observations from the Oxford Family Planning Association Study. *Br J Obstet Gynaecol* 1997;104(5):579–585.

71. Giri A, Hartmann KE, Hellwege JN, et al. Obesity and pelvic organ prolapse: A systematic review and meta-analysis of observational studies. *Am J Obstet Gynecol* 2017;217(1):11.e3–26.e3.

72. Handa VL, Garrett E, Hendrix S, et al. Progression and remission of pelvic organ prolapse: A longitudinal study of menopausal women. *Am J Obstet Gynecol* 2004;190(1):27–32.

73. Swift SE, Pound T, Dias JK. Case-control study of etiologic factors in the development of severe pelvic organ prolapse. *Int Urogynecol J Pelvic Floor Dysfunct* 2001;12(3):187–192.

74. Learman LA, Summitt RL Jr, Varner RE, et al. A randomized comparison of total or supracervical hysterectomy: Surgical complications and clinical outcomes. *Obstet Gynecol* 2003;102(3):453–462.

75. Thakar R, Ayers S, Clarkson P, et al. Outcomes after total versus subtotal abdominal hysterectomy. *N Engl J Med* 2002;347(17):1318–1325.

76. Blandon RE, Bharucha AE, Melton LJ III, et al. Incidence of pelvic floor repair after hysterectomy: A population-based cohort study. *Am J Obstet Gynecol* 2007;197(6):664.e1–664.e7.

77. Wiskind AK, Creighton SM, Stanton SL. The incidence of genital prolapse after the Burch colposuspension. *Am J Obstet Gynecol* 1992;167(2):399–404.

78. Sze EH, Miklos JR, Partoll L, et al. Sacrospinous ligament fixation with transvaginal needle suspension for advanced pelvic organ prolapse and stress incontinence. *Obstet Gynecol* 1997;89(1):94–96.

79. Arking R. *The biology of aging: Observations & principles*, 2nd ed. Massachusetts: Sinauer Associates, 1998.

80. Wang S, Lü D, Zhang A, et al. Effects of mechanical stretching on the morphology of extracellular polymers and the mRNA expression of collagens and small leucine-rich repeat proteoglycans in vaginal fibroblasts from women with pelvic organ prolapse. *PLoS One* 2018;13(4):e0193456.

CHAPTER 42

SURGICAL MANAGEMENT OF PELVIC ORGAN PROLAPSE

Kate V. Meriwether

PELVIC ORGAN PROLAPSE PATIENT BURDEN AND RELEVANT OUTCOME MEASURES

Pelvic organ prolapse (POP) has profound impacts on women's quality of life. Qualitative work in this field holds important revelations about how women are affected by this disorder.[1] Shame and silence surround POP, which creates an enormous emotional burden.[2,3] This problem is compounded by the fact that women often do not know about treatment options, including surgery.[1] Goals important to patients following surgery include relief of bulge symptoms and sense of restoration of normal anatomy, closely followed by desire to maintain or restore sexual function.[4,5] Given this context, it is of no surprise that at least 12.6% of women undergo POP surgery in their lifetime,[6,7] and that measuring the success of these surgeries is paramount, albeit varied.

Historically, success in POP surgery was measured by restoration of normal vaginal anatomy, and this was the way surgeons weighed the benefit of one surgery versus another. For years, the patient experience was not fully integrated into outcome measures for POP surgery. Fortunately, a shift has been occurring in the field that emphasizes the importance of patient-centered outcome measures, and compound measures that integrate both anatomic restoration and the patient's experience of POP-related symptoms are advocated.[1,8–11] In other words, surgeons in the field should evaluate if certain surgeries cause relief of symptoms relevant to patients and have a positive impact on patients' lives (Table 42.1).

Validated patient-centered outcomes that are commonly used to assess POP symptoms or their impact on the patient include the Pelvic Floor Distress Inventory (PFDI), the Pelvic Floor Impact Questionnaire (PFIQ), and the Pelvic Organ Prolapse/Urinary Incontinence Sexual Function Questionnaire (PISQ).[11,15–18] Other frequently used relevant outcomes includes recurrence of symptoms of prolapse after surgery and the prevalence of reoperation for recurrent prolapse or complications of the original surgery. For objective outcomes, high-quality studies often use an objective measure of vaginal anatomical failure as defined by the Pelvic Organ Prolapse Quantification (POP-Q) exam. Common examples of definitions of anatomical failure include any stage 2 or greater prolapse, prolapse beyond the hymen, or apical prolapse as measured by a vaginal apex more than one-third or one-half down its total vaginal length (Fig. 42.1).[1,8–11,19]

Anatomic success is measured by the different portions of the vagina, or compartments, including the apical, posterior, anterior, and distal/perineal compartments, and the different surgeries intended to address different compartments (Fig. 42.2).[20] For example, surgeries that address the apical compartment include sacrocolpopexy/sacrocervicopexy/sacrohysteropexy, uterosacral ligament suspension/uterosacral ligament hysteropexy, sacrospinous ligament fixation/sacrospinous ligament hysteropexy, sacrospinous ligament fixation with graft, anterior abdominal wall hysteropexy, iliococcygeal fixation, colpocleisis, and the Manchester procedure. Surgeries that address the anterior compartment include anterior vaginal repair, paravaginal repair, and anterior vaginal repair with graft. Similarly, surgeries that address the posterior compartment include posterior vaginal repair, posterior vaginal repair with graft, and levator plication. The distal or perineal compartment is addressed specifically by perineal repair.[20]

CURRENT DECISIONS IN SELECTING A PROCEDURE

In the current surgical climate, patients and surgeons are faced with several important decisions when selecting a procedure. For the most part, these decisions should be based on a combination of the patient's desires and goals as well as the surgeon's familiarity and experience with a procedure.

The first of these decisions is one to determine if the patient desires insertive vaginal intercourse in the future. This lack of desire for insertive vaginal intercourse

TABLE 42.1

Common Outcomes Used to Define Success in Pelvic Organ Prolapse Surgery

OUTCOME	TYPE OF OUTCOME (ANATOMIC/PATIENT BASED)	COMPARTMENT MEASURED	DETAILED DEFINITION
Compound outcome[12,13]	Combination	All	(1) No apical prolapse more than one-third down vaginal wall and no anterior/posterior prolapse past hymen, (2) no bothersome vaginal bulge symptoms, (3) no retreatment for prolapse (no pessary or surgery)
Apical anatomic success	Anatomic	Apical	No prolapse one-third to one-half down the vaginal wall (one-third to one-half of vaginal length)
Anterior/posterior anatomic success	Anatomic	Anterior and/or posterior	No prolapse past the hymen (POP-Q measurement of 0 for Aa/Ba or Ap/Bp)
No bothersome bulge symptoms	Subjective	N/A	No positive response (bother "not at all") to the PFDI question "Do you usually have a bulge or something falling out that you can see or feel in your vaginal area?"
PFDI[14]	Subjective	N/A	Score ranges from 0 (least distress) to 300 (most distress) and is a sum of the three subscale scores (Pelvic Organ Prolapse Distress Inventory, Urogenital Distress Inventory, and Colorectal Anal Distress Inventory), each ranging from 0 (least distress) to 100 (most distress).
PFIQ[14]	Subjective	N/A	Score ranges from 0 (least impact) to 300 (most adverse impact) and is a sum of three subscale scores (Pelvic Organ Prolapse Impact Questionnaire, Urinary Impact Questionnaire, and Colorectal Anal Impact Questionnaire), each ranging from 0 (least impact) to 100 (most adverse impact). A midrange score for these subscales implies bother from prolapse, urinary incontinence, or fecal incontinence.
PISQ, IUGA-Revised (PISQ-IR)[15,16]	Subjective	N/A	The International Urogynecological Association (IUGA) revision, which is the most current, includes four domains for nonsexually active women, where higher scores indicate more impact of the conditions on sexual function, and six domains for sexually active women, with higher scores indicating better sexual function.

N/A, not applicable.

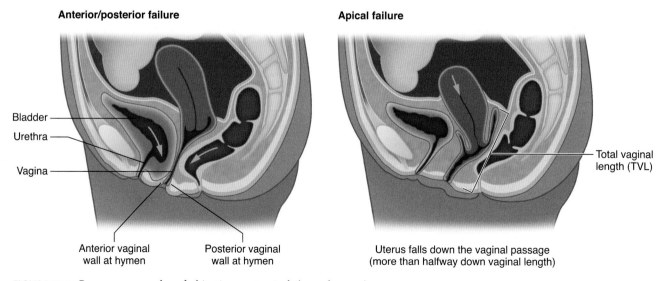

Anterior/posterior failure

Apical failure

Bladder

Urethra

Vagina

Anterior vaginal wall at hymen

Posterior vaginal wall at hymen

Total vaginal length (TVL)

Uterus falls down the vaginal passage (more than halfway down vaginal length)

FIGURE 42.1 Common examples of objective anatomic failure after prolapse surgery.

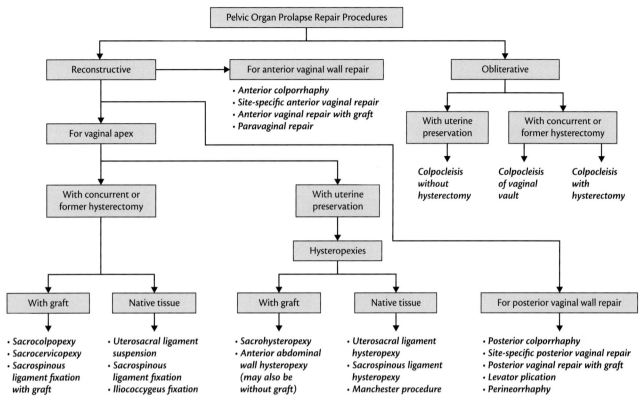

FIGURE 42.2 Types of prolapse procedures by compartment they repair or address.[20]

makes women possible candidates for an obliterative procedure. Usually, this entails a colpocleisis, where opposing vaginal walls are de-epithelialized and sutured to one another, shortening the vaginal length substantially,[71] as opposed to a reconstructive procedure, such as a vaginal apical suspension.[22–29] Of note, women consider body image, sexuality, and their sense of self when considering this decision, and even women who do not wish to engage in vaginal insertive intercourse may desire to avoid colpocleisis for a variety of reasons. It is also important to note that insertive vaginal intercourse is only a possible part of sexual activity, so the patient's range of sexual expression should be considered prior to arriving at a shared decision to perform colpocleisis. The minimal risk of recurrence after colpocleisis, as well as the minimally invasive approach,[30] should be weighed against the patient's certainty that she is amenable to this obliterative procedure.

The second important decision to be made by the patient in consultation with her surgeon is uterine preservation versus a concomitant hysterectomy during the chosen POP surgery. Clearly, this decision applies only to women with a uterus still in place (no former hysterectomy). Uterine preservation surgeries are gaining popularity among women and physicians as women consider fertility desires, menopause timing, body image, and a sense of self while making this decision.[31,32] Uterine preservation shortens operating

room time, reduces blood loss, and decreases mesh exposure risk in procedures involving permanent mesh grafts.[33,34] Contraindications to these surgeries include relatively elevated risk of cervical, uterine, or ovarian cancer; inability to comply with adequate pelvic cancer screening; genetic cancer syndromes that increase pelvic cancer risk; and current or suspected uterine or adnexal pathology.[35]

The next important decision faced by women involves use of a graft in their reconstruction versus a surgery using the patient's natural tissue. Graft reconstruction is more durable and when involving the apical/anterior compartment results in more cephalad vaginal anatomy,[36] but the reoperation rate for POP recurrence and subjective relief of POP symptoms is similar between natural tissue and graft-augmented procedures.[37–40] There is recent evidence that overall reoperation for graft-related POP surgery may be greater than natural tissue ligament surgery, even accounting for more POP recurrence, due to the large number of surgeries for graft-related complications.[41,42] Regarding biologic grafts for POP repair, it has been demonstrated that these do not improve the postoperative recurrence rate or symptoms following repair of prolapse and can have complication rates as high as those of synthetic grafts.[36,43] There are recent restrictions placed by the U.S. Food and Drug Administration (FDA) on the type and indication for which grafts can be placed in the pelvis.[44] International organizations, such as the National Institute for Health and Care Excellence, recommend that women having procedures with permanent graft should be appropriately counseled and informed and registered in a registry database to properly track outcomes.[45] Women should have specific counseling about the type of graft being used and the route of administration of that graft prior to making a decision about graft-related surgery.

Once the decision is made whether to use or not to use graft in the repair of POP, the surgeon also must decide on the route of surgery. In general, surgeons can operate laparoscopically/robotically, vaginally, or through an open abdominal incision in the repair of POP, and the choice of certain procedures (such as sacrocolpopexy) may dictate the most optimal route. Certain comorbidities held by the patient, such as an enlarged uterus that is to be removed concurrently or suspected concurrent uterine or adnexal malignancy, may entice the patient or surgeon to choose an open abdominal route or, in the case of an experienced laparoscopic surgeon, a laparoscopic or robotic route. For some surgeons, the need to remove the adnexa concurrently for malignancy risk reduction may also entice them to approach the surgery abdominally or laparoscopically/robotically. Patient comorbidities that make abdominal or laparoscopic surgery too risky, such as pulmonary compromise or heart conditions, may argue for the vaginal route to avoid Trendelenburg positioning, abdominal distension, or longer operating room times. It should be noted that laparoscopic or robotic routes are associated with less blood loss, recovery time, and pain than open abdominal procedures despite longer operating room times.[46] Regardless of the route deemed most appropriate for the patient, the surgeon should have expertise in the route chosen, the patient should have the health and lack of comorbidities to undergo that route of surgery, and the surgery should address the components of the vagina that are prolapsed.[47]

Another key decisional step in POP surgery is to decide whether to perform a concurrent stress urinary incontinence (SUI) procedure at the time of POP surgery. Women undergoing POP surgery, especially those with preexisting SUI symptoms, are at higher risk for SUI following prolapse correction if they do not undergo an anti-incontinence procedure at the time of their POP surgery.[48,49] There are many different practice patterns on concurrent SUI surgery, including performing universal concurrent SUI surgery, always doing stress incontinence surgery as an interval procedure, or basing the decision on preoperative testing including reduction cough stress testing and/or urodynamic studies. Evidence does not demonstrate any of these approaches to be superior but does indicate that women without preoperative SUI symptoms prior to POP surgery or with a negative workup for stress incontinence get less benefit from concurrent stress incontinence surgery than those who do have SUI symptoms.[49,50] Surgeons must weigh the risks of the stress incontinence surgery itself, including the increased operating room time and the risks of urinary retention, urinary tract infections, and de novo urgency symptoms, against the benefit to the individual patient.

SURGICAL OUTCOMES WITH INDIVIDUAL PROCEDURE TYPES (TABLE 42.2)

Graft-Augmented Apical Suspension Procedures: Sacrocolpopexy and Sacrohysteropexy

To many, a sacrocolpopexy is believed to be the "gold standard" of apical suspension procedures due to this procedure's increased durability and its multicompartment repair of the vagina (Fig. 42.3).[28,51] On the other hand, some debate this "gold standard" label, citing anatomic failure rates of 22% to 27% at 7 years in a large rigorous trial.[28] It is important to note, however, that reoperation for POP was small, only 5%, in the same study in the same time frame.[28] Another randomized controlled trial showed 100% success in a median follow-up of 42 months,[52] indicating how change in follow-up time and the definition of success can dramatically affect the success rate of a procedure. Similar outcomes, with low reoperation rates but substantial anatomic recurrence, were discovered for sacrohysteropexy in a recent systematic review.[34]

These procedures, however, require specialized training, expertise, and, most typically in the current climate, knowledge of a minimally invasive platform. Because minimally invasive versus abdominal procedures involve less blood loss, less time to recovery, and less hospital stay, the minimally invasive approach to this procedure is ideal, although operating room time is increased.[53-55] Despite these advantages, there are some data that the laparoscopic approach may have worse recurrence-free survival than the open approach.[52] There is no established difference in outcome comparing laparoscopic surgeries to robotic-assisted laparoscopic surgeries for sacrocolpopexy, although the robotic approach has historically been associated with higher costs.[56-58]

Sacrocolpopexy or sacrohysteropexy are demonstrated to have higher durability than vaginal native tissue repair, with less recurrence in symptoms or reoperation with longer duration following the surgery.[37] However, these surgeries have a higher prevalence of complications than transvaginal native tissue repairs, highlighting the fact that this surgery is more invasive than transvaginal native tissue repair surgeries and requires a higher level of skill and experience.[37-40] When sacrocolpopexy or sacrohysteropexy is compared to

TABLE 42.2

Surgical Outcomes with Individual Procedure Types

SURGERY	DEFINITION OF PROCEDURE[a]	OUTCOMES IN RIGOROUS TRIALS[b]	IMPORTANT EVIDENCE-BASED KNOWLEDGE
Sacrocolpopexy/ sacrohysteropexy	Suspension of the vaginal apex to the anterior longitudinal ligament of the sacrum using a graft, with possible incorporation of the graft into the fibromuscular layer of the anterior and/or posterior vaginal walls	Success 73%–78% at 7 y	• Similar outcomes between sacrocolpopexy and uterine preservation (sacrohysteropexy) • More durable than vaginal native tissue repair • Better sexual function and anatomic outcomes than vaginal graft procedures
Uterosacral ligament suspension	Suspension of the vaginal apex to the ipsilateral uterosacral ligament and/ or plication across the midline incorporating the uterosacral ligaments	Success 30%–38% at 5 y	• Similar outcomes with uterine preservation • Similar outcomes to sacrospinous ligament fixation
Sacrospinous ligament fixation	Suspension of the vaginal apex to the unilateral or bilateral sacrospinous ligament(s) using suture	Success 30%–38% at 5 y	• Similar outcomes with uterine preservation • Similar outcomes to uterosacral ligament fixation
Anterior vaginal repair	Repair of the fibromuscular layer of the anterior vaginal wall	Success 30%–82% at 2 y	• Improved anatomic outcomes with graft augmentation
Posterior vaginal repair	Repair of the fibromuscular layer of the posterior vaginal wall	Success 54%–93% at 1 y	• Improved anatomic and subjective outcomes with vaginal/perineal route vs. transanal • No improvement with graft augmentation
Colpocleisis	Obliteration of the vaginal canal by partial removal of the vaginal epithelium on the anterior and posterior vaginal walls and suturing together the fibromuscular layers of the anterior and posterior vaginal walls within these wounds with or without the creation of bilateral tunnels from the cervix to the introitus if a uterus is being left in place	Success 73%–100% at 1–5 y	• No evidence on difference in success with or without uterine preservation • Highest durability and success of POP procedures • Cannot have insertive vaginal intercourse following performance of this procedure; regret rate up to 13% • Study with only 73% success at 1 year after colpocleisis was based on criteria of stage 1 or less being success[85]

[a]According to American Urogynecologic Society/International Urogynecological Association joint terminology document.[20]
[b]Depends on definition of success.

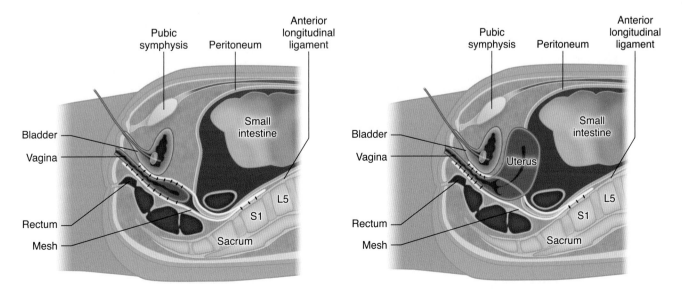

FIGURE 42.3 Multicompartment repair of the vagina using sacrocolpopexy (without uterine preservation, **left**) or sacrohysteropexy (with uterine preservation, **right**).[20]

transvaginal graft procedures, sacrocolpopexy or sacrohysteropexy has similar patient satisfaction and symptoms relief but may have better sexual function and anatomic outcomes than transvaginal graft procedures.[59-61] Important to note is that sacrocolpopexy or sacrohysteropexy, although still a procedure that usually involve permanent graft placement, has substantially lower permanent graft exposure than transvaginal graft.[36,43] This explains why the sacrocolpopexy or sacrohysteropexy procedures, and the permanent grafts used for them, are still in wide use, although the United States has banned the use of "transvaginal mesh" for anterior/apical compartment POP repair.[62]

Apical Native Tissue Vaginal Suspension Procedures

Uterosacral ligament suspension and sacrospinous ligament suspension are the mainstays of transvaginal native tissue repair. Uterosacral suspension can be performed either by plicating the lateral vaginal apex to the ipsilateral uterosacral ligament bilaterally or by plicating across the midline with circular sutures across the midline (Fig. 42.4), two methods that have never been compared in a randomized trial setting.[63-66] Both methods appear to have moderate success in rigorous trials,[13] but failure is as high as 62% to 70% at 5 years.[27] Uterosacral suspension enjoys the benefits of restoring a more "natural" apical axis[67] but has the disadvantages

of often requiring entry into the peritoneum and having relatively high rates of ureteral injury.[68]

Sacrospinous ligament fixation, which has a similar general success rate to uterosacral ligament suspension in a large randomized trial,[19] can be performed unilaterally or bilaterally.[27,69,70] The unilateral and bilateral methods produce similar outcomes in a single study of this comparison.[71] Benefits to sacrospinous ligament fixation include not having to enter the peritoneum and preservation of a fast, vaginal surgical approach (Fig. 42.5),[69,72] although risks include relatively high rates of buttock pain and neurologic injury with this surgery.[73]

Native tissue suspension of the uterus, or native tissue hysteropexy, involves either uterosacral or sacrospinous hysteropexy or a Manchester procedure.[70,74,75] Recurrence and reoperation rates are similar to the corresponding procedures involving a hysterectomy or the vaginal vault, whereas the Manchester has no corresponding uterine removal because of its unique nature (Fig. 42.6).

Native Tissue Vaginal Procedures for Other Compartments

Anterior vaginal repair, the plication of the anterior vaginal wall,[76] has general success rates that are as low at 30% to 46% in one randomized trial[77] but as high as 82% at 2 years in another.[78] In addition, in comparison to anterior vaginal repair with graft, anterior vaginal

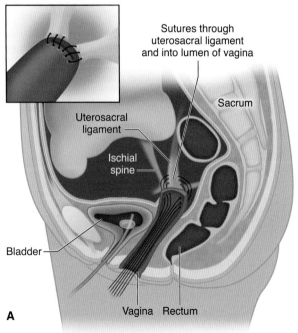

Cuff of vagina and tied down
sutures plicating uterosacral ligaments

Sutures through
uterosacral ligament
and into lumen of vagina

Sacrum

Uterosacral
ligament

Ischial
spine

Bladder

A   Vagina   Rectum

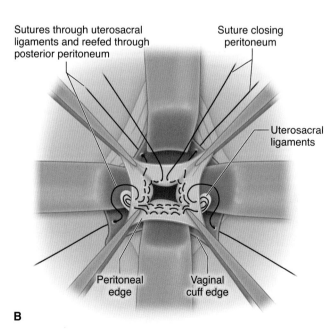

Sutures through uterosacral
ligaments and reefed through
posterior peritoneum

Suture closing
peritoneum

Uterosacral
ligaments

Peritoneal
edge

Vaginal
cuff edge

B

FIGURE 42.4 Side-by-side comparison of the ipsilateral method of uterosacral ligament suspension (**left**) versus the method across the midline (**right**).[20]

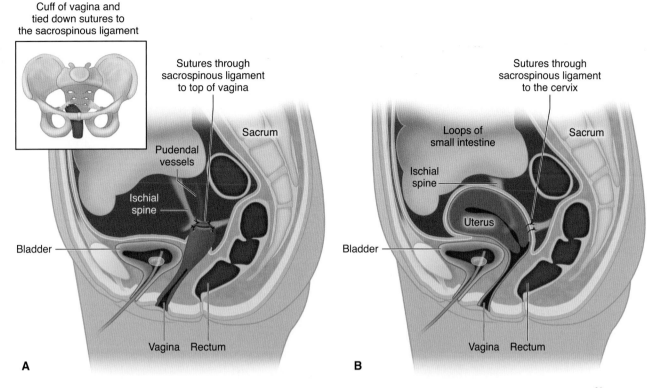

FIGURE 42.5 Unilateral sacrospinous fixation without uterine preservation (**left**) or with uterine preservation (**right**).[20]

repair without graft is shown to have less objective or anatomic success than graft-augmented procedures but similar subjective and reoperation outcomes.[76,78–80] Posterior vaginal repair also demonstrates a wide range of success varying from 54% in one randomized trial[81] to as much as 93%,[8,82–84] again depending highly on the definition of success. It is known that transvaginal or transperineal repair improves outcomes over transanal repair,[83,84] but it has not been demonstrated

that posterior vaginal repair outcomes are improved by the augmentation of graft in several randomized trials.[81,82,85–88]

Perineal Repair

These surgeries vary widely in how perineal repairs are performed,[89] but, in general, they restore the muscular tendons of the perineal body toward the central

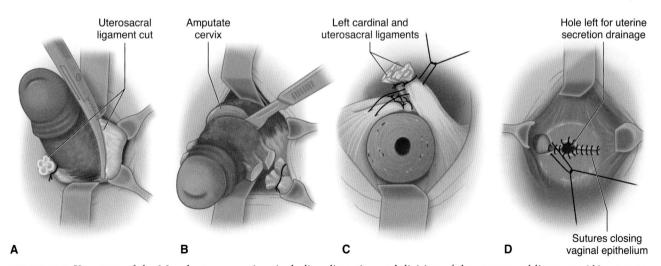

FIGURE 42.6 Key steps of the Manchester operation, including dissection and division of the uterosacral ligaments (**A**), amputation of the cervix (**B**), plication of the uterosacral ligaments across the cervical stump (**C**), and closure of the vaginal epithelium with canal left for uterine drainage (**D**).

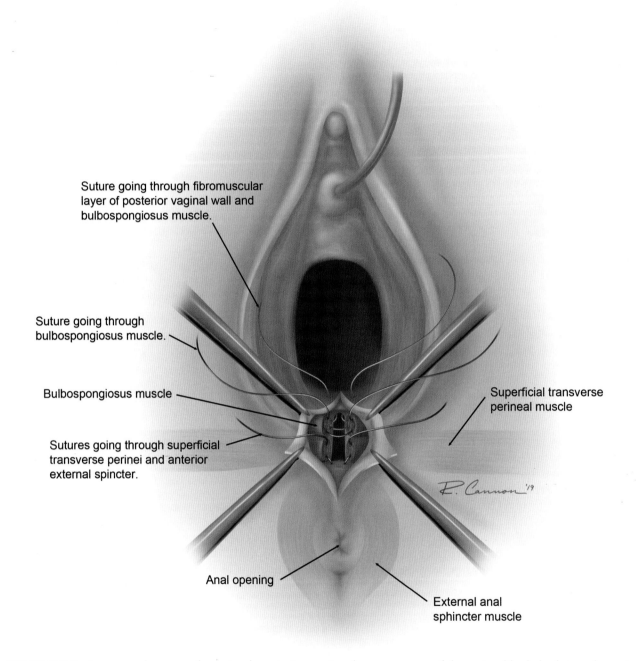

Suture going through fibromuscular layer of posterior vaginal wall and bulbospongiosus muscle.

Suture going through bulbospongiosus muscle.

Bulbospongiosus muscle

Sutures going through superficial transverse perinei and anterior external spincter.

Superficial transverse perineal muscle

Anal opening

External anal sphincter muscle

FIGURE 42.7 Basic steps and sutures of a perineal repair, integrating the components of the perineal body back into the perineal anatomy.[20]

conjoined tendon in an attempt to restore perineal anatomy (Fig. 42.7).[20] There is a remarkable dearth of evidence for the role of perineal repair in prolapse outcomes. One randomized trial demonstrated that they did not improve body image when added to apical prolapse surgery.[90] Another randomized study compared perineal repair to physical therapy for delayed repair of second-degree lacerations in childbirth and found that surgical treatment was more effective at relieving symptoms.[91] Despite emerging evidence that a smaller genital

hiatus is protective for prolapse recurrence following prolapse surgery,[92–94] little is known about long-term outcomes of prolapse surgeries when perineal repair is (or is not) performed.

Obliterative Vaginal Procedures

Colpocleisis (Fig. 42.8), which involves closure of the inner vaginal vault or significant shortening of the vagina,[95–97] is an excellent choice for women who no

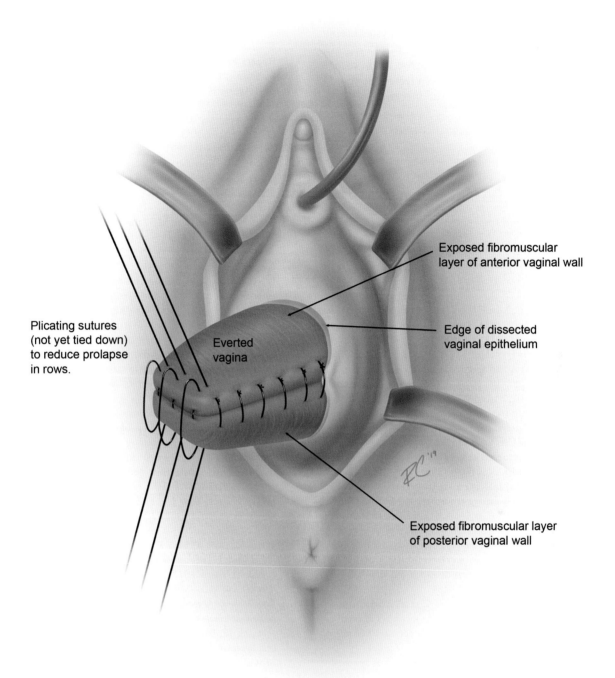

Plicating sutures (not yet tied down) to reduce prolapse in rows.

Everted vagina

Exposed fibromuscular layer of anterior vaginal wall

Edge of dissected vaginal epithelium

Exposed fibromuscular layer of posterior vaginal wall

FIGURE 42.8 Closure of the anterior and posterior muscularis layers of the vaginal wall together with sutures in a colpocleisis procedure.[20]

longer desire a patent vagina receptive to insertive vaginal intercourse. Colpocleisis without a hysterectomy that preserved the uterus, traditionally referred to as a LeFort colpocleisis, has high anatomical success of 98.9% to 100% with rare need for reoperation[24,25,98] and relatively few complications given the elderly populations on which this is usually performed.[99,100] Colpocleisis of the vaginal vault or colpocleisis with a hysterectomy, traditionally referred to as a partial colpectomy, appears to have similar outcomes[101] despite the fact that there are no directly comparative

data comparing POP outcomes of a colpocleisis with or without a concurrent hysterectomy.[33,102] However, the regret associated with this procedure is reported as up to 13%.[23,26]

CONCLUSION

POP procedures available for surgical repair are widely varied, and approach depends largely on patient goals and risks to which they are most averse. Current salient decisions to make with the patient include route of approach (based also on expertise of surgeon), to have hysterectomy or uterine preservation, to have a mesh graft or no graft, and to have or not have a concurrent stress incontinence procedures. Surgeons employing a given technique should know the particular risks, benefits, and techniques of the approach they have chosen with their patient in order to assure informed consent and shared decision-making.

References

1. Rada MP, Jones S, Falconi G, et al. A systematic review and meta-synthesis of qualitative studies on pelvic organ prolapse for the development of core outcome sets. *Neurourol Urodyn* 2020;39(3):880–889.

2. Ghetti C, Skoczylas LC, Oliphant SS, et al. The emotional burden of pelvic organ prolapse in women seeking treatment: A qualitative study. *Female Pelvic Med Reconstr Surg* 2015;21(6):332–338.

3. Lowder JL, Ghetti C, Moalli P, et al. Body image in women before and after reconstructive surgery for pelvic organ prolapse. *Int Urogynecol J* 2010;21(8):919–925.

4. Baskayne K, Willars J, Pitchforth E, et al. Women's expectations of prolapse surgery: A retrospective qualitative study. *Neurourol Urodyn* 2014;33(1):85–89.

5. Sung VW, Rogers RG, Barber MD, et al. Conceptual framework for patient-important treatment outcomes for pelvic organ prolapse. *Neurourol Urodyn* 2014;33(4):414–419.

6. Wu JM, Matthews CA, Conover MM, et al. Lifetime risk of stress urinary incontinence or pelvic organ prolapse surgery. *Obstet Gynecol* 2014;123(6):1201–1206.

7. Wilkins MF, Wu JM. Lifetime risk of surgery for stress urinary incontinence or pelvic organ prolapse. *Minerva Ginecol* 2017;69(2):171–177.

8. Lourenço TRM, Pergialiotis V, Durnea CM, et al. A systematic review of reported outcomes and outcome measures in randomized trials evaluating surgical interventions for posterior vaginal prolapse to aid development of a core outcome set. *Int J Gynaecol Obstet* 2020;148(3):271–281.

9. Lourenço TRM, Pergialiotis V, Durnea C, et al. A systematic review of reported outcomes and outcome measures in randomized controlled trials on apical prolapse surgery. *Int J Gynaecol Obstet* 2019;145(1):4–11.

10. Lourenço TRM, Pergialiotis V, Duffy JMN, et al. A systematic review on reporting outcomes and outcome measures in trials on synthetic mesh procedures for pelvic organ prolapse: Urgent action is needed to improve quality of research. *Neurourol Urodyn* 2019;38(2):509–524.

11. Barber MD, Brubaker L, Nygaard I, et al. Defining success after surgery for pelvic organ prolapse. *Obstet Gynecol* 2009;114(3):600–609.

12. Nager CW, Visco AG, Richter HE, et al. Effect of vaginal mesh hysteropexy vs vaginal hysterectomy with uterosacral ligament suspension on treatment failure in women with uterovaginal prolapse: A randomized clinical trial. *JAMA* 2019;322(11):1054–1065.

13. Barber MD, Brubaker L, Burgio KL, et al. Comparison of 2 transvaginal surgical approaches and perioperative behavioral therapy for apical vaginal prolapse: The OPTIMAL randomized trial. *JAMA* 2014;311(10):1023–1034.

14. Barber MD, Chen Z, Lukacz E, et al. Further validation of the short form versions of the Pelvic Floor Distress Inventory (PFDI)

15. Rogers RG, Espuña Pons ME. The Pelvic Organ Prolapse Incontinence Sexual Questionnaire, IUGA-Revised (PISQ-IR). *Int Urogynecol J* 2013;24(7):1063–1064.

16. Constantine ML, Pauls RN, Rogers RR, et al. Validation of a single summary score for the Prolapse/Incontinence Sexual Questionnaire-IUGA revised (PISQ-IR). *Int Urogynecol J* 2017;28(12):1901–1907.

17. Barber MD, Kuchibhatla MN, Pieper CF, et al. Psychometric evaluation of 2 comprehensive condition-specific quality of life instruments for women with pelvic floor disorders. *Am J Obstet Gynecol* 2001;185(6):1388–1395.

18. Barber MD, Walters MD, Bump RC. Short forms of two condition-specific quality-of-life questionnaires for women with pelvic floor disorders (PFDI-20 and PFIQ-7). *Am J Obstet Gynecol* 2005;193(1):103–113.

19. Lee U, Raz S. Emerging concepts for pelvic organ prolapse surgery: What is cure? *Curr Urol Rep* 2011;12(1):62–67.

20. Developed by the Joint Writing Group of the American Urogynecologic Society, International Urogynecological Association. Joint report on terminology for surgical procedures to treat pelvic organ prolapse. *Int Urogynecol J* 2020;31(3):429–463.

21. Joint report on terminology for surgical procedures to treat pelvic organ prolapse. *Female Pelvic Med Reconstr Surg* 2020;26(3):173–201.

22. Crisp CC, Book NM, Cunkelman JA, et al. Body image, regret, and satisfaction 24 weeks after colpocleisis: A multicenter study. *Female Pelvic Med Reconstr Surg* 2016;22(3):132–135.

23. Katsara A, Wight E, Heinzelmann-Schwarz V, et al. Long-term quality of life, satisfaction, pelvic floor symptoms and regret after colpocleisis. *Arch Gynecol Obstet* 2016;294(5):999–1003.

24. Song X, Zhu L, Ding J, et al. Long-term follow-up after LeFort colpocleisis: Patient satisfaction, regret rate, and pelvic symptoms. *Menopause* 2016;23(6):621–625.

25. Wang X, Chen Y, Hua K. Pelvic symptoms, body image, and regret after LeFort colpocleisis: A long-term follow-up. *J Minim Invasive Gynecol* 2017;24(3):415–419.

26. Winkelman WD, Haviland MJ, Elkadry EA. Long-term pelvic floor symptoms, recurrence, satisfaction, and regret following colpocleisis. *Female Pelvic Med Reconstr Surg* 2020;26(9):558–562.

27. Jelovsek JE, Barber MD, Brubaker L, et al. Effect of uterosacral ligament suspension vs sacrospinous ligament fixation with or without perioperative behavioral therapy for pelvic organ vaginal prolapse on surgical outcomes and prolapse symptoms at 5 years in the OPTIMAL randomized clinical trial. *JAMA* 2018;319(15):1554–1565.

28. Nygaard I, Brubaker L, Zyczynski HM, et al. Long-term outcomes following abdominal sacrocolpopexy for pelvic organ prolapse. *JAMA* 2013;309(19):2016–2024.

29. Wadsworth K, Lovatsis D. A qualitative study of women's values and decision-making surrounding LeFort colpocleisis. *Int Urogynecol J* 2020;31(6):1099–1103.

30. Buchsbaum GM, Lee TG. Vaginal obliterative procedures for pelvic organ prolapse: A systematic review. *Obstet Gynecol Surv* 2017;72(3):175–183.

31. Ridgeway B, Frick AC, Walter MD. Hysteropexy. A review. *Minerva Ginecol* 2008;60(6):509–528.

32. Korbly NB, Kassis NC, Good MM, et al. Patient preferences for uterine preservation and hysterectomy in women with pelvic organ prolapse. *Am J Obstet Gynecol* 2013;209(5):470.e1–470.e6.

33. Meriwether KV, Antosh DD, Olivera CK, et al. Uterine preservation vs hysterectomy in pelvic organ prolapse surgery: A systematic review with meta-analysis and clinical practice guidelines. *Am J Obstet Gynecol* 2018;219(2):129–146e.2.

34. Meriwether KV, Balk EM, Antosh DD, et al. Uterine-preserving surgeries for the repair of pelvic organ prolapse: A systematic review with meta-analysis and clinical practice guidelines. *Int Urogynecol J* 2019;30(4):505–522.

35. Gutman R, Maher C. Uterine-preserving POP surgery. *Int Urogynecol J* 2013;24(11):1803–1813.

36. Schimpf MO, Abed H, Sanses T, et al. Graft and mesh use in transvaginal prolapse repair: A systematic review. *Obstet Gynecol* 2016;128(1):81–91.

37. Rogers RG, Nolen TL, Weidner AC, et al. Open sacrocolpopexy and vaginal apical repair: Retrospective comparison of success and serious complications. *Int Urogynecol J* 2018;29(8):1101–1110.

38. Coolen AWM, Bui BN, Dietz V, et al. The treatment of posthysterectomy vaginal vault prolapse: A systematic review and meta-analysis. *Int Urogynecol J* 2017;28(12):1767–1783.

39. Coolen AWM, van IJsselmuiden MN, van Oudheusden AMJ, et al. Laparoscopic sacrocolpopexy versus vaginal sacrospinous fixation for vaginal vault prolapse, a randomized controlled trial: SALTO-2 trial, study protocol. *BMC Womens Health* 2017;17(1):52.

40. Siddiqui NY, Grimes CL, Casiano ER, et al. Mesh sacrocolpopexy compared with native tissue vaginal repair: A systematic review and meta-analysis. *Obstet Gynecol* 2015;125(1):44–55.

41. Dallas KB, Rogo-Gupta L, Elliott CS. What impacts the all cause risk of reoperation after pelvic organ prolapse repair? A comparison of mesh and native tissue approaches in 110,329 women. *J Urol* 2018;200(2):389–396.

42. Dieter AA, Willis-Gray MG, Weidner AC, et al. Vaginal native tissue repair versus transvaginal mesh repair for apical prolapse: How utilizing different methods of analysis affects the estimated trade-off between reoperation for mesh exposure/erosion and reoperation for recurrent prolapse. *Int Urogynecol J* 2015;26(5):721–727.

43. Abed H, Rahn DD, Lowenstein L, et al. Incidence and management of graft erosion, wound granulation, and dyspareunia following vaginal prolapse repair with graft materials: A systematic review. *Int Urogynecol J* 2011;22(7):789–798.

44. Hanno P. Toward optimal health: Philip Hanno, M.D., M.P.H., discusses improved management of painful bladder syndrome (interstitial cystitis). Interview by Jodi R. Godfrey. *J Womens Health (Larchmt)* 2007;16(1):3–8.

45. Urinary incontinence and pelvic organ prolapse in women: Management. Published April 2, 2019. Updated June 24, 2019. Accessed January 20, 2021. https://www.nice.org.uk/guidance/ng123/chapter/Recommendations#surgical-management-of-pelvic-organ-prolapse

46. Pelvic organ prolapse: ACOG Practice Bulletin, Number 214. *Obstet Gynecol* 2019;134(5):e126–e142.

47. Walters MD, Ridgeway BM. Surgical treatment of vaginal apex prolapse. *Obstet Gynecol* 2013;121(2 Pt 1):354–374.

48. Brubaker L, Cundiff GW, Fine P, et al. Abdominal sacrocolpopexy with Burch colposuspension to reduce urinary stress incontinence. *N Engl J Med* 2006;354(15):1557–1566.

49. Wei JT, Nygaard I, Richter HE, et al. A midurethral sling to reduce incontinence after vaginal prolapse repair. *N Engl J Med* 2012;366(25):2358–2367.

50. Brubaker L, Nygaard I, Richter HE, et al. Two-year outcomes after sacrocolpopexy with and without Burch to prevent stress urinary incontinence. *Obstet Gynecol* 2008;112(1):49–55.

51. Maher C, Feiner B, Baessler K, et al. Surgical management of pelvic organ prolapse in women. *Cochrane Database Syst Rev* 2010;(4):CD004014.

52. Costantini E, Mearini L, Lazzeri M, et al. Laparoscopic versus abdominal sacrocolpopexy: A randomized, controlled trial. *J Urol* 2016;196(1):159–165.

53. Coolen AWM, van Oudheusden AMJ, Mol BWJ, et al. Laparoscopic sacrocolpopexy compared with open abdominal sacrocolpopexy for vault prolapse repair: A randomised controlled trial. *Int Urogynecol J* 2017;28(10):1469–1479.

54. Khan A, Alperin M, Wu N, et al. Comparative outcomes of open versus laparoscopic sacrocolpopexy among Medicare beneficiaries. *Int Urogynecol J* 2013;24(11):1883–1891.

55. De Gouveia De Sa M, Claydon LS, Whitlow B, et al. Laparoscopic versus open sacrocolpopexy for treatment of prolapse of the apical segment of the vagina: A systematic review and meta-analysis. *Int Urogynecol J* 2016;27(1):3–17.

56. Anger JT, Mueller ER, Tarnay C, et al. Robotic compared with laparoscopic sacrocolpopexy: A randomized controlled trial. *Obstet Gynecol* 2014;123(1):5–12.

57. Paraiso MF, Jelovsek JE, Frick A, et al. Laparoscopic compared with robotic sacrocolpopexy for vaginal prolapse: A randomized controlled trial. *Obstet Gynecol* 2011;118(5):1005–1013.

58. Tan-Kim J, Menefee SA, Luber KM, et al. Robotic-assisted and laparoscopic sacrocolpopexy: Comparing operative times, costs and outcomes. *Female Pelvic Med Reconstr Surg* 2011;17(1):44–49.

59. Jambusaria LH, Murphy M, Lucente VR. One-year functional and anatomic outcomes of robotic sacrocolpopexy versus vaginal extraperitoneal colpopexy with mesh. *Female Pelvic Med Reconstr Surg* 2015;21(2):87–92.

60. Kanasaki H, Oride A, Hara T, et al. Comparative retrospective study of tension-free vaginal mesh surgery, native tissue repair, and laparoscopic sacrocolpopexy for pelvic organ prolapse repair. *Obstet Gynecol Int* 2020;2020·7367403.

61. Gutman RE, Rardin CR, Sokol ER, et al. Vaginal and laparoscopic mesh hysteropexy for uterovaginal prolapse: A parallel cohort study. *Am J Obstet Gynecol* 2017;216(1):38.e1–38.e11.

62. U.S. Food and Drug Administration. Urogynecologic surgical mesh implants. Accessed July 3, 2019. https://www.fda.gov/medical-devices/implants-and-prosthetics/urogynecologic-surgical-mesh-implants

63. Shull BL, Bachofen C, Coates KW, et al. A transvaginal approach to repair of apical and other associated sites of pelvic organ prolapse with uterosacral ligaments. *Am J Obstet Gynecol* 2000;183(6):1365–1374.

64. Parisi S, Novelli A, Olearo E, et al. Traditional McCall culdoplasty compared to a modified McCall technique with double ligament suspension: Anatomical and clinical outcomes. *Int Urogynecol J* 2020;31(10):2147–2153.

65. Spelzini F, Frigerio M, Manodoro S, et al. Modified McCall culdoplasty versus Shull suspension in pelvic prolapse primary repair: A retrospective study. *Int Urogynecol J* 2017;28(1):65–71.

66. Wall LL. A technique for modified McCall culdeplasty at the time of abdominal hysterectomy. *J Am Coll Surg* 1994;178(5):507–509.

67. Barber MD, Visco AG, Weidner AC, et al. Bilateral uterosacral ligament vaginal vault suspension with site-specific endopelvic fascia defect repair for treatment of pelvic organ prolapse. *Am J Obstet Gynecol* 2000;183(6):1402–1411.

68. Manodoro S, Frigerio M, Milani R, et al. Tips and tricks for uterosacral ligament suspension: How to avoid ureteral injury. *Int Urogynecol J* 2018;29(1):161–163.

69. Morgan DM, Larson K. Uterosacral and sacrospinous ligament suspension for restoration of apical vaginal support. *Clin Obstet Gynecol* 2010;53(1):72–85.

70. Schulten SFM, Detollenaere RJ, Stekelenburg J, et al. Sacrospinous hysteropexy versus vaginal hysterectomy with uterosacral ligament suspension in women with uterine prolapse stage 2 or higher: Observational follow-up of a multicentre randomised trial. *BMJ* 2019;366:l5149.

71. Salman S, Babaoglu B, Kumbasar S, et al. Comparison of unilateral and bilateral sacrospinous ligament fixation using minimally invasive anchorage. *Geburtshilfe Frauenheilkd* 2019;79(9):976–982.

72. Doğanay M, Aksakal O. Minimally invasive sacrospinous ligament suspension: Perioperative morbidity and review of the literature. *Arch Gynecol Obstet* 2014;289(2):235.

73. Ferrando CA, Walters MD. A randomized double-blind placebo-controlled trial on the effect of local analgesia on postoperative gluteal pain in patients undergoing sacrospinous ligament colpopexy. *Am J Obstet Gynecol* 2018;218(6):599.e1–599.e8.

74. Schulten SFM, Enklaar RA, Kluivers KB, et al. Evaluation of two vaginal, uterus sparing operations for pelvic organ prolapse: Modified Manchester operation (MM) and sacrospinous hysteropexy (SSH), a study protocol for a multicentre randomized non-inferiority trial (the SAM study). *BMC Womens Health* 2019;19(1):49.

75. Detollenaere RJ, den Boon J, Stekelenburg J, et al. Sacrospinous hysteropexy versus vaginal hysterectomy with suspension of the uterosacral ligaments in women with uterine prolapse stage 2 or higher: Multicentre randomised non-inferiority trial. *BMJ* 2015;351:h3717.

76. Maher C, Feiner B, Baessler K, et al. Surgery for women with anterior compartment prolapse. *Cochrane Database Syst Rev* 2016;(11):CD004014.

77. Weber AM, Walters MD, Piedmonte MR, et al. Anterior colporrhaphy: A randomized trial of three surgical techniques. *Am J Obstet Gynecol* 2001;185(6):1299–1306.

78. Menefee SA, Dyer KY, Lukacz ES, et al. Colporrhaphy compared with mesh or graft-reinforced vaginal paravaginal repair for anterior vaginal wall prolapse: A randomized controlled trial. *Obstet Gynecol* 2011;118(6):1337–1344.

79. Gutman RE, Nosti PA, Sokol AI, et al. Three-year outcomes of vaginal mesh for prolapse: A randomized controlled trial. *Obstet Gynecol* 2013;122(4):770–777.

80. Feldner PC Jr, Castro RA, Cipolotti LA, et al. Anterior vaginal wall prolapse: A randomized controlled trial of SIS graft versus traditional colporrhaphy. *Int Urogynecol J* 2010;21(9):1057–1063.

81. Paraiso MF, Barber MD, Muir TW, et al. Rectocele repair: A randomized trial of three surgical techniques including graft augmentation. *Am J Obstet Gynecol* 2006;195(6):1762–1771.

82. Mowat A, Maher D, Baessler K, et al. Surgery for women with posterior compartment prolapse. *Cochrane Database Syst Rev* 2018;3(3):CD012975.

83. Nieminen K, Hiltunen K-M, Laitinen J, et al. Transanal or vaginal approach to rectocele repair: A prospective, randomized pilot study. *Dis Colon Rectum* 2004;47(10):1636–1642.

84. Farid M, Madbouly KM, Hussein A, et al. Randomized controlled trial between perineal and anal repairs of rectocele in obstructed defecation. *World J Surg* 2010;34(4):822–829.

85. Gustilo-Ashby AM, Paraiso MF, Jelovsek JE, et al. Bowel symptoms 1 year after surgery for prolapse: Further analysis of a randomized trial of rectocele repair. *Am J Obstet Gynecol* 2007;197(1):76.e1–76.e5.

86. Sung VW, Rardin CR, Raker CA, et al. Porcine subintestinal submucosal graft augmentation for rectocele repair: A randomized controlled trial. *Obstet Gynecol* 2012;119(1):125–133.

87. Nüssler E, Granåsen G, Nüssler EK, et al. Repair of recurrent rectocele with posterior colporrhaphy or non-absorbable polypropylene mesh-patient-reported outcomes at 1-year follow-up. *Int Urogynecol J* 2019;30(10):1679–1687.

88. Madsen LD, Nüssler E, Kesmodel US, et al. Native-tissue repair of isolated primary rectocele compared with nonabsorbable mesh: Patient-reported outcomes. *Int Urogynecol J* 2017;28(1):49–57.

89. Kanter G, Jeppson PC, McGuire BL, et al. Perineorrhaphy: Commonly performed yet poorly understood. A survey of surgeons. *Int Urogynecol J* 2015;26(12):1797–1801.

90. Ninivaggio CS, Komesu YM, Jeppson PC, et al. Perineorrhaphy outcomes related to body imagery: A randomized trial of body image perception. *Female Pelvic Med Reconstr Surg* 2021;27(5):281–288.

91. Bergman I, Söderberg MW, Ek M. Perineorrhaphy compared with pelvic floor muscle therapy in women with late consequences of a poorly healed second-degree perineal tear: A randomized controlled trial. *Obstet Gynecol* 2020;135(2):341–351.

92. Hill AM, Shatkin-Margolis A, Smith BC, et al. Associating genital hiatus size with long-term outcomes after apical suspension. *Int Urogynecol J* 2020;31(8):1537–1544.

93. Medina CA, Candiotti K, Takacs P. Wide genital hiatus is a risk factor for recurrence following anterior vaginal repair. *Int J Gynaecol Obstet* 2008;101(2):184–187.

94. Bradley MS, Askew AL, Vaughan MH, et al. Robotic-assisted sacrocolpopexy: Early postoperative outcomes after surgical reduction of enlarged genital hiatus. *Am J Obstet Gynecol* 2018;218(5):514.e1–514.e8.

95. FitzGerald MP, Richter HE, Siddique S, et al; for the Pelvic Floor Disorders Network. Colpocleisis: A review. *Int Urogynecol J Pelvic Floor Dysfunct* 2006;17(3):261–271.

96. Fitzgerald MP, Richter HE, Bradley CS, et al. Pelvic support, pelvic symptoms, and patient satisfaction after colpocleisis. *Int Urogynecol J Pelvic Floor Dysfunct* 2008;19(12):1603–1609.

97. Gutman RE, Bradley CS, Ye W, et al. Effects of colpocleisis on bowel symptoms among women with severe pelvic organ prolapse. *Int Urogynecol J* 2010;21(4):461–466.

98. Park JY, Han SJ, Kim JH, et al. Le Fort partial colpocleisis as an effective treatment option for advanced apical prolapse in elderly women. *Taiwan J Obstet Gynecol* 2019;58(2):206–211.

99. Mueller MG, Ellimootil C, Abernethy MG, et al. Colpocleisis: A safe, minimally invasive option for pelvic organ prolapse. *Female Pelvic Med Reconstr Surg* 2015;21(1):30–33.

100. Catanzarite T, Rambachan A, Mueller MG, et al. Risk factors for 30-day perioperative complications after Le Fort colpocleisis. *J Urol* 2014;192(3):788–792.

101. Lu M, Zeng W, Ju R, et al. Long-term clinical outcomes, recurrence, satisfaction, and regret after total colpocleisis with concomitant vaginal hysterectomy: A retrospective single-center study. *Female Pelvic Med Reconstr Surg* 2021;27(4):e510–e515.

102. Bochenska K, Leader-Cramer A, Mueller M, et al. Perioperative complications following colpocleisis with and without concomitant vaginal hysterectomy. *Int Urogynecol J* 2017;28(11):1671–1675.

CHAPTER 43

ANTERIOR WALL SUPPORT DEFECTS

Joseph B. Pincus • Peter K. Sand

Introduction

The International Urogynecological Association and International Continence Society defined anterior vaginal wall (compartment) prolapse as the "observation of descent of the anterior vaginal wall (compartment)."[1] Most commonly, this might represent bladder prolapse (cystocele). Higher stage anterior vaginal wall prolapse will generally involve descent of the uterus or vaginal vault (if the uterus is absent). Occasionally, there might be an anterior enterocele (hernia of peritoneum and possibly abdominal contents), most commonly after prior reconstructive surgery.

This definition serves as a starting place for understanding anterior vaginal wall support and the defects in that support that can lead to prolapse. After reviewing the anatomy and histology of the anterior compartment, we review the epidemiology, workup, and treatment of anterior vaginal compartment support defects.

ANATOMY

The vaginal canal has been described by DeLancey[2] as having three levels of support. Level 1 supports of the upper 2 to 3 cm of the vagina are composed of the cardinal–uterosacral ligament complex. At level 2, the vaginal canal is attached laterally to the arcus tendineus fascia pelvis (ATFP). The endopelvic connective tissue often called "pubocervical fascia" stretches from one ATFP laterally to the other. Finally, level 3 supports include the attachments of the vagina to the pelvic floor, levator ani, and urethra in the distal 2 to 3 cm of the vagina.

A defect in the midline of the endopelvic connective tissue may lead to a midline cystocele. This central defect had been previously described by Richardson et al.[3] Alternatively, a disruption in the endopelvic connective tissue laterally at the point of attachment to the ATFP may lead to paravaginal support defects. Richardson popularized this terminology in 1981,[4] but it was first described by White[5] in 1912. This prolapse in the anterior compartment was reported to be related to descent of the lateral attachments of the anterior vaginal wall to the ATFP.[6] Larson et al.[7] described this paravaginal support defect using dynamic magnetic resonance imaging (MRI) and showed that women who had anterior compartment prolapse also had descent of the paravaginal tissues.

Anterior compartment prolapse is also highly associated with apical prolapse.[8] Hsu et al.[9] were able to explain up to 77% of anterior wall prolapse by relating it to the apical descent of the vagina. This relationship is important in considering treatment, as anterior compartment surgical procedures are often paired with apical procedures with improved outcomes. In 2020, Moalli et al.[10] laid out a study to evaluate the mechanism of anterior vaginal compartment prolapse based on MRI after surgical repair. These results are eagerly anticipated and will serve to further the understanding of the pathophysiology of descent of the anterior vaginal wall.[10]

Histologically, the vaginal canal is a hollow fibromuscular organ (Fig. 43.1). The walls of the vagina have four layers: a nonkeratinized squamous epithelium, a dense connective tissue layer of the lamina propria, the smooth muscle layer of the muscularis, and the loose connective tissue of the adventitia.[11] There is no fascia in the vaginal wall. The epithelial layer overlies the lamina propria, neither of which contain glandular elements. This is why it is a misnomer to describe the vaginal epithelium as a mucosa. Within the muscularis layer is a network of blood vessels. The vaginal lubrication is not exudative in nature; rather, it is a transudate from these vessels together with secretions from the cervix and other glands at the introitus, such as the Bartholin and Skene glands. Finally, the adventitial layer is shared with the bladder adventitia, essentially forming the endopelvic connective tissue often called the "pubocervical fascia" or "endopelvic fascia."

EPIDEMIOLOGY

Because anterior vaginal wall prolapse symptoms overlap with the symptoms of other types of pelvic organ prolapse, patient survey is not a reliable way to assess prevalence. As such, prevalence must be estimated using studies that rely on physical examination. When evaluating the literature, anterior vaginal wall support defects are the most common location for pelvic organ prolapse to occur.[12]

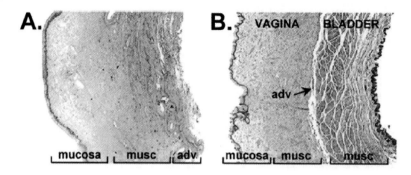

FIGURE 43.1 Anatomic/histologic layers of vagina and bladder. Both (**A**) and (**B**) are full-thickness, cross-sectional anterior vaginal wall specimens. (**A**) taken at hysterectomy, (**B**) cadaveric and containing bladder wall. Both show vagina contains squamous epithelium, muscularis (musc), and adventitia (adv). Deep to this is only bladder muscularis and bladder mucosa. No fascia is seen. (Reprinted from Boreham MK, Wai CY, Miller RT, et al. Morphometric analysis of smooth muscle in the anterior vaginal wall of women with pelvic organ prolapse. *Am J Obstet Gynecol* 2002;187[1]:56–63, Fig. 2. Copyright © 2002, with permission from Elsevier.)

Handa et al.[12] studied a cohort that had a baseline cystocele prevalence of 24.6%. They found that anterior vaginal wall prolapse was associated with increasing parity (odds ratio of 1.3 per pregnancy) and increasing waist circumference.[12] Hendrix et al.[13] corroborated these findings with an incidence of anterior compartment prolapse of 34.3% in the Women's Health Initiative trial. Although Hendrix et al.[13] found similar risk factors to Handa et al.'s[12] study, this study also identified the body mass index as a significant risk factor.

Other risk factors for pelvic organ prolapse have not been studied independently for anterior vaginal prolapse. These include Latina or white race, chronically elevated intra-abdominal pressures, connective tissue disease, and family history.[14–17] The role of genetics in pelvic organ prolapse remains unclear.[18,19]

PRESENTATION AND EVALUATION

A thorough history and physical examination is critical to evaluate a patient with anterior compartment prolapse. Symptoms of anterior vaginal wall prolapse are often nonspecific and include vaginal pressure, sensation of a bulge, vaginal fullness, low back pain, difficulty sitting, spotting, and dyspareunia.[20] Although nonspecific for anterior compartment prolapse, vaginal bulge symptoms are highly predictive of vaginal prolapse.

Anterior vaginal wall prolapse is often accompanied by urinary symptoms. Women may experience difficulty voiding due to a kinking of the urethra with advanced prolapse. The reduction of the prolapse may unmask "occult" stress urinary incontinence.[21] Inquiry about urgency, frequency, nocturia, postmicturition dribbling, insensible loss, and nocturnal enuresis may prove helpful. Women with prolapse should be questioned about sexual function because pelvic organ prolapse is highly associated with sexual dysfunction.[22]

The medical history should include a review of the patient's prior surgical procedures. Knowledge of prior surgical procedures, including if there is mesh in the

pelvis, is critical to accurately counsel the patient on the best treatment options.

As with all pelvic organ prolapse, treatment is contingent on patient satisfaction outcomes.[23] As such, a detailed discussion of the goals of care should be discussed at the initial patient encounter. This discussion may be paired with validated standardized questionnaires, which are calibrated to reflect small changes in symptoms. Although not specific to anterior compartment defects, the Pelvic Floor Distress Inventory (PFDI) and the shortened version, PFDI-20, are often used to assess prolapse symptoms.

The physical examination for evaluation of the anterior compartment is comparable to the examination of patients with all types of pelvic organ prolapse. The examination begins with inspection, followed by a speculum examination, and a bimanual examination. When evaluating the anterior compartment only, a rectovaginal examination is not helpful. The inspection phase of the exam is a careful observation of the vulva, labia, perineum, and perianal skin. The patient should be relaxed at first, followed by maximum Valsalva. The posterior blade of a bivalve speculum or a Sims speculum may be used to isolate the various compartments of the vagina. To evaluate the anterior wall and its supports, the posterior blade of the speculum should be placed posteriorly and the patient should be asked to Valsalva and/or cough strongly. The Baden-Walker or Pelvic Organ Prolapse Quantification system may be used to quantify the points of maximum descent (see Chapter 9). A scored popsicle stick, tongue depressor, ring forceps, or landmarks on the examiner's finger may be used to measure points in relation to the hymen. This should be performed during maximum Valsalva. Finally, the bimanual exam is performed to assess the tone, tenderness and strength of the pelvic floor musculature, the adnexa, the uterus, the bladder, and the urethra. The exam may be repeated with the patient standing to evaluate the prolapse on a different axis with the assistance of gravity to help reveal the full extent of the prolapse. This will often reveal greater degrees of prolapse compared to examination in the supine position.

The role of imaging in the evaluation of pelvic organ prolapse remains unclear in routine clinical care. Pelvic floor ultrasonography gives further texture to the diagnosis by evaluating the levator defects in pelvic floor support. Ultrasonography may also diagnose anterior compartment defects with a high correlation to the physical examination.[24] However, these added parameters, including the measurement of the levator hiatus, have yet to be proven clinically useful and at this time, routine ultrasound to image anterior compartment prolapse is not indicated.[25] MRI may also be used to evaluate pelvic organ prolapse, with a detailed view of support defects and the pelvic floor musculature.[26] However, routine dynamic MRI use is not indicated at this time and this modality should be reserved for research or complex patients. Ultrasonography and MRI may be useful in women who have recurrent anterior compartment prolapse after failed surgical reconstruction.

Adjunct testing may be necessary depending on the symptoms at the time of presentation. For example, if a patient presents with symptoms of incomplete emptying, a postvoid residual, uroflowmetry, or even multichannel urodynamics with support of the prolapse may be indicated. If pain or pressure is associated, cystoscopy may be useful as well. Sometimes, cystourethroscopy may help to clarify if the prolapsing viscus is the bladder and/or an anterior enterocele.

OUTCOMES

Anterior vaginal wall prolapse has been historically challenging to treat surgically.[27] When considering pelvic floor diseases, one must look through three lenses to evaluate success (or failure). Firstly, anatomic success may be measured by physical exam, but this does not always correlate with patient symptoms. Anatomic and symptomatic outcomes are often aligned but may be divergent. Symptomatic or patient-defined success is more important than anatomic success. An interdisciplinary American working group highlighted the importance of this truism.[28] Their review explained that pelvic floor disorders are uniquely positioned to benefit from an assessment of patient-reported outcomes. As such, when evaluating surgeries for the repair of anterior vaginal wall compartment defects, it is critical to use patient-reported outcomes as part of the overall evaluation of outcomes.

Finally, the outcome of "reoperation rates" provides another window into treatment success. Using this metric serves as a measure of patients who are symptomatic enough from their recurrent prolapse to seek further surgical intervention. However, this measure may be significantly influenced by cultural bias, age, income, and surgeon influence.

NATIVE TISSUE ANTERIOR COLPORRHAPHY

The anterior colporrhaphy is the most standard repair of an anterior vaginal wall defect. Chapter 44 contains a detailed surgical review of the procedure and its techniques. This chapter focuses on the outcomes.

Outcomes of isolated anterior repairs are difficult to report on, as so frequently they are paired with apical support procedures. As mentioned earlier, apical prolapse and anterior vaginal wall prolapse can be intimately linked and, thus, their surgical outcomes can be related.

Historically, the published success rates of native tissue anterior colporrhaphies in cohort studies ranged from 80% to 100%.[29] However, in the first and second prospective randomized controlled trials from Sand et al.[30] and Weber et al.,[31] they cited success rates of 52% and 30%, respectively, for the native tissue arms, which demonstrated that success rates were not as high as historical reports. Guerette et al.[32] reported a 78.4% success in the native tissue arm of their study.

NATIVE TISSUE PARAVAGINAL DEFECT REPAIR

Paravaginal defect repairs may be performed either independently or together with an anterior colporrhaphy. The purpose of this procedure is to reattach the pubocervical "fascia" to the arcus tendinous fascia pelvis to resupport the lateral vagina. This procedure may be performed using an open or laparoscopic approach to access the retropubic space or transvaginally to access

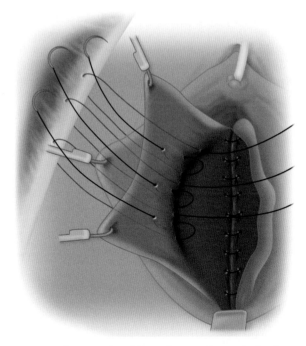

FIGURE 43.2 Sutures placed from the superior vaginal sulcus to the lateral pelvic wall at the level of the iliopectineal ligament.

the ATFP. The surgical techniques are described thoroughly in Chapter 44. As explained in Chapter 2, the ATFP goes from the ischial spine to the pubic tubercle. By attaching the vagina to this support, the anterior vaginal wall is tethered bilaterally to recreate normal lateral vaginal support as seen in Figure 43.2.

The outcomes of native tissue paravaginal defect repairs are difficult to assess. There are no randomized trials that have evaluated the success of paravaginal defect repairs in isolation. However, Shippey et al.[33] retrospectively assessed the addition of a paravaginal repair at the time of a sacrocolpopexy. The group noted a trend toward improved outcomes at 1 year, although the difference did not reach statistical significance.[33] Due to the improved success of apical support procedures in combination with midline anterior colporrhaphy, the native tissue paravaginal defect repair has become less popular. Additionally, there is no evidence that it is a critical part of prolapse repair surgery when good apical support is present.

BIOLOGIC GRAFT AND MESH TECHNIQUES AND OUTCOMES

Due to the historical native tissue failures of anterior vaginal wall defect repairs, surgical innovation has been focused on improving outcomes in the anterior compartment. This led to the integration of mesh and biologic grafts to augment traditional native tissue anterior colporrhaphies (and potentially apical suspensions).

Due to variations in design, application, and materials in these products, one cannot form wide sweeping conclusions about these techniques. Rather, one must individually appraise each individual product and technique. Generally, these adjuvant grafts are intended to strengthen the endopelvic connective tissue lying underneath the vaginal epithelium.

Synthetic mesh may serve as a scaffold for the ingrowth of a patient's own connective tissue. The science of understanding mesh properties has evolved significantly since the first products were available. Pore size and porosity are noted to be the most important properties. Increased pore size and higher porosity both allow for increased tissue ingrowth and a reduced inflammatory response.[34] Additionally, lower stiffness mesh protects against "stress shielding," a response when the tissues surrounding a stiff prosthetic weaken when they undergo remodeling and atrophy.

In 2019, the U.S. Food and Drug Administration ordered medical device companies to cease selling nonabsorbable synthetic vaginal mesh kits in the United States.[35] Since then, the use of nonabsorbable synthetic mesh as an augmentation device, even outside of "kits," has fallen out of practice in the United States.[36] Although ongoing National Institutes of Health–funded trials with evidence to suggest that a mesh-augmented sacrospinous hysteropexy is equivalent to a native tissue uterosacral suspension, mesh kits remain off the market at this time in the United States and throughout most of the world.[37]

Additionally, there are absorbable mesh products that can be used to augment anterior compartment surgery. Sand et al.[30] described the use of polyglactin 912 (Vicryl) (Ethicon, NJ, United States) mesh underneath the anterior colporrhaphy mattress sutures to augment the anterior vaginal wall repair (Fig. 43.3). In their randomized controlled trial, the addition of Vicryl mesh to the anterior colporrhaphy was protective against the recurrence of anterior vaginal wall defects at 1 year, with the failure rate of 25% in the mesh group versus 43% in the control group ($P = .02$).[30] Despite this study, due to the popularity of polypropylene mesh at the time, this technique did not gain widespread popularity.

Biologic grafts may act as regenerative grafts or as scaffolds to allow for scar tissue formation. There are both xenograft (from another species) and allografts (from another human) that have been studied for this purpose. The biografts serve as a scaffolding for the ingrowth of host tissue. Both xenografts and allografts are acellular. Human dermal grafts are often impregnated with growth factors and antibiotics to encourage incorporation into the patient's tissue.

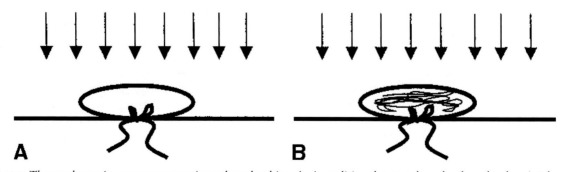

FIGURE 43.3 These schematics represent anterior colporrhaphies. **A:** A traditional suture-based colporrhaphy. A "dead space" is left between the layers of the repair. **B:** An anterior colporrhaphy with insertion of polyglactin 910 mesh. The "dead space" has been filled by mesh. (Reprinted from Sand PK, Koduri S, Lobel RW, et al. Prospective randomized trial of polyglactin 910 mesh to prevent recurrence of cystoceles and rectoceles. *Am J Obstet Gynecol* 2001;184[7]:1357–1364. Copyright © 2001, with permission from Elsevier.)

Early studies with biologic grafts did not support their routine use in prolapse repair surgery. Several of these early studies focused on xenografts, specifically on hexamethylene diisocyanate (HMDI)-cross-linked, porcine collagen matrix (Pelvicol). Dahlgren et al.,[38] reporting outcomes for the European Pelvicol Study Group, presented a negative study with no benefits over native tissue repairs seen at 3 years in 132 patients. Hviid et al.[39] saw no difference between Pelvicol use and native tissue anterior repair at 1 year in 31 patients. An earlier randomized controlled trial with 206 patients in 2007 from Meschia et al.[40] demonstrated a benefit to using Pelvicol to augment anterior vaginal wall prolapse repairs. These conflicting data were possibly related to differing techniques between the surgeons; the surgeons in the negative studies did not perform a traditional anterior colporrhaphy prior to placing the Pelvicol. However, in the positive study, the surgeons performed an anterior repair prior to placement of the biograft. We have shown that HMDI-cross-linked porcine dermis releases HMDI in the surrounding host tissues eliciting a severe inflammatory response with early resorption of the graft.[41] Due to the marginal success and the controversial findings, porcine biografts are not commonly used in pelvic organ prolapse surgery. Small intestine submucosa (SIS) grafts has also been investigated as a potential material to serve to bolster repair strength. Feldner et al.[42] ran a small randomized trial which demonstrated a significant difference in anatomic outcome with the use of SIS (86% success) versus traditional colporrhaphy (59% success). There was no difference in quality-of-life outcomes.

In 2019, Iyer et al.[43] published a small prospective randomized controlled trial comparing the use of human dermal allograft–augmented anterior repair versus native tissue anterior colporrhaphy. The study found no difference in failure rates, both at 1-year and at 7- to 10-year long-term follow-up. In a retrospective cohort, Botros et al.[44] found a significant benefit to human dermal allograft. In their study, there was a 19% anatomic failure rate in the dermal graft group compared to 43% in the control group.[44] As such, further information is still needed on the benefits of dermal allograft usage in augmentation of anterior colporrhaphies (Fig. 43.4).

The Cochrane Library published a definitive systematic review in 2016, examining various surgeries for anterior compartment prolapse.[45] Thirty-three trials were assessed with a total of 3,332 patients. The authors compared native tissue repairs to biologic grafts, nonabsorbable mesh, and absorbable mesh. They concluded that biologic graft repair and absorbable mesh provided minimal benefit as compared to native tissue repair. When they compared native tissue repairs to polypropylene mesh-augmented repairs, they concluded that native tissue repairs had lower anatomic success rates with a higher rate of surgery for recurrence (risk ratio [RR] 3.01, 95% confidence interval [CI] 2.52 to 3.60). However, polypropylene mesh was associated

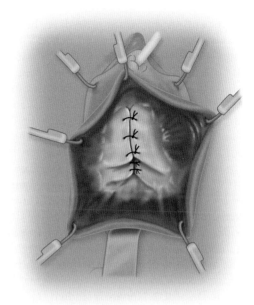

FIGURE 43.4 Anterior colporrhaphy with dermal graft augmentation.

with an increased risk of de novo stress urinary incontinence (RR 0.67, 95% CI 0.44 to 1.01), an increased risk of bladder injury (RR 0.21, 95% CI 0.06 to 0.82), and an increased risk for further surgery if mesh exposure is included in the composite outcome (RR 0.59, 95% CI 0.41 to 0.83). The Cochrane review concluded "current evidence does not support the use of (nonabsorbable) mesh repair compared with native tissue repair for anterior compartment prolapse owing to increased morbidity."

IMPACT ON URINARY SYMPTOMS

Surgery to correct anterior vaginal compartment defects is known to impact urinary symptoms. In fact, early anti-incontinence procedures included elements of surgeries in the anterior compartment, such as the Kelly-Kennedy plication and paravaginal defect repair.[46]

Anterior compartment surgery may also affect detrusor overactivity. It is well known that prolapse of the anterior compartment is strongly associated with detrusor overactivity and overactive bladder symptoms.[21] Kim et al.[47] found that patients with pelvic organ prolapse and overactive bladder syndrome symptoms had a statistically significant improvement after surgery. Therefore, it is suggested that surgical repair of anterior compartment prolapse can have rehabilitative effects on urgency urinary incontinence and overactive bladder syndrome symptoms.

The impact on stress urinary incontinence of surgical repair of an anterior compartment defect has been well established. Firstly, patients with pelvic organ prolapse often have the same anatomic structural defects in the support of the urethra and sphincter.[48] Repair of prolapse, whether anterior or apical, without a concomitant anti-incontinence procedure, bears a risk of unmasking stress urinary incontinence.[49] The prevailing current theory is that the prolapsed state causes a type of "urethral kinking" that prevents clinical stress urinary incontinence. Relief of that obstruction can reveal "occult" stress urinary incontinence.[50] Wen et al.[51] demonstrated a reduction in "urethral kinking" following prolapse repair, which was theorized to be due to the repair of the anterior vaginal wall defect. For this reason, patients with advanced prolapse can have a progression of stress urinary incontinence symptoms, followed by a complete cessation of these symptoms as the kinked urethra prevents passage of urine.

Preoperative planning for anterior compartment surgery should include stress testing with vaginal support or urodynamic testing with vaginal support to evaluate for occult stress urinary incontinence. The Pelvic Floor Disorders Network studied this question via the Colpopexy and Urinary Reduction Efforts randomized surgical trial.[50] In this trial, the researchers sought to evaluate the efficacy of an anti-incontinence procedure (Burch) at the time of a prolapse surgery (sacrocolpopexy). Patients were randomized either to receive the anti-incontinence procedure or not to receive it when undergoing the prolapse repair. The study concluded that patients who underwent a concomitant anti-incontinence procedure experienced significantly lower rates of stress urinary incontinence with similar adverse events. Secondary reporting from this study demonstrated that women who demonstrated urodynamic stress incontinence on urodynamics evaluation with vaginal support were more likely to experience stress urinary incontinence post-operatively, regardless of whether they underwent a Burch procedure.[52] For these reasons, preoperative evaluation with support of the prolapse during stress testing or urodynamics is important for all women planning to undergo a prolapse repair surgery, regardless of current continence status.

COMPLICATIONS

The risks related to anterior compartment surgery are limited in nature. Intraoperative surgical risks include excessive bleeding or injury to the bladder, urethra, or ureters. Hemorrhage requiring blood transfusion is rare in urogynecologic surgeries.[53]

Intraoperative cystotomy and urethrotomy are real but uncommon complications in surgery in the anterior compartment. Anterior colporrhaphy is the most common surgery to have an unrecognized ureteral injury.[54] For these reasons, cystourethroscopy at the conclusion of the procedure is absolutely necessary.[55] Gustilo-Ashby et al.[56] demonstrated that cystourethroscopy is 94.4% sensitive and 99.5% specific for detecting an intraoperative bladder or urethral injury.

Use of mesh carries another set of postsurgical risks. Mesh may cause pain; dyspareunia; vaginal bleeding associated with mesh exposure in the vagina; and/or erosion into the bladder, urethra, or other adjacent organs. Mesh and mesh complications are discussed further in Chapters 51 and 53.

Urinary symptoms including voiding dysfunction, irritative voiding symptoms, and de novo stress urinary incontinence can all occur as a result of surgical intervention in the anterior vaginal compartment, as addressed in the earlier section.

Sexual function may also be impacted by surgical repair of the anterior compartment. Sexual function improves in the majority of cases, and dyspareunia related to pelvic organ prolapse is reduced after anterior compartment surgery.[57] However, in an individual patient, prolapse repair surgery might cause narrowing of the vagina and dyspareunia if excessive scar tissue forms or if overcorrection or excessive excision of redundant vaginal epithelium occurs. These symptoms are more often associated with posterior colporrhaphies and perineorrhaphies, but the surgeon must be cautious not to overly narrow the introitus or cause scar tissue bands that will lead to de novo dyspareunia.

References

1. Haylen BT, de Ridder D, Freeman RM, et al. An International Urogynecological Association (IUGA)/International Continence Society (ICS) joint report on the terminology for female pelvic floor dysfunction. *Int Urogynecol J* 2010;21(1):5–26.
2. DeLancey JO. Anatomic aspects of vaginal eversion after hysterectomy. *Am J Obstet Gynecol* 1992;166(6 Pt 1):1717–1728.
3. Richardson AC, Lyon JB, Williams NL. A new look at pelvic relaxation. *Am J Obstet Gynecol* 1976;126(5):568–573.
4. Richardson AC, Edmonds PB, Williams NL. Treatment of stress urinary incontinence due to paravaginal fascial defect. *Obstet Gynecol* 1981;57(3):357–362.
5. White GR. An anatomical operation for the cure of cystocele. *Am J Obstet Dis Women Child* 1912;65(2):286.
6. Arenholt LTS, Pedersen BG, Glavind K, et al. Paravaginal defect: Anatomy, clinical findings, and imaging. *Int Urogynecol J* 2017;28(5):661–673.
7. Larson KA, Luo J, Guire KE, et al. 3D analysis of cystoceles using magnetic resonance imaging assessing midline, paravaginal, and apical defects. *Int Urogynecol J* 2012;23(3):285–293.
8. Rooney K, Kenton K, Mueller ER, et al. Advanced anterior vaginal wall prolapse is highly correlated with apical prolapse. *Am J Obstet Gynecol* 2006;195(6):1837–1840.
9. Hsu Y, Chen L, Summers A, et al. Anterior vaginal wall length and degree of anterior compartment prolapse seen on dynamic MRI. *Int Urogynecol J Pelvic Floor Dysfunct* 2008;19(1):137–142.
10. Moalli PA, Bowen ST, Abramowitch SD, et al. Methods for the Defining Mechanisms of Anterior Vaginal Wall Descent (DEMAND) study. *Int Urogynecol J* 2021;32(4):809–818.
11. De Landsheere L, Munaut C, Nusgens B, et al. Histology of the vaginal wall in women with pelvic organ prolapse: A literature review. *Int Urogynecol J* 2013;24(12):2011–2020.
12. Handa VL, Garrett E, Hendrix S, et al. Progression and remission of pelvic organ prolapse: A longitudinal study of menopausal women. *Am J Obstet Gynecol* 2004;190(1):27–32.

13. Hendrix SL, Clark A, Nygaard I, et al. Pelvic organ prolapse in the Women's Health Initiative: Gravity and gravidity. *Am J Obstet Gynecol* 2002;186(6):1160–1166.

14. Whitcomb EL, Rortveit G, Brown JS, et al. Racial differences in pelvic organ prolapse. *Obstet Gynecol* 2009;114(6):1271–1277.

15. Spence-Jones C, Kamm MA, Henry MM, et al. Bowel dysfunction: A pathogenic factor in uterovaginal prolapse and urinary stress incontinence. *Br J Obstet Gynaecol* 1994;101(2):147–152.

16. Carley ME, Schaffer J. Urinary incontinence and pelvic organ prolapse in women with Marfan or Ehlers Danlos syndrome. *Am J Obstet Gynecol* 2000;182(5):1021–1023.

17. Lince SL, van Kempen LC, Vierhout ME, et al. A systematic review of clinical studies on hereditary factors in pelvic organ prolapse. *Int Urogynecol J*. 2012;23(10):1327–1336.

18. Ward RM, Velez Edwards DR, Edwards T, et al. Genetic epidemiology of pelvic organ prolapse: A systematic review. *Am J Obstet Gynecol* 2014;211(4):326–335.

19. Li L, Sun Z, Chen J, et al. Genetic polymorphisms in collagen-related genes are associated with pelvic organ prolapse. *Menopause* 2020;27(2):223–229.

20. Ellerkmann RM, Cundiff GW, Melick CF, et al. Correlation of symptoms with location and severity of pelvic organ prolapse. *Am J Obstet Gynecol* 2001;185(6):1332–1338.

21. Romanzi LJ, Chaikin DC, Blaivas JG. The effect of genital prolapse on voiding. *J Urol* 1999;161(2):581–586.

22. Zielinski R, Miller J, Low LK, et al. The relationship between pelvic organ prolapse, genital body image, and sexual health. *Neurourol Urodyn* 2012;31(7):1145–1148.

23. Mahajan ST, Elkadry EA, Kenton KS, et al. Patient-centered surgical outcomes: The impact of goal achievement and urge incontinence on patient satisfaction one year after surgery. *Am J Obstet Gynecol* 2006;194(3):722–728.

24. Majida M, Braekken I, Bø K, et al. Anterior but not posterior compartment prolapse is associated with levator hiatus area: A three- and four-dimensional transperineal ultrasound study. *BJOG* 2011;118(3):329–337.

25. Gao Y, Zhao Z, Yang Y, et al. Diagnostic value of pelvic floor ultrasonography for diagnosis of pelvic organ prolapse: A systematic review. *Int Urogynecol J* 2020;31(1):15–33.

26. Berger MB, Kolenic GE, Fenner DE, et al. Structural, functional, and symptomatic differences between women with rectocele versus cystocele and normal support. *Am J Obstet Gynecol*. 2018;218(5):510.e1–510.e8.

27. Houman J, Weinberger JM, Eilber KS. Native tissue repairs for pelvic organ prolapse. *Curr Urol Rep* 2017;18(1):6.

28. Bordeianou LG, Anger JT, Boutros M, et al. Measuring pelvic floor disorder symptoms using patient-reported instruments: Proceedings of the consensus meeting of the Pelvic Floor Consortium of the American Society of Colon and Rectal Surgeons, the International Continence Society, the American Urogynecologic Society, and the Society of Urodynamics, Female Pelvic Medicine and Urogenital Reconstruction. *Female Pelvic Med Reconstr Surg* 2020;26(1):1–15.

29. Maher C. Anterior vaginal compartment surgery. *Int Urogynecol J* 2013;24(11):1791–1802.

30. Sand PK, Koduri S, Lobel RW, et al. Prospective randomized trial of polyglactin 910 mesh to prevent recurrence of cystoceles and rectoceles. *Am J Obstet Gynecol* 2001;184(7):1357–1364.

31. Weber AM, Walters MD, Piedmonte MR, et al. Anterior colporrhaphy: A randomized trial of three surgical techniques. *Am J Obstet Gynecol* 2001;185(6):1299–1306.

32. Guerette NL, Peterson TV, Aguirre OA, et al. Anterior repair with or without collagen matrix reinforcement: A randomized controlled trial. *Obstet Gynecol* 2009;114(1):59–65.

33. Shippey SH, Quiroz LH, Sanses TVD, et al. Anatomic outcomes of abdominal sacrocolpopexy with or without paravaginal repair. *Int Urogynecol J* 2010;21(3):279–283.

34. Liang R, Knight K, Abramowitch S, et al. Exploring the basic science of prolapse meshes. *Curr Opin Obstet Gynecol* 2016;28(5):413–419.

35. U.S. Food and Drug Administration. Urogynecologic surgical mesh implants. Published October 14, 2020. Accessed November 6, 2020. https://www.fda.gov/medical-devices/implants-and-prosthetics/urogynecologic-surgical-mesh-implants

36. Hudson PL, DeAndrade SP, Weinstein MM. It's not that mesh, is it? What providers should know about the transvaginal mesh controversy. *Menopause* 2020;27(11):1330–1335.

37. Nager CW, Visco AG, Richter HE, et al. Effect of vaginal mesh hysteropexy vs vaginal hysterectomy with uterosacral ligament suspension on treatment failure in women with uterovaginal prolapse: A randomized clinical trial. *JAMA* 2019;322(11):1054–1065.

38. Dahlgren E, Kjølhede P, RPOP-PELVICOL Study Group. Long-term outcome of porcine skin graft in surgical treatment of recurrent pelvic organ prolapse. An open randomized controlled multicenter study. *Acta Obstet Gynecol Scand* 2011;90(12):1393–1401.

39. Hviid U, Hviid TVF, Rudnicki M. Porcine skin collagen implants for anterior vaginal wall prolapse: A randomised prospective controlled study. *Int Urogynecol J* 2010;21(5):529–534.

40. Meschia M, Pifarotti P, Bernasconi F, et al. Porcine skin collagen implants to prevent anterior vaginal wall prolapse recurrence: A multicenter, randomized study. *J Urol* 2007;177(1):192–195.

41. Gandhi S, Kubba LM, Abramov Y, et al. Histopathologic changes of porcine dermis xenografts for transvaginal suburethral slings. *Am J Obstet Gynecol* 2005;192(5):1643–1648.

42. Feldner PC Jr, Castro RA, Cipolotti LA, et al. Anterior vaginal wall prolapse: A randomized controlled trial of SIS graft versus traditional colporrhaphy. *Int Urogynecol J* 2010;21(9):1057–1063.

43. Iyer S, Seitz M, Tran A, et al. Anterior colporrhaphy with and without dermal allograft: A randomized control trial with long-term follow-up. *Female Pelvic Med Reconstr Surg* 2019;25(3):206–212.

44. Botros SM, Sand PK, Beaumont JL, et al. Arcus-anchored acellular dermal graft compared to anterior colporrhaphy for stage II cystoceles and beyond. *Int Urogynecol J Pelvic Floor Dysfunct* 2009;20(10):1265–1271.

45. Maher C, Feiner B, Baessler K, et al. Surgery for women with anterior compartment prolapse. *Cochrane Database Syst Rev* 2016;11(11):CD004014.

46. Shull BL, Baden WF. A six-year experience with paravaginal defect repair for stress urinary incontinence. *Am J Obstet Gynecol* 1989;160(6):1432–1440.

47. Kim MS, Lee GH, Na ED, et al. The association of pelvic organ prolapse severity and improvement in overactive bladder symptoms after surgery for pelvic organ prolapse. *Obstet Gynecol Sci* 2016;59(3):214–219.

48. Rosenzweig BA, Pushkin S, Blumenfeld D, et al. Prevalence of abnormal urodynamic test results in continent women with severe genitourinary prolapse. *Obstet Gynecol* 1992;79(4):539–542.

49. Gallentine ML, Cespedes RD. Occult stress urinary incontinence and the effect of vaginal vault prolapse on abdominal leak point pressures. *Urology* 2001;57(1):40–44.

50. Brubaker L, Cundiff GW, Fine P, et al. Abdominal sacrocolpopexy with Burch colposuspension to reduce urinary stress incontinence. *N Engl J Med* 2006;354(15):1557–1566.

51. Wen L, Shek KL, Dietz HP. Changes in urethral mobility and configuration after prolapse repair. *Ultrasound Obstet Gynecol* 2019;53(1):124–128.

52. Visco AG, Brubaker L, Nygaard I, et al. The role of preoperative urodynamic testing in stress-continent women undergoing sacrocolpopexy: The Colpopexy and Urinary Reduction Efforts (CARE) randomized surgical trial. *Int Urogynecol J Pelvic Floor Dysfunct* 2008;19(5):607–614.

53. Bretschneider CE, Sheyn D, Mahajan S, et al. Complications following vaginal colpopexy for the repair of pelvic organ prolapse. *Int Urogynecol J* 2021;32(4):993–999.

54. Kwon CH, Goldberg RP, Koduri S, Sand PK. The use of intraoperative cystoscopy in major vaginal and urogynecologic surgeries. *Am J Obstet Gynecol* 2002;187(6):1466–1472.

55. Cohen SA, Carberry CL, Smilen SW. American Urogynecologic Society Consensus Statement: Cystoscopy at the time of prolapse repair. *Female Pelvic Med Reconstr Surg* 2018;24(4):258–259.

56. Gustilo-Ashby AM, Jelovsek JE, Barber MD, et al. The incidence of ureteral obstruction and the value of intraoperative cystoscopy during vaginal surgery for pelvic organ prolapse. *Am J Obstet Gynecol* 2006;194(5):1478–1485.

57. Jha S, Gray T. A systematic review and meta-analysis of the impact of native tissue repair for pelvic organ prolapse on sexual function. *Int Urogynecol J.* 2015;26(3):321–327.

CHAPTER 44

ANTERIOR AND POSTERIOR COLPORRHAPHY

Sarah E. Eckhardt • Tajnoos Yazdany

ANTERIOR WALL PROLAPSE AND REPAIR

Anatomy and Pathology

Anterior vaginal wall prolapse (AVP) is defined as the herniation of bladder through the anterior vagina wall. It is the most common site of pelvic organ prolapse and also has the highest rate of recurrence after surgical repair.[1,2]

The pathophysiology and etiology of anterior wall support defects is reviewed in detail in Chapters 41 and 43 and is only briefly reviewed here. Normal anterior vaginal wall anatomy is best understood by the three levels of support described by Delancey. All three levels are interconnected and crucial to maintaining normal pelvic anatomy. Level 1 includes the cardinal and uterosacral ligaments and supports the cervix and upper vagina, providing vaginal length. Level 2 includes the lateral vaginal attachments of the midvagina, including the arcus tendineus fasciae pelvis (ATFP) and the arcus tendineus fasciae rectovaginalis (ATFR). Both levels 1 and 2 serve to stabilize the proximal two-thirds of the vagina while maintaining the vaginal axis in a horizontal plane that rests on the levator plate. Level 3 is the perineum and includes the perineal body, perineal membrane, superficial and deep perineal muscles, and the surrounding connective tissue. Level 3 and the distal ATFR serve to create the vertical axis of the distal vagina. Interruption in support at levels 1 and 2 plays a large role in the development of AVP. Level 3 also contributes to anterior support but is much more important to the anatomy of the posterior compartment.

The layer of connective tissue between the vagina and bladder that is damaged and attenuated in anterior vaginal prolapse has historically been referred to as pubocervical or endocervical "fascia." However, anatomical and histologic studies have confirmed the tissue between bladder and vagina is not a true fascial layer but a layer of vaginal epithelium, muscularis, and adventitia overlying the bladder muscularis (Fig. 44.1).[3] Rather than using the term *fascia*, we instead refer to the fibromuscular layer of the vagina, composed of vaginal muscularis and adventitia, to more accurately describe the tissue overlying the bladder.

Injury can occur from distension and attenuation of the overlying fibromuscular layer or by lateral detachment from the ATFP, or level 2. Apical defects can occur from detachment at the level of the cervix, or level 1.

It is important to note the relationship between apical and anterior prolapse when considering anterior prolapse repair because it is estimated that approximately 50% of anterior wall support originates from the apex.[4] Furthermore, apical suspension will address AVP in up to 63% of cases.[5,6] Thus, the approach to AVP repair requires consideration of the origin of the defect. Apical suspension alone may be adequate for combined anterior and apical prolapse and may ultimately result in better long-term outcomes than anterior colporrhaphy or paravaginal repair alone.[6-10] However, if apical prolapse is not present or significant AVP is present after apical suspension, a midline plication-based repair with anterior colporrhaphy or repair of a paravaginal defect is necessary. This chapter focuses on technique for anterior colporrhaphy and paravaginal repair. Nonsurgical treatment of AVP is covered in Chapters 15 and 16.

History and Physical Evaluation

During physical exam, the surgeon may attempt to identify midline versus lateral defects in order to determine the optimal surgical approach. Absence of rugal folds may indicate a midline defect and distention, whereas presence of rugal folds and loss of the lateral sulcus may indicate a paravaginal defect. It is important to note, however, that data on the accuracy of these exams are limited, and exams appear to be poorly reproducible between providers.[11-13] Imaging with ultrasound or magnetic resonance imaging prior to anterior vaginal prolapse repair is not routinely recommended unless there is concern for abnormal pathology that requires further evaluation.

Anterior Colporrhaphy

The objective of anterior colporrhaphy is to plicate and reinforce the attenuated muscularis and adventitial layers overlying the bladder at the midline. This serves to reduce the vaginal defect and restore the bladder to its anterior position.

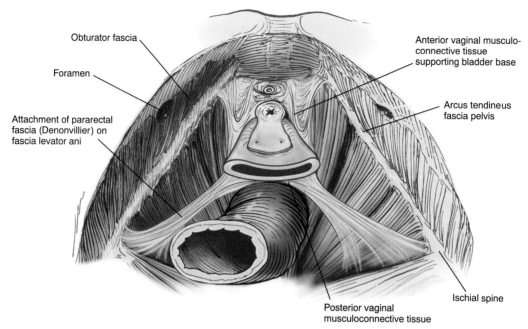

FIGURE 44.1 ATFP. ATFP extending from the posterior pubic symphysis to ischial spine, demarcated superiorly by the obturator fascia and inferiorly by the levator ani muscle. (Reprinted from Berek JS. *Berek & Novak's gynecology essentials.* Philadelphia: Wolters Kluwer, 2020.)

All patients undergoing colporrhaphy should have a catheter placed after surgical preparation is complete, typically with a 16 French Foley catheter. Patients should receive antibiotics within 60 minutes of the surgical incision. With the patient in dorsal lithotomy position, a weighted speculum is then placed in the vagina. Suture of 0-Silk or Nylon can be placed through the medial groin and labia majora to retract the labia and optimize visualization, taking care to not strangulate the tissue. A hook retractor (i.e., Lonestar) can be used for better exposure. Exam under anesthesia with the patient relaxed can help identify specific defects and confirm surgical approach.

Hydrodissection of the vaginal epithelium from the underlying muscularis layer is then performed with normal saline, plain analgesic, or a hemostatic agent. Plain anesthetic agents include 1% lidocaine and 0.25% bupivacaine and are often used in a combined solution of 1:200,000 epinephrine for hemostasis. Alternatively, vasopressin 10 units in 50 mL of normal saline can be used.

When anterior colporrhaphy is performed with an apical suspension, the anterior repair may be completed first. If a hysterectomy has been performed, two Allis clamps are placed at the anterior vaginal cuff with a third placed approximately 2 cm below the urethral meatus to mark the most distal edge of the planned dissection. If a midurethral sling is planned, the distal Allis clamp should be placed at the urethrovesical junction, or approximately 3 to 4 cm below the urethral meatus. Anterior colporrhaphy should be completed before the

midurethral sling, which is performed through a separate suburethral incision.

A midline vertical incision is made from the distal Allis clamp and carried until 1 cm distal to the vaginal cuff edge if hysterectomy has been performed or 1 cm distal to the vaginal apex if hysterectomy has not been performed. The incision is preferentially made with the 15-blade scalpel through full thickness of vaginal epithelium in order to expose the underlying vaginal muscularis layer. Alternatives include a 10-blade scalpel or Metzenbaum scissors. If using Metzenbaum scissors, dissection is carried from the vaginal apex toward the urethra. The scissor tips face away from the bladder and are placed between the vaginal epithelium and muscularis layer, gently pushing upward half-opened and half-closed. Countertraction with Allis clamps or Russian forceps along the midline can be used to help prevent cystotomy.

Allis clamps are then placed along the cut epithelial edges of the incision to facilitate traction for dissection. The vaginal epithelium is dissected off of the underlying vaginal muscularis, which serves to leave a layer of vaginal muscularis and adventitia over the bladder. This is typically performed with Metzenbaum scissors but can also be completed with a scalpel. Traction is facilitated by folding the vaginal epithelium over the surgeon's index finger of the nondominant hand where he or she is dissecting. Index finger placement also serves to communicate depth of dissection. An assistant can also hold traction of the vaginal muscularis and bladder with forceps to facilitate dissection. The technique is a combination of sharp dissection to identify the appropriate white, hypovascular plane, as well as gentle blunt dissection with an unfolded Ray-Tec sponge over the index finger to enlarge the plane of dissection. Dissection is carried out bilaterally as far as the medial aspect of the ischiopubic rami.

Hemostasis during dissection can be achieved with pressure, gentle cautery, and interrupted or figure-of-eight suture of 3-0 polyglactin on a small needle, such as an SH.

If the midline defect is very large, a purse-string or running suture can be placed first to facilitate reduction with delayed absorbable suture such as 2-0 polyglactin or polydioxanone suture (PDS).[14] Plication has been described with two different approaches by Goff and Bullard.[15] The technique described by Goff includes plication of the vaginal muscularis just medial to the vaginal flaps in a series of interrupted U-stitches of 0 or 2-0 polyglactin or PDS suture starting at the most distal portion of the dissection and moving toward the apex. Sutures are placed where the fibromuscular tissue is still connected to the vaginal epithelium.

For the Bullard approach, the surgeon can first repair site-specific defects if noted with interrupted 2-0 PDS. Midline plication of the vaginal muscularis and adventitia is then performed with interrupted or running 2-0 PDS and can be performed in multiple layers as needed for larger defects. This is distinct from the Goff approach in that plication sutures are not placed as far laterally at the junction of vaginal epithelium and muscularis layer.

During plication, it is important to remember the proximity of the ureter, particularly with large anterior defects.

After plication, excess epithelium may be trimmed, taking care to not remove too much because this will place undue tension on the epithelial closure and risk causing vaginal stenosis, narrowing, or wound breakdown in postoperative healing. Closure is performed with 2-0 polyglactin. If there is concern regarding vaginal length, interrupted sutures or running-locked sutures can help preserve length. Otherwise, running closure is appropriate. If there is additional concern for hemostasis prior to closure, a hemostatic agent such as thrombin hemostatic matrix (Floseal) or fibrin sealant (Tisseel) can be placed before closing epithelium, or vaginal packing can be placed after closure.

Cystoscopy should always be performed after anterior colporrhaphy to ensure there is no intravesical suture placement, vesical injury, ureteral kinking, or injury.

Paravaginal Repair

A significant proportion of anterior vaginal support arises from the attachment of the vaginal wall to the ATFP. The objective of paravaginal repair is to reattach lateral vaginal defects to the ATFP.

The paravaginal approach can be performed by open, vaginal, or a minimally invasive approach. This chapter reviews the vaginal and open technique. The minimally invasive technique is similar to open, but through laparoscopic ports rather than a Pfannenstiel incision.

Vaginal approach

When a paravaginal repair is performed in conjunction with an apical suspension, the paravaginal repair is completed first. Marking sutures can be placed at the urethrovesical junction and vaginal apex if concomitant hysterectomy has been performed.[16]

The techniques for hydrodissection, incision, and dissection are the same as for anterior colporrhaphy; however, the dissection is carried further laterally to the inferior and lateral edge of the ischiopubic rami. After reaching the bilateral ischiopubic rami, the surgeon's index finger palpates along the ischiopubic ramus until encountering the ischial spine, which marks the posterior boundary of the ATFP. Identifying the obturator internus and levator ani will delineate the superior and inferior border of the ATFP, respectively (see Fig. 44.1). Blunt dissection with the index finger is used to gently clear this space and better identify anatomy prior to entering the retroperitoneal space.

Retroperitoneal entry should be performed 1 to 2 cm anterior to the ischial spine, using perpendicular pressure on a closed curved Mayo scissors immediately inferior to the ischiopubic ramus. Entry can be confirmed by visualization of retroperitoneal fat, the pelvic side wall, and, occasionally, the neurovascular obturator bundle can be noted running along the superior edge of the obturator internus. After entry is confirmed, serially sized Breisky-Navratil retractors can be placed anteriorly and a lighted right-angle retractor can be placed medially to retract the bladder and optimize visualization.

Paravaginal repair requires a 3-point closure. The first suture is placed through the ATFP, the second through the vaginal muscularis, and the third through the vaginal epithelium and mucosa (Fig. 44.2). Ideally, the first suture is placed along the ATFP; however, it is often impossible to visualize if there is any previous injury. In this case, sutures can be placed at its approximate location in the obturator fascia at the junction of obturator internus and levator ani. A 0 nonabsorbable or delayed absorbable suture on a CT-1 needle is used with a long straight needle driver or the Capio device.[16,17] The angle of the needle should be perpendicular to the ATFP for adequate purchase of tissue. A total of 4 to 6 sutures are placed approximately 1 cm apart, starting 1 to 2 cm anterior to the ischial spine and carried up to the level of the urethrovesical junction (see Fig. 44.2A). Sutures can be tagged with a hemostat along the drape in order to prevent tangling and confusion.

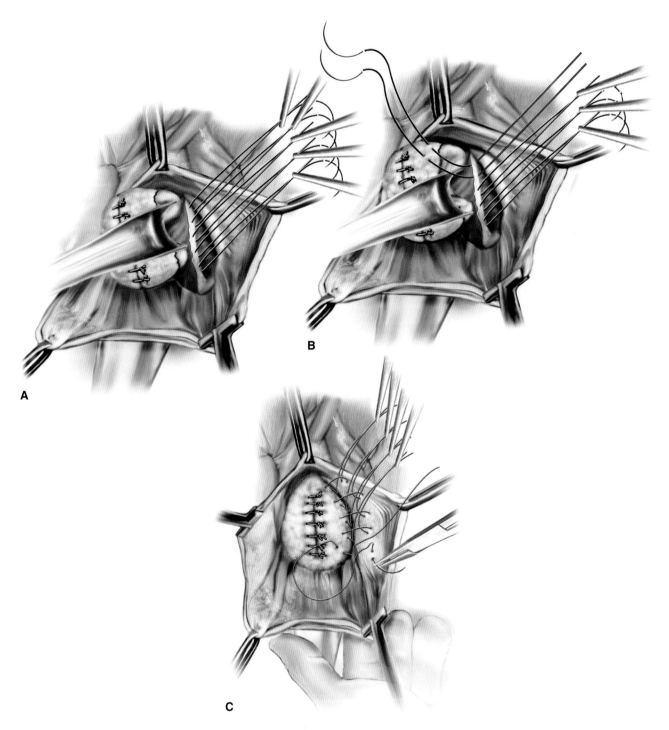

FIGURE 44.2 Paravaginal repair: three-step vaginal approach. **A:** Sutures placed along the ATFP *(white line)* between urethrovesical junction and pubic symphysis. **B:** Sutures placed in the vaginal muscularis approximately halfway between pubic ramus and bladder midline. **C:** Sutures are carried through vaginal mucosa and deep epithelial layer, avoiding superficial vaginal epithelium. (Reprinted from Handa VL, Van Le L. *Te Linde's operative gynecology*, 12th ed. Philadelphia: Wolters Kluwer, 2019.)

If midline anterior colporrhaphy is also indicated, this should be performed prior to placing the second set of paravaginal sutures along the vaginal muscularis. Sutures in the vaginal muscularis should be placed approximately halfway between the pubic ramus and bladder midline. Sutures placed too medially will place

undue tension on the repair and sutures too lateral will not adequately address the defect.[14] Suturing is started anteriorly at the level of the urethrovesical junction and carried posteriorly toward the ischial spine (see Fig. 44.2B). The previously placed marking sutures at the urethrovesical junction and vaginal apex serve as guidance for correct suture placement. Finally, in the third step, the sutures are carried through the previously dissected vaginal mucosa and deep epithelial layer, taking care to avoid the superficial vaginal epithelium (see Fig. 44.2C). This is then repeated on the contralateral side prior to tying sutures. Sutures are then tied proximal to distal, alternating sides with each suture and taking care to avoid suture bridges.

Excess vaginal epithelium is trimmed. Technique for closure of the epithelium is the same as for anterior colporrhaphy. Cystoscopy is always recommended after paravaginal repair.

Open approach

An open paravaginal repair is often done in conjunction with a Burch colposuspension or if a persistent defect is noted during sacral colpopexy. An open approach is described in this chapter, but a similar technique can be applied to the laparoscopic approach.

Abdominal incision is typically made through a small Pfannenstiel approach. A Foley catheter is placed prior to incision. If a Burch is planned, this is typically an 18 or a 20 French Foley catheter with a 30-mL balloon. If only performing a paravaginal repair with or without a concomitant Burch, there is no need to enter the peritoneal cavity. For patients with no previous surgeries, retroperitoneal dissection can be performed mostly in a blunt fashion, using the index finger to brush along the posterior pubic symphysis until reaching the ischial spine. If there is scarring from previous surgeries, sharp dissection should be used to open the retroperitoneal space. The borders of the retroperitoneal space are marked anteriorly by the pubic symphysis, medially by the bladder, laterally by the obturator internus, and posteriorly by the retropubic space of the vagina.[14]

The patient should be placed in the Trendelenburg position, and Breisky or Deaver retractors can deviate the bladder medially to optimize visualization. A vaginal hand can serve to elevate the vaginal vault and further delineate the anatomy and the defect. The ATFP should be observed at the junction of the obturator internus and pubococcygeus muscle of the levator ani, extending along the ischiopubic ramus from the posterior pubic symphysis to ischial spine; however, previous injury often precludes adequate visualization. The objective of the repair is to reattach the lateral vaginal sulcus to the fascia overlying the obturator internus and levator ani, incorporating the ATFP if visualized (Fig. 44.3). Suture is typically 0-nonabsorbable but delayed absorbable can be used. Suturing is started at 1 to 2 cm anterior to the ischial spine and placed 1 cm apart until reaching the urethrovesical junction. Sutures are tied posteriorly to anteriorly.

Cystoscopy is then performed before the procedure is terminated and the abdomen is closed.

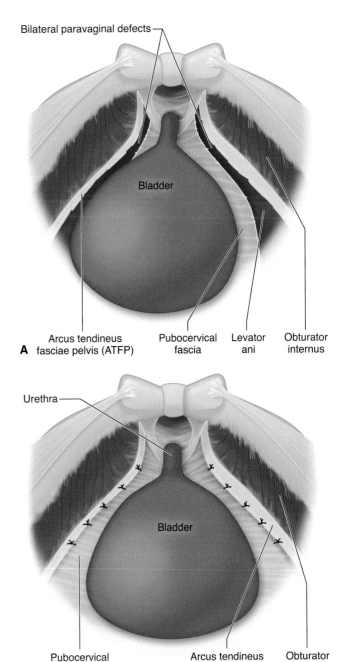

FIGURE 44.3 Open paravaginal repair. The detached paravaginal defect is reattached to the ATFP in a series of interrupted permanent or delayed absorbable suture.

Graft Augmentation

The objective of graft augmentation is to replace the weakened fibromuscular layer between vagina and bladder with a permanent implant to prevent future herniation. Alternatively, some grafts serve as a nonpermanent scaffold for fibroblast infiltration and scarring to reinforce the attenuated fibromuscular layer.[14] Implants can be allografts (human donor), autografts (self-donor), xenografts (animal donor), or synthetic.

In a large 2016 Cochrane review of 33 randomized controlled trials (RCTs) on anterior colporrhaphy using native tissue, biologic grafts, and synthetic grafts, anterior compartment repair with permanent mesh resulted in decreased rates of prolapse recurrence, awareness of prolapse, and reoperation.[3] However, permanent mesh was associated with higher rates of adverse events, including increased operating time, blood loss, transfusion, cystotomy, de novo stress incontinence, and de novo dyspareunia when compared to native tissue repair. Mesh exposure rate was 11.3% with a 7% reoperation rate for mesh removal. Furthermore, in 2019, the U.S. Food and Drug Administration[18] removed vaginal mesh from the market.

The same Cochrane review demonstrated that absorbable mesh and biologic grafts were not superior to native tissue repair in preventing recurrence of prolapse, and there were no advantages to employ these grafts over native tissue repair.

The authors conclude that grafts should not be considered as first-line management. Despite transvaginal mesh demonstrating improved anatomical outcomes, the disadvantages and adverse events appear to outweigh these benefits. If considering graft augmentation, the physician should have a detailed conversation of the risks and benefits with the patient before proceeding.

Given the findings of the Cochrane review as well as the removal of vaginal mesh from the market, we do not review surgical technique for graft augmentation in this chapter.

Postoperative Care

After surgery is complete, the decision to remove the indwelling catheter depends on the extent of surgery. For example, if only anterior colporrhaphy or vaginal paravaginal repair was performed, then the catheter can be removed in the operating room followed by an active or passive voiding trial in postoperative recovery prior to discharge. However, if the patient has also undergone an anti-incontinence procedure and/or hysterectomy with apical suspension and is being admitted, it is reasonable to leave the catheter in place for 6 to 24 hours depending on patient status and recovery. A postvoid residual greater than 100 to 200 mL is considered elevated. Depending on surgeon preference, the patient can be discharged home with a Foley catheter for several days or taught how to perform clean intermittent catheterization depending on preference. A voiding trial can be performed in the office several days postoperatively.

For anterior colporrhaphy alone with or without midurethral sling, hospital admission is typically unnecessary. If the patient has undergone more extensive surgery, such as hysterectomy and apical suspension, admission requirements vary across hospitals and providers; however, if meeting postoperative milestones, same-day discharge is reasonable.

Open approach to paravaginal repair often requires hospital admission for pain control due to the Pfannenstiel incision. Foley catheter is not indicated for paravaginal repair alone, but if the patient has had a Burch procedure or a more extensive surgery such as sacral colpopexy, the catheter is often left in place in postoperative recovery until the patient is able to undergo a passive or active voiding trial.

Complications

Serious complications following anterior colporrhaphy and vaginal paravaginal repair are rare. Abdominal paravaginal repairs via laparotomy have a higher rate of complication related specifically to the laparotomy, such as higher blood loss, more postoperative pain, longer postoperative recovery, and higher risk of incisional complications such as seroma and infection.

Blood loss during anterior colporrhaphy is typically low, and need for transfusion is rare. Paravaginal repairs may have higher blood loss due to the close proximity of dissection to the fragile venous plexus of Santorini in the retroperitoneal space, with one study reporting hemorrhage in 3% of patients.[19] Hematomas were not reported in the majority of studies reviewed but can occur in up to 4% of cases[19–22] and are typically self-limited in the vagina and vulva; however, retroperitoneal hematomas after paravaginal repair may be more serious and require intervention if expanding and the patient is hemodynamically unstable. Adequate hemostasis intraoperatively helps to prevent hematoma formation.

Cystotomy may occur during anterior colporrhaphy and paravaginal repair but is rare (0.5% to 2.3%).[21,23–25] In addition, there are case reports on vesicovaginal fistula formation after undiagnosed bladder injury at the time of anterior repair.

Ureteral injury is also uncommon, but ureteral kinking may occur after aggressive plications for large cystoceles. Cystoscopy should always be performed in order to confirm ureteral integrity. Ureteral injury was not reported in any of the trials reviewed on anterior colporrhaphy but was reported in two studies on paravaginal repair in 1.9% and 2.2% of patients.[21,22] If ureteral kinking is suspected, suture should be removed in an attempt to release the ureter. Ureteral stenting may be indicated for 4 to 6 weeks if there is concern for crush injury or interruption of ureteral blood supply.

Urinary tract infection (UTI) is among the most common complications after anterior colporrhaphy and paravaginal repair, occurring in as many as 13% to 18% of women.[26–28] Although it is recommended that women receive antibiotic prophylaxis intraoperatively, postoperative prophylaxis to prevent UTI is not indicated. Vaginal incisional infections and incisional dehiscence are rare, particularly if caution has been taken intraoperatively to not place excessive tension on the epithelial closure.

Postoperatively, voiding dysfunction and urinary retention is also relatively common, particularly if concomitant procedures have been performed such as midurethral sling. New voiding dysfunction may affect as many as 3% to 11% of patients.[24,29,30] Urinary retention is reported to occur in up to 11% of patients postoperatively, although in many of these trials, women underwent multiple additional prolapse procedures and urinary retention may not be attributable to anterior repair alone.[20,26,28,29,31,32]

De novo urinary incontinence is a known risk after anterior repair. It is important to note, however, that some patients report improvement in both stress urinary incontinence (SUI) and urge urinary incontinence (UUI) after AVP repair. A 2016 Cochrane review found that risk of de novo SUI was less after native tissue repair than mesh augmented repair and similar to repair with biologic graft.[3] De novo SUI rates occur in up to 9.4% of women postoperatively after native repair[17,27,30,31,33]; however, not all women pursue treatment for their SUI or require future surgical interventions. De novo urgency incontinence has been reported in as many as 14% of patients postoperatively.[33]

Like SUI and UUI, dyspareunia will often improve for patients postoperatively; however, there is a subset of women who will experience new dyspareunia. De novo dyspareunia has been reported in various studies and ranges between 5% and 20% of women.[20,23,26,28,31,33–35] Similarly, new chronic pelvic pain has been reported in 5% to 18% of patients postoperatively after native tissue repair but details on pain duration and severity was limited.[29,36,37] Thorough patient counseling preoperatively is important to set appropriate expectations with patients on the risks of voiding dysfunction, retention, incontinence, dyspareunia, and pain postoperatively.

Surgical Outcomes

The anterior vaginal wall is not only the most common site of prolapse, but it is also the most common site to recur after repair.[3] Surgical failure rates vary between 3% and 70% among clinical trials.[6] This may, in part, be due to a lack of standardized approach to anterior colporrhaphy and paravaginal repair. In a systematic review of 40 RCT, there was no single RCT that provided a detailed description of each step of the procedure, and the steps that were described were highly variable between studies.[38] A separate study by the Dutch Urogynecologic Society similarly found that even within a small group of FPMRS providers, operative technique varied greatly, possibly explaining some of the discrepant outcomes among studies.[39]

Interpretation of RCT outcomes is further confounded by the presence of multiple other concomitant prolapse procedures at the time of anterior repair such as apical suspension. Definitions of success also vary across studies and impact outcomes. The majority of RCTs define success as stage 1 pelvic organ prolapse or less using the Pelvic Organ Prolapse Quantification (POP-Q) system, but others define it as point Ba on POP-Q of −1 cm or less. Not surprisingly, trials that use the definition of Ba of −1 cm or less have better outcomes than those that use stage 1 or less (61% to 80% success vs. 30% to 80% success).[20,23,24,26–37,40–45] It is important to note that despite high failure rates in the majority of trials (Table 44.1), subjective outcome was often better than anatomical outcome, and most women did not elect for repeat surgery even if anatomical failure was noted. However, most trials did not follow patients past 12 months; thus, it is impossible to say if any of those women went on to undergo additional surgery in the future.

Data on paravaginal repairs is much more limited (Table 44.2). There is only one RCT directly comparing abdominal paravaginal repair to anterior colporrhaphy with permanent mesh. Success rates at 2 years were not different between paravaginal and anterior repair groups (60% vs. 68%, $P = .56$).[47] The remaining studies on paravaginal repair are observational and cohort studies and quote success rates of 69.5% to 97% for vaginal repair, 60% to 88.5% for abdominal repair, and 64% for laparoscopic (see Table 44.2).[17,19,21,22,46,48,49] Although the fairly high success rates of vaginal paravaginal repair are encouraging, high-quality RCTs are needed to truly evaluate success of paravaginal repair compared to anterior colporrhaphy. More data is also needed on abdominal and minimally invasive approaches.

The high rates of recurrence of anterior vaginal prolapse with anterior repair alone highlights the importance of concomitant apical suspension. As mentioned earlier in this chapter, approximately 50% of anterior wall support originates from the apex and apical suspension will address AVP in up to 63% of cases.[4,5] Women who undergo apical suspension in addition to anterior repair are less likely to experience recurrence than women who undergo treatment of AVP alone (11.6% vs. 20.2%).[50]

Conclusion

AVP typically occurs due to midline defects in the vaginal fibromuscular layer overlying the bladder or from lateral detachment of vaginal support from the ATFP secondary to trauma such as childbirth. Outcomes of native tissue repair of the anterior vaginal wall through anterior colporrhaphy or paravaginal repair alone demonstrates a wide range of success rates, and recurrence rates are relatively high. Apical suspension can help prevent anterior recurrence and is reviewed in Chapters 46 to 48. Complications after anterior colporrhaphy and paravaginal repair are rare, the most common of which are UTI, short-term urinary retention, de novo SUI and UUI, and de novo dyspareunia.

TABLE 44.1

Outcomes and Complications of Anterior Colporrhaphy Randomized Controlled Trials

AUTHOR	COMPARISON GROUP	PRIMARY OUTCOME	FOLLOW-UP (mo)	NATIVE TISSUE SUCCESS (%, N)	COMPARISON SUCCESS (%, N)	NATIVE TISSUE COMPLICATIONS
Altman et al.[24]	Mesh	Stage 1 prolapse or less	12	48 (87/183)	82 (153/186)	Bladder perforation 0.5% UTI 2.1% Voiding dysfunction 3.2% Urinary retention 1.1% Pelvic pain 0.5% Dehiscence 0.5%
Carey et al.[23]	Mesh	Stage 1 prolapse or less	12	66 (40/61)	81 (51/63)	De novo dyspareunia 15.2% Bladder perforation 1.45%
Delroy et al.[28]	Mesh	Stage 1 prolapse or less	12	56 (22/39)	83 (33/40)	Blood transfusion 5.1% UTI 13.8% Urinary retention 5.1% Dyspareunia 10.2%
de Tayrac et al.[20]	Mesh	Stage 1 prolapse or less	12	64 (43/67)	89 (59/66)	Reoperation 2.8% De novo dyspareunia 7.1% Vaginal hematoma 4.2% Urinary retention 11.1%
Feldner et al.[40]	Biologic graft	Stage 1 prolapse or less	12	59 (16/27)	86 (25/29)	UTI 7.4% Urinary retention 7.4% Dyspareunia 15%
Gandhi et al.[37]	Biologic graft	Stage 1 prolapse or less	12	71 (55/78)	79 (60/76)	De novo pelvic pain 18% Resolved pelvic pain 78%
Guerette et al.[35]	Biologic graft	Ba −1 or less	12, 24	12 mo: 78 (29/37) 24 mo: 63 (17/27)	12 mo: 86 (30/35) 24 mo: 77 (13/17)	Dyspareunia 20%
Iyer et al.[41]	Biologic graft	Ba −1 or less	12, 7–10 y	12 mo: 61 (35/57) 7–10 y: 29 (10/34)	12 mo: 78 (28/36) 7–10 y: 47 (9/19)	Not reported
Menefee et al.[42]	Mesh, biologic graft	Stage 1 prolapse or less	24	42 (10/24)	Mesh: 82 (23/28) Biologic: 54 (14/26)	De novo SUI 4.2% De novo dyspareunia 12.5%
Meschia et al.[43]	Biologic graft	Ba −1 or less	12	80 (78/98)	93 (96/103)	Urinary retention or voiding difficulty 15%
Nguyen and Burchette[26]	Mesh	Stage 1 prolapse or less	12	55 (21/38)	87 (33/38)	De novo dyspareunia 9% Blood transfusion 3% Urinary retention 5% UTI 18%
Hiltunen et al.[30] and Nieminen et al.[44]	Mesh	Stage 1 prolapse or less	12, 36	12 mo: 62 (60/97) 36 mo: 59 (57/97)	12 mo: 93 (97/104) 36 mo: 87 (90/104)	De novo SUI 9.4% New voiding dysfunction 11% (combined)
Robert et al.[36]	Absorbable mesh	Ba −1 or less	12	61 (17/28)	56 (15/27)	Pelvic pain 7%
Rudnicki et al.[27,45]	Mesh	Stage 1 prolapse or less	12, 36	12 mo: 40 (32/78) 36 mo: 41 (28/68)	12 mo: 88 (67/76) 36 mo: 86 (60/70)	UTI 13% De novo UUI 1.3%
Tamanini et al.[32]	Mesh	Ba −1 or less	24	86 (43/50)	95 (40/42)	Voiding dysfunction 3.6%

TABLE 44.1 *(Continued)*

Outcomes and Complications of Anterior Colporrhaphy Randomized Controlled Trials

AUTHOR	COMPARISON GROUP	PRIMARY OUTCOME	FOLLOW-UP (mo)	NATIVE TISSUE SUCCESS (%, N)	COMPARISON SUCCESS (%, N)	NATIVE TISSUE COMPLICATIONS
Turgal et al.[29]	Mesh	Ba −1 or less	12	75 (15/20)	95 (19/20)	Voiding dysfunction 5% Pelvic pain 5% UI 10%
Vollebregt et al.[34]	Mesh	Stage 1 prolapse or less	12	41 (23/56)	91 (53/58)	De novo dyspareunia 9% TVT 2%
Weber et al.[33]	Mesh, Ultralateral anterior colporrhaphy	Stage 1 prolapse or less	23 (median)	30 (10/33)	Mesh: 42 (11/26) Ultralateral: 46 (11/24)	De novo UUI 14% De novo SUI 8% De novo dyspareunia 5%
Withagen et al.[31]	Mesh	Stage 1 prolapse or less	12	55 (46/84)	90 (75/83)	Urinary retention 5% De novo dyspareunia 10% De novo SUI 9%

UTI, urinary tract infection; SUI, stress urinary incontinence; UUI, urge urinary incontinence.

TABLE 44.2

Paravaginal Repair Outcomes and Complications

AUTHOR	STUDY TYPE	APPROACH	PRIMARY OUTCOME	FOLLOW-UP (mo)	SUCCESS RATE (%)	COMPLICATIONS
Bedford et al.[46]	Case series	Laparoscopic	Stage 1 prolapse or less	62 (median)	64 (142/223)	Repeat operation 30% UTI 6.7%
Maggiore et al.[17]	Case series	Vaginal with Capio device	Stage 1 prolapse or less	24	92 (33/36)	De novo SUI 5.6% De novo dyspareunia 5.6%
Mallipeddi et al.[22]	Case series	Vaginal	Baden-Walker grade 0	20 (mean)	91 (32/35)	Ureteral obstruction 2.2% Retropubic hematoma 2.2% Vaginal abscess 4.4% Mild dyspareunia 5.7%
Minassian et al.[47]	RCT[a]	Abdominal	Stage 1 prolapse or less	24	Abdominal: 60 (15/25) AC w/ mesh: 68 (17/25)	Complications related to associated surgical procedures only
Reid et al.[21]	Retrospective cohort[b]	Vaginal	Baden-Walker grade 1 or less	72 (mean)	Vaginal: 70 (41/59) Abdominal: 89 (46/52)	Vaginal: Hematoma 1.7% Abdominal: Obturator nerve avulsion 1.9% Ureteric occlusion 1.9% Cystotomy 1.9%
Shull et al.[48]	Case series	Vaginal	Baden-Walker grade 0	19 (mean)	73 (41/56)	Complications related to associated surgical procedures only
Viana et al.[49]	Case series	Vaginal	Baden-Walker grade 0	12	92 (54/59)	Complications related to associated surgical procedures only
Young et al.[19]	Case series	Vaginal	Baden-Walker grade 0	3–11	78 (78/100)	Hemorrhage 3% Hematoma 1%

UTI, urinary tract infection; SUI, stress urinary incontinence; RCT, randomized controlled trial; AC, anterior colporrhaphy.
[a]Comparison group: anterior colporrhaphy with mesh.
[b]Comparison group: abdominal paravaginal repair.

POSTERIOR WALL PROLAPSE AND REPAIR

Anatomy

Posterior vaginal wall prolapse (PVP) is defined as herniation of either the rectum or small bowel into the vagina, defined as rectocele and enterocele, respectively. This chapter focuses specifically on surgical management of posterior prolapse. The pathophysiology of PVP is reviewed in Chapter 41. Similar to the anterior vaginal wall, loss of apical support also affects support of the posterior vaginal wall.[51] Thus, it is always important to consider the need for concomitant apical suspension when approaching surgical repair of posterior prolapse.

Posterior Colporrhaphy

Midline plication

The objective of posterior colporrhaphy is to plicate the fibromuscular layer of the posterior vaginal wall in order to alleviate an existing rectocele as well as to narrow the width of the posterior vaginal wall.[14,16]

Surgical preparation and positioning is the same as for anterior colporrhaphy. Bowel preparation is not indicated. Visualization is optimized with labial retraction sutures and/or hook retractors. A right-angle retractor is placed along the anterior vaginal wall to visualize the posterior vaginal wall and perineum.

The posterior vaginal wall and perineum are then injected with a hemostatic agent, preferentially vasopressin 10 units in 50 mL normal saline, 1% lidocaine with 1:200,000 epinephrine or 0.25% bupivacaine with 1:200,000 epinephrine. Injection should hydrodissect the vaginal epithelium from the underlying fibromuscularis layer.

Incision for posterior repair can be accomplished using various techniques and depends, in part, on if perineorrhaphy is also planned. For an isolated posterior repair, a horizontal incision can be made immediately proximal to the posterior hymenal ring.

If perineorrhaphy is planned, an inverse triangle incision or diamond incision can be made. For an inverted triangle incision, two Allis clamps are placed along the hymenal ring at approximately the 4 and 8 o'clock position (Fig. 44.4). The base of the triangle is along the posterior hymenal ring, with the point of the triangle at the inferior perineal body. Incision is made with a 15-blade scalpel and is also used to clear off the perineal epithelium from the underlying perineum. A diamond incision will carry the incision into the vagina along the posterior vaginal wall and is a good approach for posterior repair with perineorrhaphy.

The posterior vaginal wall is then examined to identify extent of the rectocele, which can be aided with a rectal finger. Allis or Allis Adair clamp is placed just cephalad of the superior edge of the rectocele. Starting from the distal incision at the hymen, midline incision of the vaginal epithelium is made with Metzenbaum or curved Mayo scissors. First, a small incision is made with the scissors to identify the appropriate layer. Then, with the tips of the scissors facing up and away from the rectum, the epithelium is sharply dissected from the underlying fibromuscularis with tips half-opened, half-closed (see Fig. 44.4). Like with anterior colporrhaphy, Allis clamps can be placed along the midline or an assistant can use Russian forceps to create tension and countertraction along the midline to avoid injury to the rectum. Alternatively, the midline incision can be made with the 15-blade scalpel.

Like in anterior colporrhaphy, Allis clamps are placed along the incised epithelial edge to facilitate traction during dissection. The vaginal epithelium is dissected off of the underlying fibromuscularis layer with the Metzenbaum scissors. Traction is facilitated by folding the vaginal epithelium over the surgeon's nondominant index finger during dissection. An assistant can also use smooth forceps to hold traction of the fibromuscular tissue during dissection. Technique is a combination of sharp dissection and gentle blunt dissection with an unfolded Ray-Tec sponge to enlarge potential planes. The correct plane should be white and hypovascular. Dissection is carried out bilaterally to the pelvic side walls and superiorly to the Allis clamp demarcating the superior border of the rectocele.

Although dissection in the correct plane is typically hypovascular, enlarged veins and venous sinuses are encountered more frequently during posterior repair than anterior repair. Hemostasis can be achieved with gentle cautery, pressure, or interrupted 3-0 polyglactin suture on a small needle such as an SH.

Plication of the fibromuscularis layer is performed using delayed absorbable suture such as 2-0 polyglactin or 2-0 PDS (see Fig. 44.4). It can be performed in a running or interrupted fashion, with interrupted recommended if vaginal length is a concern. Plication begins proximally and is carried toward the hymenal ring. Each plication suture should be placed in continuity with the previous suture to avoid creating a ridge along the posterior wall. Suture placement can be done with the nondominant index finger in the rectum to ensure appropriate depth of suture placement. Otherwise, it is crucial to perform a digital rectal exam after plication is complete to ensure no suture is in the rectum.

Levator ani plication can be considered in women who are no longer sexually active but is otherwise not recommended due to risk of overconstricting the vagina and subsequent dyspareunia. If performing, interrupted sutures of 0-polyglactin are placed in the levator ani muscle along the muscular sidewall and brought to midline prior to completing perineorrhaphy and closing the vaginal epithelium.

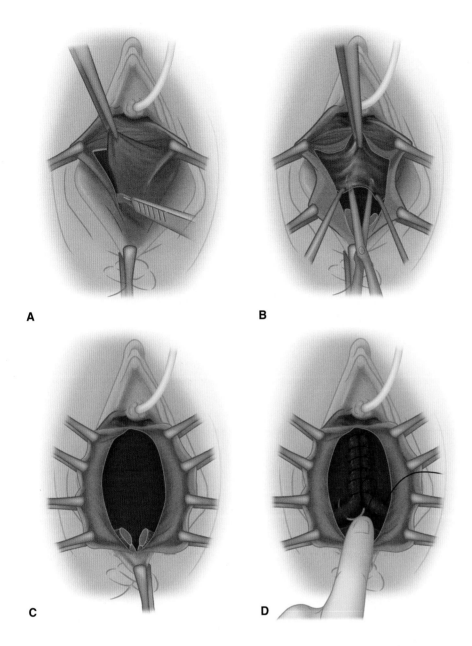

FIGURE 44.4 Posterior colporrhaphy. **A:** Inverted triangle incision over the posterior hymenal ring and perineal body. **B:** Sharp dissection of the vaginal epithelium from the underlying fibromuscularis layer. **C:** Completed dissection of vaginal epithelium from the underlying rectovaginal septum to bilateral pelvic side walls. **D:** Midline fibromuscular plication.

A   B

C   D

Excess vaginal epithelium is then trimmed, and epithelium is closed with 2-0 polyglactin. Prior to closure, a hemostatic agent such as thrombin tissue matrix or fibrin sealant can be placed for additional hemostasis.

Site-specific repair

The objective of site-specific posterior repair is to identify discrete defects in the rectovaginal septum and address each isolated defect individually. This can be done alone, or in combination, with a traditional posterior colporrhaphy. Advocates for this approach argue that a defect-directed method over midline plication may result in better functional outcomes, such as less dyspareunia. Critics argue that it is at times difficult to differentiate if the surgeon has created the defect in the

fibromuscularis during his or her dissection or if the defect previously existed. Thorough rectovaginal exam with the index finger in the rectum can help determine location of the defect prior to dissection.

The incision is the same as for posterior colporrhaphy and depends on whether concomitant perineorrhaphy is planned. The incision is carried to the cephalad border of the noted defect and carried out laterally to the pelvic sidewalls. Careful inspection of the rectovaginal septum is performed to identify defects in the fibromuscularis layer (Fig. 44.5).

Once specific defects have been identified, they can be repaired with interrupted or running 2-0 delayed-absorbable sutures. Permanent sutures are not recommended because they can increase the risk of postoperative dyspareunia.

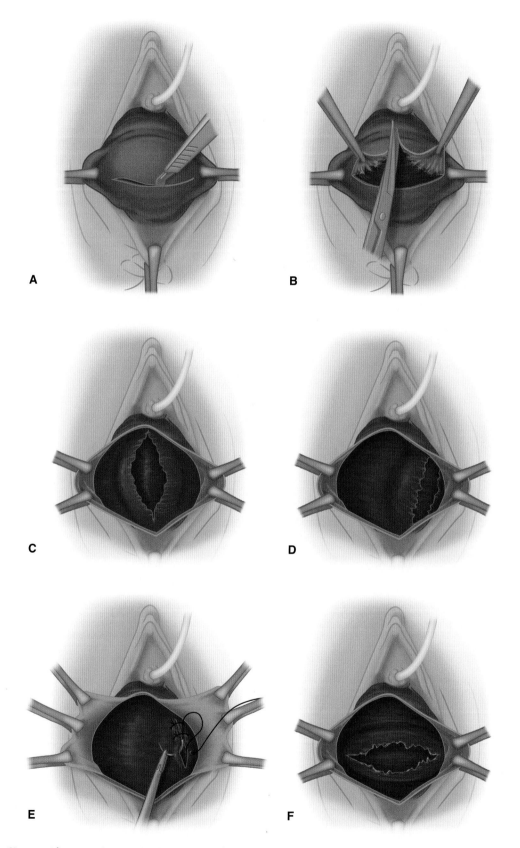

FIGURE 44.5 Site-specific posterior repair. **A:** Horizontal epithelial incision superior to posterior hymenal ring. **B:** Dissection of vaginal epithelium from underlying fibromuscularis. **C–F:** Examples of site-specific defects and repair.

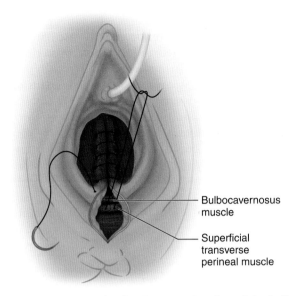

Bulbocavernosus
muscle

Superficial
transverse
perineal muscle

FIGURE 44.6 Perineorrhaphy. Reapproximation of the bulbo-cavernosus and superficial transverse perineal muscle.

Perineorrhaphy

The objective of the perineorrhaphy, or perineoplasty, is to reapproximate the bulbocavernosus and superficial transverse perineal muscles of the perineal body and re-store the appropriate caliber of the genital hiatus. The vaginal caliber at the end of the procedure should be 3 loose fingerbreadths, or approximately 5 cm, to avoid postoperative dyspareunia.

Two allis clamps are placed at 4 and 8 o'clock along the posterior hymenal ring and can be used to approximate the new desired vaginal caliber. As dis-cussed for posterior repair, an inverted triangle incision is made along the posterior hymenal ring and carried to the desired point along the perineal body (Fig. 44.6). This should be completed with the 15-blade scalpel, fol-lowed by removal of the overlying perineal epithelium with the scalpel.

Although ideally, during dissection, the surgeon will identify remnants of atrophied bulbocavernosus or trans-verse perineal muscles to reapproximate, this is often unrealistic due to severe atrophy and damage from pre-vious trauma such as childbirth. Using Metzenbaum or curved Mayo scissors, and with the nondominant index finger in the rectum for tactile depth, dissection is carried laterally and posteriorly in attempt to mobilize the free ends of the previously atrophied and/or avulsed mus-cles. Alternatively to placing a finger in the rectum, the surgeon can fold the vaginal epithelium grasped by the Allis clamps at the posterior hymenal ring over his or her nondominant index finger for traction while dissecting posterolaterally.

Plication is performed with 0-polyglactin or other delayed absorbable suture on a large needle such as a CT-1. Delayed absorbable is preferred due to concern

for increased rates of dyspareunia with permanent su-ture. A deep U-stitch is placed horizontally along the parallel plane of the posterior vagina in order to pli-cate the bulbocavernosus muscles. The suture should be tagged with a hemostat while placing the next stitch. If also performing a posterior repair, care should be taken to incorporate the distal portion of the posterior repair to avoid creating a "shelf" that will increase risk of postoperative dyspareunia. Next, a more distal, vertical U-stitch serves to plicate the superficial transverse peri-neal muscles and is tagged with a hemostat. The proxi-mal stitch is tied first, followed by the more distal stich (see Fig. 44.6).

Perineal closure is similar to a second-degree obstet-ric laceration. If a posterior repair has been performed, closure can be carried down to the perineum with the same suture of 2-0 polyglactin but requires changing di-rection with a crown stitch once at the hymenal ring. If only perineorrhaphy has been performed, the suture is anchored just inside of the hymenal ring. The underly-ing fibromuscular layer of the perineal body is closed in a running fashion, exiting at the posterior edge of the incision and returning in a subcuticular fashion toward the hymenal ring. The suture knot should be tied inside the hymenal ring for patient comfort.

Enterocele Repair

Enteroceles are defined as herniation of small bowel through defects in the fibromuscular layer of the vag-inal wall and can be anterior, apical, or posterior in lo-cation. It is often difficult to differentiate an enterocele from a rectocele posteriorly if both are present, and en-teroceles do not usually occur in isolation. The patient will frequently need a concomitant apical suspension or culdoplasty as well.

If an enterocele is suspected posteriorly, it is im-portant to first perform a thorough rectal exam to at-tempt to differentiate the rectocele from the enterocele sac. Once identified, a posterior vertical midline inci-sion can be carried over the enterocele sac toward the vaginal apex, just past the superior edge of the entero-cele. Dissection is then carried laterally in order to mo-bilize the enterocele sac from the vagina and underlying rectum. Once the sac has been identified, a finger in the rectum can help differentiate the peritoneal sac and avoid damage to the rectum. The sac is sharply incised, followed by gentle digital inspection for adhesions.

The sac is then closed in 2 to 3 circumferential lay-ers of delayed absorbable or nonabsorbable purse string sutures and any excess peritoneum is ligated. A delayed absorbable suture of material such as 2-0 PDS should then incorporate the posterior apical vaginal wall, the anterior rectum and the bilateral uterosacral ligaments to obliterate any potential space.[16] Epithelial closure is the same as for posterior colporrhaphy.

Postoperative Care

For posterior colporrhaphy and perineorrhaphy alone, the Foley catheter does not need to remain in place at the end of the procedure; however, if a more extensive surgery with an anti-incontinence procedure, hysterectomy, apical suspension, and/or anterior colporrhaphy has been performed, then the Foley catheter should be left based on surgeon discretion. Same day discharge is acceptable for posterior colporrhaphy and perineorrhaphy alone.

During healing, it is imperative that constipation be treated adequately, as defecation may be painful in the postoperative period and chronic constipation will increase the risk of recurrence. All patients should be discharged home with a stool softener and laxative to take as needed.

Alternative Surgical Approaches to Posterior Vaginal Wall Prolapse

Although transanal approach to rectocele repair has been described in the literature, a 2018 Cochrane review on posterior repair demonstrated level 1 evidence that vaginal approach is superior.[52] Awareness of prolapse, recurrent PVP, and postoperative obstructed defecation were all higher after transanal repair. A 2019 systematic review similarly found that anatomical outcomes and defecatory symptoms showed greater improvement after transvaginal over the transanal approach.[53] Given the evidence in favor of transvaginal repair, the transanal approach is not covered in this chapter.

The 2018 Cochrane review also demonstrated no difference between native tissue repair and augmentation with biologic grafts in rates of prolapse awareness, repeat surgery for prolapse, rates of recurrence, postobstructive defecation, or dyspareunia. Postoperative complications were more common after repair with biologic graft. The authors concluded that the current evidence does not support the use of biologic or synthetic grafts, and graft augmentation is not be reviewed in this chapter.

Complications

Serious complications after posterior colporrhaphy and perineorrhaphy such as hemorrhage requiring transfusion, abscess, and rectovaginal fistula are extremely rare. However, less severe complications such as rectovaginal hematoma, proctotomy, incisional infections, and dehiscence can occur.

Intraoperatively, adequate hemostasis is important to avoid a postoperative hematoma, particularly if a hemostatic agent is used for hydrodissection. Hemorrhage requiring transfusion during posterior colporrhaphy is rare but can occur, particularly in patients with enlarged and engorged posterior vaginal vasculature that can form with prolonged and advanced posterior prolapse. Rectovaginal hematomas can typically be observed unless there is concern for rapid expansion or the patient is hemodynamically unstable.

It is not uncommon to place a suture through rectal mucosa, which is why it is imperative to perform a thorough rectal exam after posterior repair. Alternatively, plication can be performed with one finger in the rectum to ensure appropriate depth of suture placement throughout the repair. Any suture in the rectal mucosa should be removed. Proctotomy is rare but should be repaired in layers if noted, using 4-0 or 5-0 polyglactin to repair the rectal mucosa and 3-0 polyglactin for the rectal muscularis and serosa. Large injuries or thermal injuries may require colorectal surgery consultation intraoperatively, depending on surgeon preference. Undiagnosed suture or injury, as well as an improperly repaired injury, can lead to rectovaginal fistula formation, which is a rare but serious complication of posterior repair.

Postoperative incisional infections were not reported in the majority of studies reviewed for this chapter. Incisional infection was noted in 2.4% and 5.3% of patients in two separate studies.[54,55]

Although constipation is common in the immediate postoperative period, defecatory dysfunction often improves after surgery. Many patients who report defecatory dysfunction preoperatively ultimately experience improvement in symptoms such as constipation, digitation, splinting, and incontinence postoperatively.[53] For example, defecatory dysfunction has been reported to improve by 23% to 90% of patients.[54,56–61] However, persistent or de novo defecatory dysfunction has been reported in up to 34% of patients.[59,62–66]

Dyspareunia is also a concern for patients after posterior repair. Many women report improvement in their preoperative dyspareunia by rates of 33% to 92%[54,57,60,63]; however, de novo dyspareunia may occur in up to 19% of women.[57,59,61–63,67]

Thus, for patients with both defecatory dysfunction and dyspareunia, it is important to set realistic expectations during preoperative counseling. Although in most patients defecatory issues and dyspareunia will improve, it may stay the same, worsen, or form de novo in a subset of patients.

Surgical Outcomes

Like anterior vaginal prolapse, the posterior vaginal wall receives substantial support from the apex, or level 1 support. In a patient with concomitant apical prolapse, apical suspension will often improve posterior prolapse and require a smaller posterior colporrhaphy or eliminate the need for repair altogether. Furthermore, much of the literature reporting outcomes of standard colporrhaphy and site-specific repair must be interpreted with some caution, as patients in many of these studies underwent additional concomitant prolapse procedures, including apical suspension.

Like in studies on anterior repair, outcome definitions vary across trials and can influence reported success rates. Overall, native tissue repair in the posterior compartment has higher success rates than anterior colporrhaphy. Anatomical success rates

for standard posterior colporrhaphy fall between 80% and 92% in studies with at least 12-month follow-up (Table 44.3).[55-57,61,62,66-70] Site-specific repairs have slightly lower success rates between 56% and 86% at 12-month follow-up or greater (Table 44.4).[54,59,60,63,64,66,69] A review article by Karram et al.[71] concluded that level 1 and level 2 evidence supported that standard colporrhaphy was superior to site-specific repair[53]; however, the 2018 Cochrane review of posterior repair was unable to make a definitive conclusion based on very limited evidence from RCTs.[52]

TABLE 44.3

Standard Posterior Colporrhaphy Outcomes and Complications

AUTHOR	STUDY TYPE	COMPARISON GROUP	PRIMARY OUTCOME	FOLLOW-UP (mo)	SUCCESS RATES (%)	COMPLICATIONS (STANDARD COLPORRHAPHY GROUP ONLY)
Abramov et al.[63]	Retrospective cohort	Site-specific repair	Baden-Walker grade 1 or less	12	Standard: 90 (165/183) Site-specific: 65 (80/124)	De novo dyspareunia 11% De novo constipation 10% De novo fecal incontinence 4%
Glazener et al.[62]	RCT	Mesh; biologic graft	Ap/Bp less than 0 cm	12	Standard: 85 (547/641) Mesh: 84 (282/336) Biologic: 82 (244/298)	Reoperation 2.5% Severe dyspareunia 5.1% Fecal incontinence 27.3%
Grimes et al.[68]	Retrospective cohort	Biologic graft	Bp less than −1 cm	35.8	86 (107/124)	Persistent dyspareunia 36% Persistent constipation 34%
Madsen et al.[61]	Retrospective cohort	Mesh	Awareness of bulge	12	61 (853/1,408)	De novo dyspareunia 15% De novo defecatory dysfunction 5% Reoperation 1.1%
Maher et al.[56]	Case series	None	Bp stage 1 or less	12.5 (median)	87 (33/38)	Proctotomy 2.6% Rectovaginal hematoma 2.6%
Milani et al.[57]	Case series	None	Ap/Bp stage 1 or less	14 (median)	80 (167/208)	De novo dyspareunia 19%
Paraiso et al.[69]	RCT	Site-specific repair, biologic graft	Bp less than −2 cm	12	Standard: 86 (24/28) Site-specific: 78 (21/27) Graft: 54 (14/26)	Reoperation 3%
Sand et al.[70]	RCT	Mesh	Baden-Walker grade 1 or less	12	90 (63/70)	Not documented
Schmidlin-Enderli et al.[67]	Case series	None	Ap/Bp stage 1 or less	22 (median)	92 (35/38)	De novo dyspareunia 5.2% Persistent defecatory dysfunction 27.8%
Sung et al.[55]	RCT	Biologic graft	Ap/Bp stage 1 or less	12	Standard: 91 (64/70) Graft: 88 (59/67)	Wound separation 6.2% Wound infection 5.3%

RCT, randomized controlled trial.

TABLE 44.4

Site-Specific Repair Outcomes and Complications

AUTHOR	STUDY TYPE	PRIMARY OUTCOME	FOLLOW-UP (mo)	SUCCESS RATES (%)	COMPLICATIONS
Abramov et al.[63]	Retrospective cohort[a]	Baden-Walker grade 1 or less	12	Site-specific: 56 (69/124) Standard: 82 (150/183)	De novo dyspareunia 11% De novo constipation 11% De novo fecal incontinence 7%
Cundiff et al.[66]	Case series	Ap/Bp stage 1 or less	12 (median)	86 (37/43)	De novo constipation 4% De novo fecal incontinence 3%
Rojas et al.[64]	Case series	Bp less than −1	17 (mean)	86 (118/137)	Persistent obstructed defecation 34% De novo dyspareunia 11%
Kenton et al.[60]	Case series	Bp −2 or less	12	77 (34/44)	De novo dyspareunia 7% De novo constipation 3%
Paraiso et al.[69]	RCT[b]	Bp less than −2	12	Site-specific: 78 (21/27) Graft: 54 (14/26) Standard: 86 (24/28)	Site-specific reoperation 5%
Sardeli et al.[59]	Case series	Bp less than −1	27 (mean)	69 (35/51)	De novo dyspareunia 4%
Singh et al.[54]	Case series	Ap/Bp stage 1 or less	18	73 (24/33)	Incisional infection 2.4%

[a]Comparison group: standard posterior colporrhaphy.
[b]Comparison groups: standard posterior colporrhaphy, biologic graft.

Subjective improvement is also typically equivalent to or higher than objective success rates, and patients often do not complain of bulge even if anatomical failure is diagnosed. This is, in part, why rates of reoperation for recurrent prolapse are relatively low. Many studies reviewed for this chapter reported no reoperation for prolapse recurrence, but those that did reported rates between 1.1% and 5%.[61,62,69]

Conclusion

PVP typically arises from a defect in the fibromuscular layer of the rectovaginal septum or lateral detachment from the ATFR secondary to trauma or injury such as previous childbirth, previous surgery, and chronic constipation. Graft augmentation has not been demonstrated to be superior to native tissue repair and is not recommended given the higher risk of complications and removal of synthetic vaginal mesh from the market in the United States. Standard posterior colporrhaphy appears to be slightly superior to site-specific repair, but both approaches have relatively high success rates. Perineorrhaphy is frequently performed with posterior repair, and care must be taken to avoid overnarrowing the genital hiatus which increases the risk of postoperative dyspareunia. Patients should be counseled that defecatory dysfunction and dyspareunia will often improve but in a subset of patients it can persist, worsen, or occur de novo.

References

1. Barber MD, Maher C. Epidemiology and outcome assessment of pelvic organ prolapse. *Int Urogynecol J* 2013;24(11):1783–1790.
2. Olsen AL, Smith VJ, Bergstrom JO, et al. Epidemiology of surgically managed pelvic organ prolapse and urinary incontinence. *Obstet Gynecol* 1997;89(4):501–506.
3. Maher C, Feiner B, Baessler K, et al. Surgery for women with anterior compartment prolapse. *Cochrane Database Syst Rev* 2016;(11):CD004014.
4. DeLancey JO. Anatomy of the female pelvis. In: Jones HW, Rock JA, eds. *Te Linde's operative gynecology*, 7th ed. Philadelphia: JB Lippincott, 1992:33–65.
5. Lowder JL, Park AJ, Ellison R, et al. The role of apical vaginal support in the appearance of anterior and posterior vaginal prolapse. *Obstet Gynecol* 2008;111(1):152–157.
6. Lang P, Whiteside JL. Anterior compartment prolapse: What's new? *Curr Open Obstet Gynecol* 2017;29(5):337–342.
7. Margulies RU, Rogers MA, Morgan DM. Outcomes of transvaginal uterosacral ligament suspension: Systematic review and metaanalysis. *Am J Obstet Gynecol* 2010;202(2):124–134.
8. Beer M, Kuhn A. Surgical techniques for vault prolapse: A review of the literature. *Eur J Obstet Gynecol Reprod Biol* 2005;119(2):144–155.
9. Maher CF, Murray CJ, Carey MP, et al. Iliococcygeus or sacrospinous fixation for vaginal vault prolapse. *Obstet Gynecol* 2001;98(1):40–44.
10. Nygaard IE, McCreery R, Brubaker L, et al. Abdominal sacrocolpopexy: A comprehensive review. *Obstet Gynecol* 2004;104(4):805–823.
11. Whiteside JL, Barber MD, Paraiso MF, et al. Clinical evaluation of anterior vaginal wall support defects: Interexaminer and

intraexaminer reliability. *Am J Obstet Gynecol* 2004;191(1): 100–104.

12. Segal JL, Vassallo BJ, Kleeman SD, et al. Paravaginal defects: Prevalence and accuracy of preoperative detection. *Int Urogynecol J Pelvic Floor Dysfunct* 2004;15(6):378–383.

13. Arenholt LTS, Pedersen BG, Glavind K, et al. Paravaginal defect: Anatomy, clinical findings, and imaging. *Int Urogynecol J* 2017;28(5):661–673.

14. Young SB, Kambiss SM. Anterior wall support defects. In: Ostergard DR, Bent AE, Cundiff G, et al, eds. *Ostergard's urogynecology and pelvic floor dysfunction*. Philadelphia: Lippincott Williams & Wilkins, 2008:463–478.

15. Nichols D, Randall CL. *Vaginal surgery*, 4th ed. Baltimore: Williams & Wilkins, 1996.

16. Walters MD, Barber MD. Surgical treatment of anterior vaginal wall prolapse. In: Walters MD, Karram MM, eds. *Urogynecology and reconstructive pelvic surgery*. Philadelphia: Elsevier/Saunders, 2015:327–341.

17. Maggiore ULR, Ferrero S, Mancuso S, et al. Feasibility and outcome of vaginal paravaginal repair using the Capio suture-capturing device. *Int Urogynecol J* 2012;23(3):341–347.

18. U.S. Food and Drug Administration. Urogynecologic surgical mesh implants. Published 2019. Updated July 10, 2019. Accessed September 25, 2020. https://www.fda.gov/medical-devices /implants-and-prosthetics/urogynecologic-surgical-mesh-implants

19. Young SB, Daman JJ, Bony LG. Vaginal paravaginal repair: One-year outcomes. *Am J Obstet Gynecol* 2001;185(6):1360–1367.

20. de Tayrac R, Cornille A, Eglin G, et al. Comparison between trans-obturator trans-vaginal mesh and traditional anterior colporrhaphy in the treatment of anterior vaginal wall prolapse: Results of a French RCT. *Int Urogynecol J* 2013;24(10):1651–1661.

21. Reid RI, You H, Luo K. Site-specific prolapse surgery. I. Reliability and durability of native tissue paravaginal repair. *Int Urogynecol J* 2011;22(5):591–599.

22. Mallipeddi PK, Steele AC, Kohli N, et al. Anatomic and functional outcome of vaginal paravaginal repair in the correction of anterior vaginal wall prolapse. *Int Urogynecol J Pelvic Floor Dysfunct* 2001;12(2):83–88.

23. Carey M, Higgs P, Goh J, et al. Vaginal repair with mesh versus colporrhaphy for prolapse: A randomised controlled trial. *BJOG* 2009;116(10):1380–1386.

24. Altman D, Väyrynen T, Engh ME, et al. Anterior colporrhaphy versus transvaginal mesh for pelvic-organ prolapse. *N Engl J Med* 2011;364(19):1826–1836.

25. Speights SE, Moore RD, Miklos JR. Frequency of lower urinary tract injury at laparoscopic Burch and paravaginal repair. *J Am Assoc Gynecol Laparosc* 2000;7(4):515–518.

26. Nguyen JN, Burchette RJ. Outcome after anterior vaginal prolapse repair: A randomized controlled trial. *Obstet Gynecol* 2008;111(4):891–898.

27. Rudnicki M, Laurikainen E, Pogosean R, et al. Anterior colporrhaphy compared with collagen-coated transvaginal mesh for anterior vaginal wall prolapse: A randomised controlled trial. *BJOG* 2014;121(1):102–101.

28. Delroy CA, de Castro AR, Dias MM, et al. The use of transvaginal synthetic mesh for anterior vaginal wall prolapse repair: A randomized controlled trial. *Int Urogynecol J* 2013;24(11):1899–1907.

29. Turgal M, Sivaslioglu A, Yildiz A, et al. Anatomical and functional assessment of anterior colporrhaphy versus polypropylene mesh surgery in cystocele treatment. *Eur J Obstet Gynecol Reprod Biol* 2013;170(2):555–558.

30. Hiltunen R, Nieminen K, Takala T, et al. Low-weight polypropylene mesh for anterior vaginal wall prolapse: A randomized controlled trial. *Obstet Gynecol* 2007;110(2 Pt 2):455–462.

31. Withagen MI, Milani AL, den Boon J, et al. Trocar-guided mesh compared with conventional vaginal repair in recurrent prolapse: A randomized controlled trial. *Obstet Gynecol* 2011;117(2 Pt 1):242–250.

32. Tamanini JT, de Oliveira Souza Castro RC, Tamanini JM, et al. A prospective, randomized, controlled trial of the treatment of anterior vaginal wall prolapse: Medium term followup. *J Urol* 2015;193(4):1298–1304.

33. Weber AM, Walters MD, Piedmonte MR, et al. Anterior colporrhaphy: A randomized trial of three surgical techniques. *Am J Obstet Gynecol* 2001;185(6):1299–1306.

34. Vollebregt A, Fischer K, Gietelink D, et al. Primary surgical repair of anterior vaginal prolapse: A randomised trial comparing anatomical and functional outcome between anterior colporrhaphy and trocar-guided transobturator anterior mesh. *BJOG* 2011;118(12):1518–1527.

35. Guerette NL, Peterson TV, Aguirre OA, et al. Anterior repair with or without collagen matrix reinforcement: A randomized controlled trial. *Obstet Gynecol* 2009;114(1):59–65.

36. Robert M, Girard I, Brennand E, et al. Absorbable mesh augmentation compared with no mesh for anterior prolapse: A randomized controlled trial. *Obstet Gynecol* 2014;123(2 Pt 1):288–294.

37. Gandhi S, Goldberg RP, Kwon C, et al. A prospective randomized trial using solvent dehydrated fascia lata for the prevention of recurrent anterior vaginal wall prolapse. *Am J Obstet Gynecol* 2005;192(5):1649–1654.

38. Halpern-Elenskaia K, Umek W, Bodner-Adler B, et al. Anterior colporrhaphy: A standard operation? Systematic review of the technical aspects of a common procedure in randomized controlled trials. *Int Urogynecol J* 2018;29(6):781–788.

39. Lensen EJ, Stoutjesdijk JA, Withagen MI, et al. Technique of anterior colporrhaphy: A Dutch evaluation. *Int Urogynecol J* 2011;22(5):557–561.

40. Feldner PC Jr, Castro RA, Cipolotti LA, et al. Anterior vaginal wall prolapse: A randomized controlled trial of SIS graft versus traditional colporrhaphy. *Int Urogynecol J* 2010;21(9):1057–1063.

41. Iyer S, Seitz M, Tran A, et al. Anterior colporrhaphy with and without dermal allograft: A randomized control trial with long-term follow-up. *Female Pelvic Med Reconstr Surg* 2019;25(3):206–212.

42. Menefee SA, Dyer KY, Lukacz ES, et al. Colporrhaphy compared with mesh or graft-reinforced vaginal paravaginal repair for anterior vaginal wall prolapse: A randomized controlled trial. *Obstet Gynecol* 2011;118(6):1337–1344.

43. Meschia M, Pifarotti P, Bernasconi F, et al. Porcine skin collagen implants to prevent anterior vaginal wall prolapse recurrence: A multicenter, randomized study. *J Urol* 2007;177(1):192–195.

44. Nieminen K, Hiltunen R, Takala T, et al. Outcomes after anterior vaginal wall repair with mesh: A randomized, controlled trial with a 3 year follow-up. *Am J Obstet Gynecol* 2010;203(3): 235.e1–235.e8.

45. Rudnicki M, Laurikainen E, Pogosean R, et al. A 3-year follow-up after anterior colporrhaphy compared with collagen-coated transvaginal mesh for anterior vaginal wall prolapse: A randomised controlled trial. *BJOG* 2016;123(1):136–142.

46. Bedford ND, Seman EI, O'Shea R T, et al. Long-term outcomes of laparoscopic repair of cystocoele. *Aust N Z J Obstet Gynaecol* 2015;55(6):588–592.

47. Minassian VA, Parekh M, Poplawsky D, et al. Randomized controlled trial comparing two procedures for anterior vaginal wall prolapse. *Neurourol Urodyn* 2014;33(1):72–77.

48. Shull BL, Benn SJ, Kuehl TJ. Surgical management of prolapse of the anterior vaginal segment: An analysis of support defects, operative morbidity, and anatomic outcome. *Am J Obstet Gynecol* 1994;171(6):1429–1439.

49. Viana R, Colaço J, Vieira A, et al. Cystocele—Vaginal approach to repairing paravaginal fascial defects. *Int Urogynecol J Pelvic Floor Dysfunct* 2006;17(6):621–623.

50. Eilber KS, Alperin M, Khan A, et al. Outcomes of vaginal prolapse surgery among female Medicare beneficiaries: The role of apical support. *Obstet Gynecol* 2013;122(5):981–987.

51. Luo J, Larson KA, Fenner DE, et al. Posterior vaginal prolapse shape and position changes at maximal Valsalva seen in 3-D MRI-based models. *Int Urogynecol J* 2012;23(9):1301–1306.

52. Mowat A, Maher D, Baessler K, et al. Surgery for women with posterior compartment prolapse. *Cochrane Database Syst Rev* 2018;(3):CD012975.

53. Grimes CL, Schimpf MO, Wieslander CK, et al. Surgical interventions for posterior compartment prolapse and obstructed defecation symptoms: A systematic review with clinical practice recommendations. *Int Urogynecol J* 2019;30(9):1433–1454.

54. Singh K, Cortes E, Reid WM. Evaluation of the fascial technique for surgical repair of isolated posterior vaginal wall prolapse. *Obstet Gynecol* 2003;101(2):320–324.

55. Sung VW, Rardin CR, Raker CA, et al. Porcine subintestinal submucosal graft augmentation for rectocele repair: A randomized controlled trial. *Obstet Gynecol* 2012;119(1):125–133.

56. Maher CF, Qatawneh AM, Baessler K, et al. Midline rectovaginal fascial plication for repair of rectocele and obstructed defecation. *Obstet Gynecol* 2004;104(4):685–689.

57. Milani AL, Withagen MI, Schweitzer KJ, et al. Midline fascial plication under continuous digital transrectal control: Which factors determine anatomic outcome? *Int Urogynecol J* 2010;21(6):623–630.

58. Yamana T, Takahashi T, Iwadare J. Clinical and physiologic outcomes after transvaginal rectocele repair. *Dis Colon Rectum* 2006;49(5):661–667.

59. Sardeli C, Axelsen SM, Kjaer D, et al. Outcome of site-specific fascia repair for rectocele. *Acta Obstet Gynecol Scand* 2007;86(8):973–977.

60. Kenton K, Shott S, Brubaker L. Outcome after rectovaginal fascia reattachment for rectocele repair. *Am J Obstet Gynecol* 1999;181(6):1360–1364.

61. Madsen LD, Nüssler E, Kesmodel US, et al. Native-tissue repair of isolated primary rectocele compared with nonabsorbable mesh: Patient-reported outcomes. *Int Urogynecol J* 2017;28(1):49–57.

62. Glazener CM, Breeman S, Elders A, et al. Mesh, graft, or standard repair for women having primary transvaginal anterior or posterior compartment prolapse surgery: Two parallel-group, multicentre, randomised, controlled trials (PROSPECT). *Lancet* 2017;389(10067):381–392.

63. Abramov Y, Gandhi S, Goldberg RP, et al. Site-specific rectocele repair compared with standard posterior colporrhaphy. *Obstet Gynecol* 2005;105(2):314–318.

64. Rojas RG, Atan IK, Shek KL, et al. Defect-specific rectocele repair: Medium-term anatomical, functional and subjective outcomes. *Aust N Z J Obstet Gynaecol* 2015;55(5):487–492.

65. Gillor M, Langer S, Dietz HP. Long-term subjective, clinical and sonographic outcomes after native-tissue and mesh-augmented posterior colporrhaphy. *Int Urogynecol J* 2019;30(9):1581–1585.

66. Cundiff GW, Weidner AC, Visco AG, et al. An anatomic and functional assessment of the discrete defect rectocele repair. *Am J Obstet Gynecol* 1998;179(6 Pt 1):1451–1457.

67. Schmidlin-Enderli K, Schuessler B. A new rectovaginal fascial plication technique for treatment of rectocele with obstructed defecation: A proof of concept study. *Int Urogynecol J* 2013;24(4):613–619.

68. Grimes CL, Tan-Kim J, Whitcomb EL, et al. Long-term outcomes after native tissue vs. biological graft-augmented repair in the posterior compartment. *Int Urogynecol J* 2012;23(5):597–604.

69. Paraiso MF, Barber MD, Muir TW, et al. Rectocele repair: A randomized trial of three surgical techniques including graft augmentation. *Am J Obstet Gynecol* 2006;195(6):1762–1771.

70. Sand PK, Koduri S, Lobel RW, et al. Prospective randomized trial of polyglactin 910 mesh to prevent recurrence of cystoceles and rectoceles. *Am J Obstet Gynecol* 2001;184(7):1357–13654.

71. Karram M, Maher C. Surgery for posterior vaginal wall prolapse. *Int Urogynecol J* 2013;24(11):1835–1841.

CHAPTER 45

APICAL SUPPORT DEFECTS

Zhuoran Chen • Christopher Maher

Introduction

Pelvic organ prolapse is a common condition that affects up to 50% of parous women, increases with age,[1] and has an 11% to 20% lifetime risk of surgical intervention.[1,2] Apical prolapse which is the descent of the uterus or the vault (post-hysterectomy) results from loss of level 1 support from the uterosacral and cardinal ligament complex.[3] Although not as common as anterior or posterior vaginal wall defects, apical prolapse rarely occurs in isolation and is typically seen in prolapse beyond the hymen.[4,5] Recognition of apical defects on clinical assessment and recreating adequate apical support at the time of midvaginal repair is important for the successful surgical treatment of advanced prolapse[6,7] and reduces cystocele recurrence in the long term.[8–10]

TYPES OF APICAL PROCEDURES

Surgical repair for the apex, both uterine and vault, has several options with high success rates and can be broadly divided into reconstructive or obliterative surgery (Fig. 45.1). Obliterative approaches such as total colpocleisis or LeFort partial colpocleisis have success rates of greater than 90%,[11] with low morbidity, short operative time, and high patient satisfaction.[12] However, due to loss of coital function, it is generally reserved for the frail or elderly and/or those unable to tolerate the surgical morbidity of hysterectomy and repairs.

In those undergoing reconstructive apical suspensions, the surgical options and data supporting the options vary with those having vault and uterine prolapse which are evaluated separately.

Vault Prolapse (Post-hysterectomy)

Vaginal versus abdominal apical suspension

Reconstructive surgery for vaginal vault prolapse can be performed either transvaginally or transabdominally via open, laparoscopic or robotically assisted approaches. Vaginal apical suspension includes both native tissue repair (i.e., sacrospinous colpopexy, uterosacral ligament suspension, McCall culdoplasty, or iliococcygeus

fixation) and mesh augmentation with commercially available kits aimed at concurrent apical and anterior or posterior vaginal wall support. These kits are no longer available in some countries. Transabdominally, sacrocolpopexy for post-hysterectomy vault prolapse is the most commonly performed apical suspension.[13]

Level 1 evidence comparing the success of these two approaches have been reported in various studies. In the 2016 Cochrane review, six randomized trials (n = 583) compared sacrocolpopexy to vaginal prolapse repair for a predominately vault prolapse cohort. These include three trials comparing abdominal sacrocolpopexy to sacrospinous ligament suspension,[14–16] one trial comparing abdominal sacrocolpopexy to uterosacral ligament suspension,[17] one trial comparing laparoscopic sacrocolpopexy to transvaginal mesh repair,[18] and one comparing abdominal or laparoscopic sacrocolpopexy to uterosacral ligament suspension with mesh augmentation.[19] On meta-analysis, sacrocolpopexy when compared to the vaginal approach with or without mesh was associated with a lower risk of awareness of prolapse, less recurrent prolapse on examination, less reoperation for prolapse, and less postoperative stress incontinence and dyspareunia.[19] Complications of mesh erosion were similar between the groups at 3% to 4%.

Subsequent to the Cochrane publication, Lucot et al.[20] reported the outcomes of a large French multicenter randomized trial comparing laparoscopic sacrocolpopexy (n = 130) and transvaginal mesh (n = 129) for those presenting with cystocele with uterus present. They demonstrated no difference between the groups in symptoms of prolapse, reoperation for prolapse, or validated satisfaction or quality-of-life outcomes. However, laparoscopic sacrocolpopexy had higher elevation of point C on examination, a longer total vaginal length, lower risk of reoperation, and dyspareunia compared to the transvaginal mesh group.[20]

Furthermore, a systematic review by the Society of Gynecologic Surgeons Systematic Review Group evaluated both uterine and vault prolapse with randomized and nonrandomized comparative trials and noncomparative studies comparing sacrocolpopexy to native tissue vaginal repairs. They reported improved anatomical outcomes with sacrocolpopexy with no difference in reoperation rates or postoperative sexual function.[21]

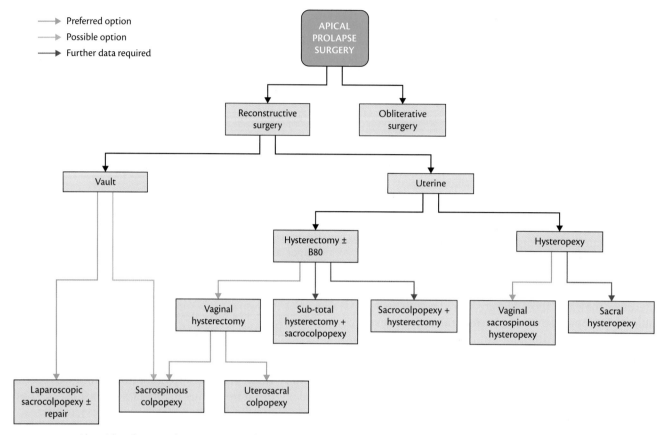

FIGURE 45.1 Algorithm for apical support procedures. (Adapted from Abrams P, Cardozo L, Wagg A, et al. *Incontinence*, 6th ed. Bristol: International Continence Society, 2017.)

Although sacrocolpopexy clearly provides better anatomical and functional outcomes in randomized controlled trial for vault prolapse, the open procedure is associated with a longer operative time, slower recovery, and increased cost when compared to vaginal approach.[19] The laparoscopic technique has been adopted by many surgeons over the last decade with a reduction in postoperative recovery and blood loss without compromising surgical outcome.[22,23] One limitation to widespread uptake is the steep learning curve associated with laparoscopic suturing; hence, the robotic approach was developed.[24] However, robotic sacrocolpopexy has a longer operative time, more postoperative pain and bleeding,[25] slower recovery, and significantly greater cost than the laparoscopic route[26] with equivalence in all other outcomes.[27] More recently, several units have reported the learning curve to minimizing intraoperative and postoperative complications using the robotic approach to sacrocolpopexy was longer than anticipated and the learning curve was 80 cases.[28,29]

Vaginal native tissue versus vaginal mesh apical suspension

Vaginal native tissue apical suspension procedures have been compared to mesh augmentation in various randomized trials, with vaginal mesh conferring no additional benefit. In the 2016 Cochrane review, six randomized trials ($n = 589$) comparing sacrospinous ligament suspension to first generation polypropylene mesh (either monofilament Prolift, Ethicon, or multifilament weave) were combined for meta-analysis. By 3 years, no difference was observed between mesh and nonmesh repair in awareness of prolapse, recurrent prolapse on examination, reoperation for prolapse, or postoperative stress incontinence and dyspareunia.[19] There was a trend toward higher bladder injury in the mesh group (risk ratio 3; 95% confidence interval 0.91 to 9.89) and high mesh erosion rate of 18%, with 9.5% reoperation for mesh exposure.

Since the 2011 U.S. Food and Drug Administration public health notification regarding transvaginal meshes, most first-generation vaginal mesh kits are no longer marketed. Furthermore, between 2016 and 2019, countries such as United Kingdom, Australia, and United States have banned the use of all transvaginal mesh kits outside the context of clinical trials.[30] Thus, these results serve as only historic reading for a large portion of clinicians.

Different types of vaginal native tissue apical suspension

To date, only one randomized trial (OPTIMAL trial, $n = 374$)[31] has compared the two most commonly performed apical suspension procedures: sacrospinous ligament and uterosacral ligament suspension. In both groups, post-hysterectomy vault prolapse and uterine prolapse (which were the minority) were included, but all patients underwent a concurrent vaginal hysterectomy if the uterus was present.

At 2 years follow-up, there were no differences between the groups on composite outcome of success, defined as the absence of (1) descent of the vaginal apex more than one-third of the vaginal canal, (2) anterior or posterior vaginal wall descent beyond the hymen, (3) bothersome vaginal bulge symptoms as reported by the Pelvic Floor Distress Inventory, and (4) retreatment with surgery or a pessary. Nor were there any differences in quality-of-life and functional outcomes, with both procedures recording high patient satisfaction and low reoperation rate of 5% at 2 years. However, robustness of the surgery steadily declined in both groups by 5 years with only 30% of sacrospinous ligament suspension and 38% of uterosacral ligament suspension meeting the primary outcome of success. Reoperation and reintervention rates also increased to 8% to 11.9% with no difference between groups. Based on the available evidence, either procedure is suitable for vaginal apical suspension, should sacrocolpopexy not be appropriate or feasible for vault prolapse.

Uterine Prolapse

Decision for hysterectomy or uterine preservation at the time of uterine prolapse surgery is an important consideration with both pros and cons and patient treatment is best individualized. Although hysterectomy +/− salpingo-oophorectomy in the postmenopausal women reduces the long-term risk of uterine, cervical, or ovarian pathology without adverse effects on sexual function,[32,33] there has been growing interest in uterine preservation apical suspension due to less operative time and blood loss[34] with similar short-term success[34,35] when compared to hysterectomy. When considering and counseling for uterine preservation, contraindications must first be excluded (Table 45.1) and the malignant risks of uterine preservation discussed.

Vaginal versus abdominal surgery for uterine prolapse

Although the role and benefit of sacrocolpopexy in post-hysterectomy prolapse is well established, the evidence is less clear for uterine prolapse. There is a paucity of evidence for the superiority of sacrohysteropexy, supracervical, or total hysterectomy with concurrent sacrocolpopexy when compared to vaginal based interventions.

Total laparoscopic hysterectomy and sacrocolpopexy for uterine prolapse is associated with significantly increased risk of mesh erosion when compared to sacrocolpopexy alone for vault prolapse (7% vs. 2%) and is thus not recommended.[38] Although supracervical

TABLE 45.1	
Relative Contraindications for Uterine Preservation	
Cervical pathology	CIN/AIS
	Cervical cancer
	Unable to follow up with cervical screening
Uterine pathology	Postmenopausal bleeding
	Dysfunctional uterine bleeding
	Known hyperplasia
	Large fibroid uterus
	Lynch syndrome[a]
Ovarian pathology	BRCA1 and BRCA2 genes
	Risk of ovarian cancer or large ovarian mass
	Elective salpingectomy/salpingo-oophorectomy for ovarian cancer risk–reducing surgery[36,37]
Other	Tamoxifen therapy
	Unable to follow up with gynecologic surveillance or cervical screening

CIN, cervical intraepithelial neoplasia; AIS, adenocarcinoma in situ.
[a]Defined as hereditary nonpolyposis colorectal cancer syndrome; have increased risk of colorectal and endometrial cancer.
Bonadona V, Bonaïti B, Olschwang S, et al. Cancer risks associated with germline mutations in *MLH1*, *MSH2*, and *MSH6* genes in Lynch syndrome. *JAMA* 2011; 305(22):2304–2310.

hysterectomy and sacrocolpopexy reduces the risk of mesh exposure, observational data suggest higher recurrent prolapse rates.[39] The data to date is supportive of neither sacrocolpopexy with total nor subtotal hysterectomy. Furthermore, uterine morcellation is banned in many US states due to the unknown risk of leiomyosarcoma.

When sacrocolpopexy with total or subtotal hysterectomy was compared to sacrohysteropexy (either open or laparoscopic), uterine preservation option was associated with less mesh erosion, less blood loss, shorter operative time, and similar objective success rates.[34] However, one study at 3 years suggested a higher symptomatic recurrence associated with sacrohysteropexy.[40]

The high rate of recurrent prolapse with sacrohysteropexy when compared to abdominal hysterectomy and sacrocolpopexy seen above was also demonstrated in two separate randomized trials when sacrohysteropexy was compared to vaginal hysterectomy and uterosacral ligament suspension.[41–43] The findings favored the vaginal approach with less operative time and less operative pain. Furthermore, by 8 years follow-up,[42] despite similar anatomical success and reoperation rate for recurrent prolapse between interventions, the quality of life, urinary distress inventory, and overactive bladder (OAB) scores significantly favored the hysterectomy group. Rahmanou et al.[41] also demonstrated a higher reoperation rate in the laparoscopic hysteropexy group, again questioning the efficacy of this as a reasonable option for uterine preservation.

Lastly, a recent randomized trial (LAVA trial, $n = 126$) comparing laparoscopic sacrohysteropexy to vaginal sacrospinous hysteropexy[44] showed no difference in recurrent prolapse or composite outcome (defined as recurrence of uterine prolapse; Pelvic Organ Prolapse Quantification [POP-Q] ≥ 2) with bothersome bulging/protrusion symptoms and/or repeat surgery or pessary at 12 months. However, 1 in 10 sacrohysteropexy were converted to vaginal hysteropexy due to technical challenges. The sacrohysteropexy was also associated with more bothersome OAB symptoms, higher posterior wall anatomical recurrence, and increased fecal incontinence compared to vaginal hysteropexy.

The minimally invasive abdominal uterosacral ligament plication for uterine prolapse has attracted some support, but with very limited long-term data on efficacy and variable results, it has not seen a dramatic uptake clinically. Thus, without strong evidence to support any of the abdominal interventions (sacrocolpopexy with total or subtotal hysterectomy or sacrohysteropexy), the vaginal approach to uterine prolapse appears to be the more sensible first-line surgical intervention on balance of the risk of and benefits. This allows for sacrocolpopexy to be reserved as a successful option for recurrent prolapse in the future.

In the United States, the most common vaginal approach for uterine prolapse is a hysterectomy with apical suspension; however, uterine preservation with its lower perioperative morbidity is an attractive surgical option for some women.[45] This chapter explores the evidence and the role of uterine preservation surgery.

Vaginal uterine preservation

The surgical options for vaginal uterine preservation include a native tissue hysteropexy, Manchester, or mesh hysteropexy. Vaginal hysteropexy is typically performed with unilateral fixation of the cervix to the sacrospinous ligament via absorbable or nonabsorbable sutures and can be combined with concurrent anterior or posterior repairs. In the short term, a meta-analysis of 13 randomized and nonrandomized trials[34] comparing sacrospinous hysteropexy to hysterectomy +/− sacrospinous ligament or uterosacral ligament suspension found no difference in recurrent prolapse between the procedures. In addition, patient satisfaction was similar, but the hysteropexy group had less blood loss by 90 mL and 18 minutes less operative time and less perioperative morbidity.[46]

Outcomes beyond 12 months are more controversial. To date, there is only one randomized trial

that reported 5-year outcomes of sacrospinous hysteropexy versus hysterectomy and high uterosacral ligament suspension ($n = 204$).[35] Although the Schulten et al.[35] concluded that hysteropexy was associated with lower surgical failure rate (1% vs. 7.8%), the results need to be interpreted with caution as this statement was drawn from a composite finding which can exaggerate the effect size. When the outcomes were reviewed individually, there was no difference in the anatomical apical recurrence, repeat surgery for apical prolapse, or any other secondary outcomes. Differences in anterior and posterior compartment reoperation were what contributed to the positive composite outcome, but these procedures were performed at the clinician's discretion in the original prolapse repair. Attribution bias due to unequal follow-up and observer bias due to the presence of a cervix in the hysteropexy group also overshadow the conclusion of uterine preservation as a more successful operation. In addition, endometrial cancer was reported in the hysteropexy group, further highlighted the need for appropriate patient selection and counseling regarding the cancer minimizing role of hysterectomy and salpingectomy.

In contrast to Schulten et al.,[35] a large cohort study of 100,000 women 4 years postprolapse surgery with or without hysterectomy[46] found that hysterectomy was associated with a 1% to 3% decrease in risk of future prolapse surgery on multivariant analysis. Importantly, the overall risk of repeat surgery in both groups was relatively low at 3% to 4.4%.

Thus, in the medium term, the current data on vaginal uterine preserving surgery is conflicting. Further long-term trials evaluating function and reintervention outcomes for prolapse and malignancy are required to fully inform the debate regarding hysterectomy versus hysteropexy.

Vaginal mesh surgery for uterine prolapse

Vaginal mesh surgery remains a viable surgical option in some countries and as such is evaluated. Mesh hysteropexy has a more favorable perioperative morbidity profile[34] when compared to vaginal hysterectomy and concurrent vaginal mesh. However, vaginal mesh surgery is still associated with a higher overall mesh erosion and revision rate when compared to native tissue repairs.

In 2019 Nager et al.[47] reported on the outcomes of a randomized trial comparing mesh hysteropexy (Uphold, Boston Scientific, Marlborough, MA) to vaginal hysterectomy with uterosacral ligament suspension. At 3 years, there was no difference in the primary composite outcome of failure (defined as combination of [1] retreatment for prolapse either pessary fitting or surgery; [2] anatomical outcomes, defined as any POP-Q measure beyond the hymen; and [3] symptomatic outcomes) between the mesh (26%) and nonmesh repair (38%). Although the mesh hysteropexy group had longer total vaginal length and higher C point on examination, no additional benefit was seen in functional and quality-of-life outcomes or any differences in the recurrent prolapse rate. More importantly, the mesh erosion rate was still 8% for the hysteropexy group, and the mesh within this randomized trial as well as all other vaginal mesh kits are no longer commercially available in the United Kingdom, Australia, and United States.

Currently, with limited evidence on superior patient outcomes, mesh erosion risk, and restricted use of vaginal mesh kits worldwide, the role of vaginal mesh in uterine preservation remains unclear.

Other uterine-sparing procedures

In the recent decade, with the decline of vaginal mesh use, the Manchester repair classically used to treat prolapse in context of cervical elongation has seen some support as an alternative surgical option. There is low-quality evidence from retrospective series that demonstrate a shorter operative time, less blood loss, and longer return of prolapse with the Manchester repair[48,49] but no difference in repeat surgery rates[34] when compared to hysterectomy. Its benefits are offset by the risk of subsequent uterine malignancy, dysmenorrhea in event of cervical stenosis, risk of preterm delivery in the event of unexpected pregnancy, and more challenging hysterectomy in the future.

Furthermore, level 1 evidence supporting its use is still lacking. The results of the randomized SAM trial (SAM study: Manchester vs. sacrospinous hysteropexy currently still in recruitment)[50] may yield more information and clarify the role of this procedure in the patients' treatment pathway.

CONCLUSION

The evidence supports sacrocolpopexy as the gold standard treatment of post-hysterectomy vault prolapse. In contrast to this, the data supporting the use of sacrocolpopexy (either with total or with subtotal hysterectomy or sacrohysteropexy) for the management of uterine prolapse is lacking. The 2017 International Consultation on Incontinence (ICI) report on the surgical management of prolapse preferences the vaginal approach for the management of uterine prolapse.[38] For both uterine and vault prolapse vaginal mesh kits offer very little additional benefit when compared to native tissue repair or sacrocolpopexy and are currently unable to be performed in many countries throughout the world.

References

1. Wu JM, Matthews CA, Conover MM, et al. Lifetime risk of stress urinary incontinence or pelvic organ prolapse surgery. *Obstet Gynecol* 2014;123(6):1201–1206.
2. Nygaard I, Bradley C, Brandt D, et al. Pelvic organ prolapse in older women: Prevalence and risk factors. *Obstet Gynecol* 2004;104(3):489–497.
3. Ashton-Miller JA, DeLancey JO. Functional anatomy of the female pelvic floor. *Ann N Y Acad Sci* 2007;1101:266–296.
4. Swift SE. The distribution of pelvic organ support in a population of female subjects seen for routine gynecologic health care. *Am J Obstet Gynecol* 2000;183(2):277–285.
5. Delancey JO. Fascial and muscular abnormalities in women with urethral hypermobility and anterior vaginal wall prolapse. *Am J Obstet Gynecol* 2002;187(1):93–98.
6. Rooney K, Kenton K, Mueller ER, et al. Advanced anterior vaginal wall prolapse is highly correlated with apical prolapse. *Am J Obstet Gynecol* 2006;195(6):1837–1840.
7. Summers A, Winkel LA, Hussain HK, et al. The relationship between anterior and apical compartment support. *Am J Obstet Gynecol* 2006;194(5):1438–1443.
8. Eilber KS, Alperin M, Khan A, et al. Outcomes of vaginal prolapse surgery among female Medicare beneficiaries: The role of apical support. *Obstet Gynecol* 2013;122(5):981–987.
9. Elliott CS, Yeh J, Comiter CV, et al. The predictive value of a cystocele for concomitant vaginal apical prolapse. *J Urol* 2013;189(1):200–203.
10. Lowder JL, Park AJ, Ellison R, et al. The role of apical vaginal support in the appearance of anterior and posterior vaginal prolapse. *Obstet Gynecol* 2008;111(1):152–157.
11. FitzGerald MP, Richter HE, Siddique S, et al. Colpocleisis: A review. *Int Urogynecol J Pelvic Floor Dysfunct* 2006;17(3):261–271.
12. Buchsbaum GM, Lee TG. Vaginal obliterative procedures for pelvic organ prolapse: A systematic review. *Obstet Gynecol Surv* 2017;72(3):175–183.
13. Ilaya N, Baessler K, Christmann-Schmid C, et al. Prolapse and continence surgery in countries of the Organization for Economic Cooperation and Development in 2012. *Am J Obstet Gynecol* 2015;212(6):755.e1–755.e27.
14. Benson JT, Lucente V, McClellan E. Vaginal versus abdominal reconstructive surgery for the treatment of pelvic support defects: A prospective randomized study with long-term outcome evaluation. *Am J Obstet Gynecol* 1996;175(6):1418–1421.
15. Lo TS, Wang AC. Abdominal colposacropexy and sacrospinous ligament suspension for severe uterovaginal prolapse: A comparison. *J Gynecol Surg* 1998;14:59–64.
16. Maher CF, Qatawneh A, Dwyer P, et al. Abdominal sacral colpopexy or vaginal sacrospinous colpopexy for vaginal vault prolapse: A prospective randomized trial. *Am J Obstet Gynecol* 2004;190(1):20–26.
17. Rondini C, Braun H, Alvarez J, et al. High uterosacral vault suspension vs sacrocolpopexy for treating apical defects: A randomized controlled trial with twelve months follow-up. *Int Urogynecol J* 2015;26(8):1131–1138.
18. Maher C, Feiner B, DeCuyper E, et al. Laparoscopic sacral colpopexy versus total vaginal mesh for vaginal vault prolapse: A randomized trial. *Am J Obstet Gynecol* 2011;204(4):360.e1–360.e7.
19. Maher C, Feiner B, Baessler K, et al. Surgery for women with apical vaginal prolapse. *Cochrane Database Syst Rev* 2016;(10):CD012376.

20. Lucot J-P, Cosson M, Bader G, et al. Safety of vaginal mesh surgery versus laparoscopic mesh sacropexy for cystocele repair: Results of the prosthetic pelvic floor repair randomized controlled trial. *Eur Urol* 2018;74(2):167–176.

21. Siddiqui NY, Grimes CL, Casiano ER, et al. Mesh sacrocolpopexy compared with native tissue vaginal repair: A systematic review and meta-analysis. *Obstet Gynecol* 2015;125(1):44–55.

22. Freeman RM, Pantazis K, Thomson A, et al. A randomised controlled trial of abdominal versus laparoscopic sacrocolpopexy for the treatment of post-hysterectomy vaginal vault prolapse: LAS study. *Int Urogynecol J* 2013;24(3):377–384.

23. Tyson MD, Wolter CE. A comparison of 30-day surgical outcomes for minimally invasive and open sacrocolpopexy. *Neurourol Urodyn* 2015;34(2):151–155.

24. Claerhout F, Roovers JP, Lewi P, et al. Implementation of laparoscopic sacrocolpopexy—A single centre's experience. *Int Urogynecol J Pelvic Floor Dysfunct* 2009;20(9):1119–1125.

25. Paraiso MF, Jelovsek JE, Frick A, et al. Laparoscopic compared with robotic sacrocolpopexy for vaginal prolapse: A randomized controlled trial. *Obstet Gynecol* 2011;118(5):1005–1013.

26. Anger JT, Mueller ER, Tarnay C, et al. Robotic compared with laparoscopic sacrocolpopexy: A randomized controlled trial. *Obstet Gynecol* 2014;123(1):5–12.

27. Pan K, Zhang Y, Wang Y, et al. A systematic review and meta-analysis of conventional laparoscopic sacrocolpopexy versus robot-assisted laparoscopic sacrocolpopexy. *Int J Gynaecol Obstet* 2016;132(3):284–291.

28. van Zanten F, Schraffordt Koops SE, Pasker-de Jong PCM, et al. Learning curve of robot-assisted laparoscopic sacrocolpo(recto)pexy: A cumulative sum analysis. *Am J Obstet Gynecol* 2019;221(5):483.e1–483.e11.

29. Linder BJ, Anand M, Weaver AL, et al. Assessing the learning curve of robotic sacrocolpopexy. *Int Urogynecol J* 2016;27(2):239–246.

30. U.S. Food and Drug Administration. Urogynecologic surgical mesh implants. Updated August 16, 2021. Accessed November 10, 2020. https://www.fda.gov/medical-devices/implants-and-prosthetics/urogynecologic-surgical-mesh-implants#:~:text=On%20April%2C016%2C%202019%2C%20the,and%20distributing%20their%20products%20immediately.&text=The%20companies%20will%20have%2010,these%20products%20from%20the%20market

31. Jelovsek JE, Barber MD, Brubaker L, et al. Effect of uterosacral ligament suspension vs sacrospinous ligament fixation with or without perioperative behavioral therapy for pelvic organ vaginal prolapse on surgical outcomes and prolapse symptoms at 5 years in the OPTIMAL randomized clinical trial. *JAMA* 2018;319(15):1554–1565.

32. Lethaby A, Mukhopadhyay A, Naik R. Total versus subtotal hysterectomy for benign gynaecological conditions. *Cochrane Database Syst Rev* 2012;(4):CD004993.

33. Andersen LL, Zobbe V, Ottesen B, et al. Five-year follow up of a randomised controlled trial comparing subtotal with total abdominal hysterectomy. *BJOG* 2015;122(6):851–857.

34. Meriwether KV, Antosh DD, Olivera CK, et al. Uterine preservation vs hysterectomy in pelvic organ prolapse surgery: A systematic review with meta-analysis and clinical practice guidelines. *Am J Obstet Gynecol* 2018;219(2):129.e2–146.e2.

35. Schulten SFM, Detollenaere RJ, Stekelenburg J, et al. Sacrospinous hysteropexy versus vaginal hysterectomy with

36. uterosacral ligament suspension in women with uterine prolapse stage 2 or higher: Observational follow-up of a multicentre randomised trial. *BMJ* 2019;366:l5149.

36. Salvador S, Scott S, Francis JA, et al. No. 344-opportunistic salpingectomy and other methods of risk reduction for ovarian/fallopian tube/peritoneal cancer in the general population. *J Obstet Gynaecol Can* 2017;39(6):480–493.

37. ACOG Committee Opinion No. 774: Opportunistic salpingectomy as a strategy for epithelial ovarian cancer prevention. *Obstet Gynecol* 2019;133:e279–e284.

38. Abrams P, Cardozo L, Wagg A, et al. *Incontinence*, 6th ed. Bristol: International Continence Society, 2017.

39. Myers EM, Siff L, Osmundsen B, et al. Differences in recurrent prolapse at 1 year after total vs supracervical hysterectomy and robotic sacrocolpopexy. *Int Urogynecol J* 2015;26(4):585–589.

40. Pan K, Cao L, Ryan NA, et al. Laparoscopic sacral hysteropexy versus laparoscopic sacrocolpopexy with hysterectomy for pelvic organ prolapse. *Int Urogynecol J* 2016;27(1):93–101.

41. Rahmanou P, White B, Price N, et al. Laparoscopic hysteropexy: 1- to 4-year follow-up of women postoperatively. *Int Urogynecol J* 2014;25(1):131–138.

42. Roovers J-P, van der Vaart CH, van der Bom JG, et al. A randomised controlled trial comparing abdominal and vaginal prolapse surgery: Effects on urogenital function. *BJOG* 2004;111(1):50–56.

43. Roovers JP, van der Bom JG, van der Vaart CH, et al. A randomized comparison of post-operative pain, quality of life, and physical performance during the first 6 weeks after abdominal or vaginal surgical correction of descensus uteri. *Neurourol Urodyn* 2005;24(4):334–340.

44. van IJsselmuiden MN, van Oudheusden A, Veen J, et al. Hysteropexy in the treatment of uterine prolapse stage 2 or higher: Laparoscopic sacrohysteropexy versus sacrospinous hysteropexy—A multicentre randomised controlled trial (LAVA trial). *BJOG* 2020;127(10):1284–1293.

45. Madsen AM, Raker C, Sung VW. Trends in hysteropexy and apical support for uterovaginal prolapse in the United States from 2002 to 2012. *Female Pelvic Med Reconstr Surg* 2017;23(6):365–371.

46. Dallas K, Elliott CS, Syan R, et al. Association between concomitant hysterectomy and repeat surgery for pelvic organ prolapse repair in a cohort of nearly 100,000 women. *Obstet Gynecol* 2018;132(6):1328–1336.

47. Nager CW, Visco AG, Richter HE, et al. Effect of vaginal mesh hysteropexy vs vaginal hysterectomy with uterosacral ligament suspension on treatment failure in women with uterovaginal prolapse: A randomized clinical trial. *JAMA* 2019;322(11):1054–1065.

48. Thys SD, Coolen A-L, Martens IR, et al. A comparison of long-term outcome between Manchester Fothergill and vaginal hysterectomy as treatment for uterine descent. *Int Urogynecol J* 2011;22:1171–1178.

49. Tolstrup CK, Lose G, Klarskov N. The Manchester procedure versus vaginal hysterectomy in the treatment of uterine prolapse: A review. *Int Urogynecol J* 2017;28(1):33–40.

50. Schulten SFM, Enklaar RA, Kluivers KB, et al. Evaluation of two vaginal, uterus sparing operations for pelvic organ prolapse: Modified Manchester operation (MM) and sacrospinous hysteropexy (SSH), a study protocol for a multicentre randomized non-inferiority trial (the SAM study). *BMC Womens Health* 2019;19(1):49.

CHAPTER 46

SACROCOLPOPEXY

Ali Azadi • Polina Sawyer • Patrick Culligan

Introduction

Symptomatic pelvic organ prolapse is a common condition affecting women. Currently, it is estimated that 13% to 19% of women in the United States will undergo at least one surgical procedure to repair pelvic organ prolapse in their lifetimes.[1,2] Some studies have shown that up to 30% of these patients will require at least one additional surgical repair due to surgical failure and prolapse recurrence.[3]

The International Continence Society (ICS) defines "apical prolapse" as any descent of the vaginal cuff or cervix, below a point which is 2 cm less than the total vaginal length above the plane of the hymen.[4] Sacrocolpopexy is an abdominal procedure in which the apex of the vagina is affixed to the anterior longitudinal ligament overlying the sacral promontory of the sacral hollow at the level of the S1 vertebra using an intervening piece of mesh or graft material. This procedure functionally restores support of the vaginal apex and was originally described as a method specific to addressing prolapse of the apical compartment. Figure 46.1A shows normal pelvic organ anatomy in the sagittal view with Figures 46.1B and 46.1C demonstrating uterovaginal and posthysterectomy vaginal prolapse, respectively.

Sacral hysteropexy is the predecessor to the sacrocolpopexy and was first described in 1957 by Humphrey and colleagues[5] (Fig. 46.2). Posthysterectomy abdominal sacrocolpopexy (ASC) for vaginal vault prolapse was then described by Lane[6] in 1962. This version of the procedure has been widely adopted and is the most studied, although several other important modifications have been introduced over the years. For example, later authors described the attachment of the mesh material along the full length of the anterior vaginal wall as well as down to the level of the perineal body.[7] One important modification, the laparoscopic sacrocolpopexy, was first described in 1994 by Nezhat.[8] Currently, minimally invasive approaches using laparoscopy or robotic assistance are commonly adopted to perform sacrocolpopexy.

Regardless of the approach, the procedure uses a suspensory bridge of graft or mesh to attach the vaginal wall to the anterior longitudinal ligament of sacrum in order to suspend the vagina to the sacral promontory (see Fig. 46.2).

Sacrocolpopexy is considered to be the most durable surgical procedure for anatomic support of vaginal apex and has reported reoperation rates of less than 5%.[9,10] Although support of the vaginal apex can be provided by vaginal approach procedures such as the uterosacral ligament suspension or sacrospinous ligament fixation, sacrocolpopexy has several distinct advantages over these procedures. Specifically, sacrocolpopexy preserves vaginal length, provides support to anterior and posterior compartment, and reestablishes the anatomic vaginal axis. This is supported by several randomized control trials which suggest better objective anatomic outcomes with ASC as opposed to vaginal native tissue repair.[11,12]

ANATOMY

Knowledge of pelvic anatomy is critical to the surgeon performing sacrocolpopexy.

First, the surgeon should be familiar with the presacral space, which is a potential retroperitoneal space beginning below the bifurcation of the aorta. This space is bounded laterally by the common and internal iliac vessels and extends inferiorly to the superior fascia of the levator muscles.[13] Figure 46.3 shows the typical view encountered laparoscopically of the sacral promontory with an artistic rendering showing the structures typically located within close proximity to this space.

The sacral promontory represents the most superior aspect of the anterior surface of the first sacral vertebra and is a commonly used bony landmark in gynecologic surgery. The fifth lumbar intervertebral disc is found just superior to the sacral promontory. The anterior longitudinal ligament, which overlies the vertebra, is a common anchoring site for the sacral end of mesh during sacrocolpopexy. Several important structures run within close proximity to this space. The sacral promontory and presacral space are partially covered by the sigmoid colon and the ureters and common iliac and internal iliac vessels lie within close proximity to the midpoint of the sacral promontory.

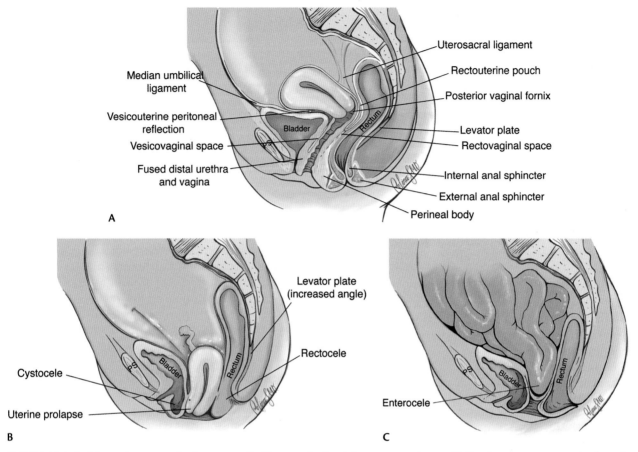

FIGURE 46.1 A: Normal uterovaginal support. **B:** Uterovaginal pelvic organ prolapse. **C:** Posthysterectomy vaginal prolapse. PS, pubic symphysis.

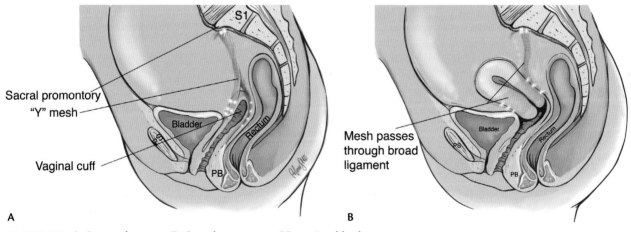

FIGURE 46.2 A: Sacrocolpopexy. **B:** Sacrohysteropexy. PB, perineal body.

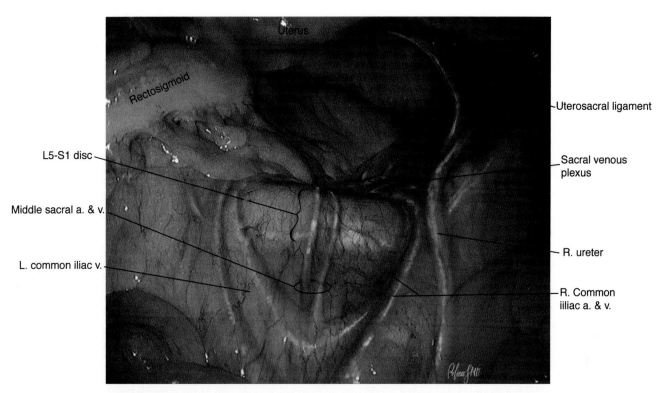

FIGURE 46.3 Laparoscopic view of sacral promontory with superimposed artistic rendering showing the relative proximity of important anatomic structures. a, artery; v, vein; R, right; L, left.

Identification of the major vessels within the lateral boundaries of the presacral space is essential during dissection as inadvertent injury to these vascular structures can lead to catastrophic bleeding. The aortic bifurcation generally occurs at the level of L4 with an average distance of 5.3 cm above the sacral promontory (Fig. 46.4). The left common iliac vein is the closest large vascular structure to the midpoint of the sacral promontory with a mean reported distance of 27 mm (9 to 52 mm).[14]

Other important vascular structures within this area include the middle sacral artery, which branches from the posterior surface of the aorta and travels inferiorly within the areolar tissue of the presacral space. Likewise, its partner, the middle sacral vein,

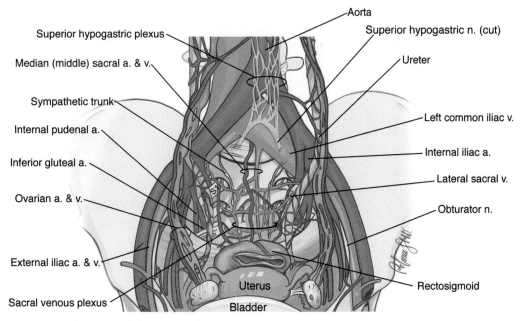

FIGURE 46.4 Anatomy of the presacral space. a, artery; n, nerve; v, vein.

arises from the vessels emerging beneath the common iliac veins and drains into the inferior vena cava. Both the middle sacral artery and vein can be easily identified lying directly on the midpoint of the sacral promontory.

The presacral venous plexus is another important anatomical structure that should be identified and avoided as damage to these structures could result in disastrous blood loss. This vascular plexus is composed of anastomoses between the lateral and median sacral veins from which blood courses into the pelvic fascia covering the body of sacrum. Surgeons should be careful to avoid injuring these vascular vessels during dissection and suturing around the sacral promontory.

The hypogastric plexus carries autonomic innervation to the pelvic viscera and descends into the pelvis anterior to the bifurcation of the aorta. In the presacral space, it is located anterior to the middle sacral artery and vein. Because the two trunks of the hypogastric nerves run within the uterosacral ligaments, the right uterosacral ligament remnant can be used as a landmark by surgeons to help to identify the hypogastric nerve as it enters the presacral space. Damage to the hypogastric plexus can result in bladder, bowel, and sexual dysfunction and should be avoided during the procedure.

The course of the ureters should be carefully considered as they descend from kidneys to enter the pelvis. This anatomy is particularly relevant during dissection of the peritoneum over the sacrum as well as extension of this peritoneal dissection inferiorly toward the posterior vaginal cuff.

The ureters exit the medial aspect of the renal pelvis and course inferiorly and medially over the psoas muscles in the retroperitoneal space of the upper pelvis. Surgically, they are most easily identified at the pelvic brim, where they course over the bifurcation of the internal and external iliac arteries. Here, they are within relatively close proximity to the midpoint of the sacral promontory. From here, the ureters follow the branches of the internal iliac arteries as they course along the medial leaflet of the posterior broad ligament within the pararectal space (Fig. 46.5).

The blood supply of the ureter changes as it courses from proximal to distal (see Fig. 46.4). In addition to being retroperitoneal, they are enveloped by an endopelvic fascial covering that is closely adherent to the peritoneum. Small arterioles travel through in this adventitial endopelvic fascial layer and provide the ureter with its blood supply. The upper ureters closest to the kidneys receive blood supply directly from the renal arteries. The middle ureter receives blood supply from the ovarian vessels and from direct branches of the internal iliac arteries. However, once the ureter crosses the bifurcation of the common iliac vessels as it enters the pelvis, it receives blood supply on its lateral side, from branches of the internal iliac vessels (superior vesical, uterine, middle rectal, vaginal, and inferior vesical arteries).

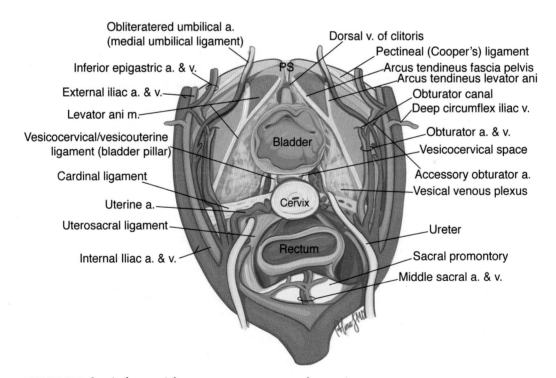

FIGURE 46.5 Surgical potential spaces. a, artery; m, muscle; v, vein.

CHOICE OF MESH/GRAFT

Different types of materials have been used as grafts in sacrocolpopexy. These include autologous and cadaveric fascia, xenograft, as well as synthetic materials. Graft materials should have several important general properties.

First, the ideal graft material should be chemically and physically inert while remaining biocompatible and noncarcinogenic. Secondly, an ideal graft material should be sterilizable and resistant to infection. Also, because the material is used to elevate the vaginal apex and is subject to fluctuations in intra-abdominal pressures, the material should be durable and strong while still maintaining some degree of flexibility. Finally, the material should be affordable and easily manufactured. With these properties in mind, the ideal mesh used in ASC surgery should restore normal anatomy and allow for normal function of the vagina and pelvic organs.

Permanent synthetic mesh has the highest success rates and is the best studied of all of the graft materials used in sacrocolpopexy. Although there are several different types of synthetic meshes that have been used, type 1 mesh is currently the most commonly used and associated with the lowest rates of adverse clinical outcomes. Type 1 mesh consists of light weight monofilament polypropylene with large-pore sizes (>75 μm). Type 1 mesh is commercially available in both Y-shaped and single-stranded configurations, with selection being dependent on surgeon preference (Fig. 46.6).[15]

Knitted mesh is preferred over woven mesh as it allows macrophages to traverse the mesh (except at the interstices where the spaces are too small for a macrophage to enter) and allows for the deposition of the most ideal collagen type.

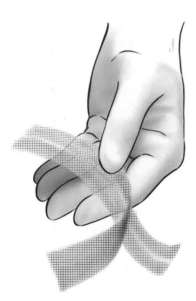

FIGURE 46.6 Typical appearance of a Y-shaped mesh used for sacrocolpopexy.

Ultralightweight (i.e., ≤25 grams/meter^2) loosely knitted polypropylene mesh is currently the best available choice for sacrocolpopexy. The long-term safety and efficacy of this mesh have been well studied.[16,17]

Besides synthetic meshes, autologous as well as xenograft materials have been used in sacrocolpopexy. A 2005 double-blinded randomized clinical trial comparing the surgical outcomes of solvent dehydrated cadaveric fascia lata with synthetic polypropylene mesh in sacrocolpopexy found improved outcomes with synthetic mesh.[18] In this study, 91% of the patients who received synthetic mesh ($n = 54$) were classified as clinically cured at 1 year as compared to 68% of the fascia lata ($n = 46$) group. However, a 2013 study comparing the 12-month surgical outcomes of porcine dermis to polypropylene mesh for laparoscopic sacrocolpopexy found no statistically significant difference in "clinical cure" between the two groups.[19]

EFFICACY AND COMPARATIVE OUTCOMES

ASC is an effective surgical procedure for the treatment of apical prolapse.[11]

A comprehensive review of outcome of ASC studies has been published by Nygaard.[9] The study looked at outcomes of sacrocolpopexy in the time period ranging from 1966 to 2004. Key findings of the study were that success rate, when defined as lack of apical prolapse postoperatively, ranged from 78% to 100%. The median reoperation rates for pelvic organ prolapse and for stress urinary incontinence were 4.4% (range 0% to 18.2%) and 4.9% (range 1.2% to 30.9%), respectively. The study also found relatively low rates of mesh exposure with an overall rate of 3.4%. However, the study found that functional outcomes such as the effect of ASC on bowel or bladder function were not well studied (Table 46.1).

In addition to the aforementioned study, the Colpopexy and Urinary Reduction Efforts (CARE) trial is a landmark study which has provided significant insights into the long-term surgical outcomes of sacrocolpopexy procedures. The study was designed to assess the utility of retropubic urethropexy, or Burch, performed at the time of sacrocolpopexy. Initial 2-year outcome data showed that ASC was associated with very low rates of surgical failure.[24] However, a secondary analysis evaluating surgical outcomes at 7 years (the extended-CARE or "e-CARE" trial) reported much higher failure rates ranging from 34% to 48%. Notably, the study used composite outcomes including both subjective and anatomic findings to define success. Consequently, one of the criticisms of this paper is that this strategy of defining failure may not have fully captured the scope of patient bother, which is reflected in the finding that ultimately only 5% of patients underwent reoperation for recurrent prolapse. Another criticism of the e-CARE study was the high rate of attrition because

TABLE 46.1
Landmark Studies of Abdominal Sacrocolpopexy

LANDMARK STUDIES OF ABDOMINAL SACROCOLPOPEXY

REFERENCE	STUDY DESIGN	FOLLOW-UP	CRITERIA	COMMENTS
1996 Benson et al.[20]	RCT comparing outcomes of vaginal repair[a] vs. abdominal sacrocolpopexy	Mean 2.5 y	88 women with cervical prolapse to or beyond the hymen or with vaginal vault inversion >50% of its length and anterior vaginal wall descent to or beyond the hymen were randomized to a vaginal ($n = 48$) vs. abdominal surgical approach ($n = 40$).	The relative risk (RR) of optimal effectiveness by the abdominal route was 2.03 (95% confidence interval [CI] 1.22–9.83), and the RR of unsatisfactory outcome by the vaginal route was 2.11 (95% CI 0.90–4.94).
2004 Nygaard et al.[9]	Cochrane Database Systematic Review looking at outcomes of abdominal sacrocolpopexy	6 mo–3 y	Included seven studies which defined "success" using variable anatomic and subjective symptomatic outcomes	Success rate for apical support 78%–100% Success in all compartments 58%–100% Mean rate of mesh exposure was 3.4%. Median reoperation rate for prolapse and SUI 4.4% and 4.9% respectively
2011 Culligan et al.[21]	RCT comparing use of autologous fascia vs. synthetic mesh in ASC	5 y	Primary outcome was objective anatomic failure: any Pelvic Organ Prolapse Quantification (POP-Q) point ≥ -1. Secondary outcome was clinical failure—presence of bulge or prolapse symptoms and either a POP-Q point C $\geq \frac{1}{2}$ TVL or any POP-Q point >0—and interim surgical retreatment.	Objective anatomic success rates were: mesh 93% (27/29) and fascia 62% (18/29) ($P = .02$). Clinical success rates were: mesh 97% (28/29) and fascia 90% (26/29) ($P = .61$).
2013 Nygaard et al.[22]	PFDN multicenter study of Colpopexy and Urinary Reduction Efforts (CARE) trial of women with stress continence who underwent abdominal sacrocolpopexy between 2002 and 2005 for symptomatic POP and also received either concomitant Burch urethropexy or no urethropexy	7 y	Women without SUI undergoing abdominal sacrocolpopexy for POP between 2001 and 2006 (CARE trial) to study whether adding a prophylactic anti-incontinence procedure (Burch urethropexy) effects de novo SUI, a common adverse event after POP surgery.	7-year failure was 34% in the urethropexy group and was 48% in the no-urethropexy group. Only 5% underwent reoperation for failure. Mesh exposure probability at 7 y was 10.5%.
2016 Maher et al.[23]	Cochrane Database Systematic Review	Mean 2 y	Included six RCTs comparing outcomes of vaginal–based apical prolapse repair with sacral colpopexy for apical prolapse repair in women with at least stage 2 apical prolapse	Awareness of prolapse: RR 2.11 (CI 1.06–4.21) for vaginal approach at 2 y Repeat surgery for prolapse: RR 2.28 (CI 1.20–4.32) for vaginal approach at 2 y Risk of repeat surgery for incontinence was not significantly increased in the vaginal approach compared with sacrocolpopexy RR 1.87 (CI 0.72–4.86).

[a]Vaginal repair was a performed via a bilateral sacrospinous vault suspension and paravaginal repair.
ASC, abdominal sacrocolpopexy; CI, confidence interval; mo, months; n, nerve; PFDN, Pelvic Floor Disorders Network; POP, pelvic organ prolapse; RCT, randomized controlled trial; SSLF, sacrospinous ligament fixation; SUI, stress urinary incontinence; TVL, total vaginal length; y, year.

less than 40% of the original study group completed long-term subjective and objective follow-up.

In the CARE trial, mesh exposures occurred in 5% of patients at 7 years. Here, it is important to note that the majority of mesh-related complications were associated with the use of a nonpolypropylene (Teflon) mesh material, which is no longer used in practice. The use of contemporary type 1 surgical mesh products seems to be associated with significantly lower rates of mesh exposures.

Studies comparing ASC with vaginal approaches to prolapse repair have shown that ASC is associated with higher intraoperative morbidity, longer operating time, higher blood loss, and longer hospital stay. However, several randomized controlled trials and Cochrane reviews have shown superiority of the ASC when compared to vaginal reconstructive techniques. In contrast, the Operations and Pelvic Muscle Training in the Management of Apical Support Loss (OPTIMAL) trial, which looked at outcomes from two common vaginal reconstructive techniques found failure rates of around 25% at 2 years and near 47% at 5 years for both procedures.[25]

The majority of the studies cited in this chapter evaluated the outcomes of ASC using an open technique. This fails to address the question of outcomes from laparoscopic and robotic-assisted procedures, which are techniques more commonly employed in ASC today. The data that is available has shown that minimally invasive techniques are associated with similar success rates with advantages of decreased intraoperative blood loss, rapid postoperative recovery, and reduced pain.[26,35]

Likewise, in a randomized controlled trial in which women were assigned to laparoscopic versus open ASC, no differences were demonstrated between recurrence of apical prolapse, surgical complications, or mesh exposure at a mean of 41 months of follow-up. In one study, significantly higher numbers of anterior compartment prolapse recurrences were encountered in the laparoscopic compared with the abdominal group (18% vs. 2%).[27]

Studies comparing the mode of minimally invasive techniques have shown no differences in anatomical or subjective outcomes between laparoscopic or robotic-assisted techniques. Most of these studies did show that robotic assistance was associated with higher costs.[28]

Although short-term studies show upwards of 95% success rates with minimally invasive techniques, reported long-term follow-up of patients following minimally invasive versus open surgical techniques did note an increase in rate of recurrent prolapse; however, these differences were small.[26]

IMPACT OF FDA ADVISORY ON USE OF TRANSVAGINAL MESH

The use of sacrocolpopexy to treat pelvic organ prolapse has increased in recent years, and the popularity of these procedures coincides with a decline in the use of transvaginal mesh as a result of a recent U.S. Food and Drug Administration (FDA) Notification.[29]

Midurethral slings and mesh used for sacrocolpopexy were not included in this recommendation and thus have remained on the market. Consequently, surgeons looking for durable repair options for pelvic organ prolapse are more frequently looking to the sacrocolpopexy as a surgical treatment option.

This coupled with better anatomic success, increased resilience, high patient satisfaction, and increased use of minimally invasive modalities explains why sacrocolpopexy has been increasingly considered as a primary surgical option for women who present with vaginal vault or uterovaginal prolapse.[30,31]

PREOPERATIVE CONSIDERATIONS

The decision to proceed with an abdominal versus vaginal approach is affected by multiple factors including patient preference; surgeon experience; degree and severity of prolapse; patient age and level of physical activity; as well as patient weight, surgical history, presence of urinary and defecatory symptoms, and presence of concurrent pathology such as ovarian cysts, cervical dysplasia, or abnormal uterine bleeding.

During the preoperative evaluation, a detailed physical examination with assessment of each vaginal compartment for support defects is essential. Because isolated apical prolapse is rare, careful assessment of the anterior and posterior wall is important.[32] Physical examination findings should be correlated to patient symptoms because this will help to set realistic expectations and postoperative goals. Correction of prolapse without alleviation of symptoms is clearly not productive and places patients under unjustified harm with minimal benefit. Several validated questionnaires have been developed to assist the clinician in assessing the presence and severity of subjective symptomatology and their impact on the patient's quality of life.

Apical prolapse frequently coexists with voiding dysfunction. For women undergoing repair of apical prolapse, a concomitant continence procedure is often performed if indicated to treat or prevent stress urinary incontinence.

Studies have reported various percentages of continent women developing symptoms of stress urinary incontinence after surgical correction of prolapse, also called "de novo" stress incontinence.[33] Preoperative evaluation for occult stress urinary incontinence can be performed through an office cough stress test with reduction of prolapse or with multichannel urodynamics.

Consent

Informed consent and shared decision-making are important when discussing surgical options with patients. Physicians should make efforts to establish appropriate postoperative expectations with their patients regarding symptom resolution as well as the impact of surgery on their quality of life. Postoperative satisfaction scores after surgery correlate highly with the patient's perceived achievement of self-described preoperative goals but poorly with objective outcome measures.[34]

The informed consent should include a discussion of surgical risks and a discussion of options for alternative surgical as well as conservative treatment options. Physicians should strive to provide evidence-based expectations for short- as well as long-term clinical outcomes including overall success rates, potential complications such as mesh complications, and risk of adverse postoperative symptoms including dyspareunia, pelvic pain, new or worsening urinary symptoms including urinary incontinence, and risk of reoperation. For minimally invasive procedures, the risk of conversion to laparotomy should be discussed.

Women undergoing a sacrocolpopexy should particularly be counseled regarding the potential short- and long-term risks of mesh.

SACROCOLPOPEXY (OPEN ABDOMINAL, LAPAROSCOPY, ROBOTIC ASSISTED)

Robotic-assisted sacrocolpopexy is performed similarly to the laparoscopic approach; however, there are some important modifications.

First, trocar placement in robotic surgery should allow for proper docking to enable the surgeon to perform all of the required steps of the operation without redocking. Figure 46.7 shows a typical trocar placement scheme for the da Vinci Xi robotics system. This configuration has been simplified into a straight-across scheme from the previous "W" shaped scheme used in the older Si system.

Several trials evaluating robotic-assisted versus laparoscopic sacrocolpopexy have shown that robotic assistance is associated with acceptable complication rates and a relatively short learning curve as compared to the laparoscopic sacrocolpopexy.[35,36] Surgically, potential advantages of robotic surgery include three-dimensional (3-D) magnified visualization as well as improved dexterity and ergonomics. The advantages particularly relevant to sacrocolpopexy include the availability of an additional robotic arm, which allows surgeons to retract and manipulate the mesh for themselves, as opposed to relying on a trained assistant as they would in "straight-stick" laparoscopy. Additionally, articulation of the surgical instruments close

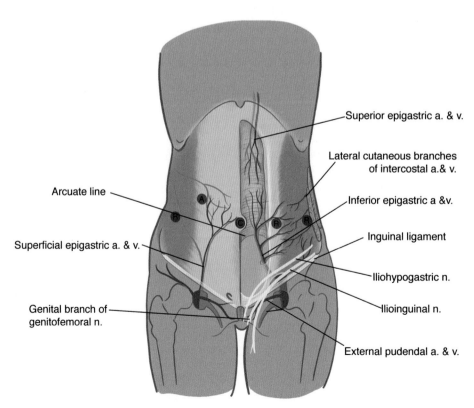

FIGURE 46.7 Typical port placement for robotic systems. A, assistant port; R, robotic port; C, camera port

to their tips allows the instruments to operate within the presacral space at an angle that provides an option with appropriate distance to major vessels.

SACROCOLPOPEXY WITH UTERINE PRESERVATION (SACROHYSTEROPEXY)

Although hysterectomy has traditionally been performed at the time of surgeries for prolapse repair, there is little evidence to support such practice. Uterine preservation during prolapse surgery has been considered with growing emphasis on patient-centered shared decision-making.

Meta-analysis studies have shown that uterine-preserving prolapse repair procedures are associated with decreased operative time, decreased blood loss, and decreased risk of mesh exposure when compared with similar surgical routes with concomitant hysterectomy. Data has also suggested that uterine preservation does not significantly change short-term prolapse outcomes. Although it is suggested that surgeons discuss uterine preservation as an option to appropriate candidates, patients should be counseled regarding the lack of long-term data pertaining to the outcomes and risks of hysteropexy procedures.[37,38] They particularly need to be counseled regarding the challenges of future pelvic surgeries if mesh is used for hysteropexy.

In cases where patients elect uterine preservation, it is essential that cervical and uterine pathologies are excluded prior to surgery. Women at high risk for endometrial carcinoma may not be ideal candidates for uterine preservation, and thorough counseling is imperative.

Women who choose uterine preservation for fertility should be counseled about the lack of strong data regarding pregnancy outcomes as well as the possible effect of prior hysteropexy on mode of delivery and uncertain effect of pregnancy on prolapse outcomes.

During sacrohysteropexy, the graft is attached to the posterior vaginal wall and cervix. Then, similar to sacrocolpopexy, the mesh is attached to the anterior longitudinal ligament of sacrum (see Fig. 46.2B). The anterior graft can be attached to the anterior surface of the cervix and anterior vaginal wall and brought to the sacrum through an opening created in the broad ligament.

Data regarding surgical outcomes of sacrohysteropexy have been promising with the majority of studies demonstrating good outcomes for apical support. Studies have been conflicting, however, regarding outcomes within the anterior and posterior compartments.[39,40]

SACROCOLPOPEXY WITH TOTAL HYSTERECTOMY VERSUS SUPRA CERVICAL HYSTERECTOMY

Because the majority of the studies show increased risk of mesh exposure with concomitant total hysterectomy, some surgeons adopt supracervical hysterectomy as the preferred method. By leaving the cervix in-situ, it is theorized that the cervix acts as a buffer and decreases potential exposure of the mesh to vagina.

The ICS released a proposed surgical decision-making algorithm in 2019 which recommended that physicians perform a supracervical hysterectomy in all cases where women elect a sacrocolpopexy and do not desire uterine preservation.

In the case of supracervical hysterectomy, the surgeon should consider anterior and posterior compartment defects carefully with proper dissection and mesh attachment in these compartments. The risk of future trachelectomy in the presence of mesh should be carefully considered in the decision making process as this surgery may be particularly challenging.

SACRAL COLPOPERINEOPEXY

Sacral colpoperineopexy is a modification of sacral colpopexy aimed at correcting a combination of conditions including apical prolapse, rectocele, and perineal descent.

One theory suggests that excessive perineal descent occurs due to detachment of the "rectovaginal septum" from the perineal body. Although the presence of the rectovaginal septum has been debated among experts, it is known that regardless of etiology, perineal descent may be associated with variety of defecatory disorders. Additionally, with progressive descent of the perineum, stretch injuries can occur to the pudendal nerve, resulting in neuropathic symptoms.[41–43]

During sacral colpoperineopexy, a continuous graft is placed from the anterior longitudinal ligament to the perineal body. This can be accomplished either through an abdominal or combined abdominal and vaginal approach.

With the abdominal approach, the rectovaginal space is dissected toward the perineal body and the posterior mesh is sutured to it.

With the combined abdominal and vaginal approach, the posterior vaginal wall is opened, and a rectocele repair is completed. Then, the vaginal and abdominal dissections are connected, and mesh is anchored inferiorly to the perineal body and laterally to the arcus tendineus fascia rectovaginalis.

COMPLICATIONS OF SACROCOLPOPEXY

Presacral Hemorrhage/Blood Transfusion

Presacral hemorrhage and blood transfusion has been reported to complicate 4.4% of ASC procedures (Table 46.2). Due to the venous nature of the bleeding in this type of injury, pressure should be applied to obtain hemostasis. Other methods may include use of bone wax, titanium thumb tacks, topical hemostatics, or a portion of rectus muscle applied to the bleeding sacrum and then deeply coagulated to stop bleeding. Conversion to laparotomy should be considered if required to obtain hemostasis.

TABLE 46.2

Complication Rates Associated with Abdominal Sacrocolpopexy

COMPLICATION	REPORTED RATE
Urinary tract infection (UTI)	~10%
Mesh complications	0%–27%
Presacral hemorrhage	4.4%
Wound infection	4.6%
Port site hernia	0.3%
Thromboembolic event	3.3%
Cystotomy	3.1%
Ureteral injury	1.0%
Enterotomy/proctotomy	0.3% (LSC)–1.6% (open)
Ileus	3.6%
Small bowel obstruction	0.7%

LSC, laparoscopic sacrocolpopexy.

Complications of Mesh

In order to achieve a consensus on terminology and severity of mesh-related complications, the International Urogynecological Association (IUGA) and ICS convened an expert panel to recommend appropriate terminology to report on mesh complications. This group recommended the term *exposure* be used to describe "vaginal mesh visualized through separated vaginal epithelium." They likewise recommended that the term *erosion* be avoided and be replaced by terms with greater physical specificity and clarity. Although the term erosion was used in earlier studies, the authors of this chapter have purposely avoided the use of this term in accordance with the IUGA and ICS recommendations.[44]

Vaginal mesh exposure is the most commonly identified mesh complication following ASC with a widely reported range of 0% to 27%.[45,46] Non-type 1 polypropylene mesh, smoking, and concomitant total hysterectomy have been identified as risk factors that increase the risk of mesh exposure.[29,47–50] Seven-year follow-up of the CARE trial showed a 10% mesh exposure rate and was a rate that was higher than previous reports. It is important to note that older mesh types (including Teflon) were included in this study group.

Retrospective analysis of Mersilene mesh showed that this type of mesh was associated with about a 4% risk of mesh exposure.[51]

The data regarding mesh exposure rate with concurrent hysterectomy is controversial. Whereas some authors have shown no increased risk of mesh exposure with hysterectomy, many others have shown increased risk of exposure in sacrocolpopexy if done at the same time of total hysterectomy.[52–54]

Theoretically, placement of synthetic mesh over a healing sutured incision with exposure to vaginal microbial flora can increase the risk of exposure. Consequently, some suggest that supracervical hysterectomy may leave the cervix as a barrier and therefore decrease risk of mesh exposure.

Finally, studies on lightweight mesh have suggested that mesh exposure rates may be lower with these mesh types when compared with heavier mesh types.[55]

Incisional Problems

Wound infection and dehiscence have been reported up to 4.6%. With widespread use of minimally invasive approaches, incisional problems are less frequently encountered. Some studies report port site hernias as 0.3%.

Discitis and Osteomyelitis

Few case reports have been published regarding the risk of osteomyelitis and discitis following sacrocolpopexy. These complications may arise shortly after surgery, or may arise several years after the procedure. Available evidence suggests that this is a rare complication with an incidence of less than 1 per 1000 cases.[56]

Gastrointestinal Complications and UTI

Studies report that gastrointestinal complications, such as small bowel obstruction or ileus, occur after 0.1% to 5% of open ASCs and after 0.7% to 2.5% of minimally invasive sacrocolpopexies.[57]

In the CARE trial, 4 of 322 women required reoperation for small bowel obstruction, and all were associated with incisional problems. No intraoperative bowel injuries were reported.

Urinary tract infections are the most common complications reported after surgery with up a 10% reported incidence cited in the literature.

SURGICAL TECHNIQUE (TABLE 46.3)

ASC can be performed through a laparotomy incision, by laparoscopy or robotic-assisted laparoscopy. Despite differences in the surgical approach, the principles of the procedure should remain the same.

Positioning

The patient is placed in dorsal lithotomy position (Fig. 46.8). Laparoscopic and robotic-assisted approaches require placing the patient in steep Trendelenburg position to allow small bowel and redundant colon to move out of the pelvis. It is the responsibility of the surgeon to check the position in order to avoid any injuries. Potential sites of injury include the femoral, tibial, sacral, and ulnar nerves as well as the brachial plexus if undue stretch is inadvertently placed on the neck during

TABLE 46.3

Suggested Steps of Abdominal Sacrocolpopexy

SURGICAL STEP	DESCRIPTION
Step 1	Patient positioning
Step 2	Abdominal entry
Step 3	Development of the presacral space and the peritoneal incision with visualization of the anterior longitudinal ligament. Peritoneal incision extends to the posterior vaginal cuff.
Step 4	Dissection of the rectovaginal space
Step 5	Dissection of the vesicovaginal space
Step 6	Attachment of the anterior and posterior arms of the mesh
Step 7	Attachment of the mesh to the anterior longitudinal ligament overlying S1 vertebra
Step 8	Closure of the peritoneum over the mesh
Step 9	Cystourethroscopy

positioning. The patient's arms are usually tucked into her sides to allow the surgeon to maneuver around the patient. Care should be taken during positioning to pad the arms and ensure anatomic position of the arms with thumbs facing up toward the ceiling.

After prepping the patient's abdomen, perineum, and vagina and after completion of draping, a urethral catheter will be inserted prior to starting surgery. Prophylactic antibiotics, usually with a second-generation cephalosporin, are administered prior to the surgical incision.

If hysterectomy is done concomitantly, a uterine manipulator can be placed.

Abdominal Incision/Trocar Placement

A lower transverse abdominal or a vertical incision can provide adequate exposure for open ASC.

The choice of incision is based on surgeon's preference, patient's anatomy, and coexisting pathologies.

For laparoscopic or robotic procedures, trocar placement can be done by several different methods. For the initial trocar insertion, using Veress needle, open technique, and entry via visual access trocars are among the most common methods.

All the other trocars should be placed under direct visualization and with care to avoid injury to superficial and inferior epigastric vessels. The locations of trocar placement vary according to surgeon's preference. The goal is to provide adequate access to perform all of the required steps of the procedure (see Fig. 46.7).

Dissection

- Vesicovaginal dissection
- Rectovaginal dissection
- Dissection over the sacral promontory
- Peritoneal dissection over the uterosacral ligaments

Lysis of adhesions will be done if adhesions of the bowel to the pelvis are encountered to restore normal anatomy and obtain optimal exposure. Key pelvic structures including major vessels over the sacrum and course of ureter should be identified.

If hysterectomy is planned, it will be completed at this point (total vs. supracervical).

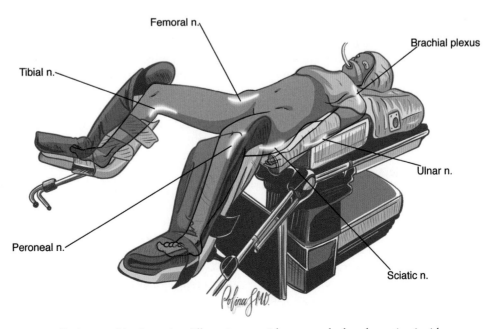

FIGURE 46.8 Patient positioning using Allen stirrups with arms tucked at the patient's sides. n, nerve.

Retraction of the small intestine out of the pelvis and to the right toward the ileocecal junction will improve the visualization of the sacrum. Retraction of the sigmoid colon to the left will facilitate the exposure over the sacrum.

Some surgeons start with dissection over the sacral promontory (Fig. 46.9A) first, whereas others start with the rectovaginal (Fig. 46.9B) and vesicovaginal (Fig. 46.9C) dissection.

After retraction of the sigmoid colon and opening the peritoneum over the sacral promontory, the presacral space is entered (see Fig. 46.9A). Then, the anterior longitudinal ligament of sacrum is exposed by gentle blunt dissection and minimal use of cautery if needed to clear the sacral promontory. Excellent visualization is essential for dissection of the sacral promontory. After the sigmoid colon is retracted to the left and the right ureter is identified, the peritoneal incision is made by elevating the peritoneum covering the sacral promontory medial to the right ureter.

After opening the peritoneum, the vesicovaginal (see Fig. 46.9C) and the rectovaginal (see Fig. 46.9B) dissections are performed using a combination of sharp and blunt dissection techniques.

The vesicovaginal dissection is performed to mobilize the bladder from the anterior vaginal wall and to expose an adequate portion of the vaginal wall for attachment of the mesh (see Fig. 46.9C).

The rectovaginal dissection is continued until the rectal reflection or perineal body reached (see Fig. 46.9B).

Placing a vaginal manipulator provides adequate exposure and countertraction which facilitates the dissection. There are variety of instruments and commercially made devices that can be used for this purpose (Fig. 46.10).

Identifying the border of the bladder and rectum may be difficult in some cases. Surgeons use techniques such as backfilling the bladder and simultaneous placement of a rectal probe (EEA sizer) to identify these structures.

The extent of dissection on the anterior and posterior vaginal walls depends on the extent of the defect present in different compartments involved. In most cases, inadequate dissection and suboptimal attachment of the mesh may increase the failure rate with recurrent prolapse of the anterior or posterior vaginal walls. If excessive perineal descent exists, the rectovaginal dissection is extended and the distal portion of the mesh is attached to the perineal body (sacrocolpoperineopexy).

Attachment of Graft (Fig. 46.9D,E)

There is no consensus regarding the ideal method and material used to attach the mesh to vaginal tissue and the anterior longitudinal ligament of sacrum.

Traditionally, permanent sutures have been used for the attachment of mesh to the vagina and sacrum. Passage through vaginal epithelium should be avoided if permanent material is used.

There has been a trend toward the use of delayed absorbable material to suture the graft to the vagina. Studies have shown that the suture type used for vaginal graft attachment did not influence mesh or suture exposure rates or composite success.[58]

Typically, a series of interrupted sutures attach the mesh to the vagina. The sutures are typically placed laterally. Some surgeons recommend incorporating the mesh onto the levator ani muscle at the attachment of rectovaginal fascia.

A variety of techniques and materials have been described. Some surgeons use a running barbed suture to minimize the operating time; however, these sutures have an increased risk of bacterial colonization, biologic tissue ingrowth response, and higher tissue reactivity.[59]

After mesh is attached to the endopelvic fascia of the vaginal wall, the tension of the mesh is adjusted prior to suturing to the anterior longitudinal ligament of the sacrum. One should avoid excessive tension during adjustment. Postimplant shrinkage of the mesh should be considered. Overtension may increase the risk of developing de novo stress urinary incontinence postoperatively by changing the angle of urethrovesical junction.

The mesh arms then are attached to the anterior longitudinal ligament of the sacrum just below the most prominent point of the sacral promontory (Fig. 46.9F). These sutures are placed at the S1 to S2 level.

Attachment of the mesh to higher areas of the sacral promontory is not consistent with the original description of the procedure. However, many use a higher attachment to avoid the bleeding which can be profuse.

Higher attachments may theoretically increase the risk of discitis and osteomyelitis. The L5 to S1 disc is situated at the sacral prominence in the majority of cases.

Peritoneal Closure

Vaginal examination to confirm proper tension of the mesh and to ensure lack of suture in the vagina can be done after attachment of the mesh to the sacrum.

Peritoneal closure using running or interrupted sutures is done to avoid entrapment of the sigmoid colon and adhesion of the bowel to the mesh as well as the risk of small bowel obstruction.

Cystourethroscopy

Evaluation of the urethra and bladder is essential at the end of the procedure to confirm the integrity of the bladder and urethra.

Cystoscopy also confirms lack of bladder damage and presence of any mesh or suture placed inadvertently in the bladder during the dissection and suturing.

Patency of the ureters is supported by the finding of ureteral efflux during cystoscopy.

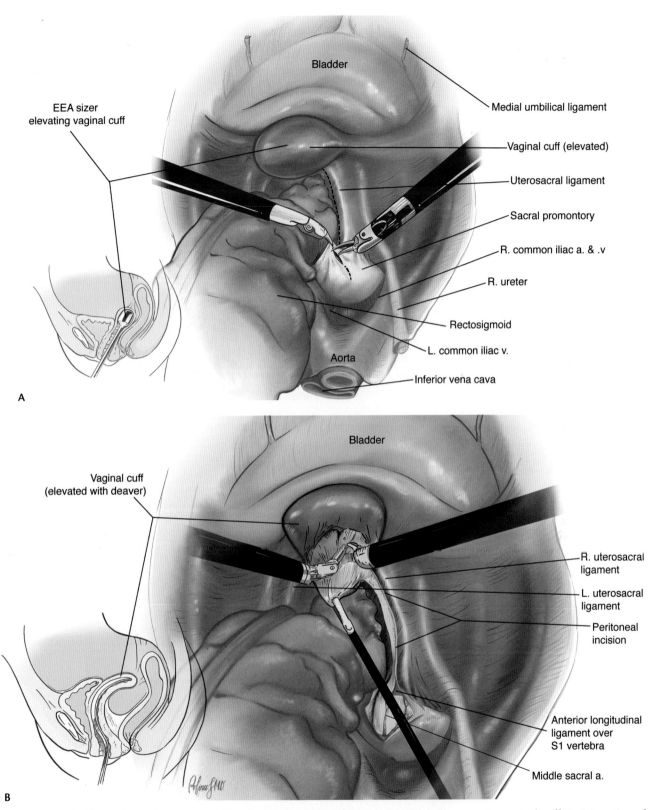

A: EEA sizer elevating vaginal cuff

Bladder

Medial umbilical ligament

Vaginal cuff (elevated)

Uterosacral ligament

Sacral promontory

R. common iliac a. & .v

R. ureter

Rectosigmoid

L. common iliac v.

Aorta

Inferior vena cava

A

Vaginal cuff (elevated with deaver)

Bladder

R. uterosacral ligament

L. uterosacral ligament

Peritoneal incision

Anterior longitudinal ligament over S1 vertebra

Middle sacral a.

B

FIGURE 46.9 **A:** The peritoneal incision overlies the sacral promontory and extends to the posterior vaginal cuff. **B:** Dissection of the rectovaginal space. a, artery; *dashed line*, extends to the posterior vaginal cuff; EEA, end to end anastomosis sizer; IVC, inferior vena cava, L, left; R, right; S1, first sacral vertebra; v, vein. *(Continued)*

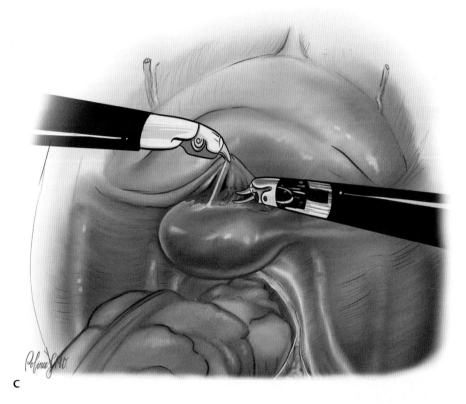

C

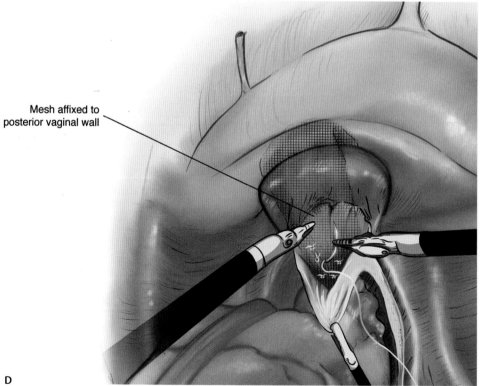

Mesh affixed to
posterior vaginal wall

D

FIGURE 46.9 *(Continued)* C: Dissection of vesicovaginal space. D: Attachment of posterior mesh arm.

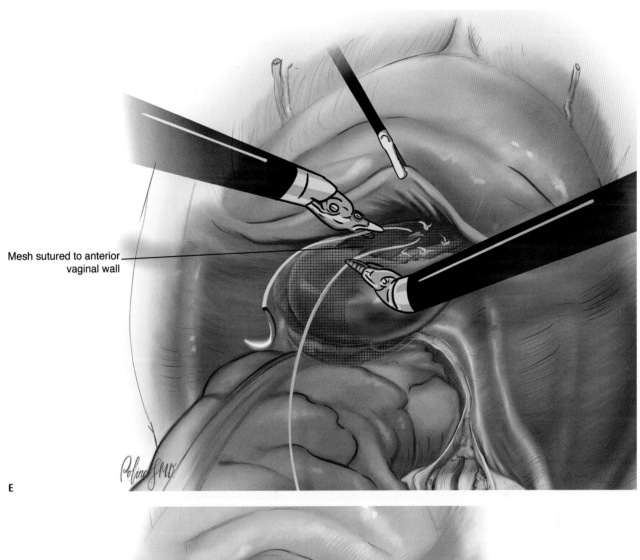

Mesh sutured to anterior
vaginal wall

E

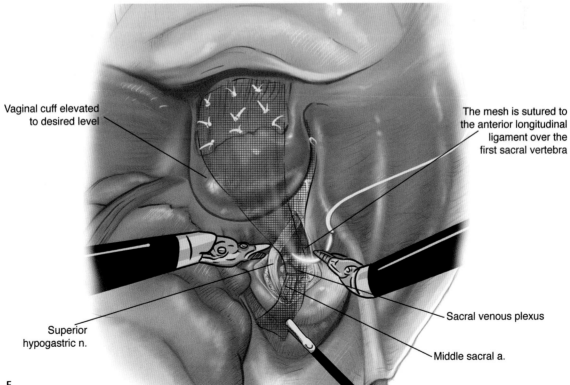

Vaginal cuff elevated
to desired level

The mesh is sutured to
the anterior longitudinal
ligament over the
first sacral vertebra

Sacral venous plexus

Superior
hypogastric n.

Middle sacral a.

F

FIGURE 46.9 *(Continued)* **E:** Attachment of anterior mesh arm. **F:** Attachment of mesh to the anterior longitudinal ligament.
a, artery; n, nerve.

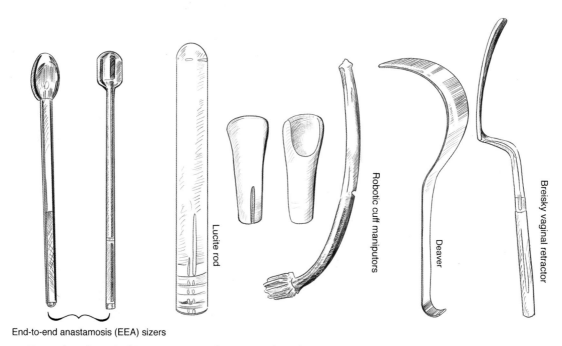

End-to-end anastamosis (EEA) sizers

FIGURE 46.10 Examples of surgical instruments used to manipulate the vaginal cuff during sacrocolpopexy procedure.

References

1. Wu JM, Matthews CA, Conover MM, et al. Lifetime risk of stress urinary incontinence or pelvic organ prolapse surgery. *Obstet Gynecol* 2014;123 (6):1201–1206.

2. Smith FJ, Holman CD, Moorin RE, et al. Lifetime risk of undergoing surgery for pelvic organ prolapse. *Obstet Gynecol* 2010;116(5):1096–1100.

3. Olsen AL, Smith VJ, Bergstrom JO, et al. Epidemiology of surgically managed pelvic organ prolapse and urinary incontinence. *Obstet Gynecol* 1997;89(4):501–506.

4. Abrams P, Cardozo L, Fall M, et al. The standardisation of terminology of lower urinary tract function: Report from the Standardisation Sub-Committee of the International Continence Society. *Neurourol Urodyn* 2002;21(2):167–178.

5. Humphrey A, Savage D. Uterine prolapse and prolapse of the vaginal vault treated by sacral hysteropexy. *BJOG* 1957;64(3): 355–360.

6. Lane FE. Repair of posthysterectomy vaginal-vault prolapse. *Obstet Gynecol* 1962;20:72–77.

7. Addison WA, Livengood CH, Sutton GP, et al. Abdominal sacral colpopexy with Mersilene mesh in the retroperitoneal position in the management of posthysterectomy vaginal vault prolapse and enterocele. *Obstet Gynecol* 1985;153(2):140–146.

8. Nezhat CH, Nezhat F, Nezhat C. Laparoscopic sacral colpopexy for vaginal vault prolapse. *Obstet Gynecol* 1994;84(5):885–888.

9. Nygaard IE, McCreery R, Brubaker L, et al. Abdominal sacrocolpopexy: A comprehensive review. *Obstet Gynecol* 2004;104(40):805–823.

10. Nygaard I, Brubaker L, Zyczynski HM, et al. Long-term outcomes following abdominal sacrocolpopexy for pelvic organ prolapse. *JAMA* 2013;309(19):2016–2024.

11. Maher C, Feiner B, Baessler K, et al. Surgical management of pelvic organ prolapse in women. *Cochrane Database Syst Rev* 2013;(4):CD004014.

12. Siddiqui NY, Grimes CL, Casiano ER, et al. Mesh sacrocolpopexy compared with native tissue vaginal repair: A systematic review and meta-analysis. *Obstet Gynecol* 2015;125(1):44–55.

13. Handa V, Van Le L. *Te Linde's operative gynecology*, 12th ed. Philadelphia: Wolters Kluwer, 2019.

14. Wieslander CK, Rahn DD, McIntire DD, et al. Vascular anatomy of the presacral space in unembalmed female cadavers. *Am J Obstet Gynecol* 2006;195(6):1736–1741.

15. Ostergard DR. Degradation, infection and heat effects on polypropylene mesh for pelvic implantation: What was known and when it was known. *Int Urogynecol J* 2011;22(7):771–774.

16. Culligan PJ, Lewis C, Priestley JL, et al. Long-term outcomes of robotic-assisted laparoscopic sacrocolpopexy using lightweight Y-mesh. *Female Pelvic Med Reconstr Surg* 2020;26(3):202–206.

17. Askew AL, Visco AG, Weidner AC, et al. Does mesh weight affect time to failure after robotic assisted laparoscopic sacrocolpopexy? *Female Pelvic Med Reconstr Surg* 2020;26(9):536–540.

18. Culligan PJ, Blackwell L, Goldsmith LJ, et al. A randomized controlled trial comparing fascia lata and synthetic mesh for sacral colpopexy. *Obstet Gynecol* 2005;106(1):29–37.

19. Culligan PJ, Salamon C, Priestley JL, et al. Porcine dermis compared with polypropylene mesh for laparoscopic sacrocolpopexy: A randomized controlled trial. *Obstet Gynecol* 2013;121(1): 143–151.

20. Benson JT, Lucente V, McClellan E. Vaginal versus abdominal reconstructive surgery for the treatment of pelvic support defects: A prospective randomized study with long-term outcome evaluation. *Am J Obstet Gynecol* 1996;175:1418–1422.

21. Tate SB, Blackwell L, Lorenz DJ, et al. Randomized trial of fascia lata and polypropylene mesh for abdominal sacrocolpopexy: 5-year follow-up. *Int Urogynecol J* 2011;22(2):137–143.

22. Nygaard I, Brubaker L, Zyczynski HM, et al. Long-term outcomes following abdominal sacrocolpopexy for pelvic organ prolapse. *JAMA* 2013;309(19):2016–2024.

23. Maher C, Feiner B, Baessler K, et al. Surgery for women with apical prolapse. *Cochrane Database Syst Rev* 2016;10(10):CD012376.

24. Brubaker L, Cundiff G, Fine P, et al. A randomized trial of Colpopexy and Urinary Reduction Efforts (CARE): Design and methods. *Control Clin Trials* 2003;24(5):629–642.

25. Jelovsek JE, Barber MD, Brubaker L, et al; for the NICHD Pelvic Floor Disorders Network. Effect of uterosacral ligament suspension vs sacrospinous ligament fixation with or without perioperative behavioral therapy for pelvic organ vaginal prolapse on surgical outcomes and prolapse symptoms at 5 years in the OPTIMAL randomized clinical trial. *JAMA* 2018;319(15):1554–1565.

26. Freeman RM, Pantazis K, Thomson A, et al. A randomised controlled trial of abdominal versus laparoscopic sacrocolpopexy for the treatment of post-hysterectomy vaginal vault prolapse: LAS study. *Int Urogynecol J* 2013;24(3):377–384.

27. Constantini E, Mearini LL, Lazzeri M, et al. Laparoscopic versus abdominal sacrocolpopexy: A randomized, controlled trial. *J Urol* 2016;196(1):159–165.

28. Paraiso MFR, Jelovsek JE, Frick A, et al. Laparoscopic compared with robotic sacrocolpopexy for vaginal prolapse: a randomized controlled trial. *Obstet Gynecol* 2011;118(5):1005–1013.

29. Skoczylas LC, Turner LC, Wang L, et al. Changes in prolapse surgery trends relative to FDA notifications regarding vaginal mesh. *Int Urogynecol J* 2014;25(4):471–477.

30. Wang LC, AlHussein Al Awamlh B, et al. Trends in mesh use for pelvic organ prolapse repair from the Medicare database. *Urology* 2015;86(5):885–891.

31. Wihersaari O, Karjalainen P, Tolppanen AM. Complications of Pelvic Organ Prolapse Surgery in the 2015 Finnish Pelvic Organ Prolapse Surgery Survey Study. *Obstet Gynecol* 2020;136(6):1135–1144.

32. Rooney K, Mueller E, Kenton K, et al. Can advanced stages of anterior or posterior vaginal wall prolapse occur without apical involvement. *J Pelvic Surg* 2006;12:70.

33. Swift S, Woodman P, O'Boyle A, et al. Pelvic Organ Support Study (POSST): The distribution, clinical definition, and epidemiologic condition of pelvic organ support defects. *Am J Obstet Gynecol* 2005;192(3):795–806.

34. Hullfish KL, Bovbejerg VE, Steers WD. Patient-centered goals for pelvic floor dysfunction surgery: Long-term follow up. *Am J Obstet Gynecol* 2004;191(1):201–205.

35. Paraiso MF, Walters MD, Rackley RR, et al. Laparoscopic and abdominal sacral colpopexies: A comparative cohort study. *Am J Obstet Gynecol* 2005;192(5):1752–1758.

36. Akl MN, Long JB, Giles DL, et al. Robotic assisted sacrocolpopexy: Technique and learning curve. *Surg Endosc* 2009;23(10):2390–2394.

37. Meriwether KV, Antosh DD, Olivera CK, et al. Uterine preservation vs. hysterectomy in pelvic organ prolapse surgery: A systematic review with meta-analysis and clinical practice guidelines. *Am J Obstet Gynecol* 2018;219(2):129–146.

38. Meriwether KV, Balk EM, Antosh DD, et al. Uterine-preserving surgeries for the repair of pelvic organ prolapse: A systematic review with meta-analysis and clinical practice guidelines. *Int Urogynecol J* 2019;30(4):505–522.

39. Barranger E, Fritel X, Pigne A. Abdominal sacrohysteropexy in young women with uterovaginal prolapse: Long-term follow-up. *Am J Obstet Gynecol* 2003;189(5):1245–1250.

40. Costantini E, Lazzeri M, Zucchi A, et al. Five-year outcome of uterus sparing surgery for pelvic organ prolapse repair: A single-center experience. *Int Urogynecol J* 2011;22(3):287–292.

41. Cundiff GW, Harris RL, Coates K, et al. Abdominal sacral colpoperineopexy: A new approach for correction of posterior compartment defects and perineal descent associated with vaginal vault prolapse. *Am J Obstet Gynecol* 1997;177(6):1345–1355.

42. Parks AG, Porter NH, Hardcastle J. The syndrome of the descending perineum. *Proc R Soc Med* 1966;59(6):477–482.

43. Henry MM, Parks AG, Swash M. The pelvic floor musculature in the descending perineum syndrome. *Br J Surg* 1982;69(8):470–472.

44. Haylen BT, Freeman RM, Swift SE, et al. An International Urogynecological Association (IUGA)/International Continence Society (ICS) joint terminology and classification of the complications related directly to the insertion of prostheses (meshes, implants, tapes) and grafts in female pelvic floor surgery. *Int Urogynecol J Pelvic Floor Dysfunct* 2011;22(1):3–15.

45. Borahay MA, Oge T, Walsh TM, et al. Outcomes of robotic sacrocolpopexy using barbed delayed absorbable sutures. *J Minim Invasive Gynecol* 2014;21(3):412–416.

46. Culligan PJ, Murphy M, Blackwell L, et al. Long-term success of abdominal sacral colpopexy using synthetic mesh. *Am J Obstet Gynecol* 2002;187(6):1473–1482.

47. Visco AG, Weidner AC, Barber MD, et al. Vaginal mesh erosion after abdominal sacral colpopexy. *Am J Obstet Gynecol* 2001;184(3):297–302.

48. Cundiff GW, Varner E, Visco AG, et al. Risk factors for mesh/suture erosion following sacral colpopexy. *Am J Obstet Gynecol* 2008;199(6):688.e1–688.e5.

49. Akyol A, Akca A, Ulker V, et al. Additional surgical risk factors and patient characteristics for mesh erosion after abdominal sacrocolpopexy. *J Obstet Gynaecol Res* 2014;40(5):1368–1374.

50. Bensinger G, Lind L, Lesser M, et al. Abdominal sacral suspensions: Analysis of complications using permanent mesh. *Am J Obstet Gynecol* 2005;193(6):2094–2098.

51. Visco AG, Weidner A, Barber MD, et al. Vaginal mesh erosion after abdominal sacral colpopexy. *Am J Obstet Gynecol* 2001;183(3):297.

52. Brizzolara S, Pillai-Allen A. Risk of mesh erosion with sacral colpopexy and concurrent hysterectomy. *Obstet Gynecol* 2003;102(2):306–310.

53. Culligan PJ, Murphy M, Blackwell L, et al. Long-term success of abdominal sacral colpopexy using synthetic mesh. *Am J Obstet Gynecol* 2002;187(6):1473–1482.

54. Wu JM, Wells EC, Hundley AF, et al. Mesh erosion in abdominal sacral colpopexy with and without concomitant hysterectomy. *Am J Obstet Gynecol* 2006;194(5):1418–1422.

55. Salamon CG, Lewis C, Priestley J, et al. Prospective study of an ultra-lightweight polypropylene Y mesh for robotic sacrocolpopexy. *Int Urogynecol J* 2013;24(8):1371–1375.

56. Stork AM, Giugale LE, Bradley MS, et al. Incidence of sacral osteomyelitis and discitis after minimally invasive sacrocolpopexy. *Female Pelvic Med Reconstr Surg* 2021;27(11):672–675.

57. Whitehead WE, Bradley CS, Brown MB, et al. Gastrointestinal complications following abdominal sacrocolpopexy for advanced pelvic organ prolapse. *Am J Obstet Gynecol* 2007;197(1):78.e1–78.e7.

58. Matthews CA, Geller EJ, Henley BR, et al. Permanent compared with absorbable suture for vaginal mesh fixation during total hysterectomy and sacrocolpopexy: A randomized controlled rial. *Obstet Gynecol* 2020;136(2):355–364.

59. Shepherd JP, Higdon HL III, Stanford EJ, et al. Effect of suture selection on the rate of suture or mesh erosion and surgery failure in abdominal sacrocolpopexy. *Female Pelvic Med Reconstr Surg* 2010;16(4):229–233.

CHAPTER 47

UTEROSACRAL/CARDINAL LIGAMENT SUSPENSION FOR UTEROVAGINAL AND POSTHYSTERECTOMY VAGINAL VAULT PROLAPSE

Peter L. Dwyer • Ariel Zilberlicht

Introduction

The uterosacral/lateral cervical ligament complex is the cornerstone of apical support of the uterus, cervix, and upper vagina and is an important element in the prevention of pelvic organ prolapse (POP). Loss of apical support will lead to uterovaginal and vaginal vault prolapse but is also a major etiologic factor in most cystoceles and enteroceles. Assessment and diagnosis of support defects causing POP is necessary prior to surgical treatment. In this chapter, we review the role of the uterosacral–cardinal ligament complex (UCC) in the maintenance of pelvic organ support and their place in the surgical treatment of both uterovaginal and vaginal vault prolapse post hysterectomy.

DeLancey[1] has categorized three levels of support. Level 1 support is the vaginal apex of the cervix and upper vagina by the parametrium and the paracolpium. Level 2 supports the anterior and posterior vaginal walls with the attachments of the endopelvic fascia and vagina to the arcus tendinous fascia pelvis, and level 3 provides the support of the distal vaginal and the perineal body. Denervation and injury to the levator muscles and pelvic ligaments during childbirth together with the secondary aggravating factors of aging and lifestyle factors (e.g., obesity, heavy lifting) frequently result in uterovaginal prolapse later in life.

ANATOMY OF UTEROSACRAL LIGAMENTS AND RELATED STRUCTURES

The pelvic organs are supported to the sacrum and lateral pelvis sidewall of the bony pelvis by the pelvic floor muscles and endopelvic fascial and ligamentous connective tissues. Level 1 support is achieved by the intermingling of the uterosacral ligament (USL) and the cardinal ligament (CL) attaching the cervix and upper vagina

to the sacrum and lateral pelvic sidewalls maintaining the vaginal length and the cervix at the level of the ischial spines or above. Vu et al.[2] described the surgical anatomy; the average total length of the USL is 12 to 13 cm and can be divided into three sections according to thickness and attachments: The distal section, which attaches to the cervix and upper vagina and forms posterior-lateral aspect of the UCC, is about 2 to 3 cm in length and 5 to 20 mm thick. The intermediate portion is thick, well-defined structure that lies medially to the ureter. It is approximately 5 cm in length and 1 to 2 cm wide. The proximal sacral section is approximately 5 to 6 cm in length and has a generally thin and diffuse attachment. Histologically, the USL is composed of fibrous tissue, vessels, nerves, and fatty tissue and vary in composition at the different sections of the lament. The ligament complex originates from S2 to S4 sacral vertebrae in a fan-shaped area and runs lateral to the rectum and medially to the ureter; it has a superficial component covered by peritoneum and a deep retroperitoneal component. Finally, the USL attaches distally at the posterior-lateral aspect of the cervix and/or the upper vaginal wall where they form an integrated complex with the CL.[3] Its relation to the ureter is of a clinical and surgical significance as the distance from the ureter to the USL is greatest at the level of the sacrum (4.1 ± 0.6 cm), 2.3 ± 0.9 cm at the level of the ischial spines, and 0.9 ± 0.4 cm at the level of the cervical internal os.

Anatomically, the ligaments act in unison to provide not only apical support but also the correct vertical orientation of the vagina and uterus and other pelvic viscera (Fig. 47.1). Chen et al.[4] created 3D models of CL and deep USL from magnetic resonance images to establish ligaments line of action and load sharing to study the mechanisms of apical support. They found that the CL is relatively vertical in the standing position, whereas the deep USL is more dorsally directed. These ligaments and fascia load share with the levator

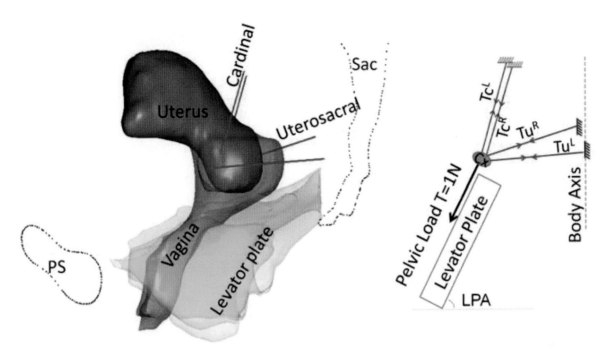

FIGURE 47.1 Diagram by Chen et al.[4] showing on the **left** the MR-based 3D model of the uterus and vagina and transparent levator ani muscle *(blue)* with lines of action of CL and USL in the right-side view. PS, pubic symphysis; Sac, sacrum. (Adapted from Chen L, Ramanah R, Hsu Y, et al. Cardinal and deep uterosacral ligament lines of action: MRI based 3D technique development and preliminary findings in normal women. *Int Urogynecol J* 2013;24[1]:37–45.)

pelvic floor musculature to provide apical support. The direction and magnitude of pelvic loading to the apex are important factors in the maintenance of support; the tension in these ligaments should be parallel and complementary to the direction of the levator plate (Fig. 47.2). Deviation of the axis by surgery either posteriorly as with sacrospinous suspension or anteriorly

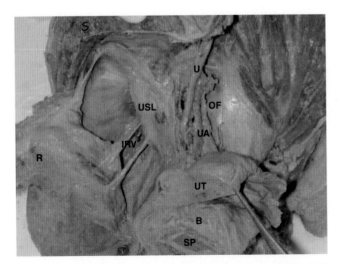

FIGURE 47.2 Left hemipelvis displaying the course of the left ureter (U) and its relationship to the uterine artery (UA) and uterosacral/lateral cervical ligament complex (USL) and uterus (UT). Other structures are sacrum (S), rectum (R), inferior rectal vessels (IRV), obturator fascia (OF), bladder (B), and pubic symphysis (SP) (Photograph of C Achtari and P Dwyer).

as in Burch colposuspension will predispose to development of prolapse in the opposing compartment. This has been known since the time of Victor Bonney. A higher incidence of postoperative compartment after Burch colposuspension compared to midurethral slings has repeatedly been shown.[5,6] The sacrospinous suspension has a high incidence of recurrent cystocele, although there was no difference in anterior wall recurrence between sacrospinous versus USL suspension at 5-year follow-up in the OPTIMAL trial.[7] A major advantage of using the UCC for apical re-support is to provide the correct alignment is maintained which will protect both the anterior and posterior compartment from developing POP.

The ureters have a close anatomical relationship to the UCC and are at significant risk when surgery is performed in this area for either hysterectomy or uterovaginal suspension procedures. A good understanding of the anatomy together with appropriate intraoperative assessment for ureteric integrity is important for pelvic surgeons performing POP surgery if ureteric injury is to be avoided.

The ureter enters the pelvis as an extraperitoneal structure crossing anterior to the common or external iliac arteries. On the pelvic sidewall, the ureter is anterior to the internal iliac artery and immediately posterior to the ovary in the peritoneum forming the posterior boundary of the ovarian fossa. The fascia of the obturator internus is situated laterally, and the ureter crosses and is medial to the umbilical artery;

the obturator nerve, artery, and vein; and the inferior vesical and middle rectal arteries.

The ureter descends into the pelvis anteriorly and superiorly to the uterosacral/lateral cervical ligament complex (see Fig. 47.1) and continues anteromedially close to the uterine artery, cervix, and vaginal fornices. The uterine artery initially lies lateral to the ureter and runs a short parallel course along the pelvic sidewall. The ureter then travels inferior medially in the broad ligament of the uterus where the uterine artery is antero-superior for approximately 2.5 cm. The uterine artery crosses the ureter to its medial side to ascend alongside the uterus. The ureter turns anteriorly approximately 2 cm above the vaginal fornix and lateral to the uterine cervix and moves medially before entering the bladder posteriorly. The ureter courses medially for 1.5 cm in the intramural and submucosal segments of the bladder wall before entering the bladder lumen via the ureteric orifices sited at the upper trigone.

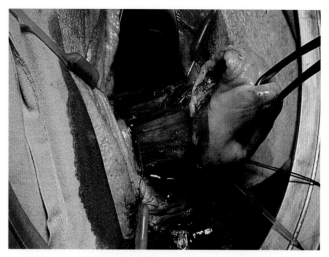

FIGURE 47.3 Vaginal incision made around the cervix exposing the uterosacral complex to the midportion. The bladder with ureters dissected off the cervix and removed from the operative field with a Breisky-Navratil retractor. The USL/CL are ready to be clamped and ligated for VH or MR.

SURGICAL SIGNIFICANCE OF THE UTEROSACRAL–CARDINAL LIGAMENT COMPLEX

The UCC is primarily important not only in uterovaginal support but also in the surgical management of hysterectomy and POP. Knowledge of the anatomy is essential to enable surgeons to perform these procedures safely and effectively. At hysterectomy, clamping and ligation of the UCC is an essential step in the mobilization of the uterus and cervix. Reattachment of the UCC to the vaginal vault is necessary to treat apical prolapse and prevent future vault prolapse whether the hysterectomy is performed vaginally or abdominally. Correcting apical descent during POP surgery for cystocele significantly reduces anterior compartment reoperation rates.[8] Unfortunately, the UCC reattachment is frequently not performed at the time of hysterectomy and is a major factor in the subsequent development of vaginal vault prolapse.

When the hysterectomy is performed vaginally, an incision is made circumferentially around the cervix to reflect the vagina off the UCC ligaments laterally and the bladder and ureters anteriorly. The bladder and ureters can then be removed from the operative field using a Breisky-Navratil retractor (Fig. 47.3), so dissection of and identification of the UCC is important to prevent ureteric injury and to identify the ligaments for suture placement. By pushing the vaginal tissue laterally, the UCC ligament can be exposed up to its intermediate portion, enabling a higher suspension suture placement.

There is a worldwide trend away from vaginal hysterectomy (VH) to abdominal hysterectomy either by robotic or laparoscopic surgery particularly in the United States, United Kingdom, and other developed countries.

The popularity of robotic and laparoscopic surgery among gynecologists is occurring despite the vaginal approach being shown to be a safer and less expensive alternative.[9] The American College of Obstetricians and Gynecologists[10] in a Committee Opinion stated in 2017 that

> *"the vaginal approach is preferred among the minimally invasive approaches. Laparoscopic hysterectomy is a preferable alternative to open abdominal hysterectomy for those patients in whom a vaginal hysterectomy is not indicated or feasible. Although minimally invasive approaches to hysterectomy are the preferred route, open abdominal hysterectomy remains an important surgical option for some patients."*

Gynecologists may feel more comfortable performing the surgery abdominally because of their training and experience and feel less familiar performing vaginal surgery particularly where the uterus is well supported with little prolapse. However, once the uterosacral cardinal ligament has been exposed and uterus mobilized as described earlier (see Fig. 47.3), VH can be performed without difficulty if there is adequate vaginal access, even in nulliparous women with previous cesarean sections or large uteri. Increasing the VH rate can be achieved by education and reemphasis on the vaginal route.[11] In Finland, VH rate was as low as 7% in the 1980s. Following annual meetings on gynecologic surgery where vaginal and laparoscopic surgery were encouraged, and individual training provided, the VH rate increased to 44% in 2006 and the rate of laparoscopic hysterectomy increased from 24% to 36%. Over this time, the complication rates including ureteric injuries decreased.[12]

CHOICE OF SURGERY

The aim of surgical repair is to restore the anatomical support while maintaining or restoring normal bowel and bladder functions and maintaining normal sexual and reproductive function if desired. Surgery is an effective treatment for POP but has operative morbidity and a recurrence rate. The risks of surgery will vary with the type of operation performed and experience of the surgeon. Surgical selection should be based on what suits the needs of the patient best: what is the most effective and safest way to surgically correct her POP. The operation and its benefits and risks to the patient should be discussed and then a joint decision made on what operation is to be performed.

In the first instance, the decision whether to operate or not should be based on the patient's symptoms, degree of bother, and her medical health. Symptoms should correlate with the examination findings of the site of prolapse and its severity. Women with marked apical loss of support with uterocervical or vaginal vault prolapse will frequently have associated cystocele and/or enterocele; the options are whether to repair this vaginally or abdominally, and if abdominally by an open, laparoscopic, or a robotic procedure. There are advantages and disadvantages of all techniques, and the decision should be based on the patient's needs. Relevant clinical factors in making this decision are the patient age and general health, whether further pregnancies are desired, the need for sexual activity, presence of dyspareunia, and vaginal length. The abdominal approach will be preferable in the presence of other abdominal pathology requiring treatment such as an ovarian cyst or when vaginal capacity is already reduced from previous surgery in a sexually active woman. However, the vaginal approach may be preferable in the presence of severe pelvic adhesions, which increase the difficulty

and risk of the abdominal approach. The risk of recurrence may influence the decision in favor of the abdominal approach and the use of synthetic mesh. Finally, the surgeon's training and experience will have an influence on the surgical choice so that the procedure can be completed. Preoperative and postoperative assessment should identify the support defects and surgical repair to the defects to minimize the surgery and therefore morbidity. Solitary rectoceles, enteroceles or cystocele where the vaginal vault is well supported do not need apical support operations, either vaginally or abdominally. Placement of synthetic mesh placed abdominally over the anterior, apical and posterior walls is unnecessary where apical support is good and increases morbidity.

SURGICAL REPAIR OF APICAL PROLAPSE USING THE UTEROSACRAL–CARDINAL LIGAMENT COMPLEX

Uterine Conservation: The Manchester Repair

The Manchester repair (MR) was first performed in 1888 and published by Donald[13] in 1908 with later modifications by Fothergill. The MR involves the clamping and mobilization of the UCC and their reattachment to the partially amputated cervix, usually with an anterior colporrhaphy. A racket-shaped vaginal incision is made around the cervix to expose the UCC with reflection of the bladder off the cervix (see Fig. 47.3), the ligament is clamped and ligated, and the two ends are sutured together to the anterior cervix with an overlapping figure-of-eight 2-0 polydioxanone (PDS) suture. The amputated cervix is reconstructed using anterior and posterior Sturmdorf sutures to re-epithelize the cervix. Video 47.1 shows the procedure.[14] Cervical elongation is frequently associated with uterine prolapse (Fig. 47.4)

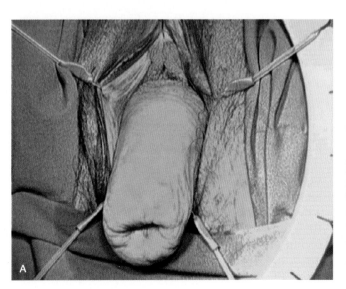
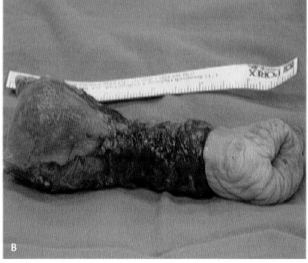

FIGURE 47.4 Stage 4 uterovaginal prolapse with elongated cervix (**A**) and following hysterectomy (**B**).

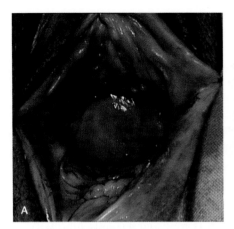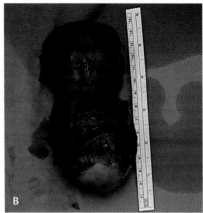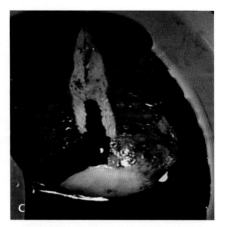

FIGURE 47.5 A 38-year-old woman with cervical stenosis from an MR (**A**) who subsequently developed an 18-week–sized hematometra requiring hysterectomy (**B,C**).

but not always. It is possible to resuspend the cervix and uterus using the UCC as described while leaving the cervix intact. This would be appropriate if fertility was important and further pregnancies desired. Cervical amputation would significantly decrease the likelihood of a woman conceiving and potentially cause cervical incompetence and preterm delivery. There are potential long-term risks with uterine conservation including the development of cancer. Hematometra (Fig. 47.5) or pyometra can result from cervical stenosis. We routinely perform a cervical dilatation to ensure that the cervix is open both before and after MR and a curettage to exclude uterine pathology.

The MR is currently not widely performed in United States but is becoming increasing popular in Europe and is the operation of choice for uterovaginal prolapse in Scandinavia. In Norway, Oversand et al.[15] recently reported excellent results with a 5-year reoperation rate of 2.8% and low surgical morbidity. These results were corroborated in a systematic review by Tolstrup et al.[16] which reported a reoperation rate for MR of symptomatic recurrence of between 3.3% and 9.5%. In a recent study by Husby et al.,[17] the modified Manchester-Fothergill operation was found to have less recurrences compared to the uterine conserving sacrospinous hysteropexy and the VH. They compared 7,247 operations for treatment of primary uterine prolapse and analyzed data from the Danish National Patient Registry. The authors found a higher reoperation rate and anterior compartment prolapse recurrence in patients who had sacrospinous hysteropexy compared to Manchester-Fothergill. The 5-year reoperation rates for Manchester-Fothergill were 7% compared to 30% of sacrospinous hysteropexy and 11% of VH.

In another study from the same department,[18] the historical cohorts of matched patients for both age and POP stage in the apical compartment were compared. Patients undergoing VH with USL suspension ($n = 295$)

were compared to those who had Manchester-Fothergill repair. Interestingly, the recurrence at any vaginal compartment was higher in the VH group as well as a higher rate of apical prolapse recurrence after VH (5.1% vs. 0.3%). There were more complications in the VH group, both perioperative (2.7% vs. 0%) and postoperative intra-abdominal bleeding (2% vs. 0%). The authors concluded that Manchester-Fothergill is superior to VH and it should be the preferred method for apical prolapse in cases there are no contraindications for hysterectomy. Additional studies are needed.

Vaginal Hysterectomy for Uterovaginal Prolapse

The VH has been the preferred option by gynecologists worldwide for woman presenting with significant uterovaginal prolapse after completion of childbearing. The removal of the uterus and tubes even with conservation of the ovaries significantly decreases the risk of subsequent genital tract cancer. Eighty percent of gynecologists surveyed in Australia, New Zealand, and the United Kingdom in 2007 said that VH was their preferred operation when a woman presented with a stage 3 symptomatic prolapse.[19] Seventy percent to 75% of gynecologists would resuture the vaginal vault to the UCC ligaments most using the McCall procedure, whereas 20% to 25% prefer to use a sacrospinous suspension with hysterectomy for vault support.

When VH is performed for POP, it is essential to support the vaginal apex. McCall[20] described his culdoplasty in 1957 which aims to correct an enterocele and a deep cul-de-sac as well to support the vaginal cuff at time of hysterectomy. In his original description, the technique uses the USL and CL which are incorporated into the peritoneum and the posterior cul-de-sac. Tying the McCall sutures will obliterate the cul-de-sac, prevent enterocele formation as well as resuspend the vaginal cuff, and restore vaginal length. This technique at the time of VH in cases of mild to moderate uterine prolapse has shown good results with relatively few complications including urinary tract and bowel injury. Chene et al.[21] reported a recurrence rate of 0.6% for the vaginal cuff; 1.5% had stage 2 cystocele or more, and 3% had stage 2 or more rectocele.

Despite apical support being essential to pelvic support, the majority of hysterectomies performed in the United States between 2004 and 2013 did not include an apical support procedure. Overall, only 3.1% of hysterectomies performed from 2004 to 2013 for nonprolapse indications and 37.1% of those with a diagnosis of prolapse used a vaginal apex suspension operation.[22] There is level 1 evidence that an apical support procedure at time of hysterectomy not for prolapse can prevent future posthysterectomy vaginal vault prolapse (PHVVP). In 1999, Cruikshank and Kovac[23] in a randomized trial found that use of a modified McCall procedure results in a significantly lower rate of recurrent prolapse than a simple Moschcowitz-type or simple peritoneal vaginal closure 3 years postoperatively.

The sacrospinous suspension is increasing being used with VH for large uterovaginal prolapse such as procidentia. Cruikshank and Cox[24] recommended that sacrospinous ligament fixation (SSF) at the time of VH should be considered when the vault descends to the introitus during closure; but is this necessary or appropriate? The Royal College of Obstetricians and Gynaecologists Green-top Guidelines recommendation is to use a prophylactic SSF in cases with advanced uterovaginal prolapse.[25] However, adding an SSF can potentially add morbidity including a risk of gluteal pain. Montoya et al.[26] reported an incidence of 6.8% new-onset buttock and/or lower extremity pain or numbness in 278 women undergoing transvaginal intraperitoneal USL suspension with 1 in 5 having suture removal. Gluteal pain has not been reported with the extraperitoneal approach either with the McCall procedure at the time of hysterectomy or the extraperitoneal USL suspension.[27] Colombo and Milani[28] retrospectively compared matched patient groups of the SSF to their modified McCall culdoplasty at time of hysterectomy for advanced POP. One-hundred and twenty-four patients were divided into two groups: 62 patients, with either stage 2 uterine prolapse (39%) or stage 3 (61%), had a VH with SSF and were compared to 62 patients with stage 2 (36%) and stage 3 (64%) who underwent a culdoplasty. Operative time and blood loss were significantly greater ($P < .001$) in the group with sacrospinous suspension. With a follow-up from 4 to 9 years, 17 (27%) patients receiving sacrospinous suspension had prolapse recurrence at any vaginal site compared with 9 (15%) patients receiving modified McCall culdoplasty ($P = .14$).

Recurrent vault prolapse was recorded in 5 (8%) and 3 (5%) subjects, respectively ($P = .72$). Thirteen (21%) and 4 (6%) patients, respectively, had recurrent cystocele (odds ratio 4.1, 95% confidence interval 1.3 to 14.2, $P = .04$). No significative difference was observed in postoperative sexual function. Their conclusion was that the SSF is not recommended as a prophylactic measure at VH in patients with significant uterovaginal prolapse.

We have recently modified the McCall culdoplasty by placing sutures higher and more lateral into the USL/CL extraperitoneally to improve support the vaginal cuff at the time of a VH in large uterovaginal prolapse and procidentia. The UCC is identified and ligated at transvaginal hysterectomy and dissected free laterally to the midportion to enable high suture placement. The bladder with ureters are removed from the operative field using a Breisky-Navratil retractor as described earlier (see Fig. 47.3), the McCall vault suspension was performed following hysterectomy using a 1.0 Vicryl suture which was passed through the posterior vaginal wall and the midportion of the UCC on both the right and left sides. This suture is tied in the midline before a second pass is made through and through the vaginal vault to re-support and close it. The last 2-0 PDS suture from the anterior repair is tied to the UCC suture at the vaginal vault to suspend and support the anterior and apical compartments. Finally, closure of any existing large levator hiatal defects using interrupted sutures of 0 and 2-0 PDS will provide further support to the levator plate and treat any posterior compartment prolapse. Video 47.2 shows the procedure.[29]

A recent study by Zilberlicht et al.[30] followed 176 women with stage 3 to 4 uterine prolapse; there were 25 cases (14%) of recurrences (stage 2 and higher), of which 19 (76%) were asymptomatic. Of all recurrences, 12 (48%) occurred at the anterior wall, 6 (25%) at the posterior wall, 3 (12%) were combined anterior and posterior wall, 2 (8%) were posterior and vault, and 1 case (4%) recurred at all three compartments. Only 6 cases (3%) were symptomatic and required further surgery; all had recurrent enterocele.

Vaginal Vault Prolapse

Vaginal vault prolapse is described as the descent of the vaginal apex after hysterectomy and is usually not a bother until the presenting prolapse comes to and beyond the vaginal introitus. High USL suspension (HUSLS) can be done vaginally, either extraperitoneally where it is not necessary to open the peritoneal pouch or intraperitoneally. USL suspension sutures are placed bilaterally below and posteriorly to the ischial spine to suspend the vaginal vault. Intraperitoneal USL suspension can also be performed abdominally either laparoscopically or as an open procedure.

Posthysterectomy Vault Suspension

Vaginal vault or apical prolapse is defined by International Urogynecological Association/International Continence Society as "descent of the apex of the vagina (vaginal vault or cuff scar after hysterectomy), where the vaginal cuff corresponds to point C on the POP-Q."[31] There is wide variation in prevalence (0.2% to 43%) following hysterectomy for all causes,[32-34] although a recent study estimated the prevalence to be 11.6% for those who had a hysterectomy performed for prolapse and only 1.8% of women with a hysterectomy for other benign disease.[35] Presumably, the reason for the difference is that the ligamentous supports and the muscular levator complex is compromised in women who had POP previously. Aigmueller et al.[36] in an Austrian study found 6% to 8% needed a surgical repair for vault prolapse post hysterectomy. Surgical correction is required when there are bothersome symptoms usually with the presenting prolapse comes to and beyond the introitus and is frequently associated with anterior or posterior compartment defects or both.

Transperitoneal USL suspension for vault prolapse is popular in the United States but performed less frequently in the United Kingdom and Australasia where the sacrospinous suspension has been the vaginal procedure of choice for vault prolapse.

Intraperitoneal Uterosacral–Cardinal Ligament Complex Vault Suspension

The first description of apical suspension using the intraperitoneal part of USL was by Miller[37] in 1927 with a further modification in 1976 by Richardson et al.[38] who introduced the HUSLS. The well-known modification of the USL suspension technique is based on the description of Shull et al.[39] who reported his results in a study of 302 consecutive women with apical and other POP defects. Out of the initial cohort, 87% had optimal anatomical outcomes, and 13% had grade 1 or more loss of support. The surgical technique involves a vertical incision in the vaginal epithelium, identification of the enterocele, and the hernia sac which is carefully opened. The bowel is then packed out of the operative field, and the USL are identified posterior and medial to the ischial spines at 4 and 8 o'clock positions. With gentle traction by an Allis clamp and retraction of the rectum medially, three sutures are placed on the medial portion of the USL at the level of the ischial spine bilaterally. These sutures are then attached to the vaginal apex and tied in order of their placement. In a large retrospective study, Karram et al.[40] used the intraperitoneal USL suspension using nonabsorbable and delayed absorbable sutures to attach the superior parts of the pubocervical and the rectovaginal fascia and vagina to the ligaments.

A total of 168 patients were followed for an average of 21.6 months, and 89% reported satisfaction with the result. The overall reoperation rate was 5.5%, and additional 5% had at least grade 2 recurrent prolapse but did not require any further treatment. In a prospective randomized controlled trial comparing abdominal sacrocolpopexy (ASC) to HUSLS for women whose point C was greater than 1 cm beyond the introitus, Rondini et al.[41] reported 100% success rate for the ASC versus 82.5% in the HUSLS group. The study had a short-term follow-up and an objective success defined as point C less than −1 cm. There were higher recurrences for both the anterior and posterior compartments in the HUSLS group (5.3% vs. 33.3% and 0% vs. 6.2%, respectively) as well as significantly lower rates of reoperation in the ASC group. Furthermore, the postoperative complications were higher in the USL group.

In their systematic review and meta-analysis, Margulies et al.[42] have reported a total of 11 studies which have used either the McCall culdoplasty or the HUSLS. They concluded that the uterosacral suspension is of highly effective procedure for apical vaginal support, with reported success rate of 98%. Another well-designed randomized controlled trial by Jelovsek et al.[7] compared the HUSLS and the SSF. With a 2-year follow-up, there were no differences in success rate (HUSLS 59.2% vs. SSF 60.5%) or serious adverse events (HUSLS 16.5% vs. SSF 16.7%).

Complications reported with intraperitoneal USL post hysterectomy vault prolapse were ureteric injury (mainly urethral kinking) with a rate between 1% and 11%.[7,43] Other complications described are bladder injuries, urinary tract infection, blood transfusion, and small bowel injury.

Extraperitoneal Uterosacral–Cardinal Ligament Complex Vault Suspension

In 2007, Dwyer and Fatton[44] described the technique and reported their experience of 123 patients with symptomatic grade 3 to 4 posthysterectomy vault prolapse.[45] In women with complete vaginal eversion (Fig. 47.6), a longitudinal midline incision is made on the vaginal epithelium extending from the urethra anteriorly onto the vault and down the posterior wall to the perineal body. The vaginal epithelium was reflected off the underlying endopelvic fascia, and the bladder is completely mobilized from the pelvic sidewall. The bladder and ureters are retracted anteriorly using a Breisky-Navratil retractor. The UCC is identified posteriorly with remnant ligament often still present at the vaginal vault where they create dimples in the vagina. The UCC can be seen and palpated running posterior-laterally on the lateral pelvic sidewall with traction of the vaginal skin. Two sutures are placed through the ligament on each side

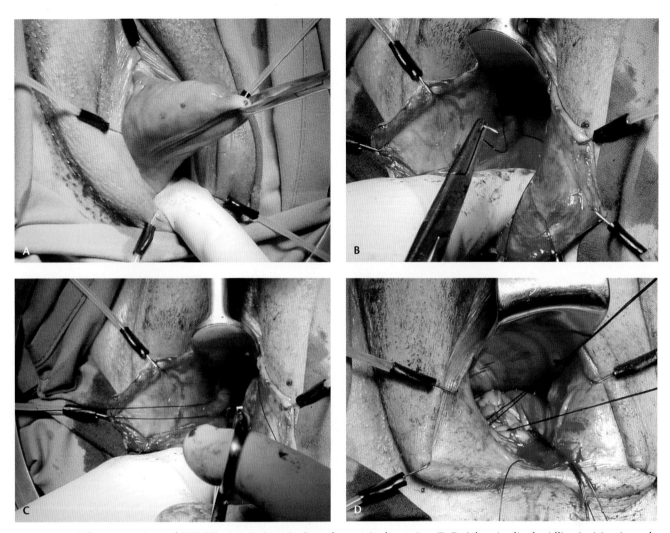

FIGURE 47.6 The extraperitoneal USL/CL suspension. **A:** Complete vaginal eversion. **B,C:** A longitudinal midline incision is made on the vaginal epithelium extending from the urethra anteriorly onto the vault and down the posterior wall to the perineal body. The vaginal epithelium was reflected off the underlying endopelvic fascia, and the bladder is completely mobilized from the pelvic sidewall. The bladder and ureters are retracted anteriorly using a Breisky-Navratil retractor. The UCC is identified posteriorly and can be seen and palpated running posterior-laterally on the lateral pelvic sidewall with traction of the vaginal skin. Two sutures are placed through the ligament on each side (delayed absorbable monofilament 00 PDS suture). **D:** These sutures are passed full thickness through the vagina at the location of the new apex where they were tied following vaginal closure.

(delayed absorbable monofilament 0 PDS suture) and provide excellent anchoring strength. These sutures are passed full thickness through the vagina at the location of the new apex where they will be tied eventually following vagina closure (Fig. 47.7A). A further 0 PDS suture is used to plicate the UCC together in the midline and also passed through the vaginal to provide extra central support so the vault is supported by five anchoring sutures across the apex (Fig. 47.7B). A concomitant repair of cystocele and rectocele is then carried out and a cystoscopy is performed to ensure ureteric patency and exclude any other bladder abnormalities. The authors reported a mean surgical time of 88 minutes and relatively low complication rates. The technique was

initially evaluated in 110 patients over a 2-year period. The authors reported a 95.4% objective success rate regarding recurrent apex prolapse and a global anatomical success rate of 85.5% with improvements of urinary, bowel, and coital symptoms. Polypropylene mesh (PPM) was placed as an overlay graft over the anterior compartment apex and posterior compartment early in the series to provide a stronger long-lasting repair but was discontinued because of a 19.3% rate of mesh exposure. All cases were treated conservatively or with local excision of the exposed mesh.[45] A longitudinal long-term follow-up of 472 patients with grade 3 to 4 posthysterectomy vault prolapse who underwent extraperitoneal UCC vault suspension was reported in

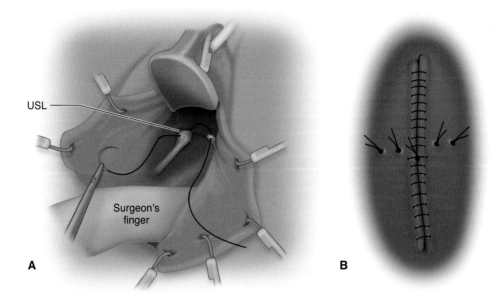

FIGURE 47.7 Drawing of extraperitoneal USL suspension following midline vaginal incision and suture placement (**A**) and with vaginal closed with continuous 2-0 Vicryl and five USL suspension sutures tied onto the vagina across the new vault (**B**).

BJOG in 2019 and showed an objective success rate for vaginal cuff support of 89% over a mean follow-up of 5 years.[27] Only 4% needed revision surgery for recurrence of vault prolapse. In this more recent series, PPM was discontinued early because of high exposure rate of 17%. The results using native tissue repair only were not significantly different to when PPM was used. One major advantage of using this technique is a low risk of ureteric injury which was 1% with the few cases occurring early in the series. Similar to VH, the bladder and ureters are moved anteriorly out of the operative field with a Breisky-Navratil retractor so the risk is minimal. Buttock and leg pain has not been reported in this cohort of patients unlike the sacrospinous ligament and iliococcygeus suspension techniques (10% to 20%)[46] and even the intraperitoneal approach. A retrospective cohort study by Mounir et al.[47] compared the intraperitoneal to the extraperitoneal approaches for the treatment of PHVVP. The authors defined the primary outcome as a composite outcome for surgical failure as either apical decent less than one-third of total vaginal length or anterior or posterior vaginal wall beyond the hymen, retreatment of prolapse, or bothersome vaginal bulge symptoms with positive response on several questionnaires. They also investigated secondary outcomes such as operative time, duration of hospitalization, blood loss, and perioperative complications. With a mean duration of 7 months follow-up in 80 patients (36 in the intraperitoneal USL vs. 44 in the extraperitoneal USL group), there were no differences in the surgical success (72% vs. 81%, $P = .307$); however, the operative time, hospitalization, and blood loss were lower in the extraperitoneal group. The authors concluded that the extraperitoneal technique for PHVVP repair has similar short-term success rate to the intraperitoneal approach.

CONCLUSION

The uterosacral/lateral cervical ligament complex provides apical support for the uterus, cervix, and upper vagina which is parallel and complementary to the direction of the levator musculature and levator plate. These ligaments are important not only in prevention of POP but also in the surgical treatment of POP. The UCC are the primary anchoring structure for the surgical treatment of POP in VH, MR, and the procedures for PHVVP with intraperitoneal and extraperitoneal vault suspension. These procedures provide good lasting support with uterine conservation or removal using native tissues.

References

1. DeLancey JO. The anatomy of the pelvic floor. *Curr Opin Obstet Gynecol* 1994;6(4):313–316.
2. Vu D, Haylen BT, Tse K, et al. Surgical anatomy of the uterosacral ligament. *Int Urogynecol J* 2010;21(9):1123–1128.
3. Ramanah R, Berger MB, Parratte BM, et al. Anatomy and histology of apical support: A literature review concerning cardinal and uterosacral ligaments. *Int Urogynecol J* 2012;23(11):1483–1494.
4. Chen L, Ramanah R, Hsu Y, et al. Cardinal and deep uterosacral ligament lines of action: MRI based 3D technique development and preliminary findings in normal women. *Int Urogynecol J* 2013;24(1):37–45.

5. Ward K, Hilton P. Tension-free vaginal tape versus colposuspension for primary urodynamic 399 stress incontinence: 5-Year follow up. *BJOG* 2008;115(2):226–233.

6. Karmakar D, Dwyer PL, Murray C, et al. Long-term effectiveness and safety of open Burch colposuspension vs retropubic midurethral sling for stress urinary incontinence—results from a large comparative study. *Am J Obstet Gynecol* 2021;224(6):593.e1–593.e8.

7. Jelovsek JE, Barber MD, Brubaker L, et al. Effect of uterosacral ligament suspension vs sacrospinous ligament fixation with or without perioperative behavioral therapy for pelvic organ vaginal prolapse on surgical outcomes and prolapse symptoms at 5 years in the OPTIMAL randomized clinical trial. *JAMA* 2018;319(15):1554–1565.

8. Eilber KS, Alperin M, Khan A, et al. Outcomes of vaginal prolapse surgery among female Medicare beneficiaries: The role of apical support. *Obstet Gynecol* 2013;122(5):981–987.

9. Aarts JW, Nieboer TE, Johnson N, et al. Surgical approach to hysterectomy for benign gynaecological disease. *Cochrane Database Syst Rev* 2015;2015(8):CD003677.

10. American College of Obstetricians and Gynecologists Committee on Gynecologic Practice. Committee Opinion No. 701: Choosing the route of hysterectomy for benign disease. *Obstet Gynecol* 2017;129(6):e155–e159.

11. Whiteside JL, Kaeser CT, Ridgeway B. Achieving high value in the surgical approach to hysterectomy. *Am J Obstet Gynecol* 2019;220(3):242–245.

12. Mäkinen J, Brummer T, Jalkanen J, et al. Ten years of progress—improved hysterectomy outcomes in Finland 1996–2006: A longitudinal observation study. *BMJ Open* 2013;3(10):e003169.

13. Donald A. Operation in cases of complete prolapse. *J Obstet Gynaecol Brit Emp* 1908;13:195–196.

14. Walsh CE, Ow LL, Rajamaheswari N, et al. The Manchester repair: An instructional video. *Int Urogynecol J* 2017;28(9):1425–1427.

15. Oversand SH, Staff AC, Spydslaug AE, et al. Long-term follow-up after native tissue repair for pelvic organ prolapse. *Int Urogynecol J* 2014;25(1):81–89.

16. Tolstrup CK, Lose G, Klarskov N. The Manchester procedure versus vaginal hysterectomy in the treatment of uterine prolapse: A review. *Int Urogynecol J* 2017;28(1):33–40.

17. Husby KR, Larsen MD, Lose G, et al. Surgical treatment of primary uterine prolapse: A comparison of vaginal native tissue surgical techniques. *Int Urogynecol J* 2019;30(11):1887–1893.

18. Tolstrup CK, Husby KR, Lose G, et al. The Manchester-Fothergill procedure versus vaginal hysterectomy with uterosacral ligament suspension: A matched historical cohort study. *Int Urogynecol J* 2018;29(3):431–440.

19. Vanspauwen R, Seman E, Dwyer PL. Survey of current management of prolapse in Australia and New Zealand. *Aust N Z J Obstet Gynaecol* 2010;50(3):262–267.

20. McCall ML. Posterior culdeplasty; surgical correction of enterocele during vaginal hysterectomy; a preliminary report. *Obstet Gynecol* 1957;10(6):595–602.

21. Chene G, Tardieu A-S, Savary D, et al. Anatomical and functional results of McCall culdoplasty in the prevention of enteroceles and vaginal vault prolapse after vaginal hysterectomy. *Int Urogynecol J Pelvic Floor Dysfunct* 2008;19(7):1007–1011.

22. Ross WT, Meister MR, Shepherd JP, et al. Utilization of apical vaginal support procedures at time of inpatient hysterectomy performed for benign conditions: A national estimate. *Am J Obstet Gynecol* 2017;217(4):436.e1–436.e8.

23. Cruikshank SH, Kovac SR. Randomized comparison of three surgical methods used at the time of vaginal hysterectomy to prevent posterior enterocele. *Am J Obstet Gynecol* 1999;180(4):859–865.

24. Cruikshank SH, Cox DW. Sacrospinous ligament fixation at the time of transvaginal hysterectomy. *Am J Obstet Gynecol* 1990;162(6):1611–1619.

25. Royal College of Obstetricians and Gynaecologists. *Posthysterectomy vaginal vault prolapse.* London: Royal College of Obstetricians and Gynaecologists, 2015. Green-top Guideline No. 46.

26. Montoya TI, Luebbehusen HI, Schaffer JI, et al. Sensory neuropathy following suspension of the vaginal apex to the proximal uterosacral ligaments. *Int Urogynecol J* 2012;23(12):1735–1740.

27. Karmakar D, Dwyer PL, Thomas E, et al. Extraperitoneal uterosacral suspension technique for post hysterectomy apical prolapse in 472 women: Results from a longitudinal clinical study. *BJOG* 2019;126(4):536–542.

28. Colombo M, Milani R. Sacrospinous ligament fixation and modified McCall culdoplasty during vaginal hysterectomy for advanced uterovaginal prolapse. *Am J Obstet Gynecol* 1998;179(1):13–20.

29. Zilberlicht A, Dwyer PL, Rajamaheswari N, et al. Video of uterovaginal procidentia repair incorporating a high extraperitoneal uterosacral vault suspension. *Int Urogynecol J* 2020;31(10):2173–2175.

30. Zilberlicht A, Dwyer PL, Karmakar D, et al. Extraperitoneal high vaginal cuff suspension at the time of vaginal hysterectomy for advanced uterovaginal prolapse: Results of a modified McCall technique from a longitudinal clinical study. *Aust N Z J Obstet Gynaecol* 2021;61(2):258–262.

31. Haylen BT, de Ridder D, Freeman RM, et al; for International Urogynecological Association, International Continence Society. An International Urogynecological Association (IUGA)/International Continence Society (ICS) joint report on the terminology for female pelvic floor dysfunction. *Neurourol Urodyn* 2010;29(1):4–20.

32. Barrington JW, Edwards G. Posthysterectomy vault prolapse. *Int Urogynecol J Pelvic Floor Dysfunct* 2000;11(4):241–245.

33. Toozs-Hobson P, Boos K, Cardozo L. Management of vaginal vault prolapse. *Br J Obstet Gynaecol* 1998;105(1):13–17.

34. Symmonds RE, Pratt JH. Vaginal prolapse following hysterectomy. *Am J Obstet Gynecol* 1960;79:899–909.

35. Marchionni M, Bracco GL, Checcucci V, et al. True incidence of vaginal vault prolapse. Thirteen years of experience. *J Reprod Med* 1999;44(8):679–684.

36. Aigmueller T, Dungl A, Hinterholzer S, et al. An estimation of the frequency of surgery for posthysterectomy vault prolapse. *Int Urogynecol J* 2010;21(3):299–302.

37. Miller N. A new method of correcting complete inversion of the vagina: With or without complete prolapse; report of two cases. *Surg Gynecol Obstet* 1927:550–555.

38. Richardson AC, Lyon JB, Williams NL. A new look at pelvic relaxation. *Am J Obstet Gynecol* 1976;126(5):568–573.

39. Shull BL, Bachofen C, Coates KW, et al. A transvaginal approach to repair of apical and other associated sites of pelvic organ prolapse with uterosacral ligaments. *Am J Obstet Gynecol* 2000;183(6):1365–1374.

40. Karram M, Goldwasser S, Kleeman S, et al. High uterosacral vaginal vault suspension with fascial reconstruction for vaginal repair of enterocele and vaginal vault prolapse. *Am J Obstet Gynecol* 2001;185(6):1339–1343.

41. Rondini C, Braun HF, Alvarez J, et al. Prospective-randomized study comparing high uterosacral vault suspension vs. abdominal sacral colpopexy for the correction of apical defects and vaginal vault prolapse. *Int Urogynecol J* 2011;22(Suppl 1): S87–S88.

42. Margulies RU, Rogers MA, Morgan DM. Outcomes of transvaginal uterosacral ligament suspension: Systematic review and metaanalysis. *Am J Obstet Gynecol* 2010;202(2):124–134.

43. Milani R, Frigerio M, Cola A, et al. Outcomes of transvaginal high uterosacral ligaments suspension: Over 500-patient single-center study. *Female Pelvic Med Reconstr Surg* 2018;24(3):39–42.

44. Dwyer PL, Fatton B. Bilateral extraperitoneal uterosacral suspension: A new approach to correct posthysterectomy vaginal vault prolapse. *Int Urogynecol J Pelvic Floor Dysfunct* 2008;19(2):283–292.

45. Fatton B, Dwyer PL, Achtari C, et al. Bilateral extraperitoneal uterosacral vaginal vault suspension: A 2-year follow-up longitudinal case series of 123 patients. *Int Urogynecol J Pelvic Floor Dysfunct* 2009;20(4):427–434.

46. Maher C, Murray C, Carey M, et al. Iliococcygeus or sacrospinous fixation for vaginal vault prolapse. *Obstet Gynecol* 2001;98(1):40–44.

47. Mounir D, Vasquez-Tran NO, Lindo FM, et al. Vaginal intraperitoneal versus extraperitoneal uterosacral ligament vault suspensions: A comparison of a standard and novel approach. *Int Urogynecol J* 2021;32(4):913–918.

CHAPTER 48

SACROSPINOUS LIGAMENT AND ILIOCOCCYGEUS MUSCLE SUSPENSIONS

J. Eric Jelovsek

Introduction

Sacrospinous ligament fixation (or "suspension") and iliococcygeus muscle suspension are common vaginal approaches for resuspending the apical or upper vagina in women with pelvic organ prolapse. They are a core part of the armamentarium of the vaginal surgeon because they allow the surgeon to resupport the vagina and do not necessarily require entry into the peritoneal cavity. Both procedures can be simultaneously performed with other procedures including hysterectomy, anterior colporrhaphy, posterior colporrhaphy, enterocele sac repair using peritoneal closures, modified Moschcowitz, or modified McCall culdoplasty.[1]

SACROSPINOUS LIGAMENT SUSPENSION

Brief History

Sacrospinous and sacrotuberous ligament fixations were introduced in Europe by Zwiefel, possibly as early as 1892. Sacrospinous ligament fixation was subsequently described by Amreich in 1950 and then modified by Richter in 1968.[2,3] In the United States, enthusiasm for the procedure progressed as a common option for correction of apical vaginal prolapse after 1971 when Randall and Nichols reported on a series of 18 patients.[3]

Relevant Anatomy

The ischial spines are an important bilateral landmark and reference point for various female pelvic reconstructive surgeries. In the upright woman, the ischial spine is a bony projection located at the level of the pubic symphysis that projects posteriorly toward the sacrum. In lithotomy, the ischial spine can be easily palpated during pelvic or rectal exam. It separates the superior greater sciatic notch and the inferior lesser

sciatic notch. The sacrospinous ligament has a triangular shape. The apex of the sacrospinous ligament attaches to the ischial spine and the wider base attaches broadly to the lower sacrum and coccyx. *An Elementary Treatise on Anatomy* (1837) describes the ligament as "a strong, flattened, vertical fasciculus, fixed on one side to the posterior-superior spine of the os ilium, and on the other to the lateral and posterior parts of the sacrum, on a level with the third sacral foramen."[4] The presence of the ligament results in the greater sciatic foramen which contains the gluteal and thigh vessels and nerves and the piriformis muscle. The inferior gluteal and the internal pudendal arteries arise from the internal iliac artery and exit through the greater sciatic foramen closest to the top of the sacrospinous ligament.[5,6] The pudendal nerve arises from sacral nerves S2, S3, and S4 and exits the greater sciatic foramen and travels through the ischioanal fossa where it branches anteriorly to innervate the perineum and posteriorly to innervate portions of the external anal sphincter. The pudendal nerves and vessels lie immediately posterior to the ischial spine, whereas the sciatic nerve is superior and lateral to the sacrospinous ligament. The nerve to coccygeus muscle arises from contributions from S3, S4, or S5 and pierces the sacrospinous ligament to reach the underlying coccygeus muscle. The nerve to levator ani muscle also arises from contributions from S3, S4, or S5 and courses over the cephalad surface of the sacrospinous ligament and give off branches to innervate iliococcygeus, pubococcygeus, and the puborectalis muscles (Fig. 48.1).

The levator ani muscles originate from a linear thickening musculofascial attachment covering the obturator internus muscle called the arcus tendinous levator ani which runs from the ischial spine to the posterior surface of the ipsilateral pubic ramus. The levator ani muscle consists of the puborectalis, pubococcygeus, and iliococcygeus muscle. This muscle's posterior boundary is the ischial spine.

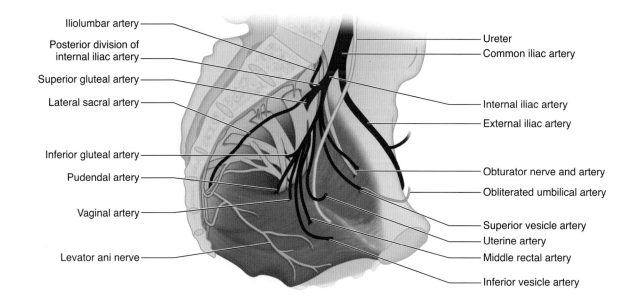

Iliolumbar artery

Posterior division of
internal iliac artery

Superior gluteal artery

Lateral sacral artery

Inferior gluteal artery

Pudendal artery

Vaginal artery

Levator ani nerve

Ureter

Common iliac artery

Internal iliac artery

External iliac artery

Obturator nerve and artery

Obliterated umbilical artery

Superior vesicle artery

Uterine artery

Middle rectal artery

Inferior vesicle artery

A

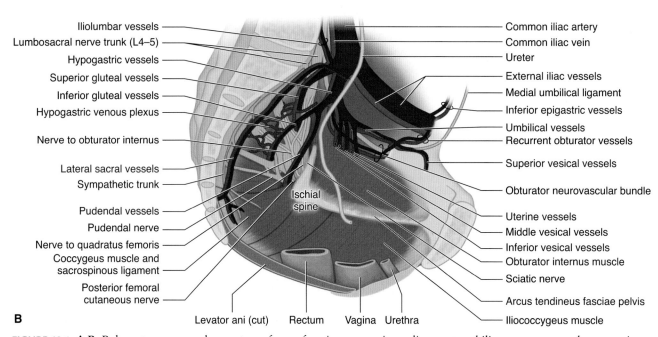

Iliolumbar vessels

Lumbosacral nerve trunk (L4–5)

Hypogastric vessels

Superior gluteal vessels

Inferior gluteal vessels

Hypogastric venous plexus

Nerve to obturator internus

Lateral sacral vessels

Sympathetic trunk

Pudendal vessels

Pudendal nerve

Nerve to quadratus femoris

Coccygeus muscle and
sacrospinous ligament

Posterior femoral
cutaneous nerve

Ischial
spine

Common iliac artery

Common iliac vein

Ureter

External iliac vessels

Medial umbilical ligament

Inferior epigastric vessels

Umbilical vessels

Recurrent obturator vessels

Superior vesical vessels

Obturator neurovascular bundle

Uterine vessels

Middle vesical vessels

Inferior vesical vessels

Obturator internus muscle

Sciatic nerve

Arcus tendineus fasciae pelvis

Iliococcygeus muscle

B   Levator ani (cut)   Rectum   Vagina   Urethra

FIGURE 48.1 **A,B:** Relevant neurovascular anatomy for performing sacrospinous ligament and iliococcygeus muscle suspension.

Surgical Technique

Sacrospinous ligament suspension

The sacrospinous ligament suspension is a popular transvaginal approach to manage posthysterectomy apical prolapse and can be performed with simultaneous hysterectomy or as a hysteropexy. It is most commonly performed by suspending the vaginal apex to the right sacrospinous ligament but can be easily performed using the woman's left sacrospinous ligament or bilaterally. The Michigan four-wall suspension described by Morely and DeLancey[7] is a modification of the original description and emphasizes the excision of excess vaginal length from the anterior, posterior, and lateral vaginal walls to prevent laxity between the suspension point at the sacrospinous ligament and the introitus.

Prior to performing a sacrospinous ligament suspension, the surgeon should be familiar with relevant pelvic anatomy including the perirectal space and ischioanal fossa. The technique is as follows:

1. Pelvic examination should be performed to identify the ischial spines.
2. It is often useful to determine whether the prolapsed vaginal apex will easily reach the sacrospinous ligament by manually reducing the prolapse to the targeted suspension site. This can be accomplished by bilaterally grasping the apex of the vagina using two or more Allis clamps. In order to obtain a more

symmetric repair, the surgeon can shift the "new" vaginal apex anteriorly for anterior wall-predominate apical prolapse or posteriorly for posterior wall-predominate prolapse. This attachment site can be tagged with suture for future identification.

3. There are two main approaches to the sacrospinous ligament fixation: posterior and anterior approach. In the posterior approach, the posterior vaginal wall is incised in the midline and ends approximately 1 to 2 cm before the vaginal apex. If an enterocele is encountered, some surgeons will dissect this sac away from the rectum, enter the peritoneum, and occlude the enterocele sac using purse-string suture. Kearney and DeLancey[8] reported that a diamond-shaped incision is performed posterior to the hysterectomy scar in 75% of patients undergoing a Michigan four-wall suspension.

4. Dissection begins into the perirectal space on the ipsilateral side of the anticipated suspension. This is usually performed using blunt dissection and facilitated while retracting the rectum medially and the bladder gently retracted upward often accomplished using one or two Breisky-Navratil vaginal retractors. Recurrent palpation of the ischial spine helps facilitate appropriate location during dissection.

5. Dissection should proceed until the ischial spine is identified. Blunt dissection may be used in a lateral to medial fashion to expose the surface of the sacrospinous ligament.

6. There are several techniques to pass sutures into the sacrospinous. Many surgeons use the Capio suture-capturing device to pass suture. The Michigan four-wall suspension that uses a Deschamps ligature carrier and others perform fixation using a Miya hook.[9,10] In our practice, we prefer the ease of placing the end of the Capio ligature carrier on the surface of the ligament. Prior to passing suture, the rectum should be retracted medially, and caution should be used in retracting the vaginal walls superiorly to prevent neurovascular damage. The left hand should palpate the right ischial spine. Holding the suture-passing device in the right hand, the notch should be placed at the middle (approximately 3 cm from ischial spine) of the sacrospinous ligament and held firmly in place using the finger of the opposing hand. With continued downward pressure, the suture is passed using the device, the device removed, and the suture tagged to the side for later use. In our practice, we place two to four sutures in the middle portion of the ligament (Fig. 48.2). There is currently

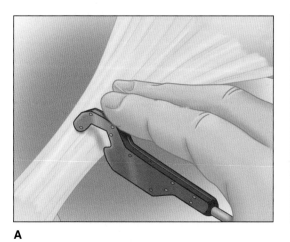

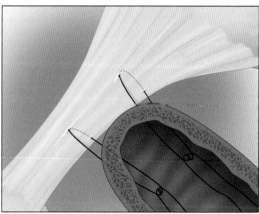

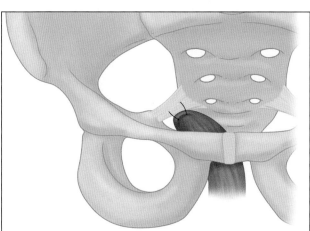

FIGURE 48.2 **A–C:** Approximate suture attachment location when performing sacrospinous ligament suspension or fixation.

a lack of consensus on the optimal number and location of sutures placed during sacrospinous ligament fixation.[11] It is possible to place sutures as far laterally as the lateral third of the ligament closest to the ischial spine and as far medially as the medial third of the ligament closest to the sacrum. Cadaveric studies suggest that the middle segment of the sacrospinous ligament has the lowest incidence of nerves and arteries located there.[11]

7. If the surgical plan includes performing an anterior colporrhaphy, our practice has been to perform this procedure at this time.

8. The suspension sutures are then anchored to the new apex of the vagina but they are not tied down. The vaginal apical incision is closed using a continuous running absorbable 2-0 suture. Using a vaginal retractor, the anterior vaginal wall and apex are elevated toward the sacral promontory and the sacrospinous sutures are tied down. It is useful to ensure that the vaginal apex comes into contact with the sacrospinous ligament.

9. Concomitant anticontinence procedure and posterior colporrhaphy can be performed.

10. Although the risk of ureteral kinking or obstruction is very low with a sacrospinous ligament fixation, the procedure is usually performed with the concomitant anterior colporrhaphy or anti-incontinence procedures warranting cystourethroscopy.

ILIOCOCCYGEUS MUSCLE SUSPENSION

Brief History

Originally described by Inmon,[12] the iliococcygeus muscle suspension served as an alternative extraperitoneal vaginal approach for surgically suspending the posthysterectomy vault prolapse when the uterosacral ligaments could not be identified. The procedure was originally described as "a chromic #1 suture begins in the left lateral angle of the vaginal cuff, enters the iliococcygeus below the ischial spine and is brought back through the cuff and tied. In like manner the right lateral angle of the vaginal cuff is attached to the right iliococcygeus."[12] A modification of the Inmon technique has also been described in which the prolapsed vaginal vault was sutured to the fascia of the coccygeal muscle.[13,14]

Surgical Technique

In our practice, the iliococcygeus muscle suspension is used for women with high apical posterior wall prolapse and is often combined with a rectocele repair. It can also be used when the vaginal length is too short to reach the sacrospinous ligament or if risk is too high to attempt the dissection required for a sacrospinous ligament fixation.

Similar to approaching a sacrospinous ligament fixation, planning an iliococcygeus muscle suspension involves being familiar with relevant perirectal space and ischioanal fossa, and pelvic examination should be performed to identify the ischial spines.

1. The surgical approach begins with dissection of the posterior vaginal wall in the midline in a similar fashion to starting a rectocele repair.

2. The perirectal spaces are widely dissected and the levator muscles are identified by palpating caudal to the ischial spine.

3. The rectum is retracted medially using a short Breisky-Navratil vaginal retractor. A finger is used to identify the ipsilateral ischial spine. An anchoring point 1 to 2 cm caudal and 1 to 2 cm medial from the ischial spine is identified in the iliococcygeus muscle (Fig. 48.3).

4. A single 0 delayed absorbable suture is placed by passing the suture from lateral to medial through the muscle with the rectum deviated medially. The ends of the suture are then passed through the vaginal apex. This is repeated on the opposite site.

5. With the ends of the suture tagged to the side, the posterior repair is completed, and the posterior vaginal wall incision is closed. With a vaginal retractor lifting the vaginal apex, the bilateral iliococcygeus sutures are tied down elevating the posterior vaginal apex.

Outcomes

Numerous observational cohort studies have been reported using sacrospinous ligament suspension and iliococcygeus muscle suspension and few high-quality randomized trials. All studies report variable rates of success largely due to how "success" was defined. A systematic review of 27 published papers from the years 1995 to 2011 of sacrospinous ligament fixation included mostly observational studies involving 3,893 participants, with only 2 being published randomized controlled trials.[15] Twenty-four studies reported an overall cure rate of 85% (range 69% to 100%), and 21 studies reported the following recurrence rates: apex—5%, range 0% to 14%; anterior—18%, range 0% to 42%; and posterior—1%, range 0% to 2%.[15] One of the longest cohort studies by Paraiso et al.[16] demonstrated that the vaginal vault remained well supported up to 5 years after sacrospinous ligament fixation, but more than one-third of patients developed postoperative cystoceles. During the same time period, Shull et al.[17] reported a 95% and Meeks et al.[18] a 100% success rate using iliococcygeus fixation in the management of vaginal vault prolapse, with low rates of postoperative cystocele. Together, these findings caused some groups to change from the sacrospinous to the iliococcygeus suspension.[16] However, there are few studies comparing

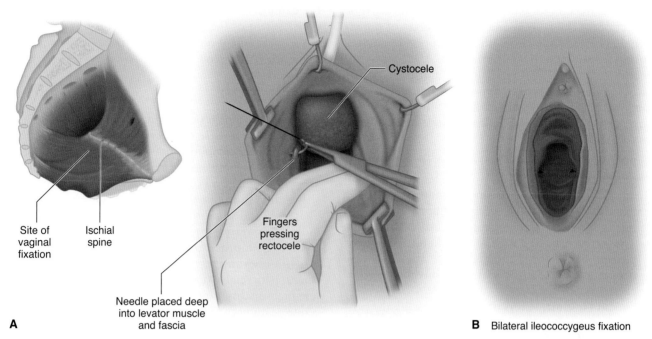

A

Site of vaginal fixation

Ischial spine

Needle placed deep into levator muscle and fascia

Cystocele

Fingers pressing rectocele

B Bilateral ileococcygeus fixation

FIGURE 48.3 Approximate suture location (**A**), technique, and final appearance (**B**) after suture attachment when performing iliococcygeus muscle suspension.

these two procedures. Maher[19] compared 78 women approximately 20 months after undergoing sacrospinous ligament fixation and 50 women who underwent iliococcygeus suspension using a matched retrospective cohort design. Out of 36 matched pairs, subjective success rate for the iliococcygeus group was 91% compared to 94% for the sacrospinous group. The objective success rate was 53% and 67%. There were no significant difference between groups in the incidence of postoperative cystoceles or damage to the pudendal neurovascular bundle.[19]

A recent systematic review identified three randomized trials comparing sacrospinous ligament fixation to sacrocolpopexy and six trials compared sacrospinous colpopexy to vaginal apical procedures with mesh.[20] The review estimated that overall awareness of prolapse, repeat surgery for prolapse, any recurrent prolapse, and postoperative dyspareunia were more common after sacrospinous ligament fixation than after sacral colpopexy. One of the longest trials of 374 women in the United States compared the sacrospinous ligament fixation to the uterosacral ligament suspension.[21] Success was defined as the absence of all of the following: (1) descent of the vaginal apex more than one-third into the vaginal canal, (2) anterior or posterior vaginal wall descent beyond the hymen, (3) bothersome vaginal bulge symptoms, or (4) re-treatment for prolapse by either surgery or pessary. At 2 years after surgery, success rates were 63% for the sacrospinous ligament fixation group compared with 65% for the uterosacral ligament suspension group and the adjusted odds ratio for the difference was

1.1 (95% confidence interval, 0.7 to 1.7). Fewer than 1 in 5 women experienced a serious adverse event over the 2-year follow-up, and less than 5% of these were directly related to the index surgery. There were more temporary ureteral obstructions after uterosacral ligament suspension (3.2%) than sacrospinous ligament fixation (0%), and all of these obstructions were detected at the time of the index surgery and released. The rate of persistent buttock pain after sacrospinous ligament fixation was 4%.[21] Compared with outcomes at 2 years, rates of surgical success decreased during the follow-up period, although prolapse symptom scores remained improved and reoperations remained low.[22]

Complications

Perioperative complications of sacrospinous ligament fixation and iliococcygeus muscle suspension may include hemorrhage, nerve entrapment resulting in buttock pain or anesthesia, cystotomy, ureteral kinking or obstruction, urinary retention, urinary tract infection, vaginal cuff infection, or enterotomy. One systematic review estimated the following complication rates after sacrospinous ligament fixation: neurovascular injury (7.4%, range 0% to 36%), urinary retention (13.4%, range 0% to 75%), urinary tract infection (8.8%, range 4% to 21%), cuff infection (5.6%, range 0% to 18%), and cystotomy or enterotomy (1.1%, range 0% to 2%).[15]

Life-threatening hemorrhage has been reported during sacrospinous ligament fixation.[5,23,24] The most likely artery to be injured during sacrospinous ligament fixation is the inferior gluteal artery based on cadaveric dissections.[5] The rectum and the tributaries of the internal iliac vein have also both been reportedly injured during sacrospinous ligament fixation. A suggested approach to control life-threatening hemorrhage during sacrospinous ligament fixation is listed as follows and modified and adapted from Barksdale.[5] To control massive intraoperative bleeding from above or below the sacrospinous ligament,

1. Pack the operative space tightly with several laparotomy packs under moderate pressure for 20 to 30 minutes. Communicate to the anesthesiologist about the expected blood loss and ensure that appropriate hemorrhage and resuscitation protocols may be triggered.
2. The packs may be gently removed and the injured portion of the vessel isolated above and below the defect. Injectable fibrin sealant or medium surgical clips may be used.
3. Should these maneuvers prove unsuccessful, the perirectal space may be packed with several moistened laparotomy packs to maintain adequate tamponade against the sacrospinous ligament and surrounding vessels. Additional vaginal packs may also be placed.
4. The patient may be taken from the operating room, and these packs may be left in place for several hours or until the patient is stable.
5. After adequate blood volume replacement, the patient may return to the operating room and the packs can be sequentially removed. The source of the bleeding should be visible at this point.
6. Alternatively, selective arterial catheterization may be performed and intraluminal embolization used. The latter technique requires a stable patient, ready access to a fluoroscopy suite, and skilled radiologists on hand to perform the procedure.

The most common postoperative complication following sacrospinous ligament fixation is short-term buttock pain. We believe that entrapping or "irritating" the nerve to the coccygeus is largely unavoidable, given the nerves' small size and anatomic course in a deep pelvic space filled with abundant loose connective tissue. Careful exposure and visualization of the anterior surface of the coccygeus–sacrospinous ligament complex may allow visualization and avoidance of larger caliber nerves. However, many surgeons prefer to limit the extent of the exposure to reduce the risk of bleeding from vessel avulsion. We continue to support suture placement at the midportion of the ligament, 2 to 3 cm from the ischial spine, because suture placement too close to the sacrum may lead to S3 and/or S4 nerve root entrapment and placement too close to the ischial spine may lead to pudendal nerve and/or vessel injury. A thorough understanding of the complex anatomy surrounding the sacrospinous ligament, limiting the depth of needle penetration into the ligament, and avoiding

the extension of needle exit or entry point above the upper extent of the sacrospinous ligament may reduce nerve entrapment and postoperative gluteal pain and other neurologic sequelae.[25]

CONCLUSION

The main advantages of the sacrospinous ligament and iliococcygeus muscle suspensions are that they allow the surgeon to resupport the vagina and do not require entry into the peritoneal cavity. The sacrospinous ligament suspension is most commonly performed by suspending the vaginal apex to the right sacrospinous ligament, and the iliococcygeus muscle suspension is most commonly performed bilaterally. Prior to performing both procedures, the surgeon should be familiar with relevant pelvic anatomy including the ischial spines, perirectal space, and ischioanal fossa. Although few high-quality randomized trials exist for both procedures, numerous observational cohort studies have been reported. Surgeons should be aware that hemorrhage and nerve entrapment resulting in buttock pain or anesthesia are just a few of the potential complications necessitating careful surgical technique.

References

1. Cruikshank SH, Muniz M. Outcomes study: A comparison of cure rates in 695 patients undergoing sacrospinous ligament fixation alone and with other site-specific procedures—A 16-year study. *Am J Obstet Gynecol* 2003;188:1509–1515.
2. Amreich J. Technic in vaginal surgery. *Arch Gynakol* 1950;178:44–57.
3. Richter K. The surgical anatomy of the vaginaefixatio sacrospinalis vaginalis. A contribution to the surgical treatment of vaginal blind pouch prolapse. *Geburtshilfe Frauenheilkd* 1968;28(4):321–327.
4. Bayle ALJ. *An elementary treatise on anatomy.* New York: Harper & Brothers, 1837.
5. Barksdale PA, Elkins TE, Sanders CK, et al. An anatomic approach to pelvic hemorrhage during sacrospinous ligament fixation of the vaginal vault. *Obstet Gynecol* 1998;91(5 Pt 1): 715–718.
6. Thompson JR, Gibb JS, Genadry R, et al. Anatomy of pelvic arteries adjacent to the sacrospinous ligament: Importance of the coccygeal branch of the inferior gluteal artery. *Obstet Gynecol* 1999;94(6):973–977.
7. Morley GW, DeLancey JO. Sacrospinous ligament fixation for eversion of the vagina. *Am J Obstet Gynecol* 1988;158(4): 872–881.
8. Kearney R, DeLancey JO. Selecting suspension points and excising the vagina during Michigan four-wall sacrospinous suspension. *Obstet Gynecol* 2003;101(2):325–330.
9. Larson KA, Smith T, Berger MB, et al. Long-term patient satisfaction with Michigan four-wall sacrospinous ligament suspension for prolapse. *Obstet Gynecol* 2013;122(5):967–975.
10. Pollak J, Takacs P, Medina C. Complications of three sacrospinous ligament fixation techniques. *Int J Gynaecol Obstet* 2007;99(1):18–22.

11. Katrikh AZ, Ettarh R, Kahn MA. Cadaveric nerve and artery proximity to sacrospinous ligament fixation sutures placed by a suture-capturing device. *Obstet Gynecol* 2017;130(5):1033–1038.

12. Inmon WB. Pelvic relaxation and repair including prolapse of vagina following hysterectomy. *South Med J* 1963;56:577–582.

13. Peters WA III, Christenson ML. Fixation of the vaginal apex to the coccygeus fascia during repair of vaginal vault eversion with enterocele. *Am J Obstet Gynecol* 1995;172(6):1894–1902.

14. Thornton WN Jr, Peters WA III. Repair of vaginal prolapse after hysterectomy. *Am J Obstet Gynecol* 1983;147(2):140–148.

15. Tseng L-H, Chen I, Chang S-D, et al. Modern role of sacrospinous ligament fixation for pelvic organ prolapse surgery—A systemic review. *Taiwan J Obstet Gynecol* 2013;52(3):311–317.

16. Paraiso MF, Ballard LA, Walters MD, et al. Pelvic support defects and visceral and sexual function in women treated with sacrospinous ligament suspension and pelvic reconstruction. *Am J Obstet Gynecol* 1996;175(6):1423–1431.

17. Shull BL, Capen CV, Riggs MW, et al. Bilateral attachment of the vaginal cuff to iliococcygeus fascia: An effective method of cuff suspension. *Am J Obstet Gynecol* 1993;168(6 Pt 1):1669–1677.

18. Meeks GR, Washburne JF, McGehee RP, et al. Repair of vaginal vault prolapse by suspension of the vagina to iliococcygeus (prespinous) fascia. *Am J Obstet Gynecol* 1994;171(16):1444–1454.

19. Maher CF, Murray CJ, Carey MP, et al. Iliococcygeus or sacrospinous fixation for vaginal vault prolapse. *Obstet Gynecol* 2001;98(1):40–44.

20. Maher C, Feiner B, Baessler K, et al. Surgery for women with apical vaginal prolapse. *Cochrane Database Syst Rev* 2016;10(10):CD012376.

21. Barber MD, Brubaker L, Burgio KL, et al. Comparison of 2 transvaginal surgical approaches and perioperative behavioral therapy for apical vaginal prolapse: The OPTIMAL randomized trial. *JAMA* 2014;311(10):1023–1034.

22. Jelovsek JE, Barber MD, Brubaker L, et al. Effect of uterosacral ligament suspension vs sacrospinous ligament fixation with or without perioperative behavioral therapy for pelvic organ vaginal prolapse on surgical outcomes and prolapse symptoms at 5 years in the OPTIMAL randomized clinical trial. *JAMA* 2018;319(15):1554–1565.

23. Jain A, Sheorain VS, Ahlawat K, et al. Vascular complication after sacrospinous ligament fixation with uterine preservation. *Int Urogynecol J* 2017;28(3):489–491.

24. Pahwa AK, Arya LA, Andy UU. Management of arterial and venous hemorrhage during sacrospinous ligament fixation: Cases and review of the literature. *Int Urogynecol J* 2016;27(3):387–391.

25. Florian-Rodriguez ME, Hare A, Chin K, et al. Inferior gluteal and other nerves associated with sacrospinous ligament: A cadaver study. *Am J Obstet Gynecol* 2016;215(5):646.e1–646.e6.

CHAPTER 49

Obliterative Procedures: LeFort Colpocleisis and Colpocleisis With Hysterectomy

Brittni A. J. Boyd • Felicia L. Lane

Introduction

Pelvic organ prolapse is a common condition, the incidence of which increases with age.[1] By the age of 80 years, 12.6% of women from the United States undergo surgery for pelvic floor disorders[2]; 61% of these surgeries include correction for pelvic organ prolapse.[3] As the elderly population continues to increase, the number of patients seeking treatment for pelvic organ prolapse will also increase, including those who do not wish to maintain the ability to have vaginal intercourse. Female pelvic medicine and reconstructive surgeons should therefore be comfortable discussing obliterative procedures such as a LeFort colpocleisis or colpocleisis with hysterectomy.

HISTORY

Throughout history, women have endured advanced pelvic organ prolapse. Early attempts at treatment included vaginal packing, crude pessaries, and instillation of caustic materials. Hippocrates describes a process called succussion, a technique to reduce prolapse by hanging the patient upside down to invert the prolapse back into the pelvis (Fig. 49.1).[4] Initial methods of surgical management involved amputation of the prolapsing segments or closure of the vaginal introitus[5] with morbid results.

The idea to surgically obliterate severe prolapse is credited to Gerardin,[6] who suggested suturing surgically denuded anterior and posterior vaginal walls together. Although he described the technique in 1823, he never attempted the procedure. Subsequently, the first known procedure was performed in 1867 by Neugebauer,[7] who waited until 1881 to publish his technique. Neugebauer[7] obliterated the vagina by denuding 6 × 3 cm anterior and posterior areas proximal to the introitus and suturing them together. The French surgeon Léon Clément LeFort[8] published his technique first in 1877 (Fig. 49.2). LeFort modifications differed in that longer and narrower areas of denudation were performed and that a

colpoperineoplasty was performed 8 days after the colpocleisis to address the widened genital hiatus. In general, an obliterative procedure in which the lateral vaginal epithelium remains in situ forming bilateral drainage tunnels is referred to as a partial, or LeFort colpocleisis, but a less common eponym is the Neugebauer-LeFort procedure. Edebohls,[9,10] in 1901, was the first to report performing a total colpocleisis with levator myorrhaphy following hysterectomy (i.e., panhysterocolpectomy). His report was followed by several case series that had comparable results to the partial colpocleisis-type procedures.[11] Although adoption of colpocleisis procedures was slow in the United States, in 1880, Berlin[12] reported a series of three cases (one of which failed) in the New England Hospital. The failure was blamed on lack of a concurrent perineorrhaphy.

To make colpocleisis a more accepted treatment option, early modifications were directed at reducing the recurrence risk and the incidence of postoperative urinary incontinence, which was as high as 25%.[13] Urinary incontinence was attributed to scarring from the distal dissection and distortion of the bladder neck. Other authors addressed postoperative urinary incontinence by sparing the distal vagina near the urethra or by supporting the bladder neck.[5,14–18] Goodall and Power[19] in 1937 tried to preserve sexual function by creating a triangular recess higher in the vagina that would allow for intercourse and potentially minimize stress urinary incontinence.

As a result of the many modifications to the colpocleisis, the American Urogynecologic Society and the International Urogynecological Association created standardized terminology for obliterative procedures. The term *colpectomy* has been used synonymously with *colpocleisis* for posthysterectomy vaginal vault prolapse. It specifically refers to the complete removal of the vaginal epithelium. Per the new standardized terminology, the terms *colpocleisis without hysterectomy*, *colpocleisis of vaginal vault*, and *colpocleisis with hysterectomy* is used throughout the remainder of this chapter. A *LeFort*

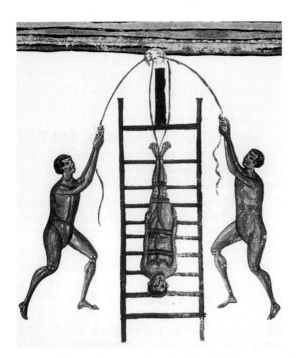

FIGURE 49.1 Succussion, as described by Hippocrates, is a technique to reduce prolapse by hanging the patient upside down to invert the prolapse back into the pelvis.

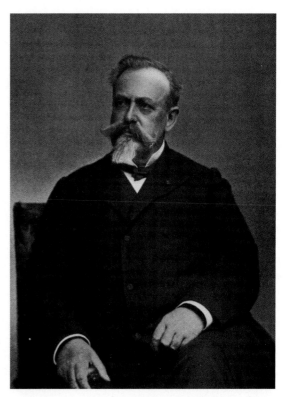

FIGURE 49.2 Léon Clément LeFort, French surgeon known for his work on uterine prolapse, specifically, LeFort colpocleisis.

colpocleisis is a term used to describe a colpocleisis without hysterectomy. It requires the obliteration of the vaginal canal by removal of panels of vaginal epithelium on the anterior and posterior vaginal walls and suturing together the fibromuscular layers of the anterior and posterior vagina with creation of bilateral tunnels from the cervix to the introitus.[20] When patients have a concurrent or history of a hysterectomy, a *colpocleisis with hysterectomy* or *colpocleisis of the vaginal vault* is performed.

PATIENT SELECTION AND CONSIDERATIONS

Colpocleisis is an effective treatment for those who no longer desire vaginal intercourse. In a multicenter study by Crisp et al.,[21] colpocleisis positively impacted bowel, bladder, and prolapse symptoms, with high satisfaction and low levels of regret. Outcome assessments repeatedly report 90% to 100% success for treatment of symptomatic pelvic organ prolapse.[22] In one retrospective cohort study of women who underwent LeFort colpocleisis, 94.3% were satisfied with the outcome. After a median follow-up of 5 years, none of the women in the cohort had prolapse recurrence.[23] In 2017, a retrospective study was conducted to evaluate the impact of LeFort colpocleisis on body image, regret, and pelvic floor symptoms long term after surgery. At a median follow-up of 3 years, 97% of the patients were satisfied with their surgery and none regretted their decision to proceed with colpocleisis.[24] Body image was assessed using the modified Body Image Scale (BIS), a tool validated for subjects with pelvic organ prolapse.[25]

The mean and total body image scores improved significantly postoperatively ($P < .001$).[24]

Traditionally, colpocleisis has been reserved for older patient populations with multiple comorbidities. However, it may be an ideal surgery for anyone who no longer desires vaginal penetrative intercourse and/or has significant medical comorbidities and does not tolerate or desire a pessary. The preoperative assessment of patients includes informed consent, a discussion of patient goals, history, physical exam, and evaluation of urinary dysfunction such as incontinence or retention. The actual procedure may be conducted under local, general, or regional anesthesia after an assessment of the patient's anesthesia risk. Enhanced Recovery after Surgery (ERAS) pathways are encouraged because elderly patients are particularly sensitive to fluid imbalances, falls, and opioid side effects. Such pathways include preoperative counseling, no bowel preparation, an opioid-sparing multimodal approach to pain management, goal-directed fluid management, and early mobilization and feeding.[26]

Urinary Incontinence

Similar to reconstructive approaches of treating prolapse, obliterative procedures carry a risk of worsening or unmasking of occult urinary incontinence. Such postoperative incontinence may be mitigated with inclusion of a concomitant anti-incontinence procedure, and a 2017 survey found that 94% of respondents routinely performed concurrent anti-incontinence procedures with colpocleisis.[27]

The strongest evidence to support a concomitant midurethral sling derives from the Outcomes following vaginal Prolapse repair and mid Urethral Sling (OPUS) trial. Published in 2012, this multicenter, randomized, single-blinded, sham-controlled, surgical-intervention trial analyzed 337 participants, including 24 who underwent colpocleisis.[28] The study demonstrated that a midurethral sling at the time of prolapse repair in women without symptoms of urinary incontinence resulted in a lower rate of postoperative urinary incontinence. The number needed to treat to prevent one case of urinary incontinence at 12 months was 6.3. These findings are likely applicable to patients undergoing colpocleisis, although they may enjoy a more modest benefit. In a retrospective cohort study comparing patient-reported outcomes after combined surgery for pelvic organ prolapse and stress urinary incontinence between older and younger women, women younger than 65 years old had higher odds of stress urinary incontinence treatment failure but not pelvic organ prolapse treatment failure.[29] In addition to the decreased benefit, elderly patients also experience increased risk of bladder perforation, de novo urgency incontinence, and postoperative voiding dysfunction.[30] Given that those undergoing obliterative procedures skew older and more frail, the surgeon and patient must weigh the potential morbidity and operative time of anti-incontinence procedures against the benefits.

Bowel Symptoms

It is important to adequately assess bowel symptoms in women with severe pelvic organ prolapse. Gutman et al. demonstrated in a prospective cohort study of 152 women that many bothersome bowel symptoms resolve after colpocleisis. Specifically, patients experience diminished obstructive and incontinence symptoms with low rates of de novo bowel symptoms.[31] Patients should also be evaluated for rectal mucosal prolapse as it may coexist with pelvic organ prolapse. If identified preoperatively, abdominal or perineal approaches such as a rectopexy, Altemeier or Delorme operations can be concomitantly performed. A rectopexy corrects rectal prolapse by affixing a suture or piece of mesh from the pararectal tissue to the presacral periosteum along the sacral promontory and may be performed with or without sigmoid resection and reanastomosis. The Altemeier procedure is a perineal rectosigmoidectomy to reduce rectal procidentia. The Delorme procedure is used to correct rectal prolapse by stripping the mucosa and plicating the muscle. In a series of case reports by Karateke et al.,[32] they performed LeFort and Delorme operations, demonstrating the safety and feasibility of addressing both pelvic floor disorders simultaneously under local anesthesia with sedation.

Special Considerations of the Geriatric Patient

Advanced age alone is not a contraindication to any type of surgery, including colpocleisis. However, surgeons who perform colpocleisis need to be adept at surgical care of the frail and geriatric patient.

In addition to open communication with the anesthesiologist regarding the optimal method of anesthesia, underlying medical conditions should be reviewed and optimized prior to surgery. Conditions meriting particular attention include those with cardiac, pulmonary, nutritional, cognitive, and functional status implications. The goal is to minimize risk factors for the occurrence of complications. From a cardiac standpoint, a diastolic blood pressure greater than 110 mm Hg should postpone surgery. Many antihypertensives should be given the day of surgery and restarted immediately after surgery because the risk of severe hypertension outweighs the risk posed by giving medicine prior to anesthesia induction. Consultation with an internist or cardiologist should be considered for patients on multiple classes of antihypertensive medications. Poor functional status, as shown by decreased activities of daily living, is predictive of pulmonary complications and should prompt a rigorous preoperative assessment.[33] Poor nutrition inhibits wound healing, and a serum albumin may be checked to assess preoperative nutritional status.[33] A history of alcohol abuse should be queried, and smoking should be stopped. Routine laboratory studies include hematocrit, electrolytes, blood urea nitrogen, and creatinine, whereas other studies to be considered are complete blood cell count, arterial blood gases, and prothrombin time and partial thromboplastin time.[33]

Falls are a leading cause of death in the geriatric population. Those recovering from falls suffer from mobility limitations associated with depression, social isolation, and decreased quality of life.[34] Fall risk can be determined preoperatively with the Timed Up and Go test, which further assesses one's mobility. The patient goes from sitting in a chair to standing and then walking 10 feet or 3 meters away. They then turn around, walk back to the chair, and sit down. An adult who takes longer than or equal to 12 seconds to complete the Timed Up and Go test is at risk for falling.[35] These patients are at greater risk for subsequent postoperative complications.

Postoperative delirium may be seen in up to 10% of older surgical patients and is often misdiagnosed, leading to longer hospital stays, nursing home admissions, and morbidity. Baseline dementia increases the incidence of acute postoperative delirium and adverse outcomes. A basic check of cognitive function should be performed in older surgical candidates, and if cognitive processes are impaired, consultation with an internist, geriatrician, neurologist, or other individual skilled in dementia management should be considered perioperatively to reduce the risk of postoperative delirium. Delirium occurrence is reduced by improving orientation, decreasing sensory overload or deprivation, and providing reassurance.

Perioperative and postoperative care are tailored for a speedy recovery and avoidance of a decline in functional status. After colpocleisis, early ambulation is vital. Hypertensive episodes can be managed by identifying an underlying cause such as pain or lack of medications. Potent direct vasodilators are contraindicated because of the potential exacerbation of diastolic dysfunction commonly found in the elderly; therefore, volume overload should be avoided. Adequate pain control must be ensured, along with avoidance of common drug–drug interactions in this population. Atelectasis is a common postoperative occurrence; therefore, incentive spirometry should be initiated immediately after surgery with turning, coughing, and deep breathing to prevent increased respiratory compromise. Prophylaxis should also be employed against deep venous thrombosis, infection, and constipation.[33]

As previously mentioned, age is not a contraindication to colpocleisis. However, there are certain preoperative factors to consider that may preclude a patient from proceeding with surgery. Although a minimally invasive surgery, patients with severe cardiovascular or pulmonary risk factors may not be able to undergo the necessary anesthesia for surgery. LeFort colpocleisis is also contraindicated in patients with a history of uterine or cervical pathology that warrants surveillance or staging of disease. Therefore, confirmation of negative cervical cancer screening and absence of postmenopausal bleeding with uterine pathology is an essential part of the preoperative evaluation. Literature suggests that "there is a 1.1% risk of missing an early endometrial carcinoma in postmenopausal women when preserving the uterus for prolapse surgery."[36] In 2010, Frick et al. conducted a retrospective analysis of pathology findings after hysterectomy during female pelvic medicine and reconstructive surgery. They found that approximately 2.6% had unanticipated endometrial hyperplasia or malignancy.[37] Jones et al. found in their 2017 survey of 322 physicians who perform colpocleisis, 68% routinely performed an endometrial evaluation prior to proceeding with surgery. Of those, approximately 81% proceeded with transvaginal ultrasound versus 14% who conducted dilation and curettage (with or without hysteroscopy) during their preoperative evaluation.[27] Despite these data, there is no consensus about the necessity for a transvaginal ultrasound or endometrial sampling prior to proceeding with colpocleisis. In fact, a decision analysis model that compared uterine evaluation to no evaluation in women undergoing LeFort colpocleisis found that no evaluation was superior to either biopsy or ultrasound. Endometrial evaluation was not deemed cost-effective in low-risk populations.[38]

TECHNIQUES

LeFort Colpocleisis

The cervix or vaginal cuff is grasped and brought out through the introitus (Fig. 49.3). A marking pen is used to outline two rectangular areas along the vaginal

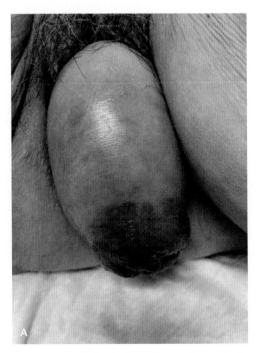
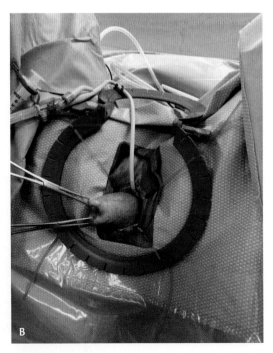

FIGURE 49.3 **A:** Stage 4 uterine prolapse. **B:** Long allis clamps applied to the cervix to exteriorize the uterine body.

FIGURE 49.4 LeFort colpocleisis. One rectangular areas along the anterior vaginal wall and one on the posterior wall are demarcated.

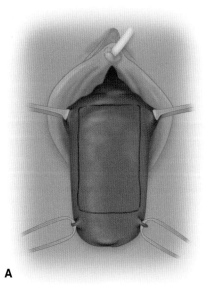

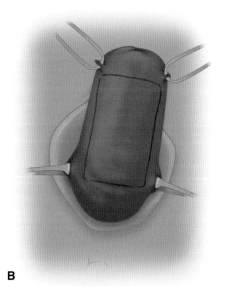

A

B

epithelium for incision, one on the anterior vaginal wall and one on the posterior wall (Fig. 49.4). When the cervix is present, the incision borders closest to the cervix are demarcated approximately 1 cm from the cervical vaginal reflection. The border of the rectangle closest to the bladder neck is placed approximately 1 to 2 cm proximal to the urethrovesical junction in order to allow for minimal traction on the bladder neck. Surgeons may prefer to use the LeFort technique in patients with a previous hysterectomy. In the case of vaginal vault prolapse, the anterior and posterior rectangles begin approximately 1 cm from the cuff in order to create an apical tunnel as is typical for the LeFort technique (Video 49.1). The inferior border of the posterior rectangle terminates approximately 2 cm proximal to the hymenal remnant. The lateral lines should leave approximately 2 to 3 cm between the anterior rectangle and posterior rectangle to allow for adequate lateral tunnels. The outlined nonkeratinized stratified

squamous epithelium can be infiltrated with saline or a vasoconstrictor of choice. It is then incised and dissected off the underlying lamina propria, including the basal cell layer in the excision is important to decrease the risk of reepithelialization. Sharp dissection is performed to leave as much vaginal adventitia and muscularis tissue overlying these structures as possible while maintaining an avascular plane of dissection (Fig. 49.5). The enterocele, if encountered, is not entered.

The lateral tunnels can be created first or in a stepwise fashion as each imbricating layer of the LeFort is tied. To create the tunnels, the proximal anterior epithelial edges are grasped and approximated with a series of interrupted or running sutures to the posterior edges of the epithelium. The reapproximation of all the epithelial strips covers the cervix or cuff and creates the apical and lateral channels (Fig. 49.6). These stitches can be tagged and held long to aid in procedural orientation. In order to ensure tunnel patency during the

FIGURE 49.5 **A,B:** Sharp dissection of the previously demarcated rectangles of vaginal epithelium. The demarcated anterior and posterior vaginal rectangles of stratified squamous epithelium are dissected off the underlying lamina propria layer.

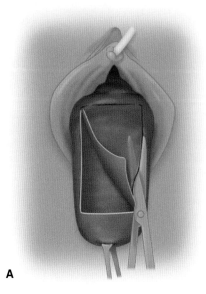

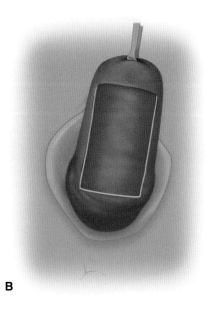

A

B

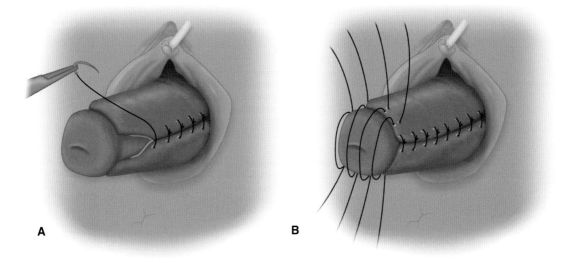

A   **B**

FIGURE 49.6 **A,B:** Lateral and apical drainage channels. The reapproximation of all the epithelial strips covers the cervix or cuff and creates the apical and lateral channels.

procedure, there have been case reports of using a vessel loop during LeFort colpocleisis.[39]

Next, the reapproximation of the anterior to posterior vaginal muscularis is accomplished with 2-0 delayed absorbable suture. Several horizontal side-by-side sutures approximately 1 cm apart are placed anterior to the cervix or vaginal cuff and then brought across the cervix or cuff to the corresponding edge of the posterior rectangle. When these sutures are tied, the cervix or vaginal cuff is thereby pushed cephalad. This is repeated in sequential rows inverting the prolapsed apex. This affords multiple points of attachment and a shelf of support (note this can

be accomplished in horizontal rows as described earlier or purse string) (Fig. 49.7). At completion of the procedure, the vaginal depth is typically 2 to 3 cm (Fig. 49.8). Cystoscopy is performed to assess for ureteral patency.

Colpocleisis with Hysterectomy or Vaginal Vault

For patients without a uterus, there is less need to leave lateral drainage channels and a total colpocleisis can be performed. The vaginal epithelium can be divided into four quadrants or removed en bloc. As in the LeFort colpocleisis, the dissection is terminated 1 to 2 cm proximal to the urethrovesical junction (Fig. 49.9). Placing Allis clamps on the edge of the epithelium being

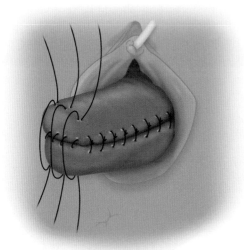

FIGURE 49.7 Inversion of uterine prolapse with side-by-side sutures. Several horizontal side-by-side sutures are placed anterior to the cervix or vaginal cuff and then brought across the cervix or cuff to the corresponding edge of the posterior rectangle to push the prolapsing part cephalad.

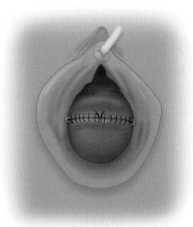

FIGURE 49.8 Reapproximated vaginal epithelium and patent lateral drainage channels. After the prolapse is reduced, the final edges of the rectangles are closed, leaving patent lateral drainage channels.

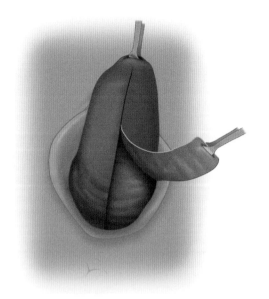

FIGURE 49.9 Colpocleisis with hysterectomy or colpocleisis of the vaginal vault. The entire vaginal epithelium is removed.

removed will aid in the dissection. Once the vaginal epithelium is denuded, the vaginal canal is then obliterated with sequential purse-string sutures (or interrupted sutures) through the fibromuscular adventitia and the distal vaginal epithelium is reapproximated. (Fig. 49.10).

Perineal Repair

The perineal repair, also known as a perineorrhaphy or perineal plication, includes the approximation of any or all of the following: the transverse perineal, bulbospongiosus, and anterior muscle fibers of the external anal sphincter to the distal end of the fibromuscular layer of the posterior vaginal wall and perineal body (Fig. 49.11). Restriction of the genital hiatus with a perineal repair is thought to be an important step in reducing the risk of prolapse recurrence.

Suture going through fibromuscular layer of posterior vaginal wall and bulbospongiosus muscle

Suture going through bulbospongiosus muscle

Bulbospongiosus muscle

Sutures going through superficial transverse perineal and anterior external sphincter

External anal sphincter muscle

Anal opening

Superficial transverse perineal muscle

FIGURE 49.11 Perineal repair or perineorrhaphy. Approximation of the transverse perineal, bulbospongiosus, and anterior muscle fibers of the external anal sphincter to the distal end of the fibromuscular layer of the posterior vaginal wall and perineal body.

Therefore, colpocleisis success is secondary to the amount of denuded tissue sutured in apposition and an adequate perineal repair.[22]

CONCURRENT HYSTERECTOMY

In general, hysterectomy should be reserved for pathologic indications or if a total colpocleisis is planned. The main benefit of hysterectomy is the prevention of endometrial or cervical cancer, in addition to the rare

FIGURE 49.10 **A,B:** Inversion of prolapse using purse-string approach. Sequential purse-string delayed absorbable sutures are placed through the fibromuscular adventitia and the distal vagina is reapproximated.

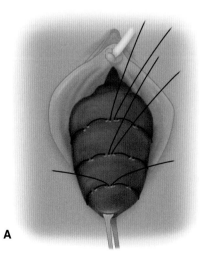

A

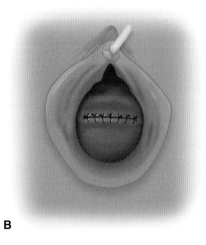

B

event of pyometra after LeFort colpocleisis secondary to occluded lateral channels.[40] The main argument against routine hysterectomy is that the advantages of less operative time and a less invasive technique with LeFort colpocleisis are compromised. Several observational studies showed longer operating times,[41] with one of these studies showing increased blood loss and longer hospital stay.[42,43] Similar findings were seen in a retrospective review by Hill et al.,[44] in which patients undergoing concurrent hysterectomy were more likely to experience postoperative venous thromboembolism when compared to those undergoing LeFort colpocleisis alone (4.6% vs. 0%, $P = .01$), in addition to longer operating times and estimated blood loss. After controlling for various demographics, comorbidities, and surgical factors, the risk of venous thromboembolism was no longer significant. Although overall complication rates are low, concomitant vaginal hysterectomy has been shown to increase the risk of serious medical complications (e.g., sepsis, cerebral vascular accident [CVA], organ space infection, myocardial infarction [MI], cardiac arrest, ventilator dependence greater than 48 hours).[41] Accordingly, vaginal hysterectomy is not routinely indicated at the time of LeFort colpocleisis unless there is uterine or cervical pathology.

In a retrospective single-center study, Lu et al.[45] sought to investigate long-term clinical outcomes, recurrence, satisfaction, and regret after total colpocleisis with concomitant vaginal hysterectomy. They found that the subjective satisfaction rate was greater than 98% and regret rate was less than 1% in both the hysterectomy and LeFort groups, leading to a conclusion of no patient perceived difference between the two procedures.[45]

COMPLICATIONS

Several large national database studies have demonstrated that colpocleisis is a safe surgery with rare serious adverse events. In one retrospective cohort study with 283 women, 8.1% had a complication within 30 days of colpocleisis, more than three quarters of which were urinary tract infections.[46] Approximately 2.1% of patients required reoperation, and a single death yielded a mortality of 0.4%. Risk factors for increased complication rates were associated with "age less than 75 years (p = 0.03), chronic obstructive pulmonary disease (p = 0.03), hemiplegia (p = 0.03), disseminated cancer (p = 0.03) and open wound infection (p = 0.02)."[46] Zebede et al.[47] described a retrospective cohort of LeFort colpocleisis patients with similar findings: 15.2% had a minor complication and a 1.3% mortality risk within 3 months. This further demonstrates that the morbidity and mortality associated with colpocleisis is low even in this high-risk population.

CONCLUSION

Colpocleisis for advanced pelvic organ prolapse remains a highly effective treatment option for patients who no longer wish to have vaginal penetrative intercourse and desire a procedure with a high rate of success, high patient satisfaction, low risk of regret, and low complication rates. Female pelvic medicine and reconstructive surgeons should ensure this underused procedure is offered to appropriate patients during surgical counseling.

ACKNOWLEDGMENT

We would like to acknowledge Lauren Anne Cadish M.D. Her contributions to the content and editing made this chapter entirely more readable.

References

1. Nygaard I, Barber MD, Burgio KL, et al. Prevalence of symptomatic pelvic floor disorders in US women. *JAMA* 2008;300(11):1311–1306.
2. Wu JM, Matthews CA, Conover MM, et al. Lifetime risk of stress urinary incontinence or pelvic organ prolapse surgery. *Obstet Gynecol* 2014;123(6):1201–1206.
3. Buchsbaum GM, Lee TG. Vaginal obliterative procedures for pelvic organ prolapse: A systematic review. *Obstet Gynecol Surv* 2017;72(3):175–183.
4. Bradbury WC. Subtotal vaginectomy. Present status in treating uterovaginal prolapse, with modified technique. *Am J Obstet Gynecol* 1963;86:663–671.
5. Adair F, DaSef L. The Le Fort colpocleisis. *Am J Obstet Gynecol* 1936;32:218–226.
6. Gerardin R. Memoire presente a la Societe Medicale de Metz en 1823. *Arch Gen Med* 1825;8:1825.
7. Neugebauer IA. Einige worte uber die mediane vaginalnaht als mittel zur beseitgung des gebarmuttervorfalls. *Zentralbl Gynaekol* 1881;3:25–33.
8. Le Fort L. Nouveau procede pour la guerison du prolapsus uterin. *Bull Gen Therap* 1877;92:337–346.
9. Edebohls GM. Panhysterokolpectomy: A new prolapsus operation. *Med Rec NY* 1901;60(15):561–564.
10. Edebohls GM. Panhysterokolpectomy: A new prolapsus operation. *Trans Am Gynecol Soc* 1901;26:150–162.
11. Hayden RC, Levinson JM. Total vaginectomy, vaginal hysterectomy, and colpocleisis for advanced procidentia. *Obstet Gynecol* 1960;16:564–566.
12. Berlin F. Three cases of complete prolapus uteri operated upon according to the method of Leon Le Fort. *Am J Obstet Gynecol* 1881;14:866.
13. FitzGerald MP, Brubaker L. Colpocleisis and urinary incontinence. *Am J Obstet Gynecol* 2003;189(5):1241–1244.
14. Wyatt J. LeFort's operation for prolapse, with an account of eight cases. *J Obstet Gynaecol Brit Emp* 1912;22:266–269.
15. Mazer C, Isral SL. The Le Fort colpocleisis: An analysis of 43 operations. *Am J Obstet Gynecol* 1948;56(5):944–949.
16. Falk HC, Kaufman SA. Partial colpocleisis: The Le Fort procedure; analysis of 100 cases. *Obstet Gynecol* 1955;5(5):617–627.
17. Hanson GE, Keettel WC. The Neugebauer–Le Fort operation. A review of 288 colpocleises. *Obstet Gynecol* 1969;34(3):352–357.

18. Ubachs JM, van Sante TJ, Schellekens LA. Partial colpocleisis by a modification of LeFort's operation. *Obstet Gynecol* 1973;42(3): 415–420.

19. Goodall JR, Power R. A modification of the Le Fort operation for increasing its scope. *Am J Obstet Gynecol* 1937;34:968–976.

20. American Urogynecologic Society, International Urogynecological Association. Joint report on terminology for surgical procedures to treat pelvic organ prolapse. *Female Pelvic Med Reconstr Surg* 2020;26(3):173–201.

21. Crisp CC, Book NM, Smith AL, et al. Body image, regret, and satisfaction following colpocleisis. *Am J Obstet Gynecol* 2013;209(5):473.e1–473.e7.

22. FitzGerald MP, Richter HE, Siddique S, et al. Colpocleisis: A review. *Int Urogynecol J Pelvic Floor Dysfunct* 2006;17(3):261–271.

23. Song X, Zhu L, Ding J, et al. Long-term follow-up after LeFort colpocleisis: Patient satisfaction, regret rate, and pelvic symptoms. *Menopause* 2016;23(6):621–625.

24. Wang X, Chen Y, Hua K. Pelvic symptoms, body image, and regret after LeFort colpocleisis: A long-term follow-up. *J Minim Invasive Gynecol* 2017;24(3):415–419.

25. Crisp CC, Book NM, Cunkelman JA, et al; Society of Gynecologic Surgeons' Fellows' Pelvic Research Network. Body image, regret, and satisfaction 24 weeks after colpocleisis: A multicenter study. *Female Pelvic Med Reconstr Surg* 2016;22(3):132–135.

26. Scheib SA, Thomassee M, Kenner JL. Enhanced recovery after surgery in gynecology: A review of the literature. *J Minim Invasive Gynecol* 2019;26(2):327–343.

27. Jones K, Wang G, Romano R, et al. Colpocleisis: A survey of current practice patterns. *Female Pelvic Med Reconstr Surg* 2017;23(4):276–280.

28. Wei JT, Nygaard I, Richter HE, et al. A midurethral sling to reduce incontinence after vaginal prolapse repair. *N Engl J Med* 2012;366(25):2358–2367.

29. Sung VW, Joo K, Marques F, et al. Patient-reported outcomes after combined surgery for pelvic floor disorders in older compared to younger women. *Am J Obstet Gynecol* 2009;201(5): 534.e1–534.e5.

30. Engen M, Svenningsen R, Schiotz HA, et al. Mid-urethral slings in young, middle-aged, and older women. *Neurourol Urodyn* 2018;37(8):2578–2585.

31. Gutman RE, Bradley CS, Ye W, et al. Effects of colpocleisis on bowel symptoms among women with severe pelvic organ prolapse. *Int Urogynecol J* 2010;21(4):461–466.

32. Karateke A, Batu P, Asoglu MR, et al. Approach to concomitant rectal and uterine prolapse: Case report. *J Turk Ger Gynecol Assoc* 2012;13(1):70–73.

33. Katz PR, Grossberg G, Potter JF, et al. *Geriatric syllabus for specialists.* New York: American Geriatrics Society, 2002.

34. Kumar C, Salzman B, Colburn JL. Preoperative assessment in older adults: A comprehensive approach. *Am Fam Physician* 2018;98(4):214–220.

35. Centers for Disease Control and Prevention. *Timed Up & Go (TUG) assessment.* Atlanta: Centers for Disease Control and Prevention; 2017.

36. Elkattah R, Brooks A, Huffaker RK. Gynecologic malignancies post-LeFort colpocleisis. *Case Rep Obstet Gynecol* 2014;2014:846745.

37. Frick AC, Walters MD, Larkin KS, et al. Risk of unanticipated abnormal gynecologic pathology at the time of hysterectomy for uterovaginal prolapse. *Am J Obstet Gynecol* 2010;202(5): 507.e1–507.e4.

38. Kandadai P, Flynn M, Zweizig S, et al. Cost-utility of routine endometrial evaluation before Le Fort colpocleisis. *Female Pelvic Med Reconstr Surg* 2014;20(3):168–173.

39. Dessie SG, Rosenblatt PL. Use of a vessel loop to ensure tunnel patency during LeFort colpocleisis. *Int Urogynecol J* 2015;26(10):1541–1543.

40. Kohli N, Sze E, Karram M. Pyometra following Le Fort colpocleisis. *Int Urogynecol J Pelvic Floor Dysfunct* 1996;7(5):264–266.

41. Bochenska K, Leader-Cramer A, Mueller M, et al. Perioperative complications following colpocleisis with and without concomitant vaginal hysterectomy. *Int Urogynecol J* 2017;28(11):1671–1675.

42. von Pechmann WS, Mutone M, Fyffe J, et al. Total colpocleisis with high levator plication for the treatment of advanced pelvic organ prolapse. *Am J Obstet Gynecol* 2003;189(1):121–126.

43. Hoffman MS, Cardosi RJ, Lockhart J, et al. Vaginectomy with pelvic herniorrhaphy for prolapse. *Am J Obstet Gynecol* 2003;189(2):364–371.

44. Hill AJ, Walters MD, Unger CA. Perioperative adverse events associated with colpocleisis for uterovaginal and posthysterectomy vaginal vault prolapse. *Am J Obstet Gynecol* 2016;214(4): 501.e1–501.e6.

45. Lu M, Zeng W, Ju R, et al. Long-term clinical outcomes, recurrence, satisfaction, and regret after total colpocleisis with concomitant vaginal hysterectomy: A retrospective single-center study. *Female Pelvic Med Reconstr Surg* 2020;27(4):e510–e515.

46. Catanzarite T, Rambachan A, Mueller MG, et al. Risk factors for 30-day perioperative complications after Le Fort colpocleisis. *J Urol* 2014;192(3):788–792.

47. Zebede S, Smith AL, Plowright LN, et al. Obliterative LeFort colpocleisis in a large group of elderly women. *Obstet Gynecol* 2013;121(2 pt 1):279–284.

CHAPTER 50

UTERINE PRESERVATION DURING PELVIC RECONSTRUCTIVE SURGERY

Robert E. Gutman • Katherine L. Woodburn

Introduction

Pelvic organ prolapse is one of the most common indications for hysterectomy in the United States, although the uterus is a passive structure in the development of prolapse.[1-3] In recent years, there has been a growing acknowledgment of the desire of many patients for uterine preservation, or hysteropexy, at the time of prolapse surgery. Patient surveys have demonstrated that, assuming equal surgical outcomes, 36% to 60% of women undergoing prolapse surgery in the United States would choose uterine preservation.[4,5] International patient surveys show similar rates of interest in uterine preservation.[6,7] Patient demographics are associated with preference for hysteropexy, with college-educated women 3 times more likely to choose uterine preservation, whereas women living in the Southern United States were less likely to request hysteropexy (odds ratio 0.7).[5]

There are a variety of reasons that patients are interested in uterine preservation including concerns about decreased libido, weight gain, hormonal changes, sense of feminine identity, cultural importance, and increased risk for hysterectomy complications. Interestingly, many reasons that patients report interest in uterine preservation are more closely related to ovarian function and conservation.[4] Proven benefits of uterine preserving surgery compared to hysterectomy include decreased blood loss, shorter operating room time, and a decreased risk of early menopause.[2,8,9] Consequently, it is important to fully elicit patient goals and their understanding of the surgical risks, benefits, and alternatives to provide patient-centered counseling during the informed consent process.

Uterine conservation may not be the best surgical options for many patients, and strict selection criteria should be maintained. Given the limited outcomes data, we prefer to avoid hysteropexy procedures for patients who desire future fertility. Instead, we encourage conservative management with observation, physical therapy, or a pessary until childbearing is complete. Additionally, uterine preservation is not recommended when there is an increased risk of subsequent cervical, uterine, or endometrial pathology, given the potential technical challenges of a subsequent hysterectomy. Women with recent or current cervical dysplasia should not be considered hysteropexy candidates, and patients undergoing hysteropexy should be up-to-date on cervical screening. Those with increased risks for endometrial cancer due to obesity, genetic syndromes such as Lynch syndrome, endometrial hyperplasia, or current tamoxifen use are also poor candidates for uterine preservation. Even with a negative workup, uterine preservation in patients with postmenopausal bleeding is discouraged because there remains a 13% lifetime risk of endometrial pathology, which may impact subsequent treatment.[10] Current estimates of overall rates of endometrial cancer in patients who have undergone uterine preservation during prolapse surgery is 0.3% to 0.8%.[10,11] Additionally, there is limited to no access to adnexal structures during the majority of hysteropexy procedures; thus, women who have BRCA1 or BRCA2 mutations or a history of estrogen receptor–positive breast cancer should be offered hysterectomy and bilateral salpingo-oophorectomy. Patients should also be counseled on the inability to perform opportunistic salpingectomy at the time of most hysteropexy procedures, which decreases ovarian cancer risk up to 20%.[12] Lastly, there are anatomic factors to consider; women with abnormal uterine bleeding, fibroids, or adenomyosis are at a higher potential risk for future interventions, whereas women with cervical elongation may experience worse outcomes in uterine preserving prolapse procedures unless a partial trachelectomy is performed.[13]

As hysteropexy procedures and patient desire for uterine preservation increases, it is important to determine patient goals and expectations while maintaining strict selection criteria to limit potential surgical risks, uterine or cervical pathology, and recurrent prolapse.

TRANSVAGINAL PROCEDURES

LeFort Colpocleisis

LeFort colpocleisis is one of the oldest and most successful prolapse repairs. Patient selection is extremely important for women undergoing a LeFort colpocleisis given that the proximal vagina is closed and the vaginal introitus is shortened and narrowed, limiting access for future uterine evaluation. Specifics regarding the technique are covered elsewhere in the textbook. Colpocleisis is intended for women who are no longer sexually active and are not interested in preserving the option for penetrative intercourse. With a high success rate and low morbidity, this procedure is ideal for an older population with advanced prolapse and multiple medical comorbidities. There are two retrospective cohort studies comparing LeFort colpocleisis to total vaginal hysterectomy (TVH) with colpocleisis, showing no overall difference in adverse events except for urinary tract infections.[14,15] A study using the National Surgical Quality Improvement Program database demonstrated a shorter operating time and fewer serious medical complications in patients undergoing LeFort colpocleisis compared to vaginal hysterectomy and colpocleisis.[15]

Manchester

The Manchester procedure is an older hysteropexy procedure with a recent resurgence, especially in Europe. It is primarily a treatment for cervical elongation. During this procedure, the cervix is amputated and the uterus reattached to the cardinal ligaments. A modified Manchester includes the plication of the uterosacral ligaments posteriorly and the cardinal ligaments anteriorly. Frequently, Sturmdorf sutures are used to close the amputated cervical stump, which can lead to problems related to cervical stenosis. The literature supporting the use of the Manchester procedure is dated and limited, with only retrospective studies that include short-term follow-up, heterogenous anatomic outcomes, and inadequate comparison groups lacking apical support procedures performed at the time of vaginal hysterectomy. These studies generally demonstrated no difference in anatomic or symptomatic outcomes, with shorter operative time and decreased estimated blood loss in the Manchester group.[16–18] A systematic review estimated the rate of repeat surgery for prolapse to be 1.1% to 5.4% with recurrent prolapse from 5.4% to 19.4%.[19] An ongoing multicenter randomized controlled trial in the Netherlands comparing the Manchester procedure to sacrospinous hysteropexy (SSHP) for milder uterine prolapse should provide valuable information about the role of this procedure for uterine conservation.[20]

Vaginal Mesh Hysteropexy

Although vaginal mesh hysteropexy products are no longer on the market in the United States, this procedure is reviewed for historical purposes. Originally developed in an effort to decrease recurrent prolapse after vaginal native tissue repairs, vaginal mesh hysteropexy was performed with mesh placed vaginally, anchored to the sacrospinous ligament (SSL) to provide apical support and then attached to the anterior cervix and fibromuscular layer overlying the bladder (Fig. 50.1). A variety of mesh kits were available, with varying delivery systems, anchor points, and mesh types. Although overall mesh complication rates were lower in mesh procedures with uterine preservation, the rate of mesh-associated complications such as erosion, exposure, bleeding, pain, contractures, and scaring was high enough to prompt reclassification of the devices by the U.S. Food and Drug Administration[21] and eventual complete removal from the United States marketplace in April 2019. When compared to vaginal native tissue repairs, vaginal mesh prolapse repairs resulted in less prolapse awareness (relative risk [RR] 0.66, 95% confidence interval [CI] 0.54 to 0.81), fewer anatomic recurrences (RR 0.4, 95% CI 0.30 to 0.53), and fewer reoperations for prolapse (RR 0.53, 95% CI 0.31 to 0.88) in a Cochrane review. Unfortunately, overall reoperations were more common (RR 2.4, 95% CI 1.51 to 3.81) due to an 8% reoperation rate for mesh complications, leading the Cochrane review to not support vaginal mesh repairs for apical prolapse.[22]

Uterosacral Hysteropexy

Similar to a uterosacral suspension for vaginal vault prolapse or after concomitant hysterectomy, uterosacral hysteropexy (USHP) can be performed vaginally or laparoscopically. When being performed vaginally, the uterosacral ligaments are accessed via posterior colpotomy either via transverse incision between the uterosacral ligaments at the cervicovaginal junction (Fig. 50.2A) or a midline posterior vaginal wall incision (Fig. 50.2B,C). Two or three sutures are placed through the uterosacral ligaments in a similar fashion to posthysterectomy uterosacral suspension and then anchored to the posterior cervix (Fig. 50.2D). We prefer using delayed absorbable sutures through a transverse incision and close the colpotomy epithelium with these stitches (Fig. 50.2E). We perform the anterior repair and sling, if indicated, prior to tying these sutures and elevating the uterus/cervix. For laparoscopic USHP, the uterosacral suspension sutures are placed laparoscopically, and the ligament is plicated and anchored into the posterior cervix. The majority of the current literature contains few prospective and retrospective cohorts, with no randomized controlled trials. The USHP studies are a mix of the mostly laparoscopic approaches with only two vaginal cohorts. The limited data for vaginal USHP appears more favorable, whereas the laparoscopic USHP data is mixed with some studies reporting low success rates and high

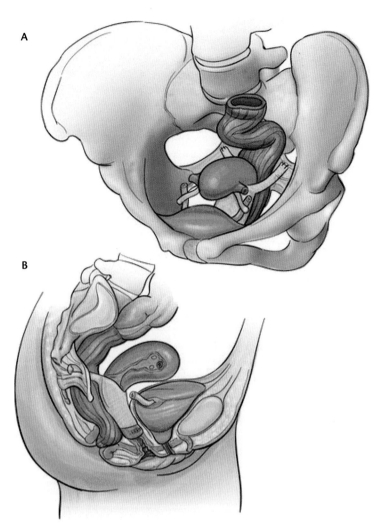

A

B

FIGURE 50.1 Vaginal mesh hysteropexy. **A:** Intra-abdominal view of the anterior mesh in the vesico-vaginal space with arms that anchor laterally to the SSLs. **B:** Sagittal view, mesh inserted between the bladder and anterior vaginal wall through an inverted U-shaped incision. Mesh is secured to the anterior cervix in the midline and lateral arms attach to each SSL providing apical support. (Reprinted from Handa VL, Van Le L. *Te Linde's operative gynecology*, 12th ed. Philadelphia: Wolters Kluwer, 2020.)

reoperation rates.[23–25] More high-quality studies are needed to determine the role of USHP for native tissue uterine conservation surgery relative to SSHP.

Sacrospinous Hysteropexy

SSHP is one of the best studied prolapse surgeries with uterine preservation and has demonstrated 5-year postoperative efficacy when compared to vaginal hysterectomy and colpopexy.[26–28] The SSL can be approached anteriorly similar to the trocarless vaginal mesh repairs (Fig. 50.3A,B), posteriorly through a posterior midline vaginal incision (Fig. 50.3C), or apically through a transverse incision in the posterior fornix at the cervicovaginal junction (see Fig. 50.2A) We prefer an apical or posterior approach under normal circumstances but have increasingly used an anterior approach when there is more severe anterior vaginal wall prolapse because this may provide better support to the proximal anterior wall and cervix. After the SSL is identified and cleared off bluntly, the procedure is similar to a posthysterectomy SSL fixation (SSLF). We use a disposable

suture capture device to place two or three delayed absorbable sutures unilaterally through the midportion of the right SSL approximately 2 to 3 cm medial to the ischial spine. For an apical approach, the anterior suture tails are then anchored to the cervix–uterosacral ligament complex on each side, whereas the posterior suture tails are secured to the distal edge of the posterior fornix incision. For an anterior approach, the posterior suture tails are anchored to the cervix on the ipsilateral side and in the midline, whereas the anterior suture tails are secured to the proximal anterior vaginal wall incision. When an anterior repair, enterocele repair, and/or sling is indicated, we typically perform these before tying down the SSHP sutures. When performing the SSHP via a posterior midline approach in anticipation of a posterior vaginal wall repair, it is our practice to begin the proximal portion of the posterior repair and closure of the vaginal epithelium before tying the SSHP sutures.

In patients with cervical elongation, a partial trachelectomy should be strongly considered. In a prospective two-part study by Lin et al.,[13] there was an

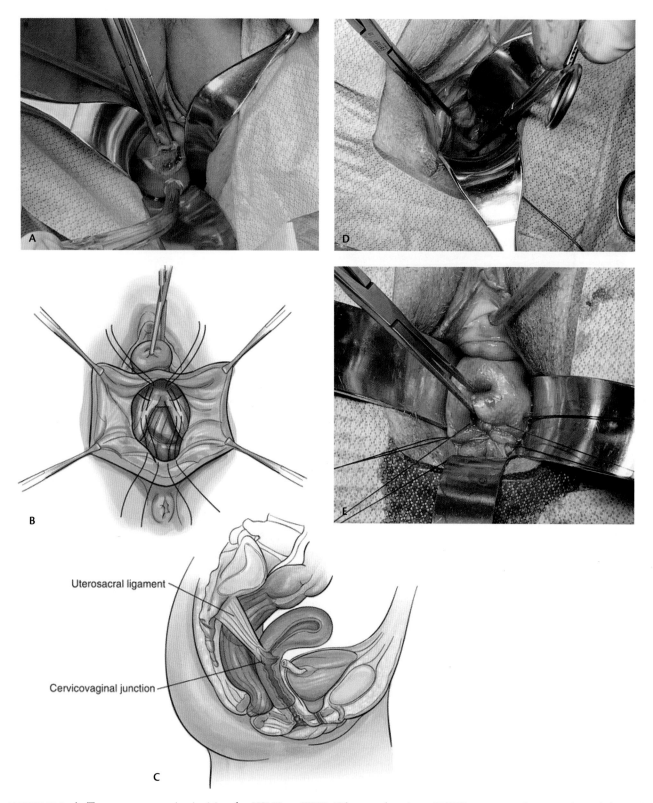

FIGURE 50.2 A: Transverse posterior incision for USHP or SSHP. When performing a USHP, access to the posterior cul-de-sac is obtained similar to a vaginal hysterectomy. **B,C:** Vaginal USHP. **B:** Uterosacral ligaments are accessed via a posterior colpotomy incision, in a modification of classic Shull technique. Two sutures have been placed on each side. **C:** Sagittal view, showing the posterior vaginal fornix and cervix supported to the uterosacral ligaments. **D:** Vaginal USHP suture placement. Breisky–Navratil retractors are used to aid in exposure. The ligament is grasped at the cuff using a Kocher clamp and proximally with a long Allis clamp for suture placement. **E:** Transverse posterior incision closure for USHP. Two delayed absorbable sutures are used to close the lateral aspects of the posterior colpotomy incision bilaterally. A figure-of-eight absorbable suture is used to close the midline. (**B,C:** Reprinted from Handa VL, Van Le L. *Te Linde's operative gynecology*, 12th ed. Philadelphia: Wolters Kluwer, 2020.)

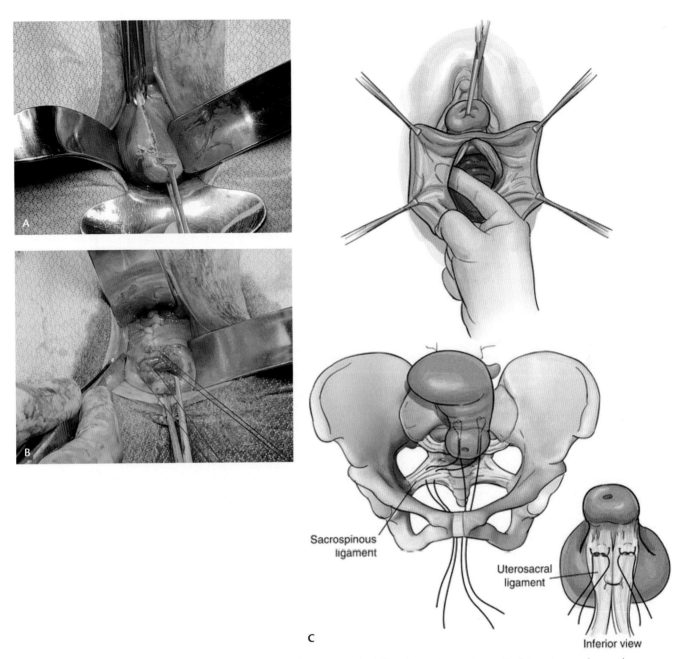

FIGURE 50.3 **A:** Anterior approach, SSHP. The incision line is scored midline from the cervicovaginal junction to the urethrovaginal junction and transversely along the cervicovaginal junction. **B:** The two delayed absorbable sutures anchored into the lateral and anterior midline cervix and vaginal epithelium. **C:** Posterior midline vertical approach for SSHP. The posterior fornix is opened through a vertical midline incision and finger dissection performed into the right pararectal space toward the SSL. Two sutures are attached to the middle third of the SSL and each side of the posterior cervix near the uterosacral ligament insertion. (**C:** Reprinted from Handa VL, Van Le L. *Te Linde's operative gynecology,* 12th ed. Philadelphia: Wolters Kluwer, 2020.)

almost 11-fold risk of failure after SSHP for patients with cervical elongation that was mitigated through performance of concomitant partial trachelectomy. Transient buttock pain has been seen at the same rates as posthysterectomy SSLF and infrequently requires suture removal for severe, intractable pain. Risks of hematoma, bleeding, and rectal injury remain rare.[26,29,30] There are two randomized controlled trials comparing

SSHP to TVH/colpopexy and four cohort studies which show similar anatomic apical success and low reoperation rates when cervical elongation is treated or excluded.[26,28] Additionally, two randomized controlled trials showed no difference in sexual function, with low rates of dyspareunia.[29,31] There is limited data regarding the possible benefits of an anterior approach SSHP, and future studies comparing approach would be useful.

TRANSVAGINAL ROUTE COMPARISONS

Overall, the data comparing routes of transvaginal hysteropexy is heterogenous and of low quality, especially when excluding vaginal mesh hysteropexy. A systematic review estimated that the range of repeat surgery for vaginal native tissue hysteropexy was 0% to 12% and recurrent prolapse ranged from 0% to 50% but with varying definitions of recurrence.[19]

ABDOMINAL SACROHYSTEROPEXY

Abdominal sacrohysteropexy can be performed via laparotomy or laparoscopically, with or without robotic assistance. The laparoscopic approach displayed similar safety and efficacy when compared to open abdominal sacrohysteropexy.[19] During this procedure, a mesh graft is attached to the anterior longitudinal ligament near the sacral promontory similar to posthysterectomy sacrocolpopexy. The mesh graft is then attached to the cervix and uterus. The most common technique uses a single polypropylene mesh strap with a bifurcation in the end of the graft, allowing the two mesh arms to be passed through windows in the broad ligament and secured to the anterior cervix. However, a wide variety of graft configurations, materials, and operative techniques have been described. We prefer to attach an anterior ultralightweight polypropylene mesh graft to the anterior vaginal wall and cervix, similar as to when performing a sacrocervicopexy. We then pass the lateral arms of the graft through windows in the broad ligaments. We also recommend a second posterior graft that is attached to the midposterior vaginal wall and uterosacral ligament–cervix complex. All three of these arms are then anchored into the anterior longitudinal ligament and the peritoneum closed over the grafts (Fig. 50.4).

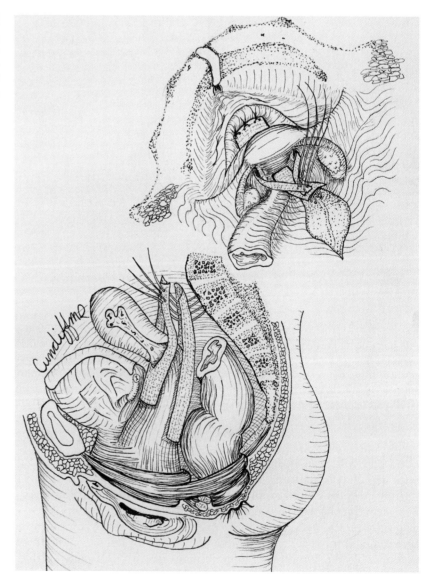

FIGURE 50.4 Sacrohysteropexy: oblique and sagittal views. (Reprinted from Gutman RE, Rardin CR, Sokol ER, et al. Vaginal and laparoscopic mesh hysteropexy for uterovaginal prolapse: A parallel cohort study. *Am J Obstet Gynecol* 2017;216[1]:38.e1–38.e11.)

These variations in technique make it difficult to meaningfully compare the available literature and outcomes. When compared to hysterectomy with native tissue apical suspension in meta-analysis, laparoscopic sacrohysteropexy (LSHP) displayed similar anatomic success and reoperation rate.[2] Although no randomized controlled trials comparing LSHP to hysterectomy with sacrocolpopexy exist, a meta-analysis of eight comparative studies suggests LSHP may have a lower anatomic success and higher reoperation rate; however, the hysterectomy group had a higher rate of mesh exposure when total hysterectomy was performed compared to supracervical hysterectomy.[2]

HYSTEROPEXY COMPARISONS

Given the wide variation in procedures, there is limited quality data comparing the route of hysteropexy. In a retrospective cohort study comparing laparoscopic USHP to LSHP, LSHP patients demonstrated more bulge symptoms and/or retreatment at 6 months, although these findings were not significant after controlling for baseline differences.[32] In one of the most rigorous comparisons, LSHP was compared to SSHP in a randomized control trial out of the Netherlands. In this study by van IJsselmuiden et al.,[33] at 12 months, LSHP was noninferior to SSHP for anatomic or surgical failure and there was no difference in quality of life or sexual function, although dyspareunia was more frequent after SSHP. Although no longer available in the United States, SSHP with anterior graft was compared to LSHP in a multicenter prospective cohort trial. At 1-year follow-up, there were no significant differences in composite success or overall satisfaction.[34]

CONCLUSION

There is growing interest for both patients and providers in uterine preservation that is supported by higher quality short- and longer-term safety and efficacy data, with SSHP being the best studied procedure. Patient selection and patient-centered counseling is crucial in order to decrease risks and reoperations while maintaining high success and satisfaction. Unfortunately, there is no strong evidence to determine the best route of hysteropexy when choosing uterine preservation at the time of prolapse procedure.

References

1. Wright JD, Herzog TJ, Tsui J, et al. Nationwide trends in the performance of inpatient hysterectomy in the United States. *Obstet Gynecol* 2013;122(2 Pt 1):233–241.
2. Gutman R, Maher C. Uterine-preserving POP surgery. *Int Urogynecol J* 2013;24(11):1803–1813.
3. DeLancey JO. Anatomic aspects of vaginal eversion after hysterectomy. *Am J Obstet Gynecol* 1992;166(6 Pt 1):1717–1728.
4. Frick AC, Barber MD, Paraiso MFR, et al. Attitudes toward hysterectomy in women undergoing evaluation for uterovaginal prolapse. *Female Pelvic Med Reconstr Surg* 2013;19(2):103–109.
5. Korbly NB, Kassis NC, Good MM, et al. Patient preferences for uterine preservation and hysterectomy in women with pelvic organ prolapse. *Am J Obstet Gynecol* 2013;209(5):470.e1–470.e6.
6. van IJsselmuiden MN, Detollenaere RJ, Gerritse MBE, et al. Dutch women's attitudes towards hysterectomy and uterus preservation in surgical treatment of pelvic organ prolapse. *Eur J Obstet Gynecol Reprod Biol* 2018;220:79–83.
7. Lyatoshinsky P, Fünfgeld C, Popov A, et al. Pelvic organ prolapse patients' attitudes and preferences regarding their uterus: Comparing German- and Russian-speaking women. *Int Urogynecol J* 2019;30(12):2077–2083.
8. Ridgeway B, Frick AC, Walter MD. Hysteropexy. A review. *Minerva Ginecol* 2008;60(6):509–528.
9. Meriwether KV, Antosh DD, Olivera CK, et al. Uterine preservation vs hysterectomy in pelvic organ prolapse surgery: A systematic review with meta-analysis and clinical practice guidelines. *Am J Obstet Gynecol* 2018;219(2):129–146.e2.
10. Frick AC, Walters MD, Larkin KS, et al. Risk of unanticipated abnormal gynecologic pathology at the time of hysterectomy for uterovaginal prolapse. *Am J Obstet Gynecol* 2010;202(5):507.e1–507.e4.
11. Renganathan A, Edwards R, Duckett JRA. Uterus conserving prolapse surgery—What is the chance of missing a malignancy? *Int Urogynecol J* 2010;21(7):819–821.
12. ACOG Committee Opinion No. 774: Opportunistic salpingectomy as a strategy for epithelial ovarian cancer prevention. *Obstet Gynecol* 2019;133(4):e279–e284.
13. Lin T, Su T, Wang Y, et al. Risk factors for failure of transvaginal sacrospinous uterine suspension in the treatment of uterovaginal prolapse. *J Formos Med Assoc* 2005;104(4):249–253.
14. Hill AJ, Walters MD, Unger CA. Perioperative adverse events associated with colpocleisis for uterovaginal and posthysterectomy vaginal vault prolapse. *Am J Obstet Gynecol* 2016;214(4):501.e1–501.e6.
15. Bochenska K, Leader-Cramer A, Mueller M, et al. Perioperative complications following colpocleisis with and without concomitant vaginal hysterectomy. *Int Urogynecol J* 2017;28(11):1671–1675.
16. Thys SD, Coolen A, Martens IR, et al. A comparison of long-term outcome between Manchester Fothergill and vaginal hysterectomy as treatment for uterine descent. *Int Urogynecol J* 2011;22(9):1171–1178.
17. Kalogirou D, Antoniou G, Karakitsos P, et al. Comparison of surgical and postoperative complications of vaginal hysterectomy and Manchester procedure. *Eur J Gynaecol Oncol* 1996;17(4):278–280.
18. Thomas AG, Brodman ML, Dottino PR, et al. Manchester procedure vs. vaginal hysterectomy for uterine prolapse. A comparison. *J Reprod Med* 1995;40(4):299–304.
19. Meriwether KV, Balk EM, Antosh DD, et al. Uterine-preserving surgeries for the repair of pelvic organ prolapse: A systematic review with meta-analysis and clinical practice guidelines. *Int Urogynecol J* 2019;30(4):505–522.
20. Schulten SFM, Enklaar RA, Kluivers KB, et al. Evaluation of two vaginal, uterus sparing operations for pelvic organ prolapse: Modified Manchester operation (MM) and sacrospinous hysteropexy (SSH), a study protocol for a multicentre randomized non-inferiority trial (the SAM study). *BMC Womens Health* 2019;19(1):49.

21. U.S. Food and Drug Administration. Urogynecologic surgical mesh implants. Accessed October 1, 2020. https://www.fda.gov/medical-devices/implants-and-prosthetics/urogynecologic-surgical-mesh-implants

22. Maher C, Feiner B, Baessler K, et al. Transvaginal mesh or grafts compared with native tissue repair for vaginal prolapse. *Cochrane Database Syst Rev* 2016;2(2):CD012079.

23. Romanzi LJ, Tyagi R. Hysteropexy compared to hysterectomy for uterine prolapse surgery: Does durability differ? *Int Urogynecol J* 2012;23(5):625–631.

24. Milani R, Manodoro S, Cola A, et al. Transvaginal uterosacral ligament hysteropexy versus hysterectomy plus uterosacral ligament suspension: A matched cohort study. *Int Urogynecol J* 2020;31(9):1867–1872.

25. Haj-Yahya R, Chill HH, Levin G, et al. Laparoscopic uterosacral ligament hysteropexy vs total vaginal hysterectomy with uterosacral ligament suspension for anterior and apical prolapse: Surgical outcome and patient satisfaction. *J Minim Invasive Gynecol* 2020;27(1):88–93.

26. Detollenaere RJ, den Boon J, Stekelenburg J, et al. Sacrospinous hysteropexy versus vaginal hysterectomy with suspension of the uterosacral ligaments in women with uterine prolapse stage 2 or higher: Multicentre randomised non-inferiority trial. *BMJ* 2015;351:h3717.

27. Schulten SFM, Detollenaere RJ, Stekelenburg J, et al. Sacrospinous hysteropexy versus vaginal hysterectomy with uterosacral ligament suspension in women with uterine prolapse stage 2 or higher: Observational follow-up of a multicentre randomised trial. *BMJ* 2019;366:l5149.

28. Dietz V, van der Vaart CH, van der Graaf Y, et al. One-year follow-up after sacrospinous hysteropexy and vaginal hysterectomy for uterine descent: A randomized study. *Int Urogynecol J* 2010;21(2):209–216.

29. Jeng C, Yang Y, Tzeng C, et al. Sexual functioning after vaginal hysterectomy or transvaginal sacrospinous uterine suspension for uterine prolapse: A comparison. *J Reprod Med* 2005;50(9):669–674.

30. Maher CF, Cary MP, Slack MC, et al. Uterine preservation or hysterectomy at sacrospinous colpopexy for uterovaginal prolapse? *Int Urogynecol J Pelvic Floor Dysfunct* 2001;12(6):381–385.

31. Detollenaere RJ, Kreuwel IAM, Dijkstra JR, et al. The impact of sacrospinous hysteropexy and vaginal hysterectomy with suspension of the uterosacral ligaments on sexual function in women with uterine prolapse: A secondary analysis of a randomized comparative study. *J Sex Med* 2016;13(2):213–219.

32. Davidson ERW, Thomas TN, Lampert EJ, et al. Route of hysterectomy during minimally invasive sacrocolpopexy does not affect postoperative outcomes. *Int Urogynecol J* 2019;30(4):649–655.

33. van IJsselmuiden MN, van Oudheusden A, Veen J, et al. Hysteropexy in the treatment of uterine prolapse stage 2 or higher: Laparoscopic sacrohysteropexy versus sacrospinous hysteropexy—A multicentre randomised controlled trial (LAVA trial). *BJOG* 2020; 127(10):1284–1293.

34. Gutman RE, Rardin CR, Sokol ER, et al. Vaginal and laparoscopic mesh hysteropexy for uterovaginal prolapse: A parallel cohort study. *Am J Obstet Gynecol* 2017;216(1):38.e1–38.e11.

Materials, Grafts, and Innovations in Pelvic Reconstructive Surgery

CHAPTER 51

SUTURES AND SYNTHETIC MATERIAL IN RECONSTRUCTIVE PELVIC SURGERY

Rubin Raju • Olivia O. Cardenas-Trowers • Emanuel C. Trabuco

Introduction

Pelvic organ prolapse affects approximately 25% of women in the United States with a 13% lifetime risk of undergoing surgery for pelvic organ prolapse.[1] Trauma to the pelvic floor associated with childbirth, chronic straining, or as a result of inherent or acquired connective tissue disorders are the main risk factors for developing this condition. When patient fails conservative therapy, native tissue repair using suture or mesh-based abdominal repairs are the main procedures available to address prolapse. Understanding suture and mesh properties is fundamentally important for pelvic surgeons to optimize functional outcomes while minimizing morbidity with the repair.

In this chapter, we review how suture and mesh biology, and the inciting host response they trigger, are key determinants of outcome and types and frequency of encountered complications.

SUTURES IN PELVIC RECONSTRUCTIVE SURGERY

Suture is an indispensable material used in female pelvic medicine and reconstructive surgery (FPMRS). The most common sutures used in FPMRS are synthetic and classified as either absorbable or nonabsorbable. Table 51.1 lists common sutures used in FPMRS. Suture selection is important as suture properties (e.g., absorption rate, filament composition, etc.) may influence surgical outcomes.

Suture Biology

The primary goal of suture material is to approximate tissues until wound healing takes place. Wound healing is usually divided into three phases: initial lag phase, fibroblastic phase, and maturation phase. In the initial lag phase (the first 5 days), sutures provide the main structural integrity for the wound. When tissue is disrupted or injured, there is an immediate response of vasospasm and clot formation at the site. At the time of

the initial incident, peaking at 24 hours, and continuing for approximately 4 days, granulocytes are active at the wound site. Epithelial cell growth begins 6 hours after injury and peaks by 24 hours. During this time and continuing up to 30 days postinjury, there is continuous macrophage activity. During the fibroblastic phase (days 5 to 15), local fibroblast growth leads to collagen deposition that leads to rapid increase in wound strength; fibroblast activity and collagen formation continue at a high level for several months. Neovascularization begins 3 days after injury with new vessel formation peaking at 7 days and scar revascularization completing by 30 days. It is during the maturation phase (day 14 and beyond) that connective tissue remodeling leads to formation of a mature, type I collagen-rich scar. Wound tensile strength increases throughout this process; from 3% to 7% at the end of the second week to 50% by 4 weeks. At best, a wound will heal to achieve approximately 80% of its preinjury strength once healing is completed.[2]

Sutures are divided into absorbable and nonabsorbable.[3] Absorbable sutures made from animal sources (e.g., purified bovine intestinal serosa, sheep submucosa) are degraded via proteolysis (broken down by the body's enzymatic systems), whereas synthetic sutures undergo hydrolysis (broken down by fluid penetration). Proteolysis causes more inflammation than hydrolysis which can lead to more scarring; hence, chromic catgut suture (which degrades by proteolysis) is not typically used to close epithelial tissue. Delayed absorbable sutures (polydioxanone [PDS II, Maxon]) take longer to be absorbed compared to other sutures in this category (Table 51.2). Nonabsorbable sutures resist enzymatic action and remain in the body permanently. The exception to this rule is silk, which resorbed within 2 years.[3]

The filamentous property of suture is also important to consider. Monofilament suture is composed of one filament and has a smaller surface area than multifilament suture. The weave, or spaces between fibers, in the multifilament sutures enable bacteria (<1 micrometer) to avoid immune cell (>20 micrometers) clearance. Although associated with increased infection risk,

TABLE 51.1

Synthetic Sutures Commonly Used in Female Pelvic Medicine and Reconstructive Surgery

SUTURE	COMPOSITION	COLOR	FILAMENT	TENSILE STRENGTH	FULL ABSORPTION	COMMENT
Absorbable						
Vicryl (Ethicon)	Polyglactin 910	Undyed (white), dyed (violet)	Braided	50% at 21 d	56–70 d	Has coated and antibacterial versions
Monocryl (Ethicon)	Poliglecaprone 25	Undyed (white), dyed (violet)	Monofilament	2 wk: 20%–30% undyed, 30%–40% dyed	90–120 d	Has antibacterial version
PDS II (Ethicon)	Polydioxanone	Undyed (white), dyed (violet)	Monofilament	60% at 6 wk	182–238 d	Has antibacterial version
Barbed						
Stratafix (Ethicon)	Polydioxanone; PGA-PCL; Monocryl; PDS	Undyed (white), dyed (violet)	Monofilament	Variable	120–180 d; 90–120 d; 182–238 d	Mono- or bidirectional barbs
V-Loc (Covidien)	Glycolide, dioxanone, and trimethylene carbonate; copolymer of glycolic acid and trimethylene carbonate	Undyed (white), dyed (violet); Undyed (clear), dyed (green)	Monofilament	7 d, 90%; 14 d, 75%; 7 d, 80%; 14 d, 75%; 21 d, 65%	90–110 d; 180 d	—
Quill (Surgical Specialties)	PGA-PCL; Polydioxanone	Undyed (clear), dyed (violet)	Monofilament	7 d, 42%–76%; 14 d, 36%–52%; 14 d, 80%–90%; 28 d, 60%–82%; 42 d, 47%–79%	90 d; 180–220 d	Uni- or bidirectional barbs
Nonabsorbable						
Gore-Tex (Gore Medical)	ePTFE	White	Monofilament	—	—	—
Ethibond (Ethicon)	Polyester	Green or white	Braided	—	—	—
Prolene (Ethicon)	Polypropylene	Blue	Monofilament	—	—	—
Barbed						
V-Loc (Covidien)	Polybutester	Blue	Monofilament	—	—	—
Stratafix (Ethicon)	Polypropylene	Undyed	Monofilament	—	—	—
Quill (Surgical specialties)	Polypropylene	Blue	Monofilament	—	—	—

PGA, polyglycolic acid; PGL, polycaprolactone.

Adapted from CP Medical Australia. Suture comparison charts. Accessed September 30, 2020. https://cpmedical.com.au/suture-comparison-charts/; Ethicon. PDS® II (polydioxanone) Suture. Accessed September 30, 2020. https://www.ethicon.com/na/epc/search/keyword/suture?lang=en-default&page=5; W. L. Gore & Associates. GORE-TEX®Suture. Accessed September 30, 2020. https://www.goremedical.com/products/suture; DemeTECH. Veterinary orthopedic implants: Suture comparison chart. Accessed September 30, 2020. https://vetimplants.com/content/Wall%20Charts/SUTURE%20COMPARISON%20CHART.pdf; Medtronic. Nonabsorbable sutures. Accessed September 30, 2020. https://www.medtronic.com/covidien/en-us/products/wound-closure/non-absorbable-sutures.html; and Surgical Specialties Corporation. Quill™ barbed sutures. Accessed September 30, 2020. https://www.surgicalspecialties.com/suture-wound-closure-brands/quill-barbed-sutures/.

Suture Material and Degradation Time

SUTURE TYPE	DEGRADATION TIME
Plain gut	7–10 d
Chromic gut	12–24 d
Vicryl (coated, braided, polyglactin)	50% tensile strength at 3 wk; all lost by 5 wk
Polydioxanone monofilament (PDS II, Maxon)	50% tensile strength at 4 wk; 25% by 6 wk

Reprinted from Table 2: Baggish MS. Suture material, suturing techniques, and knot tying. In: Baggish MS, Karram MM, eds. *Atlas of pelvic anatomy and gynecologic surgery*, 4th ed. Philadelphia: Elsevier, 2016:109–128. Copyright © 2016, with permission from Elsevier.

multifilament suture are easier to handle. In particular, multifilament suture has less memory than monofilament suture and therefore is more pliable requiring less knots to secure it. Monofilament suture, conversely, passes through tissue easier than multifilament and typically with less of an inflammatory reaction.

Suture Selection

The choice of suture should be based on the volume of tissue needed to be secured, the tensile strength of the tissue being reapproximated, and the potential for bacterial contamination. The smallest suture that can adequately accomplish tissue approximation should be selected.[3] If more healing time (e.g., fascia) is required, a suture with a delayed absorption profile (e.g., polydioxanone) should be used.[4] Multifilament sutures (e.g., Vicryl or braided silk) have a greater potential for infection compared to monofilament sutures (e.g., Monocryl or Prolene) and should not be used in areas prone to infection, e.g., skin.[4] Although there are antibiotic-infused sutures available in the market, there is no evidence that use of these sutures decreases the risk of infection from FPMRS procedures. Silk suture is made from natural material, it is easy to handle and tie secure knots. Silk and nonabsorbable sutures should not be used in the bladder.[3] Polypropylene (Prolene) cause less tissue reactive than silk and nylon and hence is ideal for repair of infected or contaminated tissues.[3] Coated suture may decrease the friction of the suture when reapproximating tissue. The barbed or "knot-less" sutures have been shown to decrease operative time and is available as an absorbable or nonabsorbable configurations.

Potential Complications of Permanent Suture

Suture erosion, diskitis, osteomyelitis, sinus tract formation, and abscesses are rare but potential complications of permanent suture use in FPMRS.[5,6,7] To minimize

the risk of diskitis and osteomyelitis during sacrocolpopexy, suture placement should not penetrate deeper than 1.9 mm into the anterior longitudinal ligament of the sacrum (the median thickness of this ligament)[8] and should avoid the disk space at the promontory. To decrease the risk of sinus tract formation and infection, permanent braided sutures (e.g., Gore-Tex or Teflon) should not penetrate the vaginal epithelium.

Sacrocolpopexy

Optimal suture selection has been most extensively studied in sacrocolpopexy. A sacrocolpopexy involves suspending the vagina to the sacrum, typically with mesh secured with suture. Minimally invasive sacrocolpopexy, which is sacrocolpopexy performed laparoscopically or with robotic assistance, has been shown to result in improved outcomes such as decreased blood loss, infection, and pain and faster recovery time compared to abdominal sacrocolpopexy.[9,10] As a result, studies have primarily evaluated different suture materials in the outcomes of minimally invasive sacrocolpopexy.[11] A multicenter randomized trial comparing the use of nonabsorbable suture (Gore-Tex) with delayed-absorbable monofilament suture (polydioxanone) for vaginal attachment of the Y-shaped lightweight mesh found no differences in mesh or permanent suture exposure rates (5.1% vs. 7.0%, respectively; risk ratio 0.73, 95% confidence interval [CI] 0.24 to 2.22).[12] A limitation of the study was that it did not standardize vaginal cuff closure, which was performed with various absorbable sutures. Most patients (9/12, 75%) with mesh or suture exposure were asymptomatic.[12] Retrospective studies have similarly found that absorbable suture appears to yield equivalent anatomical outcomes with lower risk of suture erosion compared to permanent suture for vaginal attachment of mesh during sacrocolpopexy.[13,14] However, the use of nonabsorbable, braided suture for vaginal mesh attachment to the vagina was found to be an independent and significant risk factor for mesh or suture exposure (odds ratio, 4.52; 95% CI 1.53 to 15.37)[15] and should be avoided.

The data on the use of bidirectional, barbed, self-anchoring, delayed absorbable suture for vaginal attachment of sacrocolpopexy mesh, is controversial with some studies showing no differences in anatomical recurrences and others finding increased recurrence for mesh attachment with interrupted delayed absorbable suture.[16] Further study in this topic is warranted as self-anchoring suture use is associated with significantly faster mesh attachment compared to interrupted suture use (29 minutes vs. 42 minutes, respectively, $P < .001$).[16] Noncomparative studies evaluating self-anchoring suture use in sacrocolpopexy have found this approach to be safe and effective.[17–19]

Mesh attachment to the anterior longitudinal ligament has traditionally used nonabsorbable suture.

The necessity of this practice has been questioned by a retrospective cohort study of robotic sacrocolpopexy using absorbable suture (polyglactin 910) for sacral attachment. At a median follow-up of 33 months 10 patients (7.6%) had prolapse recurrence, however, only 2 had apical failure (only 1 of which appeared to have mesh detached from the sacrum). This finding suggests that nonabsorbable suture may be utilized for sacral attachment.[14]

Hysterectomy

Hysterectomy is often performed concurrently with vaginal and abdominal prolapse repair procedures. Absorbable suture is most often used to close the vaginal cuff. However, the delayed absorbable barbed suture has gained popularity in minimally invasive hysterectomy. A 2015 systematic review[20] and a 2019 randomized controlled trial[21] comparing conventional suture to barbed suture for vaginal cuff closure during minimally invasive hysterectomy found that both suture materials are equally efficacious and safe for vaginal cuff closure with shorter operative times for the barbed suture.

Vaginal Apical Suspension

As an alternative to sacrocolpopexy, the apex of the vagina can be suspended to uterosacral ligaments or to the sacrospinous ligament. There is no difference in anatomical success between uterosacral ligament suspension performed with absorbable and nonabsorbable sutures; however, use of nonabsorbable suture increases the risk of suture exposure.[22-24] In fact, the use of braided nonabsorbable suture in sacrospinous ligament fixation resulted in suture-related complications in 36% (23/64) of patients, with 70% (16/23) requiring suture removal.[25] Even though there is presently no comparative data available to guide suture selection for sacrospinous apical suspension, the use of nonabsorbable braided suture should be avoided for both commonly used of apical suture repairs.

Vaginal Wall Repairs

The literature comparing suture material for vaginal wall repairs (i.e., colporrhaphy) is limited. There is no difference in anterior prolapse support between anterior colporrhaphy repaired with nonabsorbable or absorbable suture; with suture exposure being observed in 15% of the patients in the nonabsorbable suture arm.[26] The literature is also inconsistent regarding the benefits of delayed absorbable suture for anterior colporrhaphy; with some studies showing improved anatomical results and others showing no difference compared to rapidly absorbable sutures.[27,28] Note, however, that the use of delayed absorbable suture was associated with significantly higher rates of urinary urgency.[27] There is no benefit for the use of delayed absorbable suture in the posterior compartment.[27]

SYNTHETIC MESH AND BIOLOGIC MATERIAL USED IN PELVIC RECONSTRUCTIVE SURGERY

Mesh is defined by the International Urogynecological Association/International Continence Society as "a (prosthetic) network fabric or structure; open spaces or interstices between strands of the net"[29] that are used in prolapse repairs. Graft on the other hand refers to "any tissue or organ for transplantation."[29] In pelvic surgery, "graft" is a general term that refers to three types of materials: autografts (derived from patient), allograft (derived from cadaver), and xenografts (derived from nonhuman sources). Surgical repair of pelvic organ prolapse can involve placement of mesh or graft to reinforce the native connective tissue and restore prolapsed organs to their anatomical position. There has been controversy surrounding vaginal mesh use for pelvic organ prolapse repair, and recently on April 16, 2019, the U.S. Food and Drug Administration (FDA) ordered manufacturers of mesh for transvaginal repair of anterior compartment prolapse to stop selling their products.[30] The FDA's response stems from increased number of severe mesh-related complications reported to Manufacturer and User Facility Device Experience (MAUDE) and to FDA with no significant improvement in clinical outcomes. Yet, it is critical to understand that the FDA's recommendation was explicitly directed toward vaginal mesh kits and do not apply to mesh use for midurethral slings and for abdominal prolapse repair. Because these remain commonly performed procedures, it is imperative that the pelvic surgeon understand mesh biology and how intrinsic material characteristic impacts healing and complications.

Mesh and Graft Biology

Materials used for pelvic reconstruction can be classified into (1) synthetic mesh, (2) biologics also known as grafts (autografts, allografts, xenografts), and (3) composite material. Table 51.3 is a summary of the advantages and disadvantages of these different kinds of mesh.[31]

Synthetic materials

Synthetic mesh used can be absorbable, nonabsorbable, or a combination of absorbable and nonabsorbable material.

Absorbable mesh

Absorbable mesh (polygalactin 910 [Vicryl], polyglycolic acid [Dexon]) will degrade over time (polygalactin 30 days; polyglycolic acid 90 days) through a process called hydrolysis and is replaced by a collagen-rich scar

TABLE 51.3		
Comparison of Reconstructive Materials		
GRAFT TYPE	**ADVANTAGES**	**DISADVANTAGES**
Synthetic	Cheaper and easy to manufacture	Infection
	Reproducible	Erosion
Autograft	No risk of rejection or erosion	Variable tissue quantity and quality of harvest graft
	Cost-effective	Harvest morbidity
Allograft	Available in larger quantities than autografts; however, donor supply not reliable	Theoretical risk of infection
	No harvest morbidity	Potential for rejection
	Low-erosion risk	Inconsistent graft strength (processing of graft can weaken material), more expensive
Xenograft	Available in larger quantities; no harvest morbidity	Theoretical risk of infection
	Low-erosion risk	Potential for rejection
		Inconsistent graft strength (processing of graft can weaken material)
		Cultural barriers with porcine and bovine grafts; more expensive

From Trabuco EC, Klingele CJ, Gebhart JB. Xenograft use in reconstructive pelvic surgery: A reviewed of the literature. *Int Urogynecol J* 2007;18:555–563.

tissue that provides strength to the site of repair.[32] They have a lower risk of infection, mesh exposure, or erosion.[33,34] The resultant scar tissue, however, has less mechanical stability when compared to scar tissue containing nonabsorbable mesh.[33,35] This theoretically can lead to an increased risk of recurrent pelvic organ prolapse.

Nonabsorbable mesh

Nonabsorbable mesh such as polypropylene (Prolene) and expanded polytetrafluoroethylene (ePTFE, Gore-Tex) remain indefinitely at the site of repair and are considered permanent implants. The persistence of nonabsorbable mesh allows for better tensile support[33] and decreases the risk of pelvic organ prolapse recurrence. Polypropylene is the most widely used nonabsorbable material due to its relatively inert nature, easy of tailoring, and cheap cost.[36] Nonabsorbable mesh were initially classified by Amid[37] based on pore size and filament type (Table 51.4). Type I mesh (macroporous >75 micrometers), with large pore size, allows for collagen deposition and neovascularization throughout the mesh and results in incorporation of the material

TABLE 51.4		
Amid Classification of Synthetic Mesh		
TYPE	**PORE SIZE**	**DESCRIPTION AND EXAMPLES**
I	**Macroporous (>75 micrometers)**	Monofilament polypropylene (Prolene, Marlex, Gynemesh, Marlex, Restorelle, UltraPro) NOTE: further subdivided into heavy-, mid-, and lightweight materials
II	**Microporous (<10 micrometers)**	ePTFE (Gore-Tex)
III	**Macroporous (>75 micrometers) with multifilamentous or microporous components** NOTE: Histologic behavior is similar to type II material.	Polyethylene (Mersilene, Vypro II, eTFE, Surgipro, and Parietex) Polypropylene (ObTape, IVS Tunneler); ObTape, a heat bonded polypropylene mesh with microporous components and IVS Tunneler, multifilament polypropylene had increased rates of infections and erosion and have been removed from the market.[91]
IV	**Submicroporous (<1 micrometer)**	Polypropylene sheet [Celgard] Not used in gynecologic surgery

From Amid PK. Classification of biomaterials and their related complications in abdominal wall hernia surgery. *Hernia* 1997;1:15–21.

with the surrounding tissues.[38,39] Moreover, the large pore size allows for immune cells (>20 micrometers) to phagocytize bacteria throughout the mesh field. Type 1 mesh is currently the preferred choice for pelvic reconstructive surgery as it is associated with fewer complications compared to type 2 and 3 meshes.[40] Specifically, as discussed in detail in the following text, lightweight type 1 materials (pore sizes greater than 1 mm in diameter) are less stiff and more suitable for use in the vagina given vaginal requirements to accommodate change in volume with stooling and intimacy.[41]

Combination absorbable and nonabsorbable mesh

Combination of absorbable and nonabsorbable mesh material (e.g., polypropylene with polygalactin [Vypro] or with poliglecaprone [UltraPro]) attempts to further minimize the risk of mesh exposure. Theoretically, the absorbable component of the mesh provides temporary wound integrity and strength while lowering the permanent mesh load. As a result, these materials have functionally larger pore size (as the absorbable component eventually is resorbed), lower stiffness, less long-term inflammation; characteristics which may lead to improved outcome with lower complications.[32]

Biologic graft material

Biologics are further classified into autologous, allografts, and xenografts.[29] Allografts and xenografts are also referred to as heterologous grafts. Allografts and xenografts are acellular extracellular matrices harvested from cadavers or animal sources, respectively. Regardless, each undergoes proprietary postharvesting processes to render the material nonimmunogenic and sterile.[42] They may also be fenestrated to enhance tissue in growth.[43]

Autologous grafts

Autologous grafts are derived from the patient's own tissue,[29] commonly the fascia lata or rectus sheath. Their main advantage is that they incorporate well into native tissue and have no risk of disease transmission or rejection.[43] However, the fascial harvest procedure adds morbidity (increased patient discomfort, bleeding, infection, or hernia formation) and size of graft harvest is limited.[42]

Allografts

Allografts are connective tissue scaffolds harvested from cadaveric dermis, fascia lata, or dura mater[29] and thereby eliminate harvest related morbidity and graft size constraints associated with autografts. Human tissue bank donors are screened for blood-borne pathogens (HIV, syphilis, human T-lymphotropic virus, or hepatitis B or C)[42] and there have been no reported cases of donor-related viral infection associated with the use of allografts. The material is rendered nonimmunogenic by proprietary washing processes, which are designed to remove cellular debris without permanently damaging the connective tissue scaffold. As allografts have consistently underperformed compared to autograft and synthetic mesh, it is unclear if the structural integrity is truly preserved by these proprietary processes. Processing and sterilization techniques vary by manufacture, giving allografts varying biomechanical properties and further complicating comparisons.[42]

Xenografts

Xenografts are acellular collagen scaffolds, with or without additional extracellular matrix components that are harvested from porcine or bovine sources.[29] They differ in the source species (bovine or porcine), site of harvest (pericardium, dermis, bladder, or small intestine submucosa), and by whether or not chemical cross-linking is used in the processing to render the material nonimmunogenic. Bovine-derived xenografts pose a theoretical risk of infection with bovine spongiform encephalopathy.[36] It is not clear whether architectural differences due to harvest site (e.g., dermis with high elastin content vs. intestinal submucosa with no elastin content) affects if In vivo performance. Patients may object to use of porcine or bovine implants due to religious or cultural issues.

Composite mesh

Composite mesh combine a layer of extracellular matrix with permanent synthetic mesh (MatriStem Surgical matrix; acellular porcine urinary bladder matrix) to mitigate mesh-related complications. Although there is limited clinical data on composite meshes, animal studies have shown that the use of composite mesh attenuates the proinflammatory response and foreign body reaction elicited by noncoated mesh without affecting its biomechanical properties.[44,45] Moreover, extracellular matrix bioscaffolds promote tissue remodeling and facilitate regeneration through immune modulatory effects.[46] Composite mesh designs are also being studied for delivery of autologous mesenchymal stem cells due to the immune modulatory effects of stems cells.[47]

Host Response

Host response to a given material is a key determinant of mesh-related complications and outcomes following pelvic organ prolapse surgery.

The host response to foreign materials has been well described. Initially, there is an infiltration of neutrophils that is followed by macrophages. There are two types of macrophages, M1 (proinflammatory) and M2 (involved with remodeling and wound healing). Persistence of

M1 macrophages leads to tissue damage and destruction due to persistent inflammation. In women with complications, mesh-induced M1 response persists years after implantation. On the other hand, M2 macrophages secrete growth factors and anti-inflammatory immune modulators that result in tissue deposition and in-growth. An extensive M2 response can lead to extensive fibrosis.[48] Growing evidence shows that T cells regulate this macrophage response and in turn play a critical response in the host response to biomaterials. T cells, usually a transiently detected cell population at the mesh implantation site, remain elevated in women with mesh-related complication.[49]

Histologically, there are four host responses to mesh implantation:

- Incorporation: The mesh is infiltrated by host cells, allowing neovascularization and collagen deposition throughout the material.
- Encapsulation: Collagen and connective tissue deposition occurs only at the periphery of the mesh so that the mesh is surrounded by a connective tissue sheath.
- Mixed response: a combination of incorporation at the mesh pores and encapsulation around the remainder of the mesh
- Resorption: The mesh is replaced by host neoconnective tissue.

Materials which undergo encapsulation or mixed response are at increased risk for infection, exposure, sinus tract development, and erosion into genitourinary tract.

Mesh and graft factors influencing host response (Table 51.5)

Host response is dependent on the following factors:

- Synthetic mesh: pore size, weave, weight, and stiffness
- Autografts: autologous tissue; host response is rarely problematic.
- Allografts: Key factor(s) have not been elucidated.
- Xenografts: removal of host cellular components and chemically cross-linking

Synthetic materials

Host response to synthetic prosthetic materials depends on pore size (space between fibrils), weave (mono- or multifilament), and weight (density).

Pore size and weave

Pore size is a critical determinant of the host response. Nonabsorbable polypropylene meshes designed with pores larger than 75 micrometers undergo incorporation; a healing response whereby neovascularization and de novo collagen deposition is observed throughout the material. The large interstice, spaces between the mesh fibers, allows for immune cell to readily neutralize bacteria and limits the risk of infection. Materials with pore size less than 10 micrometers undergo an encapsulation response with fibroblast and immune cell colonization restricted to the material surface[50] and are at increased risk of infection as large immune cells (macrophages and natural killer cells) cannot infiltrate interstices to phagocytose bacteria.[51] Mesh weave also plays an important role in host response because the microporous space between fibers restricts immune cell access similar to what is observed for microporous mesh.[52]

Even though all material with pores sizes greater than 75 micrometers are incorporated, the quality of the neoconnective tissue that form between mesh fibers is optimal for mesh with pores size greater than 1 mm. Materials with pore size less than 1 mm have less effective tissue in-growth, elicit chronic inflammatory changes and can undergo fibrotic encapsulation. As a result, most contemporary polypropylene mesh have pore size ≥1 mm.[53]

Weight

Mesh weight, or density, is a measure of the spacing between polypropylene fibers in a given material (Fig. 51.1). All other things being constant, the larger the pore size, the less total material needed to make a given size of mesh and the more flexible the graft and resulting scar.[54] It has been postulated that lightweight materials may be less prone to infection and exposure compared to heavyweight materials. The density or stiffness of a given material appears to impact vaginal smooth muscle in a process called *stress shielding*. Stress shielding occurs when the stiff mesh (e.g., Marlex) shields the softer vaginal tissues from force transmission resulting in maladaptive remodeling leading to vaginal atrophy and degeneration. Gynemesh (Ethicon) has been associated with greater negative impact on vaginal smooth muscle compared to the less stiff mesh (e.g., UltraPro and Restorelle [Coloplast]).[55] Emerging data suggests that pore size distortion during tensioning can alter the effective pore size to <1 mm and lead to poor tissue ingrowth and fibrotic encapsulation despite the mesh preimplantation dimensions.[41,53]

Other potential factors

Square pore geometry may be more stable with less distortion during tensioning compared to diamond pores geometry.[56] Polypropylene, a dense stiff material originally employed in abdominal wall hernia repair had poorer incorporation and more exposure compared to polyamide mesh when used in vaginal ovine model; suggesting that material type and density may be important determinants of mesh response.[47]

TABLE 51.5

Contemporary Mesh Products and Their Properties

SLING PRODUCT	MATERIAL	COLOR	TYPE AND APPROACH	PORE SIZE	WEIGHT	PORE GEOMETRY
Advantage (Boston Scientific)[a,b]	Polypropylene Monofilament	Blue or white	Retropubic, transvaginal bottom-up approach	1,182 micrometers	100 g/m^2	Nonsquare
Advantage Fit (Boston Scientific)[a,b]	Polypropylene Monofilament	Blue or white	Retropubic, transvaginal bottom-up approach	1,182 micrometers	100 g/m^2	Nonsquare
Lynx (Boston Scientific)[a,c]	Polypropylene Monofilament	Blue or white	Retropubic, suprapubic top-down approach	1,182 micrometers	100 g/m^2	Nonsquare
Obtryx (Boston Scientific)[a]	Polypropylene Monofilament	White	Transobturator, outside-in approach	1,182 micrometers	100 g/m^2	Non Square
Obtryx II (Boston Scientific)[a,d]	Polypropylene Monofilament	Blue	Transobturator, outside-in approach	1,182 micrometers	100 g/m^2	Nonsquare
Solyx (Boston Scientific)[a,e]	Polypropylene Monofilament	Blue or white	Single-incision system, anchoring hooks that attach to obturator membrane	1,182 micrometers	100 g/m^2	Nonsquare
Altis (Coloplast)	Polypropylene Monofilament	White with blue at suture attached sites	Single-incision system, polypropylene anchors that attach to obturator membrane	374 micrometers	70 g/m^2	Square
Supris (Coloplast)	Polypropylene Monofilament	White	Retropubic, top-down or bottom-up approach	374 micrometers	70 g/m^2	Square
Aris (Coloplast)	Polypropylene Monofilament	White	Transobturator, outside-in approach	374 micrometers	70 g/m^2	Square
Align (Bard)	Polypropylene Monofilament	White	Transobturator, outside-in approach	1,160 micrometers	81 g/m^2	Nonsquare
Desara Sling (Caldera)	Polypropylene Monofilament	Blue or white	Retropubic, bottom-up approach	1,000 micrometers	140 g/m^2	Non Square
Desara SL Sling (Caldera)	Polypropylene Monofilament	Blue or white	Transobturator, both outside-in and inside-out approach	1,000 micrometers	140 g/m^2	Nonsquare
Desara One Sling (Caldera)[f]	Polypropylene Monofilament	Blue or white	Single-incision system, anchoring hooks that attach to obturator membrane	1,000 micrometers	140 g/m^2	Nonsquare
Gynecare TVT Abbrevo (Ethicon)	Polypropylene Monofilament	Blue	Transobturator, inside-out approach	1,379 micrometers	100 g/m^2	Nonsquare
Gynecare TVT –O Transobturator (Ethicon)	Polypropylene Monofilament	Blue	Transobturator, inside-out approach	1,379 micrometers	100 g/m^2	Nonsquare
Gynecare TVT Exact (Ethicon)	Polypropylene Monofilament	Blue	Retropubic, bottom-up approach	1,379 micrometers	100 g/m^2	Nonsquare
Gynecare TVT Sling (Ethicon)	Polypropylene Monofilament	Blue	Retropubic, bottom-up approach	1,379 micrometers	100 g/m^2	Nonsquare

(continued)

TABLE 51.5 *(Continued)*

Contemporary Mesh Products and Their Properties

COLPOPEXY MESH PRODUCT	MESH MATERIAL	COLOR	PORE SIZE	WEIGHT	PORE GEOMETRY
Upsylon Y-Mesh (Boston Scientific)[g,h]	Polypropylene Y-mesh, lightweight	Blue with white midline stripe	2,800 micrometers	25 g/m^2	Nonsquare
Vertessa Lite (Caldera)[h,i]	Polypropylene Y-shaped mesh, lightweight, and single sheet	Blue	1,500 micrometers	20.9 g/m^2	Square
Restorelle Y (Coloplast)[h,j,k]	Polypropylene Y-shaped mesh, ultralightweight mesh	White	1,800 micrometers	20 g/m^2	Square
Restorelle Flat Mesh (Coloplast)[l]	Polypropylene, ultralightweight mesh	White	1,800–1,830 micrometers	19 g/m^2	Nonsquare
Artisyn Y (Gynecare)[l]	Polypropylene Y-shaped mesh, partially absorbable (poliglecaprone 25)	White with blue lines	3,900 micrometers	28[m] g/m^2	Nonsquare
UltraPro (Ethicon)[l]	Partially absorbable, lightweight mesh, polyglactin 910	White with blue lines	3,000–4,000 micrometers	28[m] g/m^2	Nonsquare
Gynemesh PS (Ethicon)[l]	Polypropylene mesh, heavier weight	White with blue lines	2,500 micrometers	42 g/m^2	Nonsquare

[a]https://www.cmeinfo.com/wp-content/uploads/2021/02/Pelvic-Floor-Portfolio-Brochure.pdf.

[b]https://www.bostonscientific.com/content/dam/bostonscientific/uro-wh/portfolio-group/sling-systems/advantage-fit/pdf/WH-465202-AD-adv-adv-fit-brochure.pdf.

[c]https://www.bostonscientific.com/content/dam/bostonscientific/uro-wh/portfolio-group/sling-systems/lynx/pdf/WH-489506-AD-lynx-brochure.pdf.

[d]https://www.bostonscientific.com/content/dam/bostonscientific/uro-wh/portfolio-group/sling-systems/obtryx-II/pdf/WH-118616-AG-obtryx-II-brochure.pdf.

[e]https://www.bostonscientific.com/content/dam/bostonscientific/uro-wh/portfolio-group/sling-systems/solyx/pdf/WH-413614-AD-solyx-brochure.pdf.

[f]https://calderamedical.com/desaraone/.

[g]http://comequi.com/wp-content/uploads/2020/06/Upsylon-Y-Mesh-PDF.pdf.

[h]https://www.pfdweek.org/assets/3/6/AUGS_Sacrocolpopexy_Course_2017.pdf.

[i]https://www.calderamedical.com/products/vertessa-family/.

[j]https://www.coloplast.us/restorelle-y-en-us.aspx#section=product-description_3.

[k]https://fda.report/PMN/K123914/12/K123914.pdf.

[l]Barone WR, Moalli PA, Abramowitch SD. Textile properties of synthetic prolapse mesh in response to uniaxial loading. *Am J Obstet Gynecol* 2016;215(3):326.e1–326.e3269.
[m]After hydrolysis of absorbable component.

From Mesh app (https://meshcatalogue.glideapp.io/), individual company brochures, and research paper (Moalli PA, Papas N, Menefee S, et al. Tensile properties of five commonly used mid urethral slings relative to the TVT. *Int Urogynecol J Pelvic Floor Dysfunct* 2008;19[5]:655–663.)

CLINICAL OUTCOMES FOR MESH AND GRAFT MATERIALS USED IN PELVIC RECONSTRUCTIVE SURGERY

Suburethral Slings for Stress Urinary Incontinence

Synthetic midurethral slings (retropubic or transobturator approach) are the gold standard operation to treat stress urinary incontinence. Women with primary stress urinary incontinence treated with retropubic sling procedures have significantly lower cumulative incidence of reoperation for recurrent stress urinary incontinence compared to the transobturator approach, especially in women with concomitant prolapse.[50] Retropubic midurethral slings are associated with higher risk for voiding dysfunction compared to the transobturator approach.[57] A meta-analysis of 11 trials and 5 studies

Heavy   Medium   Light weight

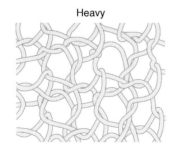
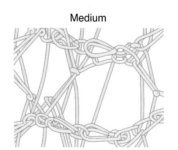
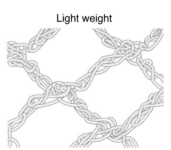

FIGURE 51.1 Macroporous mesh with varying weights. (Used with permission of Mayo Foundation for Medical Education and Research. All rights reserved.)

showed that the combined mesh erosion rates for ret-ropubic and transobturator sling ranged from 0% to 15%.[58] A subsequent study of 1,881 women under-going a sling procedure for primary stress urinary in-continence showed that reintervention rates for mesh exposure was 2% to 3% at 8 years of follow-up.[50] Autologous pubovaginal slings are not associated with mesh-related complication and may be a viable non–mesh-based option; however, these procedures are as-sociated with an increased risk of voiding dysfunction requiring surgical intervention.[59]

Mesh Use in Sacrocolpopexy for Apical Prolapse

Sacrocolpopexy is considered the gold standard oper-ation to treat apical prolapse as it achieves high success (ranging from 78% to 100%) with lower complication rates (3.4% to 6 %).[60] Importantly, the exposure rate was 4-fold higher for ePTFE (Gore-Tex; type II microporous) compared to polypropylene mesh and suggest that Gore-Tex mesh should be avoided.[5] Xenografts have been asso-ciated with a higher risk of apical failure (11%) compared to synthetic mesh (1%) and autologous grafts (1%).[61] Autologous fascial grafts may reduce the risk of synthetic mesh-related complications; however, long-term follow-up is limited.[62,63]

Transvaginal Mesh for Pelvic Organ Prolapse

Although transvaginally placed mesh has been shown to yield improved anatomical outcomes, they are associated with an array of complications ranging from asymp-tomatic mesh exposure to rare life-threatening compli-cations.[64,65] In a systematic review of 11 randomized controlled and 9 prospective studies of 2,289 patients who underwent transvaginal mesh repair, the mean total complication rate was 27% for anterior repairs, 20% for posterior repairs, and 40% for combined mesh repair.[66] As a result of these high complication rates and sever-ity of mesh-related morbidity, the FDA banned the sale of transvaginal mesh in the United States in April 2019. However, the ban did not apply to mesh use for stress urinary incontinence or transabdominal prolapse repair.[30]

COMMON MESH-RELATED COMPLICATIONS

Mesh Exposure

A common complication with nonabsorbable mesh is exposure; a condition whereby the material protrudes through the vaginal epithelial wall into the vaginal canal.[29] Symptoms range from incidental mesh detected on an asymptomatic patient during routine follow-up

exam to chronic discharge, spotting, patient and part-ner dyspareunia, or pain. Although commonly rec-ommended, there is little evidence that local estrogen therapy is effective in the management of mesh exposure with successful reepithelization observed in between 0% and 33% of patients following estrogen therapy. Regardless, a short course of vaginal estrogen therapy may be reasonable for small (<2 cm), flat (with plain of exposure parallel to the vaginal epithelial axis) non-infected mesh exposures in asymptomatic patients.[64,67] For patients with persistent exposure or who are symp-tomatic, excision is recommended. If the area of expo-sure is small and easily accessible, an in-office excision may be attempted. If mesh exposure is large or difficult to access, excision in the operating room is warranted. During excision of the exposed mesh the surrounding vaginal epithelium should be widely mobilized to allow for a tension-free closure. Additionally, the epithe-lial edges should be resected to promote healing, and closure with interrupted delayed absorbable sutures is recommended.

Mesh Erosion

Erosion refers to protrusion of mesh into the urethra, bladder, or the anorectum.[29] Urethra or bladder perfo-rations are rare impacting <1% of midurethral sling.[68] Women with these complications are often diagnosed during cystoscopy and may present with pelvic pain, recurrent urinary tract infections, hematuria, irrita-tive voiding symptoms, fistula, or bladder calculi.[69] Treatment requires removing of the intraluminal mesh. Large urethral defects during removal may require re-construction with graft augmentation (e.g., Martius). If severe stress incontinence symptoms are present, we suggest a concomitant autologous fascia sling. Holmium laser has been used to successfully excise ex-posed mesh especially in the bladder.[70]

Infection

Mesh-related infections are rare and impact less than 1% of women undergoing sacrocolpopexy or trans-vaginal mesh repairs.[71] When there is suspicion for mesh infection the mesh should be excised, especially if the implanted material induces an encapsulation response. The incidence of urinary tract infections after midurethral sling placement ranges between 12% and 33%.[72]

Mesh Contraction

Focal areas of tension detected on tight vaginal bands in areas corresponding to the trajectory of the arms of vaginal mesh kit. Whether mesh contraction is re-lated to postimplantation shrinkage of the mesh or overtensioning of the arms during index implantation is not known. Regardless of the underlying pathophysiology, excision of the tight band or removal of the arms leads to significant improvement in pelvic pain and dyspareunia.[73]

Pelvic Pain or Dyspareunia

Pelvic pain in the absence of mesh contraction has also been reported. In fact, pelvic pain has been noted in up to 16% of women undergoing mesh-based pelvic organ prolapse or stress urinary incontinence surgeries within 1 year of the index procedure.[74] Risk factors for pain included a younger age, history of fibromyalgia, worse physical health, lower surgery satisfaction, and higher somatization.[74] The etiology of pelvic pain is complex and often not clear. It is important to rule out nonmesh causes for pain and dyspareunia including vulvodynia and pelvic floor muscle spasticity. Mesh excision may be attempted following thorough patient counseling regarding possible persistence of pain despite mesh removal and treatment of non–mesh-related causes of pain.

Voiding Dysfunction

Voiding dysfunction is one of the most common complications following midurethral sling placement, occurring in 20% to 47% of patients. It is often transient, with less than 3% of patients requiring sling revision.[68]

Defecatory Dysfunction

Posterior compartment prolapse repair with nonabsorbable mesh has been associated with defecatory dysfunction in 1% to 10% of women.[75,76]

Classifying Mesh-Related Complications

Please see Table 51.6.[29]

MODIFIABLE RISK FACTORS FOR MESH COMPLICATIONS

There are several modifiable risk factors that may mitigate the risks of mesh-related complications. One of the most important modifiable risk factor is the

---

TABLE 51.6

International Urogynecological Association/International Continence Society Classification of Complications Related Directly to the Insertion of a Prosthesis in Female Pelvic Surgery

CATEGORY	TIME	SITE	PAIN
1. Vaginal: no epithelial separation	T1: intraoperative to 48 h	S1: vaginal: area of suture line	U: unspecified
2. Vaginal: smaller ≤1 exposure	T2: 48 h–2 mo	S1: vaginal: away from suture line	a: asymptomatic or no pain
3. Vaginal: large >1 cm exposure or any extension	T3: 2–12 mo	S3: trocar passage	b: provoked pain only
4. Urinary tract: compromise or perforation including prosthesis (graft) perforation or fistula	T4: over 12 mo	S4: intra-abdominal	c: pain during sexual intercourse
5. Rectal or bowel: compromise or perforation including prosthesis (graft) perforation or fistula			d: pain during physical activities
6. Skin or musculoskeletal: complications including discharge, pain, lump or sinus tract formation			e: spontaneous pain
7. Patient: compromise including hematoma or systemic compromise			

From Haylen BT, Freeman RM, Swift SE, et al. An International Urogynecological Association (IUGA)/International Continence Society (ICS) joint terminology and classification of the complications related directly to the insertion of prostheses (meshes, implants, tapes) & grafts in female pelvic floor surgery. *Int Urogynecol J* 2011;22(1):3–15.

material selection. Materials eliciting an encapsulation response (type II [microporous] or type III [macroporous with microporous/multifilament components]) preclude large immune cells (greater than 20 micrometers) from accessing small interstices between the mesh filaments and small pores (both less than 10 micrometers). As a result, this type of histologic response is associated with higher risk of mesh-related complications including exposure, erosion, and sinus tract formation. In fact, every material eliciting this response that has been used for midurethral slings has been since removed from the market because of unacceptably high complication rates. Moreover, as reviewed earlier, Gore-Tex mesh use in sacrocolpopexy is associated with a 4.5 times higher risk for mesh exposure compared to type 1 macroporous polypropylene mesh.[5] Smoking increases the risk of mesh erosion by 5-fold; with current smokers having 5.2- and a 3.2-fold increased risk of mesh exposure following sacrocolpopexy and transvaginal mesh surgery, respectively.[77] Encouraging patients to quit smoking for at least 4 weeks prior to surgery minimizes the risk of wound healing complications[78] and should be encouraged. Another modifiable risk factor is estimated blood loss during reconstructive surgery, with patient's experiencing increased blood loss having a 7.3-fold increased risk of mesh exposure compared to those who did not.[77] Lastly, women with a history of bariatric surgery are seven times more likely to have mesh exposure following midurethral sling compared to those without prior bariatric surgery.[79] Optimization of nutritional deficiencies may be beneficial to minimize this risk. Pre- and postoperative vaginal estrogen therapy has been use anecdotally to minimize the risk of mesh-related complications; however, there are some studies that question this benefit.[80,81]

SURGICAL TECHNIQUE

The pelvic surgeon should receive specialized training that allows for thorough preoperative counseling, understanding of mesh biology, and recognition and management of mesh-related complications. In a study of 198 patients treated with mesh for pelvic organ prolapse, experienced surgeons had fewer mesh exposure compared to less experience providers.[82]

Adequate dissection of the vaginal epithelium, with development of a deeper surgical plane leaving the pubocervical connective tissue attached to the vaginal epithelium, maintains the vascular supply and improves healing. The additional layer of protection and improved vascularization of the epithelium may lower the risk of mesh exposure during slings. Lastly, slings should be deployed in a tension-free fashion while avoiding rolling or bunching of the mesh. These factors may improve mesh incorporation and

minimize the risk of tight vaginal bands, pain, and mesh exposure.[73,83,84]

There is no difference in the rate of mesh exposure between abdominal and minimal invasive sacrocolpopexy (laparoscopic or robotic).[9,85] In 2017, the National Institute for Health and Care Excellence found the available data on whether or not to perform a concomitant hysterectomy at the time of sacrocolpopexy indeterminate.[86] Some studies have shown lower risk of mesh exposure in women undergoing hysterectomy compared to those who had a hysteropexy or supracervical hysterectomy.[87] On the other hand, other investigators have shown an increase in mesh exposure in women undergoing concomitant hysterectomy only during robotic but not open procedures.[88] Noncomparative studies have shown that cuff closure technique is another important factor; with series in which the cuff is closed in two layers having no increased risk of mesh exposure. Regardless, the potential improvement in mesh exposure following sacrocolpopexy with cervical or uterine preservation, needs to be counterbalanced with the risk of persistent cyclical bleeding in premenopausal women, need for cervical cancer surveillance, risk with uterine morcellation and potential morbidity with subsequent reoperation for uterine or cervical pathology.[89,90]

CONCLUSION

Surgical repair of pelvic organ prolapse involves reapproximating endopelvic fascia with sutures or with the interposition of mesh between the vaginal epithelium and the prolapsed organs. An understanding of the complex interaction between the host and biomaterial enables surgeons to choose materials that improve surgical outcomes while minimizing complications.

Absorbable suture appears to have equivalent surgical outcomes to nonabsorbable sutures for vaginal and sacral attachment of mesh used for sacrocolpopexy. Absorbable sutures, regardless if barbed, are equally effective for vaginal cuff closure following laparoscopic hysterectomy. There was no difference in prolapse outcomes for absorbable, delayed absorbable, and permanent suture for transvaginal repair of pelvic organ prolapse, with higher rates of suture exposure when permanent sutures were used.

Monofilament macroporous polypropylene nonabsorbable mesh should be used for midurethral slings and transabdominal prolapse repairs because they have been associated with improved success with the lowest complication rates. The type of mesh material used (macroporous vs. microporous and mixed), smoking cessation, meticulous hemostasis, optimizing nutritional deficiencies in patients with a history of bariatric surgery and surgical technique are modifiable risks factors that may further reduce the risk of mesh-related complications.

References

1. Wu JM, Vaughan CP, Goode PS, et al. Prevalence and trends of symptomatic pelvic floor disorders in U.S. women. *Obstet Gynecol* 2014;123(1):141–148.

2. Fonseca R, Dexter Barber H, Powers MP, et al. Management of soft tissue injuries. In: Fonseca R, Dexter Barber H, Powers MP, eds. *Oral & maxillofacial trauma.* St. Louis: Elsevier, 2013:506–565.

3. Baggish MS, Karram MM. Suture material, suturing techniques, and knot tying. In: Baggish MS, Karram MM, eds. *Atlas of pelvic anatomy and gynecologic surgery*, 4th ed. Philadelphia: Elsevier, 2016:109–128.

4. Rose J, Tuma F. *Sutures and needles.* Florida: StatPearls Publishing, 2021.

5. Cundiff GW, Varner E, Visco AG, et al. Risk factors for mesh/suture erosion following sacral colpopexy. *Am J Obstet Gynecol* 2008;199(6):688.e1–688.e5.

6. Downing KT. Vertebral osteomyelitis and epidural abscess after laparoscopic uterus-preserving cervicosacropexy. *J Minim Invasive Gynecol* 2008;15(3):370–372.

7. Hart SR, Weiser EB. Abdominal sacral colpopexy mesh erosion resulting in a sinus tract formation and sacral abscess. *Obstet Gynecol* 2004;103(5 Pt 2):1037–1040.

8. Florian-Rodriguez ME, Hamner JJ, Corton MM. First sacral nerve and anterior longitudinal ligament anatomy: Clinical applications during sacrocolpopexy. *Am J Obstet Gynecol* 2017;217(5):607.e1–607.e4.

9. Geller EJ, Siddiqui NY, Wu JM, et al. Short-term outcomes of robotic sacrocolpopexy compared with abdominal sacrocolpopexy. *Obstet Gynecol* 2008;112(6):1201–1206.

10. Linder BJ, Occhino JA, Habermann EB, et al. A national contemporary analysis of perioperative outcomes of open versus minimally invasive sacrocolpopexy. *J Urol* 2018;200(4):862–867.

11. Shepherd JP, Higdon HL III, Stanford EJ, et al. Effect of suture selection on the rate of suture or mesh erosion and surgery failure in abdominal sacrocolpopexy. *Female Pelvic Med Reconstr Surg* 2010;16(4):229–233.

12. Matthews CA, Geller EJ, Henley BR, et al. Permanent compared with absorbable suture for vaginal mesh fixation during total hysterectomy and sacrocolpopexy: A randomized controlled trial. *Obstet Gynecol* 2020;136(2):355–364.

13. Tan-Kim J, Menefee SA, Lippmann Q, et al. A pilot study comparing anatomic failure after sacrocolpopexy with absorbable or permanent sutures for vaginal mesh attachment. *Perm J* 2014;18(4):40–44.

14. Linder BJ, Anand M, Klingele CJ, et al. Outcomes of robotic sacrocolpopexy using only absorbable suture for mesh fixation. *Female Pelvic Med Reconstr Surg* 2017;23(1):13–16.

15. Durst PJ, Heit MH. Polypropylene mesh predicts mesh/suture exposure after sacrocolpopexy independent of known risk factors: A retrospective case-control study. *Female Pelvic Med Reconstr Surg* 2018;24(5):360–366.

16. Tan-Kim J, Nager CW, Grimes CL, et al. A randomized trial of vaginal mesh attachment techniques for minimally invasive sacrocolpopexy. *Int Urogynecol J* 2015;26(5):649–656.

17. Stubbs JT III. Short-term results of robotic sacrocolpopexy using the Quill SRS bi-directional polydioxanone (PDO) suture. *J Robot Surg* 2011;5(4):259–265.

18. Borahay MA, Oge T, Walsh TM, et al. Outcomes of robotic sacrocolpopexy using barbed delayed absorbable sutures. *J Minim Invasive Gynecol* 2014;21(3):412–416.

19. Kallidonis P, Al-Aown A, Vasilas M, et al. Laparoscopic sacrocolpopexy using barbed sutures for mesh fixation and peritoneal closure: A safe option to reduce operational times. *Urol Ann* 2017;9(2):159–165.

20. Bogliolo S, Musacchi V, Dominoni M, et al. Barbed suture in minimally invasive hysterectomy: A systematic review and meta-analysis. *Arch Gynecol Obstet* 2015;292(3):489–497.

21. López CC, Ríos JFL, González Y, et al. Barbed suture versus conventional suture for vaginal cuff closure in total laparoscopic hysterectomy: Randomized controlled clinical trial. *J Minim Invasive Gynecol* 2019;26(6):1104–1109.

22. Bradley MS, Bickhaus JA, Amundsen CL, et al. Vaginal uterosacral ligament suspension: A retrospective cohort of absorbable and permanent suture groups. *Female Pelvic Med Reconstr Surg* 2018;24(3):207–212.

23. Kowalski JT, Genadry R, Ten Eyck P, et al. A randomized controlled trial of permanent vs absorbable suture for uterosacral ligament suspension. *Int Urogynecol J* 2021;32(4):785–790.

24. Peng L, Liu YH, He SX, et al. Is absorbable suture superior to permanent suture for uterosacral ligament suspension? *Neurourol Urodyn* 2020;39(7):1958–1965.

25. Toglia MR, Fagan MJ. Suture erosion rates and long-term surgical outcomes in patients undergoing sacrospinous ligament suspension with braided polyester suture. *Am J Obstet Gynecol* 2008;198(5):600.e1–600.e4.

26. Zebede S, Smith AL, Lefevre R, et al. Reattachment of the endopelvic fascia to the apex during anterior colporrhaphy: Does the type of suture matter? *Int Urogynecol J* 2013;24(1):141–145.

27. Bergman I, Söderberg MW, Kjaeldgaard A, et al. Does the choice of suture material matter in anterior and posterior colporrhaphy? *Int Urogynecol J* 2016;27(9):1357–1365.

28. Valtersson E, Husby KR, Elmelund M, et al. Evaluation of suture material used in anterior colporrhaphy and the risk of recurrence. *Int Urogynecol J* 2020;31(10):2011–2018.

29. Haylen BT, Freeman RM, Swift SE, et al. An International Urogynecological Association (IUGA)/International Continence Society (ICS) joint terminology and classification of the complications related directly to the insertion of prostheses (meshes, implants, tapes) & grafts in female pelvic floor surgery. *Int Urogynecol J* 2011;22(1):3–15.

30. U.S. Food and Drug Administration. Urogynecologic surgical mesh implants. Updated July 10, 2019. Accessed September 30, 2020. https://www.fda.gov/medical-devices/implants-and-prosthetics/urogynecologic-surgical-mesh-implants

31. Trabuco EC, Klingele CJ, Gebhart JB. Xenograft use in reconstructive pelvic surgery: A review of the literature. *Int Urogynecol J Pelvic Floor Dysfunct* 2007;18(5):555–563.

32. Elango S, Perumalsamy S, Ramachandran K, et al. Mesh materials and hernia repair. *Biomedicine (Taipei)* 2017;7(3):16.

33. Lamb JP, Vitale T, Kaminski DL. Comparative evaluation of synthetic meshes used for abdominal wall replacement. *Surgery* 1983;93(5):643–648.

34. Chen CC, Ridgeway B, Paraiso MF. Biologic grafts and synthetic meshes in pelvic reconstructive surgery. *Clin Obstet Gynecol* 2007;50(2):383–411.

35. Klinge U, Schumpelick V, Klosterhalfen B. Functional assessment and tissue response of short- and long-term absorbable surgical meshes. *Biomaterials* 2001;22(11):1415–1424.

36. Deprest J, Zheng F, Konstantinovic M, et al. The biology behind fascial defects and the use of implants in pelvic organ prolapse repair. *Int Urogynecol J Pelvic Floor Dysfunct* 2006;17(Suppl 1):S16–S25.

37. Amid PK. Classification of biomaterials and their related complications in abdominal wall hernia surgery. *Hernia* 1997;1:15–21.

38. Bobyn JD, Wilson GJ, MacGregor DC, et al. Effect of pore size on the peel strength of attachment of fibrous tissue to porous-surfaced implants. *J Biomed Mater Res* 1982;16(5):571–584.

39. White RA. The effect of porosity and biomaterial on the healing and long-term mechanical properties of vascular prostheses. *ASAIO Trans* 1988;34(2):95–100.

40. Campbell P, Jha S, Cutner A. Vaginal mesh in prolapse surgery. *Obstet Gynaecol* 2018;20(1):49–56.

41. Barone WR, Knight KM, Moalli PA, et al. Deformation of transvaginal mesh in response to multiaxial loading. *J Biomech Eng* 2019;141(2):0210011–0210018.

42. Nazemi TM, Kobashi KC. Complications of grafts used in female pelvic floor reconstruction: Mesh erosion and extrusion. *Indian J Urol* 2007;23(2):153–160.

43. Cox A, Herschorn S. Evaluation of current biologic meshes in pelvic organ prolapse repair. *Curr Urol Rep* 2012;13(3):247–255.

44. Wolf MT, Carruthers CA, Dearth CL, et al. Polypropylene surgical mesh coated with extracellular matrix mitigates the host foreign body response. *J Biomed Mater Res A* 2014;102(1):234–246.

45. Wolf MT, Dearth CL, Ranallo CA, et al. Macrophage polarization in response to ECM coated polypropylene mesh. *Biomaterials* 2014;35(25):6838–6849.

46. Liang R, Knight K, Barone W, et al. Extracellular matrix regenerative graft attenuates the negative impact of polypropylene prolapse mesh on vagina in rhesus macaque. *Am J Obstet Gynecol* 2017;216(2):153.e1–153.e9.

47. Emmerson S, Mukherjee S, Melendez-Munoz J, et al. Composite mesh design for delivery of autologous mesenchymal stem cells influences mesh integration, exposure and biocompatibility in an ovine model of pelvic organ prolapse. *Biomaterials* 2019;225:119495.

48. Nolfi AL, Brown BN, Liang R, et al. Host response to synthetic mesh in women with mesh complications. *Am J Obstet Gynecol* 2016;215(2):206.e1–206.e8.

49. Tennyson L, Rytel M, Palcsey S, et al. Characterization of the T-cell response to polypropylene mesh in women with complications. *Am J Obstet Gynecol* 2019;220(2):187.e1–187.e8.

50. Trabuco EC, Carranza D, El Nashar SA, et al. Reoperation for urinary incontinence after retropubic and transobturator sling procedures. *Obstet Gynecol* 2019;134(2):333–342.

51. Iglesia CB, Fenner DE, Brubaker L. The use of mesh in gynecologic surgery. *Int Urogynecol J Pelvic Floor Dysfunct* 1997;8(2):105–115.

52. Dias FG, Dias PH, Prudente A, et al. New strategies to improve results of mesh surgeries for vaginal prolapses repair—An update. *Int Braz J Urol* 2015;41(4):623–634.

53. Barone WR, Moalli PA, Abramowitch SD. Textile properties of synthetic prolapse mesh in response to uniaxial loading. *Am J Obstet Gynecol* 2016;215(3):326.e1–326.e9.

54. Klinge U, Klosterhalfen B, Birkenhauer V, et al. Impact of polymer pore size on the interface scar formation in a rat model. *J Surg Res* 2002;103(2):208–214.

55. Jallah Z, Liang R, Feola A, et al. The impact of prolapse mesh on vaginal smooth muscle structure and function. *BJOG* 2016;123(7):1076–1085.

56. Knight KM, Liang R, King GE, et al. Altered mesh geometry: A pathway to reproducible mesh complications *in vivo. Female Pelvic Med Reconstr Surg* 2020;26(10 Suppl 1):s18.

57. Schimpf MO, Rahn DD, Wheeler TL, et al. Sling surgery for stress urinary incontinence in women: A systematic review and metaanalysis. *Am J Obstet Gynecol* 2014;211(1):71.e1–71.e27.

58. Maggiore ULR, Finazzi Agrò E, Soligo M, et al. Long-term outcomes of TOT and TVT procedures for the treatment of female stress urinary incontinence: A systematic review and meta-analysis. *Int Urogynecol J* 2017;28(8):1119–1130.

59. Morgan TO Jr, Westney OL, McGuire EJ. Pubovaginal sling: 4-YEAR outcome analysis and quality of life assessment. *J Urol* 2000;163(6):1845–1848.

60. Nygaard IE, McCreery R, Brubaker L, et al. Abdominal sacrocolpopexy: A comprehensive review. *Obstet Gynecol* 2004;104(4):805–823.

61. Quiroz LH, Gutman RE, Shippey S, et al. Abdominal sacrocolpopexy: Anatomic outcomes and complications with Pelvicol, autologous and synthetic graft materials. *Am J Obstet Gynecol* 2008;198(5):557.e1–557.e5.

62. Abraham N, Quirouet A, Goldman HB. Transabdominal sacrocolpopexy with autologous rectus fascia graft. *Int Urogynecol J* 2016;27(8):1273–1275.

63. Seth J, Toia B, Ecclestone H, et al. The autologous rectus fascia sheath sacrocolpopexy and sacrohysteropexy, a mesh free alternative in patients with recurrent uterine and vault prolapse: A contemporary series and literature review. *Urol Ann* 2019;11(2):193–197.

64. Hiltunen R, Nieminen K, Takala T, et al. Low-weight polypropylene mesh for anterior vaginal wall prolapse: A randomized controlled trial. *Obstet Gynecol* 2007;110(2 Pt 2):455–462.

65. Nguyen JN, Burchette RJ. Outcome after anterior vaginal prolapse repair: A randomized controlled trial. *Obstet Gynecol* 2008;111(4):891–898.

66. Barski D, Otto T, Gerullis H. Systematic review and classification of complications after anterior, posterior, apical, and total vaginal mesh implantation for prolapse repair. *Surg Technol Int* 2014;24:217–224.

67. Abdel-Fattah M, Ramsay I; for West of Scotland Study Group. Retrospective multicentre study of the new minimally invasive mesh repair devices for pelvic organ prolapse. *BJOG* 2008;115(1):22–30.

68. Richter HE, Albo ME, Zyczynski HM, et al. Retropubic versus transobturator midurethral slings for stress incontinence. *N Engl J Med* 2010;362(22):2066–2076.

69. Cohen SA, Goldman HB. Mesh perforation into a viscus in the setting of pelvic floor surgery—Presentation and management. *Curr Urol Rep* 2016;17(9):64.

70. Ogle CA, Linder BJ, Elliott DS. Holmium laser excision for urinary mesh erosion: A minimally invasive treatment with favorable long-term results. *Int Urogynecol J* 2015;26(11):1645–1648.

71. de Tayrac R, Sentilhes L. Complications of pelvic organ prolapse surgery and methods of prevention. *Int Urogynecol J* 2013;24(11):1859–1872.

72. Hammett J, Lukman R, Oakes M, et al. Recurrent urinary tract infection after midurethral sling: A retrospective study. *Female Pelvic Med Reconstr Surg* 2016;22(6):438–441.

73. Feiner B, Maher C. Vaginal mesh contraction: Definition, clinical presentation, and management. *Obstet Gynecol* 2010;115(2 Pt 1):325–330.

74. Geller EJ, Babb E, Nackley AG, et al. Incidence and risk factors for pelvic pain after mesh implant surgery for the treatment of pelvic floor disorders. *J Minim Invasive Gynecol* 2017;24(1):67–73.

75. Fatton B, Amblard J, Debodinance P, et al. Transvaginal repair of genital prolapse: Preliminary results of a new tension-free vaginal mesh (Prolift technique)—A case series multicentric study. *Int Urogynecol J Pelvic Floor Dysfunct* 2007;18(7):743–752.

76. Dwyer PL, O'Reilly BA. Transvaginal repair of anterior and posterior compartment prolapse with Atrium polypropylene mesh. *BJOG* 2004;111(8):831–836.

77. Gold KP, Ward RM, Zimmerman CW, et al. Factors associated with exposure of transvaginally placed polypropylene mesh for pelvic organ prolapse. *Int Urogynecol J* 2012;23(10):1461–1466.

78. Mills E, Eyawo O, Lockhart I, et al. Smoking cessation reduces postoperative complications: A systematic review and meta-analysis. *Am J Med* 2011;124(2):144–154.e8.

79. Linder BJ, El-Nashar SA, Carranza Leon DA, et al. Predictors of vaginal mesh exposure after midurethral sling placement: A case-control study. *Int Urogynecol J* 2016;27(9):1321–1326.

80. Cadish LA, West EH, Sisto J, et al. Preoperative vaginal estrogen and midurethral sling exposure: A retrospective cohort study. *Int Urogynecol J* 2016;27(3):413–417.

81. Sun Z, Zhu L, Xu T, et al. Effects of preoperative vaginal estrogen therapy for the incidence of mesh complication after pelvic organ prolapse surgery in postmenopausal women: Is it helpful or a myth? A 1-year randomized controlled trial. *Menopause* 2016;23(7):740–748.

82. Achtari C, Hiscock R, O'Reilly BA, et al. Risk factors for mesh erosion after transvaginal surgery using polypropylene (Atrium) or composite polypropylene/polyglactin 910 (Vypro II) mesh. *Int Urogynecol J Pelvic Floor Dysfunct* 2005;16(5):389–394.

83. Hurtado EA, Appell RA. Management of complications arising from transvaginal mesh kit procedures: A tertiary referral center's experience. *Int Urogynecol J Pelvic Floor Dysfunct* 2009;20(1):11–17.

84. Margulies RU, Lewicky-Gaupp C, Fenner DE, et al. Complications requiring reoperation following vaginal mesh kit procedures for prolapse. *Am J Obstet Gynecol* 2008;199(6):678.e1–678.e4.

85. Campbell P, Cloney L, Jha S. Abdominal versus laparoscopic sacrocolpopexy: A systematic review and meta-analysis. *Obstet Gynecol Surv* 2016;71(7):435–442.

86. National Institute for Health and Care Excellence. *Sacrocolpopexy with hysterectomy using mesh to repair uterine prolapse.* London: National Institute for Health and Care Excellence, 2017.

87. Abrams P, Andersson KE, Apostolidis A, et al. 6th International Consultation on Incontinence. Recommendations of the International Scientific Committee: Evaluation and treatment of urinary incontinence, pelvic organ prolapse and faecal incontinence. *Neurourol Urodyn* 2018;37(7):2271–2272.

88. Baker MV, Weaver A, Tamhane P, et al. 85: Mesh erosion after robotic and abdominal sacrocolpopexy with and without hysterectomy. *Am J Obstet Gynecol* 2019;220(3):S759.

89. Ala-Nissilä S, Haarala M, Järvenpää T, et al. Long-term follow-up of the outcome of supracervical versus total abdominal hysterectomy. *Int Urogynecol J* 2017;28(2):299–306.

90. Lethaby A, Mukhopadhyay A, Naik R. Total versus subtotal hysterectomy for benign gynaecological conditions. *Cochrane Database Syst Rev* 2012;(4):CD004993.

91. Baessler K, Hewson AD, Tunn R, et al. Severe mesh complications following intravaginal slingplasty. *Obstet Gynecol* 2005;106(4):713–716.

CHAPTER 52

THE USE OF AUTOLOGOUS FLAPS IN PELVIC RECONSTRUCTIVE SURGERY

Johnny Yi • Alanna Rebecca

Introduction

In female pelvic and reconstructive surgery, pedicled autologous tissue flaps provide the benefits of tissue volume and structural reconstruction. Autologous tissue flaps have been used in complex reconstruction as interposition flaps which increase bulk and augment vascular supply to a needed area. Interposition flaps have typically been reserved for multifaceted or recurrent conditions such as complex or radiation-induced fistulas. Flaps can also be used as tissue replacement where surgical extirpation or congenital absence creates a structural need. Autologous tissue flaps can also be used to provide volume and fill space after an exenterative procedure, such as a pelvic exenteration for malignancy. Alternatively, they can also be used to create a neovagina due to congenital absence, atresia due to radiation damage, or iatrogenic extirpation due to malignancy.

Prior to the advent of synthetic materials, the need for tissue augmentation in pelvic reconstructive surgery was recognized. As far back as 1928, Heinrich Martius,[1] described the bulbocavernosus flap as an interposition pedicled, vascularized flap for repair of vesicovaginal fistula. Alternatively, interposition flaps for abdominal surgery have commonly used pedicled omentum or rectus abdominis flaps. Both have the robust vascular supply and bulk needed to apply as an interposition when an abdominal approach is preferred or required. A flap is tissue which maintains its blood supply but is mobilized to a different location. For pelvic reconstructive surgery, the majority of flaps described are pedicled flaps which maintain an identified vascular pedicle while the tissue supplied by that blood flow is mobilized to a different location around a fulcrum. Alternatively, free flaps can also be used. This involves transecting the artery and vein supplying the tissue and performing a microvascular anastomosis at a distant location to reestablish blood flow. Free flap reconstruction is not typically used in urogynecologic surgery. This chapter focuses on pelvic floor conditions which benefit from the utilization of pedicled autologous tissue flaps.

INDICATIONS

Fistula

The most common surgical scenarios for interposition flaps in urogynecology are fistulas. Fistulas are described as an aberrant connection between two viscera. The most common fistulas of the reproductive tract include vesicovaginal and rectovaginal fistula (Fig. 52.1). Fistulas, although rare in the United States, are debilitating and significantly diminish the quality of life of women. They are most commonly found as a result of gynecologic surgery, although in the developing world are primarily associated with obstetric injury. Success rates with surgical correction for vesicovaginal fistula are high, 70% to 100%.[2,3] Although two approaches are described, vaginal and abdominal, there is a lack of comparative studies to show superiority of one modality, although the vaginal approach, by definition, has less morbidity due to the lack of abdominal incisions. The open abdominal approach has been shown to have increased hospitalization time and cost as compared to vaginal approach in one cost-effectiveness study.[4] However, with complex or recurrent vesicovaginal fistula, interposition flaps can be considered to improve vascular supply and healing. There is a lack of comparative data guiding when to use interposition flaps for fistula. Singh et al.[5] performed a randomized controlled trial of obstetric and gynecologic fistulas with randomization with or without interposition flaps. Overall success was 97% with or without interposition whether vaginal or abdominal approach. Given the high success, standard utilization of interposition flap is not recommended, although larger studies would likely be necessary to show a statistical difference. Therefore, surgeons should consider interposition flaps for fistula in cases of recurrent fistula, prior surgery with failure, and complex fistulas, such as radiation fistulas or large fistulas, which may lack adequate vascular supply for proper healing. Placing an interposition flap would provide increased vascular supply and avoiding apposing suture lines, which may benefit surgical outcome.

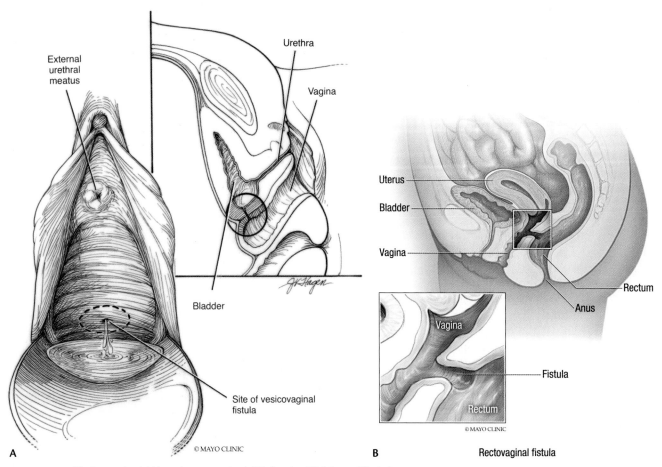

FIGURE 52.1 Vesicovaginal (**A**) and rectovaginal (**B**) fistula. (© Mayo Clinic.)

EXENTERATIVE PROCEDURES

Pelvic exenterative procedures are typically performed in cases of gynecologic, urologic, or colorectal malignancy. Following extirpation of pelvic organs, bulky interposition can be used to decrease the risk of seroma and abscess formation. Omental interposition may be adequate, but a larger flap may be necessary depending on the patient's body habitus, and if the omentum is not available or robust. Alternatively, a myocutaneous flap may assist in closing a perineal skin defect and in addition can be used to create a neovagina following pelvic exenteration procedures, if a patient desires preservation of sexual function. A recent systematic review comparing primary closure and myocutaneous flap evaluated outcomes in 566 patients.[6] Devulapalli et al.[6] described significantly increased risk of a perineal wound complication when a myocutaneous flap was not used. When the patient has desire for sexual function following exenteration, the myocutaneous flap can be mobilized to create a vaginal canal and provide a patent vagina for intercourse. Dilation and/or vaginal intercourse is likely necessary to maintain vaginal caliber. Casey et al.[7] and Scott et al.[8] described

postoperative sexual function after neovagina use. Evaluating multiple different routes of neovagina creation, overall sexual function with vaginal intercourse was approximately 47%. When the cutaneous portion is not required, a less complicated rectus abdominis interposition flap can be performed to fill dead space following exenterative procedures.

Vaginal Approach

Knowledge of the perineal anatomy and vascular supply is critical when considering the use of a perineal approach to a flap. The vascular supply to the perineum originates from branches of the internal iliac artery and the femoral artery. The anterior perineum is supplied by the external pudendal artery, superficial, and deep, originating from the femoral artery. The more robust internal pudendal artery supplies the blood supply mainly to the posterior perineum, although distal branches including the dorsal clitoral artery supply portions of the anterior perineum.[9] Interposition pedicled flaps require an intact blood supply to survive, and therefore, a thorough understanding of this anatomy is important.

Martius labial fat pad flap

Vesicovaginal fistula repair can be approached either vaginally or abdominally. Vaginal approach is less invasive and amenable when there is adequate vaginal caliber and distal location of the fistula. With this approach, the most amenable interposition flap is the Martius flap, or bulbocavernosus flap. The original description of the Martius flap included the bulbocavernosus muscle, and the dissection was performed more medially.[1] However, modification of this flap moved to exclusion of the muscle and utilization of the labial fat pad lateral to the muscle. This may decrease the risk of hemorrhage and damage to surrounding structures, such as the erectile function of the vestibular bulb.[10] Despite the lack of muscular tissue, the fat pad carries adequate vascular supply for an interposition flap as demonstrated by multiple clinical studies.

Knowledge of surgical anatomy is critical for successful performance of this procedure. A vertical incision is made lateral to the bulbocavernosus muscle along the labia majora. The medial border of the dissection is the fascia of the bulbocavernosus muscle, whereas the deep dissection is the urogenital diaphragm. Laterally, the labiocrural fold is identified separating the fat from the lateral fascial connections to the ischiopubic ramus and fascia lata. (Fig. 52.2).[10,11]

For vesicovaginal fistula, the posterior aspect of the flap is clamped and released, leaving the anterior vascular supply coming from the external pudendal artery branches along with the distal branches of the internal pudendal artery. For posterior use such as rectovaginal fistula, the anterior aspect is released, and the vascular supply is from the internal pudendal artery branches. Excision of the fistulous tract and mobilization of the vagina allows space for the flap to be laid in a tension-free manner (Fig. 52.3).

Benefits of this procedure are its less invasive approach, avoiding intra-abdominal surgery, and adequate tissue supply with a locally advanced interposition flap. Risks and morbidity associated with the Martius flap can include distortion of the labial anatomy due to dissection of the labial fat pad, leading to asymmetry with reported poor cosmetic outcomes ranging from 0.6% to 12.5%.[11,12] Further, the distal branches of the pudendal nerve, including the dorsal clitoral nerve can be damaged, leading to pain and neurologic symptoms. Numbness or decreased sensation is common, ranging from 14% to 62%, and pain at the harvest site is

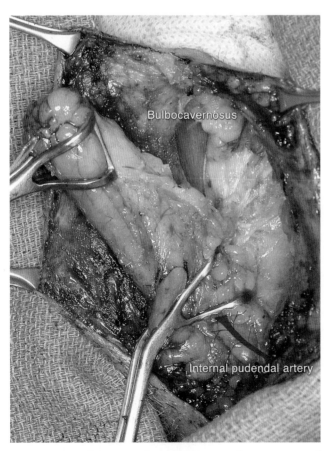

FIGURE 52.2 Left Martius flap. The Martius flap is composed of a fat pad lateral to the bulbocavernosus muscle and supplied by the internal pudendal artery.

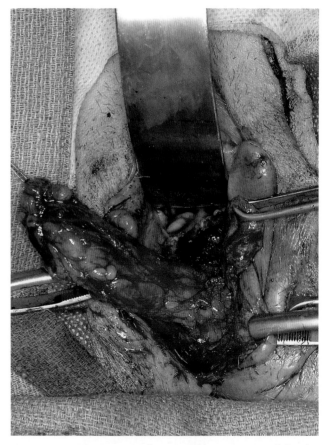

FIGURE 52.3 The Martius flap used for rectovaginal fistula. Martius flap is mobilized with a posterior vascular pedicle, placed through a lateral tunnel to overlay the fistula repair.

also not rare, 5% to 37%.[11,13] Finally, perioperative bleeding and infection are risks, and temporary drain placement can be considered. Use of the Martius flap in urologic conditions has shown high success rates, ranging from 80% to 100%.[3,11] However, given the high success rates of primary repair of urologic fistula, and due to the more invasive nature of this operation, use of the Martius flap should be individualized for cases of complex or recurrent fistula.

Gracilis muscle flap

If there is concern for lack of tissue volume or integrity with the Martius flap, an alternative flap for the vaginal approach can include the gracilis muscle or myocutaneous flap. The gracilis muscle originates along the ischiopubic ramus and courses down the medial aspect of the thigh, inserting into the medial tibia at the pes anserine. By detaching the insertion from the tibia or with division of the musculotendinous junction, the gracilis muscle can be mobilized along the medial thigh for use as an interposition flap in vaginal surgery (Fig. 52.4). The vascular pedicle reliably originates from the medial circumflex femoral artery and courses through the adductor magnus and longus to perfuse the gracilis muscle. This muscle can be easily mobilized from distal to proximal leaving the origin and vascular supply intact while maintaining ease of rotation into the defect. This interposition flap is more robust than the Martius flap, but requires further dissection from the leg, which may require a multidisciplinary approach with plastic and reconstructive

surgeons. Reported clinical outcomes from this approach are limited with described success rates about 75%, in rectovaginal fistula in women without Crohn disease, but much lower success with the disease.[14,15] This lower success rate may be explained by the higher mean number of prior operations, and underlying inflammatory conditions affecting healing, explaining a more complex clinical scenario. Benefits to this approach include more bulk of tissue, perineal approach, and avoidance of the radiated field in patients that may have had prior perineal or pelvic radiation for malignancy.

Abdominal Approach

An abdominal approach to repair may be necessary when the fistula is located high in the vaginal canal, with limited exposure, or when there is a complex fistula with ureteral or bowel involvement. When considering an abdominal approach, the same principles apply as the perineal approach. Bulk of tissue, vascular pedicle, and mobilization to reach the target to act as an interposition are key factors when considering this approach. Simple interposition flaps via the abdominal approach for pelvic surgery include a peritoneal or sigmoid epiploica flap. The peritoneal flap does not have a discrete or robust vascular supply, but does provide tissue interposition, which prevents apposing suture lines. For situations that are less complicated, such as primary cystotomy repair, this is a tool that surgeons can consider. The sigmoid epiploica is also abundant and convenient for use in pelvic surgery. Given its location and blood supply from the

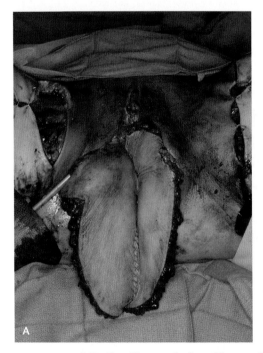
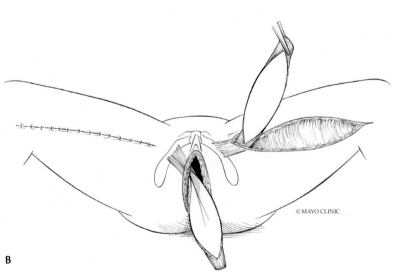

FIGURE 52.4 **A,B:** Gracilis muscle flap. The gracilis flap is a large volume interposition flap of muscle only, or myocutaneous interposition. The flap is supplied by the medial circumflex femoral artery. (**B,** Used with permission of Mayo Foundation for Medical Education and Research. All rights reserved.)

sigmoid mesentery, it may provide a more robust tissue interposition as compared to a peritoneal flap. However, this flap may still be limited in the volume and mobility needed for certain pelvic operations. More robust interposition flaps described in the literature include an omental pedicled flap and the rectus abdominis muscular or myocutaneous flap. Traditionally described via open laparotomy, advancements in minimally invasive surgery now allow most genital fistula repair to be completed with laparoscopic or robotic assistance.[16] Given this move toward minimally invasive approach, surgeons should also familiarize themselves with techniques to perform interposition flaps via laparoscopy with or without robotic assistance. Given the increase in morbidity and cost, efforts should be made to perform minimally invasive surgery if the abdominal approach is performed.

Omental flap

In an abdominal approach to vesicovaginal fistula repair, excision of the fistulous tract and repair of the bladder and vagina in layers is performed. Critical concepts to successful fistula repair include a tension-free repair that is watertight. Interposition can be performed as needed. When an abdominal approach is indicated, a pedicled omental flap is a robust interposition flap to consider. The omentum is an organ composed mainly of adipose and has a rich vascular supply. Attached to the greater curvature of the stomach, its vascular supply is from the right and left gastroepiploic arteries and has important functions in immune regulation and healing.

In order to mobilize the omentum for a pelvic interposition, the omentum can be transected below the level of the right gastroepiploic artery and vein, allowing for more length while maintaining vascular supply. Maintaining an adequate blood supply is critical, and large arteries and veins are maintained through this dissection. Once the flap is mobilized, it typically has adequate length for placement into the pelvis, although the patient may need to be taken out of the Trendelenburg position, typically used in pelvic laparoscopy and robotic surgery, to decrease tension on the flap and aide in placement of the flap (Video 52.1). With the vagina and bladder mobilized and repaired, the interposition is then sutured between the vagina and bladder. Dissection well beyond the fistulous tract is necessary to ensure the interposition flap provides a tissue barrier between the two layers. The flap is then sutured into place, typically with an absorbable suture.

Rectus abdominis interposition flap

Rectus abdominis muscle interposition flap can be used as muscle only or as a myocutaneous flap. This is a reliably long muscle and can provide a voluminous interposition flap for utilization in pelvic surgery. This approach may be warranted when larger bulk is required such as

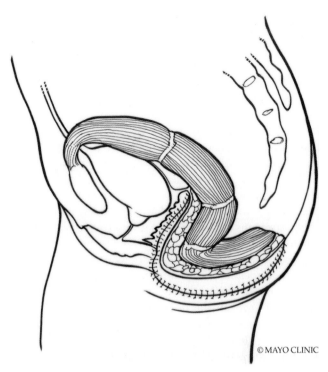

FIGURE 52.5 Rectus abdominis flap. The rectus abdominis flap is transected at the superior margin and mobilized to the pelvis. Adequate length is noted while maintaining insertion on the pubic symphysis. The flap is supplied by the inferior epigastric vessels. (Used with permission of Mayo Foundation for Medical Education and Research. All rights reserved.)

in exenterative procedures for cancer, or when alternative interposition flaps have failed. Either the right or left rectus abdominis muscle can be used when given consideration of other comorbidities such as an ostomy (Fig. 52.5). When using a muscle only flap, dissection begins by entering the posterior sheath and dissecting superficially over the muscle belly to free the muscle from the anterior fascial sheath to maintain abdominal fascial integrity. Transverse tendinous inscriptions are released from the anterior fascial sheath, mobilizing the entire rectus muscle superiorly to its insertion at the costal margin. The superior portion of the muscle is then transected, taking care to seal the superior epigastric vessels, which are the superior vascular supply. The inferior epigastric artery and its accompanying veins are then identified and preserved for flap perfusion. The muscle can be left adherent to the insertion at the pubic symphysis when mobilized as a pedicled flap or released from this attachment as an island flap if further mobilization is necessary. Again this provides a robust, well-vascularized muscle flap for interposition (Video 52.2). Leaving the posterior sheath attached to the muscle body allows for ease of suturing to inlay the flap into the desired location. The myocutaneous flap has been traditionally used, and is still considered when the skin is required, for example, in an infralevator pelvic exenteration, where the vulva and perineum are resected for cancer. Primary closure in this situation may not be possible without tension, creating the need for a skin flap. Further, the myocutaneous flap can be implemented in women for whom continued sexual function is desired, and neovaginal creation is warranted.

The omental flap generally has less morbidity and should be preferentially used if available for an interposition flap in the treatment of fistulas or pelvic reconstructive surgery. Although rectus abdominis flaps have been traditionally performed via midline vertical laparotomy, recent advances have been reported in robotic-assisted approach when rectus muscle alone is needed.[17,18] Robotic surgery has been widely adopted by pelvic surgeons and recently is of interest to plastic and reconstructive surgeons to minimize morbidity. The robotic approach allows the multidisciplinary team to complete the procedure via a minimally invasive approach. Further outcomes studies are needed to guide clinical practice. However, this approach minimizes blood loss, hospital stay, and infection as with most minimally invasive surgery; it also preserves the anterior fascial sheath and may lead to decreased risk of hernia formation. Due to the nature of the flap, myocutaneous flaps cannot be approached via minimally invasive techniques.

CONCLUSIONS

Autologous flaps are used in complex pelvic reconstructive surgery. Depending on the desired and chosen approach, vaginal or abdominal, different interposition flaps are available to the reconstructive surgeon to increase tissue bulk and vascular supply. An advanced knowledge of surrounding anatomy is necessary to choose and perform these complex surgeries and multidisciplinary approach may include not only urogynecologic surgeons but also plastic and reconstructive surgeons. Novel approaches may allow for the minimally invasive nature to provide interposition flaps; further prospective studies are required to understand the indications and benefits this provides over traditional approaches.

References

1. Martius H. Die operative Wiederherstellung der vollkommen fehlenden Harnrohre und des Schiessmuskels derselben. *Zentralbl Gynakol* 1928;52(7):480.
2. Tatar B, Oksay T, Selcen Cebe F, et al. Management of vesicovaginal fistulas after gynecologic surgery. *Turk J Obstet Gynecol* 2017;14(1):45–51.
3. Kumar M, Agarwal S, Goel A, et al. Transvaginal repair of vesico vaginal fistula: A 10- year experience with analysis of factors affecting outcomes. *Urol Int* 2019;103(2):218–222.
4. Warner R, Beardmore-Gray A, Pakzad M, et al. The cost effectiveness of vaginal versus abdominal repair of vesicovaginal fistulae. *Int Urogynecol J* 2020;31(7):1363–1369.
5. Singh V, Mehrotra S, Bansal A, et al. Prospective randomized comparison of repairing vesicovaginal fistula with or without the interposition flap: Result from a tertiary care Institute in Northern India. *Turk J Urol* 2019;45(5):377–383.
6. Devulapalli C, Jia Wei AT, DiBiagio JR, et al. Primary versus flap closure of perineal defects following oncologic resection: A systematic review and meta-analysis. *Plast Reconstr Surg* 2016;137(5):1602–1613.
7. Casey WJ III, Tran NV, Petty PM, et al. A comparison of 99 consecutive vaginal reconstructions: An outcome study. *Ann Plast Surg* 2004;52(1):27–30.
8. Scott JR, Liu D, Mathes DW. Patient-reported outcomes and sexual function in vaginal reconstruction: A 17-year review, survey, and review of the literature. *Ann Plast Surg* 2010;64(3):311–314.
9. Niranjan NS. Perforator flaps for perineal reconstructions. *Semin Plast Surg* 2006;20(2):133–144.
10. Elkins TE, DeLancey JO, McGuire EJ. The use of modified Martius graft as an adjunctive technique in vesicovaginal and rectovaginal fistula repair. *Obstet Gynecol* 1990;75(4):727–733.
11. Malde S, Spilotros M, Wilson A, et al. The uses and outcomes of the Martius fat pad in female urology. *World J Urol* 2017;35(3):473–478.
12. Petrou SP, Jones J, Parra RO. Martius flap harvest site: Patient self-perception. *J Urol* 2002;167(5):2098–2099.
13. Lee D, Dillon BE, Zimmern PE. Long-term morbidity of Martius labial fat pad graft in vaginal reconstruction surgery. *Urology* 2013;82(6):1261–1266.
14. Wexner SD, Ruiz DE, Genua J, et al. Gracilis muscle interposition for the treatment of rectourethral, rectovaginal, and pouch-vaginal fistulas: Results in 53 patients. *Ann Surg* 2008;248(1):39–43.
15. Park SO, Hong KY, Park KJ, et al. Treatment of rectovaginal fistula with gracilis muscle flap transposition: Long-term follow-up. *Int J Colorectal Dis* 2017;32(7):1029–1032.
16. Miklos JR, Moore RD, Chinthakanan O. Laparoscopic and robotic-assisted vesicovaginal fistula repair: A systematic review of the literature. *J Minim Invasive Gynecol* 2015;22(5):727–736.
17. Hammond JB, Howarth AL, Haverland RA, et al. Robotic harvest of a rectus abdominis muscle flap after abdominoperineal resection. *Dis Colon Rectum* 2020;63(9):1334–1337.
18. Haverland R, Rebecca AM, Hammond J, et al. A case series of robot-assisted rectus abdominis flap harvest for pelvic reconstruction: A single institution experience. *J Minim Invasive Gynecol* 2021;28(2):245–248.

CHAPTER 53

MANAGEMENT OF MESH COMPLICATIONS

Taylor John Brueseke • Daniel Jacob Meller

HISTORICAL PERSPECTIVE

The potential value of surgical mesh can be traced to the late 19th century. In 1890, Viennese surgeon Theodor Billroth theorized that a new prosthetic material could efficiently close hernia defects.[1] In the following years, unsuccessful attempts were made to create such a mesh from a wide variety of naturally occurring surgical materials (e.g., cotton, silk); however, these procedures failed due to infection, rejection, or recurrence.[2] It was not until 1955 that Francis Usher at Baylor College developed the first successful mesh. The group evaluated new synthetic materials developed in the post-World War II period, including nylon, Orlon, Dacron, and Teflon. Shortcomings, including foreign body reaction, sepsis, rigidity, fragmentation, loss of tensile strength, and encapsulation, were noted in their work. One material made of polyethylene, Marlex, was discovered to be suitable for implantation. Over the next 2 years, the team worked to develop a safe and effective product, eventually settling on a woven mesh with large pores. This key feature encouraged interstitial growth of the tissue through the mesh. The team finally switched to knitted polypropylene, which could be autoclaved, had firm borders, permitted two-way stretching, and could be rapidly incorporated, and published their findings in 1958.[2] This work was foundational for the development of modern mesh hernia repair techniques, the precursor to mesh-augmented vaginal prolapse repairs. History specific to sacrocolpopexy began in the late 19th century when Freund (1889) and Kustner (1890) described procedures in which the vaginal vault was fixed to the anterior longitudinal ligament by the interposition of an autologous graft. In 1958, Huguier and Scali used cutaneous flaps to successfully complete a similar procedure. Finally, in 1974, Scali was the first to report the use of a synthetic graft for abdominal repair of pelvic organ prolapse (POP).[3,4]

The modern era of pelvic mesh began in the 1990s and was defined by the meteoric rise and fall of vaginally placed mesh for the treatment of urinary incontinence and prolapse. In 1996, Boston Scientific received U.S. Food and Drug Administration (FDA) premarket approval for the ProteGen Sling, the first transvaginal mesh to be approved for marketing in the United States. By citing ProteGen as a direct or indirect predicate device, Mentor, Ethicon, American Medical Systems, Gyne Ideas, Tyco, and Caldera all gained approval for marketing under the FDA's fast track 510(k) system which did not require any form of human study to gain marketing approval. In March of 1999, Boston Scientific pulled ProteGen from the market citing higher than expected vaginal erosion and dehiscence rates. However, devices that obtained FDA approval by using ProteGen as a predicate device were not required to be removed from the market, and numerous additional devices continued to be developed. In 2002, Ethicon began marketing Gynemesh PS, the first preconfigured surgical mesh for POP, opening the gates for wide-spread adoption of nearly 100 different "mesh kits" all marketed as less invasive alternatives to abdominal surgery but ultimately found to have high complication rates when brought into general use.

U.S. FOOD AND DRUG ADMINISTRATION RESPONSES TO COMPLICATIONS ASSOCIATED WITH VAGINAL MESH

The rapid and widespread adoption of mesh kits brought mesh-augmented pelvic floor disorder surgery to large number of surgeons with varying degrees of reconstructive surgical experience. This brought with it a growing concern for complications both within the medical community and literature. Between 2005 and 2007, the FDA received over 1,000 vaginal mesh–related medical device reports adverse events to the Manufacturer and User Facility Device Experience (MAUDE) database.[5] As word spread and skepticism of safety claims by manufacturers grew, the FDA[6] released a safety communication on October 20, 2008, calling attention to "rare but serious consequences" associated with transvaginal placement of surgical mesh to treat POP and stress urinary incontinence. These complications included erosion (more currently referred to as exposure) through vaginal epithelium, infection, pain, urinary problems, and recurrence of prolapse and/or incontinence. Initial recommendations to physicians included calls to obtain specialized training before implanting mesh kits for POP and recommendations for heightened vigilance for adverse effects.

Concerns continued to grow between January 1, 2008, and December 31, 2010, as the FDA's MAUDE database received 2,874 additional reports of complications associated with vaginal mesh devices. On July 13, 2011, the FDA[7] released a safety communication and a white paper citing surgical mesh for transvaginal repair of POP as an area of "continuing serious concern." The most notable changes from their 2008 report include the statements: (1) Serious complications associated with surgical mesh for vaginal repair of POP are not rare and (2) it is not clear that transvaginal POP repair with mesh is more effective than traditional nonmesh repair. As such, the panel concluded in January 2012 (1) the risk/benefit profile of surgical mesh for transvaginal POP repair was not well established, (2) vaginally placed mesh for prolapse should be reclassified from class II (low- to moderate-risk devices) to class III (high-risk devices), and (3) companies must conduct postmarket surveillance studies to establish safety and effectiveness. Ultimately, 131 postmarket 522 study orders to 34 manufacturers of vaginal mesh were issued. Most manufacturers elected to cease marketing vaginal mesh after receiving the 522 orders, although Boston Scientific and Coloplast committed to women's health by investing in the performance of these studies. Finally, on April 16, 2019, citing insufficient evidence "that the probable benefits of these devices outweigh their probable risks," the FDA ordered all manufacturers of "surgical mesh intended for transvaginal repair of anterior compartment prolapse (cystocele)" to stop selling and distributing their products immediately.[8] It is difficult to overstate the impact this regulation has had on the surgical management of pelvic floor conditions, but it is a strong reminder of the need to establish the safety and efficacy of medical devices prior to their widespread adoption.

The FDA's willingness to grant premarket approval to dozens of new devices deemed "substantially equivalent" to existing products had a significant influence on the decisions of medical societies and governing bodies around the globe and international use of the procedures quickly became widespread in the late 2000s. However, regulation began to be imposed in the United Kingdom, Scotland, Wales, and Ireland soon after release of the influential 2017 PROSPECT study,[9] in which patients with primary POP were randomized to conventional anterior colporrhaphy, anterior colporrhaphy with synthetic mesh implant, and anterior mesh repair with biologic implant. Although the procedures resulted in similar patient-oriented subjective treatment success, 12% of patients undergoing mesh-augmented repairs experienced a mesh-related complication. After publication, the United Kingdom, through the National Institute for Care and Health Excellence (NICE) committee, drafted new guidance recommending that mesh-augmented POP repair be restricted to clinical studies. In 2019, NICE expanded opportunities for mesh surgery providing certain requirements are met including (1) women be informed about the type of mesh to be used

and whether or not it is permanent; (2) details of the procedure and its subsequent short- and long-term outcomes are recorded in a national registry; and (3) written information about the implant, including its name, manufacturer, and date of insertion, are provided to the patient.[10] Responses in other countries have varied widely.[11]

CLASSIFICATION AND TERMINOLOGY OF VAGINAL MESH COMPLICATIONS

The use of commonly agreed on terms is critical to the expansion of standardized research into the causes and treatments for vaginal mesh complications. Currently, some terms have entered the common vernacular that may not accurately reflect the pathophysiology involved. For example, the term mesh "erosion" is commonly used to describe mesh that is visible in the vagina. However, the word *erosion* implies that friction or pressure has caused the tissue covering the mesh to wear away. Current evidence suggests exposure of mesh into the vagina is the result of a significantly more complex pathophysiologic host response to the graft that involves upregulation of matrix metalloproteinases and collagenases (see "Pathophysiology of Mesh Exposure" section). As such, the use of standardized terminology should be employed to accurately describe the complication that is present and terms that imply causation should be avoided unless accurately descriptive. American Urogynecologic Society/International Urogynecological Association (AUGS/IUGA) have developed a consensus-based terminology and classification report for prosthesis and graft complications that aims to improve clinical practice and research.[12] That work is summarized in Table 53.1.

In addition to the anatomical mesh complications listed earlier, functional complications have been reported after the placement of vaginal mesh. These include the following:

- Pain
  - Acute and chronic pelvic pain
    - Provoked and unprovoked
  - Dyspareunia
  - Partner dyspareunia
- Vaginal bleeding/discharge
- Infection of the implant
- Fistula formation
- Recurrent POP
- Recurrent stress urinary incontinence

RISK FACTORS FOR VAGINAL MESH COMPLICATIONS

As described earlier, there are multiple potential complications that can result from the implantation of vaginal mesh, the most common of which is exposure of mesh into the vagina. Multiple risk factors for vaginal mesh exposure have been studied and is briefly reviewed here.

TABLE 53.1

AUGS/IUGA Definitions and Descriptions for Anatomical Mesh Complications

TYPE OF COMPLICATION	DEFINITION
Separation	Physically disconnected (vaginal epithelium)
Exposure	A condition of displaying, revealing, exhibiting, or making accessible (vaginal mesh visualized through separated epithelium)
Extrusion	Passage gradually out of body structure or tissue (a loop of tape protruding into the vaginal cavity)
Perforation	Abnormal opening into a hollow organ or viscous
Dehiscence	A bursting open or gaping along natural or sutured line
Contraction	Shrinkage or reduction in size
Prominence	Parts that protrude beyond the surface (wrinkling or folding with no epithelial separation)

AUGS/IUGA recommends against using the generic term *erosion* because this implies tissue being worn away by friction or pressure, and current evidence suggests more complex biochemical mechanisms are involved.

Graft Material

As recognized from the inception of graft-augmented reconstructive surgery, the material used in surgical management of POP has been shown to directly influence risk of exposure. Perhaps the most widely cited complication rates for various mesh types are published in the Colpopexy and Urinary Reduction Efforts (CARE) trial,[13] a randomized surgical trial of 322 stress-continent women with stages 2 to 4 POP that investigated the benefit of an adjuvant Burch colposuspension at the time of open sacral colpopexy. In addition to allograft material (cadaveric rectus facia or fascia lata), and xenograft material (hexamethylene diisocyanate cross-linked porcine dermis [Pelvicol, CR Bard, Murray Hill, NJ]), a variety of synthetic materials were used in the study. These include woven polyester (Mersilene, Ethicon, Somerville, NJ), polypropylene (Prolene, Ethicon, Somerville, NJ), soft weave polypropylene (Gynemesh, Ethicon Women's Health & Urology, Cincinnati, OH), and expanded polytrafluoroethylene (ePTFE, Gore-Tex, GORE Medical, Newark, DE). Synthetic mesh was the most common graft, used in 92% of trial procedures. Of those cases, the most commonly used materials were woven polyester (42%) (Mersilene, Ethicon, Somerville, NJ) and polypropylene (48%), with minimal usage of ePTFE (6%). At 2 years after surgery, the study found a significantly

higher risk of mesh erosion in women who had ePTFE mesh (alone or in combination) compared to those without ePTFE mesh (4 of 21 [19%] vs. 16 of 301 [5.3%]; odds ratio [OR] 4.2, 95% confidence interval [CI] 1.3 to 13.9). The extended CARE study[13] reported 7-year follow-up data, including mesh exposure rates, but unfortunately, loss to follow-up was high. Of the originally enrolled 322 women, only 122 were available for data collection at 7 years. Given the high loss to follow-up, the authors employed modeling with right censoring and projected that 10.5% of patients would have experienced mesh exposure by 7 years postsurgery. Although this is the most robust data available regarding mesh exposure rates, debate continues among surgeons regarding how to apply it when counseling patients given that many of the meshes used in this study are no longer in clinical use and the right censoring employed in the model development may inherently exclude patients less likely to have had a mesh-related complication.

In additional to material type, most surgeons recognize that higher mesh burden (mesh implanted into multiple compartments or the use of larger pieces of mesh) is associated with increased risk of mesh exposure.[14,15]

Concomitant Hysterectomy

Concomitant hysterectomy at the time of mesh-augmented prolapse repair is a debated risk factor for vaginal mesh exposure in patients undergoing sacrocolpopexy. In the CARE trial,[13] concurrent hysterectomy was performed in 83 of 322 (26%) of participants and the risk of mesh/suture exposure was higher in this group (60% exposure rate in patients with concomitant hysterectomy vs. 24% in those with prior hysterectomy [OR 4.9, CI 1.9 to 12.4]). Hysterectomy was also associated with increased risk of mesh exposure in a retrospective cohort study of 188 women who underwent minimally invasive sacrocolpopexy between November 2004 and January 2009 at the University of California, San Diego or Kaiser Southern California.[16] Nineteen (10%) of these women experienced mesh erosion with a higher rate seen in patients who underwent concomitant total vaginal hysterectomy compared with women who had a prior hysterectomy (23% vs. 5%, $P = .003$). In contrast, other studies suggest that concomitant hysterectomy with robotic sacrocolpopexy (RSCP) may be protective or not associated with mesh exposure. In a study comparing mesh exposure rates 6 weeks after surgery that included 230 participants, 118 (51.7%) had RSCP only, and 112 (48.7%) had RSCP with hysterectomy.[17] Of the nine mesh exposures identified, three occurred in the concomitant hysterectomy with RSCP group, whereas six occurred in the RSCP only group. There was no significant difference in the mesh exposure rate between total and supracervical hysterectomy. Similarly, in a retrospective comparison of exposure rates between commercial mesh kits and surgeon-fashioned mesh-augmented vaginal repairs, no significant difference in exposure rate was seen between patients who underwent concomitant hysterectomy compared to previous hysterectomy.[18]

Although the debate continues over whether performing hysterectomy at the time of prolapse repair increases the risk of mesh exposure, this potentially increased risk of mesh exposure should be used for counseling and not preclude apical suspension in patients with indications for graft-augmented apical prolapse repair.

Surgeon Volume and Intraoperative Complications

Among the multitude of factors that influence adverse outcomes after mesh surgery, the most striking may be the risk of complication stratified by low-, intermediate-, and high-volume surgeons. In a 5% random national sample of female Medicare beneficiaries obtained from the Centers for Medicare and Medicaid Services, medium- and high-volume surgeons performed only 25% and 22% of the cases, respectively, but had rates of reoperation of 2% and 3%. However, low-volume surgeons performed the majority of cases (53%) and had the highest rates of reoperation (6%).[19] The high relative risk of complication seen in low- versus high-volume surgeons has been identified repeatedly in other publications.[20-23] On a related note, intraoperative complications, such as organ perforation, have been associated with mesh complications. In a study of 77 patients experiencing vaginal mesh exposure or bladder/urethra mesh perforation, trocar injury during surgery was associated with an increased risk of mesh perforation.[24] This concern requires the surgeon to thoughtfully consider how to manage complications such as trocar perforation during midurethral sling placement or cystotomy during sacrocolpopexy. Intraoperative factors will guide high-volume surgeons in determining if a midurethral sling mesh can still be placed and the trocar safely repositioned away from the perforation site during midurethral sling placement and that sacrocolpopexy mesh can be placed if the cystotomy can be closed in a tension-free manner with overlapping layers and not in juxtaposition to the mesh. For surgeons with limited experience in these procedures, data suggest that graft placement should be deferred in the event of an intraoperative complication.

Radiation

Pelvic floor disorders are common in gynecologic cancer survivors,[25] and radiation therapy is frequently indicated to obtain cure or remission of these malignancies. The long-term effects of radiation include progressive vascular damage, obliterative arteritis, ischemia, and fibrosis.[26] Intuitively, this reduction in tissue quality is thought to predispose women to developing vaginal

mesh exposure, but limited data exist to guide reconstructive surgeons when counseling patients on the degree of increased relative risk of complication in this scenario.[27,28]

Vaginal Estrogen Exposure

Vaginal estrogen (VE) exposure is known to stimulate growth of the stratified squamous epithelium resulting in a thickening of the vaginal wall.[29] Despite these observations, perioperative estrogen exposure has not been shown to be protective against vaginal mesh exposure. A randomized controlled trial of 186 women who underwent a single surgeon noninferiority study compared 93 women who received twice weekly VE cream with 93 women who did not. Mesh exposure was documented in 16.1% (15 of 93) in the VE group versus 12.9% (12 of 93) in the non-VE group. At 1 year, the study concluded that no VE therapy before surgery was noninferior to VE therapy.[30] Similar findings were observed in a retrospective study of 1,544 patients, of which 248 (16%) used estrogen preoperatively. Thirty-seven (2.4%) of total patients experienced mesh exposure, but no significant difference was seen in the mesh exposure rate between women who used estrogen preoperatively compared to those who did not (OR 0.79, CI 0.26 to 2.38).[31] It is not clear why preoperative estrogen treatment does not reduce the risk of mesh exposure; however, the explanation is likely multifactorial.

Age

Age is an interesting risk factor for mesh exposure. As vaginal atrophy becomes more prevalent with age,[32] one may expect that older patients would be more likely to experience mesh exposure. However, studies of women undergoing transvaginal mesh-augmented prolapse repair[33] and midurethral mesh slings[34] have shown that younger age is associated with an increased risk of mesh exposure. Although the reasons for this observation are not certain, it is possible that younger patients are more likely to engage in sexual activity and that this activity may introduce a mechanical stress on the tissues. Alternatively, it has been hypothesized that the increased vascularity present in younger women may predispose to hematoma formation which impairs wound healing.

Smoking

Although studies have reported differing associations between smoking and mesh exposure,[14,16,20,24,31,34–37] most surgeons agree that smoking is a risk factor for mesh exposure. Smoking is well known to cause microvascular dysfunction which impairs wound healing[38] presumably promoting epithelial degradation of vaginal tissue overlying vaginal mesh.

PATHOPHYSIOLOGY OF MESH EXPOSURE

Although multiple mechanisms for mesh exposure have been proposed, including mechanical erosion, infection, or hematoma formation, it is likely that the full explanation of vaginal mesh exposure is complex and multifactorial. A detailed explanation of the cellular response to graft implantation is beyond the scope of this chapter, but one key element may be macrophage invasion, which is a common host response to the implantation of a foreign body, including polypropylene. Two major macrophage subtypes that are involved in the response to vaginal mesh include the M1 and M2 subtypes. The M1 macrophage response results in chronic inflammation which can result in tissue damage and destruction. M2 macrophage activity results in chronic fibrosis and encapsulation of the mesh. Current research suggests that placement of polypropylene vaginal mesh can alter the balance of the M1 versus M2 macrophage activity[39] and that this disruption of homeostasis contributes to the degradation of vaginal epithelium overlying vaginal mesh. T cells also appear to play a critical role in the long-term host response and may be a central pathway that leads to complications.[40] Additional basic science research is needed to more fully elucidate the cellular and molecular host response to the implantation of vaginal mesh.

INNERVATION OF MESH PAIN

An understanding of pelvic neuroanatomy is crucial to the prevention of neurologic injury during reconstructive surgery as well as the evaluation and management of patients with postoperative pelvic pain. The pelvic structures contain both somatic and autonomic innervation. The vulva and distal vagina receive sensory innervation via the pudendal nerve. Sensory nerves map to specific locations on the sensory cortex and offer focused localization of pain signals. In contrast, the proximal vagina transmits efferent signals to the brain via autonomic nerves, including the sympathetic hypogastric nerve. Innervation via autonomic pathways provides a more diffuse sensation that patients may have trouble localizing. Pelvic reconstructive surgery, particularly in the case of trocar-based mesh prolapse kits, can result in injury to one or more these nerve pathways (Fig. 53.1).

EVALUATION OF MESH COMPLICATIONS

The clinical evaluation of a patient presenting with a vaginal mesh-related complication requires a systematic approach to be effective. Complications of vaginal mesh bear a wide range of symptoms. Some complications are straightforward, for example, a vaginal mesh exposure causing vaginal bleeding that is otherwise asymptomatic. However, other complications are more complex and are potentially influenced by other factors present in the patient's life, for example, acute onset of new vaginal pain in a patient with chronic pelvic pain. This complex symptomatology can be difficult for patients to relate fully; thus, the practitioner caring for the patient must have a robust clinical approach to the patient interview. These encounters often take more time than is available in a standard office visit template.

Evaluation of mesh-related complications begins with a detailed history. Review of the patient's symptomatology should include an assessment of the patient's pain, presence of dyspareunia and partner dyspareunia, and vaginal bleeding. Although difficult to characterize, some patients will report other vague symptoms to which the clinician should be attentive. The duration of the patient's symptoms should be assessed. Anecdotally, pain present for many years or initiating remote from the time of mesh implantation has a lower likelihood of resolving with mesh excision and understanding the chronicity of the problem is helpful with determining the prognosis. Although many patients have a limited understanding of the differences between meshes placed for prolapse versus incontinence, asking what symptom was being addressed at the time of surgery can provide insight to the type of mesh that may be present. It is important to assess the efficacy of the mesh surgery in resolving their original complaint. For example, patients with mixed incontinence may have resolution of their stress urinary incontinence while urgency incontinence persists. The goal is to understand how the chief complaint impacts the patient's quality of life or, more specifically, how it is limiting their ability to function. An effective line of questioning will also provide insight into the patient's coping skills and social support structures. The remainder of the medical and surgical history should also be elicited with attention paid to coexisting pain disorders and psychiatric conditions.

The physical exam of a patient with vaginal mesh complications begins before the provider picks up the speculum. The patient's gait should be assessed while she is entering the exam area as well as how she sits during the history. Examination of the pelvis starts with assessment of the vulvar skin for comorbid dermatologic conditions. In patients presenting with a primary complaint of pain, a musculoskeletal and neurologic exam[41] should be performed to distinguish if the pain is centralized versus peripheral. Although the ideal technique for examining pelvic pain is not well established,[42] our approach to the internal exam begins with a small cotton swab on a stick. This instrument is smaller than a digit and more sensitive than a speculum and allows for focused examination of specific components of the vagina and its surrounding structures. The cotton swab is covered

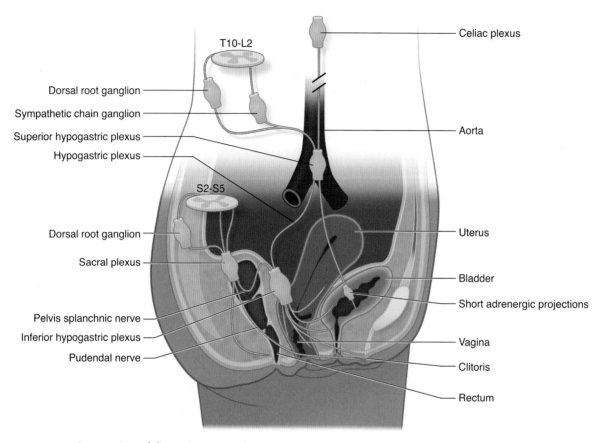

FIGURE 53.1 Innervation of the vagina.

in lubricating jelly and superficial assessment of the epithelium is done by gently brushing the skin to assess for elicited pain suggestive of a dermatologic (e.g., dermatitis) or neurologic (e.g., neuroma) condition followed by deeper palpation with the cotton swab to assess for muscular involvement. Use of the cotton swab begins at the introitus and then progresses internally within the vagina following a systematic approach that includes superficial and deep palpation of the levator ani, obturator internus, and if desired more proximal muscles such as the pyriformis. The examiner should identify if the patient's pain is reproducible and if it localizes to a specific location in the vagina. Importantly, the area of the vagina that contains mesh should be specifically examined. Many patients with pelvic pain will have pain on exam that does not localize to the mesh, and it is likely that such pain will not resolve with mesh excision.[43] After the cotton swab evaluation is complete, a similar exam is performed digitally which allows for assessment of larger structures such as the uterus, adnexa, bladder, and rectovaginal septum. A Pelvic Organ Prolapse Quantification system exam is performed with attention toward assessment of vaginal shortening (total vaginal length <7 cm) and narrowing which is a known complication of vaginal mesh surgery.[44,45] Visual assessment of the cervix and

vaginal epithelium is then performed. In patients presenting with vaginal mesh exposures, examiners should have a high index of suspicion for unrecognized concurrent bladder and rectal involvement. Retrospective series of vaginal mesh excision surgeries have reported unexpected bladder and bowel involvement in 1% and 2% of cases, respectively.[46] Practitioners should have a low threshold to perform cystoscopy and/or proctoscopy particularly in patients with hematuria/hematochezia. Microscopic urinalysis should be performed to assess for hematuria and stool guaiac to assess for rectal bleeding. In unusual circumstances where an adequate office examination cannot be performed, consideration may be given to examination under anesthesia.[43] Additional imaging modalities such as ultrasound or magnetic resonance imaging (MRI) may have utility is select situations. Consultative services should be readily employed in cases with a suspicion of bladder or intestinal involvement.

MANAGEMENT OF MESH COMPLICATIONS

Management of mesh complications depends on the presence of symptoms and the nature of the complication, and it is important to recognize that there are many potential management strategies. Conservative options should be exhausted before surgical intervention is undertaken.

Management of Mesh-Related Complications—Other Than Mesh Exposure

Management strategies for mesh-related pelvic pain

The incidence of pelvic pain after placement of vaginal mesh has been reported to affect as many as 1 in 6 women.[47] Pelvic pain is complex, and full discussion of its etiology, evaluation, and treatment is beyond the scope of this chapter. However, as it relates to implanted vaginal mesh, pelvic pain has been hypothesized to have several possible etiologies. These include musculoskeletal, mechanical (e.g., contracture), neurologic, host rejection of the graft (i.e., inflammatory), and infection.

The evaluation and management of the pain is dependent on the presumed etiology. Musculoskeletal pain can be identified with a detailed assessment of pelvic floor tone and identification of tender pelvic muscles that is reproducible on examination. Likewise, mesh contracture can be identified via palpation during pelvic examination. Neurologic examination can be used to identify potential nerve entrapment from vaginally placed mesh. In addition to potential injury to large named nerves in the pelvis (e.g., obturator, pudendal), injury to nerve branches with subsequent neuroma formation has been reported after reconstructive pelvic surgery and hysterectomy[48,49] and a case series of perineal nerve neuroma resection has been reported to be successful in reducing perineal pain in men.[50] Management of pelvic pain after vaginal mesh placement often requires a multidisciplinary team including pelvic floor physical therapy, pain management, psychiatry, and pelvic floor reconstructive surgeons.

Pelvic floor physical therapy

Pelvic floor physical therapy is an appropriate first-line treatment for patients with a musculoskeletal component to mesh-related pain. However, additional treatments should not be delayed if pain is significant or progressive.[43]

Trigger point injection

Trigger point injections using local anesthetic and/or steroid solutions can be both diagnostic and therapeutic, although the role for injections in this patient population is not well defined. Additional treatments should not be delayed if repetitive injections become necessary.[51]

Medical management

Medical management of mesh-related pain is directed toward reduction of centralized pain processes. Long-term pain can become centralized, meaning that upregulation of sensory pathways within the central nervous system results in allodynia and hyperalgesia that does not localize to peripheral anatomy. Centralized pain is unlikely to respond to peripheral interventions such as trigger point injections and mesh excision but can be treated with centrally acting medications such as gabapentin or duloxetine. Surgeons should thoroughly evaluate and manage anatomical complications of mesh implantation, recognize centralized pain, and have a low threshold for consulting pain medicine specialists for assistance as needed.

Management strategies for mesh-related vaginal constriction or shortening

Mesh contraction or overzealous plication of vaginal tissues at the time of reconstructive surgery can lead to vaginal constriction and shortening. Treatment of these conditions can be challenging and often requires prolonged therapy. Much of the literature on the treatment of vaginal constriction/shortening comes from the neovagina literature for patients with congenital vaginal atresia; however, many of the principles of epithelial grafting are applicable to management of vaginal constriction/shortening after pelvic reconstructive surgery where insufficient epithelial tissue is available to close a wound after mesh excision has been performed.

Manual vaginal dilators

Manual vaginal dilators are widely available in online stores in individual sizes or kits that include multiple sizes. Whereas vaginal dilators can be effective for treatment of vaginal constriction and shortening, compliance with their use is unfortunately low.[52] When prescribing vaginal dilator use, physicians should explore potential barriers to dilator use with the patient or refer patients to practitioners (including pelvic floor physical therapists) comfortable assisting the patient. There are multiple potential barriers to dilator use including cost because these devices are not generally covered by insurance. Embarrassment is another potential barrier as patients need to undress and many lay down during dilator insertion and may not have privacy to do this at times that would be convenient for dilator use. Furthermore, lack of patient understanding of the need for consistent and sometimes prolonged usage of dilators may lead to patients to stop usage prematurely.

Patients beginning manual vaginal dilator use are generally instructed to insert the largest diameter dilator that can comfortably be fit as deeply into the vagina as possible without pain. The ideal length of time the dilator should be left in place has not been well established, but experts agree that longer duration and increased frequency is more likely to result in resolution of constriction/shortening. The patient should progressively increase the size of the dilator and depth of penetration over time.

Surgical (Vecchietti procedure) vaginal elongation

The Vecchietti procedure is a form of vaginal elongation that employs the principle of prolonged traction to stretch the vaginal tissue.[53] This technique was developed in the 1960s. An olive-shaped plug is placed at the vaginal apex and connected to a pully system that is anchored to the anterior abdominal wall. Traction is placed on the vaginal plug and the tension adjusted over time. This allows for slow continuous stretching that is not dependent on patient compliance. However, this approach requires a degree of vaginal elasticity and thus may not be effective where scaring is present.

Graft-augmented repair of vaginal shortening

Autograft of buccal mucosa

Buccal epithelium shares many histologic similarities with vaginal epithelium. Buccal epithelium is hairless, distensible, secretory, and has a similar color and texture as vaginal epithelium. Whereas not germane to gynecologic practice, buccal graft harvesting is familiar to most pediatric urologists and oral maxillofacial surgeons. Bilateral buccal epithelium grafts can be harvested and then fenestrated to provide coverage of a wide area of deficient vaginal epithelium and has been reported as a successful treatment of vaginal atresia.[54,55]

Skin flap (full or split thickness) (McIndoe procedure)

Interpositional autogenic flaps can be used to augment a narrow or shortened vagina. Options include rotational flaps (gracilis, rectus abdominus, bulbocavernosus) and free flaps (full- and split-thickness skin). The McIndoe procedure involves harvest of skin flaps from the patient's buttocks or abdomen that are then fastened around a stent that is inserted into a surgically opened but epithelially deficient vesicorectal space.[56]

Xenograft

Xenografts provide a readily available alternative to autografts for repair of large vaginal defects after vaginal mesh excision. Use of an absorbable graft purportedly provides tissue growth factors and extracellular scaffolding that supports development of replacement vaginal epithelium. Porcine small intestinal submucosa has been used in the reconstruction of large epithelial defects after vaginal mesh excision.[57,58]

Management of Mesh-Related Complications—Mesh Exposure

Expectant management

Expectant management is an appropriate option for patients with asymptomatic mesh exposures.[59] Patients electing to pursue this management plan should be made aware of common presenting symptoms associated with mesh complications. Follow-up, including repeat pelvic examination, can be offered at regular intervals. Alternatively, patients who are truly asymptomatic can defer follow-up until symptoms develop.

Mesh excision

The decision to remove vaginal mesh is made in shared decision making with the patient. The FDA, American College of Obstetricians and Gynecologists, and AUGS have stated that mesh that is asymptomatic does not need to be removed.[8,59] Symptoms of mesh exposure where excision may be indicated include the following:

- Vaginal bleeding
- Vaginal discharge
- Dyspareunia/partner dyspareunia
- Pain that is reproducible with palpation of the mesh
- Urinary retention/obstructed voiding
- Infection
- Exposure of mesh into viscera
- Recurrent urinary tract infections with exposure of mesh into the urinary tract

Every effort to obtain and review the operative note of the index mesh implantation surgery should be made. The operative note should be examined to identify the following:

- Type of mesh implanted
- Type of suture used to fix mesh to the vagina and/ or supporting ligaments (permanent vs. absorbable)
- Color of mesh implanted
- Route of insertion
- Compartment the implant was placed
- Structures the mesh was anchored into
- Time since implantation
- Complications noted during insertion

Review of these items aids in surgical planning and allows the physician to effectively counsel the patient regarding treatment options and prognosis.

Approaches to Surgical Mesh Revision

The AUGS/IUGA have published joint guidelines and treatment algorithms for management of mesh complications.[43] Importantly, these guidelines recommend a progression from conservative to invasive treatment options. They emphasize avoidance of repeating steps. For example, repeated attempts at partial mesh excision are unlikely to provide additional benefit and may preclude the ability to perform a complete resection.

Patients electing to pursue surgical revision of vaginal mesh should be fully counseled on the risks, benefits, and alternatives of the procedure. Although excision of small exposures of mesh are relatively low-risk procedures, full excision of vaginal mesh has high risk of morbidity. These risks include the following:

- Injury to bowel or bladder
- Persistent pain
- Hemorrhage
- Recurrent urinary incontinence
- Recurrent POP
- That complete removal of the mesh may not be possible
- Vaginal shortening/narrowing
- De novo dyspareunia

Terminology

When performing surgical procedures to correct mesh complications, the use of standardized terminology is strongly encouraged. Using standardized terminology increases uniformity in documentation which allows for rapid understanding of what was performed intraoperatively. As patients with mesh complications are inherently complex and care is frequently provided by a multidisciplinary team, uniformity in terminology will increase intraprovider communication. Additionally, using standardized terms supports the development of research and treatment protocols as well as decision-support tools. AUGS/IUGA have developed standardized terminology to describe surgical procedures used in the management of mesh complications (Table 53.2).[43]

Technique for Mesh Removal

Given the high degree of risk associated with surgical excision of vaginal mesh, these procedures should be performed by a female pelvic medicine and reconstructive surgeon or similarly trained high-volume surgeon with deep anatomical and histologic understanding of the compartments of the vagina and its surrounding structures. The surgeon should be prepared to employ reconstructive surgical techniques such as advancement flaps, rotational tissue grafts, and xenograft placement to ensure that adequate vaginal length and patency remains at the completion of the procedure. Preparation for the procedure includes review of the index operative note to aid in surgical

TABLE 53.2	
AUGS/IUGA Description of Surgical Procedures for Management of Mesh Complications	
SURGICAL PROCEDURE	**DESCRIPTION**
Mesh revision	Either no mesh is removed (e.g., dissecting and primarily closing vaginal epithelium) or a small edge of mesh is removed such that the structural integrity of the implant is left intact.
Partial vaginal mesh excision	A segment/component of the mesh is removed or transected such that the structural integrity of the implant is altered.
Complete vaginal mesh excision	The entirety of the mesh that is in contact with the vagina is excised.
Extravaginal mesh excision	This involves removal of segments or components of mesh beyond, or not in contact with, the vagina. Note the following: • Because of the wide variation of devices and approaches, this category should include additional description of which mesh segments were removed. • This term should be used in addition to any relevant vaginal mesh excision, if performed.
Total mesh excision	The surgical goal is the removal of 100% of the implant (extirpation).

The use of standardized terminology in describing surgical management of mesh complications is encouraged to (1) provide complete documentation of procedures performed, (2) increase intraprovider communication, and (3) support development of treatment protocols and decision-support tools.

planning. During the surgical procedure, maximal exposure and visualization are critical to successful mesh excision. Visualization can be optimized with utilization of self-retaining retractors (e.g., LoneStar, vaginal Bookwalter), fixation sutures, and use of a head lamp or self-lighting retractors.

Effective identification of tissue planes is critical to safe mobilization of vaginal mesh and its excision. Histologically, the vaginal wall is a multilaminar structure composed of nonkeratinized stratified squamous epithelium, lamina propria, muscularis, and adventitia (Video 53.1). The index placement of vaginal mesh is performed via a partial-thickness (deep to the stratified squamous epithelium) or full-thickness (entering the adventitia) dissection. Vaginal mesh becomes exposed when overlying tissue planes degenerate and the removing surgeon must be prepared to identify the surrounding remnant of these planes during excision, so they can be safely reapproximated after mesh removal.

Removal of vaginal mesh begins by grasping the exposed mesh with a tonsil clamp. Some surgeons will inject local anesthetic/vasoconstrictive agents at this point; however, care should be taken not to obscure the identification of tissue planes during this step. Wide mobilization of the surrounding epithelium is then performed by sharply dissecting tissue off the underlying mesh. The mesh can be used as a backboard and the scissors tips gently pushed against the mesh to release the surrounding tissue superficial to the mesh. Care must be taken not to incise the mesh during this mobilization. After adequate mobilization has been achieved, the mesh is incised at the point of greatest visibility and the mesh is reflected off the underlying tissue. A combination of meticulous sharp and blunt dissection is further employed to release the undersurface of the mesh from the underlying tissue with care taken to dissect as close to the mesh as possible. In cases with planned partial mesh resection, the mesh can now be amputated without injury to surrounding organs and the tissue planes closed in layers. In cases with planned complete mesh resection, the dissection is carried further to the ligamentous structure that was used to anchor the mesh. Deep dissections to the sacrospinous or sacrotuberous ligament (pararectal space), obturator membrane (paravesical space), are technically challenging and bring a high risk of vascular injury. Evaluation of the surrounding organs (e.g., cystoscopy, rectal exam) should be employed liberally (Fig. 53.2).

Management of Rare Complications

Osteomyelitis

Special mention should be made of a rare but debilitating complication that has been associated with mesh-augmented repair of POP: osteomyelitis. When present, osteomyelitis requires extensive evaluation and management. In a review of published case studies, back pain was the most common presenting symptom and occurred in 85% of cases.[60] The AUGS/IUGA Joint Writing Group on management of mesh complications[43] recommends that patients with persistent back pain should be evaluated for signs of systemic infection including serologic markers of infection (white blood cell count, erythrocyte sedimentation rate, and C-reactive protein) and imaging (MRI). Direct aspiration should be performed when possible. Intravenous antibiotics should be employed as first-line treatment. However, most cases will

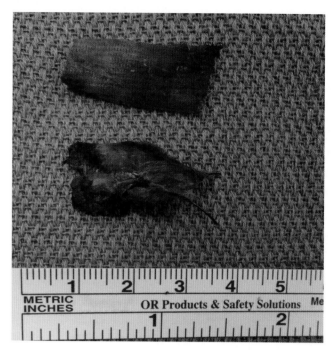

FIGURE 53.2 Explanted transobturator sling.

require surgical intervention to remove the infected implants (including mesh, permanent suture, tacks, etc.). Furthermore, surgeons should be aware that in cases where surgical intervention is required, 40% may require multiple surgeries. Additionally, neurosurgical/orthopedic consultation may be required in severe cases where discectomy or joint stabilization is needed.

Urethral exposures

Urethral exposure of vaginal mesh is a rare but potentially devastating complication of mesh-augmented incontinence surgery. Traditionally, management of urethral mesh exposure has been performed via a vaginal approach. This technique can result in surgical disruption of the sphincter mechanism which can result in profound incontinence. Endoscopic removal has been suggested as a sphincter-sparing alternative, and the use of a pediatric nasal speculum has been reported to facilitate visualization and exposure of the urethral mesh.[61,62] Expert opinion suggests that concomitant placement of new surgical mesh at the time of urethral mesh excision (e.g., to prevent worsening stress incontinence) should be avoided which leads some surgeons to offer an autologous fascial sling at the time of urethral mesh excision. An open discussion with the patient regarding potential risks of surgical exploration and planned interventions to reduce this risk should occur preoperatively.

Bladder exposures

Exposure of vaginal mesh into the bladder is a challenging complication which is often low on the provider's differential diagnosis often resulting in a delayed diagnosis. Presenting symptoms include hematuria, urinary tract infections, urinary retention, bladder calculi, and urogenital fistula formation.[36] Management of this condition is dependent on location of the exposure within the bladder. Exposures at the bladder dome have a relatively good prognosis with minimal expected morbidity. Exposures into the trigone or bladder neck are anatomically challenging to access and have a high chance of disrupting the urethral sphincter which can result in profound postoperative incontinence. Endoscopic approaches with cystoscopic resection or holmium laser ablation of the mesh has been reported with lower morbidity but may be associated with a high chance of recurrence of the mesh exposure.[63-66]

Rectal exposures

Rectal exposures are likewise complex conditions that require consultation with a colorectal surgeon for effective management. Rectal bleeding, tenesmus, and pelvic pain are possible presenting symptoms. Complications have been reported as much as 20 years after mesh implantation.[67] Both abdominal and transanal approaches to mesh excision can be employed to manage the exposure.[68-70]

OUTCOMES OF MESH EXCISION

Patient-centered outcomes after mesh removal are variable and depend on the indication for mesh removal and the metric examined postoperatively. For example, simple small mesh exposures are likely to be cured with excision alone, whereas complex conditions like chronic pain have more mixed outcomes and often require additional therapy. The guiding factor in determining whether to excise vaginal mesh should be to improve a specific aspect of a patient's quality of life, and therefore, success should be measured based on achievement of this goal. This expected benefit is to be tempered against the fact that mesh excision is not a low-risk procedure (with likely under reporting of complication rates) and patients should be advised on the possible outcomes associated with mesh excision. Additionally, many patients require multiple surgeries to manage recurrent (e.g., repeat mesh exposure) or de novo symptoms (e.g., stress incontinence) after mesh excision.

Surgical Complications

Surgical complications are not uncommon after excision of vaginal mesh. Multiple types of complications have been reported ranging from minor to severe. In a retrospective review of 277 patients who underwent primarily partial mesh excision via a vaginal approach, 115 (55%) experienced a minor complication (Clavien-Dindo grades 1 to 2), whereas 37 (13%) experienced a significant complication (grade 3). These high-grade complications included de novo stress urinary incontinence, persistent urgency incontinence, bladder outlet obstruction, seroma, hematuria, de novo POP, bowel injury, ureteral injury, and dyspareunia. Importantly, two cases of severe (grade 4) complications occurred, and these include respiratory failure and iliac vein injury. Intuitively, additional studies have shown that complication rates are higher when mesh is removed from multiple compartments concurrently. In another retrospective review of 398 procedures performed for the removal of vaginally placed mesh, 326 patients (82%) underwent single compartment excision and 48 (12%) multicompartment surgery.[15] Bleeding complications were significantly higher in surgeries with concomitant removal of mesh from multiple vaginal compartments. Estimated blood loss was 3 times higher in multicompartment versus single compartment surgeries ($P < .001$) and odds of blood transfusion were 9 times higher (OR 9.7, 2.1 to 44.6, $P < .01$). Other surgical complications including need for reoperation due to unrecognized bladder injury,[71] ureteral injury,[72] rectal injury,[73] and vesicovaginal fistula formation[74] have been reported.

Pelvic Organ Prolapse Recurrence

Recurrent POP is a known possible outcome after mesh removal with the likelihood of recurrence likely influenced by the amount of mesh removed. Prolapse recurrence rates range from 15% to 46%. Although prolapse recurrence rates are relatively high, retreatment rates are lower and range from 1.4% to 30.8%.[74-77] Retreatment rates are likely lower than recurrence rates due several factors including varying definitions of recurrence, that many recurrences are not bothersome from a patient perspective, and that there are patient barriers to returning to the operating room including time away from work/family.

Stress Urinary Incontinence Recurrence

Recurrence of stress urinary incontinence after mesh revision again varies, likely based on the amount of mesh removed. Recurrence ranges from 16% to 35% after division of mesh slings and from 36% to 69% after removal of mesh slings.[74,78,79] The lower risk of recurrent stress urinary incontinence associated with sling release compared to mesh excision needs to be balanced against the risk of recurrent mesh exposure which is presumably higher if the mesh is not excised. Some have proposed the performance of a repeat concomitant anti-incontinence procedure at the time of mesh revision as a mechanism to reduce de novo stress incontinence; however, this remains controversial.

Pain Resolution

A detailed review of pain outcomes after mesh removal is beyond the scope of this chapter. However, because the pathophysiologic mechanism of mesh-induced pain is poorly understood, it is not surprising that studies report widely differing degrees of pain resolution after mesh removal.[74,77,80] It is important to recognize that surgical intervention can have a strong impact on short-term pain outcomes, whereas pain can recur or persist in the long term. Additionally, interpretation of the literature requires a detailed understanding of the type (e.g., pain at rest, during activity, dyspareunia) of pain being studied. The authors recommend cautious counseling when prognosticating pain resolution after mesh removal, with higher likelihood of success expected in acute cases where palpation of the mesh clearly reproduces the patient's pain and lower expectations in scenarios of chronic pain.

Voiding and Storage Symptom Resolution

Voiding symptoms such as incomplete micturition with elevated postvoid residual and straining to void as well as storage symptoms such as frequency and urgency with or without incontinence are known complications of midurethral sling placement. The etiology of these symptoms is variable and may include mechanical obstruction of the urethra, an inflammatory response from surgery, and host reaction to graft placement. As such, management of these lower urinary tract symptoms varies based on the presumed etiology. When mechanical obstruction is thought to be the cause, revision of midurethral sling has been reported to resolve symptoms in 30% to 70% of cases.[74,79]

CONCLUSION

Complications associated with vaginal mesh vary widely ranging from asymptomatic mesh exposures into the vagina to recalcitrant chronic pain. Several risk factors for mesh exposure have been identified, although more research is needed to further elucidate the cause of this complex phenomenon. A wide evidence base exists to guide physicians in the management of these complications, but effective intervention requires a comprehensive approach to the patient assessment, deep knowledge of management strategies, use of standardized terminology, and a robust understanding of potential outcomes.

References

1. Buklijas T. Surgery and national identity in late nineteenth-century Vienna. *Stud Hist Philos Biol Biomed Sci* 2007;38(4):756–774.
2. Baylón K, Rodríguez-Camarillo P, Elías-Zúñiga A, et al. Past, present and future of surgical meshes: A review. *Membranes (Basel)* 2017;7(3):1–23.
3. Barbalat Y, Tunuguntla HSGR. Surgery for pelvic organ prolapse: A historical perspective. *Curr Urol Rep* 2012;13(3):256–261.
4. Manodoro S, Werbrouck E, Veldman J, et al. Laparoscopic sacrocolpopexy. *Facts Views Vis Obgyn* 2011;3(3):151–158.
5. U.S. Food and Drug Administration. MAUDE—Manufacturer and User Facility Device Experience. Accessed May 31, 2020. https://www.accessdata.fda.gov/scripts/cdrh/cfdocs/cfmaude/search.cfm#fn1
6. U.S. Food and Drug Administration. FDA public health notification: Serious complications associated with transvaginal placement of surgical mesh in repair of pelvic organ prolapse and stress urinary incontinence. Accessed June 24, 2015. http://www.fda.gov/MedicalDevices/Safety/AlertsandNotices/ucm262435.htm
7. U.S. Food and Drug Administration. FDA safety communication: Urogynecologic surgical mesh: Update on the safety and effectiveness of transvaginal placement for pelvic organ prolapse. Accessed May 31, 2020. http://www.fda.gov/downloads/medical
8. U.S. Food and Drug Administration. Urogynecologic surgical mesh implants. Published 2019. Accessed May 31, 2020. https://www.fda.gov/medical-devices/implants-and-prosthetics/urogynecologic-surgical-mesh-implants
9. Glazener CM, Breeman S, Elders A, et al. Mesh, graft, or standard repair for women having primary transvaginal anterior or posterior compartment prolapse surgery: Two parallel-group, multicentre, randomised, controlled trials (PROSPECT). *Lancet* 2017;389(10067):381–392.
10. National Institute for Health Care and Excellence. Urinary incontinence and pelvic organ prolapse in women: Management. Published April 2, 2019. Accessed May 31, 2020. https://www.nice.org.uk/guidance/ng123/resources/urinary-incontinence-and-pelvic-organ-prolapse-in-women-management-pdf-66141657205189
11. Ng-Stollmann N, Fünfgeld C, Gabriel B, et al. The international discussion and the new regulations concerning transvaginal mesh implants in pelvic organ prolapse surgery. *Int Urogynecol J* 2020;31(10):1997–2002.
12. Haylen BT, Freeman RM, Swift SE, et al. An International Urogynecological Association (IUGA)/International Continence Society (ICS) joint terminology and classification of the complications related directly to the insertion of prostheses (meshes, implants, tapes) and grafts in female pelvic floor surgery. *Int Urogynecol J* 2011;22(1):3–15.
13. Nygaard I, Brubaker L, Zyczynski HM, et al. Long-term outcomes following abdominal sacrocolpopexy for pelvic organ prolapse. *JAMA* 2013;309(19):2016–2024.
14. Khrucharoen U, Ramart P, Choi J, et al. Clinical predictors and risk factors for vaginal mesh extrusion. *World J Urol* 2018;36(2):299–304.
15. Pickett SD, Barenberg B, Quiroz LH, et al. The significant morbidity of removing pelvic mesh from multiple vaginal compartments. *Obstet Gynecol* 2015;125(6):1418–1422.

16. Tan-Kim J, Menefee SA, Luber KM, et al. Prevalence and risk factors for mesh erosion after laparoscopic-assisted sacrocolpopexy. *Int Urogynecol J* 2011;22(2):205–212.

17. Crane AK, Geller EJ, Sullivan S, et al. Short-term mesh exposure after robotic sacrocolpopexy with and without concomitant hysterectomy. *South Med J* 2014;107(10):603–606.

18. Finamore PS, Echols KT, Hunter K, et al. Risk factors for mesh erosion 3 months following vaginal reconstructive surgery using commercial kits vs. fashioned mesh-augmented vaginal repairs. *Int Urogynecol J* 2010;21(3):285–291.

19. Eilber KS, Alperin M, Khan A, et al. The role of the surgeon on outcomes of vaginal prolapse surgery with mesh. *Female Pelvic Med Reconstr Surg* 2017;23(5):293–296.

20. Withagen MI, Vierhout ME, Hendriks JC, et al. Risk factors for exposure, pain, and dyspareunia after tension-free vaginal mesh procedure. *Obstet Gynecol* 2011;118(3):629–636.

21. Welk B, Al-Hothi H, Winick-Ng J. Removal or revision of vaginal mesh used for the treatment of stress urinary incontinence. *JAMA Surg* 2015;150(12):1167–1175.

22. Bristow RE, Zahurak ML, Diaz-Montes TP, et al. Impact of surgeon and hospital ovarian cancer surgical case volume on in-hospital mortality and related short-term outcomes. *Gynecol Oncol* 2009;115(3):334–338.

23. Adams-Piper ER, Guaderrama NM, Chen Q, et al. Impact of surgical training on the performance of proposed quality measures for hysterectomy for pelvic organ prolapse. *Am J Obstet Gynecol* 2017;216(6):588.e1–588.e5.

24. Osborn DJ, Dmochowski RR, Harris CJ, et al. Analysis of patient and technical factors associated with midurethral sling mesh exposure and perforation. *Int J Urol* 2014;21(11):1167–1170.

25. Bochenska K, Mueller M, Geynisman-Tan J, et al. Concomitant repair of pelvic floor disorders in women undergoing surgery for gynecologic malignancies. *Female Pelvic Med Reconstr Surg* 2020;25(5):362–364.

26. Dobberfuhl AD. Evaluation and treatment of female stress urinary incontinence after pelvic radiotherapy. *Neurourol Urodyn* 2019;38(Suppl 4):S59–S69.

27. Lee J, Eddib A, Eddib A. The impact of radiation treatment on the mid-urethral sling in women with gynecology malignancies: Experience in a large urology/urogynecology practice. Published 2020. Accessed May 31, 2020. https://www.ics.org/2020/abstract/596

28. Leow JJ, Gurbani C, Yeow S, et al. Autologous pubovaginal sling for the treatment of stress urinary incontinence in a patient with high risk of mesh erosion. *Urology* 2020;143:266.

29. Rahn DD, Good MM, Roshanravan SM, et al. Effects of preoperative local estrogen in postmenopausal women with prolapse: A randomized trial. *J Clin Endocrinol Metab* 2014;99(10):3728–3736.

30. Sun Z, Zhu L, Xu T, et al. Effects of preoperative vaginal estrogen therapy for the incidence of mesh complication after pelvic organ prolapse surgery in postmenopausal women: Is it helpful or a myth? A 1-year randomized controlled trial. *Menopause* 2016;23(7):740–748.

31. Cadish LA, West EH, Sisto J, et al. Preoperative vaginal estrogen and midurethral sling exposure: A retrospective cohort study. *Int Urogynecol J* 2016;27(3):413–417.

32. Versi E, Harvey MA, Cardozo L, et al. Urogenital prolapse and atrophy at menopause: A prevalence study. *Int Urogynecol J Pelvic Floor Dysfunct* 2001;12(2):107–110.

33. Kaufman Y, Singh SS, Alturki H, et al. Age and sexual activity are risk factors for mesh exposure following transvaginal mesh repair. *Int Urogynecol J* 2011;22(3):307–313.

34. Linder BJ, El-Nashar SA, Carranza Leon DA, et al. Predictors of vaginal mesh exposure after midurethral sling placement: A case–control study. *Int Urogynecol J* 2016;27(9):1321–1326.

35. Cundiff GW, Varner E, Visco AG, et al. Risk factors for mesh/suture erosion following sacral colpopexy. *Am J Obstet Gynecol* 2008;199(6):688.e1–688.e5.

36. Zambon JP, Badlani GH. Vaginal mesh exposure presentation, evaluation, and management. *Curr Urol Rep* 2016;17(9):1–8.

37. El-Khawand D, Wehbe SA, O'Hare PG, et al. Risk factors for vaginal mesh exposure after mesh-augmented anterior repair: A retrospective cohort study. *Female Pelvic Med Reconstr Surg* 2014;20(6):305–309.

38. Fawcett A, Shembekar M, Church JS, et al. Smoking, hypertension, and colonic anastomotic healing; a combined clinical and histopathological study. *Gut* 1996;38(5):714–718.

39. Nolfi AL, Brown BN, Liang R, et al. Host response to synthetic mesh in women with mesh complications. *Am J Obstet Gynecol* 2016;215(2):206.e1–206.e8.

40. Tennyson L, Rytel M, Palcsey S, et al. Characterization of the T-cell response to polypropylene mesh in women with complications. *Am J Obstet Gynecol* 2019;220(2):187.e1–187.e8.

41. Zolnoun D, Bair E, Essick G, et al. Reliability and reproducibility of novel methodology for assessment of pressure pain sensitivity in pelvis. *J Pain* 2012;13(9):910–920.

42. Meister MRL, Sutcliffe S, Lowder JL. Definitions of apical vaginal support loss: A systematic review. *Am J Obstet Gynecol* 2017;216(3):232.e1–232.e14.

43. Joint Writing Group of the American Urogynecologic Society and the International Urogynecological Association. Joint position statement on the management of mesh-related complications for the FPMRS specialist. *Int Urogynecol J* 2020;31(4):679–694.

44. Blandon RE, Gebhart JB, Trabuco EC, et al. Complications from vaginally placed mesh in pelvic reconstructive surgery. *Int Urogynecol J Pelvic Floor Dysfunct* 2009;20(5):523–531.

45. U.S. Food and Drug Administration. Surgical mesh for transvaginal repair of pelvic organ prolapse in the anterior vaginal compartment. FDA executive summary. Accessed May 31, 2020. https://www.fda.gov/downloads/AdvisoryCommittees/CommitteesMeetingMaterials/MedicalDevices/MedicalDevicesAdvisoryCommittee/ObstetricsandGynecologyDevices/UCM630949.pdf

46. Crosby EC, Abernethy M, Berger MB, et al. Symptom resolution after operative management of complications from transvaginal mesh. *Obstet Gynecol* 2014;123(1):134–139.

47. Geller EJ, Babb E, Nackley AG, et al. Incidence and risk factors for pelvic pain after mesh implant surgery for the treatment of pelvic floor disorders. *J Minim Invasive Gynecol* 2017;24(1):67–73.

48. Millheiser LS, Chen B. Severe vaginal pain caused by a neuroma in the rectovaginal septum after posterior colporrhaphy. *Obstet Gynecol* 2006;108(3 II):809–811.

49. Sunderji Z, Buitenhuis D, Lee G, et al. Vaginal vault traumatic neuromas. *J Minim Invasive Gynecol* 26(7):1219–1220.

50. Wan EL, Dellon AL. Injury to the perineal branch of the pudendal nerve in men: Outcomes from surgical resection of the perineal branches. *Microsurgery* 2018;38(2):172–176.

51. Duckett JRA, Jain S. Groin pain after a tension-free vaginal tape or similar suburethral sling: Management strategies. *BJU Int* 2005;95(1):95–97.

52. Liu M, Juravic M, Mazza G, et al. Vaginal dilators: Issues and answers. *Sex Med Rev* 2021;9(2):212–220.

53. Kölle A, Taran FA, Rall K, et al. Neovagina creation methods and their potential impact on subsequent uterus transplantation: A review. *BJOG* 2019;126(11):1328–1335.

54. Chan JL, Levin PJ, Ford BP, et al. Vaginoplasty with an autologous buccal mucosa fenestrated graft in two patients with vaginal agenesis: A multidisciplinary approach and literature review. *J Minim Invasive Gynecol* 2018;24(4):670–676.

55. Wu M, Wang Y, Xu J, et al. Vaginoplasty with mesh autologous buccal mucosa in vaginal agenesis: A multidisciplinary approach and literature review. *Aesthetic Surg J* 2020;40(12):1–9.

56. Michala L, Cutner A, Creighton SM. Surgical approaches to treating vaginal agenesis. *BJOG* 2007;114(12):1455–1459.

57. Alperin M. Collagen scaffold: A treatment for large mesh exposure following vaginal prolapse repair. *Int Urogynecol J* 2014;25(11):1597–1599.

58. Khong SY, Lam A. Use of Surgisis mesh in the management of polypropylene mesh erosion into the vagina. *Int Urogynecol J* 2011;22(1):41–46.

59. American College of Obstetricians and Gynecologists. Committee Opinion 694: Management of mesh and graft complications in gynecologic surgery. *Obstet Gynecol* 2017;129(4):e102–e108.

60. Müller PC, Berchtold C, Kuemmerli C, et al. Spondylodiscitis after minimally invasive recto- and colpo-sacropexy: Report of a case and systematic review of the literature. *J Minim Access Surg* 2020;16(1):5–12.

61. Wijffels SAM, Elzevier HW, Lycklama a Nijeholt AA. Transurethral mesh resection after urethral erosion of tension-free vaginal tape: Report of three cases and review of literature. *Int Urogynecol J Pelvic Floor Dysfunct* 2009;20(2):261–263.

62. Plowright LN, Duggal B, Aguilar VC, et al. Endoscopic transurethral resection of urethral mesh erosion with the use of a pediatric nasal speculum. *Obstet Gynecol* 2013;121(2 Part 2):440–443.

63. Karim SS, Pietropaolo A, Skolarikos A, et al. Role of endoscopic management in synthetic sling/mesh erosion following previous incontinence surgery: A systematic review from European Association of Urologists Young Academic Urologists (YAU) and Uro-technology (ESUT) groups. *Int Urogynecol J* 2020;31(1):45–53.

64. Grange P, Kouriefs C, Georgiades F, et al. Eroded tape: A case of an early vesicoscopy rather than laser melting. *Urology* 2017;102:247–251.

65. Doumouchtsis SK, Lee FYK, Bramwell D, et al. Evaluation of holmium laser for managing mesh/suture complications of continence surgery. *BJU Int* 2011;108(9):1472–1478.

66. Sakalis VI, Gkotsi AC, Triantafyllidis A, et al. Transurethral holmium laser intravesical tape excision following TVT procedure: Results from seven patients in a 12-month follow-up. *Int Urogynecol J* 2012;23(6):769–777.

67. Ratneswaren A, Laskaratos F-M, Kumar A, et al. Rectal bleeding due to rectal erosion of vaginal mesh. *Ann Gastroenterol* 2015;28(4):498.

68. Campagna G, Panico G, Caramazza D, et al. Rectal mesh erosion after posterior vaginal kit repair. *Int Urogynecol J* 2019;30(3):499–500.

69. Ferry P, Sedille L, Roncheau V. Rectal mesh exposure after laparoscopic sacrocolpopexy. *J Minim Invasive Gynecol* 21(2):311–313.

70. Hirai C-A, Bohrer JC, Ruel M, et al. Rectal mesh erosion after robotic sacrocolpopexy. *Female Pelvic Med Reconstr Surg* 19(5):298–300.

71. Rigaud J, Pothin P, Labat JJ, et al. Functional results after tape removal for chronic pelvic pain following tension-free vaginal tape or transobturator tape. *J Urol* 2010;184(2):610–615.

72. Miklos JR, Chinthakanan O, Moore RD, et al. Indications and complications associated with the removal of 506 pieces of vaginal mesh used in pelvic floor reconstruction: A multicenter study. *Surg Technol Int* 2016;29:185–189.

73. Gluck O, Grinstein E, Blaganje M, et al. Rectal injury during laparoscopic mesh removal after sacrocervicopexy. *Int Urogynecol J* 2020;31(4):835–837.

74. Ismail S, Chartier-Kastler E, Reus C, et al. Functional outcomes of synthetic tape and mesh revision surgeries: A monocentric experience. *Int Urogynecol J* 2019;30(5):805–813.

75. Sassani JC, Ross JH, Lopa S, et al. Prolapse recurrence after sacrocolpopexy mesh removal: A retrospective cohort study. *Female Pelvic Med Reconstr Surg* 2020;26(2):92–96.

76. George A, Mattingly M, Woodman P, et al. Recurrence of prolapse after transvaginal mesh excision. *Female Pelvic Med Reconstr Surg* 2020;19(4):202–205.

77. Bergersen A, Price E, Callegari M, et al. Pain resolution and recurrent prolapse rates following vaginal mesh removal. *Urology* 2021;150:134–138.

78. Jambusaria LH, Heft J, Reynolds WS, et al. Incontinence rates after midurethral sling revision for vaginal exposure or pain. *Am J Obstet Gynecol* 2016;215(6):764.e1–764.e5.

79. Rardin CR, Rosenblatt PL, Kohli N, et al. Release of tension-free vaginal tape for the treatment of refractory postoperative voiding dysfunction. *Obstet Gynecol* 2002;100(5 Pt 1):898–902.

80. Hou JC, Alhalabi F, Lemack GE, et al. Outcome of transvaginal mesh and tape removed for pain only. *J Urol* 2014;192(3):856–860.

CHAPTER 54

INNOVATION AND EVOLUTION OF MEDICAL DEVICES: THE CASE OF SURGICAL ROBOTS

Jonia Alshiek • S. Abbās Shobeiri

Introduction

Innovating even the most straightforward device requires time, energy, patience, and much money. Innovation in the medical device industry does not require inventing something completely new. It may involve applying the already available idea or product in a new setting or a unique "innovative" manner from an entrepreneurship perspective. In such an environment, (1) quick release of new medical devices and services backed with (2) scientific support of key opinion leaders, followed by (3) robust clinical education of practitioners in the field, with (4) clear communication of problems and flaws to the designers while (5) building and protecting brand equity and value, forms the five pillars of successful medical device launch.

Innovation is influenced by the patients, the care providers, the doctors, the payers, the policymaking groups, and the manufacturers or suppliers who can all affect real-world health care decision-making. Once a device is ready to be released to the market, the company has to tackle the country-specific regulatory requirements, which are in place to protect patient safety and guarantee the local markets' efficiency. The regulatory process creates a fundamental bottleneck in time and cost for any medical device or biomaterial-based therapy.[1] Forces behind device innovation, the methods of disruptive innovations, the patenting process, marketing, and economic considerations, along with regulatory considerations, is the focus of this chapter.

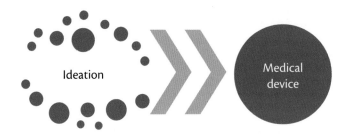

FACTORS THAT DETERMINE SUCCESS OR FAILURE OF MEDICAL DEVICES

Wieringa et al. state that "innovation in medical technology is a critical chain of events, ideally leading to an improved situation for patient and staff as well as a profit for the supplier of the innovation. Many innovative ideas are not successful in practice."[2] The failure of an idea to become a medical device may frequently be because of the lack of one of the following elements[3]:

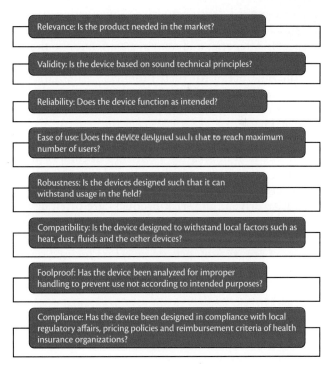

Relevance: Is the product needed in the market?

Validity: Is the device based on sound technical principles?

Reliability: Does the device function as intended?

Ease of use: Does the device designed such that to reach maximum number of users?

Robustness: Is the devices designed such that it can withstand usage in the field?

Compatibility: Is the device designed to withstand local factors such as heat, dust, fluids and the other devices?

Foolproof: Has the device been analyzed for improper handling to prevent use not according to intended purposes?

Compliance: Has the device been designed in compliance with local regulatory affairs, pricing policies and reimbursement criteria of health insurance organizations?

Medical devices can form a "converging technology" that crosses borders between already established medical devices. Converging technologies may combine medical devices, pharmaceutical products, or human tissues. The medical products may be from the same or different categories.[4] Such convergent technologies may be both more acceptable to the users and more adaptable to a marketplace niche. Such technologies are generally not viewed as breakthrough technologies. Bringing separate technology silos with different processes together to create a convergent product requires communication.[5] After a device manufacturer bridges the divide between an idea and a certified product, the clinical introduction stage will prove if and how the projected innovation becomes widespread use in a harsh clinical environment.

THE FORCES BEHIND DISRUPTIVE DEVICE INNOVATION

Disruptive innovations are socially relevant. Disruptive innovations are market-driven because of (1) increasing demand for health care services, (2) increasing demand for higher efficiency, (3) increasing empowerment of the patient, and (4) increase in the effect of market forces.[6]

Companies with mature and productive market positions may benefit from improvements of existing products rather than genuinely new disruptive innovations that disturb their markets, challenge their recognized status, and at times, render their hard-earned production facilities without utility.[3] Frequently "market-driven" research will find industry-funded "curiosity-driven" innovation riskier. This mindset of maintaining a company's dominance in specific categories and not paying attention to the alternatives leaves the door open to the competition seeking the blue ocean for their products.[7] Alternatively, companies with market dominance may purchase and buy out emerging technologies to maintain the status quo. A blend of curiosity-driven and market-driven inventions creates a balanced portfolio for a company.[8] Medical innovation flourishes in clinical (doctors and nurses) watersheds and academic (scientists, engineers, and human factors experts) confluences. Curiosity-driven, high-risk products are often developed with support from government grants or angel investors who are willing to sustain high risk. Angel investors are wealthy private investors focused on financing small business ventures in exchange for equity.

Unlike a venture capital firm that uses an investment fund, angels use their own net worth.

INNOVATIONS THAT DISRUPT THE MARKET

Christensen et al.[13] argue that disruptive innovations are generally more straightforward products than all the customers' need. The disruptive innovations are generally more straightforward, more convenient, and less costly offerings initially designed to appeal to the market's low end. Figure 54.1 illustrates this dynamic.[13] The *top blue arrow* depicts the speed of sustaining technologic innovations. The enhancements an industry creates as it introduces new and more progressive products to serve the more sophisticated customers at the high end of the market. The *shaded area* is the degree of improvement the market can absorb over a specified period.[9] Because the sustaining innovations nearly consistently outperform even the most demanding customers' dimensions, and because the existing market leaders want to meet and exceed the demands of the most demanding customers, there is a window of opportunity to introduce lower or higher performance products. Suppose one views the performance of a physician as a time-dependent product. In that case, it generally takes 13 years of higher education for a surgeon to be board eligible or, in other words, have minimum performance criteria. A surgeon with 20 years of experience generally outperforms a younger colleague. The exception to this is when a new surgeon boosts their performance with the latest technology.

Similarly, prominent health care institutions such as medical schools, general hospitals, specialist physician groups, and research organizations have overdelivered on the level of care required to keep the vast majority of patients healthy. But at the same time, the industry creates demands in the areas previously untapped. Although our medical education system has churned out specialists and subspecialists with extraordinary capabilities to attend to the new markets such as erectile dysfunction in men, in the third-world countries, the patients are afflicted with emergencies and relatively

FIGURE 54.1 The progress of disruptive innovation.

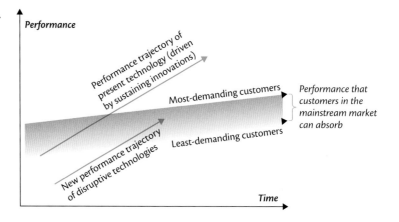

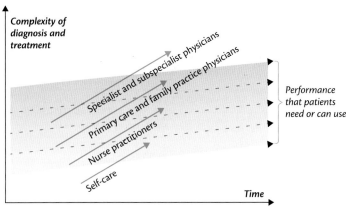

Disruptions of Health Care Professions

FIGURE 54.2 The graph delineates how in each industry the market can be segmented among various health care providers with different skill sets.

specific disorders such as diabetes and hypertension, whose diagnoses and treatments most often do not require physician expertise. In the United States, the number of patients asking for new advanced surgical treatments, coupled with low reimbursement to the primary care physicians, has left the door open for mid-level providers such as nurse practitioners and physician assistants to serve the primary care markets, whereas the primary care physicians have been fleeing these markets in search of more profitable business models.[9] Similarly, the medical device industry could profit if a larger population of less-skilled people performed in a convenient, economical way that previously were only performed by costly specialists in centralized and inconvenient locations.[9] The industry actively searches for the blue ocean opportunities to create solutions from the least to most complex solutions addressed by self-care and telemedicine to highly specialized care offered only at major hospital settings. (Blue Ocean Strategy is the simultaneous pursuit of differentiation and low cost to open up a new market space and create new demand. It is about creating and capturing uncontested market space, thereby making the competition irrelevant.) By simplifying the procedures such that they can be done in the office setting more conveniently and cost-effectively, the physicians can provide new innovative, disruptive

technologies (Figs. 54.2 and 54.3).[13] The industry focuses on creating procedures that are easily done as simple outpatient procedures with cheaper devices and equipment. An example of this is introducing small vaginal robots such as Hominis® by Memic Innovative Surgery (Or Yehuda, Israel) which uses a transvaginal route to efficiently and economically perform a hysterectomy.

THE PATENTING PROCESS

In principle, the patent owner has the right to exclusively prevent or stop others from commercially exploiting the patented invention. Patent protection dictates that the invention cannot be commercially made, distributed, imported, used, or sold by others without the patent owner's consent. The patent process generally occurs early on at the concept and design stage.[10] Patents are territorial rights. The exclusive rights are applicable only in the region or the country in which a patent has been granted and filed, following the law of that region or country.[11] Medical patents, are defined broadly to include patents that relate to pharmaceuticals; methods of making and using them; medical treatment regimens; surgical procedures; medical devices; health care information technology for hospital and health care management systems (including software for managing hospital bed utilization,

FIGURE 54.3 By providing simple to use solutions, the medical device industry strives to enable lower skilled health care providers to accomplish more complex tasks.

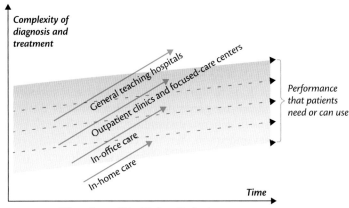

Disruptions of Health Care Professions

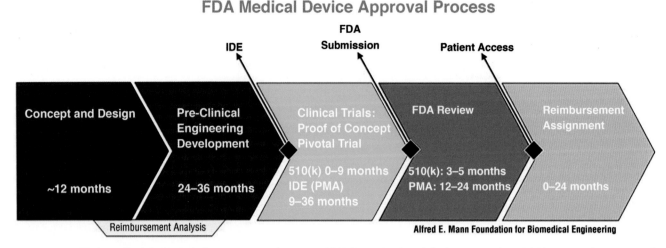

FIGURE 54.4 FDA medical device regulatory approval process. IDE, investigational device exemption; PMA, premarket approval. (From U.S. Food and Drug Administration.)

care distribution, medical staff allocation, and cost containment), and combinations of these (Fig. 54.4).[12] In the United States, the main categories of patents are (medical) utility patents (machines, processes/methods, and manufactured objects), design patents (ornamentation), and plant patents (under the Plant Variety Protection Act, not to be confused with a plant utility patent).[12]

A 510(k) is a premarket submission made to U.S. Food and Drug Administration (FDA) to demonstrate that the device to be marketed is as safe and effective, that is, substantially equivalent, to a legally marketed device, which cannot be one that is in violation of the Federal Food, Drug, and Cosmetic Act. The 510(k) allows manufacturers to apply for marketing clearance without any studies in humans of the device in question. All that needs to be done is to say that the product is substantially equivalent, the predicate, to a product previously cleared by the FDA. The 510(K) process does not necessarily address safety and efficacy of the product. For example, the currently marked polypropylene slings were cleared for marketing by using as a predicate a sling (ProteGen) that was significantly different in design and had many problems, prompting its recall from the market.

The FDA, upon approval of a new drug application, provides medical product applicants, perhaps the most essential element needed to bring the product to the public. The FDA is responsible for assuring that a new drug or new product is safe and effective. The FDA-approval process requires compliance with rigorous testing programs (clinical trials) and compliance with a lengthy administrative approval process and is often very costly. The FDA-approval process frequently runs concurrently with the patent application procurement process before the United States Patent and Trademark Office (USPTO). Because of lengthy time frame involved in obtaining FDA approval, the period during which a patented device may be commercialized under the effective patent term may be shortened. To correct the delay, the patent

term restoration provision was created. This provision grants patent term extensions for patents on human drug products, medical devices, food and color additives, and processes for making or using such products. This provision serves to restore a part of the patent term to the patentee for the period over which the patentee could not sell or market a product while awaiting FDA approval. The Hatch-Waxman Act also provides a "safe harbor" provision for patentees.[1] It serves to shield a party from a charge of patent infringement for making, using, and offering to sell another's patented product/process.[12]

The first step toward obtaining a patent is to file a patent application with the USPTO. With the implementation of the America Invents Act (AIA), the first inventor to file a patent application has priority over another person who gets a patent application filed after that initial date, but who nonetheless may assert he or she was the first to "invent" the technology covered in the patent application. With this change in the law (before AIA, the race to get a patent application on file was not paramount to establishing the right of priority), the potential patentee needs to expedite the filing of his or her patent application on the earliest date possible.

THE ECONOMIC PERSPECTIVE

The hospitals continuously look for ways to trim medical expenditure. The number one expense for hospitals is labor, followed by supply chain management. What has been done traditionally by specialists, if simplified, can be done by generalists, and what was done by physicians in general, if simplified, can now be done by the nurses and so on. Yet, this constant downmarketing has not decreased the United States gross domestic product expenditure on health care. The savings from such equipment and personnel innovations do not necessarily translate to better care for the patients. It has resulted in more top-heavy hospital management, healthier

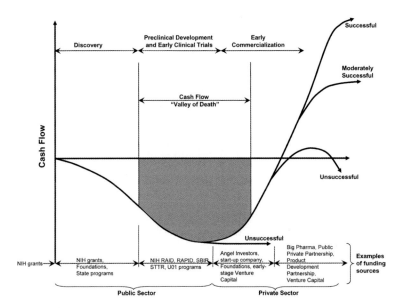

FIGURE 54.5 Cash flow "valley of death" diagram. The cash flow "valley of death" as a function of development stage (time) with typical funding sources at various stages (Adapted from Bridging the Valley of Death: Transitioning from Public to Private Sector, Lynne M. Murphy and Phillip Edwards, 2003). NIH, National Institutes of Health; RAID, Rapid Access to Interventional Development; SBIR, Small Business Innovation Research; RAPID, Rapid Access to Preventive Intervention Development; STTR, Small Business Technology Transfer. (From Steinmetz KL, Spack EG. The basics of preclinical drug development for neurodegenerative disease indications. *BMC Neurol* 2009;9[Suppl 1]:S2.)

instrument manufacturer stocks, and flat physician salaries, but it has not resulted in less health care spending.

The Valley of Death for Medical Device Development

Between the stages of the research and development process in which the industry predominantly invests (commercialization of reliably profitable products) and the government predominantly invests (fundamental research), lies the technology's "valley of death" (Fig. 54.5). That is the gap where private investment markets fail to finance the research needed to support the so-called

"platform" technologies. This investment failure occurs because generic technologies are either expensive or risky or both for the industry to independently develop the product. Ironically, it is these platform technologies that jumpstart new devices and products and, in many cases, entire new market categories.[13,14] Before becoming commercially available in the market, a medical device must first achieve standards and comply with regulations designated by its class. Class, I, II, or III device classification is based on the device's risk and the level of control needed to ensure efficacy and safety (Fig. 54.6).[1] Low-risk devices are designated class I and are subjected to general controls only. Conversely, most

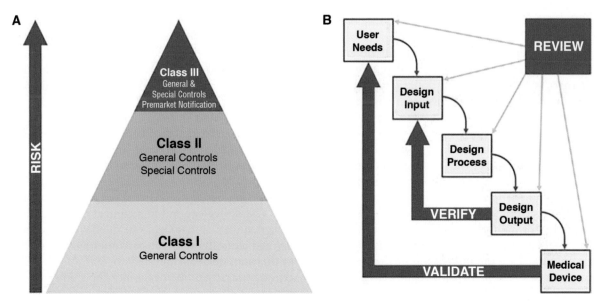

FIGURE 54.6 Classification of medical devices and the design control process for device design. **A:** Classification of medical devices is based on the degree of risk to the patient. Greater risk necessitates a greater degree of regulatory control for device market approval. **B:** The design control model is suggested by the FDA for medical device development. (Adapted from U.S. Food and Drug Administration. *Design control guidance for medical device manufacturers.* Silver Spring: FDA Center for Devices and Radiological Health, 1997.)

implants are considered high-risk class III and are subject to the most complete and stringent standards. They are granted a preliminary investigational device exemption to use the device in an FDA-regulated clinical trial to assemble the required safety and efficacy data needed to justify safe introduction to markets.[1]

A problem for the developers may be that although the academic demands require publication of one's findings, in reality, this will leave the idea for others to develop. It is essential to differentiate a marketable idea from academic work and obtain a patent as soon as possible. An alternative is to obtain a patent in one country first, to get 1-year protection because the first-to-invent system has been substituted with the first-to-file-a patent system since 2013. The first-to-file-a patent system allows the inventor to further evaluate the idea and see if it is worth obtaining the next level of patent protection afforded at the international level.[1]

Medical Device Good Manufacturing Practice

FDA was first to mandate medical device quality system requirements to ensure the safety and effectiveness of medical devices. The FDA issued a ruling, prescribing current good manufacturing practice requirements for medical devices that required establishing a documentation and record-keeping method to investigate quality problems and patient injuries associated with medical devices. The government and industry use this quality assurance system to ensure that medical devices are manufactured to comply with the already established specifications and a continuous improvement strategy.

Postmarket surveillance programs instituted by medical device companies are vital to capturing unforeseen hazards and proper device performance. When a medical device fails expectations and regulations once in widespread use, a worldwide recall might cost a manufacturer at least 50 million dollars, not counting future income loss. The direct litigation costs are formidable, and indirect litigation costs such as loss of reputation and market share loss can drive the products out of the market. In calculating a medical device's profitability, the manufacturers often include the cost of future litigation as a cost of doing business. Because the more prominent manufacturers generally choose to avoid the development of newer products with the high regulatory or liability risks, this leaves the market open for small- and medium-sized enterprises (SMEs) that not only navigate the innovation process and regulatory processes (e.g., 510[k], premarket approval, combination product) toward market approval but also if the innovation fails, it will be easier for an SME to dissolve. The customer and the continually changing regulatory environment represent both innovation challenges and opportunities for small- and medium-sized

medical device companies because the larger companies are more resistant to exposing themselves to risk.[1] Conversely, a small company can conveniently go bankrupt if the litigation burden is too severe, conversely, companies with a large and diverse portfolio can weathered the burden of litigations better. Many larger companies are not interested in purchasing a proof of concept. Small- and medium-sized companies use alternative funding concepts, technology transfer, and licensing methods to move scientific medical device innovation through an increasingly challenging and uncertain regulatory environment. The larger companies subsequently take over the successful SME product launchers as their competitive threat becomes evident. Therefore, a market derive is the incentive for a successful SME to be bought up for many folds the initial investment to either be dismantled or incorporated into a larger company's product line. Of all the ideas in all the world, in all the countries, in all the companies, only a tiny fraction become products, and only 1 in 10 of those medical devices launched will succeed, and very few will be a best seller.

The innovative landscape in medical devices is mostly made of SMEs. In Europe, for example, 95% of the 25,000 medical technology companies are SMEs that employ less than 50 people (small- and micro-sized companies).[15] The early-stage innovations, which are primarily financed at an SME level, focus on a single product with high liability risk.[16] In this environment, the quality aspects are at a low standard combined with high manufacturing optimization. The cost of goods sold is high, which makes the initial SME devices expensive. When there is a successful disruptive technology/product, the large companies may adopt the innovation to make products through an already established reliable and cost-effective manufacturing methods. These devices and products may be additionally upgraded by the acquired technology by developing line extensions and second-generation incremental inventions.[1]

In the United States, a significant hurdle to a device approval is presented during the clinical trials. The trials are performed at a high cost, and as such, upfront laboratory testing and preclinical evaluation reduce the risk of failure. Mimicking the disease process in the laboratory setting better predicts the device's behavior in real life. The device can fail in a clinical trial. Still, a poorly designed clinical trial can fail the device due to poorly defined clinically relevant outcomes and/or quantifiable evaluation, unclear intermediate end points, and vague criteria for patient inclusion into the study.[1]

Reimbursement Challenge

Medical device development pro forma should take into account the reimbursement for the device and the service provided. Even under the best circumstances, the prices and reimbursement are not as predicted. According to Advanced Medical Technology Association, a U.S. medical device trade association, medical device average prices have decreased in the United States. For example, drug-eluted stents decreased by 34% from 2007 to 2011. Although the reimbursement pressure may partially explain the price decrease of medical devices, a new successful device should expect competition closing in in reality. The medical device has a finite time to become profitable, improve, and dominate the market.[17] A successful device that provides a robust solution should reduce cost by developing value-for-money propositions for payers to achieve acceptance. The current economic pressures dictate to do more with less.

Expanding Portfolio Challenge

Because of the advance of technology and new needs posed by a changing and aging population, the medical device industry has more opportunities in areas previously unavailable such as personalized, integrative, complementary, or regenerative medicine, advanced therapy medicinal products, three-dimensional (3D) printers, new biomaterials, and the internet of things. The same fields create new challenges as a product that previously could have a 20-year lifespan could be obsolete because of new solutions previously unimaginable.

COST-EFFECTIVENESS RESEARCH

The inventor and the manufacturing company cannot determine if their product benefits society as a whole. Comparative effectiveness research (CER), a broad term encompassing many concepts, is used loosely as an essential tool to lower costs and improve patient outcomes by the policymakers. CER research compares population outcomes, risks, and benefits when two or more therapies or devices are used. Policymakers who are entities with access to large data banks set goals for payers, physicians, and patients. This data in CER is used to make clinical and health care choices. From the medical device perspective, there is also the time required for the device to evolve through feedback and continuous improvement. Continuous improvement and evolution of the technology, procedure techniques, and physician skills influence clinical data end points to be considered in a CER setting.[18]

INNOVATION CLUSTERS

The commercial success of a medical device is not exclusively technology driven. It requires presenting cost-effective solutions to the market, ease of use for customers (e.g., doctors), robust clinical evidence, regulatory compliance, and effective marketing.[1]

Commercial translation of a medical device can also be costly because larger companies may not invest in newer technologies. A growing trend is the SME incubators in significant clinical and universities, collaborative agreements, or larger companies' investments and joint ventures. Universities create incubators where the companies are present on campuses. Once an innovative idea is identified, the patent and intellectual property issues, the execution of business agreements (nondisclosure, collaborative research, material transfer) need to be instituted to have a meaningful sense of the costs and realistic expectations of the revenue generated.[1] Just like the concept of IDEO, a collaborative environment including inventors, investors, hospitals, universities, companies need to come together to make the magic happen in the right place and the right time. The timing of innovation is crucial to a successful launch.

CASE STUDY: SURGICAL ROBOT INNOVATION AND EVOLUTION

The use of robotics in gynecology, gynecologic oncology, and urogynecology has been heavily driven by rapid technologic developments that capitalized on adaptations to laparoscopic procedures.[19] There are three main types of robotic surgical systems: active, semiactive, and master-slave. Each of these types is categorized by how the surgeon interacts with each system.

Active systems: a fully autonomous system that runs preprogrammed tasks under the surgeon's control

Semiactive systems: runs preprogrammed tasks, but instead of having an entire autonomous property, the surgeon completes the preprogrammed functions to perform the surgery fully

Master-slave system: a complete lack of autonomous properties and preprogrammed tasks entirely in the surgeon's control. Quickly, the importance of telepresence allowed master-slave systems to begin to take hold of the market. Telepresence demonstrated recognition of a surgeon's potential significance linked up to a robotic system by reducing the mortality and morbidity rates. From here, two rival master-slave surgical systems emerged as competitors, the ZEUS and da Vinci.[19] The ZEUS robotic surgical system was a medical robot designed to assist in surgery, initially produced by the American robotics company "Computer Motion." Its predecessor, automated endoscopic system for optimal positioning (AESOP), was cleared by the FDA in 1994 to assist surgeons in minimally invasive surgery. The ZEUS itself was cleared by the FDA 7 years later, in 2001. ZEUS had three robotic arms, which were remotely controlled by the surgeon. The first arm, AESOP, was a voice-activated endoscope, allowing the surgeon to see inside the patient's body. The other two robotic arms mimicked the surgeon's movements to make precise incisions and extractions. ZEUS was discontinued in 2003, following the merger of Computer Motion with its rival Intuitive Surgical (Sunnyville, CA); the merged company instead developed the da Vinci surgical system.[20] The da Vinci surgical system is a master-slave system that allows the surgeon to use an advanced set of instruments to perform minimally invasive surgery with robotic assistance. The system has three components that all work together to give the surgeon the ability to operate through small incisions. The first component is the surgeon console. The next component is the patient cart. The cart is positioned alongside the patient bed, where it is then aligned and remains in position during surgery. The cart includes three to four robotic arms that are controlled by the surgeon console. These arms move around fixed pivot points and contain safety checks to ensure no independent movement is made from the surgeon's movements. The third and last component of this system is the vision cart with a high-definition 3D endoscope and an imaging processing unit to allow real-time images to appear. The vision cart is responsible for the communication between the various components and ensures a reliable vision system.[21]

The Senhance surgical system (Morrisville, NC), the competitor to da Vinci, boasts a console center that includes eye-tracking camera control, which allows the system to sense the surgeon's eye activity, which stabilizes the camera control. High-definition 3D visualization provides the surgeon with the additional depth and spatial relation of the anatomy.[22] This system's pros include the fully reusable aspect that the Senhance instruments with haptic feedback and familiar laparoscopic motions and technique.

The da Vinci surgical system and the Senhance system have improved surgeons' dexterity, surgical precision, visualization, and ergonomics. Crowding, while improved, remained prominent in conjunction with the bulky robotic system components.[23] To address these limitations, the fourth-generation model, the da Vinci SP surgical system, was developed. The system provided necessary articulation, good power, and less crowding. Senhance differentiated itself from da Vinci by robot by aiming to assist in the accurate control of laparoscopic instruments for visualization and endoscopic manipulation of tissue including grasping, cutting, blunt and sharp dissection, approximation, ligation, electrocautery, suturing, mobilization, and retraction. The Senhance surgical system is intended for laparoscopic gynecologic surgery, colorectal surgery, cholecystectomy, and inguinal hernia repair. In its first-quarter 2020 earnings report, the company noted just $600,000 in revenue, following up on a lackluster 2019 that saw the company's stock drop from a $2.41 per share in

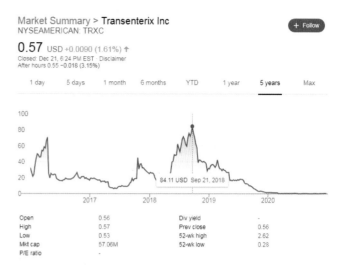

FIGURE 54.7 The stock market performance of the TransEnterix publically traded shares. (From New York Stock Exchange information.)

January 2019 to less than $0.24 late in the year 2020, as investors worried about the lack of sales of the company's robotic surgical system (Fig. 54.7).[24]

The Hominis surgical system (Or Yehuda, Israel) is a master-slave system that emulates human dexterity by using humanoid-designed robotic arms (Fig. 54.8) with access to 360° articulation (Fig. 54.9).[25] The design also includes an endoscopic instrument control

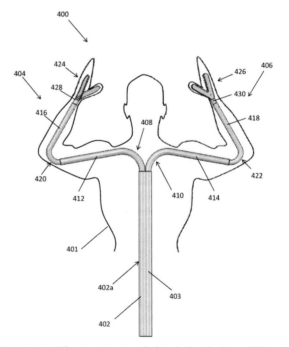

FIGURE 54.8 The inspiration behind the design of Hominis robot demonstrating the human-like arms. (Courtesy of Hominis.)

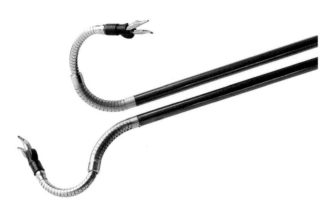

FIGURE 54.9 The Hominis Instrument ARMS demonstrating the 360° articulation. (Courtesy of Hominis.)

system used for transvaginal surgical procedures and disposable and reusable components. The sterile components consist of the "Hominis Instrument ARMS" and a "Vaginal Access Kit," while nonsterile features include the "Hominis Surgeon Console," the "Hominis Robotic Control Unit," and "Retroflex ARMS Controllers" (Fig. 54.10).[25] The surgeon console acts as the human interface by providing the surgeon a seated area to access the instrument ARMS through the Hominis Robotic Control Unit, which contains sensors and drivers to allow the electronic board to interact with the ARMS. The movement of the ARMS is operated via the "Surgeon ARMS Controller." The

motor unit is either attached to the surgical table using the "Robotic Control Unit Support System," or in the future, it may be attached to a pedestal cart as a floor-mounted system.[26,27] An exciting pro about the Hominis system is that it allows for a single port approach through the rectouterine pouch to accomplish the hysterectomy with the assistance of minimal abdominal laparoscopic view because of the motor unit's small footprint. The system allows for improved ergonomics, lower costs, a smaller footprint, and a different type of robotic surgery. The company prides itself on patient safety and has completed many animal feasibility studies,[26,27] along with the use of the Hominis robot in Israel and Belgium for salpingo-oophorectomy[25] and hysterectomy.[28] In the Hominis human studies, no severe intraoperative complications were observed, and the feedback from the surgeons has been favorable.[28] In these studies, surgeons had a fast learnings curve and felt that the Hominis surgical approach could make gynecologic surgeries accessible to more women.[8]

ASSESSMENT OF MEDICAL INNOVATIONS

The investors would like to know if a medical device would succeed and the likelihood of success. As such, there are many models in use as an assessment tool. The payers may use a similar mechanism because they would like to know the likelihood of adverse events and

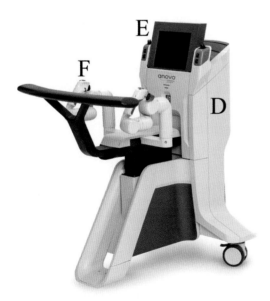

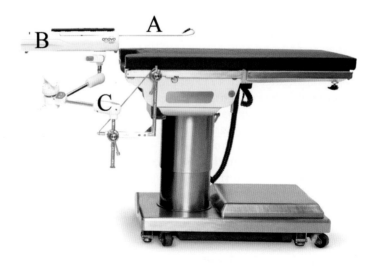

FIGURE 54.10 The Anovo System: *A*, Anovo Instrument ARMS; *B*, Anovo Robotic Control Unit; *C*, Robotic Control Unit Support System; *D*, Anovo Surgeon Console; *E*, Retroflex ARMS Controllers; *F*, Surgeon ARMS Controller. (Courtesy of Momentis Surgical.)

how much they will cost. The Health technology assessment (HTA) discipline was initiated about 30 years ago to evaluate how the development, diffusion, and use of health technology impacted the economic, social, medical, and ethical aspects of the environment in which it was introduced. In the era of CER and evidence-based medicine, the HTA has become widely used to determine which health technologies may provide value for money.[29] Such models have proven to be complicated and as good as the data entered into them. For example, the cost-effectiveness assessment of diagnostic rather than treatment tools can be tricky because they do not directly treat disease parameters but influence mortality.[3]

An interesting recurrent scenario for medical devices is that while the financial analysis for an SME may indicate that a device is not cost-effective to develop from a health care perspective, the SMEs are not in the business of deciding if technology is cost-effective from a societal perspective. For example, a laparoscopic donor nephrectomy is much more cost-effective from a societal perspective than from a health care perspective.[3] Although it is common sense that CER and HTA should be concerned with societal perspective, in countries such as the United States with free-market health care, the decisions about the appropriateness of devices and technologies are made in silos. The patient advocacy organizations, the hospital associations, industry, and the other health care sectors lobby for their financial benefit, which is not necessarily the societal benefit. The more centralized societies such as those in Europe have a two-perspective approach for medical technology assessment. They calculate cost-effectiveness ratios for both the health care perspective and the common societal perspective.[30]

Using HTA should not be a one-time exercise but rather as part of a continuous improvement process as the data parameters entered into the models are constantly changing. Once a technology or medical device is employed, periodic assessments based on original assumptions used for modeling should be used. If the outcome of interest was used in the model, these need to be assessed. For example, many slings have been withdrawn from the market because they did not meet the efficacy end point. If there is a substantial negative variance from the anticipated outcome, consideration should be given to forsaking the technology in favor of the assessment model.[31]

The Importance of Clear, Concise, and Closed-Loop Communication about Medical Device Adverse Events

Meager education of the users, poor implementation of a product, and the lack of a feedback loop mechanism form profound and commonly observed pitfalls in the road to the successful evolution of innovation.

Human lack of acceptance of feedback and reluctance to acknowledge an incorrect choice should not be a part of an objective assessment mechanism. For this reason, the inventors and investors should be separated from the assessment mechanism.[3] What fuels the medicolegal industry is a cycle of rushed products to the market and withdrawn only after their complications become evident too late due to poor feedback loop mechanism. Innovations in medical devices do not automatically translate into medical practice advances.[32] Positive technology impact in medicine requires human factor engineering to augment the health care team's skills, rather than seek the providers entirely with technology.[33] With human factor engineering, it is vital to recognize the nurses as crucial in the acceptance, application, and routine use of medical technologic devices.[3] Medical devices can help doctors and their teams to be more efficient. Like automobiles that have undergone continuous improvement, medical devices require several reiterations via technologic advancement, only possible by an efficient feedback loop. The input of the whole team is a crucial component for such improvements. Ideally, medical representative in the operating room should close the loop between the developers and users, but because of the incentive mechanisms in place, most instrument representatives are most concerned with their items' sales.[3] In this phase of innovation, many medical device start-up companies under economic pressure do not form the communication loop. They market their products widely to a large number of novice users to demonstrate profitability. A large number of problems occur in the field, and this will not translate to better product design because of a lack of feedback loop. Although we have stated that good communication between physicians and industry is essential, the physician payments sunshine act was created to increase transparency around the financial relationships between the physicians, teaching hospitals, and the device manufacturers.[34]

Investigating Incidents and Their Contributing Factors

Although medical device–related adverse events can be divided to "device" or "operator" failure, this categorization is an oversimplification of an often difficult diagnostic issue. An objective structured approach is advocated, and the team can use Shepherd global patterns of causes.[35]

The general evaluation of medical device failures fall under **five failure types or groups**:

1. **Equipment.** The number of medical devices that may have the same function, availability of equipment, and service readiness requirements for maintenance and repair should be evaluated.[3] Does the facility have many types of equipment for the same function with different operability? An example of

this is stocking various trocars for laparoscopy procedures. Each may have different resistance during abdominal entry, which may increase the risk of viscus injury.

2. **Operator**. Analysis of possible device errors should include evaluation of improper handling. This aspect of evaluation may be challenging, which is why medical devices should be used on a trial basis to evaluate human factors to predict improper handling that can occur during normal intended use or reasonably foreseeable off-label use. It would be perhaps impossible for the manufacturer to indicate how a medical device may be used in a not reasonably foreseeable off-label use.[3]

3. **Facility**. This concerns the physical building and the organization, management, training, and culture of a health service. To maximize the best possible care for the patients, it may be essential to provide specialty care. In a recent study of high-scoring hospitals, four out of five top-scoring hospitals were specialty facilities—surgical hospitals, orthopedics hospitals, or heart hospitals. And of the remainder, nearly all were small hospitals that were nominally general-purpose but in practice provided the same kind of focused care that the specialty hospitals did.[36] Using a device in a facility not suited for it reduces the patients' chances of a better outcome. For example, a competent surgeon performing urogynecology surgery in an orthopedic hospital will introduce the patient to many sources of errors that would have been eliminated if the patient was operated on by an experienced cohesive specialty women's team.

4. **Environment**. Facility and environment go hand in hand. The physical design of the health care environment should enhance the operations of the health services. The aspects, such as illumination, heating/cooling, sounds, adequate work and storage space, elevators, utilities, pagers, phones, etc., should be thought through carefully. Defects within the device or the installations can remain undetected if only relied on end-user input. Conducting regular inspections, accessibility, availability, or the absence of policy or guidelines are essential. Even when there are written policies, there can be misinterpretation or noncompliance with policies, procedures, or established practices. Once there are set policies and protocols, the availability and flow path of information (verbal, written, or electronic) among staff and the patient and family members should be regularly evaluated. Documentation of activities by the team as well as activities and communication with the patients should be standardized. For example, the chronologic documentation and surgery timing can convey much about the operating room efficiency and the team dynamics (Fig. 54.11).[3]

5. **Patient**. When pursuing medical care, a patient's physical or mental health status will chiefly

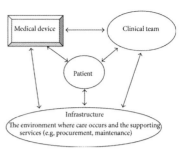

FIGURE 54.11 Diagram summarizing the interactions between a medical device, the clinical team, and the patient within an infrastructure that includes both the physical environment and the supporting services. Each of the elements (device, clinical team, patient, and infrastructure) interacts and depends on each other. (From Amoore JN. A structured approach for investigating the causes of medical device adverse events. *J Med Eng* 2014;2014:314138.)

determine the outcome of treatment in contrast to the typically expected outcome. Although predictive models can identify subgroups of patients with a very high risk of dying before hospital discharge (e.g., old intensive care unit patients),[3] these models may not be validated for a new medical device. For example, using mesh in a patient with severely uncontrolled diabetes will increase the risk of mesh infection, erosion, or extrusion. Or, using mesh in a pelvic cavity of a patient with underlying pelvic pain may exacerbate the pain. The instructions for use by the manufacturers are meant to be a comprehensive guide for patient selection when a physician is being oriented to the new device.

FEDERAL REGULATIONS IN THE UNITED STATES TO MONITOR ADVERSE EVENTS AND RECALLS

The Center for Devices and Radiological Health (CDRH) is the regulatory entity that reviews and systematically evaluates medical device recall data. As defined at Title 21, Code of Federal Regulations, 7.3(g), "*Recall* means a firm's removal or correction of a marketed product that the FDA considers violating the laws it administers and against which the agency would initiate legal action, e.g., seizure." The recalls are divided into three classes as "there is a reasonable probability that use of or exposure to a violative product":

Class I	**will cause** serious adverse health consequences or death
Class II	**may cause** temporary or medically reversible adverse health consequences or where the probability of serious adverse health consequences is remote
Class III	**is not likely** to cause adverse health consequences

Combating Unsafe or Defective Medical Devices Public Health Risks

The FDA is engaged in continuous improvement of the device monitoring process. Although there were 18 high-risk medical device recalls in 2008, this rate increased by 350% in 2013 when 63 high-risk devices were recalled by the FDA.[37] The annual number of medical device recalls increased by 97% between 2003 and 2012, which was attributed to enhanced cognizance by device firms, especially those previously named for reporting violations, and exact CDRH initiatives to improve medical device safety. The annual number of class I device recalls historically associated with high numbers of device problems, such as ventilators, infusion pumps, and external defibrillators, increased partly because of joint CDRH and industry efforts to enhance safe device performance. Per CDRH reports between 2009 and 2012 that medical device problems were effectively addressed and underlying issues resolved as evidenced by the average classification times for high-risk class I and II, recalls were reduced by 9 and 26 days, respectively.

The top reasons for recalls were related to device design, software, and nonconforming material or component issues. If industry and CDRH could successfully address these problems, as many as 400 recalls could be prevented annually.

The medical device firms, U.S. Food and Drug Administration's Office of Regulatory Affairs (ORA), and CDRH interact and collaborate to initiate, classify, and terminate the process of medical device recalls (Fig. 54.12).

The recall process typically relies on the device manufacturer acknowledging an issue that warrants a recall action. In initiating a recall, the FDA's ORA district office is notified. Although it typically takes the FDA 1 day to post the classification, the annual average time from firm awareness of the problem to acknowledging the problem by recall posting between 2010 and 2012 ranged from 233.7 days to 256.6 days.

Once the firm notifies the FDA (phase I in Fig. 54.12), the ORA district office issues a 24-hour alert to CDRH and a recall classification recommendation (phase II). CDRH conducts a final review and classification (phase III). Recalls are publicly posted online within a day of classification.

CDRH recall of radiation-emitting products and medical devices were studied in a 10-year study period. According to the FDA, between 2003 and 2012, there was an increase in the overall annual recall counts from 604 recalls to 1,190 recalls representing a 97% increase in both class I and II recalls. Class I recalls increased from 7 (1%) in fiscal year (FY) 2003 to 57 (5%) in FY 2012. Between 2003 and 2012, annually class II recalls more than doubled, whereas the number of class III recalls declined by approximately 35%. Recalls were associated with distinct medical specialties. Radiology, cardiovascular, general hospital, general surgery, orthopedics, and chemistry were the six specialties representing the majority of recalls. The radiology medical devices' use of identified media was the top recall item, which resulted in focusing and better monitoring for and reporting problems by the radiology industry.[37]

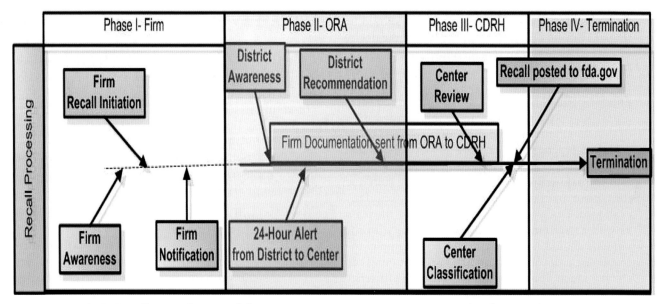

FIGURE 54.12 CDRH recall counts by FY and class (FY 2003 to FY 2012). (From U.S. Food and Drug Administration.)

Device Procodes

The FDA uses a device, "procode" composed of five components: industry, class, subclass, Process Indicator Code (PIC), and product. This is a useful method of cataloging and monitoring medical devices to report industry-wide product performance problems and barriers that impact device quality, safety, and effectiveness. Between 2004 and 2012, the top ten device procodes associated with recalls (0.15% of all procodes) resulted in 20% of device recall events. Given this system, the CDRH can conduct a more detailed analysis of recall data to identify trends. Between 2004 and 2012, the percentage of recalls affecting medical devices within 1 year of FDA marketing approval held constant at around 10%. Likewise, medical devices that had been on the market for more than 15 years consistently represented around 10% of recalled devices, proving that the proportion of recalls had not increased. No trends were recognized with respect to the time on the market and medical device recalls.

Recall and Regulatory Violations

For each medical device recall, the FDA decides the related Federal Food, Drug, and Cosmetic Act violations. A medical device recall may be assigned one or more regulatory violations. The top ten regulatory violations for medical device recalls classified between 2010 and 2012 were all linked to quality system regulations. An increase in the number of recalls between 2003 and 2012 was credited to better reporting by manufacturers that were named in 806 reporting violations and by producers of radiologic devices. There has been better reporting by industry and also determined exertion by CDRH and manufacturers to collaborate to increase the quality and safety of medical devices.

The regulatory requirements for the market introduction of new medical devices differ radically around the globe. Notwithstanding a wide range of various initiatives aiming at regulatory synchronization, opposing regulatory standards for approval continue, with a rising number of countries demanding local testing before local approval. Just to give an example of differing standards and timelines, it was 10 years between European regulatory approval of the Watchman left atrial appendage closure device and FDA 2015 approval in the United States, and it was just in 2017 that a clinical trial was finally initiated in Japan to secure device regulatory endorsement in that country.[38]

MARKETING OF MEDICAL DEVICES

During the 1997 and 2006 periods, given the evolution of market dynamics, the frequency and type of financial content observed in pharmaceutical versus medical device commercials changed. The scarcity of supportive proof in medical device ads and pharmaceutical formulary assertions is a potential area of worry that needs further analysis by watchdogs, policymakers, and academia.[39] Interestingly, the types of financial assertions in pharmaceutical versus medical device commercials differed considerably. The pharmaceuticals frequently presented market share claims (12.8%), whereas medical device commercials seldom made such claims (1.1%) ($P < .01$). Additionally, assertions other than market share claims were more numerous for medical devices than pharmaceuticals (28.3% vs. 11.4%; $P < .01$). For example, claims concerning compensation were encountered frequently in medical device advertisements (4.9% vs. 0.8%; $P < .01$), as were cost-effectiveness claims (6.5% vs. 0.6%; $P < .01$). Price claims were more common for medical devices (10.3%) compared with pharmaceuticals (6.9%).[39] Of the 561 distinctive commercials with economic content, 408 (73%) supported the assertions. Although proof was commonly given in pharmaceuticals, it was not provided for medical device ads. Just one medical device ad that made a financial claim gave no proof.[39]

CONCLUSION

Advances in medical device innovations often propagate from profound clinical acumens and a needs-based approach to providing more efficient clinical care. It can be argued that there is a significant role for incremental improvements to existing solutions, but what if the paradigm for existing solutions is wrong? Then real shifts in clinical outcomes, population health, patient satisfaction, surgical efficiency, and better use of economic resources dictate a transformational paradigm shift, which in the case of medical devices can only be achieved by thinking outside the box by disruptive innovations.[40] From the medical device industry's perspective, successful innovation and marketing require collaborations both with customers (patients and surgeons) and technology providers (academia, SMEs, and large companies). The patients and surgeons' needs should be identified, and the innovations should translate into commercially feasible solutions by using existing or evolving technologies.[1]

Before introducing a medical device into the market or producing a device, all technologic, societal, economic, and administrative challenges and "side effects" of the medical device from the design phase on should be thoroughly studied. A medical device is not passive because just one end-user in the organization uses it. On the contrary, a device affects the immediate team and impacts organizations' social contexts and supporting mechanisms. A value analysis to assess milestones to be achieved at specific times is essential from the financial perspective. Adaptation of the medical device by insurance providers and appropriate reimbursement is a crucial milestone before mass production. There are systematic methods for performing these tasks.[41] Although the history of other disruptive revolutions suggests systemic transformation is occurring in health care, there is a medical instrument industry crisis that requires "responsible innovation" for a medical device to succeed in the market.[9] The term "responsible" is used to denote the manufacturers' responsibility to adequately educate and provide a continuous quality control feedback loop mechanism in the field once the product is released. Many companies today provide physicians with medical devices without proper training. Although disruptive technologies enable caregivers to move competently upward, education is needed to reach competence.

Intuitive (Sunnyville, CA) placed a costly technology into the hands of highly skilled physicians in urology and other subspecialties. Once these markets saturated, they expanded their device into the hands of some highly skilled generalist surgeons. Robotic innovations have transformed health care by allowing the surgeries to be performed more safely and efficiently but perhaps at a high financial cost that is negated by patients' lower length of stay and fewer complications. Many endometrial cancer surgeries performed in morbidly obese women resulted in chronic wound infections and various complications. These surgeries are now often performed in an outpatient setting. The economic analysis of robots is mixed, but the patients are undoubtedly doing better. The robot technology's success flies in the face of the general belief that the blue ocean growth markets merge when the alterations are made to products, processes, or technologies to let less highly compensated individuals perform tasks in more expedient settings. The surgical robot technology has gone through many revisions through the years but still uses a highly trained, expensive workforce to deliver consistent clinical outcomes. What has made a difference in the robot's case was that the manufacturer was calculated and methodical in introducing the robot. The technology was placed in highly trained professional hands after intensive training followed by close follow-up by proctors and robot reps. This prevented numerous early complications and scrutiny of the technology, which would have prevented it from revision and adaptation by slightly less highly trained physicians.

How can the health care instrument industry, venture capital, entrepreneurial energy, and technology development interface with the regulators, insurers, physicians, hospitals, and medical schools so they will not end up in litigation? The medical institutions are certainly no match for goliaths such as Johnson & Johnson, Bard, and Boston Scientific. Still, they do have the responsibility to educate the next generation of surgeons to practice evidence-based medicine and ask for long-term safety and efficacy data for a new product.

However, patients' and physicians' frustration should not be directed at the FDA alone. The agency does not bear sole responsibility for the current lack of sufficient data to support and inform the use of many high-risk and implanted devices. Responsibility is shared with the clinical community, which often resists requirements to report data; with manufacturers, which often oppose substantial premarketing and postmarketing requirements; and with payers, which often do little with the significant data assets control.[42]

Currently, there is a significant divide in the information accessible to evaluate the value, safety, efficacy, or quality of medical devices.[43] The reporting of medical device issues are voluntary, and there is no centralized data source to obtain the details on the specific brand or model of medical devices in use. It is postulated that if health insurance claims included device-identifying tracking information, researchers could gauge the incidence of device malfunctions and failures to evaluate further the total costs of care connected with various medical device products.[44] The insurance claims databases are currently used in a similar manner to monitor prescription drugs' safety.[45] A nongovernmental organization called X12 manages the data submitted in typical insurance claims forms used by hospitals or health insurers. (The Accredited Standards Committee X12 is a standards organization. Chartered by the American National Standards Institute in 1979, it develops and maintains the X12 Electronic Data Interchange.) The X12 has published a draft recommendation to include in claims the device identifiers that implanted device manufacturers have been placing on their packaging since early 2015. The claim forms are updated very infrequently, and the current environment provides an optimal timing for introducing this revision. A delay would mean an additional decade or more before changes can be instituted.[46] Integrating unique device identifier for medical devices is supported by the health insurers, hospitals, medical societies, the Medicare Payment Advisory Commission, the FDA, Centers for Medicare & Medicaid Services (CMS), and the Office of Inspector General of the U.S. Department of Health and Human Services.[46]

It is unlikely that the medical device industry can be liable solely for patient safety. It is doubtful that governments can effectively regulate medical device manufacturers without suffocating innovation. Although some of the responsibility lies with the medical educators and can teach the evidence-based practice of medicine in medical schools and the residency programs, the innovation, evolution, and marketing of medical devices often affects surgeons in clinical practice and not subservient to medical schools. The credentialing committees at the hospitals ask for certificates of training, which are issued by the manufacturers. Which surgeon or health care team member may competently use a medical device depends on the education provided by the manufacturers, the facility credentialing process, the surgeon expertise and volume, and the proctorship for the cases until the operator reaches the minimum competency. In summary, medical device innovation is a dynamic field with unique complexities and interactions involving innovator, manufacturers, investors, regulators, hospitals, educators, surgeons, sales, and marketing which has made much of the progress in modern medicine possible.

References

1. Bayon Y, Bohner M, Eglin D, et al. Innovating in the medical device industry—Challenges & opportunities ESB 2015 translational research symposium. *J Mater Sci Mater Med* 2016;27(9):144.

2. Wieringa FP, Poley MJ, Dumay ACM, et al. Avoiding pitfalls in the road from the idea to certified product (and the harsh clinical environment thereafter) when innovating medical devices. In: *Proceedings of the IEEE EMBS Benelux Symposium/Belgian Day on Biomedical Engineering.* TNO Industrie en Techniek; 2007.

3. Wieringa FP, Poley MJ, Dumay ACM, et al. Avoiding pitfalls in the road from the idea to certified product (and the harsh clinical environment thereafter) when innovating medical devices. In: *Proceedings of the IEEE Benelux EMBS Symposium/Belgian Day on Biomedical Engineering.* TNO Industrie en Techniek, 2007.

4. Geertsma RE, de Bruijn ACP, Hilbers-Modderman ESM. *New and emerging medical technologies—A horizon scan of opportunities and risks.* Bilthoven: National Institute for Public Health and the Environment, 2007.

5. National Health Service. *Design for patient safety—A system-wide design-led approach to tackling patient safety in the NHS.* London: Department of Health, Design Council, 2003.

6. Dumay ACM. Innovating eHealth in the Netherlands. In: Bos L BB, ed. *Conference of the International Committee on Medical and Care Compunetics,* 2007:157–165.

7. Kim WC, Mauborgne RA. *Blue ocean strategy: How to create uncontested market space and make the competition irrelevant.* Boston: Harvard Business Review Press, 2014.

8. Innovation versus science? Harder economic times will force governments to ask tough questions about their investments in research. *Nature* 2007;448(7156):839.

9. Christensen CM, Bohmer R, Kenagy J. Will disruptive innovations cure health care? *Harv Bus Rev* 2000;78(5):102–112, 199.

10. U.S. Food and Drug Administration. US FDA medical device regulatory approval process. Accessed January 24, 2018. https://libguides.nccuslis.org/c.php?g=766608&p=5500348

11. World Intellectual Property Organization. Patents. Accessed January 14, 2018. http://www.wipo.int/patents/en/2018

12. Mayfield DL. Medical patents and how new instruments or medications might be patented. *Mo Med* 2016;113(6):456–462.

13. Bingaman J, Simon RM, Rosenberg AL. Needed: A revitalized national S&T policy. *Issues Sci Technol* 2004;20(3):21–22.

14. Steinmetz KL, Spack EG. The basics of preclinical drug development for neurodegenerative disease indications. *BMC Neurol* 2009;9(Suppl 1):S2.

15. MedTech Europe. The European medical industry: In figures. Accessed January 24, 2018. http://www.medtecheurope.org/sites/default/files/resource_items/files/MEDTECH_FactFigures_ONLINE3.pdf

16. Roberts EB. Technological innovation and medical devices. *Symposium on New Medical Devices: Factors Influencing Invention, Development, and Use.* National Academy of Engineering/Institute of Medicine. 1987. http://dspace.mit.edu/bitstream/handle/1721.1/2183/SWP-1930-18388674.pdf?sequence=1

17. Market Realist. Must-know: Dropping medical device prices suggest a strong market. Accessed January 25, 2018. https://marketrealist.com/2013/09/must-know-device-prices-dropping-suggests-strong-market

18. Sharma A, Blank A, Patel P, et al. Health care policy and regulatory implications on medical device innovations: A cardiac rhythm medical device industry perspective. *J Interv Card Electrophysiol* 2013;36(2):107–117.

19. Kalan S, Chauhan S, Coelho RF, et al. History of robotic surgery. *J Robot Surg* 2010;4(3):141–147.

20. Wikipedia. ZEUS robotic surgical system. Accessed February 21, 2022. https://en.wikipedia.org/wiki/ZEUS_robotic_surgical_system

21. Harmanli O, Solak S, Bayram A, et al. Optimizing the robotic surgery team: An operations management perspective. *Int Urogynecol J* 2021;32(6):1379–1385.

22. Pappas T, Fernando A, Nathan M. Senhance surgical system: Robotic-assisted digital laparoscopy for abdominal, pelvic, and thoracoscopic procedures. In: Abedin-Nasab M. *Handbook of robotic and image-guided surgery.* New York: Elsevier, 2020:1–14.

23. Shin HJ, Yoo HK, Lee JH, et al. Robotic single-port surgery using the da Vinci SP® surgical system for benign gynecologic disease: A preliminary report. *Taiwan J Obstet Gynecol* 2020;59(2):243–247.

24. Google Finance. TransEnterix stock trend. Accessed February 21, 2022. https://www.google.com/finance/quote/TRXC:NYSEAMERICAN?sa=X&ved=2ahUKEwiDgtvwnuDtAhVCwVkKHawKDb8Q3ecFMAB6BAgOEBk

25. Lowenstein L, Matanes E, Weiner Z, et al. Robotic transvaginal natural orifice transluminal endoscopic surgery for bilateral salpingo oophorectomy. *Eur J Obstet Gynecol Reprod Biol X* 2020;7:100113.

26. Alshiek J, Marroquin J, Shobeiri SA. The Fresh Frozen Cadaveric Study of Direct Pouch of Douglas laparoscopic and robotic trocar insertion for vaginal natural orifice transluminal endoscopic surgery. *J Minim Invasive Gynecol* 2021;28(2):320–324.

27. Alshiek J, Bar-El L, Shobeiri SA. Vaginal robotic supracervical hysterectomy in an ovine animal model: The proof of concept. *Open J Obstet Gynecol* 2019;9(8):1114–1129.

28. Lowenstein L, Mor O, Matanes E, et al. Robotic vaginal natural orifice transluminal endoscopic hysterectomy for benign indications. *J Minim Invasive Gynecol* 2021;28(5):1101–1106.

29. Drummond M, Weatherly H. Implementing the findings of health technology assessments. If the CAT got out of the bag, can the TAIL wag the dog? *Int J Technol Assess Health Care* 2000;16(1):1–12.

30. Brouwer WB, van Exel NJ, Baltussen RM, et al. A dollar is a dollar is a dollar—Or is it? *Value Health* 2006;9(5):341–347.

31. Abenstein JP. Technology assessment for the anesthesiologist. *Anesthesiol Clin* 2006;24(4):677–696.

32. Wieringa FP. *Pulse oxigraphy: And other new in-depth perspectives through the near infrared window.* Rotterdam: Erasmus University Rotterdam, 2007.

33. Vosburgh KG, Newbower RS. Moore's law, disruptive technologies, and the clinician. *Stud Health Technol Inform* 2002;85(85):8–13.

34. Baim DS, Donovan A, Smith JJ, et al. Medical device development: Managing conflicts of interest encountered by physicians. *Catheter Cardiovasc Interv* 2007;69(5):655–664.

35. Amoore JN. A structured approach for investigating the causes of medical device adverse events. *J Med Eng* 2014;2014:314138.

36. Advisory Board. Want to please patients? Maybe you should start a specialty hospital. Accessed January 13, 2018. https://www.advisory.com/research/health-care-advisory-board/blogs/at-the-helm/2015/04/patient-experience-and-specialty-hospitals

37. Ferriter A. *Medical device recall report FY 2003–FY 2012*. Silver Spring: U.S. Food and Drug Administration, 2013.

38. Stein KM. The long and winding road after FDA approval: A medical device industry perspective. *Circulation* 2017;135(20):1877–1878.

39. Ackerly DC, Glickman SW, Schulman KA. Economic content in medical journal advertisements for medical devices and prescription drugs. *Pharmacoeconomics* 2010;28(5):429–438.

40. Ray PP, Amaral JF, Hinoul P. Innovation best practices in the medical device industry. *Tech Vasc Interv Radiol* 2017;20(2):90–93.

41. van Boxsel J, Schoone M. Tertz: Een technologietoets voor de zorgsector. *Health Manag Forum* 2005;1:36–37.

42. Redberg RF, Jacoby AF, Sharfstein JM. Power morcellators, postmarketing surveillance, and the US Food and Drug Administration. *JAMA* 2017;318(4):325–326.

43. Ibrahim AM, Dimick JB. Monitoring medical devices: Missed warning signs within existing data. *JAMA* 2017;318(4):327–328.

44. Reed TL, Levy D, Steen LT, et al. Adverse event triggered event reporting for devices: Report of a Food and Drug Administration–supported feasibility pilot of automated adverse event reporting. *J Clinic Eng* 2016;41(2):83–89.

45. Moscovitch B, Rising J, Daniel G, et al. Time to fix the black hole in Medicare data. Accessed July 6, 2017. https://www.healthaffairs.org/do/10.1377/forefront.20160629.055612/full/

46. Moscovitch B, Rising JP. Medical device identification in claims data. *JAMA* 2017;318(19):1936–1937.

Disorders of Anus and Rectum

CHAPTER 55

EVALUATION AND MANAGEMENT OF COLORECTAL DYSFUNCTION

Tisha N. Lunsford • Michael D. Crowell

EPIDEMIOLOGY

Constipation is a term often used to describe a constellation of symptoms, including decreased frequency of bowel movements, a sensation of incomplete evacuation, significant straining with defecation, and prolonged toilet time. This spectrum of variable symptoms is often accompanied by abdominal discomfort or pain, a sensation of fullness, heaviness, and bloating, and can be coexistent with anorectal disease such as symptomatic hemorrhoidal disease, rectal prolapse, and anal fissure. Constipation prevalence is estimated to impact at least 10% of the population and is nearly twice as common in women compared to men, increasing with advancing age.[1] About one-third of chronic constipation cases in tertiary referral centers are due to rectal evacuation disorders,[2] whereas the majority do not involve a motility or evacuation disturbance and are referred to as normal transit (functional) constipation. Normal transit constipation is frequently termed chronic constipation and, if abdominal pain is relieved or exacerbated by bowel movements, is diagnosed as constipation-predominant irritable bowel syndrome (IBS-C). For research purposes, the Rome criteria, developed by expert consensus and validated in large populations, define constipation as having two or more characteristic features relating to frequency less than three bowel movements in a week and relationship of bowel movements to pain and sensation. Criteria include hard or lumpy stools, straining, a sense of incomplete evacuation, feeling of anorectal blockage or obstruction, or the need for digital maneuvers to assist defecation.[3] Although a sudden change in bowel habits with a change in frequency or caliber of stools or the presence of symptoms such as unintentional weight loss or gastrointestinal (GI) bleeding warrants prompt evaluation for mechanical obstruction or luminal narrowing, the majority of patients experience chronic (defined as at least greater than 3 to 6 months and often years) symptoms that are not explained by biochemical assessment, cross-sectional imaging, or endoscopic evaluation. Constipation is often secondary in that it is a result of insufficient dietary fiber, a side-effect of medications (such as antihypertensives, antidepressants, antihistamines, or analgesics), diminished mobility (sedentary lifestyle), metabolic disorders (diabetes mellitus, chronic renal insufficiency), hormonal states (pregnancy), connective tissue disorders (scleroderma, Ehlers-Danlos), or neuropathic degeneration (Parkinson disease, multiple sclerosis).[4] Rarely, constipation is a primary disorder related to slow transit such as chronic intestinal pseudo-obstruction or autoimmune gastrointestinal dysmotility. If primary, it is usually more prominently accompanied by upper GI and systemic symptoms including early satiety, weight loss, nausea, and vomiting. If slow transit constipation is suspected, before investigating a rare underlying primary disorder, it is imperative that a careful screening for secondary causes is completed and a disorder of rectal evacuation considered and treated if present because these may be the true explanations for the proximal motility disturbance phenotype.[5] For this reason, as well as for guiding diagnostic and therapeutic interventions, constipation is typically categorized into subtypes (normal transit, slow transit, and defecatory dysfunction (also known as dyssynergia) based on an assessment of clinical or physiologic motility or transit evaluation and ease of evacuation. As diagnostic testing for assessments of physiologic function may not be widely available and as the approach to chronic constipation in clinical practice is algorithmic and fairly well-standardized independent of physiologic testing, the majority of patients are treated empirically based on a careful history and physical examination. Laboratory, radiographic, and endoscopic evaluation may be warranted. Regardless of etiology, chronic constipation has been shown to result in impaired quality of life, diminished work productivity and school attendance, and considerable economic and health care burden.[4]

DIAGNOSTIC ASSESSMENT

When available, diagnostic testing can be beneficial. The two categories typically used to guide intervention are assessment for rectal evacuation disorders and assessment for slow transit constipation via colonic transit assessment. Symptoms associated with chronic constipation are vague and variable, and it is essential to clarify what the patient is describing as constipation. In certain instances, the patient will complain of upper or middle GI symptoms such as bloating, nausea, and vomiting that may have their true origin in constipation. If constipation is suspected, in addition to inquiring about the frequency of bowel movements, patients should be asked about their sense of completeness of evacuation, degree of strain (if any), feeling like they "want to but can't," time spent on the toilet, use of digital maneuvers including stimulation and splinting the perineum as well as a description of stool form and caliber. The Bristol Stool Scale is a validated measure with varying pictorial stool consistencies ranging from small hard lumps (type 1) to liquid void of solid components (type 7) and may offer insight into the underlying issue and surrogate measure of motility (Fig. 55.1).[6] Just as hard, separate lumps may represent slow transit, and watery stools may represent diarrhea or, conversely, liquid overflow around stool impacted in the rectum, or "pseudodiarrhea". This heterogeneity of etiologies of loose stools highlights the importance of the digital rectal exam (DRE) and clarification of the patient's sense of complete evacuation, experience of anorectal obstruction, or need for digital maneuvers.

Digital Rectal Exam

Visual and digital inspection of rectum both at rest and with request to simulate defecation are essential in the evaluation of chronic constipation because it

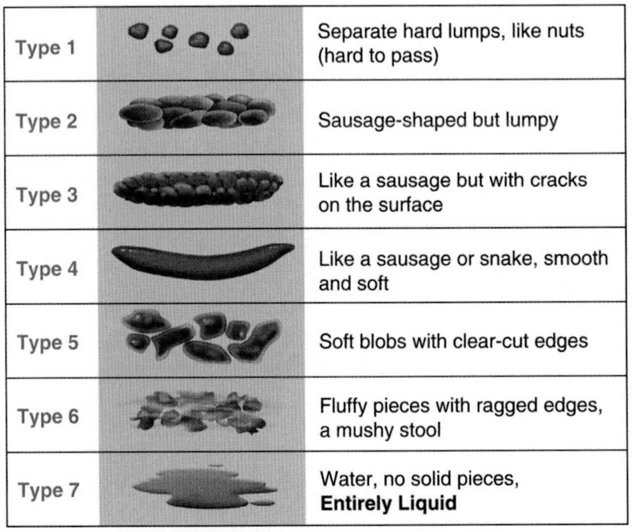

FIGURE 55.1 Bristol Stool Scale Chart. (Reprinted with permission from Baskin LS. *Handbook of pediatric urology*, 3rd ed. Philadelphia: Wolters Kluwer, 2018.)

may reveal grade III and IV internal hemorrhoids, perirectal excoriation or fecal matter suspicious for leakage or incontinence, rectal prolapse, an anal fissure with spasm and sphincteric hypertonicity with or without myalgia, impacted stool or stricture in the setting of previous surgery, radiation stricturing, or stigmata suspicious for inflammatory bowel disease such as anal fistula. Request for the patient to simulate defecation may produce either impaired or inadequate anal relaxation or may produce a paradoxical contraction moving the examiner's finger toward the umbilicus as opposed to generating adequate abdominal propulsive forces and synchronous anal relaxation necessary for defecation.[7] These findings are collectively referred to as defecatory dysfunction. Despite the widely held belief that anorectal dysfunction is most often related to obstetric trauma, defecatory dysfunction is often diagnosed in young nulliparous women. Although the pathophysiology remains poorly understood, it is felt to be related to maladaptive learning in response to psychological factors unique to the patient or symptomatic anorectal disorders such as anal fissure.[8] Other functional disorders of evacuation that are poorly understood can coexist and complicate defecatory dysfunction include rectocele, descending perineum syndrome, and rectal intussusception. Although there is no gold standard for diagnosing defecatory dysfunction, studies suggest that careful and expert DRE is 93% sensitive.[9,10]

Balloon Expulsion Test

Balloon expulsion test (BET) with or without anorectal manometry (ARM) is another noninvasive test often used to complement the DRE during assessment for defecatory dysfunction. Although testing parameters are poorly standardized and comparative performance with ARM and defecography is unknown, the BET is a simple, reliable test to screen for rectal evacuation dysfunction.[11] Optimal testing parameters include placing the deflated balloon in the rectum and inflating with water from 50 to 60 mL with subsequent time taken to expulsion in the left lateral or seated position in a private setting documented with a stopwatch. An expulsion time of greater than 1 minute suggests defecatory dysfunction.[12] The BET does not distinguish between functional and mechanical or anatomical causes of disordered defecation and abnormal results may warrant further testing.[13]

Electromyography

Electromyography (EMG) by surface intra-anal EMG tracings provides a unique opportunity for real-time visual feedback to the provider and patient on the movement and responses of the puborectalis muscle and external anal sphincter during simulated defecation.

If a sustained increase in EMG response greater than 50% above resting levels is noted on the recordings, a diagnosis of dyssynergic defecation with a visual goal to relaxation is provided.[14]

Anorectal Manometry

A test often performed to complement findings from DRE, BET, and EMG is ARM. ARM is available with the use of both conventional water-perfused catheters or high-resolution and high-definition solid-state catheters. Although a high-resolution ARM may provide greater constancy and spatiotemporal topography with closely arranged solid-state sensors than conventional manometry, both are minimally invasive, well-tolerated, and reliable methods for evaluating disorders of pelvic floor dysfunction.[15,16] Both techniques are designed to assess anal sphincter tone at rest and during squeeze, rectal sensation at different rectal volumes, rectoanal reflexes, and intrarectal pressure and coordination involved during attempted defecation.[17] Both conventional and high-resolution manometry are acceptable for evaluation for defecatory dysfunction as long as the data interpreter is facile in standardized values for the type of catheter used. Although they provide a unique synchronous visual, there is some concern that high-resolution and high-definition ARM recordings may overdiagnose dyssynergia, even in healthy controls.[18] Four subtypes of dyssynergia have been described with the use of ARM

in its diagnostic assessment of constipation. A normal response consists of an increase in intrarectal pressure combined with a relaxation of the anal sphincter with simulated defecation. Type I dyssynergic defecation is described as intrarectal pressure increasing appropriately but with paradoxical anal sphincter contraction resulting in a functional obstruction (Fig. 55.2).[19] Type II is when there is both paradoxical anal sphincter contraction and no increase in intrarectal pressure to promote evacuation. Type III differs from type I only in that rather than paradoxical, relaxation of the anal sphincter is absent or inadequate. Type IV is defined as both rectal relaxation and sphincter contraction are absent or inadequate. Traditionally, paradoxical contraction pattern with simulated defecation is felt to have high reproducibility and interobserver agreement for the diagnosis of defecatory dysfunction. The goal of classifying the subtype of dyssynergic defecation is to identify a treatment goal for pelvic floor retraining to improve or resolve any component of impaired evacuation contributing to the patient's constipation. This pelvic floor rehabilitation/retraining is often referred to as biofeedback.

ANORECTAL BIOFEEDBACK THERAPY

Pelvic floor retraining by biofeedback therapy is a valuable tool in the management of constipation due to disordered defecation. A behavioral training technique introduced in 1987, biofeedback incorporates exercises,

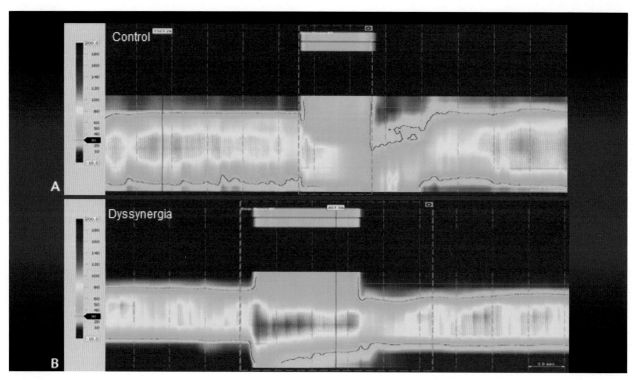

FIGURE 55.2 High-Resolution ARM: control compared to dyssynergia during simulated defecation. Areas in green represent lowering pressure (relaxation) while areas in red represent paradoxical increased pressure. **A:** Control. **B:** Dyssynergia. (Courtesy of Michael D. Crowell, PhD).

repetition, and auditory and/or visual cues to optimize abdominopelvic coordination during simulated defecation. Biofeedback training includes an instrument in situ for an objective measure of physiologic functioning such as a manometry system, an air-filled balloon, EMG, ultrasound, or digital palpation with the aim of instructing the patient in coordinating abdominal and rectal propulsive force generation and puborectalis/sphincteric relaxation.[20] The goal of biofeedback is to correct and improve muscle control, which translates into actual function.[21] Biofeedback should be carried out by an experienced physician, physiotherapist, or nurse with expertise in pelvic floor dysfunction. Exercises and simulation are repeated, modified, and corrected until the patient is able to perform successful maneuvers independently. In addition to biofeedback, patients should also be counseled comprehensively on bowel management techniques, including the physiology of the pelvic floor, diaphragmatic breathing and behavioral, nutritional, and lifestyle techniques, and nonpharmacologic options for treatment. Patients with hyposensitivity on initial evaluation may benefit from sensory retraining with a water-filled balloon, in which patients learn to discriminate lower sensations of rectal distension with filling. Most biofeedback sessions are 30 to 60 minutes every 1 to 2 weeks and duration is variable over 5 to 6 sessions depending on patient progress. Contraindications to biofeedback therapy include impaired mobility or cognition, pregnancy, active rectal inflammation or anal fissure, as well as skepticism of its utility as this has also been shown to predict suboptimal outcomes. Overall, 70% of patients will respond to biofeedback therapy and bowel management counseling.[22] Often, patients with defecatory dysfunction may also have an epiphenomenon or coexistent slow transit constipation and diagnosis and treatments for those disorders may need to be combined with biofeedback.[23,24]

For further assessment and management of defecatory dysfunction that does not respond to anorectal biofeedback therapy, there may be a role for defecography for diagnostic purposes as well as the use of valium orally or as a suppository, transanal injection of botulinum toxin type A (BTX-A), and bilateral partial division of puborectalis for therapy.

Defecography

Contrast defecography using barium or functional magnetic resonance imaging provides information about the function or completeness of evacuation as well as about other coexistent conditions such as rectocele, enterocele, or intussusception. Defecography is complicated by some potentially confounding variables that can be misleading, including patient factors such as embarrassment that may favor contrast retention or supine positioning for evacuation, which is not physiologic.[25]

Alternatives to Anorectal Biofeedback Therapy

In patients who have failed biofeedback therapy for dyssynergic defecation, injection via transanal approach, most commonly using digital palpation for guidance, of up to 100 units of BTX-A has been shown to result in clinical improvements; however, high-quality evidence is lacking.[26] Although invasive and with a risk of incontinence, bilateral partial division of puborectalis has been found to be an effective method in treating patients suffering from an inability to evacuate due to dyssynergia.[27] Another option for patients for use in conjunction with biofeedback or if biofeedback fails, is a trial of diazepam either in oral or per rectal/per vaginal suppositories. The concept of this therapy has been trailed in high-tone pelvic floor dysfunction, and although successful in the area of pelvic floor tension myalgia, the data for defecatory function are lacking.[28] Caution must be used in the elderly and those prone to risk with the use of benzodiazepines. Antegrade colonic enemas and sacral nerve stimulation for refractory dyssynergia are options that have been trialed but are not currently endorsed. Further studies are needed to address these modalities as options are limited if biofeedback therapy fails and potential risks of fecal incontinence may outweigh benefits.

SLOW TRANSIT CONSTIPATION

If defecatory dysfunction has been excluded or treated, the approach to therapy for constipation is fairly well standardized. Although a subset of patients who suffer from chronic constipation will have slow transit, patients may be diagnosed incorrectly if defecatory dysfunction is present as functional outlet obstruction may result in more proximal delays interpreted on physiologic testing. As the approach to the treatment of chronic constipation is essentially the same, it is usually not necessary to assess colonic transit unless therapies have failed, prompting the practitioner to contemplate colectomy or assess for whole gut motility disturbance as would be seen in some primary autoimmune and connective tissue disorders. Tests of colonic transit include an evaluation with the transit of radiopaque markers, wireless motility capsule, scintigraphy, and colonic manometry. All three modalities are clinically useful for the detection of altered colonic transit, although scintigraphy is only available in limited centers.

Radiopaque Marker Test

This standardized, simple, noninvasive test most commonly performed in the Hinton method, involves oral intake of 20 to 24 tiny ring-like radiopaque markers given to a patient to swallow on day 1 with subsequent imaging on day 5. Retention of more than 5 (20%) on day 5 is supportive of slow colonic transit.[29]

Wireless Motility Capsule

Ingestion of a pH- and temperature-sensitive capsule is able to detect segmental and whole-gut transit time by determination of changes in intraluminal pH. The patient is asked to discontinue all acid-suppressing medications 1 week before the test so that the capsule will detect a fall in intraluminal pH below 4 consistent with the low gastric pH and a rise in the pH by 3 units indicative of entry into the small bowl to be followed by a decrease in 1 unit when the capsule enters the cecum. The capsule is also able to detect amplitude of contractions throughout the GI tract that can be seen to increase after meals. Capsule studies have shown that more than one-third of patients with chronic constipation have transit abnormalities more proximally than the colon that may give pause to consideration for colectomy if study abnormalities and proximal symptoms coexist.[30]

Scintigraphy

Specialized centers use radioisotopes ingested with a standard meal or bound to capsules that undergo pH-sensitive release in the terminal ileum. Scintigraphy at 24 and 48 hours may be determined along with gastric emptying and small bowel transit to assess for a more global dysmotility underlying symptoms, similar to the role of wireless capsule endoscopy.[31]

MANAGEMENT

The importance of assessing for and treating dyssynergic defecation if present and the controversial need for assessing colonic transit arguably do not influence the standard approach to patients with constipation. The approach to the management of slow transit and normal transit constipation with or without abdominal pain and with or without evidence of pelvic floor dysfunction often overlaps because etiology is often multifactorial (Fig. 55.3).

Lifestyle and Dietary Modifications

The safest and most well-tolerated therapy includes lifestyle and dietary modifications, although many recommendations are not supported by high-quality evidence.[4] As mentioned previously, counsel from an expert nurse or advanced practitioner on behavioral changes that may benefit constipation, including educating patients on the anatomy and physiology of defecation and diaphragmatic breathing, may be the

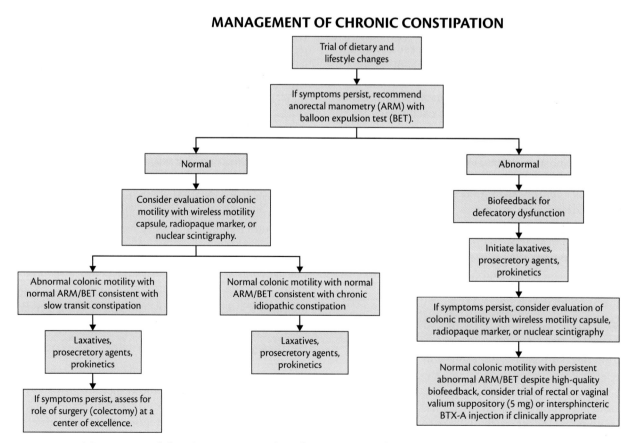

MANAGEMENT OF CHRONIC CONSTIPATION

FIGURE 55.3 Management of chronic constipation algorithm. (Courtesy of Tisha Lunsford, MD.)

first step in empowering the patient to understand their condition.[24] Patients are encouraged to set up a schedule for evacuation and take advantage of the stronger propagating contractions that occur early in the morning. These can be amplified by physical activity and eating a meal that includes fiber and a hot beverage with caffeine (if appropriate), which can intensify the gastrocolic reflex. Dietary fiber in the average Western diet is often inadequate, and usually about half the recommended dose.[32] Current recommendations suggest the intake of at least 25 to 30 g of fiber daily.[33] Patients should be encouraged to increase fiber slowly by no more than 5 g per week and to increase it as tolerated to avoid unpleasant bloating, flatulence, and discomfort. Patients with slow transit or IBS-C predominant may have a paradoxical worsening of symptoms, especially with insoluble forms of fiber.[34] Soluble fiber in the form of pectins and gums present in oats, peas, beans, apples, citrus fruits, carrots, barley, and psyllium is recommended and creates less gas and bloating than insoluble fiber. Soluble fiber can also be purchased as a supplement, and synthetic bulking agents include psyllium, methylcellulose, calcium polycarbophil, and wheat dextrin (U.S. trade name Benefiber®). Despite the widespread use of bulking agents, the evidence regarding their efficacy has been inconsistent.[35,36] Although increased fluid intake is often recommended, unless there is overt evidence of ongoing dehydration, there is little evidence that it is beneficial.[37] Increasing physical activity has had a variable impact on constipation symptoms but has been shown to have a positive effect on overall GI symptoms and well-being in patients with IBS independent of bowel habit.[38] Currently, although scientific evidence regarding dietary eliminations/simplifications is of variable quality for common diets implemented by patients with IBS, namely, low fermentable oligo-, di-, and monosaccharides and polyols (FODMAP) diet and gluten-free diet, the low FODMAP diet is included in the most updated guidelines as the most effective among the dietary interventions suggested for treating IBS.[39] A low FODMAP diet involves phases of elimination and reintroduction of poorly absorbed fermentable carbohydrates and, although the consensus is that it is somewhat effective for IBS, it can be difficult to follow and can contribute to disordered eating, highlighting benefit from the close supervision of a skilled nutritionist.

Pharmacologic Treatments for Chronic Constipation

Osmotic laxatives

If dietary and lifestyle modifications are ineffective or only partially effective, the introduction of osmotic laxatives should be considered as a next step. High-molecular-weight polyethylene glycol (PEG) is a large polymer with substantial osmotic activity that holds on to intraluminal water creating an osmotic gradient by retaining or drawing water into the gut lumen leading to increased bowel motility.[40] PEG has been proven to be effective and safe with the major side effect being bloating and flatulence. Lactulose is another osmotic laxative to relieve mild to moderate constipation. A prescription osmotic laxative that has been in use since the 1950s, it is a nonabsorbable carbohydrate that exerts its effect by altering intestinal osmolality. It is safe at a dose of 20 g (30 ml) once daily but can cause significant abdominal bloating, discomfort, and flatulence, which may decrease patient acceptance and, as it contains lactose and galactose, caution must be used in patients with diabetes.[41] Osmotic laxatives, which contain a small quantity of poorly absorbable ions, such as magnesium and phosphate available in multiple modalities from supplements to mineral water, work by an osmotic effect with retention of fluid to increase stool frequency and consistency.[42] Magnesium-based laxatives should be used with caution in patients with kidney disease because they may develop hypermagnesemia, which may lead to adverse cardiac effects such as prolongation of the QT interval with increased risk of dysrhythmia, bradycardia, and hypotension.[43]

Stimulant laxatives

In patients who do not significantly respond to osmotic laxatives, stimulant laxatives are frequently recommended. Stimulant laxatives such as bisacodyl exert their primary effects through alteration of electrolyte transport in intestinal mucosa and enhancement of colonic motility. They can be used safely for up to 4 weeks; however, the long-term safety of stimulant laxatives has not been confirmed.[44] Side effects include abdominal cramping, distension, nausea, and diarrhea. Bisacodyl or glycerin suppositories may be helpful if there is a coexistent defecation disorder to aid in evacuation. The suppository should be given 30 minutes after breakfast in order to take advantage of the gastrocolic reflex.[45]

Prosecrecretory agents

Several prescription therapies are available for the treatment of both chronic idiopathic constipation and IBS-C. Current prescription and U.S. Food and Drug Administration (FDA)-approved pharmacologic treatments for chronic constipation are listed in Table 55.1. Intestinal secretagogues (prosecretory agents) include lubiprostone, linaclotide, and plecanatide; linaclotide and plecanatide are minimally absorbed peptide agonists of guanylate cyclase-C receptor that exhibit their action through direct action upon intestinal epithelial cells resulting in the generation of cyclic guanosine monophosphate (cGMP). The increase of cGMP within the intestinal cells triggers the secretion of chloride and

TABLE 55.1			
Pharmacotherapy for Constipation			
TREATMENT	**MECHANISM OF ACTION**	**RECOMMENDED DOSE**	**POTENTIAL SIDE EFFECTS**
High-molecular-weight PEG	Osmotic	17 g daily	Nausea, bloating, abdominal cramps, flatulence, diarrhea
Lactulose	Osmotic	20 g daily	Nausea, bloating, cramping, diarrhea, flatulence
Bisacodyl	Stimulant	5–15 mg once daily	Nausea, cramping, diarrhea
Linaclotide	Prosecretory Guanylate cyclase-C receptor agonist	72, 145, or 290 μg daily	Diarrhea, cramping, flatulence, headache
Plecanatide	Prosecretory Guanylate cyclase-C receptor agonist	3 mg daily	Diarrhea
Lubiprostone	Prosecretory Chloride channel activator	8 μg BID (IBS-C—women only) 24 μg BID (CIC)	Nausea, diarrhea, shortness of breath
Prucalopride	Serotonergic Serotonin (5-HT$_4$) receptor agonist	2 mg daily, 1 mg for severe renal disease or ESRD	Diarrhea, headache, <1% suicidal ideation/ exacerbation of depression
Tegaserod	Serotonergic Serotonin (5-HT$_4$) receptor agonist	6 mg BID	Diarrhea, headache, <1% suicidal ideation/ exacerbation of depression
Tepanor	Modulating ion/exchange transporter Inhibitor of Na–hydrogen exchanger 3	50 mg BID (IBS-C only)	Diarrhea, bloating, flatulence

CIC, chronic idiopathic constipation; ESRD, end-stage renal disease; Na, sodium.

Reprinted from Lucak S, Lunsford TN, Harris LA. Evaluation and treatment of constipation in the geriatric population. *Clin Geriatr Med* 2021;37(1):85–102. Copyright © 2021, with permission from Elsevier.

bicarbonate into the intestinal lumen, increasing luminal fluid secretion, and accelerating intestinal transit.[46] Linaclotide works in a pH-independent manner and is active in both the small and large intestines at a broad pH of 5 to 8, whereas plecanatide works in a pH-dependent way at a more acidic pH of 5.5 to 7 and causes fluid secretion mostly in the upper small intestine.[47] Linaclotide is available in three doses, 72, 145, and 290 μg daily, and plecanatide is available in a single dose of 3 mg daily. The main adverse reaction to both linaclotide and plecanatide is diarrhea. Lubiprostone, another intestinal prosecretory agent, approved by the FDA for chronic constipation and opioid-induced constipation at a dose of 24 μg BID and IBS-C 8 μg BID, is a bicyclic fatty acid derivative of prostaglandin E1 which increases fluid secretion into the lumen of the intestine by activating apical chloride channel 2. Secondary to increasing intestinal fluid secretion, transit time in both small and large intestines is accelerated.[48] The main side effect of lubiprostone is nausea, which can be mitigated when the medication is taken with meals.

Serotonergic agonists

In 2018, the FDA-approved prucalopride, a highly selective serotonin 5-hydroxytryptamine 4 (5-HT$_4$) receptor agonist that increases the release of serotonin (5-HT) by the enterochromaffin cells in the intestinal mucosa activating neurons for the treatment of chronic constipation. It acts on neurons along with the enteric nervous system and stimulates intestinal motility directly by releasing acetylcholine. In addition, it secretes fluid into the intestines, which has an additional prokinetic effect. Prucalopride at a dose of 1 and 4 mg once daily was found to be superior to placebo in 4- and 12-week trials. In the United States, the recommended dose in adults is 2 mg once daily, with a lower dose (1 mg daily) recommended for patients with kidney disease. Adverse events include abdominal pain, nausea, diarrhea, abdominal bloating, flatulence, headache, dizziness, and fatigue. Uncommon but potentially serious adverse events include exacerbation of depression and suicidality warranting extreme caution in at-risk patients.[49] Prucalopride has not been associated with any cardiovascular adverse events to date.

Two 5-HT$_4$ receptor agonists were approved for the treatment of chronic constipation in the past (cisapride 1993, tegaserod 2002), but both were subsequently withdrawn from general use because of serious cardiovascular events, including cardiac ischemia, strokes, cardiac arrhythmias, and prolongation of the QTc interval. Tegaserod became available again in 2019 but is only recommended for those between the age of 18 and 65 years.[50] Like prucalopride, tegaserod also carries a warning about potential neuropsychiatric events (suicide, suicidality, depression) in at-risk patients.

Modulating ion exchangers/transporters

Tenapanor, a first-in-its-class agent also approved to treat hyperphosphatemia in patients with chronic kidney disease, is a first in class agent, a selective sodium–hydrogen exchanger 3 inhibitor that was improved in 2019 for the treatment of IBS-C. The mechanism of action is decreasing the absorption of sodium from the intestines, resulting in water secretion in the lumen, which subsequently causes softer stool attributed to increased intestinal transit. In phase III, double-blind placebo-controlled trials, tenapanor 50 mg twice daily met the combined primary end point of ≥30% reduction in abdominal pain and an increase in ≥1 completed spontaneous bowel movements in the same week for ≥6 of 12 treatment weeks. Chief side effects were diarrhea and abdominal distension.[51]

Novel therapies: bile acid modulators

Based on the natural side effect of diarrhea with use attributed to the enhancement of colonic secretion and motility and identification of a subgroup of patients with IBS-C with a deficiency of bile acids in the colon, bile acid modulators are being investigated for their possible use in the treatment of IBS-C and chronic constipation.[52] These modulators would be attractive for use given the lack of systemic absorption but may be limited by side effects such as diarrhea.[53]

Surgical intervention for slow transit constipation is rarely indicated; however, laparoscopic colectomy felt to be due to delayed transit of the colon and in the absence of defecatory dysfunction may benefit from laparoscopic total colectomy with ileorectal anastomosis by an experienced colorectal surgeon at a center of excellence. Patients with a more diffuse clinical picture and upper GI symptoms have poorer outcomes than those with isolated slow transit constipation.[54]

References

1. Suares NC, Ford AC. Prevalence of, and risk factors for, chronic idiopathic constipation in the community: Systematic review and meta-analysis. *Am J Gastroenterol* 2011;106(9):1582–1591.

2. Rao SSC, Patcharatrakul T. Diagnosis and treatment of dyssynergic defecation. *J Neurogastroenterol Motil* 2016;22(3):423–435.

3. Mearin F, Lacy BE, Chang L, et al. Bowel disorders. *Gastroenterology* 2016;150(6):1393–1407.E5.

4. Camilleri M, Ford AC, Mawe GM, et al. Chronic constipation. *Nat Rev Dis Primers* 2017;14(3):17095.

5. Lacy BE, Levenick JM, Crowell MD. Chronic constipation: New diagnostic and treatment approaches. *Therap Adv Gastroenterol* 2012;5(4):233–247.

6. Lewis SJ, Heaton KW. Stool form scale as a useful guide to intestinal transit time. *Scand J Gastroenterol* 1997;32(9):920–924.

7. Rao SSC. Rectal exam: Yes, it can and should be done in a busy practice! *Am J Gastroenterol* 2018;113(5):635–638.

8. Rao SSC, Bharucha AE, Chiarioni G, et al. Functional anorectal disorders. *Gastroenterology* 2016;150(6):1430–1442.

9. Tantiphlachiva K, Rao P, Attaluri A, et al. Digital rectal examination is a useful tool for identifying patients with dyssynergia. *Clin Gastroenterol Hepatol* 2010;8(11):955–960.

10. Neshatian L. The assessment and management of defecatory dysfunction: A critical appraisal. *Curr Opin Gastroenterol* 2018;34(1):31–37.

11. Caetano AC, Costa D, Gonçalves R, et al. Does sequential balloon expulsion test improve the screening of defecation disorders? *BMC Gastroenterol* 2020;20(1):338.

12. Shah ED, Farida JD, Menees S, et al. Examining balloon expulsion testing as an office-based, screening test for dyssynergic defecation: A systematic review and meta-analysis. *Am J Gastroenterol* 2018;113(11):1613–1620.

13. Minguez M, Herreros B, Sanchiz V, et al. Predictive value of the balloon expulsion test for excluding the diagnosis of pelvic floor dyssynergia in constipation. *Gastroenterology* 2004;126(1):57–62.

14. Chiarioni G, Kim SM, Vantini I, et al. Validation of the balloon evacuation test: Reproducibility and agreement with findings from anorectal manometry and electromyography. *Clin Gastroenterol Hepatol* 2014;12(12):2049–2054.

15. Kang HR, Lee JE, Lee JS, et al. Comparison of high-resolution anorectal manometry with water-perfused anorectal manometry. *J Neurogastroenterol Motil* 2015;21(1):126–132.

16. Seo M, Joo S, Jung KW, et al. New metrics in high-resolution and high-definition anorectal manometry. *Curr Gastroenterol Rep* 2018;20(12):57.

17. Bharucha AE, Rao SSC. An update on anorectal disorders for gastroenterologists. *Gastroenterology* 2014;146(1):37–45.e2.

18. Grossi U, Carrington EV, Bharucha AE, et al. Diagnostic accuracy study of anorectal manometry for diagnosis of dyssynergic defecation. *Gut* 2016;65(3):447–455.

19. Patcharatrakul T, Rao SSC. Update on the pathophysiology and management of anorectal disorders. *Gut Liver* 2018;12(4):375–384.

20. Enck P, Van der Voort IR, Klosterhalfen S. Biofeedback therapy in fecal incontinence and constipation. *Neurogastroenterol Motil* 2009;21(11):1133–1141.

21. Rao SSC. Dyssynergic defecation and biofeedback therapy. *Gastroenterol Clin North Am* 2008;37(3):569–586.

22. Skardoon GR, Khera AJ, Emmanuel AV, et al. Review article: Dyssynergic defaecation and biofeedback therapy in the pathophysiology and management of functional constipation. *Aliment Pharmacol Ther* 2017;46(4):410–423.

23. Aziz I, Whitehead WE, Palsson OS, et al. An approach to the diagnosis and management of Rome IV functional disorders of chronic constipation. *Expert Rev Gastroenterol Hepatol* 2020;14(1):39–46.

24. Lucak S, Lunsford TN, Harris LA. Evaluation and treatment of constipation in the geriatric population. *Clin Geriatr Med* 2021;37(1):85–102.

25. Foti PV, Farina R, Riva G, et al. Pelvic floor imaging: Comparison between magnetic resonance imaging and conventional defecography in studying outlet obstruction syndrome. *Radiol Med* 2013;118(1):23–39.

26. Chaichanavichkij P, Vollebregt PF, Scott SM, et al. Botulinum toxin type A for the treatment of dyssynergic defaecation

in adults: A systematic review. *Colorectal Dis* 2020;22(12): 1832–1841.

27. Faried M, El Nakeeb A, Youssef M, et al. Comparative study between surgical and non-surgical treatment of anismus in patients with symptoms of obstructed defecation: A prospective randomized study. *J Gastrointest Surg* 2010;14(8):1235–1243.

28. Rogalski MJ, Kellogg-Spadt S, Hoffmann AR, et al. Retrospective chart review of vaginal diazepam suppository use in high-tone pelvic floor dysfunction. *Int Urogynecol J* 2010;21(7): 895–899.

29. Rao SSC, Camilleri M, Hasler WL, et al. Evaluation of gastrointestinal transit in clinical practice: Position paper of the American and European Neurogastroenterology and Motility Societies. *Neurogastroenterol Motil* 2011;23(1):8–23.

30. Kuo B, Maneerattanaporn M, Lee AA, et al. Generalized transit delay on wireless motility capsule testing in patients with clinical suspicion of gastroparesis, small intestinal dysmotility, or slow transit constipation. *Dig Dis Sci* 2011;56(10):2928–2938.

31. Parkman HP. Scintigraphy for evaluation of patients for GI motility disorders—The referring physician's perspective. *Semin Nucl Med* 2012;42(2):76–78.

32. Storey M, Anderson P. Intake and race/ethnicity influence dietary fiber intake and vegetable consumption. *Nutr Res* 2014;34(10):844–850.

33. U.S. Department of Health and Human Services, U.S. Department of Agriculture. *2015–2020 dietary guidelines for Americans*, 8th ed. Washington: U.S. Department of Health and Human Services, U.S. Department of Agriculture, 2015.

34. Bijkerk CJ, Muris JW, Knottnerus JA, et al. Systematic review: The role of different types of fibre in the treatment of irritable bowel syndrome. *Aliment Pharmacol Ther* 2004;19(3): 245–251.

35. American College of Gastroenterology Chronic Constipation Task Force. An evidence-based approach to the management of chronic constipation in North America. *Am J Gastroenterol* 2005;100(Suppl 1):S1–S4.

36. Ramkumar D, Rao SSC. Efficacy and safety of traditional medical therapies for chronic constipation: Systematic review. *Am J Gastroenterol* 2005;100(4):936–971.

37. Müller-Lissner SA, Kamm MA, Scarpignato C, et al. Myths and misconceptions about chronic constipation. *Am J Gastroenterol* 2005;100(1):232–242.

38. Johannesson E, Jakobsson Ung E, Sadik R, et al. Experiences of the effects of physical activity in persons with irritable bowel syndrome (IBS): A qualitative content analysis. *Scand J Gastroenterol* 2018;53(10–11):1194–1200.

39. Bellini M, Tonarelli S, Mumolo MG, et al. Low fermentable oligo- di- and mono-saccharides and polyols (FODMAPs) or gluten free diet: What is best for irritable bowel syndrome? *Nutrients* 2020;12(11):3368.

40. Katelaris P, Naganathan V, Liu K, et al. Comparison of the effectiveness of polyethylene glycol with and without electrolytes in constipation: A systematic review and network meta-analysis. *BMC Gastroenterol* 2016;16:42.

41. Ford AC, Moayyedi P, Lacy BE, et al; for the Task Force on the Management of Functional Bowel Disorders. American College of Gastroenterology monograph on the management of irritable bowel syndrome and chronic idiopathic constipation. *Am J Gastroenterol* 2014;109(Suppl 1):S2–S26.

42. Dupont C, Campagne A, Constant F. Efficacy and safety of a magnesium sulfate-rich natural mineral water for patients with functional constipation. *Clin Gastroenterol Hepatol* 2014;12(8):1280–1287.

43. Bokhari SR, Siriki R, Teran FJ, et al. Fatal hypermagnesemia due to laxative use. *Am J Med Sci* 2018;355(4):390–395.

44. Noergaard M, Traerup Andersen J, Jimenez-Solem E, et al. Long term treatment with stimulant laxatives—Clinical evidence for effectiveness and safety? *Scand J Gastroenterol* 2019;54(1):27–34.

45. Bharucha AE, Wald A. Chronic constipation. *Mayo Clin Proc* 2019;94(11):2340–2357.

46. Bassotti G, Usai-Satta P, Bellini M. Linaclotide for the treatment of chronic constipation. *Expert Opin Pharmacother* 2018;19(11):1261–1266.

47. Sharma A, Herekar AA, Bhagatwala J, et al. Profile of plecanatide in the treatment of chronic idiopathic constipation: Design, development, and place in therapy. *Clin Exp Gastroenterol* 2019;12:31–36.

48. Li F, Fu T, Tong WD, et al. Lubiprostone is effective in the treatment of chronic idiopathic constipation and irritable bowel syndrome: A systematic review and meta-analysis of randomized controlled trials. *Mayo Clin Proc* 2016;91(4):456–468.

49. Omer A, Quigley EMM. An update on prucalopride in the treatment of chronic constipation. *Therap Adv Gastroenterol* 2017;10(11):877–887.

50. Madia VN, Messore A, Saccoliti F, et al. Tegaserod for the treatment of irritable bowel syndrome. *Antiinflamm Antiallergy Agents Med Chem* 2020;19(4):342–369.

51. Chey WD, Lembo AJ, Rosenbaum DP. Efficacy of tenapanor in treating patients with irritable bowel syndrome with constipation: A 12-week, placebo-controlled phase 3 trial (T3MPO-1). *Am J Gastroenterol* 2020;115(2):281–293.

52. Vijayvargiya P, Busciglio I, Burton D, et al. Bile acid deficiency in a subgroup of patients with irritable bowel syndrome with constipation based on biomarkers in serum and fecal samples. *Clin Gastroenterol Hepatol* 2018;16(4):522–527.

53. Camilleri M. What's in the pipeline for lower functional gastrointestinal disorders in the next 5 years? *Am J Physiol Gastrointest Liver Physiol* 2019;317(5):G640–G650.

54. Bharucha AE, Pemberton JH, Locke GR III. American Gastroenterological Association technical review on constipation. *Gastroenterology* 2013;144(1):218–238.

CHAPTER 56

ANAL INCONTINENCE

Frida Carswell • James Oliver Keck • Peter L. Dwyer

Introduction

Anal incontinence (AI) is defined as involuntary loss of flatus and/or feces.[1] Although it may affect men, it is generally more common and more severe in women. It is often underdiagnosed and may result in depression, anxiety, and impaired sexual function and has significant impact on women's quality of life. The most common cause of AI in women is obstetric trauma, including obstetric anal sphincter injury (OASI). The sphincter injury may not be symptomatic or recognized at birth termed occult OASI. Investigation and management of AI should be targeted at finding and treating reversible causes. Many women can be managed conservatively, but a proportion of women will require surgical management. Primary anal sphincter repair following delivery with OASI may fail in up to 30% of cases, and some women will require a second repair.

EPIDEMIOLOGY AND ETIOLOGY

AI has been estimated to occur in 15% of women,[2] but the true incidence may be more as only a third of women with incontinence ever mention this to their physician.[3] AI may be caused by a complex interplay of numerous pathophysiologic factors including aberrant anorectal sensation or innervation, colorectal motility, consistency and volume of stool, as well as structural changes or damage to the pelvic floor and sphincter complex. Indeed, women who sustain obstetric trauma often do not present with symptoms of AI until many years postpartum with the added atrophy of aging and denervation of the smooth and striated musculature of the anal sphincters and pelvic floor.[4]

Anatomy and Physiology of Defecation

The internal anal sphincter (IAS) and the external anal sphincter (EAS) encircle the anal canal and maintain continence together with the puborectalis muscle.

The IAS is a continuation of the circular rectal smooth muscle layer and generates most of the anal resting pressure and helps prevent AI at rest.[5] The IAS is under reflex control. The EAS muscle is composed

of striated muscle cells, is continuous with the levator ani and pelvic floor, and is partially under voluntary control. The EAS contributes to the anal resting pressure, but its main function is to generate anal squeeze pressure (Fig. 56.1).

The puborectalis muscle forms a sling around the upper part of the anal canal. The tone of the puborectalis muscle creates the anorectal angle, which prevents movement of feces from the rectum to the anal canal between defecations (Fig. 56.2).[3,4] The puborectalis is a 0.5- to 1.0-cm thick u-shaped muscle that forms a flap-like valve that creates a forward pull and reinforces the anorectal angle (Fig. 56.3). Recent work using transperineal ultrasound has shown that all three muscles contribute to a mechanical barrier to flatus and stool.[6]

Etiology

A common cause of AI in women is anal sphincter dysfunction from obstetric injury to the pudendal nerve, anal sphincter muscle, or both. Another common cause of fecal incontinence is remnant feces in the rectum from obstructed defecation, for example, due to rectocele or simple constipation. Stool left in the rectum may trigger the rectal-anal inhibitory reflex (RAIR) causing the sphincter to relax. If the sphincter is relaxed, soiling and incontinence can occur. Soiling can also result from incomplete closure of the sphincter due to a full-thickness rectal prolapse, rectal mucosal prolapse, or hemorrhoids. Large anal tags may interfere with cleaning (Table 56.1).

Anal sphincter dysfunction

Disruption of the anal sphincter caused by obstetric injury, as well as by anorectal surgery or less commonly external trauma, is the most common cause of AI.[7] OASI is a major risk factor for AI. Sultan and Thakar recently reviewed the literature and found 35 studies reporting outcomes of primary sphincter repair after delivery and found a prevalence of AI of 39% (range, 15% to 61%) over the long term.[8] The severity of incontinence was related to the degree of the injury with women who had a minor (grade 3a/3b) tear having a

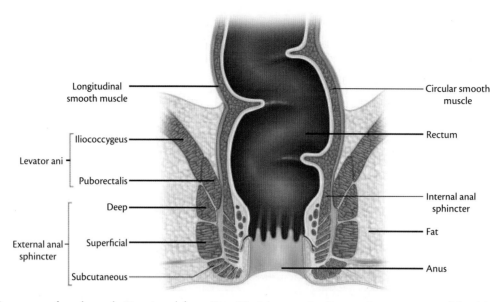

FIGURE 56.1 Anatomy of anal canal. (Reprinted from Rao SS. Advances in diagnostic assessment of fecal incontinence and dyssynergic defecation. *Clin Gastroenterol Hepatol* 2010;8[11]:910–919. Copyright © 2010, with permission from Elsevier.)

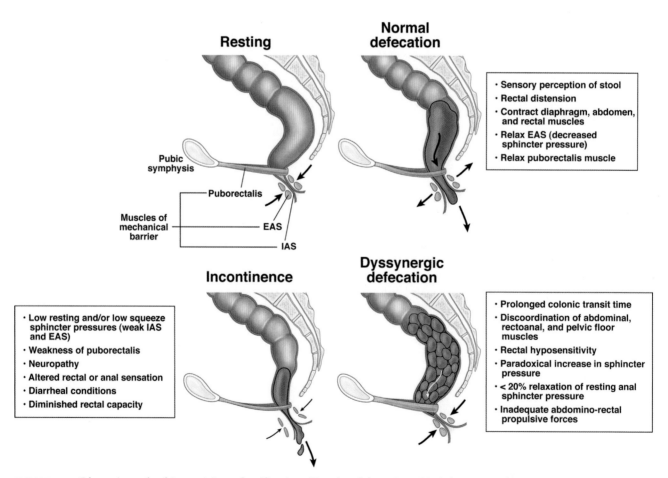

FIGURE 56.2 Obstetric anal sphincter injury classification. (Reprinted from Rao SS. Advances in diagnostic assessment of fecal incontinence and dyssynergic defecation. *Clin Gastroenterol Hepatol* 2010;8[11]:910–919. Copyright © 2010, with permission from Elsevier.)

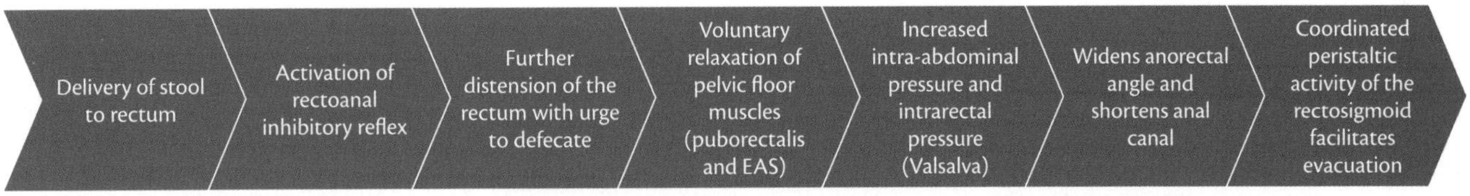

| Delivery of stool to rectum | Activation of rectoanal inhibitory reflex | Further distension of the rectum with urge to defecate | Voluntary relaxation of pelvic floor muscles (puborectalis and EAS) | Increased intra-abdominal pressure and intrarectal pressure (Valsalva) | Widens anorectal angle and shortens anal canal | Coordinated peristaltic activity of the rectosigmoid facilitates evacuation |

FIGURE 56.3 Obstetric anal sphincter injury bundle at time of delivery.

better outcome than those with a major (grade 3c/4) tear ($P < .05$) in terms of defecatory symptoms, associated quality of life, and anal manometry.[8]

The OASI classification described by Sultan and Thakar[8] has been adopted by the International Consultation on Incontinence and the Royal College of Obstetricians and Gynaecologists (Table 56.2).

Third-degree tears occur in around 6% (1.8% in 2000 to 5.9% in 2011) of vaginal deliveries with the incidence increasing. This may be due to improved reporting as well as an increase in maternal and fetal birth weight.[9] Occult sphincter injury has been reported in one-third of deliveries and may be significant cause of AI in later life.[10,11] Another contributing factor to AI is levator ani avulsion and pudendal nerve denervation, which occurs more frequently during prolonged vaginal deliveries or when forceps are used.[11]

The most common finding is a defect in the anterior EAS, which manifests clinically as urgency of defecation and urge AI. Associated disruption of the internal sphincter may cause additional symptoms of passive or stress fecal incontinence.[12]

However, even after fourth-degree tears, women with complete disruption of the anal sphincter complex fecal control may have reasonable fecal control, emphasizing the importance of the puborectalis and levator muscles in AI (Fig. 56.4).

TABLE 56.1

Causes of Anal Incontinence

Anal sphincter dysfunction (congenital malformation, radiation, OASI, anal surgery, perianal fistulas, sexual abuse)

Rectal disorders (IBS, radiation, rectocele, rectal intussusception, rectal prolapse, fecal impaction)

Neurologic disorders (spinal cord, stroke, MS, spina bifida, diabetic neuropathy, obstetric nerve damage)

Myopathy (systemic scleroderma)

Fast colorectal transit time (chronic diarrhea, IBS)

Psychological (encopresis, dementia)

MS, multiple sclerosis.
From Sultan AH, Monga A, Lee J, et al. An International Urogynecological Association (IUGA)/International Continence Society (ICS) joint report on the terminology for female anorectal dysfunction. *Neurourol Urodyn* 2017;36(1):10–34.

Anorectal disease

Anorectal disease as well as anorectal surgery is a significant risk factor for AI. Surgery for anal fistula may involve injury to the internal sphincter, external sphincter, or both. Lateral sphincterotomy for anal fissure is done rarely in modern colorectal practice but involves deliberate partial division of the internal sphincter. Perianal Crohn disease results in fistulas, ulcers, tags, and anal stenosis, which may all cause anal leakage or soiling. Prolapsing hemorrhoids as well as full-thickness and mucosal rectal prolapse may affect closure of the anal canal and cause stretching of the internal sphincter leading to incontinence. Scleroderma is a systemic disease which often involves IAS dysfunction, minor degrees of mucosal prolapse, and fecal leakage.

Fast colorectal transit time

Women with intact continence mechanisms will sometimes leak if bowel movements are loose. Common causes of loose stools include dietary intolerances, celiac disease, irritable bowel syndrome (IBS), inflammatory bowel disease (IBD—such as Crohn and ulcerative colitis), and small intestinal bacterial overgrowth SIBO.

The majority of patients with IBS experience worsening of symptoms related to carbohydrate malabsorption and ingestion of foods high in dietary *FODMAPs* (fermentable oligo-, di-, and monosaccharides and polyols).[13] FODMAPs are naturally occurring sugars such as lactose, fructose, sorbitol, mannitol, and sucrose found in milk and dairy products, fruits and vegetables,

TABLE 56.2

Obstetric Anal Sphincter Injury Classification

First-degree tear	Injury to perineal skin and/or vaginal mucosa
Second-degree tear	Injury to perineum involving perineal muscles but not involving the anal sphincter
Third-degree tear	Injury to perineum involving the anal sphincter complex: grade 3a tear: less than 50% of EAS thickness torn; grade 3b tear: more than 50% of EAS thickness torn; grade 3c tear: both EAS and IAS torn
Fourth-degree tear	Injury to perineum involving the anal sphincter complex (EAS and IAS) and anorectal mucosa

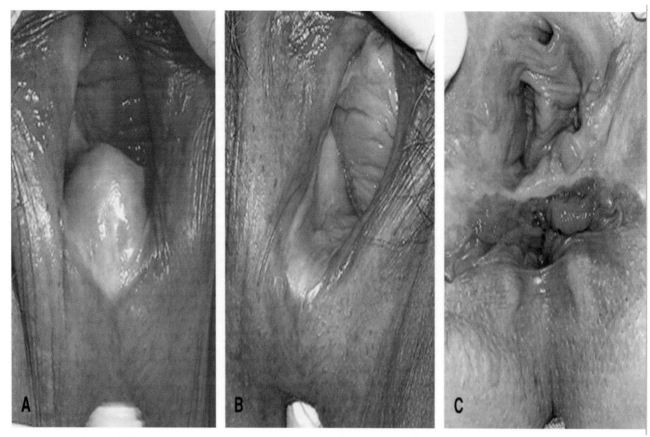

FIGURE 56.4 Sphincter defect on per rectum (PR) (**A** and **B**). Sphincter defect on visual inspection (**C**).

cereals, and processed foods. These dietary sugars are poorly absorbed in the gut, and fermentation of the sugar by colonic flora results in an osmotic effect and gas production. In IBS sufferers, this causes functional gut symptoms such as bloating, pain, and diarrhea. Restricted intake of FODMAPs has been shown in randomized controlled trials (RCTs) to relieve symptoms of IBS in up to 75% of patients.[14]

Small intestinal bacterial overgrowth in certain individuals causes symptoms almost identical to IBS. Patients with SIBO may also have unexplained weight loss and less frequently, nutritional deficiencies (such as vitamin B$_{12}$ and vitamin D deficiency). This condition can be treated with prolonged courses of antibiotics.[13,14]

Neurologic disorders

A wide variety of neurologic diseases of the central and peripheral nervous system can affect colonic and anorectal function and are associated with AI including cerbrovascular accident, multiple sclerosis, spina bifida, and diabetic neuropathy.

PREVENTION

Obstetric trauma resulting in OASI is one of the most important etiologic factors in the pathogenesis of AI.

Improved Detection of Occult Obstetric Anal Sphincter Injury

A prospective cohort study by Andrews et al.[15] of 254 primiparous women showed that the prevalence of OASI increased significantly from 11% to 24.5% when women were more carefully examined. In this study, 98.8% of the missed OASI were subsequently detected on clinical examination by a trained research fellow prior to endoanal ultrasound.[15] A Cochrane review from 2015 included a large RCT from a single center that showed a reduction of severe AI postpartum with the use of endoanal ultrasound of all second-degree tears.[16] There has been reported a reduction in the rate of third- and fourth-degree tears with a care bundle involving perineal support, perineal massage, warm compresses, and medical and midwife education in in the detection and suturing of OASI[17] (Table 56.3).

Forceps versus Vacuum Delivery

Forceps is an established risk factor for both anal sphincter and levator trauma. Although such trauma also occurs after normal vaginal delivery and vacuum extraction, it is much more likely after forceps.[18]

Forceps have shown to almost double the risk of fecal incontinence compared to vaginal birth and

TABLE 56.3

Obstetric Anal Sphincter Injury Bundle at Time of Delivery

Left hand slowing down the delivery of the head
Right hand protecting the perineum
Mother NOT pushing when head is crowning (communicate)
Think about episiotomy (risk groups and correct angle)

cesarean section (Table 56.4).[19] This may also be related to obstetrics factors that often lead to use of forceps such as macrosomia and OP position with prolonged labor rather than the forceps per se.

Cesarean Section versus Vaginal Birth

A Cochrane review in 2010 concluded that cesarean section was not protective for AI, although one trial showed a possible benefit in the long term.[20] In another meta-analysis in 2008 at 1 year postpartum in 12,237 women, cesarean was protective over vaginal birth with an odds ratio of 1.47.[21]

Women at high risk for pelvic floor dysfunction postpartum can be identified using the UR-CHOICE calculator developed by Drs. Bob Freeman and Don Wilson.[22] The calculator is based on three large pelvic floor epidemiologic studies (SWEdish Pregnancy, Obesity, and Pelvic floor [SWEPOP] and PROlapse and incontinence LONG-term research [PROLONG] Cleveland Clinic) and gives women an individual score of their risk of urinary incontinence, prolapse, and AI for each particular pregnancy.

Subsequent Delivery following Overt or Occult Obstetric Anal Sphincter Injury

Women who have already sustained a third-degree tear have a 17% risk of developing worsening symptoms after subsequent vaginal delivery.[23]

There are no systematic reviews or RCTs to suggest the best method of delivery following OASI. Scheer et al. performed a prospective study of pregnant women with a history of OASI. Women who had a sonographic defect of the external sphincter of more than 30° and with a squeeze pressure of less than 20 mm Hg were offered a cesarean section. All other women were advised to have a vaginal delivery. Short-term follow-up of this cohort of 73 women showed that the women who underwent vaginal delivery suffered no significant deterioration in anal sphincter function or quality of life.[24]

Women with OASI at high risk for AI should ideally be followed up in a dedicated perineal clinic with the availability of endoanal ultrasound and manometry and be managed by a multidisciplinary team with colorectal surgeons, physiotherapists, and urogynecologists.

CLINICAL EVALUATION

Symptoms

AI can be classified as either active or passive. Active incontinence involves severe urgency, often brought on by exercise including walking. Active incontinence is usually due to injury or dysfunction of the EAS. It is worse with loose or liquid stool but may also occur with formed or solid stool. Passive incontinence is loss of small amounts of solid or liquid stool or mucus which is often insensible. It is usually due to injury or

TABLE 56.4

Logistic Regression Subsidiary Models of More Severe Urinary Incontinence and More Severe Fecal Incontinence and Delivery Mode History

VARIABLE	TOTAL	MORE SEVERE UI SYMPTOMS n (%)	OR (95% CI)	MORE SEVERE FI SYMPTOMS n (%)	OR (95% CI)
DELIVERY MODE					
Only SVD	1852	439 (23.7)	Reference	43 (2.3)	Reference
Only CS	403	78 (19.4)	0.64 (0.48–0.84)	9 (2.2)	1.07 (0.51–2.27)
SVD + CS	293	87 (29.7)	1.24 (0.94–1.65)	8 (2.7)	1.02 (0.47–2.21)
Any forceps	956	219 (22.9)	0.87 (0.72–1.06)	40 (4.2)	1.79 (1.14–2.79)
Any vacuum, no forceps	248	66 (26.6)	1.11 (0.82–1.51)	6 (2.4)	1.14 (0.48–2.74)

Age at first birth, number of births, and body mass index not shown.

UI, urinary incontinence; OR, odds ratio; FI, fecal incontinence; SVD, spontaneous delivery; CS, cesarean section.

Reprinted from MacArthur C, Glazener C, Lancashire R, et al; for ProLong Study Group. Exclusive caesarean section delivery and subsequent urinary and faecal incontinence: A 12-year longitudinal study. *BJOG* 2011;118(8):1001–1007.

TABLE 56.5

Symptoms of Bowel Dysfunction as per International Continence Society (2017)

ANORECTAL INCONTINENCE SYMPTOMS

AI	Involuntary loss of flatus, liquid, or solid stool that is a social or hygienic problem
Fecal incontinence	Involuntary loss of liquid or solid stool that is a social or hygienic problem
Passive fecal leakage	Involuntary soiling of liquid or solid stool without sensation or warning or difficulty wiping clean
Postdefecatory soiling	Soiling occurring after defecation

ANORECTAL STORAGE SYMPTOMS

Increased daytime defecation	Complaint that defecation occurs more frequently during waking hours than previously deemed normal by the woman
Nocturnal defecation	Complaint of interruption of sleep one or more times because of the need to defecate
Tenesmus	A desire to evacuate the bowel, often accompanied by pain, cramping, and straining, in the absence of feces in the rectum
Fecal (rectal) urgency	Complaint of a sudden compelling desire to defecate that is difficult to defer
Fecal (flatal) urgency incontinence	Complaint of involuntary loss of gas or feces associated with fecal urgency

DEFECATORY AND POSTDEFECATORY SYMPTOMS

Constipation	Complaint that bowel movements are infrequent and/or incomplete and/or there is a need for frequent straining or manual assistance to defecate
Slow transit	Infrequent bowel motions due to delay in transit of bowel contents to reach rectum
Obstructed defecation	Complaint of difficulty in evacuation
Incomplete bowel evacuation	Complaint that the rectum does not feel empty after defecation and may be accompanied by a desire to defecate again
Straining to defecate	Complaint of the need to make an intensive effort (by abdominal straining or Valsalva) to either initiate, maintain, or improve defecation
Digitation	Use of fingers in rectum or vagina to manually assist in evacuation of stool contents. (1) *Rectal digitation*: use of fingers in rectum to physically extract stool contents to assist in evacuation. (2) *Vaginal digitation*: use of thumb or finger in vagina to assist in evacuation

OTHER

Rectal bleeding/mucus	Complaint of the loss of blood/mucus per rectum
Anorectal prolapse	Complaint of a "bulge" or "something coming down" toward or through the anus/rectum. The woman may state she can either feel the bulge by direct palpation or see it aided with a mirror.
Pain during straining/defecation	Complaint of pain during defecation or straining to defecate

From Sultan AH, Monga A, Lee J, et al. An International Urogynecological Association (IUGA)/International Continence Society (ICS) joint report on the terminology for female anorectal dysfunction. *Neurourol Urodyn* 2017;36(1):10–34.

dysfunction of the internal sphincter. Patients may present with mainly active or mainly passive incontinence depending on the cause of their incontinence, although a proportion will have both. Postdefecatory fecal soiling is a form of incontinence that can occur when there is incomplete closure of the anal sphincter or incomplete emptying of the rectum during defecation. This can be due to space occupying lesions such as hemorrhoids or

in functional conditions such as obstructed defecation (Table 56.5).

Questionnaires

A wide range of questionnaires and scoring systems have been developed to evaluate bowel function. The most commonly used questionnaires in clinical and research

TABLE 56.6

Patient-Reported Outcome Questionnaires for Female Anorectal Dysfunction

NAME OF SCORE	EXPLANATION OF SCORE	GRADING OF SCORE
Cleveland Clinic/Wexner score	The most widely used questionnaire. Grades the severity of AI from 0 to 20. ICI committee has not recommended a higher grade of recommendation due to the lack of more stringent validation.	Grade C
St. Mark score	Similar to Wexner + urgency use of antidiarrheals and pad use. Mark rescore showed only moderate correlation regardless of the severity of the incontinence.	Grade C
FI QoL	Quality of life only (lifestyle coping/behavior, depression, and embarrassment)	Grade B
ICIQ-B	Bowel pattern, bowel control, and quality of life	Grade B
Birmingham Bowel and Urinary Symptoms Questionnaire	Evaluates both bowel and urinary dysfunction in women (constipation, evacuatory function, AI, and urinary symptoms)	Grade B
EQ-5D	Recommended by the NICE particularly for the use of health economic analysis in calculations of quality-adjusted life-years (QALYs)	Grade B

Grading as per International Consultation on Incontinence (ICI) grading system: A = highly recommended; B = recommended; C = with potential. Other questionnaires include Fecal Incontinence Severity Index (grade B), Manchester Health Questionnaire Data (grade B), Pescatori Incontinence Score (grade C), Mayo Fecal Incontinence Survey (grade C), Elderly Bowel Symptoms Questionnaire (grade C), and the Fecal Incontinence and Constipation Assessment (grade C).
Fi QoL, Fecal Incontinence Quality of Life Scale; EQ-5D, EuroQol 5 Dimensional Questionnaire; NICE, National Institute for Health and Clinical Excellence.

practice are the "Wexner" incontinence score and the generic SF-36 quality of life questionnaire. The Cleveland Clinic, or the Wexner score, was the first attempt to have a score based on both the frequency and consistency of fecal incontinence and effect on lifestyle. Very few of the questionnaires have been validated despite their widespread use. The St. Mark score was an adaptation of the original Wexner score, adding scores for urgency and use of antidiarrheal medication. This has been found to correlate well with patients' global assessment of their bowel function.

The International Consultation on Incontinence Questionnaire (ICIQ) modular questionnaire may become the gold standard with a recent study showing promising result.[25]

A Bristol stool chart gives information on bowel consistency which should be evaluated in all patients with AI (Table 56.6).

Bowel diary

Bowel diaries are daily records of bowel consistency and frequency and have been widely used in diagnostic and intervention studies. Patient recall is less accurate than a diary and may underestimate symptom frequency by as much as 50%.[26]

Examination

Examination should aid in diagnosis of the underlying pathophysiology and identify treatable contributing factors and evaluate the strength, integrity, and function of the pelvic floor, anal sphincters, and their nerve supply (Table 56.7).

Investigations

Anorectal physiology studies are useful to complete and augment clinical evaluation. They have an important role in decision-making regarding the safety of subsequent vaginal delivery after OASI. They may a have medicolegal role confirming or excluding injury after vaginal delivery, anal surgery, or external trauma including sexual abuse. They are useful in patients who undergo surgery, particularly anal sphincter repair. The combination of both internal and external sphincter injury is likely to have a poorer outcome than injury to the external sphincter alone. Abnormal rectal compliance and pudendal nerve latency may also be poor prognostic indicators. Anorectal physiology studies are widely used in research.

Endoanal ultrasound

The structural anatomy of both the IAS and EAS can be accurately demonstrated with endoanal ultrasonography. Ultrasound has a high degree of sensitivity and specificity regarding injury to the sphincters and correlates well with manometric findings (Fig. 56.5).[27]

Anal ultrasound may be superior to clinical exam, anal manometry, and electromyography in diagnosing sphincter defects for AI.[28]

Anal physiology

Anal manometry measures the anal resting pressure and anal squeeze pressure. It can either be done with water-perfused or solid-state catheters.

TABLE 56.7

Clinical Examination in Fecal Incontinence

Abdominal exam	To be performed to rule out any masses. A neurologic exam should include extremity reflexes and sensory and muscle strength.
Inspection of vulva	Look for dermatosis (lichen sclerosis, contact dermatitis, lichen simplex chronicus) and atrophy.
Inspection of anus	Scarring from anovaginal fistula/Crohn anal tags, external hemorrhoids, fissures, rectal prolapse. A patulous anus is an indication of sphincter deficiency. Ask the patient to strain to look for rectal or uterovaginal prolapse. Also ask the patient to contract the sphincter muscles to look for symmetrical contraction and anal retraction.
POP-Q with Valsalva	To assess the extent of any uterovaginal prolapse
Speculum/bimanual	To assess the rectovaginal septum for scarring and thickness; vaginal masses
Vaginal palpation	Pelvic floor strength (Oxford), pelvic floor tenderness, levator avulsions; thickness of perineal body
PR	A digital rectal exam is performed to evaluate the anal sphincter resting tone and squeeze pressure. Proximal posterior palpation of the top of the anal sphincter complex during voluntary squeeze will assess puborectalis function. Defects of the anal sphincter may be palpated as ridges in the region of perianal scars. Rectal masses or impacted stool may be identified as well as the presence of a rectocele.
Reflexes/sensory	Pudendal nerve sensory assessment. The anal wink reflex—the presence of the anocutaneous reflex—suggests an intact sacral reflex arc and pudendal nerve innervation of the EAS.

POP-Q, Pelvic Organ Prolapse Quantification system; PR, per rectum.

Rectal capacity and compliance can be tested with a rectal balloon gradually filled with either air or water. Rectal sensibility is also assessed during balloon filling as the patient reports "first detectable sensation," "sensation of urge to defecate," and "maximum tolerable rectal volume."

Rectal capacity and rectal compliance are reduced in conditions associated with rectal fibrosis or inflammation, including scleroderma, radiation proctitis, and IBD. They are also reduced following low anterior resection. Sensory threshold and compliance values are important and may help determine whether biofeedback training can improve AI.

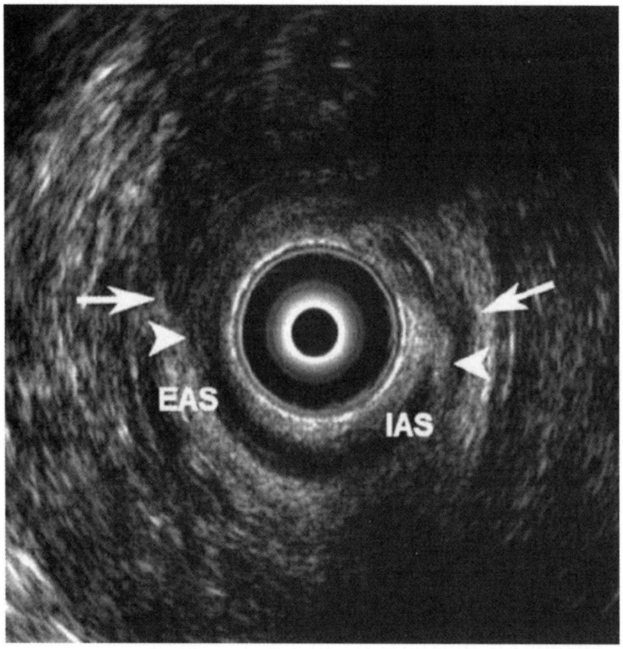

The RAIR is the relaxation of the proximal IAS in response to rectal distention. It is measured by inflating a balloon within the rectal lumen and observing a decrease in the resting anal pressure. A drop of at least 50% of the resting pressure after distention in at least one channel is considered a positive reflex. The RAIR is typically absent in patients with Hirschsprung disease and may be abnormal in patients with rectal prolapse, scleroderma, dermatomyositis, and other connective tissue disorders.

Pudendal nerve latency

This technique measures nerve conduction time in the terminal branches of the pudendal nerve just above the sphincter complex. It is thus a de facto measure of pelvic neuropathy. The clinical value of pudendal nerve latency testing is controversial. Some studies suggest that a prolonged latency is associated with poorer outcomes following anal sphincter repair.[29]

Anorectal endoscopy and other preliminary studies

Anorectal endoscopy is a simple and effective means of examining the anorectum to exclude conditions such as hemorrhoids, fissure, fistula, or abscess that may

FIGURE 56.5 Normal anal sphincter on endoanal ultrasound.

TABLE 56.8
Red Flag Symptoms for Bowel Malignancy
• Persistent unexplained change in bowel habits
• Rectal bleeding
• Unexplained weight loss
• New symptoms of wind and mucus
• Anemia
• Family history of bowel cancer

manifest as fecal soiling or passage of mucus from the anus. It allows traction on the rectal wall to diagnose early of occult rectal prolapse.

Rigid or flexible proctosigmoidoscopy, or colonoscopy should be performed to exclude malignancy, distal villous adenoma, IBD, proctitis, or proximal fecal impaction as a cause of incontinence particularly in the presence of any red flag symptoms (Table 56.8).

Diarrhea should be evaluated with specific stool studies to determine whether it is osmotic or secretory in nature. Stool culture, microscopic examination for ova and parasites, and identification of *Clostridium difficile* may also be necessary on an individual basis.

MANAGEMENT

A stepwise approach should be followed for management of fecal incontinence (Fig. 56.6). Conservative therapies with stool bulking agents, antidiarrheals, and pelvic floor exercises/biofeedback can improve continence in up to 80% of patients.[30]

Nonsurgical Therapy

The first step in the treatment of AI is regulation of diet, fluid intake, and bowel habits. Patients can be advised to avoid food or drinks that cause loose stool and frequent bowel movements.

Fiber and bulking agents, such as natural psyllium, methyl cellulose, or synthetic polycarbophil, may augment stool consistency and improve continence.[31] Loose stools can be reduced by taking psyllium/or other soluble fiber supplements. However, excessive fiber may cause increased flatus and exacerbate incontinence in some patients. Soluble fiber is generally thought to be more beneficial than insoluble fiber such as bran.

Pharmacotherapy

Constipating agents, such as loperamide, are frequently used and have been found to be effective in women with

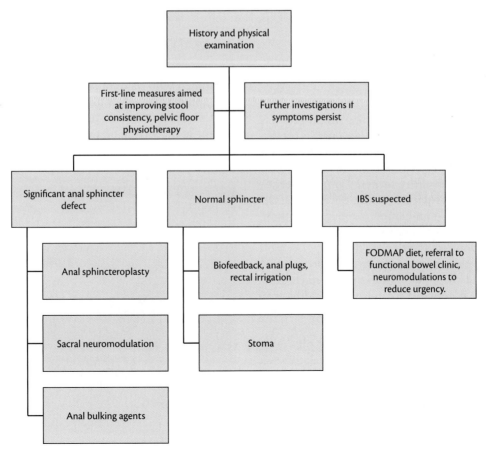

FIGURE 56.6 Stepwise management of fecal incontinence.

AI associated with loose stool.[32] Loperamide is an opiate derivate that acts by increasing transit time through the small intestine and the proximal colon, thereby promoting absorption and improving stool consistency. Furthermore, loperamide impairs the rectoanal inhibitory reflex and increases the anal resting pressure.[32]

Skin care

Perianal dermatitis has been found in 51% of older women with fecal incontinence,[33] so preventive barrier treatments should also be implemented. Generally, washable continence garments are not used because repeated cleaning is required. Disposable pads can be useful for containment but may increase the risk of dermatitis. Charcoal-based pads can be useful if fecal smearing is the primary problem.

Rectal irrigation

Transanal irrigation may reduce episodes of AI. The patient usually administers the enema or washout daily or every other day thereby obtaining a state of "pseudocontinence" because the distal colon and the rectum are empty. A number of specialized catheters can be used. Usually, body-tempered water is used. A systematic review of Peristeen system showed improvement in patients who continue to use it.[34] Laxatives, mini enemas, and suppositories can be useful, especially in those with coexisting evacuation disorders.

Pelvic floor muscle training with or without biofeedback

The aims of pelvic floor muscle training are to promote increased strength to provide more automatic protection and more effective voluntary recruitment of these muscles under times of increased abdominal pressure.

This can be achieved by targeted physiotherapy sessions to improve isolation of the correct muscle. Biofeedback, electrical stimulation, or magnetic stimulation can be used as an adjunct and is useful in patients who struggle to contract their pelvic floor.

Biofeedback therapy exercises are performed with a surface electrode or a manometric probe in the anal canal. The probe is attached to a visual or audible amplifier that gives a response proportional to the pressure delivered during squeeze.

One small trial showed that biofeedback plus exercises was better than exercises alone with a relative risk for failing to achieve full continence of 0.70.[35]

Percutaneous tibial nerve stimulation

Percutaneous tibial nerve stimulation (PTNS) involves stimulation of the tibial nerves to modify the action of the sacral nerve plexus responsible for regulation of bladder and bowel function. A mild electric current is delivered by a needle or surface electrode to the tibial nerve above the ankle, which is carried to the sacral nerves. The mechanism underlying the effect is poorly understood but is described as the modulation and stimulation of efferent and afferent nerves, with increased rectal capacity and lower sensitivity to distension have been reported.[36]

Case series data suggest beneficial outcomes in 50% to 80% of patients; however, a large double-blinded RCT in 2015 of 277 patients showed that there was no benefit compare to sham PTNS at 10 months.[37]

A systematic review comparing sacral nerve stimulation (SNS) versus PTNS found four studies that showed improvement in both groups but reduction in fecal incontinence scores greater with SNS (Fig. 56.7).[38]

Anal plugs

An anal plug can be used in patients with passive AI, especially those with soiling of small amounts of liquid stools. Plugs may be difficult to tolerate on a permanent basis, but they may be useful for occasional use.[39] Plugs come in different designs and sizes; patients are generally advised to trial the smaller size first. Anal plugs should not be retained for longer than 12 hours and need to be removed prior to defecation.[39]

Surgical Options

In the presence of a significant anal sphincter defect, in women who have failed conservative treatment, an anal sphincter repair is usually the first choice. There is, however, increasing evidence that SNS also has proven benefit in the setting of a disrupted sphincter.[40]

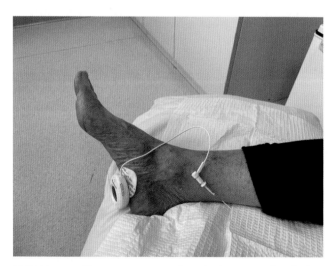

FIGURE 56.7 Transcutaneous electrical nerve stimulation treatment.

If there is an isolated defect of the IAS; anal bulking agents or SNS may be better options as the internal sphincters is difficult to access direct repair.[41]

In the absence of a repairable sphincter defect, SNS is a good option in patients who fail a nonoperative approach. Rectal prolapse is a potentially treatable cause of incontinence and may be difficult to diagnose.

Randomized controlled studies are rare, and there are very few studies comparing sphincteroplasty with other treatments. The criteria used for determining success vary considerably in the published literature and quantitative measures reporting outcomes often are not validated.

Anal sphincteroplasty with or without perineal body reconstruction

Anal sphincter repair can be performed using a transvaginal or perineal approach with few studies comparing these different techniques.

In our unit, transvaginal repair is the preferred option as a concomitant perineal repair and posterior colporrhaphy can be performed as required, although the same incision to repair any associated perineal or levator hiatal defects.

A midline incision is made on the lower posterior vaginal wall and perineum after infiltration with local anesthetic and adrenaline; the remnants of the EAS are identified and dissected out to 3 and 9 o'clock using diathermy dissection to reduce blood loss. An overlapping anal sphincter repair is then performed using 2-0 polydioxanone suture without tension. A concomitant posterior fascial plication colporrhaphy with or without a perineorrhaphy is performed when required.

A concomitant pelvic floor repair can improve AI further as the size of the perineal body thickness is a predictor of AI and the levator complex plays a part in preserving continence (Fig. 56.8).[42]

Success rates for secondary sphincter repairs are on average around 80% in the short term. Nonetheless, many studies have demonstrated deterioration in functional outcomes over time.[43] Although anal continence deteriorates over the long term following anal sphincteroplasty, patient quality of life and satisfaction remain relatively high.[43]

Barbosa et al.[44] have recently published a large cohort study with 370 patients. At 18-year follow-up, 97% of women reported flatal incontinence, 75% fecal incontinence with liquid stools, and 50% fecal incontinence with solid stools.[44]

Advanced patient age, duration of incontinence, previous surgery, and postoperative wound infection result in worse clinical outcomes.[45] Normal aging is associated with a reduction of anal resting and squeeze pressures, reduced rectal compliance, reduced rectal sensation, and perineal laxity. Therefore, asymptomatic

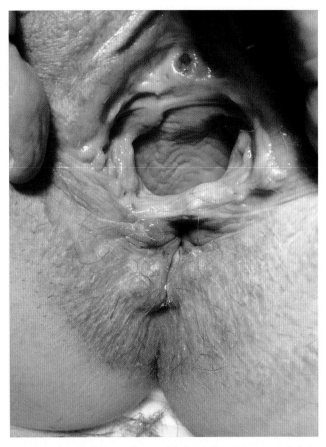

FIGURE 56.8 Patient with an old third-degree tear and deficient anal sphincter and perineum.

woman with anal sphincter injury may become symptomatic over time, particularly after menopause. A recent injury is likely to have a higher success rate following repair than an old injury, although this may relate to the age of the patient rather than the duration of the injury.[46]

If the sphincter injury affects more than one-fourth of the EAS, then a surgical repair is likely to be more beneficial.[10] Some studies show that presence of prolonged pudendal latency is associated with higher failure.[45,47] Nielsen et al.[48] suggested that early failure is usually associated with a persisting defect, identifiable using endoanal ultrasound. Performing a defunctioning colostomy in an attempt to reduce the chance of postoperative infection has not been found to improve outcomes.[47]

Overall rates of surgical complications after a sphincteroplasty range from 5% to 27%. The most common adverse event after sphincteroplasty is wound infection, which occurs in 6% to 35% of cases. Less common complications include fecal impaction, wound hematoma, urinary tract infections, and dyspareunia. Patients also may experience defecatory dysfunction, such as incomplete evacuation, straining, or the need to manually remove stool.[49]

In our department, the long-term success rate of transvaginal anal sphincter repair was 83% improvement that was sustained at 57 months follow-up and is our first-line surgical procedure used before SNS. Ultrasound of the degree of defect pre- and postoperatively did not correlate to outcomes. Wound infection and perineal breakdown occur in up to 1 in 3 women and may contribute to a less favorable outcome.[50] It is our experience that using a transvaginal approach with overlapping anal sphincter repair in a multidisciplinary team of urogynecologists and colorectal surgeons gives the best results.

Sacral neuromodulation

Another surgical option increasingly used to treat fecal incontinence is sacral neuromodulation, also termed *sacral nerve stimulation.*

SNS involves direct, chronic, low-voltage electrical stimulation of the sacral nerve roots by the siting of an electrode via a sacral foramen (S3 is the optimal site for most patients). Although there has been an evolution of systems over time, in its most common current form, SNS uses a percutaneously sited, commercially manufactured quadripolar electrode lead system connected to an implanted pulse generator buried in the subcutaneous fat of the buttock usually using local anesthetic.

A Cochrane systematic review from 2015 showed favorable mid- and long-term positive outcomes for SNS. The review reported the success rates for SNS (based on at least 50% improvement in fecal incontinence episodes per week) were 63%; furthermore, 36% of participants achieved complete fecal continence. The quality of evidence was low; there were few randomized studies with no consistent outcome reporting, and some studies did not report on adverse events.[51] These figures may be reduced further when results are reanalyzed using all available participants on an intention-to-treat basis.

A prospective study on the efficiency of SNS for fecal incontinence following OASI has shown that SNS can reduce weekly fecal incontinence episodes, regardless of the extent of the sphincter defect (Fig. 56.9).[52]

SNS has been recommended as first-line surgical treatment for fecal incontinence in people failing conservative therapies. However, the technology is expensive, and complications including infection, device migration, and device pain may occur in up to 35% of patients.[53] Newer devices on the marked are now magnetic resonance imaging (MRI)-compatible and have rechargeable batteries making SNS more favorable.[53] The ARTISAN-SNM study for the treatment of urinary urgency incontinence detailed the outcomes of one MRI-compatible rechargeable device, with 94% of participants completing the 2-year follow-up. In this cohort, only 9% needed surgical revision (lead wire, battery revision, or device explant). The as-treated analysis demonstrated an 82% responder rate.

Anal bulking

Bulking agents are a mild to moderately effective and minimally invasive method to treat incontinence.

Multiple materials have been trialed, and the most commonly used currently are currently Proctoplastique (PTQ) (a silicone biomaterial), Durasphere (pyrolytic carbon-coated beads), Solesta (dextranomer in stabilized hyaluronic acid), and implantable polyacrylonitrile, available as Gatekeeper. These agents are injected into the intersphincteric plane usually under general or spinal anesthetic with low reported complication rates.

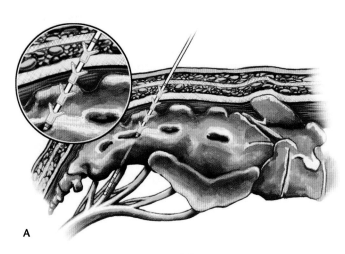
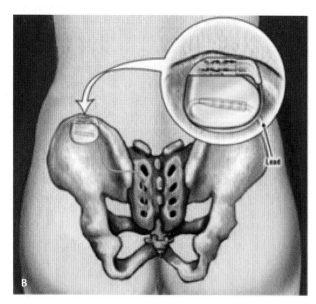

FIGURE 56.9 **A,B:** SNS. (Reprinted from Noblett KL, Cadish LA. Sacral nerve stimulation for the treatment of refractory voiding and bowel dysfunction. *Am J Obstet Gynecol* 2014;210[2]:99–106, with permission from Elsevier.)

Published data to date consists mainly of case series with few randomized trials. The results have been inconsistent and difficult to interpret owing to the multiple compounds and injection techniques that have been used. Graf et al.[54] performed a large RCT with Solesta versus sham injections, showing a 52% versus 31% improvement at 6 months. There are very few studies looking at long-term follow-up for these patients. Proctoplastique, a silicone biomaterial (PTQ), was shown to provide some advantages and was safer in treating fecal incontinence compared with carbon-coated beads (Durasphere) in the short term.[55] Gatekeeper and SphinKeeper, the latest generation of anal bulking agents, show promising results in case series from Italy. Brusciano et al.[56] followed 20 patients for 36 months, with reduction in incontinence score from 12.4 to 4.9, as well as increased resting pressure on manometry. There is a suggestion that success of bulking agents may be improved if ultrasound is used to assist with the accuracy of placement (Fig. 56.10).[55]

Miscellaneous alternative surgical options

Creating a neosphincter is reserved for circumstances where direct repair of the sphincter complex is considered inappropriate such as after extensive muscle loss due to trauma. Most commonly, the gracilis muscle is used and wrapped around the anal canal creating a new sphincter. In the past, dynamic graciloplasty was performed with electrical stimulation of the gracilis neosphincter, but this technology is no longer available. A number of other muscles have been used to create a

neosphincter including the gluteus maximus and obturator internus.

An artificial sphincter using a hydraulic silastic balloon cuff was developed in an analogous fashion to the artificial urinary sphincter, but this device is no longer marketed. More recently, there have been reports of use of a ring of miniature magnets to create an artificial sphincter (the Fenix device). This has not only shown improvement in continence scores but also may cause erosion and explanation may be close to 50%.[57]

A recent area of research that currently remains experimental is the use of progenitor cells derived from skeletal muscle myoblasts to replace or repair a damaged sphincter; a small case series of 39 patients showed decreased fecal incontinence scores and better quality of life.[58]

As a last resort, some highly symptomatic women may choose to have a colostomy. Norton et al.[59] surveyed a group of patients who had a colostomy for their incontinence, and 83% of women were happy with the outcome and did not think the colostomy restricted their life.

CONCLUSION

In conclusion, AI is a common debilitating condition. Clinicians treating pelvic floor disorders must be competent in its evaluation and management. The most important aspect of the initial workup is obtaining a thorough history. Questionnaires can be helpful for patients to explain their symptoms and for physicians to quantify their severity. Anal physiologic tests are useful adjuncts to the physical examination and are helpful in defining anatomic defects. Biofeedback in conjunction with dietary, pharmacologic, and lifestyle changes has been shown to improve AI symptoms and quality of life measures. However, if these therapies are not successful or if symptoms, sphincter injury, or neuropathy are severe, surgery can be an effective choice in the appropriately selected patient. Currently, there is a striking lack of RCTs comparing surgical options. Larger rigorous trials are still needed. However, it should be recognized that the optimal treatment regime may be a complex combination of various surgical and nonsurgical therapies.

References

1. Sultan AH, Monga A, Lee J, et al. An International Urogynecological Association (IUGA)/International Continence Society (ICS) joint report on the terminology for female anorectal dysfunction. *Int Urogynecol J* 2017;28(1):5–31.
2. Bharucha AE, Dunivan G, Goode PS, et al. Epidemiology, pathophysiology, and classification of fecal incontinence: state of the science summary for the National Institute of Diabetes and Digestive and Kidney Diseases (NIDDK) workshop. *Am J Gastroenterol* 2015;110(1):127–136.

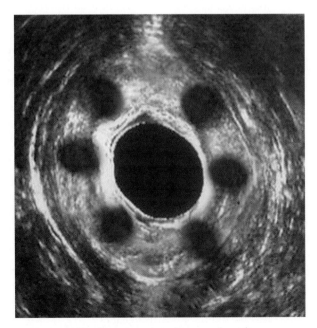

FIGURE 56.10 Gatekeeper under ultrasound guidance.

3. Johnson E, Carlsen E, Steen TB, et al. Short- and long-term results of secondary anterior sphincteroplasty in 33 patients with obstetric injury. *Acta Obstet Gynecol Scand* 2010;89:1466–1472.

4. Fox JC, Fletcher JG, Zinsmeister AR, et al. Effect of aging on anorectal and pelvic floor functions in females. *Dis Colon Rectum* 2006;49(11):1726–1735.

5. Lestar B, Penninckx F, Kerremans R. The composition of anal basal pressure. An in vivo and in vitro study in man. *Int J Colorectal Dis* 1989;4(2):118–122.

6. Fuchsjäger MH, Maier AG. Imaging fecal incontinence, *Eur J Radiol* 2003;47(2):108–116.

7. Barisic´ G, Krivokapic´ Z, Markovic´ V, et al. The role of overlapping sphincteroplasty in traumatic fecal incontinence. *Acta Chir Iugosl* 2000;47(4 suppl 1):37–41.

8. Sultan AH, Thakar R. Third and fourth degree tears. In: Sultan AH, Thakar R, Fenner DE, eds. *Perineal and anal sphincter trauma.* London: Springer; 2007:33–51.

9. Gurol-Urganci I, Cromwell DA, Edozien LC, et al. Third- and fourth-degree perineal tears among primiparous women in England between 2000 and 2012: Time trends and risk factors. *BJOG* 2013;120(12):1516–1525.

10. Malouf AJ, Norton CS, Engel AF, et al. Long-term results of overlapping anterior anal-sphincter repair for obstetric trauma. *Lancet* 2000;355(9200):260–265.

11. Cook TA, Mortensen NJ. Management of faecal incontinence following obstetric injury. *Br J Surg* 1998(3);85:293–299.

12. Madoff RD. Surgical treatment options for fecal incontinence. *Gastroenterology* 2004;126(1 suppl 1):S48–S54.

13. Barrett JS, Irving PM, Shepherd SJ, et al. Comparison of the prevalence of fructose and lactose malabsorption across chronic intestinal disorders. *Aliment Pharmacol Ther* 2009;30(2):165–174.

14. Staudacher HM, Irving PM, Lomer MC, et al. Mechanisms and efficacy of dietary FODMAP restriction in IBS. *Nat Rev Gastroenterol Hepatol* 2014;11(4):256–266.

15. Andrews V, Sultan AH, Thakar R, et al. Occult anal sphincter injuries—Myth or reality? *BJOG* 2006;113(2):195–200.

16. Walsh KA, Grivell RM. Use of endoanal ultrasound for reducing the risk of complications related to anal sphincter injury after vaginal birth. *Cochrane Database Syst Rev* 2015;(10):CD010826.

17. Gurol-Urganci I, Bidwell P, Sevdalis N. Impact of a quality improvement project to reduce the rate of obstetric anal sphincter injury: A multicentre study with a stepped-wedge design. *BJOG* 2020;128(3):584–592.

18. Friedman T, Eslick GD, Dietz HP. Delivery mode and the risk of levator muscle avulsion: A meta-analysis. *Int Urogynecol J* 2019;30(6):901–907.

19. Glazener C, Elders A, MacArthur C, et al; for ProLong Study Group. Childbirth and prolapse: Long-term associations with the symptoms and objective measurement of pelvic organ prolapse. *BJOG* 2013;120(2):161–168.

20. Nelson RL, Furner SE, Westercamp M, et al. Caesarean delivery for the prevention of anal incontinence. *Cochrane Database Syst Rev* 2010;(2):CD006756.

21. Pretlove S, Thompson P, Toosz-Hobson PM, et al. Does the mode of delivery predispose women to anal incontinence in the first year postpartum? A comparative systematic review. *BJOG* 2008;115(4):421–434.

22. Wilson D, Dornan J, Milsom I, et al. UR-CHOICE: Can we provide mothers-to-be with information about the risk of future pelvic floor dysfunction? *Int Urogynecol J* 2014;25(11):1449–1452.

23. Bek KM, Laurberg S. Risks of anal incontinence from subsequent vaginal delivery after a complete obstetric anal sphincter tear. *Br J Obstet Gynaecol* 1992;99(9):724–726.

24. Scheer I, Thakar R, Sultan AH. Mode of delivery after previous obstetric anal sphincter injuries (OASIS)—A reappraisal? *Int Urogynecol J Pelvic Floor Dysfunct* 2009;20(9):1095–1101.

25. Cotterill N, Norton C, Avery K, et al. Psychometric evaluation of a new patient-completed questionnaire for evaluating anal incontinence symptoms and impact on quality of life: The ICIQ-B. *Dis Colon Rectum* 2011;54(10):1235–1250.

26. Camilleri M, Rothman M, Ho MK, et al. Validation of a bowel function diary for assessing opioid-induced constipation. *Am J Gastroenterol* 2011;106(3):497–506.

27. Bordeianou L, Lee KY, Rockwood T, et al. Anal resting pressures at manometry correlate with the Fecal Incontinence Severity Index and with presence of sphincter defects on ultrasound. *Dis Colon Rectum* 2008;51(7):1010–1014.

28. Sultan AH, Kamm MA, Talbot IC, et al. Anal endosonography for identifying external sphincter defects confirmed histologically. *Br J Surg* 1994;81(3):463–465.

29. Ricciardi R, Mellgren AF, Madoff RD, et al. The utility of pudendal nerve terminal motor latencies in idiopathic incontinence. *Dis Colon Rectum* 2006;49(6):852–857.

30. Wald A. Update on the management of fecal incontinence for the gastroenterologist. *Gastroenterol Hepatol (N Y)* 2016;12(3):155–164.

31. Eherer AJ, Santa Ana C, Porter J, et al. Effect of psyllium, calcium polycarbophil, and wheat bran on secretory diarrhea induced by phenolphthalein. *Gastroenterology* 1992;104(4):1007–1012.

32. Read M, Read NW, Barber DC, et al. Effects of loperamide on anal sphincter function in patients complaining of chronic diarrhea with fecal incontinence and urgency. *Dig Dis Sci* 1982;27(9):807–814.

33. Bliss DZ, Zehrer C, Savik K, et al. An economic evaluation of four skin damage prevention regimens in nursing home residents with incontinence: Economics of skin damage prevention. *J Wound Ostomy Continence Nurs* 2007;34(2):143–152.

34. Dale M, Morgan H, Carter K, et al. Peristeen transanal irrigation system to manage bowel dysfunction: A NICE medical technology guidance. *Appl Health Econ Health Policy* 2019;17(1): 25–34.

35. Norton C, Cody JD. Biofeedback and/or sphincter exercises for the treatment of faecal incontinence in adults. *Cochrane Database of Syst Rev* 2012;(7):CD002111.

36. Marti L, Galata C, Beutner U, et al. Percutaneous tibial nerve stimulation (pTNS): Success rate and the role of rectal capacity. *Int J Colorectal Dis* 2017;32(6):789–796.

37. Horrocks E, Bremner SA, Stevens N, et al. Double blind randomised controlled trial of percutaneous tibial nerve stimulation (PTNS) VS. sham electrical stimulation in the treatment of faecal incontinence. *Gastroenterology* 2015;148(4):S177.

38. Simillis C, Lal N, Qiu S, et al. Sacral nerve stimulation versus percutaneous tibial nerve stimulation for faecal incontinence: A systematic review and meta-analysis. *Int J Colorectal Dis* 2018;33(5):645–648.

39. Deutekom M, Dobben AC. Plugs for containing faecal incontinence. *Cochrane Database Syst Rev* 2015;(7):CD005086.

40. Chan MK, Tjandra JJ. Sacral nerve stimulation for fecal incontinence: External anal sphincter defect vs. intact anal sphincter. *Dis Colon Rectum* 2008;51(7):1015–1025.

41. de la Portilla F. Internal anal sphincter augmentation and substitution. *Gastroenterol Rep (Oxf)* 2014;2(2):106–111.

42. Alhurry AMAH, Akool MA, Hosseini SV, et al. Does perineal body thickness affect fecal incontinence in multiparous patients? *South African J Obstet Gynaecol* 2018;24(3):57–60.

43. Glasgow SC, Lowry AC. Long-term outcomes of anal sphincter repair for fecal incontinence: A systematic review. *Dis Colon Rectum* 2012;55(4):482–490.

44. Barbosa M, Glavind-Kristensen M, Moller Soerensen M, et al. Secondary sphincter repair for anal incontinence following obstetric sphincter injury: Functional outcome and quality of life at 18 years of follow-up. *Colorectal Dis* 2020;22(1):71–79.

45. Ctercteko GC, Fazio VW, Jagelman DG, et al. Anal sphincter repair: A report of 60 cases and review of the literature. *Aust N Z J Surg* 1998;58(9):703–710.

46. Bharucha AE, Rao SSC, Shin AS. Surgical interventions and the use of device-aided therapy for the treatment of fecal incontinence and defecatory disorders. *Clin Gastroenterol Hepatol* 2017;15(12):1844–1854.

47. Young CJ, Mathur MN, Eyers AA, et al. Successful overlapping anal sphincter repair: Relationship to patient age, neuropathy, and colostomy formation. *Dis Colon Rectum* 1998;41(3):344–349.

48. Nielsen MB, Dammegaard L, Pedersen JF. Endosonographic assessment of the anal sphincter after surgical reconstruction. *Dis Colon Rectum* 1994;37(5):434–438.

49. ACOG Practice Bulletin No. 210 summary: Fecal incontinence. *Obstet Gynecol* 2019;133(4):837–839.

50. Carswell FM, Schierlitz L, Bhampiparty M, et al. Functional outcomes of secondary sphincter repair. Presented at the Annual Meeting of the International Urogynecological Association, Nashville, 2019.

51. Thaha MA, Abukar AA, Thin NN, et al. Sacral nerve stimulation for faecal incontinence and constipation in adults. *Cochrane Database Syst Rev* 2015;(8):CD004464.

52. Rydningen MB, Dehli T, Wilsgaard T, et al. Sacral neuromodulation for faecal incontinence following obstetric sphincter injury—Outcome of percutaneous nerve evaluation. *Colorectal Dis* 2017;19(3):274–282.

53. Hull T, Giese C, Wexner S, et al. Long-term durability of sacral nerve stimulation therapy for chronic fecal incontinence. *Dis Colon Rec* 2013;56(2):234–245.

54. Graf W, Mellgren A, Matzel KE, et al; for NASHA Dx Study Group. Efficacy of dextranomer in stabilised hyaluronic acid for treatment of faecal incontinence: A randomised, sham-controlled trial. *Lancet* 2011;377(9770):997–1003.

55. Maeda Y, Laurberg S, Norton C. Perianal injectable bulking agents as treatment for faecal incontinence in adults. *Cochrane Database Syst Rev* 2010;(5):CD007959.

56. Brusciano L, Tolone S, Del Genio G, et al. Middle-term outcomes of gatekeeper implantation for fecal incontinence. *Dis Colon Rectum* 2020;63(4):514–519.

57. Sugrue J, Lehur PA, Madoff RD, et al. Long-term experience of magnetic anal sphincter augmentation in patients with fecal incontinence. *Dis Colon Rectum* 2017;60(1):87–95.

58. Frudinger A, Marksteiner R, Pfeifer J, et al. Skeletal muscle-derived cell implantation for the treatment of sphincter-related faecal incontinence. *Stem Cell Res Ther* 2018;9(1):233.

59. Norton C, Burch J, Kamm MA. Patients' views of a colostomy for fecal incontinence. *Dis Colon Rectum* 2005;48(5):1062–1069.

CHAPTER 57

Rectovaginal and Anorectal Fistula

Peter L. Dwyer • Frida Carswell • James Oliver Keck

Introduction

The assessment and treatment of rectovaginal fistulae (RVFs) is an area of pelvic floor disorders where the collaboration between medical disciplines including gynecologists and colorectal surgeons will produce the best outcomes. Success rates of anatomical closure and good functional outcome can be low due to the high risk of infection and tissue breakdown when operating in an area contaminated with fecal material and on damaged denervated muscles and scarred devascularized tissue. Colorectal surgeons have experience in abdominal and rectal surgery of colorectal conditions and fistulae and diversion colostomies, whereas gynecologists have expertise in vaginal and perineal surgery and experience in obstetrics and obstetric injury; the commonest cause of RVF.

CLASSIFICATION

Rectovaginal and anorectal fistulae are abnormal epithelial communications between the rectum or anus and the vagina. The RVF can be divided into low, mid, and high fistula. The low RVF is situated between the lower third of the vaginal and the lower half of the rectum. The mid and high fistula is situated between the middle and upper rectum and the mid and upper vagina. The low RVF can be further classified whether the anal sphincter complex (ASC) is involved and the functional and anatomical state of the ASC. This is important because it decides whether the ASC needs to be reconstructed during the RVF repair.

RVF can be classified into simple and complex based on position (low mid or high vagina), size less than 2.5 cm, and causation (traumatic or infectious). Complex RVFs are larger than 2.5 cm, high vaginal position, secondary to inflammatory bowel disease, radiation, neoplasia, and had failed previous repair.[1]

ETIOLOGY

The commonest cause of anorectovaginal fistulae is obstetric trauma and are frequently associated with anal sphincter injury which potentially further contributes to the risk of fecal incontinence even after successful repair (Table 57.1). Rectal fistula may be a result of an unrecognized fourth-degree tear or a poorly repaired third- or fourth-degree tear with secondary infection and the breakdown (Fig. 57.1). The vaginal delivery may be spontaneous but more commonly associated with forceps or vacuum vaginal delivery. In developing countries, prolonged obstructed labor leading to tissue ischemia and necrosis and fistula development occur 10 to 14 days following delivery. Twenty-five percent of vesicovaginal fistula (VVF) following prolonged obstructed labor have coexisting RVF. It is rare for RVF to occur without a coexisting VVF in these circumstances.[2] In developed countries, Goldaber et al.[3] reported an incidence of 1.7% for fourth-degree perineal trauma and 0.5% for RVF in 24,000 vaginal births. This rate is now decreasing with less instrumental vaginal deliveries and a higher rate of cesarean sections.

In our experience, the second commonest cause is iatrogenic following surgery including vaginal hysterectomy, rectocele repair, hemorrhoidectomy, low anterior resection, and proctocolectomy. A contributing factor can occasional be the use of stapling devices with rectoanal resections and hemorrhoidectomy.

Trauma to the rectum can occur during posterior compartment prolapse repair; therefore, a routine postoperative rectal digital examination is essential after surgery and is also recommended after vaginal delivery, episiotomy, vaginal–perineal tears, and perineal repair. Foreign bodies inappropriately placed in the vagina and neglected vaginal pessaries are becoming more common with the more frequent use of pessaries to conservatively treat pelvic organ prolapse (POP). Synthetic mesh used for POP surgery in the posterior compartment increases the risk of fistula formation especially following a rectal injury (Fig. 57.2).

Colorectal diseases can cause fistulas from the gastrointestinal tract into the vagina. In practice, most high vaginal fistulas are secondary to diverticular disease of the sigmoid colon. Less commonly, colorectal cancer can directly invade the upper vagina. Repair of these high fistulas usually involves colonic resection and is best done abdominally.

Perianal Crohn disease may result in the formation of RVFs. Typical features of perianal Crohn such as skin tags, fissures, hidradenitis, and anal stenosis may

TABLE 57.1

Causes of Rectovaginal Fistulae

Obstetric causes	Prolonged labor, unrecognized or poorly sutured fourth-degree tears, postoperative infection causing breakdown
Iatrogenic causes	Posterior repair, hysterectomy, hemorrhoidectomy, rectal surgery
Anorectal inflammatory/infective causes	Crohn disease, ulcerative colitis, diverticular disease, cryptoglandular disease/anorectal fistula and abscess, Bartholin abscess
Postradiation	Pelvic/anorectal radiation
Foreign body	Pessaries for prolapse

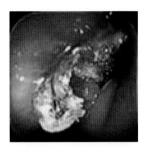

FIGURE 57.2 Proctoscopic view of RVF with mesh protrusion following transvaginal posterior colporrhaphy with mesh. RVF repaired vaginal with excision of all synthetic mesh.

or may not be present and perianal Crohn occasionally occurs without associated Crohn proctitis, colitis, or ileitis. Clinicians need to have a high index of suspicion for Crohn, and send tissue for biopsy and refer for colonoscopy as appropriate.

Injury to the gastrointestinal tract may arise following therapeutic radiotherapy with the incidence of complications increasing when the radiation dose exceeds 5,000 cGy. Ionizing radiation can cause obliterative endarteritis even when used within the therapeutic dosage and may result in urinary and RVF formation many years later.

Anal cryptoglandular fistulae arise from infection of the anal glands. Infection leads to the development of perianal and ischiorectal abscesses which spontaneously point or are drained surgically leading to fistula formation.[4] The majority of cryptoglandular fistulae extend from the anus to the perianal skin, but some can also extend from the anus into the vagina (Fig. 57.3).

A cyptoglandular abscess pointing anteriorly into the vagina can be difficult to differentiate from a Bartholin gland abscess infection. RVFs arising after drainage of a Bartholin gland abscess are more likely to be due to an underlying unexpected cryptoglandular abscess infection rather than iatrogenic injury to the rectal wall.

Bartholin cyst abscess is a common bacterial infection in women and presents as a tender right- or left-sided vulval mass anterior to the rectum. The Bartholin glands (the greater vestibular glands) are pea-sized bilateral masses of erectile tissue on either side of the vaginal opening situated in the vestibular bulbs and is surrounded by a rich plexus of veins within the spongiosis muscle. They open via a 2 cm duct into the vestibule between the hymen and labia minora. They are mucin secreting and produce copious secretions during coitus

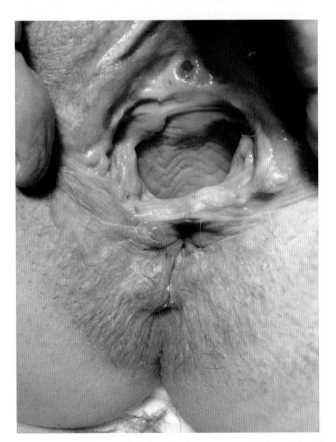

FIGURE 57.1 Old complete fourth-degree tear with loss of anal sphincter and perineal body.

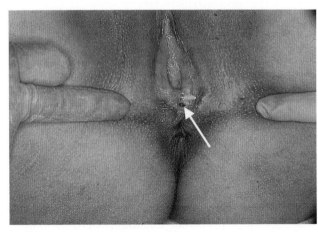

FIGURE 57.3 Small anorectal fistula.

for lubrication. The glands are anterior to the transverse perineal muscle but can extend posteriorly to be confused with perianal abscess. Injury to the rectum during surgical treatment can result in RVF and litigation.

PRESENTATION

The most common symptoms of RVF are the passage of flatus and/or liquid or solid stool into the vagina. Small fistulas may only be symptomatic when the stools are loose. Women may also report a purulent discharge from the vagina, dyspareunia, perineal pain and tenderness, along with vaginal irritation and recurrent genitourinary tract infection which is secondary to the vaginitis and dermatitis caused by the feculent discharge. There may be other symptoms present due to coexisting conditions of Crohn disease or malignancy such as bleeding. A sexual history should be taken particularly as dyspareunia can also develop after vaginal repair and perineal reconstruction.

EVALUATION

Physical examination is important to determine the location and etiology of the RVF and aid classification into simple or complex. Examination of the vagina and perineum should be performed to diagnose any associated prolapse or scarring from birth trauma and detect muscular damage to perineal and anal sphincter muscles. If small, the fistulous opening may not be easily visible on inspection of the lower anorectum and vagina, but the clinician must have a high index of suspicion when women present with signs and symptoms consistent with an RVF. Vaginal and anal examination should also assess resting and squeeze pressures of the levator and anal sphincter muscles. Perianal dimpling or the "dovetail sign" with perianal folds posterior to the anus is indicative of a disrupted anal sphincter. Women with RVF may need to be examined under anesthesia for accurate diagnosis as vaginal/rectal examination may be painful because of the scarring and infection usually present. The fistulous tracts may also require gentle probing using lacrimal duct probes to delineate the fistula or fistulae (Fig. 57.4). For pinhole fistula rectal distension with saline and with methylene blue or diluted hydrogen peroxide can be used in the evaluation of complex fistulae to visualize side tracts and areas of fluid collection.

This assessment will help to determine the best surgical approach whether transvaginal, transanal, perineal, or abdominal. We believe that this decision is best done jointly by a urogynecologist and colorectal specialist. Several imaging studies may help to identify and delineate RVF including computed tomography (CT) scan, magnetic resonance imaging (MRI), fistulography, and endoluminal ultrasound (EUS). Assessment of

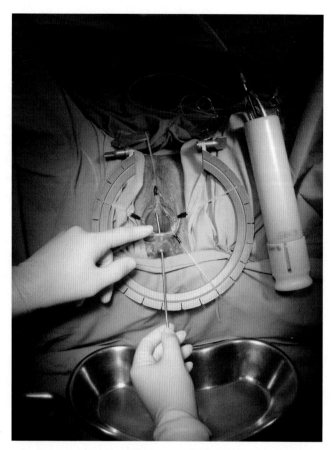

FIGURE 57.4 Small RVF demonstrated with a metal probe.

the anal sphincter complex (ASC) with EUS and manometry is frequently useful prior to surgical repair to determine the structural and functional integrity of the anal sphincter.

Preoperative Preparation

- Bowel prep
- Antibiotics
- Colonoscopy if Crohn disease is suspected
- EUA if unable to do an accurate evaluation in the rooms
- MRI/CT scan to assess extent and location. Note that these can be negative even in the presence of a fistula.
- Anal ultrasound and manometry if anal sphincter injury is suspected.
- Stomal therapy consultation if a stoma is planned.

MANAGEMENT

Patients with no or minimal bothersome symptoms may decide to have no surgical treatment especially if it is a small anovaginal fistula. Normalization of stool consistency and treatment of associated infection, and dermatitis is helpful in improving quality of life.

RVFs associated with Crohn disease require expert gastroenterologic management. Modern treatment of Crohn disease with biological disease modifying antirheumatic drugs such as Adalinumab may result in healing of fistulae.[5] A randomized, double-blinded, multicenter study[6] studied infliximab for the treatment of both abdominal and perianal fistulae from Crohn disease. After 18 weeks of infliximab treatment, the authors found significant reduction in the number of fistulae with complete closure occurring in 46% versus 13% of placebo. The follow-up was relatively short (4.5 months), and the study included all enterocutaneous fistulae, not specifically RVF.

Surgical Repair

The majority of women with RVF have severe symptoms and require surgical closure. The principals of successful surgery are careful surgical technique with RVF closure without tension with adequate interposition of well vascularized tissue to reinforce the closure and good hemostasis. Most textbooks recommend excision of the RVF and surrounding scar tissue or fibrosis. One of my mentors (P. Dwyer), Bob Zacharin[7] who learnt his fistular surgery from the Hamlins of Ethiopia was of the opinion "that excising the fistulous tract made the fistula larger and removed strong fibrous tissue useful in closure." We have always followed this advice.

Another controversial area is the timing of fistula repair. Because the symptoms are so bothersome and stressful, most women are desperate to have the repair as soon as possible, but this must be balanced against the optimal time for a successful repair. In most cases, it is beneficial to delay surgery a few months after traumatic vaginal delivery to treat associated infection and allow slough to separate and healing to occur. Obstetric RVF from obstructed labor and radiation fistulas have considerably more tissue necrosis and sloughing which should be allowed to settle before repair is undertaken, sometimes up to 12 months later.

Surgical Approach

The surgical approaches to RVF are vaginal and/or perineal, transanal, or abdominal repair. Choice of type of repair and surgical approach will depend on patient factors such as location and size of fistula, the cause of the fistula, the presence of scarring, the presence of Crohn disease or other bowel pathology, a history of radiation, and previous repairs. However, in reality the decision on surgical operation is frequently made on the surgeon's experience and their specialty. Gynecologists are experienced in the vaginal and perineal approach and colorectal surgeons the rectal and abdominal approach and may use a diversion colostomy or ileostomy. Gynecologists favor the transvaginal approach with local fat or muscle interposition. Colorectal surgeons prefer endorectal advancement flaps with or without sphincteroplasty using the transperineal or transanal approach. When the stakes are so high and success rates in most series low, there is a need for balanced consideration and a multidisciplinary approach.

There are currently no prospective, randomized, controlled trials for the surgical correction of RVF. Most studies report RVF case series usually are of low numbers and diverse etiology, using variable surgical treatments and different anatomical and functional outcome parameters. In the assessment of RVF outcomes, success can be judged by the successful closure of the RVF and longer term functional outcomes of fecal continence and associated fecal symptoms and vaginal and sexual symptoms including dyspareunia using validated standardized questionnaires.

Women with iatrogenic and obstetric fistula are more likely to have a successful outcome after surgery, whereas patients with Crohn disease and history of radiation have a less favorable success rate. Pinto et al.[8] reported an overall success rate per procedure for RVF of 60% in 125 patients caused by inflammatory bowel disease (45.6%), obstetric injury (24%), and surgical trauma (16%). The procedures performed included endorectal advancement flap (35.3%), gracilis muscle interposition (13.6%), seton placement (13.6%), transperineal (8.7%), and transvaginal repair (8.1%). They found no difference in recurrence rates based on the approach or type of repair. In this study, smoking was the only other significant patient risk factor for repair failure, especially in patients with Crohn disease.

The transvaginal approach

Transvaginal repair is the preferred method of closure in our unit. Patients are placed in a Trendelenburg position with the legs in Allen stirrups. A midline vaginal or a vaginal–perineal incision is made; the incision is extended to the perineum if the RVF is low, and reconstruction of the anal sphincters and perineum is required (Fig. 57.5). We would use a vaginal incision to treat middle or low RVF regardless of etiology in most cases. The site of the RVF is important and whether the ASC is intact and functional which is usually assessed both by clinical rectovaginal examination and endoanal ultrasound.

For RVF arising above an intact ASC, we would make a circumferential incision around the RVF usually of 1 to 2 cm diameter on the posterior vaginal wall (Fig. 57.6). The fistulous tract into the rectum is identified by a curved fistular probe which is placed transanal. The vagina is retracted using a Lonestar Brantley Scott retractor which provides excellent surgical access for complicated vaginal surgery. A 40- to 60-mL Bupivacaine and adrenaline with saline solution

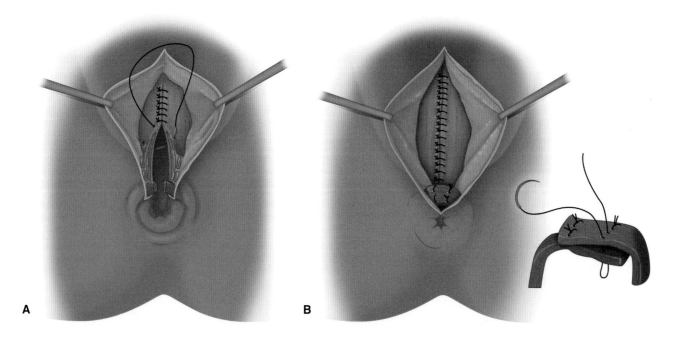

FIGURE 57.5 Transvaginal RVF repair with vaginoperineal approach with division of rectal mucosa, anal sphincter, and then layered repair and overlapping anal sphincter repair. **A:** An incision was made through the RVF, rectal mucosa, ASC, and posterior vaginal wall below the RVF, and the rectum and rectovaginal fascia were mobilized. The rectal mucosa was closed with interrupted 3/0 Vicryl sutures. **B:** The ASC is then repaired with an overlapping sphincter repair using 3/0 PDS sutures, and further interrupted fascial sutures are placed to reinforce fistula closure and treat any coexisting rectocele or perineal deficiency.

is injected circumferentially around the fistula opening into the vagina. The vaginal epithelium would be removed, and dissection is extended laterally mobilizing the vagina from the rectum and the rectovaginal fascia which will subsequently be used for tension-free fistula closure. The fistulous tract into the rectum is not excised and left intact. The size of the rectal defect is kept to a minimum and not extended unnecessarily. The smaller the defect the better the healing and less risk of subsequent infection and breakdown. The rectal mucosa is closed with interrupted 3/0 Vicryl sutures. Once the rectal closure is considered watertight on rectovaginal examination, 2 or 3 further interrupted sutures using 3/0 Vicryl or PDS are performed to provide further fascial closure and support.

When the RVF involves the ASC making surgical access difficult or there is a chronic third- or fourth-degree tear which needs repairing, the external anal sphincter will need to be repaired with an overlapping sphincter repair with 3/0 PDS sutures. If the RVF is at or above the ASC, we would cut down on the RVF probe using diathermy laying open the vagina and perineum, ASC, and rectal mucosa to the RVF. The rectal mucosa is then repaired with interrupted 3/0 Vicryl, the ASC with overlapping sphincter repair using 3/0 or 2/0 PDS, and further interrupted fascial sutures to reinforce fistula closure and treat any coexisting rectocele or perineal deficiency (Fig. 57.5A,B) (Fig. 57.7A–C) (Video 57.1).

Vascular fat pad Martius grafts can be used to reinforce this closure but is usually not needed. Exceptions would be recurrent or high RVF or radiation-induced RVF (Fig. 57.8A,B).

The use of a Martius labial fat pad (MLFP) interposition has been described by Martius[9] which he thought may improve urinary incontinence after VVF repair. Now, it is commonly used in vesico- and urethrovaginal fistula[10] and RVF to improve closure rates in cases of secondary repair where tissue quality and vascularity may be suboptimal. An incision is made on the labia majora, and a 3 × 4 cm labial fat pad graft is fashioned leaving the perineal branch of the pudendal artery entering posteriorly intact. The graft is tunnelled between the vulval skin and inferior pubic ramus into the vaginal dissection to cover the rectal closure and provides healthy tissue separating the rectal and vaginal walls; it is then secured in place by 3/0 or 2/0 Vicryl sutures (Video 57.2).

Browning and Whiteside[2] reviewed 1,057 cases of genital tract fistula in Ethiopia. VVF without RVF was present in 933 (88.3%) cases, combined VVF and RVF in 79 (7.5%), and isolated RVF in 45 (4.3%). Only 4 (0.4%) women had isolated RVFs that could be attributed to prolonged obstructed labor; the remaining 41 RVFs were due to trauma (including obstetric and sexual trauma), iatrogenic causes, infection, perineal tears, or previous failed repairs. An obstetric RVF due

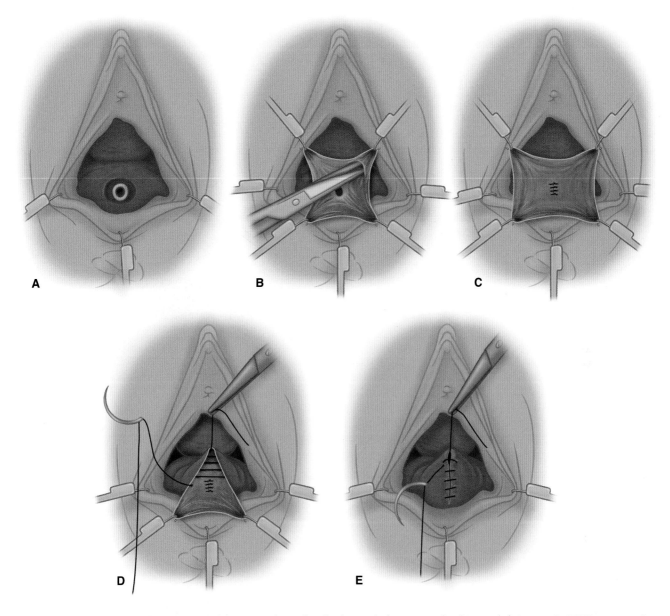

FIGURE 57.6 RVF closure though vaginal incision alone; fistular layered closure; anal sphincter left intact. **A:** RVF on posterior vaginal wall above the external anal sphincter with Brantley Scott retractor hooks in position. **B,C:** Circumferential vaginal incision with dissection and mobilization of rectum and rectovaginal fascia around the fistula to enable tension-free RVF closure. **C:** The fistula tract is not enlarged or excised; the rectal mucosa is closed with 3/0 or 4/0 interrupted Vicryl sutures. **D:** Further interrupted sutures using 2/0 Vicryl or PDS are performed to provide further fascial closure and support. **E:** The vaginal epithelium is closes with a continuous 2/0 Vicryl suture.

to obstructed labor represents a more severe injury process than does a VVF. RVFs rarely occur without a VVF in prolonged obstructed labor, and most RVF in this series were from obstetric, iatrogenic, or sexual trauma.

All RVFs in this study were managed with a transvaginal flap-splitting operative technique, without grafts or diverting colostomies. Overall, 120 (98.4%) of 122 RVFs repaired at the study hospital remained closed at discharge.

Beksac et al.[11] in a study of 19 women with RVF, successfully treated 8 women with simple RVF due to birth trauma using transvaginal sphincteroplasty and fistulectomy, 5 of the 6 cases associated with chronic inflammatory diseases (mainly Crohn disease), and only 3 of 5 cases (60%) with 1 or more failed previous repairs were cured using this surgery.

Seyfried et al.[12] reported on 424 women who underwent transvaginal fistulectomy with primary sphincter reconstruction. The primary healing rate, after a mean

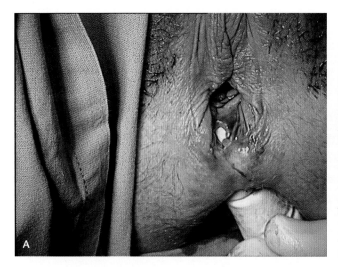

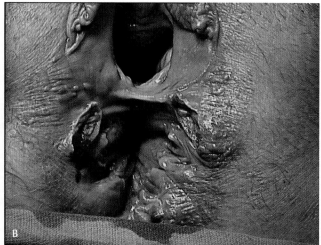

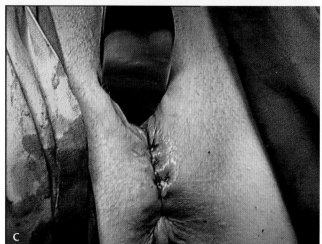

FIGURE 57.7 **A:** Two-centimeter RVF present above a nonfunctioning ASC. **B:** RVF converted to complete fourth-degree tear with diathermy dissection prior to repair. **C:** Completed repair with overlapping anal sphincter repair.

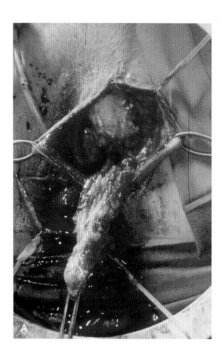

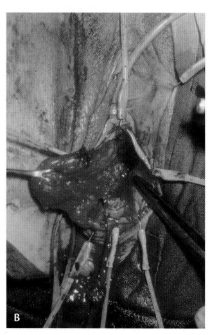

FIGURE 57.8 **A:** Martius graft used in a woman with a high RVF following rectal excision and pelvic radiation for a rectal cancer. **B:** Martius graft. A 3- × 4-cm labial fat pad graft is fashioned leaving the perineal branch of the pudendal artery entering posteriorly intact. The graft is tunnelled between the vulval skin and inferior pubic ramus into the vaginal dissection to cover the rectal closure and is secured in place by 3/0 or 2/0 Vicryl sutures placed at 6, 9, and 12 o'clock.

follow-up of 11 months (7 to 200 months), was 88.2% (374 of 424). Taking into account revisionary surgeries with secondary sphincter repair, this rate reaches 95.8% (406 of 424). After the procedure, 34 patients (23.0%) had fecal incontinence, with 23 having flatus incontinence (15.5%), 10 patients having liquid incontinence (6.8%), and 1 patient having solid fecal incontinence.

Transperineal approach

The transperineal approach uses a perineal incision to separate the rectum and vagina to repair the rectal mucosa, anal sphincter, and vaginal mucosa; the rectovaginal septum is augmented with closure of the levator muscle. A perineal incision alone can be used for low RVF repair and to perform a sphincteroplasty and even levatorplasty. Chew and Rieger[13] reported on seven women with obstetric RVF who had an operative transperitoneal repair involving division of the anovaginal fistula, closure of rectal and vaginal walls, anterior levatorplasty, and overlapping sphincteroplasty. All were successfully repaired without a stoma. However, a vaginal incision does allow better access to higher RVF and the greater mobilization of the rectovaginal fascia which can be used for tension-free fistula closure or repair of any coexisting rectocele.

Transanal rectovaginal fistula repair

First described by Noble in 1902, and then modified by Liard in 1948, the endorectal advancement flap is used for the transrectal approach to repair RVF (Fig. 57.9). A curved, broad, proximally based flap is raised consisting of mucosa and some of the underlying muscle. Once the flap is raised, there should be clear visualization of the underlying defect in the internal sphincter muscle. A probe inserted from the vaginal side or a silastic seton may aid in identifying the defect. Direct closure of the muscle defect is performed with interrupted 3/0 or 4/0 Vicryl sutures, either horizontally or vertically. The flap is then brought down as a second layer to cover this muscle closure and is sutured to the rectal mucosa and anoderm with 3/0 Vicryl sutures.

Tsang et al.[14] reported on 52 women who underwent 62 repairs of simple obstetrical RVFs. There were 27 endorectal advancement flaps and 35 mucosal flaps and sphincteroplasties (28 with and 8 without levatorplasty). Success rates were 41% with endorectal advancement flaps and 80% with sphincteroplasties (96% success with and 33% without levatorplasty.

Hull et al.[15] evaluated the results of transvaginal/perineal repair (episioproctotomy) and rectal advancement flap on 87 women with RVF of cryptoglandular or obstetrical origin. Fifty (57.5%) patients underwent transvaginal/perineal repair, and 37 (42.5%) underwent

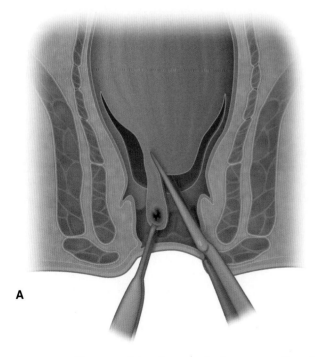
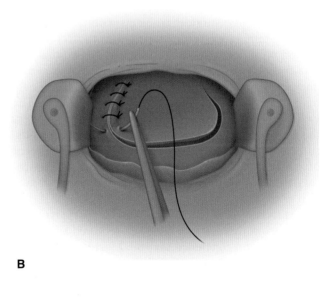

A　　　　　　　　**B**

FIGURE 57.9 Transrectal rectal mucosal advancement flap. **A:** Rectal advancement flap. A curved proximally based flap is raised consisting of mucosa and some of the underlying muscle. Once the flap is raised, there should be clear visualization of the underlying defect in the internal sphincter muscle with closure of the muscle defect is performed with interrupted horizontally or vertical 3/0 or 4/0 Vicryl sutures. **B:** The flap is then brought down as a second layer to cover this muscle closure and is sutured to the rectal mucosa and anoderm with 3/0 interrupted Vicryl sutures with exposure provided by an anal retractor.

rectal advancement flap. Thirty-nine (78%) patients had successful closure after transvaginal/perineal repair versus 23 (62.2%) patients after rectal advancement flap; the transvaginal/perineal repair was associated with significantly better fecal ($P < .001$) and sexual ($P = .04$) function. There was no significant difference in other studied variables between the two techniques on healing, postoperative continence, and sexual function.

Overview of vaginal/rectal approach for rectovaginal fistula

A German consensus group recently performed a systematic review of the literature on RVF and set guidelines.[16] In their opinion, the most common surgical treatment of most high transsphincteric anal fistulas was fistula excision with sphincter suture and closure of the ostium in the rectum by an advancement flap. "The healing rates of more recent studies range from 41% to 100% with realistic success rates are probably between 50% and 70%." They considered that the transvaginal and perineal approach studies were mainly case reports and had too few cases for analysis and comparison. It is true that the literature on transvaginal repair of RVF is not extensive; however, it would appear that the transvaginal approach is extensively used in developing countries where RVF are commonplace with good results,[2] although follow-up is limited and reporting of the results in the literature rare.

We also are of the opinion that the transvaginal approach gives good results. The realistic results of RVF repair like VVF repairs will never be 100%. Added to the technical and surgical problems with RVF, there is fecal contamination with added risks of infection and wound breakdown. In 1984, Goligher[17] stated that two disadvantages of local RVF repair were excess suture line tension and direct apposition of the rectal and vaginal suture lines without much intervening tissue. The vaginal approach allows wider tissue dissection to access the rectovaginal fascia and even ischiorectal adipose tissue, multiple layer tension-free closure, and placement of a Martius fat pad graft if required. The rectal mucosal defect is kept to a minimum. The vaginal approach also give access for rectocele repair if necessary.

McNevin et al.[18] reported on 16 patients with complex anovaginal fistulae. They reported success in 15 women and concluded that the Martius flap can be combined with an anterior sphincter repair for complex RVF with minimal morbidity. Successful use of a gracilis muscle interposition has been reported for Crohn RVF repairs, especially after other failed repairs. Wexner et al.[19] reported on their use of the gracilis flap in nine patients with RVF. Seven patients achieved successful closure with this technique. In our experience, the gracilis graft is a more morbid procedure than the Martius procedure and is rarely indicated.

There are no randomized controlled trials comparing modes of repair for RVFs. Low and superficial (anovaginal) fistulas can be laid open or excised with a simple fistulotomy with successful healing.

Abdominal approaches

Higher fistulas can also be treated abdominally as an open or laparoscopic procedure by resection of the affected segment of the intestine with primary rectal anastomosis with omental graft between the closed rectum and vagina. In one publication of 38 patients, van der Hagen et al.[20] reported a cure rates of nearly 100% in various etiologies. High fistulae are almost exclusively caused from diverticular disease and therefore have a different management and success rate to low fistulae.

Fecal Diversion

Fecal diversion in the management of RVF remains controversial but should improve healing and lower risk of infection and RVF repair breakdown. There are no set criteria regarding when and in whom proximal diversion should be performed. Furthermore, a stoma does not ensure a successful repair and requires one or two further operation to create and close the diversion. This does add to the number of operations these patients have, the morbidity and risk of legal consequences. The literature is undecided, with recommendations by some authors to routinely perform a loop ileostomy before or during a repair in all patients, whereas others recommend fecal diversion only in select situations. Without any randomized, prospective data, the creation of a stoma remains controversial and surgeons must use their best judgment in making the decision regarding diversion.

We use elective fecal diversion occasionally in complex cases where there has been extensive tissue loss, where previous attempts at repair have been unsuccessful or where there are other factors such as Crohn disease or radiation damage. Occasionally, women with RVFs come to us with a preexisting stoma performed after a major obstetric tear or after perineal wound infection and breakdown.

Future Treatments

Other grafts

A bioprosthetic fistula plug made from lyophilized porcine intestinal submucosa is a technically feasible option in closing RVF, but the data on its use is limited. Schwandner and Fuerst[21] reported using Surgisis mesh in 21 patients with RVF. After a mean follow-up of 12 months, they achieved a 78% closure rate in the Crohn group and an 83% closure rate in the non-Crohn RVF.

Stem cell transplantation

In a study by García-Olmo et al.[22] from Spain, a female with Crohn-associated RVF received autologous adipose stem cells that were injected into her RVF. At 3 months follow-up, the patient achieved successful closure of the fistula. This is an exciting potential therapy; however, larger studies with variable etiology and good follow-up are needed to justify wider usage.

CONCLUSION

The commonest causes of RVF we see are a result of childbirth and gynecologic or rectal surgery. Classification can be made into simple and complex on the etiology, size, and position of the fistula. Management is best done with gynecologic and colorectal input to improve outcomes with successful closure and a good long-term functional result. The surgical approach and use of grafts will depend on site and complexity of the RVF, although transvaginal repair with or without anal sphincter repair is an excellent option in the majority of cases. Fecal diversion is necessary in selected complex patients.

References

1. Rothenberger DA, Goldberg SM. The management of rectovaginal fistulae. *Surg Clin North Am* 1983;63(1):61–79.
2. Browning A, Whiteside S. Characteristics, management, and outcomes of repair of rectovaginal fistula among 1100 consecutive cases of female genital tract fistula in Ethiopia. *Int J Gynaecol Obstet* 2015;131(1):70–73.
3. Goldaber KG, Wendel PJ, McIntire DD, et al. Postpartum perineal morbidity after fourth-degree perineal repair. *Am J Obstet Gynecol* 1993;168(2):489–493.
4. El-Gazzaz G, Hull TL, Mignanelli E, et al. Obstetric and cryptoglandular rectovaginal fistulas: Long-term surgical outcome; quality of life; and sexual function. *J Gastrointest Surg* 2010;14(11):1758–1763.
5. Valente MA, Hull TL. Contemporary surgical management of rectovaginal fistula in Crohn's disease. *World J Gastrointest Pathophysiol* 2014;5(4):487–495.
6. Present DH, Lichtiger S. Efficacy of cyclosporine in treatment of fistula of Crohn's disease. *Dig Dis Sci* 1994;39(2):374–380.
7. Zacharin R. *Obstetric fistula.* Vienna: Springer-Verlag, 1988.
8. Pinto RA, Peterson TV, Shawki S, et al. Are there predictors of outcome following rectovaginal fistula repair? *Dis Colon Rectum* 2010;53(9):1240–1247.
9. Martius H. Uber die Behandlung von Blasenscheidenfisteln, insbesondere met Hilfe einer Lappenplastik. *Geburtshilfe Gynakol* 1932;103:22–34.
10. Dykes N, Dwyer P, Rosamilia A, et al. Video and review of the surgical management of recurrent urethral diverticulum. *Int Urogynecol J* 2020;31(12):2679–2681.
11. Beksac K, Tanacan A, Ozgul N, et al. Treatment of rectovaginal fistula using sphincteroplasty and fistulectomy. *Obstet Gynecol Int* 2018;2018:5298214.
12. Seyfried S, Bussen D, Joos A, et al. Fistulectomy with primary sphincter reconstruction. *Int J Colorectal Dis* 2018;33(7):911–918.
13. Chew SS, Rieger NA. Transperineal repair of obstetric-related anovaginal fistula. *Aust N Z J Obstet Gynaecol* 2004;44(1):68–71.
14. Tsang CB, Madoff RD, Wong WD, et al. Anal sphincter integrity and function influences outcome in rectovaginal fistula repair. *Dis Colon Rectum* 1998;41(9):1141–1146.
15. Hull TL, El-Gazzaz G, Gurland B, et al. Surgeons should not hesitate to perform episioproctotomy for rectovaginal fistula secondary to cryptoglandular or obstetrical origin. *Dis Colon Rectum* 2011;54(1):54–59.
16. Ommer A, Herold A, Berg E, et al. German S3-Guideline: Rectovaginal fistula. *GMS Ger Med Sci* 2012;10:Doc15.
17. Goligher JC. *Surgery of the anus, rectum and colon,* 5th ed. London: Bailliere Tindall, 1984:208–211.
18. McNevin MS, Lee PY, Bax TW. Martius flap: An adjunct for repair of complex, low rectovaginal fistula. *Am J Surg* 2007;193(5):597–599.
19. Wexner SD, Ruiz DE, Genua J, et al. Gracilis muscle interposition for the treatment of rectourethral, rectovaginal, and pouch-vaginal fistulas: Results in 53 patients. *Ann Surg* 2008;248(1):39–43.
20. van der Hagen SJ, Soeters PB, Baeten CG, et al. Laparoscopic fistula excision and omentoplasty for high rectovaginal fistulas: A prospective study of 40 patients. *Int J Colorectal Dis* 2011;26(11):1463–1467.
21. Schwandner O, Fuerst A. Preliminary results on efficacy in closure of transsphincteric and rectovaginal fistulas associated with Crohn's disease using new biomaterials. *Surg Innov* 2009;16(2):162–168.
22. García-Olmo D, García-Arranz M, Herreros D, et al. A phase I clinical trial of the treatment of Crohn's fistula by adipose mesenchymal stem cell transplantation. *Dis Colon Rectum* 2005;48(7):1416–1423.

CHAPTER 58

Obstetrical Anal Sphincter Injuries and Sphincteroplasty

Bhumy Dave Heliker • Afiba Arthur

EPIDEMIOLOGY

Obstetrical anal sphincter injuries (OASIS) are third- and fourth-degree lacerations that occur at the time of vaginal delivery. A third-degree perineal laceration is defined as a laceration which involves the external anal sphincter (EAS) with or without involvement of the internal anal sphincter (IAS) and a fourth-degree perineal laceration is defined as injury to EAS, IAS, and the anal mucosa.[1] In 1999, Sultan[2] published a subclassification of perineal lacerations that further delineates the extent of injury with third-degree lacerations (Table 58.1).

The prevalence of OASIS in the general population is between 0.25% and 6% and higher in primiparous women (1.4% to 16%).[3,4] In multiparous women, it is estimated to have a prevalence of 0.4% to 2.7%.[3] Significant research has been done to better understand the risk factors for OASIS. Primiparity, operative vaginal delivery with vacuum or forceps, and fetal weight greater than 4,000 g have been associated with more significant lacerations.[3–8] Other factors include a midline episiotomy at the time of delivery, persistent occiput posterior position of the fetal head, and shoulder dystocia.[8,9] Increasing maternal age has also been shown to increase the risk of OASIS during vaginal delivery.[9,10] Rahmanou et al.[10] developed a model where the odds ratio of developing pelvic floor trauma at the time of a vaginal delivery for each additional year older than age 18 years was 1.064. A long second stage of labor, specifically more than an hour, also increases the risk for a third- and fourth-degree perineal laceration.[11,12] Other factors such as epidural, induction, and increased length of labor can increase the risk for OASIS.[11,12] With regard to demographic characteristics, Meister et al.[13] reported significant risk with obesity, nonsmoking status, and other races besides black. Given the significant number of risk factors that can predispose a woman to sustaining an obstetrical anal sphincter injury, there have been attempts to develop a risk scoring system. McPherson et al.[14] created a scoring system to help practitioners determine OASIS risk with a sensitivity of 52.7% and specificity of 71%. Although this sensitivity and specificity are relatively low, this is a tool that clinicians can use to gather patient's risk factors and implement the appropriate measures to help reduce the risk of an anal sphincter injury.

The reported risk of recurrent OASIS varies between 3.2% and 10.7% depending on the population that is being studied.[3,15–17] An odds ratio of greater than 5 has been reported for recurrence.[7,18,19] Forceps delivery, birth weight greater than 4,000 g, persistent occiput posterior position, and Asian race are risk factors for sustaining a recurrent OASIS in a subsequent pregnancy.[1,11]

PATHOPHYSIOLOGY

Understanding the anatomy of the anal sphincter complex is necessary for the diagnosis and management of injuries. The anal sphincter complex consists of the EAS and IAS.

The EAS is a striated muscle and under voluntary control. The innervation comes from the inferior rectal nerve, a branch of the pudendal nerve. It is responsible for the majority of the squeeze pressure. The EAS extends to the most distal portion of the anus, whereas the IAS does not extend fully to the distal anus; thus, the very distal portion of the sphincter complex consists of the EAS alone. It is also important to understand the relationship between the EAS and other skeletal muscles of the pelvic floor. The EAS works in conjunction with one of the levator ani muscles, the puborectalis muscle, to provide anal continence. The puborectalis muscle plays a critical role in the formation of the anorectal angle and thereby contributes to the continence mechanism by helping keep the proximal anal canal closed.[20] Figure 58.1 shows the relationship between the puborectalis muscle, IAS, and EAS. In addition, 3D ultrasound shows that the EAS extends into the right and left transverse perineal muscles.[20] This means that injuries to the transverse perineal muscles or cutting an episiotomy could also compromise the full functioning of the EAS. Figure 58.2 shows the external anatomy of the pelvic floor muscles and the relation to the anal sphincter.

TABLE 58.1

Classification of Perineal Lacerations

TYPE OF LACERATION	DESCRIPTION OF LACERATION
First-degree laceration	Involves perineal skin and the vaginal epithelium
Second-degree laceration	Involves the perineal muscles but not the anal sphincter
Third-degree laceration	Involves the anal sphincter
Grade 3a	<50% of the EAS is affected
Grade 3b	>50% of the EAS is affected
Grade 3c	Involves both the EAS and the IAS
Fourth-degree laceration	Involves both the EAS and the IAS and the anal mucosa

The IAS arises from the distal thickening of the circular smooth muscles of the anal canal, and it is under the control of the autonomic nervous system.[1] It is responsible for about 80% of the resting tone of the anal sphincter complex.[1] Disruption of the EAS, the IAS, or the rectal mucosa can compromise the fecal continence mechanism.

DIAGNOSIS

OASIS should be diagnosed at the time of delivery but is occasionally diagnosed on exam remote from delivery or with an endoanal ultrasound.

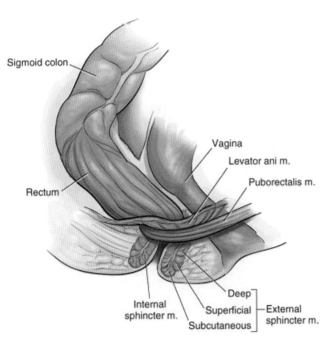

FIGURE 58.1 Sagittal view of the anal sphincter in relation to other structures of the female pelvic floor. (Reprinted from Jones HW, Rok JA. *Te Linde's operative gynecology*, 11th ed. Philadelphia: Wolters Kluwer, 2015.)

Making the diagnosis at the time of vaginal delivery is critical for ensuring immediate repair and reducing the morbidity to the patient. It is estimated that about a third of anal sphincter injuries are missed at the time of delivery, so it is important for obstetricians and midwives to be trained on how to properly identify these injuries.[21] This requires a careful examination and a rectal exam to help determine the integrity of the anal sphincter and more subtle mucosal injuries (e.g., proximal to the sphincter complex). If there is any doubt about the degree of the laceration, it is better to make a diagnosis of a higher degree laceration than a lower degree injury to ensure that an adequate repair and appropriate care is provided to the patient.[22]

Examination of the integrity of the sphincter is performed by placing the dominant index finger in the anus and the thumb of the same hand in the vagina (Fig. 58.3).[22] The two fingers are then pinched together in a side-to-side rolling motion.[22] A defect can be palpated along the EAS if there is an injury because the muscles retract to the sides. Furthermore, a half speculum can be used to retract the anterior vagina and expose the length of the posterior wall. For identification of pinpoint lacerations, one may inject gel with methylene blue into the rectum, apply gentle pressure along the rectovaginal septum, and look for extravasation through the vagina (Fig. 58.4).

For sphincter injuries are not diagnosed at the time of delivery, an endoanal ultrasound can be performed to help locate the injury, especially for patients who have symptoms of anal incontinence. Figure 58.5 demonstrates an endoanal ultrasound image of an intact anal sphincter complex juxtaposed with an image of an EAS defect from 10 to 2 o'clock.[23] Women with IAS injury compared to those who have EAS injury alone on endoanal ultrasound are more likely to have fecal incontinence.[24] Of note, 24% of women diagnosed with occult OASIS on ultrasound were found to have no evidence of injury on surgical exploration.[24] This suggests that universal ultrasound for all women with second-degree lacerations may result in a false-positive rate; further investigation about the role of universal ultrasound in asymptomatic women is needed. Currently, endoanal ultrasounds in women with second-degree perineal lacerations should be reserved for women with symptoms of anal incontinence or physical exam findings raising suspicion of occult OASIS.

MANAGEMENT

Anal sphincter injury diagnosed at the time of vaginal delivery should be properly repaired. Immediate identification and repair at the time of delivery will help reduce morbidity to the patient. Figure 58.6 outlines the muscles that are injured in third- and fourth-degree lacerations. It is important that once the diagnosis is made, the patient be given adequate pain control via epidural or pudendal block. Furthermore, the obstetrician should

FIGURE 58.2 Muscles of the female perineum. (From Toglia MR. Repair of perineal and other lacerations associated with childbirth. Accessed July 2, 2019. https://www.uptodate.com/contents /repair-of-perineal-and-other-lacerations-associated -with-childbirth. Copyright © 2019 UpToDate, Inc. and its affiliates. All rights reserved.)

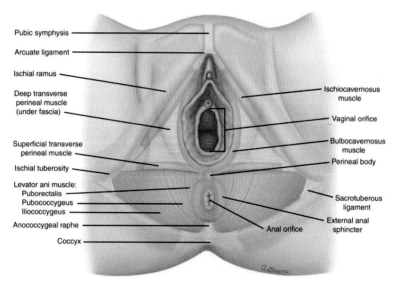

ensure there is adequate retraction, good lighting, and consider liberal irrigation with septic solutions such as dilute povidone-iodine. The patient should be moved to the operating room if better exposure and lighting is needed or adequate anesthesia cannot be achieved in the labor room. The muscles of the torn EAS may retract into ischioanal fat and may not be easily visible. Allis clamps should be used to delineate the sphincter edges and the capsule to facilitate identification during the repair.[25] Retractors such as a Gelpi retractor can be helpful to improve visibility.[25]

In cases where an ob-gyn has limited or no experience with repair, a consultant should be called, or the patient should be transferred to a facility with the appropriate expertise, so she can have the best outcome possible. Delaying the repair for a short duration of time to allow for hospital transfer or a consultant to arrive has not been associated with worse outcomes. In a Swedish study where

women who sustained anal sphincter injuries at the time of delivery were randomized to either immediate repair or delayed repair for 8 to 12 hours, there was no difference in anal incontinence between the two groups.[26]

Primary Repair of Obstetrical Anal Sphincter Injuries

Primary repair is done at the time of delivery. It is important to identify the various parts of the anal sphincter that are injured so they can be appropriately repaired. Patients who have sustained OASIS are at increased risk for anal incontinence; women who sustain a fourth-degree laceration are at about 10 times higher risk for anal incontinence compared to those with third-degree laceration injuries.[27,28]

For fourth-degree lacerations, the anal mucosa has to be identified separately and repaired. The repair can be

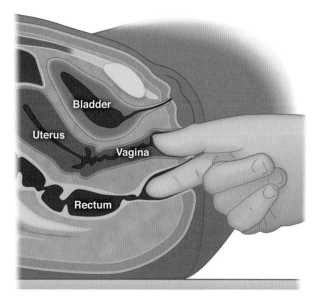

FIGURE 58.3 Illustration of how to examine for anal sphincter defects.

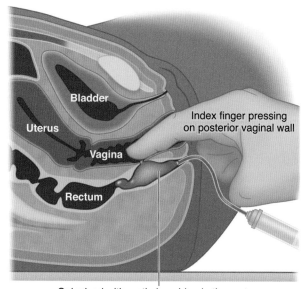

FIGURE 58.4 Injection of dye to detect anal sphincter defect.

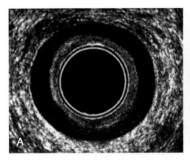
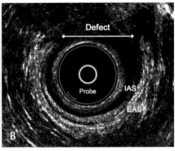

FIGURE 58.5 Endoanal ultrasound demonstrating anal sphincter ultrastructure. **A:** Intact EAS (hyperechoic ring), intact IAS (hypoechoic ring). **B:** Defect in EAS from 10 to 2 o'clock. (**A,** Reprinted from Tarnay C, ed. *Operative techniques in gynecologic surgery.* Philadelphia: Wolters Kluwer, 2018. **B,** Photograph courtesy of Justin A. Maykel, MD.)

done with 3-0 or 4-0 delayed absorbable suture such as poliglecaprone 25.[29,30] The repair can be done in a running or interrupted fashion.[29] These sutures can enter the lumen of the rectum without increasing risk for fistula. The IAS should be identified and repaired separately from the EAS to help reduce the risk of fecal incontinence post repair.[18,30] This can be done in a running or interrupted fashion using 3-0 delayed absorbable suture such as polyglactin or polydioxanone. The EAS should also be repaired separately. A 2-0 or 3-0 delayed absorbable suture should be used for both sphincters. The EAS can be repaired in an end-to-end or overlapping fashion (Fig. 58.7). In order to repair the EAS in an overlapping manner, the full thickness of the muscle must be torn and a 1- to 1.5-cm segment should overlap.[18,30] This type of EAS repair is only applicable to grade 3C and fourth-degree lacerations.[30] Three years after repair, there was no difference in the rates of anal incontinence between those with overlapping versus end-to-end sphincter repair immediately after delivery.[31]

Anal Sphincteroplasty

Anal sphincteroplasty usually refers to a delayed or secondary repair remote from delivery that is usually carried out for a primary repair that has failed or an injury

that was not diagnosed at the time of the delivery (occult OASIS). The success rate of the remote repair has been reported to decline over time. Specifically, early success rates may be 70% to 80%, but after 3 years, continence rates decline to 30% to 40%, with only 20% of patients still continent at 10 years.[32,33]

The surgery begins by making a linear or semicircular incision between the perineum and the anal edge (Fig. 58.8). The incision is then carefully taken down and the dissection is carried out laterally until the torn edges of the EAS are identified. The EAS dissection should be done carefully to avoid disruption of the inferior rectal nerve which is a branch of the pudendal nerve which innervates the anal sphincter from the lateral aspect of the anus.[29,34] In addition, care should be taken to avoid the vascular supply, inferior rectal artery and vein at 3 and 9 o'clock.[21,35] Repair of the muscles can be done in an overlapping or an end-to-end fashion.

Although studies have shown no significant long-term difference in outcomes comparing end-to-end versus overlapping repair of the anal sphincter immediately, there is limited evidence regarding the optimal method for delayed sphincteroplasty remote from delivery.[30,36–38] Some experts would advocate for an overlapping technique including surrounding scar tissue when performed

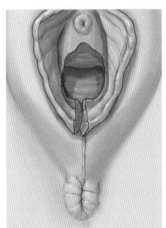
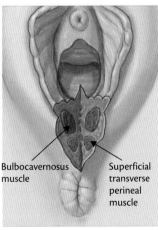
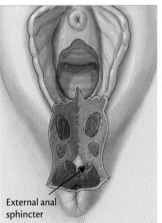
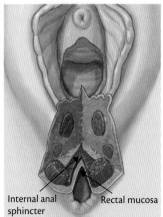

Bulbocavernosus muscle

Superficial transverse perineal muscle

External anal sphincter

Internal anal sphincter

Rectal mucosa

FIGURE 58.6 Degrees of perineal laceration. From **left** to **right:** First-degree laceration: injury to tissue of perineum and vagina, no injury to muscle; second-degree laceration: injury extends into fascia and muscle, anal sphincter intact; third-degree laceration: tearing extends into anal sphincter; fourth-degree laceration: injury extends through sphincter and rectal mucosa. (Modified from O'Meara A. *Maternity, newborn, and women's health nursing: A case-based approach.* Philadelphia: Wolters Kluwer, 2018.)

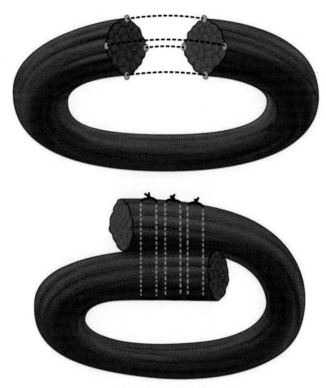

FIGURE 58.7 Anal sphincteroplasty techniques. **Top:** End-to-end repair. **Bottom:** Overlapping. (Reprinted from Tarnay C, ed. *Operative techniques in gynecologic surgery*. Philadelphia: Wolters Kluwer, 2018.)

remote from delivery.[39,40] The IAS and EAS should be repaired with delayed absorbable sutures in a tension-free manner.

Women who sustain anal sphincter injuries should be referred for pelvic floor physical therapy to help reduce symptoms of anal incontinence after delivery. This is usually done after 6 weeks postpartum, but it has been shown that it can be started sooner at 4 weeks to expedite the recovery process without affecting the laceration repair.[41]

Short-term complications

Women who sustain anal sphincter injuries during vaginal delivery are at increased risk for developing pain, bleeding, infection, and wound breakdown in the short term, immediately postpartum.[42] Some of the risk factors that have been associated with OASIS wound complications in the postpartum period are obesity, tobacco use, operative vaginal delivery, and fourth-degree laceration, although intrapartum use of antibiotics is protective against wound complications.[42] Wound breakdown is often but not always caused by an infection of the wound. A broad-spectrum antibiotic such as second-generation cephalosporin should be administered at the time of the repair.[18] This has been shown to minimize the risk of wound infection and breakdown.[42] Wound infection rates of 20% and breakdown rates of about 25% have

been reported after OASIS repair.[42] Given the high rate of complications, low suspicion for complications and early follow-up or referral to a multidisciplinary peripartum perineal clinic is suggested.[43] Patients who present with a superficial infection of their wounds can be treated with broad-spectrum antibiotics such as amoxicillin/clavulanate and metronidazole orally with very close follow-up.[42] In cases where the infection is deep, the patient should be admitted to the hospital for intravenous an- tibiotics and the wound should be surgical debrided. If the patient appears systemically ill or there is concern for necrotizing fasciitis, general surgery should be consulted and if time allows, imaging should be obtained prior to surgical exploration. Superficial breakdowns which spare the sphincter may heal by secondary intention with packing alone.[44] There is considerable debate regarding timing of surgical repair for wound breakdown—immediate versus delayed repair. Limited data suggests that early repair is feasible depending on the tissue quality. A case series of 23 women with dehiscence of third- and fourth-degree lacerations showed good outcomes with early repair.[44] These women presented between 2 and 60 days postpartum, and wound preparation via debridement was done for an average of 7 days until tissue appeared viable. Early repair was performed, and zero patients had wound breakdown, five had superficial separation, and one had a pinpoint perineal fistula that healed without operative intervention.[44] In contrast, many would advocate that if it has been greater than 10 days from delivery, waiting 3 months for repair to ensure that the inflammation has subsided and revascularization has occurred. No level 1 data exists comparing delayed versus early repair.

Constipation needs be avoided because this could put a strain on the sutures and can lead to wound breakdown. Patients should be prescribed stool softeners to achieve a Bristol type 4 stool postpartum to prevent painful passage of hard stool and suture breakdown. Of note, laxatives should be titrated to also avoid loose stool as diarrhea may contaminate the wound.[18]

Finally, a considerable amount of litigation may occur as a consequence of OASIS complications and subsequent anal incontinence. A review of 68 cases found that avoidance of episiotomy, thorough medical recordkeeping, comprehensive discharge instructions and counseling, and timely referral to a female pelvic medicine and reconstructive surgery specialist may help reduce litigation.[45]

Long-term complications

Although much attention is paid to immediate anal incontinence, a large proportion of women develop symptoms of anal incontinence (flatal incontinence, fecal incontinence and fecal urgency, fistula) later in life. The risk of anal incontinence in women who sustain anal sphincter injuries at the time of vaginal delivery has been

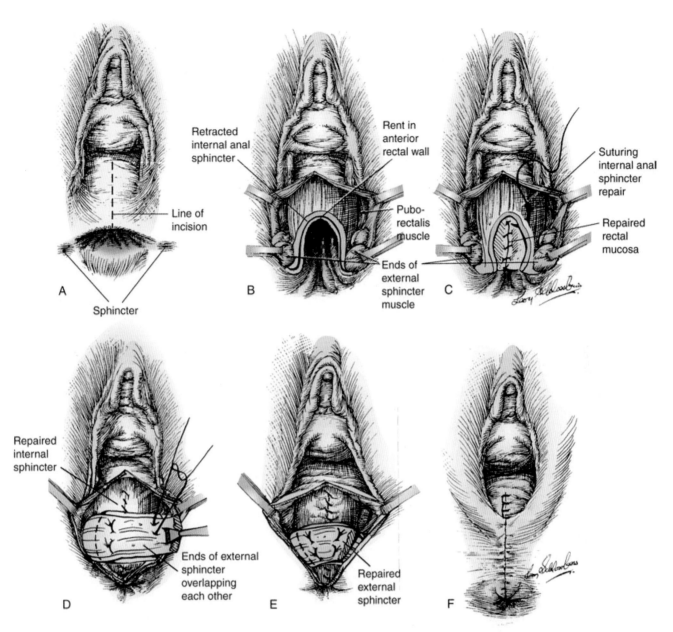

FIGURE 58.8 Layered closure of a chronic complete perineal laceration with overlapping sphincteroplasty. **A:** A transverse incision is made at the junction of the vaginal and rectal mucosa and extended up the midline of the posterior vaginal wall. **B:** The rectal wall has been separated from the posterior vaginal wall with careful sharp dissection. The ends of the EAS have been identified and grasped with Allis clamps. The IAS can be seen between the EAS and the anorectal mucosa as an area of white fibrous tissue. **C:** The defect in the anal mucosa has been closed with a continuous 3-0 delayed absorbable suture. The IAS then is reapproximated over a length of 3 to 5 cm. This layer also serves to imbricate and isolate the mucosal layer and take tension off of it to help it heal and seal against infection. **D:** The ends of the EAS are widely mobilized with the scar tissue left on. Care should be taken not to dissect beyond the 3 and 9 o'clock position as that is where the pudendal enervation to the sphincter enters laterally. The EAS then is brought together over the repaired IAS with two rows of two horizontal mattress sutures of delayed absorbable or permanent suture material. **E:** After the EAS has been repaired, the genital hiatus is narrowed by bringing the puborectalis muscles closer together with interrupted delayed absorbable sutures placed in the fascia overlying them. **F:** The bulbocavernosus and superficial transverse perineal muscles have been reattached to the perineal body, and the vaginal mucosa was closed with a continuous locking stitch of 3-0 delayed absorbable suture that was continued subcuticularly to approximate the perineal skin. (Reprinted from Jones HW, Rok JA, eds. *Te Linde's operative gynecology*, 11th ed. Philadelphia: Wolters Kluwer, 2015.)

reported to be 24% to 59% in the first 6 months, 15.4% at 6 years, and 13% at 18 years of the injury.[46-49] Long-term sequelae to OASIS also include chronic pain and dyspareunia regardless of menopausal status.[1,18,50]

Subsequent Pregnancies after Obstetrical Anal Sphincter Injuries

Women who have had previous OASIS need to be counseled about subsequent mode of delivery. The Royal College of Obstetricians and Gynaecologists and the American College of Obstetricians and Gynecologists currently recommend that women who experienced anal incontinence after their initial OASIS or have abnormal ultrasound, manometry, or wound complications from their previous injury should be offered a cesarean section.[1,18] In a prospective study from France, asymptomatic women with prior OASIS and who had injury confirmed on endoanal ultrasound were randomized to a cesarean section or vaginal delivery, and there was no significant difference in anal incontinence 6 months postpartum between the two groups.[51] Although this data suggests that asymptomatic women with prior OASIS may elect for another vaginal delivery, it is important to acknowledge the major limitation of this work: Outcomes are short term and the sequelae of neuromuscular injury and aging may not present as fecal incontinence until the fifth or sixth decade of life. Endoanal ultrasound and anal manometry are addi- tional tools that can be used in asymptomatic women who have concerns about having a vaginal delivery to determine if there is a defect in the sphincter or com- promised function before they attempt another vaginal delivery. A persistent sphincter defect may increase the risk for developing anal in- continence and further neuromuscular decline with ad- ditional pelvic floor trauma.[52-54]

For those who are symptomatic from their previous injury or asymptomatic women with two or more anal sphincter injuries, the mode of delivery should be a planned cesarean section because they are at increased risk for worsening symptoms after another vaginal delivery.[18,53] The discussion with the patient should also take into consideration the psychological impact of the previous anal sphincter injury, surgical risks of cesarean section, and most importantly the patient's desires and preferences. Studies shows that women with sphincter defects on endoanal ultrasound and high anal incontinence scores are more likely to choose a cesarean section as the mode of delivery in their subsequent pregnancy.[53]

PREVENTION

The best way to avoid the untoward sequelae of OASIS is by prevention of such injuries at the time of delivery. Although episiotomy should be limited to obstetrical indications and not used as a routine practice, certain types of episiotomies have been shown to be protective.[11,18,55] If an episiotomy must be used, a mediolateral incision is preferred because the angle of the incision is away from the midline, thereby reducing the risk of extension into a third- or fourth-degree perineal laceration.[55] Making the initial incision at 45° to 60° angle will help avoid a midline incision that could extend to the anal sphincter. Several tools such as the Episcissors-60 have been created to help practitioners achieve the correct angle of incision as swollen tissue may cause providers to underestimate the angle of their incision.[11,56,57] In contrast, midline episiotomies have been shown to be associated with an increased risk of anal sphincter injury compared to mediolateral episiotomies.[58] de Vogel et al.[58] showed in their retrospective cohort study that cutting a mediolateral episiotomy at the time of an operative vaginal delivery decreased the risk of OASIS by sixfold and this effect was strongest in forceps deliveries. The number needed to treat to prevent one OASIS with vacuum delivery was 8.64, and 5.21 with forceps delivery.[58] With regard to protecting the pelvic floor, vacuum-assisted vaginal delivery is the preferred method of operative delivery and compared to forceps has been shown to help reduce anal sphincter tears.[59] Sultan et al.[59] in their study of anal sphincter lacerations found on endoanal ultrasound that about 80% of women who had forceps vaginal delivery had anal sphincter lacerations compared to 24% of those who had vacuum-assisted deliveries.

Application of warm compresses at the time of delivery by the delivery attendant can be protective against a sphincter injury. A Cochrane review showed that the risk of anal sphincter injuries was reduced with the application of warm compresses to the perineum at the time of delivery compared to those who did not have warm compresses applied to their perineum.[1,60]

Also, perineal massage during the second stage of labor has been shown to reduce OASIS.[61]

The delivery position could play a role in reducing a woman's risk of anal sphincter injury at the time of vaginal delivery. Gottvall et al.[12] in their Swedish cohort study found that a vaginal delivery in the squatting or lithotomy position increased the risk for anal sphincter injury compared to kneeling, supine, and semirecumbent positions. In a study where patients were randomized to delayed pushing in lateral position versus early pushing in lithotomy, those in the delayed lateral pushing group were found to be more likely to deliver without perineal lacerations.[61]

There are other prevention methods that have not been shown to make a difference in the reduction of OASIS. Pelvic floor physical therapy in the antepartum period has not been shown to decrease the risk of OASIS or an episiotomy.[62,63] Wearing balloon devices, such as the Epi-No in the vagina to stretch the perineum in the antepartum period, have not been shown to reduce the risk of perineal lacerations.[11,64] Support of the perineum and the fetal head at the time of delivery has also not been clearly shown to reduce the risk of OASIS, so clinicians can either use a "hands on," where perineum is supported, or "hands off," where the delivery attendant does not support the fetal head or the perineum.[65] Finally, perineal self-massage prenatally has some benefits, but there is scant data to support its use for OASIS prevention. In a systematic review, women who massaged their perineum in the third trimester reduced the risk of an episiotomy by 16% and subjectively had more control over their child birth experience, but it did not have lower rates of perineal lacerations.[11,60]

For patients with an epidural during labor, delaying pushing compared to immediate pushing from the time of complete cervical dilation has been shown to reduce the risk of operative vaginal delivery.[66] A reduction in operative vaginal delivery could translate to a decrease in the risk of third- and fourth-degree perineal lacerations. This reduction in risk is likely because delayed pushing allows the fetal head to descend lower into the pelvis, thereby reducing the need for midpelvic operative delivery.[66] The potential benefit of delayed pushing, however, has to be weighed against the fetal and maternal risks of doing so.

CONCLUSION

OASIS is associated with significant short- and long-term sequelae for women. It is important to both diagnose and repair these injuries properly and provide appropriate postpartum support.

References

1. American College of Obstetricians and Gynecologists' Committee on Practice Bulletins—Obstetrics. Practice Bulletin No. 165: Prevention and management of obstetric lacerations at vaginal delivery. *Obstet Gynecol* 2016;128(1):e1–e15.
2. Sultan AH. Obstetrical perineal injury and anal incontinence. *AVMA Med Legal J* 1999;5(6):193–196.
3. Thubert T, Cardaillac C, Fritel X, et al. Definition, epidemiology and risk factors of obstetric anal sphincter injuries: CNGOF perineal prevention and protection in obstetrics guidelines. *Gynecol Obstet Fertil Senol* 2018;46(12):913–921.
4. Handa VL, Danielsen BH, Gilbert WM. Obstetric anal sphincter lacerations. *Obstet Gynecol* 2001;98(2):225–230.
5. Joris F, Hoesli I, Kind A, et al. Obstetrical and epidemiological factors influence the severity of anal incontinence after obstetric anal sphincter injury. *BMC Pregnancy Childbirth* 2019;19(1):94.
6. Gundabattula SR, Surampudi K. Risk factors for obstetric anal sphincter injuries (OASI) at a tertiary centre in south India. *Int Urogynecol J* 2018;29(3):391–396.
7. Pergialiotis V, Vlachos D, Protopapas A, et al. Risk factors for severe perineal lacerations during childbirth. *Int J Gynaecol Obstet* 2014;125(1):6–14.
8. FitzGerald MP, Weber AM, Howden N, et al. Risk factors for anal sphincter tear during vaginal delivery. *Obstet Gynecol* 2007;109(1):29–34.
9. Marschalek M, Worda C, Kuessel L, et al. Risk and protective factors for obstetric anal sphincter injuries: A retrospective nationwide study. *Birth* 2018;45(4):409–415.
10. Rahmanou P, Caudwell-Hall J, Kamisan Atan I, et al. The association between maternal age at first delivery and risk of obstetric trauma. *Am J Obstet Gynecol* 2016;215(4):451.e1–451.e7.
11. Wilson AN, Homer CSE. Third- and fourth-degree tears: A review of the current evidence for prevention and management. *Aust N Z J Obstet Gynaecol* 2020;60(2):175–182.
12. Gottvall K, Allebeck P, Ekéus C. Risk factors for anal sphincter tears: The importance of maternal position at birth. *BJOG* 2007;114(10):1266–1272.
13. Meister MR, Cahill AG, Conner SN, et al. Predicting obstetric anal sphincter injuries in a modern obstetric population. *Am J Obstet Gynecol* 2016;215(3):310.e1–310.e7.
14. McPherson KC, Beggs AD, Sultan AH, et al. Can the risk of obstetric anal sphincter injuries (OASIs) be predicted using a risk-scoring system? *BMC Res Notes* 2014;7(1):471.
15. Baghestan E, Irgens LM, Børdahl PE, et al. Risk of recurrence and subsequent delivery after obstetric anal sphincter injuries. *BJOG* 2012;119(1):62–69.
16. Basham E, Stock L, Lewicky-Gaupp C, et al. Subsequent pregnancy outcomes after obstetric anal sphincter injuries (OASIS). *Female Pelvic Med Reconstr Surg* 2013;19(6):328–332.
17. Boggs EW, Berger H, Urquia M, et al. Recurrence of obstetric third-degree and fourth-degree anal sphincter injuries. *Obstet Gynecol* 2014;124(6):1128–1134.
18. RJ Fernando, Sultan AH, Freeman RM, et al. *The management of third-and fourth-degree perineal tears* (Green-Top Guideline No. 29). London: Royal College of Obstetricians and Gynaecologists, 2015.
19. Jha S, Parker V. Risk factors for recurrent obstetric anal sphincter injury (rOASI): A systematic review and meta-analysis. *Int Urogynecol J* 2016;27(6):849–857.
20. Raizada V, Bhargava V, Karsten A, et al. Functional morphology of anal sphincter complex unveiled by high definition anal manometery and three dimensional ultrasound imaging. *Neurogastroenterol Motil* 2011;23(11):1013–1019, e460.
21. Sultan AH, Monga A, Lee J, et al. An International Urogynecological Association (IUGA)/International Continence Society (ICS) joint report on the terminology for female anorectal dysfunction. *Int Urogynecol J* 2017;28(1):5–31.
22. Harvey M-A, Pierce M, Walter J-E, et al. Obstetrical anal sphincter injuries (OASIS): Prevention, recognition, and repair. *J Obstet Gynaecol Can* 2015;37(12):1131–1148.
23. Sideris M, McCaughey T, Hanrahan JG, et al. Risk of obstetric anal sphincter injuries (OASIS) and anal incontinence: A meta-analysis. *Eur J Obstet Gynecol Reprod Biol* 2020;252:303–312.
24. Faltin DL, Boulvain M, Floris LA, et al. Diagnosis of anal sphincter tears to prevent fecal incontinence: A randomized controlled trial. *Obstet Gynecol* 2005;106(1):6–13.
25. Appleton S, Huguelet T. Obstetric laceration repair. Published 2017. Accessed March 10, 2022. https://www.acog.org/-/media/project/acog/acogorg/files/pdfs/education/scog/obstetric-laceration-repair.pdf?la=en&hash=3D86926B03DFC811B6E4577512427843
26. Nordenstam J, Mellgren A, Altman D, et al. Immediate or delayed repair of obstetric anal sphincter tears—A randomised controlled trial. *BJOG* 2008;115(7):857–865.
27. Fenner DE, Genberg B, Brahma P, et al. Fecal and urinary incontinence after vaginal delivery with anal sphincter disruption in an obstetrics unit in the United States. *Am J Obstet Gynecol* 2003;189(6):1543–1549.
28. Sangalli MR, Floris L, Faltin D, et al. Anal incontinence in women with third or fourth degree perineal tears and subsequent vaginal deliveries. *Aust N Z J Obstet Gynaecol* 2000;40(3):244–248.

29. Dudding TC, Vaizey CJ, Kamm MA. Obstetric anal sphincter injury: Incidence, risk factors, and management. *Ann Surg* 2008;247(2):224–237.

30. Fernando RJ, Sultan AH, Kettle C, et al. Methods of repair for obstetric anal sphincter injury. *Cochrane Database Syst Rev* 2013;(12):CD002866.

31. Tan JJY, Chan M, Tjandra JJ. Evolving therapy for fecal incontinence. *Dis Colon Rectum* 2007;50(11):1950–1967.

32. Pescatori LC, Pescatori M. Sphincteroplasty for anal incontinence. *Gastroenterology Rep* 2014;2(2):92–97.

33. Johnson E, Carlsen E, Steen TB, et al. Short- and long-term results of secondary anterior sphincteroplasty in 33 patients with obstetric injury. *Acta Obstet Gynecol Scand* 2010;89(11):1466–1472.

34. Gibbs D, Hooks V. Overlapping sphincteroplasty for acquired anal incontinence. *South Med J* 1993;86(12):1376–1380.

35. Tsakiridis I, Mamopoulos A, Athanasiadis A, et al. Obstetric anal sphincter injuries at vaginal delivery: A review of recently published national guidelines. *Obstet Gynecol Surv* 2018;73(12):695–702.

36. Tjandra JJ, Han WR, Goh J, et al. Direct repair vs. overlapping sphincter repair: A randomized, controlled trial. *Dis Colon Rectum* 2003;46(7):937–943.

37. Fitzpatrick M, Behan M, O'Connell PR, et al. A randomized clinical trial comparing primary overlap with approximation repair of third-degree obstetric tears. *Am J Obstet Gynecol* 2000;183(5):1220–1224.

38. Londono-Schimmer EE, Garcia-Duperly R, Nicholls RJ, et al. Overlapping anal sphincter repair for faecal incontinence due to sphincter trauma: Five year follow-up functional results. *Int J Colorectal Dis* 1994;9(2):110–113.

39. Walters M, Karram M. *Urogynecology and reconstructive pelvic surgery*, 4th ed. Netherlands: Elsevier, 2014.

40. Moscovitz I, Rotholtz NA, Baig MK, et al. Overlapping sphincteroplasty: Does preservation of the scar influence immediate outcome? *Colorectal Dis* 2002;4(4):275–279.

41. Mathé M, Valancogne G, Atallah A, et al. Early pelvic floor muscle training after obstetrical anal sphincter injuries for the reduction of anal incontinence. *Eur J Obstet Gynecol Reprod Biol* 2016;199:201–206.

42. Lewicky-Gaupp C, Leader-Cramer A, Johnson LL, et al. Wound complications after obstetric anal sphincter injuries. *Obstet Gynecol* 2015;125(5):1088–1093.

43. Hickman LC, Propst K, Swenson CW, et al. Subspecialty care for peripartum pelvic floor disorders. *Am J Obstet Gynecol* 2020;223(5):709–714.

44. Arona AJ, Al-Marayati L, Grimes DA, et al. Early secondary repair of third-and fourth-degree perineal lacerations after outpatient wound preparation. *Obstet Gynecol* 1995;86(2):294–296.

45. Kim EK, Lovejoy DA, Patterson D, et al. Lessons learned from a review of malpractice litigations involving obstetric anal sphincter injury in the United States. *Female Pelvic Med Reconstr Surg* 2020;26(4):249–258.

46. Richter HE, Nager CW, Burgio KL, et al. Incidence and predictors of anal incontinence after obstetric anal sphincter injury in primiparous women. *Female Pelvic Med Reconstr Surg* 2015;21(4):182–189.

47. Davé BA, Leader-Cramer A, Mueller M, et al. Anal sphincter injuries after operative vaginal versus spontaneous delivery—Is there a difference in postpartum symptoms? *Female Pelvic Med Reconstr Surg* 2016;22(4):194–198.

48. Baud D, Meyer S, Vial Y, et al. Pelvic floor dysfunction 6 years post-anal sphincter tear at the time of vaginal delivery. *Int Urogynecol J* 2011;22(9):1127–1134.

49. Faltin DL, Otero M, Petignat P, et al. Women's health 18 years after rupture of the anal sphincter during childbirth: I. Fecal incontinence. *Am J Obstet Gynecol* 2006;194(5):1255–1259.

50. Taithongchai A, Thakar R, Sultan AH. Management of subsequent pregnancies following fourth-degree obstetric anal sphincter injuries (OASIS). *Eur J Obstet Gynecol Reprod Biol* 2020;250:80–85.

51. Abramowitz L, Mandelbrot L, Bourgeois Moine A, et al. Caesarean section in the second delivery to prevent anal incontinence after asymptomatic obstetric anal sphincter injury: The EPIC multicentre randomised trial. *BJOG* 2021;128(4):685–693.

52. Cassis C, Giarenis I, Mukhopadhyay S, et al. Mode of delivery following an OASIS and caesarean section rates. *Eur J Obstet Gynecol Reprod Biol* 2018;230:28–31.

53. Cole J, Bulchandani S. Predictors of patient preference for mode of delivery following an obstetric anal sphincter injury. *Eur J Obstet Gynecol Reprod Biol* 2019;239:35–38.

54. Jangö H, Langhoff-Roos J, Rosthøj S, et al. Modifiable risk factors of obstetric anal sphincter injury in primiparous women: A population–based cohort study. *Am J Obstet Gynecol* 2014;210(1):59.e1–59.e6.

55. Kalis V, Landsmanova J, Bednarova B, et al. Evaluation of the incision angle of mediolateral episiotomy at 60 degrees. *Int J Gynaecol Obstet* 2011;112(3):220–224.

56. Pergialiotis V, Bellos I, Fanaki M, et al. Risk factors for severe perineal trauma during childbirth: An updated meta-analysis. *E Eur J Obstet Gynecol Reprod Biol* 2020;247:94–100.

57. Hartmann K, Viswanathan M, Palmieri R. Outcomes of routine episiotomy: A systematic review. *JAMA.* 2005;293(17):2141–2148.

58. de Vogel J, van der Leeuw-Van Beek A, Gietelink D, et al. The effect of a mediolateral episiotomy during operative vaginal delivery on the risk of developing obstetrical anal sphincter injuries. *Am J Obstet Gynecol* 2012;206(5):404.e1–404.e5.

59. Sultan AH, Kamm MA, Bartram CI, et al. Anal sphincter trauma during instrumental delivery. *Int J Gynaecol Obstet* 1993;43(3):263–270.

60. Aasheim V, Nilsen ABV, Reinar LM, et al. Perineal techniques during the second stage of labour for reducing perineal trauma. *Cochrane Database Syst Rev* 2017;(6):CD006672.

61. Walker C, Rodríguez T, Herranz A, et al. Alternative model of birth to reduce the risk of assisted vaginal delivery and perineal trauma. *Int Urogynecol J* 2012;23(9):1249–1256.

62. Du Y, Xu L, Ding L, et al. The effect of antenatal pelvic floor muscle training on labor and delivery outcomes: A systematic review with meta-analysis. *Int Urogynecol J* 2015;26(10):1415–1427.

63. National Institute for Health and Clinical Excellence. *2019 Surveillance of intrapartum care for health healthy women and babies.* London: National Institute for Health and Care Excellence, 2019. NICE Guideline CG190.

64. Kamisan Atan I, Langer S, Shek K, et al. Does the Epi-No® prevent pelvic floor trauma? A multicentre randomised controlled trial. *Br J Obstet Gynaecol* 2016;123(6):995–1003.

65. Bulchandani S, Watts E, Sucharitha A, et al. Manual perineal support at the time of childbirth: A systematic review and meta-analysis. *BJOG* 2015;122(9):1157–1165.

66. Roberts CL, Torvaldsen S, Cameron CA, et al. Delayed versus early pushing in women with epidural analgesia: A systematic review and meta-analysis. In: *Database of Abstracts of Reviews of Effects (DARE): Quality-assessed reviews.* United Kingdom: Centre for Reviews and Dissemination, 2004.

CHAPTER 59

Evaluation and Management of Rectal Prolapse

Meghan L. Good • Nitin Mishra

Introduction

Rectal prolapse (rectal procidentia) has been described for centuries and is defined by the circumferential full-thickness protrusion of all layers of the rectum through the anal sphincter complex beyond the anal verge. Diagnosis can be made by physical exam and must be differentiated from prolapsing hemorrhoidal tissue. Rectal intussusception, also known as occult or internal prolapse, likewise involves all layers of the rectum infolding down into the anal canal but not beyond. Therefore, rectal intussusception is not visible on inspection. Partial-thickness prolapse, or mucosal prolapse, involves protrusion of a redundant layer of rectal or anal mucosa.

The reported incidence of rectal prolapse is low at 0.25%, with a clear predominance in elderly multiparous women suffering from long-standing constipation.[1] Although its pathophysiology is not well defined, rectal prolapse is associated with attenuation of the supportive tissues surrounding the rectum. Commonly, patients are noted to have a deep peritoneal cul-de-sac, weak pelvic floor and/or sphincter musculature, and rectal redundancy. Chronic straining during defecation as a result of anatomic or functional disorders of elimination has been implicated in the etiology. A higher incidence of psychiatric disorders has been noted in patients with rectal prolapse compared to the general population.[2] Additionally, although rare, neurologic disease, connective tissue disorders, and schistosomiasis may contribute.[1]

A number of operations, from both perineal and transabdominal approaches, have been described for the treatment of rectal prolapse, alluding to the lack of an ideal procedure. A history of prior pelvic or perineal surgery increases operative risk and should be considered when determining surgical approach. Age, comorbid conditions, functional activity level, and fecal continence are also important components of decision-making for individualized treatment.

This chapter describes the clinical features, evaluation, common surgical repairs, recurrence, and outcomes of patients with rectal prolapse.

CLINICAL FEATURES

The majority of patients with rectal prolapse will present with a history of a mass protruding from the anus, or the feeling of "sitting on a ball." The prolapse is often triggered by an episode of straining during defecation, but in more severe cases can occur with prolonged standing or ambulation. The prolapsed tissue usually retracts on its own, but may require manual pressure to reduce and in more severe cases can become incarcerated. An acute rectal prolapse may present with ulceration, bleeding, incarceration, strangulation, or gangrene. Symptoms of chronic rectal prolapse include constipation, tenesmus, mucus discharge, bleeding, fecal incontinence, fecal staining, pruritus, and perianal skin excoriation due to chronic moisture. Intermittent severe pain may be present secondary to spasm of the levator ani muscles. A feeling of fullness in the pelvis or incomplete evacuation requiring splinting and positioning maneuvers to eliminate may indicate internal prolapse or other sequelae of pelvic floor dysfunction such as enterocele, cystocele, or rectocele.

Treatment should be tailored based on the physical severity as well as the psychological impact of rectal prolapse. A detailed history of bowel function is essential. Constipation, which is present in up to 70% of patients, increases the risk of recurrence.[1] It often precedes the onset of rectal prolapse by many years and may result from internal rectal intussusception leading to obstruction, pelvic floor dyssynergia, and colonic dysmotility. A thorough history may identify other causes of constipation and excessive straining, such as inadequate dietary fiber intake, sedentary lifestyle, medications, and medical conditions. Fecal incontinence can be found in the majority of patients and usually appears late in the course of rectal prolapse as a result of weakening of the anal sphincter muscles. If fecal incontinence is severe and associated with lack of anal squeeze on exam, the patient should be counselled regarding the risk of complete fecal incontinence following surgical correction of the prolapse. In such cases, creation of an ostomy should be discussed as an option.

EVALUATION

Physical Exam Findings

Patients often will present with digital photographs that allow for confirmation of the diagnosis. Otherwise, if not apparent during external exam, the prolapse can often be elicited in the office by having the patient bear down in a squatting position on the commode. Administration of a fleet enema can help protrude the prolapsed rectum. It is important to make the distinction between rectal prolapse and prolapsing internal hemorrhoids, which may mimic the appearance of rectal prolapse on physical exam. The telescopic protrusion of a single long tube with concentric mucosal folds is diagnostic of rectal prolapse, whereas prolapsing hemorrhoids will appear as separate bundles of tissue with radial invaginations (Fig. 59.1).

An anorectal exam should be performed in the prone jackknife position or lateral Sims position if the patient is unable to kneel. In the absence of grossly visible prolapse, a patulous anus, fecal smearing, and lichenification of the anoderm due to chronic perineal moisture are suggestive of rectal or mucosal prolapse. Scars due to previous perineal surgery should be noted. A digital rectal exam is crucial to assess for masses, evaluate for enterocele, cystocele, and rectocele and to determine the adequacy of anal sphincter tone.

Diagnostic Studies

Visualization of full-thickness prolapse with the presence of circumferential mucosal folds via patient photographs, or physical exam, is diagnostic of rectal prolapse. If protrusion of the rectum is not clinically evident, defecography can be useful in making the diagnosis. Defecography, using either traditional fluoroscopy or dynamic magnetic resonance imaging, can demonstrate rectal prolapse as well as outlet obstruction and is useful to assess pelvic floor function.

It is important to exclude mucosal pathologies such as rectal cancer, polyps, or a solitary rectal ulcer, which may act as lead points for rectal prolapse. Therefore, a full colonoscopy should be performed for all patients to rule out mucosal abnormalities as well as to evaluate for synchronous tumors. If a history of severe constipation is elicited, a nuclear gastrointestinal (GI) transit study should be obtained to rule out GI motility disorders. Patients with slow colonic transit may benefit from colonic resection in conjunction with rectopexy.

We do not routinely perform anorectal manometry for patients with rectal prolapse, but do provide all patients with instructions for anal sphincter strengthening exercises after surgical repair. All patients should be followed postoperatively to determine the need for any further treatment if fecal incontinence persists despite a 6-month or longer course of dietary measures and regular sphincter strengthening exercises.

COMMON SURGICAL REPAIRS

A wide variety of surgical repairs have been described for rectal prolapse, underscoring the lack of an ideal procedure. Operative techniques are traditionally divided by approach: perineal or transabdominal. The two main perineal procedures are the Delorme procedure and the Altemeier procedure (perineal rectosigmoidectomy).

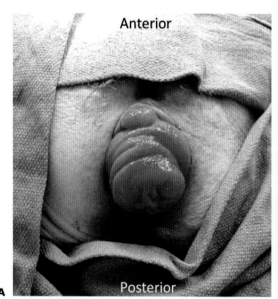
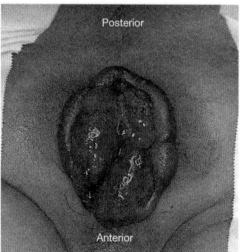

FIGURE 59.1 Rectal prolapse verses prolapsing internal hemorrhoids. **A:** Rectal prolapse is characterized by a tube of prolapsing tissue with visualization of concentric folds (patient is supine in candy canes). **B:** Separate bulges of tissue with radial folds represent prolapsed internal hemorrhoids (patient is in prone jackknife position). (Reprinted from Mulholland MW, Albo D, Dalman R, et al, eds. *Operative techniques in surgery.* Philadelphia: Wolters Kluwer, 2015.)

Mucosal prolapse and short segment full-thickness prolapse can be managed by the Delorme procedure, whereas the Altemeier procedure can be used for any degree of protrusion. Perineal stapled prolapse resection (PSPR) is a relatively new perineal procedure. Transabdominal repair can be completed via laparotomy, laparoscopy, or robotic technique and consists of fixation of the rectum in its normal anatomic position with or without colonic resection.

The first procedures described for rectal prolapse were performed via a perineal approach. With its introduction in 1955, transabdominal repair became the standard of care for patients who could tolerate laparotomy. Those who could not (frail, older adults) underwent perineal repair. The advent of laparoscopy and robotic surgery allowed for avoidance of the trauma of a laparotomy, thereby reducing surgical stress and allowing for more rapid recovery. Determination of operative approach should take into account patient age, comorbid conditions, previous abdominal or perineal operations, risk of recurrence, presence of fecal incontinence or constipation, and presence or absence of incarceration.

Perineal Approach

The ability to perform perineal repairs under local, spinal, or general anesthesia allows these procedures to be tailored according to anesthetic risk and is the reason this approach has historically been chosen for frail elderly patients with comorbidities. In addition, a perineal repair is a useful alternative to a transabdominal procedure in patients with a hostile abdomen.

Complications after perineal repairs are related to the coloanal anastomosis in the majority of cases and include bleeding, anastomotic leak/dehiscence, pelvic abscess, and stricture.

Anal encirclement

The Thiersch procedure, or anal encirclement, is reserved for extremely frail patients with limited life expectancy or prohibitive risk for anesthetic complications. First described in 1891, the Thiersch procedure involves manually reducing the prolapse, followed by narrowing of the anal canal by circumferential placement of suture, synthetic mesh, or even vascular graft. This procedure provides a mechanical barrier to further descent but does not eradicate existing prolapse and has the potential for serious morbidity including fecal impaction, erosion of the material, or pelvic sepsis.[3] When performing this procedure, it is important to place a dilator or finger in the anal canal while tying the stitch/securing the material so that stenosis and fecal impaction are avoided.

Mucosal sleeve resection (Delorme)

First described in 1900 by Delorme, a mucosal sleeve resection is a good option for patients with mucosal prolapse or minor full-thickness prolapse. A partial-thickness circumferential incision is made through the mucosa 1 to 2 cm proximal to the dentate line. The mucosa is then dissected free from the underlying muscularis to the level of the apex of the protruding bowel. The cylinder of mucosa is then excised, the denuded muscle is plicated longitudinally, and the mucosa is reapproximated.

Perineal rectosigmoidectomy (Altemeier procedure)

Although first performed in 1889 by Jan Mikulicz-Radeski, the perineal rectosigmoidectomy was popularized in the 1970s by Altemeier. Today, it is the procedure of choice for patients who cannot tolerate general anesthesia.

After applying gentle traction to completely evert the prolapse, the bowel is marked circumferentially and incised anteriorly 1 to 2 cm proximal to the dentate line (Fig. 59.2A–F). Once the inner layer of intussuscepted bowel is identified, the outer full-thickness incision is extended circumferentially, including division of the mesorectum posteriorly (Fig. 59.2G–I). The bowel is progressively exteriorized through the anus until no more redundancy exists, then resected and anastomosed to the remnant anorectum (Fig. 59.2J,K). The anastomosis can be performed either handsewn or by using a circular stapler with similar clinical and long-term functional outcomes.

Levatorplasty is often performed prior to the anastomosis as a modification to the Altemeier procedure. This involves plication of either anterior or posterior levator muscles and is associated with decreased recurrence and reduction in postoperative fecal incontinence by decreasing the pelvic outlet aperture. Posterior levatorplasty is preferred due to the increased incidence of dyspareunia associated with anterior levatorplasty.[4] To reduce the risk of outlet dysfunction, care should be taken to avoid excessive compression of the rectum during levatorplasty.

Perineal stapled prolapse resection

A relatively new procedure, the PSPR was first introduced in 2008 as an alternative to the perineal rectosigmoidectomy.[5] Although comparable to the Altemeier procedure in terms of prolapse resection, the PSPR does not allow access to the pelvic floor musculature. The operation begins by dividing the prolapsed bowel laterally with a linear stapler ending 2 cm from the dentate line. The linear stapler (a curved cutting stapler may also be used) is then inserted into the prolapsed rectum, and a resection line is created parallel to the dentate line with repeated firings circumferentially. The inability to address pelvic floor weakness may contribute to postoperative fecal incontinence

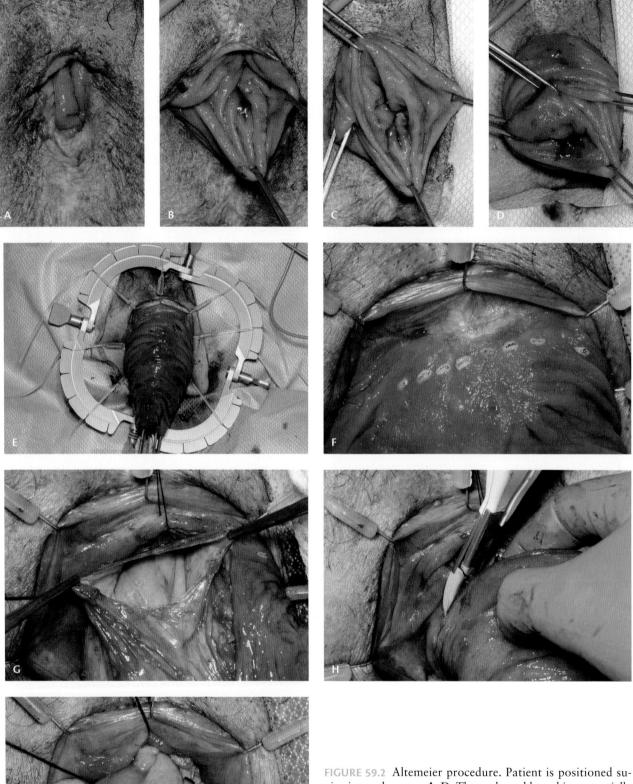

FIGURE 59.2 Altemeier procedure. Patient is positioned supine in candy canes. **A–D:** The prolapsed bowel is sequentially everted by applying gentle traction. **E:** A Lone Star retractor is placed after completely everting the prolapse. **F:** The bowel is marked circumferentially 1 to 2 cm proximal to the dentate line using electrocautery. **G:** A full-thickness incision is made in the anterior aspect of the prolapsed bowel to allow identification of the intussusceptum (inner bowel layer). **H:** The outer layer of bowel is transected circumferentially, including ligation of the mesorectum (**I**). *(Continued)*

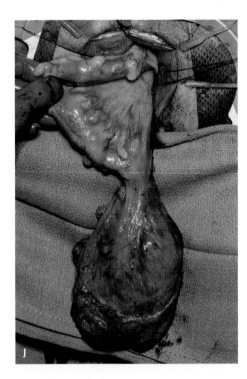

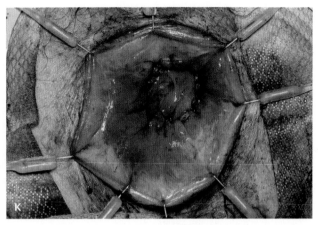

FIGURE 59.2 *(Continued)* **J**: Any additional redundancy is exteriorized. **K**: After division of the bowel, a handsewn coloanal anastomosis is performed.

and recurrent prolapse. However, recurrence rates after PSPR are comparable to those of other perineal procedures, and the technical simplicity of this procedure lends to decreased operative times.[6]

Transabdominal Approach

Repair of rectal prolapse via an open, laparoscopic, or robotic technique requires general anesthesia and is associated with the risk of future bowel obstruction secondary to adhesive disease. Various modifications of the transabdominal approach have been described, allowing for patient factors as well as surgeon preference to play a role. The goal of the described procedures is to adequately mobilize the rectum to the level of the pelvic floor musculature. Division of the lateral stalks during mobilization of the rectum has been shown to be associated with decreased prolapse recurrence but increased rates of postoperative constipation.[7] Resection should be considered when the patient is found to have very redundant sigmoid colon in the setting of severe underlying constipation. When resection rectopexy is performed, additional risks of anastomotic leak, abdominal sepsis, and anastomotic stricture must be considered. If mesh is used, there is added risk of mesh erosion, infection, and fistula formation.

Suture rectopexy

Transabdominal rectopexy involves mobilization and fixation of the rectum to the sacral promontory. Once the rectum is mobilized circumferentially, the prolapse

should be completely reduced by retracting the rectosigmoid junction cephalad. The rectal mesentery is fixated posteriorly to the presacral fascia at the level of the sacral promontory such that the rectum maintains a gentle curve as it lies in the pelvis, neither completely against the pelvic floor nor bowstringed. Fixation of the rectum can be done with suture, absorbable tacks, or a combination of the two.

Resection rectopexy

Patients with severe constipation and significant colon redundancy should be considered for sigmoid resection in addition to rectopexy. After mobilization of the rectum, sigmoid, and descending colon, resection of redundant colon is performed. The bowel should be divided distally at the top of the rectum as defined by the splaying of the taeniae coli. The proximal transection point is decided where the proximal colon reaches the rectum without tension, in the position it will lie after rectopexy. After resection and anastomosis, rectopexy is performed as described earlier. If sutures are used for fixation, they can be placed and tagged following mobilization of the rectum and tied down after the resection is completed.

Sling rectopexy

Both posterior and anterior sling rectopexy procedures were first described in the 1950s. The posterior sling rectopexy again begins with mobilization of the rectum circumferentially to the level of the pelvic floor. Mesh or

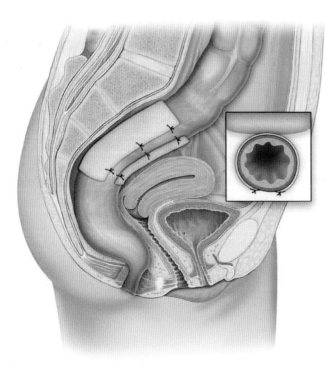

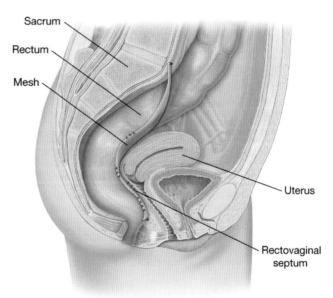

FIGURE 59.4 Ventral mesh rectopexy. Mesh is sutured along the anterior aspect of the rectum distally and fixated to the sacral promontory proximally. (Reprinted from Wexner SD, Fleshman JW. *Colon and rectal surgery: Abdominal operations*, 2nd ed. Philadelphia: Wolters Kluwer, 2018.)

FIGURE 59.3 Posterior mesh rectopexy. Mesh is wrapped posteriorly around the rectum and fixated anteriorly. *Inset* represents lateral view demonstrating incomplete cylinder of mesh anteriorly. (Reprinted from Wexner SD, Fleshman JW. *Colon and rectal surgery: Abdominal operations*. Philadelphia: Wolters Kluwer, 2011.)

polyvinyl alcohol sponge is placed posterior to the rectum and sutured at the midpoint to the presacral fascia. After straightening the rectum with cephalad retraction, the lateral ends of the mesh are wrapped around the rectum and fixated anteriorly. The mesh should create an incomplete cylinder around the rectum to avoid outlet obstruction (Fig. 59.3). The mesh is then excluded from the abdominal cavity by covering it with and securing the peritoneal fold. Anterior sling rectopexy (Ripstein procedure) has largely been abandoned due to significant risk of postoperative morbidity as well as its association with increased constipation and fecal impaction.[3]

Anterior (ventral) rectopexy

Now recognized as the anterior, or ventral rectopexy, D'Hoore et al.[8] first described a modification of the Orr-Loygue lateral mesh rectopexy in 2004. The current technique involves full mobilization of the rectum anteriorly and a limited posterior dissection only for exposure of the sacral promontory. A nonabsorbable mesh is then sutured distally along the anterior aspect of the rectum and proximally to the sacral promontory (Fig. 59.4). As with the sling rectopexy, the peritoneum is then closed over the mesh. A robotic approach may be

used to facilitate this technically demanding operation. The pelvic floor support to the rectovaginal septum potentially allows for simultaneous correction of associated genital prolapse, rectocele, and enterocele without requiring additional procedures. Another potential advantage is decreased risk of autonomic nerve injury due to the limited posterior dissection and avoidance of lateral mobilization of the rectum. The incidence of mesh-related complications, including erosion in the vagina, is low at 0% to 4.6%.[9]

RECURRENCE

Overall recurrence rates of rectal prolapse vary widely with a range of 4% to 30% following modern techniques for repair. The PROSPER trial, which was designed to evaluate recurrence rates between abdominal and perineal operations, demonstrated no significant difference in recurrence between the groups. However, due to revised patient recruitment, the study was not sufficiently powered to make this comparison.[10] Although not included in the PROSPER trial, anterior rectopexy has since been shown to have low long-term recurrence rates of 2.8% to 12.5%,[9,11] similar to other minimally invasive transabdominal repairs.

The diagnostic approach for primary rectal prolapse should again be followed for workup of recurrence with special attention to evaluate for causes of constipation, presence of pelvic floor dysfunction, and/or colorectal abnormalities.[12] There is currently no unified treatment algorithm for recurrent rectal prolapse due to the variety of surgical techniques and low level of evidence in heterogeneous studies.[13] Recurrence after rectopexy alone can be managed with repeat rectopexy with or without resection. If recurrence occurs after a previous resection, further repair must take into consideration the vascular supply of the remaining bowel. For example, a repeat perineal procedure may be performed,[14] but a sigmoid resection should be avoided in patients with previous perineal repair as blood flow to the remnant rectal segment may become compromised. Conversely, if the original procedure was a resection rectopexy, a subsequent perineal rectosigmoidectomy should only be performed if the surgeon is confident that the initial anastomosis will be included in the resection in order to avoid leaving a devascularized segment.[3] Recurrence after mesh placement may require more extensive rectal dissection and resection combined with rectopexy. It is important not to attempt removal of the mesh, as this maneuver would risk bowel injury or perforation.

Patients who recur after initial repair of rectal prolapse are at even higher risk for recurrence following subsequent procedures.[14] When planning an operation to address re-recurrence of rectal prolapse, it is especially important to adequately assess vascular supply. As with primary repair, perineal procedures for recurrent rectal prolapse have an increased risk of re-recurrence. The option of a colostomy should be discussed after multiple failures.

OUTCOMES

Long-term outcomes and recurrence rates after rectal prolapse repair have improved with modern techniques in both perineal and transabdominal procedures. Minimally invasive transabdominal repair has become the preferred approach for most patients with full-thickness rectal prolapse due to decreased recurrence rates and improved functional outcomes when compared to perineal procedures. However, most studies do not directly compare transabdominal and perineal procedures, and traditionally, patients who underwent perineal repair were older with higher number and severity of comorbidities.[13] The advent of minimally invasive techniques has increased the tolerability of transabdominal repair in a greater proportion of older, high-risk patients.

Due to the rarity of this disease, coupled with the high a number of described variations for repair, there is a paucity of evidence to suggest superiority of any one transabdominal procedure. This was highlighted in the 2000 Cochrane review as well as the 2008 update.[15] Furthermore, restoration of continence is underreported and often unpredictable with a wide range of functional outcomes.

CONCLUSION

Although a rare entity, rectal prolapse can be severely debilitating. Surgical correction is the treatment of choice. The objective of surgical treatment for full-thickness rectal prolapse is to correct the anatomic abnormality, thereby improving symptoms, with an acceptable rate of recurrence and low risk of complications.

References

1. Gallo G, Martelluci J, Pellino G, et al. Consensus statement of the Italian Society of Colorectal Surgery (SICCR): Management and treatment of complete rectal prolapse. *Tech Coloproctol* 2018;22(12):919–931.
2. Hardiman K. Operative treatment of rectal prolapse: Transabdominal approach. In: Mulholland MW, Albo D, Dalman R, et al, eds. *Operative techniques in surgery.* Philadelphia: Wolters Kluwer, 2015:1339–1348.
3. Dwyer CM, Maun DC. Pelvic floor conditions: Rectal prolapse/recurrence. In: Steele SR, Maykel JA, Wexner SD, eds. *Clinical decision making in colorectal surgery*, 2nd ed. Switzerland: Springer, 2020:219–227.
4. Bauer V. Operative treatment of rectal prolapse: Perineal approach (Altemeier and modified Delorme procedures). In: Mulholland MW, Albo D, Dalman R, et al, eds. *Operative techniques in surgery.* Philadelphia: Wolters Kluwer, 2015:1332–1338.
5. Scherer R, Marti L, Hetzer F, et al. Perineal stapled prolapse resection: A new procedure for external rectal prolapse. *Dis Colon Rectum* 2008;51(11):1727–1730.
6. Fan K, Cao A, Barto W, et al. Perineal stapled prolapse resection for external rectal prolapse: a systematic review and meta-analysis. *Colorectal Dis* 2020;22(12):1850–1861.
7. Tou S, Brown SR, Nelson RL. Surgery for complete (full-thickness) rectal prolapse in adults. *Cochrane Database Syst Rev* 2015;(11):CD001758.
8. D'Hoore A, Cadoni R, Penninckx F, et al. Long-term outcome of laparoscopic ventral rectopexy for total rectal prolapse. *Br J Surg* 2004;91(11):1500–1505.
9. Postillon A, Perrenot C, Germain A, et al. Long-term outcomes of robotic ventral mesh rectopexy for external rectal prolapse. *Surg Endosc* 2020;34:930–939.
10. Senapati A, Gray RG, Middleton LJ, et al. PROSPER: A randomised comparison of surgical treatments for rectal prolapse. *Colorectal Dis* 2013;15(7):858–868.
11. Emile SH, Elfeki H, Shalaby M, et al. Outcome of laparoscopic ventral mesh rectopexy for full-thickness external rectal prolapse: A systematic review, meta-analysis, and meta-regression analysis of the predictors for recurrence. *Surg Endosc* 2019;33(8):2444–2455.
12. Hrabe J, Gurland B. Optimizing treatment for rectal prolapse. *Clin Colon Rectal Surg* 2016;29(3):271–276.
13. Hotouras A, Ribas Y, Zakeri S, et al. A systematic review of the literature on the surgical management of recurrent rectal prolapse. *Colorectal Dis* 2015;17(8):657–664.
14. Ding JH, Canedo J, Lee SH, et al. Perineal rectosigmoidectomy for primary and recurrent rectal prolapse: Are the results comparable the second time? *Dis Colon Rectum* 2012;55(6):666–670.
15. Tou S, Brown SR, Malik AI, et al. Surgery for complete rectal prolapse in adults. *Cochrane Database Syst Rev* 2008;8(4):CD001758.

Urogenital Conditions

CHAPTER 60

COSMETIC GYNECOLOGY

Bobby Garcia • Robert D. Moore • John R. Miklos

Introduction

Cosmetic gynecology (also referred to as female genital plastic and cosmetic surgery) has garnered substantial attention and notoriety in recent years. Much of the controversy in this field can be distilled into three points. There is a concern that cosmetic gynecology procedures encourage or even pressure patients into either achieving or fitting an anatomic ideal. Critics also point to an ambiguous nomenclature, a relative paucity of data, and express concern that the quality of literature is flawed or biased. Finally, as these are elective nonmedically indicated procedures, they are generally not covered by insurance and offered on a fee-for-service model. These are valid criticisms, and although the detailed discussion necessary to adequately address each point is beyond the scope of this chapter, we hope that the evidence presented here will begin to allay some of these concerns. Despite these caveats, patient requests for cosmetic gynecology procedures are increasing dramatically with practitioners from multiple specialties offering these interventions. Between 2014 and 2018, there was a 50% increase in the number of labiaplasty procedures performed in the United States.[1] At its foundation, cosmetic gynecology is an extension of female pelvic medicine and reconstructive surgery in the same way as cosmetic surgery is subspecialty of plastic and reconstructive surgery.

In order to address the growing interest and lingering ambiguity in this subspecialty of urogynecology, the International Urogynecological Association (IUGA) and American Urogynecologic Society (AUGS) convened a joint working group to establish standardized terminology classification systems (Table 60.1) and adverse event metrics for cosmetic gynecology.[2] In addition to reviewing the information in that document, this chapter expands on the surgical techniques for each procedure.

The boundaries of cosmetic gynecology must be clearly delineated to distinguish it from either medically necessary procedures or female genital mutilation (FGM). Preoperative counseling and assessment will then be considered followed by a focused discussion on procedures of the labia majora, labia minora, clitoris, and vagina. Additionally, energy-based therapies, a new and promising treatment modality in aesthetic gynecology, is briefly surveyed. Procedures on the mons pubis are not covered in this text.

TERMINOLOGY AND SCOPE

Concomitant with development of this chapter, the American Urogynecologic Society (AUGS) and International Urogynecological Association (IUGA) developed a Joint Report on Terminology for Cosmetic Gynecology.[2] This document expands upon the terminology surveyed in this chapter along with including staging systems and an adverse event reporting scale.

Cosmetic gynecology encompasses interventions to the mons pubis, labia majora, labia minora, clitoris, and vagina. **Cosmetic gynecology can be defined as elective interventions to alter the aesthetic appearance of the external genitalia or modify the genital organs or elective functional vaginal procedures (in the absence of pathology) with the goal of improving a person's quality of life.** This definition is left intentionally broad as it is meant to include purely aesthetic procedures in addition to those that are intended to improve function. Specifically, this is in reference to vaginal tightening (either surgically or with an energy-based device [EBD]) and injections into the clitoris and anterior vaginal wall with the intent of improving sexual function. Traditionally, these interventions have been considered within the umbrella of cosmetic gynecology, and furthermore, they should be considered only in the absence of medical pathology. For example, a 66-year-old gravida 4 patient who presents with a stage III Pelvic Organ Prolapse Quantification (POP-Q) and a genital hiatus (GH) of 5 cm has a medical pathology and should be counseled on appropriate treatment options. Similarly, a woman with dyspareunia and biopsy documented endometriosis also should be offered medically indicated counseling and treatment. In both scenarios, a cosmetic gynecology procedure should not be offered as it would neither be beneficial nor indicated. To qualify this, there are some scenarios in which a woman with POP requests surgical correction for her medical condition in addition to concomitant surgical vaginal tightening; however, these should be considered as separate entities. Alternatively, if a patient presents without medically

TABLE 60.1

Cosmetic Gynecology Terminology

ANATOMIC REGION	THERAPEUTIC DESCRIPTOR[a]	THERAPEUTIC APPROACH[b]	RECOMMENDED PATIENT-CENTERED SYNONYMS	ALTERNATE SYNONYMS
Labia minora	Reduction	Surgical	Labiaplasty	Labiaplasty nymphoplasty
Clitoral frenulum	Reduction	Surgical	Frenulectomy	
Clitoral prepuce	Reduction	Surgical	Clitoral hood lift	Clitoridotomy Hoodectomy Clitoral hood resection
Clitoral	Amplification	Filler	Clitoral amplification	Platelet-rich plasma injection O-Shot
Labia majora	Augmentation	Filler	Labia majora augmentation	
Labia majora	Reduction	Surgical	Labia majoraplasty	
Labia majora	Tightening	Energy based	Labia majoraplasty	
Vaginal	Reduction	Surgical	Vaginal tightening	Vaginal rejuvenation Vagina revitalization Vaginoplasty Colpoperineoplasty
Vaginal	Tightening	Energy based	Vaginal tightening	Vaginal rejuvenating Vaginal revitalization Vaginoplasty
Vaginal	Augmentation	Filler	Vaginal augmentation	O-Shot G-Shot G-spot amplification Platelet-rich plasma injection Hyaluronic acid injection
Mons pubis	Reduction	Surgical	Monsplasty	Monspexy
Mons pubis	Reduction	Lipectomy	Monsplasty	
Mons pubis	Tightening	Energy based	Monsplasty	
Genital	Depigmentation	Energy based	Genital brightening	
Genital	Depigmentation	Topical	Genital brightening	Genital bleaching Anal bleaching

[a]Therapeutic descriptors: reduction, augmentation, amplification, tightening, depigmentation.
[b]Therapeutic approaches: S, surgical; E, energy-based therapy; L, lipectomy (liposuction); F, filler; T, topical.

significant pelvic organ prolapse (POP) on POP-Q or a diagnosis of sexual dysfunction and is requesting a procedure to narrow the vaginal caliber, this would be considered a cosmetic gynecology procedure.

There have been parallels drawn between cosmetic gynecology and FGM, so a sharp distinction should be made. FGM is defined by the World Health Organization as "all procedures involving partial or total removal of the external female genitalia or other injury to the female genital organs for non-medical reasons."[3] This is further classified into four types:

Type I: Partial or total removal of the clitoris and/or the prepuce (clitoridectomy).

Type II: Partial or total removal of the clitoris and the labia minora, with or without excision of the labia majora (excision).

Type III: Narrowing of the vaginal orifice with creation of a covering seal by cutting and appositioning the labia minora and/or the labia majora, with or without excision of the clitoris (infibulation).

Type IV: All other harmful procedures to the female genitalia for non-medical purposes for example: pricking, piercing, incising, scraping, and cauterization.[3]

The difference between FGM and cosmetic gynecology centers around both intent and patient autonomy

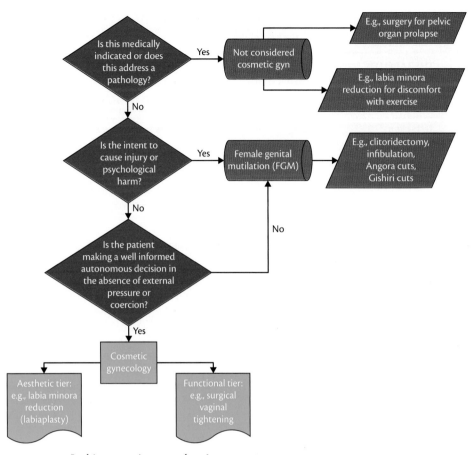

FIGURE 60.1 Is this cosmetic gynecology?

(Fig. 60.1). In FGM, procedures may be performed on children or young women without their consent in order to exert control over them or in an attempt to cause either physical or psychological harm. In cosmetic gynecology, procedures on the other hand, the patient makes the decision to proceed with intervention to improve her overall quality of life.

PREOPERATIVE CONSIDERATIONS

On consultation, a thorough history should be obtained in order to understand the patient's motivators for pursuing surgery. Why does she feel that she needs cosmetic surgery? It is of the utmost importance that she is making this decision voluntarily and without undue influence or coercion from either family members or the provider. Counseling on the wide spectrum of normal anatomic variants can help to allay concerns many patients may have about their bodies. All patients should be screened for body dysmorphic disorder (BDD) and referred for additional care as indicated. The Cosmetic Procedure Screening Scale (COPS) is a validated 9-item survey that can be used to help identify patients with BDD. Each question is scored from 0 to 8 with total ranges from 0 to 72 with scores greater than 40 suggesting possible BDD.[4] A version of this, the COPS-L, has also been validated for patients seeking labia minora reduction.[5] Additionally, the Genital Appearance

Satisfaction (GAS) scale is a validated 11-item questionnaire that assesses a subject's perception of her anatomy. On a scale of 0 to 33, higher scores suggest greater dissatisfaction (Table 60.2).[6]

During the physical examination, she should be evaluated for medical conditions such as POP, lichen sclerosus, or genitourinary syndrome of menopause (GSM), which could be contributing to some of her symptoms. In order to avoid any misunderstanding, offer the patient a hand mirror and allow her to point to any area of concern and describe how she would like this altered. If the patient is amenable, medical photographs both in lithotomy and in the standing-dependent position can help to both document and understand patient concerns. After the exam, her anatomy should be reviewed on a female pelvic anatomy illustration along with discussion of any potential interventions. Is the proposed intervention feasible and will it result in the desired outcome for the patient? A similar understanding of postoperative expectations between physician and provider is paramount.

OUTCOME METRICS

One of the most common criticisms of cosmetic gynecology is a lack of safety and efficacy data. A systematic review evaluating the peer-reviewed literature on cosmetic gynecology found that there are multiple metrics used to assess results; however, they are highly variable and

TABLE 60.2				
Genital Appearance Satisfaction Scale				
ITEM	**NEVER**	**SOMETIMES**	**OFTEN**	**ALWAYS**
1. I feel that my genitals are normal in appearance.	3	2	1	0
2. I feel that my genitals are unattractive in appearance.	0	1	2	3
3. I feel that my labia are too large.	0	1	2	3
4. I am satisfied with the appearance of my genitals.	3	2	1	0
5. I experience irritation to my labia when exercising/walking.	0	1	2	3
6. I feel, or have felt, conscious in sexual situations because of the appearance of my genitals.	0	1	2	3
7. Embarrassment about the appearance of my genitals spoils my enjoyment of sex.	0	1	2	3
8. I feel discomfort around my genitals when I wear tight clothes.	0	1	2	3
9. I feel that my genital area is visible under tight clothes.	0	1	2	3
10. I worry about the appearance of my vaginal area.	0	1	2	3
11. I feel that my genital area looks asymmetric or lopsided.	0	1	2	3

NOTE: Add all responses with total scores ranging from 0 to 33, with higher scores indicating greater dissatisfaction.
From Bramwell R, Morland C. Genital appearance satisfaction in women: The development of a questionnaire and exploration of correlates. *J Reprod Infant Psychol* 2009;27(1):15–27. doi:10.1080/02646830701759793. Copyright © 2009 Society for Reproductive and Infant Psychology, reprinted by permission of Taylor & Francis (http://www.tandfonline.com) on behalf of Society for Reproductive and Infant Psychology.

not standardized.[7] Aesthetic outcome measures can be grouped into either objective or subjective. Establishing the former is nearly impossible unless a precise anatomic metric is stipulated. For example, a sample metric could be that a labia minora reduction procedure is successful if the minora do not extend past the majora. Although these definitions can be constructed to illustrate that a procedure is successful, it does so at the expense of defining an anatomic ideal. Establishing these definitions may unduly suggest that anyone who does not meet these criteria is not normal. It should be clearly stated that in the absence of medical pathology or physical discomfort, there is no anatomic ideal for the female genitalia, and there is a wide physiologic range in the population.

A separate albeit less defined objective approach is to use photography with blinded evaluators asked to rate preoperative and postoperative photos. Although this can illustrate evidence of improved cosmesis (in the opinion of reviewers), it carries little weight if the patient is not satisfied. This leads us to patient-driven outcomes such as numeric satisfaction scales, such as the GAS described earlier which can be used both to screen patients for BDD or determine efficacy after treatment.[5] This is a good option for evaluating women who are interested in labia minora reduction. Alternatively, the Patient Global Impression of Improvement (PGI-I) is a 7-point scale that asks patients how their condition has changed since the intervention and varies from very much worse (1), through no change (4), and to very much better (7).[8] The PGI-I can be applied to any patient procedure and is well suited to cosmetic interventions to gauge patient satisfaction.

For patients requesting a vaginal tightening procedure, many sexual function questionnaires have been used such as the Female Sexual Function Index (FSFI) or the Pelvic Organ Prolapse Urinary Incontinence Sexual Questionnaire Short Form (PISQ-12). It should be noted that although improvement in many domains of these questionnaires has been shown postoperatively, they are not specifically designed to measure improvements in vaginal tightness. Vaginal laxity has been defined by an IUGA/International Continence Society joint terminology document as the "feeling of excessive vaginal looseness,"[9] and although nebulous, it truly encapsulates the condition. Given that the vagina is highly distensible and will stretch to accommodate large volumes, it is very challenging to develop objective measurements. A Brink score has been used as a proxy, but this is a much better indicator of pelvic muscular strength than resting vaginal tone. A more specific option may be the Vaginal Laxity Questionnaire (VLQ), which is a 7-point scale ranging from *very loose* to *very tight*. Along with this, the Sexual Satisfaction Questionnaire (SSQ) is a 6-point scale to assess sexual satisfaction from vaginal intercourse ranging from *none* to *excellent* (Tables 60.3 and 60.4).[10]

Ultimately for any aesthetic procedure, efficacy will ultimately be determined subjectively by the patient and results will vary substantially based on the skill and experience of the offering provider. That being said, a combination of objective and subjective outcome metrics may be employed to monitor results.

Equally important as outcome metrics, standardized reporting of complications in cosmetic gyn is paramount (Table 60.5). This table is adopted to suit cosmetic

TABLE 60.3

Vaginal Laxity Questionnaire

"How are you now (vaginal laxity/tightness) compared to before treatment?"

1	2	3	4	5	6	7
Very loose	Moderately loose	Slightly loose	Not tight or loose	Slightly tight	Moderately tight	Very tight

Reprinted from From Millheiser LS, Pauls RN, Herbst SJ, et al. Radiofrequency treatment of vaginal laxity after vaginal delivery: Nonsurgical vaginal tightening. *J Sex Med* 2010;7(9):3088–3095. doi:10.1111/j.1743-6109.2010.01910.x, with permission from Elsevier.

TABLE 60.4

Sexual Satisfaction Questionnaire

"How are you now (sexual satisfaction) compared to before treatment?"

0	1	2	3	4	5
None	Poor	Fair	Good	Very good	Excellent

Reprinted from Millheiser LS, Pauls RN, Herbst SJ, et al. Radiofrequency treatment of vaginal laxity after vaginal delivery: Nonsurgical vaginal tightening. *J Sex Med* 2010;7(9):3088–3095, with permission from Elsevier.

TABLE 60.5

Classification of Cosmetic Gynecology Revisions and Complications

GRADE	DEFINITION
Grade 0 (revision rate)	Surgical revision for aesthetic indication
Suffix "a"	Asymmetry, contour irregularities
Suffix "o"	Overcorrection
Suffix "u"	Undercorrection
Suffix "s"	Scarring
Grade I	Transient or minor complications not requiring significant medical intervention
Suffix "abx"	Antibiotics
Suffix "inj"	Injection
	Examples: urinary tract infection, steroid injection for pain, edema, seroma, superficial wound separation, granulation tissue
Grade II	Moderate complication requiring either prolonged or substantial medical intervention; any complication requiring hospitalization
Suffix "pt"	Physical therapy
Suffix "b"	Blood transfusion
	Examples: dyspareunia requiring pelvic floor physical therapy, blood transfusion for anemia, hospitalization for postoperation infection, deep venous thromboembolism
Grade III	Requiring surgical intervention for complication
	Examples: hematoma, hemorrhage, necrosis requiring resection
Grade IV	Life-threatening complication
Suffix "d"	Death of patient
	Examples: sepsis, myocardial infraction, organ failure
Grade NL	Complication profile not listed or clearly reported

gynecology procedures from the Clavien Dindo Scale, which was developed for more acute general surgical complications. Importantly, the Revision rate is defined as repeat surgical intervention for an aesthetic indication (such as inadequate or over resection). In contrast, the reoperation rate is any additional procedure needed to address a medical complication (such as bleeding or necrosis).[2]

ANATOMY (FIG. 60.2)

The mons pubis is a hair-bearing region that covers the pubic symphysis with a mound of adipose tissue. The vulva is composed of the labia majora, labia minora, clitoris, and clitoral prepuce (clitoral hood). The labia majora form the most lateral aspect of the vulva and converge anteriorly above the clitoral prepuce where they become contiguous with the mons pubis and travel posteriorly where they converge at the fourchette just anterior to the perineum. The distal tip of the clitoral glans is exposed with the rest covered by the clitoral prepuce or hood. The inferior border of the clitoral hood extends to the frenulum where the labia minora begins. Superior to the clitoris are the paired deep dorsal arteries and veins with the superficial dorsal vein superior to that. The dorsal nerves of the clitoris can be found coursing at the 11 and 1 o'clock positions just superior to the clitoral body. As they travel distally, multiple small nerve fibers branch out to innervate the glans.[11,12] Extending from the inferior aspect of the clitoris on either side is the frenulum of the clitoris, epithelial fronds, which enlarge to become the labia minora.

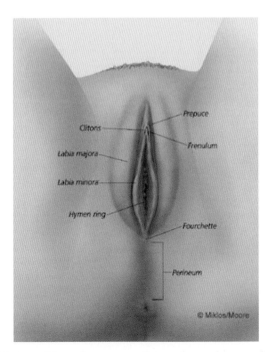

FIGURE 60.2 Normal anatomy of the vulva and external genitalia. (© John R. Miklos/Robert D. Moore.)

The labia minora are bilateral folds of keratinized squamous epithelium lying just medial to the labia majora and lateral to the vulvar vestibule. The hymen is a membranous vestige with remnants encircling the introitus.

LABIA MINORA REDUCTION (LABIAPLASTY)

Labia minora reduction surgery is one of the most commonly requested cosmetic gynecology procedures; however, this procedure is also performed for physical or functional discomfort as a medical procedure. Some of these functional symptoms may include discomfort in clothing, irritation during sports, or dyspareunia secondary to invagination of the labia minora.[13] In a survey of 131 patients undergoing labia minora reduction, the motivation for surgery was purely aesthetic in 37%, purely functional in 32%, and a combination in 31%.[14] Prior to the IUGA/AUGS terminology document, there was no well-accepted definition for elongation of the labia minora or *labia minora elongation*. This demarcation is significant as it distinguishes between an anatomic medical pathology and cosmetic desire. Of course, there are many instances in which there is overlap between pathology and cosmesis. Hodgkinson suggested that protrusion of the labia minora past the labia majora may be aesthetically displeasing.[15] Others have suggested intervention could be indicated at 3,[16] 4,[17] or 5 cm.[18] The IUGA/AUGS cosmetic terminology document defines labia minora elongation as any dimension at which the patient has functional discomfort and should be considered a medical pathology. In contrast, the desire to modify the labia minora in the absence of physical symptoms would be considered cosmetic. The term labia minora elongation is medically inaccurate and should not be used.[2]

There have been various descriptive staging systems to report the anatomy of the labia minora. The Franco classification is based on measurement of the medial aspect of the labia minora from the introitus to the most distal edge and is stratified into categories: type I (<2 cm), type II (2 to 4 cm), type III (4 to 6 cm), and type IV (>6 cm).[19] Conversely, the Motakef classification measures distance of protrusion beyond the labia majora on the lateral aspect of the labia minora: class I (0 to 2 cm), class II (2 to 4 cm), class III (>4 cm). It also includes annotations of "a" and "c" for asymmetry and involvement of the clitoral hood, respectively.[20] The classification system developed by the IUGA/AUGS Working Group incorporates aspects of both the Franco and Motakef staging. It also includes a Suffix "D" to report discomfort or functional impairment.[2] Extensive documentation of the dimensions and asymmetry of the labia minora preoperatively and postoperatively is essential.

Various surgical techniques have been introduced for labia minora reduction (Fig. 60.3). Selection of the appropriate technique will depend on the patient's anatomy,

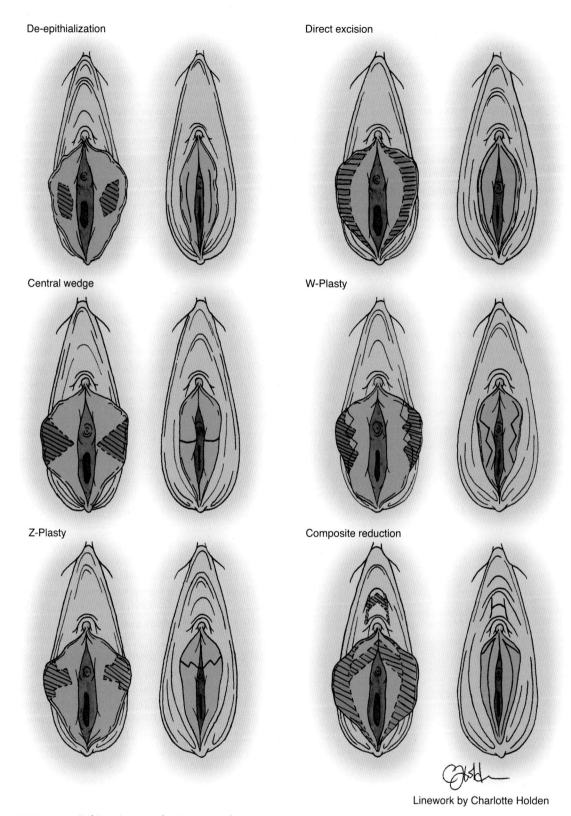

De-epithialization

Direct excision

Central wedge

W-Plasty

Z-Plasty

Composite reduction

Linework by Charlotte Holden

FIGURE 60.3 Labia minora reduction procedures.

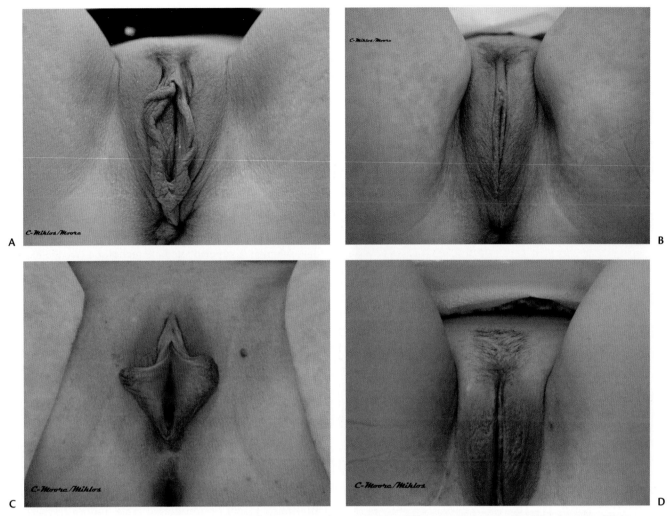

FIGURE 60.4 Linear contour or direct excision labia minora reduction in two different patients. Preop (**A**) and postop (**B**) images. Note for this patient how her anatomy with shorter but redundant labia minora folds would be best suited to this technique as opposed to the others illustrated in Figure 60.3. Preop (**C**) and postop (**D**) images. Pigmentation at the distal labia minora is excised postoperatively. If this coloration is desired, a wedge technique may be offered. (© John R. Miklos/Robert D. Moore.)

requested cosmetic outcome, and experience level of the surgeon. Regardless of technique, the amount of tissue removed should be discussed, illustrated to the patient, and agreed on preoperatively to prevent overresection or underresection. In the linear contour or direct excision (Fig. 60.4), the distal edge of the minora is resected in a curvilinear fashion. This can be accomplished with the use of an neodymium-doped yttrium aluminum garnet (Nd:YAG) contact laser[21] or a scalpel. In order to achieve a natural anatomic result, the tissue should be contoured meticulously, taking time to address the various skinfolds. Care should be taken not to "amputate" the minora in a straight line or apply a hemostat or clamp to the area to be excised, and this can lead to a suboptimal result.

A wedge resection (Fig. 60.5) is a good option if the patient prefers to keep the pigmented border on the distal edge of the labia minora. In a central wedge, a "V"-shaped mark is placed on the medial aspect of the labia minora with either a corresponding "V" or extended anterior and cephalad in a "hockey stick" formation which allows

concomitant removal of excess clitoral hood. The incision lines are closed in three layers with 5-0 monocryl.[22] With a posterior wedge on the other hand, complementary "V" incisions are generally made on the medial and lateral aspects. Preoperative marking is absolutely paramount in order to avoid irregularities and achieve symmetry as the tissue has a tendency to "roll." The use of 27 gauge needles to mark the incision site can help to maintain the correct plane during the initial incision.[23] Another technique to help operative planning involves taking a forceps at the midpoint of the labia minora and applying downward traction to the posterior fourchette. If excess skin laxity remains or if the tissue appears under too much tension, readjust the forceps anterior or posterior to determine the optimal resection.[16] A variation on the inferior wedge takes the form of a trapezoid with the long base drawn at the proximal aspect of the labia minora, the short base more distal, one leg forming the angle needed to rotate the superior flap toward the posterior fourchette, and the other leg demarcated as the labial edge.[24]

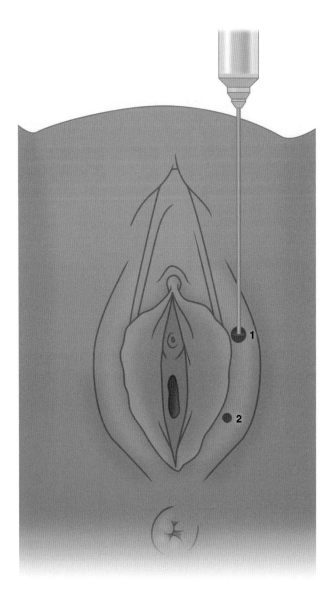

FIGURE 60.5 Wedge resection preoperative incision marking. Location and depth of resection (central vs. inferior) will depend on patient anatomy and desired result. (© John R. Miklos/Robert D. Moore.)

De-epithelialization can be used if the patient would like a more modest resection or if the labia minora are smaller and symmetric. This can be performed with "V"-shaped markings similar to the wedge; however, only the epithelium is denuded on the medial and lateral aspects leaving the underlying subcutaneous tissue which is then reapproximated with the dissected edges.[25] A variation of this involves resection of a coin-shaped area of epithelium in the central portion of the minora.

In a W-plasty offset, "W" incisions are made in the central portion of the labia minora at least a 1 cm away from the clitoris and posterior fourchette. Upon resection, the "peak and valley" tissue planes from the medial and lateral aspects of the minora are joined together with two layers of suture.[26] A Z-plasty can be thought of a modification of a central wedge wherein two "Z" lines are drawn

from a common point at the base of the minora and fanning outward to encompass the area to be resected.[27] The chief benefit of the W-plasty (and Z-Plasty) are that the nonlinear interdigitating suture lines are under less tension potentially less apt to tighten with scarring.

Although surgeons may have a preferred method of labial reduction, the ability to tailor the technique to the patient's unique anatomy and cosmetic request is paramount. Ellsworth described an algorithm for selecting the appropriate procedure based on the patient's Franco stage and desire to remove or retain the naturally pigmented edge of the labia minora. In patients with smaller labia minora a de-epithelialization was the preferred approach. With larger labia minora, the direct excision should be employed to remove the pigmented edge, whereas a superior pedicle technique (wedge excision) should be offered if this is desired.[28]

The reported complication rate for labia minora reduction is highly variable in the literature ranging from 0% to 25% with the severity Clavien-Dindo grades I to III.[7] These generally include bleeding, hematoma formation, infection, and wound breakdown. There is also a risk of postoperative pain and dyspareunia that although less common can occur, and patients should be thoroughly counseled about this before electing to proceed with surgery. This may be transient after the procedure and can be treated with a neuropathic agent such as a low-dose amitriptyline or gabapentin. Alternatively, an injection of anesthetic coupled with a corticosteroid (triamcinolone) can in some instances provide relief to patients. Overly aggressive resection can lead to absent or amputated labia minora (Fig. 60.6). For patients with overresection of the labia minora desiring reconstructive surgery, clitoral hood island flaps have been employed with success.[29]

Pending surgeon and patient preference, labia minora reduction may be performed in the outpatient clinic with local anesthetic and anxiolytics or under general anesthesia. Advantages of the latter option are that concomitant procedures may be performed, and it allows for the surgeon to proceed with a meticulous dissection that is often required to achieve the desired results. The incision site may be treated with antibiotic cream such as erythromycin to decrease the risk of postoperative infection.[25]

CLITORAL FRENULECTOMY AND CLITORAL PREPUCE (HOOD) REDUCTION

The clitoral frenulum extends inferiorly from either side of the glans clitoris and may join with the superior aspect of the labia minora. The prepuce of the clitoris or clitoral hood is the fold of skin that covers the superior and lateral aspects of the clitoral glans. Some patients may describe this tissue as redundant or bothersome on initial consultation, whereas others may just request a labia minora reduction. During counseling, the provider

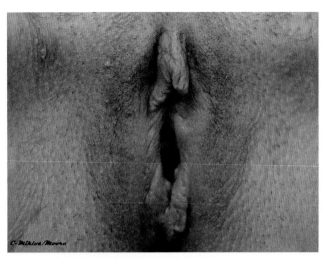
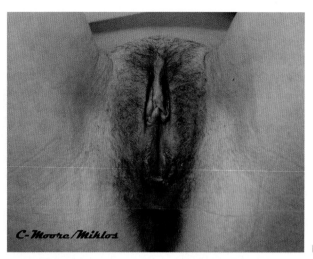

FIGURE 60.6 **A,B:** Overresection of the labia minora in two different patients. Complete amputation across the central portion of the labia with asymmetrical preservation at the fourchette and clitoral prepuce. (© John R. Miklos/Robert D. Moore.)

should convey that depending on the baseline anatomy and the degree of labia minora reduction requested, the end result could appear disproportionate if a concomitant prepuce reduction is not performed at the same time (Fig. 60.7). Additionally, a redundant prepuce may preclude the surgeon from obtaining a sufficient reduction of the labia minora. It is crucial to discuss this during the initial consultation to decrease the chance that a second surgery will be needed.

The composite reduction technique (see Fig. 60.3) simultaneously addresses both the labia minora and the clitoral hood. This is a complex procedure that involves a linear excision made down the length of the minora with the anteriormost edge preserved which functions as

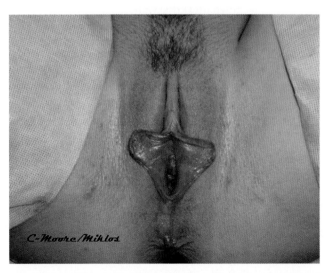

FIGURE 60.7 This patient has redundant tissue on the clitoral prepuce; however, it is in direct proportion to her labia minora, and she should be reassured that her anatomy is both physiologic and normal. If she did desire a cosmetic labia minora resection, she should be counseled that a concomitant clitoral prepuce reduction would prevent an asymmetric appearance postoperatively. (© John R. Miklos/Robert D. Moore.)

a pedicle flap. Triangular wedges of tissue anterior and posterior to the clitoris are removed, and the separated segments are joined with 5-0 Vicryl.[30] Alternatively, the labia minora and clitoris can be addressed separately during the same interaction. For example, if inferior wedge reduction is performed on the labia minora, then there may still be excess tissue from either the frenulum of the clitoris or the clitoral prepuce. A frenulectomy is performed similarly to a linear excision.

In a clitoral hood reduction, a triangular incision can be made on the prepuce superior to the glans clitoris. A clitoral hood reduction can also be performed by removing bilateral epithelial spheres on either side of the clitoris (Fig. 60.8). It is very important to remain superficial as these incisions may be very near to the dorsal nerves of the clitoris. Knowledge of the clitoral innervation and anatomy is crucial for anyone performing these procedures, and patients should be counseled that there is always a risk of nerve injury or pain postoperatively. These are elective cosmetic procedures, so patients must fully understand the anticipated risks and benefits in order to make a fully informed decision. Noting concerns about potential changes in sensitivity, Placik conducted a prospective study where he took pressure measurements of patients after labia minora reduction and clitoral hood reduction. He found there was either no change in sensitivity or an increase in sensitivity at all locations measured, and some patients reported an increase in the frequency of intercourse ($P = .011$) and orgasm frequency ($P = .013$).[31]

It should be clear that the procedures described earlier are specifically for aesthetic indications. Patients who undergo a frenulectomy or clitoral prepuce (hood) reduction may or may not experience an improvement in sexual function or orgasm; however, this should not be an indication for treatment or expected result. If a patient presents with symptoms of female sexual dysfunction (FSD), she should be worked up and treated

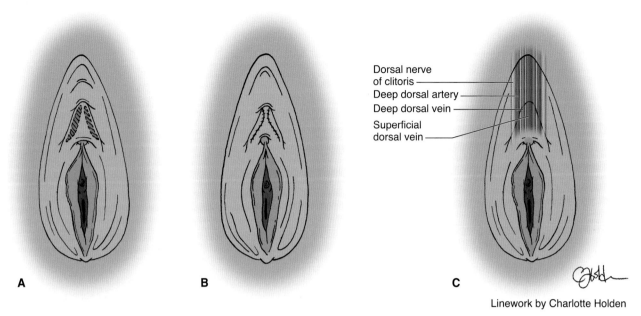

Dorsal nerve
of clitoris
Deep dorsal artery
Deep dorsal vein
Superficial
dorsal vein

A   B   C

Linework by Charlotte Holden

FIGURE 60.8 Clitoral hood reduction elliptical variant.

with appropriate medical management. Clitoral hood reduction and frenulectomy are only intended to address cosmesis.

LABIA MAJORA

In contrast to the labia minora, patients may either request labia majora augmentation or reduction. It is very important to rule out medical conditions during the history and physical exam. GSM, formerly described as vulvovaginal atrophy, is a constellation of signs and symptoms that may include genital dryness, decreased lubrication, vulvar pruritis, pallor, labia minora resorption, decreased elasticity, urinary symptoms, and dyspareunia.[32] If a patient presents with GSM, she should be treated with vaginal estrogen or medically as appropriate instead of offering a cosmetic procedure. Similarly, evaluation for lichen sclerosus or other dermatologic conditions should be ruled out during the initial physical exam.

Labia Majora Augmentation

When a patient is considering labia majora augmentation, it is crucial to understand her overall desired vulvar appearance with respect to her labia minora and entire body (Table 60.6). Is she requesting augmentation because she feels that her labia minora protrude or extend past the labia majora? If so, would she be better served by an isolated labia minora reduction? Or does she feel that her minora are too large and the labia majora are lacking fullness? Labia majora augmentation with de-epithelialized labia minora flaps could potentially address both aspects of the vulva. The epithelium from the protuberant distal ends of the labia minora are removed, leaving

a subcutaneous flap with a pedicle that can be tunneled into a precreated pocket in the labia majora. The subcutaneous tissue is temporarily held in place with stay sutures while the incisions on the labia minora are closed with delayed absorbable suture.[33] Fasciocutaneous flaps during a thigh lift[34] or dermal fat grafts from abdominoplasty[35] have also been described.

If there is no concern about the labia minora and the patient feels as though her labia majora have excess wrinkles or skin laxity (such as from weight loss), this can be addressed with either a biologic or nonbiologic filler. The most common biologic filler is adipose tissue as it is considered to be an ideal due to it being autologous, biocompatible, and easily able to integrate into the target tissue. One substantial limitation, however, is that once in the target tissue, there is a very large and unpredictable graft absorption rate. There are various techniques to harvest the adipose tissue such as vacuum-assisted or manual syringe aspiration (Coleman technique). Donor sites can be anywhere there is fat deposition such as the abdomen or inner thighs. In particular, if the patient has

TABLE 60.6
Labia Majora Classification
Stage 0: desires no alteration
Stage I: desires augmentation
Stage II: desires reduction. Distinguish between perceived skin laxity "L," an unwanted adipose tissue volume, or both

Suffixes:
   "A"—Asymmetry (specify larger side)
   "L"—Skin laxity as perceived bothersome by the patient

excess undesired adiposity on the mon pubis, this could be an ideal site as it will appear to enhance the effect of the transfer to the majora. Once obtained and prior to transfer, the graft should be processed via centrifugation or a similar method to filter out the fat from extraneous components such as blood.[36] Some authors will then combine the graft with platelet rich plasma (PRP), and injections can then be placed superficially superior lateral to the majora tracking downward. Injection volume is variable dependent on the anatomy, asymmetry, and desires of the patient but will range between 14 and 30 mL.[37] One author suggests up to 60 mL can be placed in each majora.[38]

Alternatively, nonbiologic fillers can be used to enhance the volume of the labia majora. Labia majora hypotrophy has been classified in three stages: mild, moderate, and severe, based on physical examination and symptoms experienced. Although this is helpful in the characterization of anatomy, this scale appears to have overlap with medical pathology such as GSM. A mixture of nonanimal hyaluronic acid (HA) with mannitol (to decrease degradation) can be used. The concentration of HA can vary between 19 and 21 mg/mL depending on initial anatomy and desired effect. Two-thirds of the injection are placed between the lip dartos and the fibrous tunic, with the remainder distributed in the subcutaneous tissue. Aspiration prior to injection should decrease the risk of intravascular injection. No more than 2 mL should be placed at a time, and if more is desired, the patient can return for repeat injections in 4 months.[39] Ecchymosis and erythema may be present immediately after the procedure, whereas nodules or capsule formation may occur if the area is overinjected. These nodules can be treated with injection of corticosteroids or hyaluronidase, or they may dissipate with time.[40] Providers must be familiar with the neurovascular supply of the vulva in addition to understanding potential complications of HA filler such as cutaneous or distant necrosis, herpes zoster reactivation, ischemia, granulomas, and infection. Hyaluronidase should be immediately available if needed. Finally, the provider should be aware if the HA is approved for gynecologic indication in their country or if it would be used off-label.

Labia Majora Reduction

In assessing a request for labia majora reduction, it is crucial to distinguish between excess unwanted adipose tissue, skin laxity, or a combination of the two. Along with this, did the patient have any recent weight gain or weight loss, such as from recent bariatric surgery? If there is still uncertain fluctuation in weight, it is best to defer labia majora reduction as this could affect the appearance of the vulva after the procedure. The next decision to consider is whether an energy-based or surgical approach is warranted given the patients' desired reduction and anatomy. Isolated lipectomy (liposuction) of the

labia majora is also an option, but there is a risk that this will result in skin laxity, so if adipose tissue is removed, a portion of epithelium should be resected as well.

For labia majora resection, either an elliptical or a bow-shaped incision (Fig. 60.9) should be placed medially and along the length of the labia majora with the goal of reapproximating the edges in or near the interlabial sulcus in order to minimize visualization of the resultant scar. If resection of a portion of the labial fat pad is indicated, this should be done carefully as this tissue is well vascularized. A multilayer closure with absorbable or delayed absorbable suture will help to ensure a tension-free closure.

VAGINAL CALIBER REDUCTION

Surgical vaginal caliber reduction is a broad term to describe elective nonmedically indicated procedures to narrow the diameter of the vagina based on patient request. Colloquially, this has been referred to as "vaginal rejuvenation"; however, this term is ambiguous and may refer to a procedure on the labia minora, an energy-based treatment on the genitalia, or a surgical procedure on the vagina depending on the context. As described earlier in the terminology section, procedures to address the vaginal caliber have traditionally fallen under the umbrella of cosmetic gynecology as there is no medical pathology (such as advanced POP) warranting intervention. At the same time, however, these are more appropriately described as functional as opposed to aesthetic procedures.

Herein another nuance arises surrounding overall intent, and this must be clearly parceled and delineated to offer the appropriate care to the patient. Why is the patient requesting a vaginal tightening procedure? The provider should establish that the patient is presenting of her own volition and without any undue coercion from a spouse or partner. A corollary to this is that the physician should never pressure a patient into a procedure or insinuate that her anatomy is abnormal or needs repair. The next consideration is ruling out a medical pathology. General contraindications include radiation therapy, fistula, lichen sclerosus, lichen planus, or genitourinary cancer. A history of chronic pelvic pain should also be considered a contraindication or at least a relative contraindication. In order to achieve a desired outcome with vaginal tightening, there can be considerable postoperative discomfort from muscle plication, and patients with a history of baseline pelvic pain are not ideal candidates for this procedure. If a patient presents with significant POP, she may desire surgical care to address this in addition to a vaginal tightening procedure either concomitantly or staged. The practitioner should be clear to distinguish these conditions to the patient as she may receive correction for her prolapse but still experience

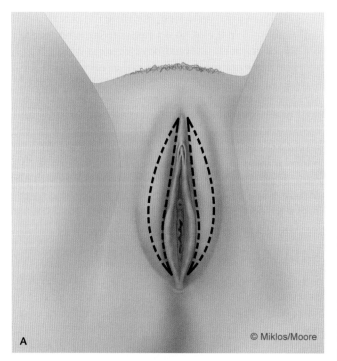

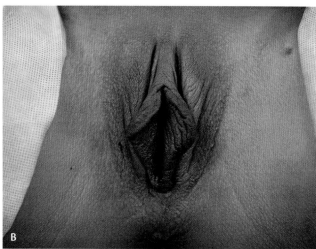

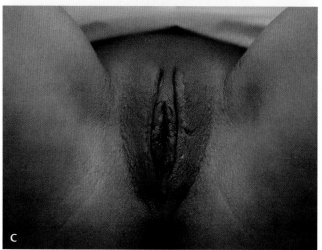

© Miklos/Moore

FIGURE 60.9 A: Elliptical incision lines on the medial aspect of the labia majora that will allow for both excision of skin and subcutaneous fat if desired. **B:** Preoperative photograph of patient desiring both a labia minora and labia majora reduction. **C:** Postoperative photograph showing a proportionate reduction of minora and majora. Note placement of majora reduction incision lines. (© John R. Miklos/Robert D. Moore.)

vaginal laxity. (A perineorrhaphy performed on the outlet at the conclusion of a POP surgery will decrease the measured GH and protect the repair; however, this is different from a vaginal tightening procedure and will not address vaginal laxity. Rather, it will result in an isolated narrowed outlet with the persistent feeling of looseness throughout the vaginal canal).

Additionally, the provider should screen for FSD. If she does exhibit symptoms of FSD, she should be treated through the appropriate medical avenues as opposed to undergoing an isolated tightening procedure. Vaginal caliber reduction should only be offered in a woman who presents complaining of vaginal laxity or reports decreased vaginal friction and sensation with intercourse.

Surgical Vaginal Caliber Reduction and Perineoplasty (Fig. 60.10)

A diamond-shaped incision is made on the perineum extending to the distal edge of the vagina, and this epithelium is removed (Fig. 60.10A,B). This incision is then extended cranially two-thirds up the length of the vagina along the midportion of the posterior vaginal

wall, and the epithelium is dissected away from the underlying rectovaginal fascia and out laterally to the levator ani muscles (Fig. 60.10C,D). This procedure is in essence an extension of the posterior repair. The rectovaginal fascia is then plicated with delayed absorbable suture in the traditional fashion (Fig. 60.10E,F). An overlapping layer of suture is then placed at the base of the wall of the vagina at the medial edge of the levator muscles which are then plicated together in the midline in a levatorplasty (Fig. 60.10G,H). When these sutures are tied down, it will distort the anatomic access of the levator muscles bringing them to the midline and result in an overall narrowing of the vaginal lumen. Depending on the baseline anatomy, multiple levator plication layers may be required to achieve the desired effect. After each layer, the vaginal diameter should be remeasured across the length to ensure an even reduction and avoid overtightening as an overly aggressive plication may result in an abnormally small vagina and dyspareunia. Once the optimal width is achieved across the distal two-thirds of the vaginal canal, the excess epithelium is trimmed and reapproximated.

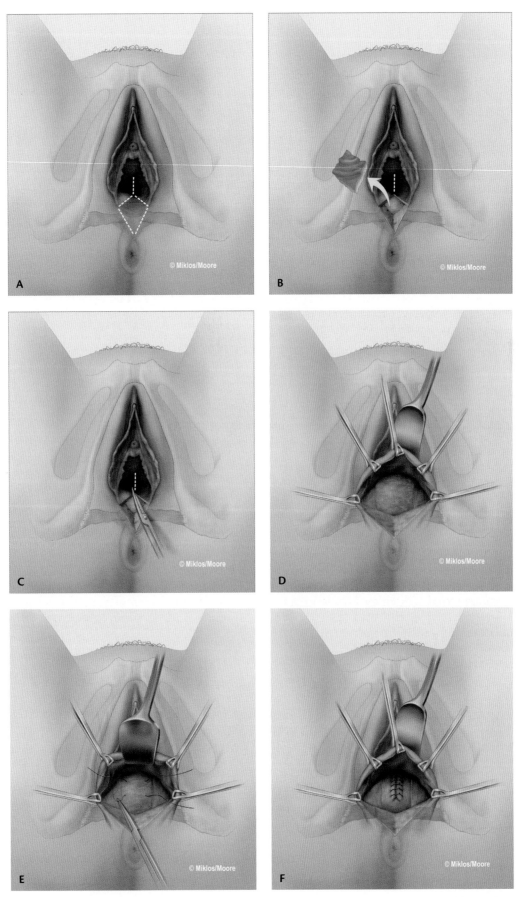

FIGURE 60.10 **A–K:** Surgical vaginal caliber reduction and perineoplasty. (© John R. Miklos/Robert D. Moore.) *(Continued)*

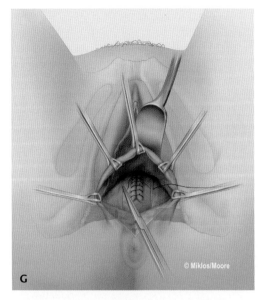

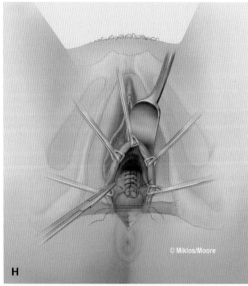

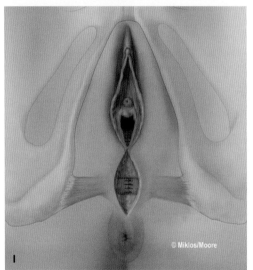

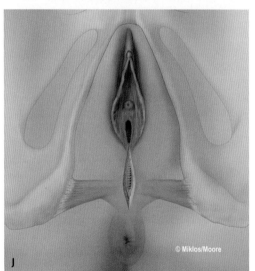

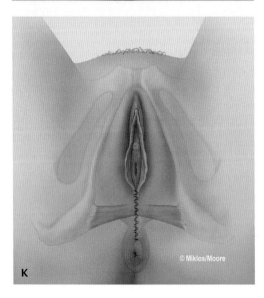

FIGURE 60.10 *(Continued)*

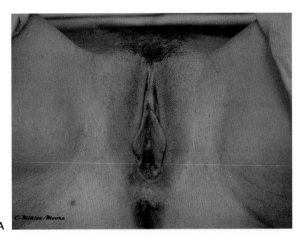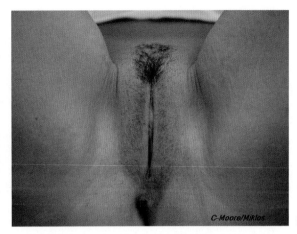

FIGURE 60.11 **A:** Preoperative photograph of a patient desiring surgical vaginal caliber reduction. **B:** Postoperative result. (© John R. Miklos/Robert D. Moore.)

The perineoplasty aims to narrow the GH via a meticulous dissection to isolate torn edges of the superficial transverse perineal muscles and plicate them along with the adjacent adventitia with 0 delayed absorbable suture in the midline and ultimately achieve uniformity with the vaginal canal (Fig. 60.10I). The skin is then closed with 2-0 delayed absorbable suture (Fig. 60.10J,K). Obtaining the ideal vaginal width is extremely challenging and will vary considerably among patients, so this must be determined during preoperative consultation physical exam and with the aid of a hand mirror. Figure 60.11 illustrates a patient prevaginal and postvaginal caliber reduction.

Postoperative Care

Postoperative management is very similar to surgery for POP. These are generally outpatient procedures that are well tolerated. Patients should be advised during initial consultation that the levatorplasty can cause moderate postoperative discomfort, and practitioners can offer a pudendal nerve block at the time of the procedure to reduce immediate postop pain. Additionally, patients can take ketorolac 10 mg every 6 hours for 3 days, followed by ibuprofen 800 mg every 8 hours as needed for pain with a small number of narcotics available for breakthrough. Scheduled polyethylene glycol can assist with normal bowel movements. The patient should avoid intercourse or excessive pressure on the operative site (riding motorcycles, bicycles, horses) for 6 weeks.

Associated risks of this procedure are also similar to those for POP and include bleeding, infection, fistula, inadequate tightening, overtightening, and dyspareunia. Risk of dyspareunia must be stressed to the patient as a poor outcome could lead to a lower quality of sexual function than prior to the procedure. This risk can be minimized with appropriate patient selection (no history of chronic pelvic pain or interstitial cystitis), a clearly defined target vaginal tightness based on preoperative exam/discussion, and avoidance of overtightening. It is always prudent to undertighten as opposed to overtighten as a revision to narrow the vagina further will be much preferred to pain that precludes intercourse.

Outcomes

As mentioned earlier, it is very challenging to show objective improvement in vaginal laxity unless the adoption of proxy metrics is employed or, alternatively, if subjective questionnaires are considered sufficient. Here, we will briefly touch on some of the supportive data. Pardo treated 53 women presenting with sexual dissatisfaction and the sensation of a wide vagina with a site-specific anterior and poster repair and paravaginal repair. Anyone with symptomatic POP, dyspareunia, or anorgasmia was excluded. At the conclusion of the procedure, the lower two-thirds of the vagina was reduced such that only two fingers could be inserted. On assessment, it was found that 96% of patients felt an adequate tightening of the vagina. Additionally, 66% of women reported sexual function "was much improved" on a 5-point rating scale.[41] Moore and colleagues[42] performed a study on 78 women undergoing vaginal rejuvenation surgery for the chief complaint of vaginal laxity resulting in decreased vaginal sensation and found that overall sexual function as measured by the PISQ-12 improved postoperatively (30.3 ± 6.6 vs. 38.2 ± 5.2; $P < .001$). In another study assessing the long-term effect of colpoperineoplasty on sexual function in 76 women, it was found that FSFI score changed from 24.19 ± 3.09 at baseline to 26.92 ± 3.41 at 6 months ($P < .001$); however, dyspareunia and dryness were also significantly increased. By 18 months, sexual function, pain, and lubrication had improved relative to 6 months postoperatively ($P < .001$).[43] Although the rate of dyspareunia in this study is not clear and appears to improve with time, this emphasizes the need for extensive preoperative counseling about risks of the procedure. In 38 patients only undergoing a perineoplasty for the sensation of a wide vagina, the dyspareunia rate was 10%.[44]

ENERGY-BASED DEVICES

EBDs are composed of carbon dioxide laser, erbium-doped yttrium aluminum garnet (Er:YAG) laser, hybrid laser, and radiofrequency (RF). EBDs have been used by multiple medical specialties including urology, gynecology, plastic surgery, and dermatology. Historically, applications centered around destructive intent with recent research being focused on regenerative applications. Within urogynecology, these technologies have been used to investigate stress urinary incontinence and overactive bladder with the most promising data emerging for the treatment of GSM. Both AUGS[45] and IUGA[46] have reviewed the existing literature and released statements advocating for increased research in this area.

Overview of Energy-Based Devices Technology

Laser is an acronym for "light amplification by simulated emission of radiation." Lasers operate at various wavelengths across the electromagnetic spectrum. Selection of the appropriate laser medium depends on the absorption characteristics of the target tissue, wavelength of emitted radiation, and time and pattern of energy application. Lasers can be characterized as ablative or nonablative. Ablative lasers heat and vaporize the top layer of tissue, whereas nonablative lasers warm the underlying tissue with minimal injury to the surface. Fractionation is the process of splitting a laser emission into multiple smaller beams which facilitates intermittent treatment across a target tissue. This functions to stimulate heat shock proteins initiating a cascade which results in the production of new collagen.[47] A variable number of "passes" with the laser are applied to the target tissue (vagina and/or vulva), over two to three treatments usually 4 to 6 weeks apart. They may then receive a maintenance treatment when desired effects abate usually every 12 months.

RF involves the transfer of electric currents from 3 kHz to 300 MHz to a target tissue where ions collide which creates a resistance that is transformed into heat. Monopolar RF involves placement of a grounding pad on the patient and may be coupled with cryogen cooling, whereas in unipolar RF, the handpiece functions as the only electrode applied to the patient. When the target temperature of 40° to 45° C is reached, collagen is stimulated by fibroblasts.[48] This will involve multiple passes with the wand to the vagina or the vulva to heat the tissue uniformly and avoiding overheating. It should be noted that although there are general treatment algorithm guidelines for EBDs provided by the manufacturers, this is not predicated on strong evidence-based data, and there is substantial variability in treatment parameters amongst devices and published literature.

Treatment of Vaginal Laxity with Energy-Based Devices

In a prospective pilot study, 24 subjects were treated with 75 to 90 J/cm^2 of RF to assess safety and tolerability. Outcome metrics included the VLQ and the SSQ. At 6-month follow-up, there were no adverse events and patients reported statistically significant improvements in sexual function and vaginal tightness.[10] Another group found similar results treating patients with RF using the same metrics at 12-month follow-up.[49] VIVIVE I was a single-blind randomized controlled trial where 186 women with vaginal laxity, defined as a score less than or equal to 3 on the VLQ, treated with either 90 J/cm^2 of monopolar RF with cryogen cooling or a sham probe with 1 J/cm^2. The primary outcome of "no vaginal laxity" as measured by the VLQ was seen in 43.5% versus 19.6% ($P = .002$) of active and sham groups at 6 months.[50] A subanalysis of this trial showed that those treated with RF noted improvement in the sexual arousal ($P = .004$), lubrication ($P = .004$), and orgasm ($P = .007$) domains of the FSFI compared to the placebo group.[51] Er:YAG laser has also been described for the treatment of "vaginal relaxation syndrome" with reported improvements in vaginal tightening[52] and sexual function[53] at 2-month follow-up.

Treatment of Vulvar Laxity with Energy-Based Devices

In a single-blind randomized controlled trial, patients were randomized to nonablative RF or heated resistor placebo probe on the labia majora over eight treatments 1 week apart. Outcome was based on evaluation of photographs before and after treatment by the subjects and blinded health care professionals, and there was noted to be a statistically significant improvement in both satisfaction ($P = .001$) and clinical improvement ($P < .01$) in the treatment group compared to placebo.[54] Similarly after four treatments with monopolar RF, blinded evaluators noted a statistically significant improvement in vulvar appearance at 1 month postprocedure.[55]

U.S. Food and Drug Administration Advisory and Complication Profile

In July of 2018, the U.S. Food and Drug Administration (FDA) released a safety communication against EBDs to alert patients and providers that the use of these devices for "vaginal rejuvenation" and to treat symptoms related to menopause, urinary incontinence, or sexual function may be associated with adverse events and that the safety and efficacy has not been established.[56] Although EBDs have been used for decades for the treatment of various body and facial skin conditions, their application for urogynecologic and cosmetic gynecologic indications are still in its infancy. The Manufacture and User Facility

Device Experience (MAUDE) database is a repository of mandatory manufacturer and voluntary provider reports concerning adverse events. In a cross sectional analysis query of the MAUDE database from 2015 to 2019, 45 distinct events were noted with pain being the most common adverse event experienced.[57] Although this is a voluntary reporting system for providers, is subject to reporting bias, and likely underestimates the total complication rate, the described events were generally mild.

VAGINAL AND CLITORAL INJECTIONS

Injections of fillers such as HA or PRP into the anterior vaginal wall and/or clitoris have been described with the intent of improving or heightening sexual stimulation. In contrast to the procedures described earlier, there is very little if any peer-reviewed literature available on these topics. A detailed discussion of this topic will be curtailed pending evidence-based data. It should be noted, however, HA pulmonary embolism has been reported after injection of this filler into the anterior vaginal wall of a patient by an unlicensed medical practitioner.[58]

CONCLUSION

Although on first glance, cosmetic gynecology may appear as an island, in reality, it is an extension of female pelvic medicine and reconstructive surgery wherein meticulous aesthetic surgical technique is applied. Although critics have argued that there is a lack of efficacy data, it should be noted that this is very difficult to objectively show for something as subjective as appearance or vaginal laxity. These are all nonmedically indicated, elective procedures, and there will likely never be extensive objective evidence in cosmetic gynecology. Although much of the published literature is retrospective, there is data to show that most patients are pleased with results, and the overall complication profile is low. One large cross-sectional study including 258 women undergoing labiaplasties, clitoral hood reductions, and surgical vaginal tightening by gynecologists, urogynecologists, and plastic surgeons showed an overall satisfaction rate of 91.6% over a 6- to 42-month follow-up.[59] Similar to other facets of urogynecology, the primary goal should be a focus on patient-centered outcomes.

References

1. Elective female genital cosmetic surgery: ACOG Committee Opinion, Number 795. *Obstet Gynecol* 2020;135(1):e36–e42.
2. Developed by the Joint Writing Group of the International Urogynecological Association and the American Urogynecologic Society. Joint report on terminology for cosmetic gynecology. *Int Urogynecol J* 2022:Epub ahead of print. doi:10.1007/s00192-021-05010-7
3. Office of the High Commissioner for Human Rights, Joint United Nations Programme on HIV/AIDS, United Nations Development Programme, et al. *Eliminating female genital mutilation: An interagency statement.* Switzerland: World Health Organization, 2008. Accessed April 18, 2019. https://apps.who.int/iris/bitstream/handle/10665/43839/9789241596442_eng.pdf;jsessionid=BB2FE2A07EE4F456DF1A221CB77469E2?sequence=1
4. Veale D, Eshkevari E, Ellison N, et al. Psychological characteristics and motivation of women seeking labiaplasty. *Psychol Med* 2014;44(3):555–566.
5. Veale D, Eshkevari E, Ellison N, et al. Validation of genital appearance satisfaction scale and the cosmetic procedure screening scale for women seeking labiaplasty. *J Psychosom Obstet Gynaecol* 2013;34(1):46–52.
6. Bramwell R, Morland C. Genital appearance satisfaction in women: The development of a questionnaire and exploration of correlates. *J Reprod Infant Psychol* 2009;27(1):15–27.
7. Garcia B, Scheib S, Hallner B, et al. Cosmetic gynecology—A systematic review and call for standardized outcome measures. *Int Urogynecol J* 2020;31(10):1979–1995.
8. Srikrishna S, Robinson D, Cardozo L. Validation of the patient global impression of improvement (PGI-I) for urogenital prolapse. *Int Urogynecol J* 2010;21(5):523–528.
9. Haylen BT, Maher CF, Barber MD, et al. An International Urogynecological Association (IUGA)/International Continence Society (ICS) joint report on the terminology for female pelvic organ prolapse (POP). *Int Urogynecol* 2016;27(4):655–684.
10. Millheiser LS, Pauls RN, Herbst SJ, et al. Radiofrequency treatment of vaginal laxity after vaginal delivery: Nonsurgical vaginal tightening. *J Sex Med* 2010;7(9):3088–3095.
11. Kelling JA, Erickson CR, Pin J, et al. Anatomical dissection of the dorsal nerve of the clitoris. *Aesthetic Surg J* 2020;40(5):541–547.
12. Ginger VAT, Cold CJ, Yang CC. Surgical anatomy of the dorsal nerve of the clitoris. *Neurourol Urodyn* 2011;30(3):412–416.
13. Rouzier R, Louis-Sylvestre C, Paniel BJ, et al. Hypertrophy of labia minora: Experience with 163 reductions. *Am J Obstet Gynecol* 2000;182(1 Pt 1):35–40.
14. Miklos JR, Moore RD. Labiaplasty of the labia minora: Patients' indications for pursuing surgery. *J Sex Med* 2008;5(6):1492–1495.
15. Hodgkinson DJ, Hait G. Aesthetic vaginal labioplasty. *Plast Reconstr Surg* 1984;74(3):414–416.
16. Munhoz AM, Filassi JR, Ricci MD, et al. Aesthetic labia minora reduction with inferior wedge resection and superior pedicle flap reconstruction. *Plast Reconstr Surg* 2006;118(5):1237–1247.
17. Jack Pardo S, Vicente Solá D, Guillermo Galán C, et al. Genital labiaplasty, experience and results in 500 consecutive cases. *Rev Chil Obstet Ginecol* 2015;80(5):394–400.
18. Fredrich E. *Vulvar disease,* 2nd ed. Philadelphia: WB Sanders, 1983.
19. Franco T, Franco D. Hipertrofia de Ninfas. *J Bras Ginecol.* 1993;103(5):163–165.
20. Motakef S, Rodriguez-Feliz J, Chung MT, et al. Vaginal labiaplasty: Current practices and a simplified classification system for labial protrusion. *Plast Reconstr Surg* 2015;135(3):774–788.
21. Pardo J, Solà V, Ricci P, et al. Laser labioplasty of labia minora. *Int J Gynaecol Obstet* 2006;93(1):38–43.
22. Alter GJ. Aesthetic labia minora and clitoral hood reduction using extended central wedge resection. *Plast Reconstr Surg* 2008;122(6):1780–1789.
23. Rauso R, Tartaro G, Salti G, et al. Utilization of needles in the surgical reduction of labia minora: A simple and cost-effective way to reduce operating time. *Aesthetic Surg J* 2016;36(10):NP310–NP312.

24. Kelishadi SS, Elston JB, Rao AJ, et al. Posterior wedge resection: A more aesthetic labiaplasty. *Aesthetic Surg J* 2013;33(6):847–853.

25. Cao YJ, Li FY, Li SK, et al. A modified method of labia minora reduction: The de-epithelialised reduction of the central and posterior labia minora. *J Plast Reconstr Aesthet Surg* 2012;65(8):1096–1102.

26. Solanki NS, Tejero-Trujeque R, Stevens-King A, et al. Aesthetic and functional reduction of the labia minora using the Maas and Hage technique. *J Plast Reconstr Aesthetic Surg* 2010;63(7):1181–1185.

27. Giraldo F, González C, de Haro F. Central wedge nymphectomy with a 90-degree Z-plasty for aesthetic reduction of the labia minora. *Plast Reconstr Surg* 2004;113(6):1820–1827.

28. Ellsworth WA, Rizvi M, Lypka M, et al. Techniques for labia minora reduction: An algorithmic approach. *Aesthetic Plast Surg.* 2010;34(1):105–110.

29. Alter GJ. Labia minora reconstruction using clitoral hood flaps, wedge excisions, and YV advancement flaps. *Plast Reconstr Surg* 2011;127(6):2356–2363.

30. Gress S. Composite reduction labiaplasty. *Aesthetic Plast Surg* 2013;37(4):674–683.

31. Placik OJ, Arkins JP. A prospective evaluation of female external genitalia sensitivity to pressure following labia minora reduction and clitoral hood reduction. *Plast Reconstr Surg* 2015;136(4):442e–452e.

32. Portman DJ, Gass MLS, Kingsberg S, et al. Genitourinary syndrome of menopause: New terminology for vulvovaginal atrophy from the International Society for the Study of Women's Sexual Health and the North American Menopause Society. *Menopause* 2014;21(10):1063–1068.

33. Karabağli Y, Kocman EA, Velipaşaoğlu M, et al. Labia majora augmentation with de-epithelialized labial rim (minora) flaps as an auxiliary procedure for labia minora reduction. *Aesthetic Plast Surg* 2015;39:289–293.

34. El Danaf AAH. Deepithelized fasciocutaneous flap for labia majora augmentation during thigh lift. *Eur J Plast Surg* 2010;33(6):373–376.

35. Salgado CJ, Tang JC, Desrosiers AE III. Use of dermal fat graft for augmentation of the labia majora. *J Plast Reconstr Aesthetic Surg* 2012;65(2):267–270.

36. Simonacci F, Bertozzi N, Grieco MP, et al. Procedure, applications, and outcomes of autologous fat grafting. *Ann Med Surg (Lond)* 2017;20:49–60.

37. Cihantimur B, Herold C. Genital beautification: A concept that offers more than reduction of the labia minora. *Aesthetic Plast Surg* 2013;37(6):1128–1133.

38. de Alencar Felicio Y. Labial surgery. *Aesthetic Surg J* 2007;27(3):322–328.

39. Fasola E, Gazzola R. Labia majora augmentation with hyaluronic acid filler: Technique and results. *Aesthetic Surg J* 2016;36(10):1155–1163.

40. Hexsel D, Dal'Forno T, Caspary P, et al. Soft-tissue augmentation with hyaluronic acid filler for labia majora and mons pubis. *Dermatol Surg* 2016;42(7):911–914.

41. Pardo JS, Solà VD, Ricci PA, et al. Colpoperineoplasty in women with a sensation of a wide vagina. *Acta Obstet Gynecol Scand* 2006;85(9):1125–1127.

42. Moore RD, Miklos JR, Chinthakanan O. Evaluation of sexual function outcomes in women undergoing vaginal rejuvenation/vaginoplasty procedures for symptoms of vaginal laxity/decreased vaginal sensation utilizing validated sexual function questionnaire (PISQ-12). *Surg Technol Int* 2014;24: 253–260.

43. Jamali S, Abedi P, Rasekh A, et al. The long term effect of elective colpoperineoplasty on sexual function in the reproductive aged women in Iran. *Int Sch Res Notices* 2014;2014:912786.

44. Ulubay M, Keskin U, Fidan U, et al. Safety, efficiency, and outcomes of perineoplasty: Treatment of the sensation of a wide vagina. *Biomed Res Int* 2016;2016:2495105.

45. Alshiek J, Garcia B, Minassian VA, et al. Vaginal energy based devices. *Female Pelvic Med Reconstr Surg* 2020;26(5):287–298.

46. Shobeiri SA, Kerkhof MH, Minassian VA, et al. IUGA committee opinion: Laser-based vaginal devices for treatment of stress urinary incontinence, genitourinary syndrome of menopause, and vaginal laxity. *Int Urogynecol J* 2019;30(3):371–376.

47. Tadir Y, Gaspar A, Lev-Sagie A, et al. Light and energy based therapeutics for genitourinary syndrome of menopause: Consensus and controversies. *Lasers Surg Med* 2017;49(2):137–159.

48. Dunbar SW, Goldberg DJ. Radiofrequency in cosmetic dermatology: An update. *J Drugs Dermatol* 2015;14(11): 1229–1238.

49. Sekiguchi Y, Utsugisawa Y, Azekosi Y, et al. Laxity of the vaginal introitus after childbirth: Nonsurgical outpatient procedure for vaginal tissue restoration and improved sexual satisfaction using low-energy radiofrequency thermal therapy. *J Womens Health (Larchmt)* 2013;22(9):775–781.

50. Krychman M, Rowan CG, Allan BB, et al. Effect of single-treatment, surface-cooled radiofrequency therapy on vaginal laxity and female sexual function: The VIVEVE I randomized controlled trial. *J Sex Med* 2017;14(2):215–225.

51. Krychman M, Rowan CG, Allan BB, et al. Effect of single-session, cryogen-cooled monopolar radiofrequency therapy on sexual function in women with vaginal laxity: The VIVEVE I Trial. *J Womens Health (Larchmt)* 2018;27(3):297–304.

52. Lee MS. Treatment of vaginal relaxation syndrome with an erbium:YAG laser using 90° and 360° scanning scopes: A pilot study & short-term results. *Laser Ther* 2014;23(2):129–138.

53. Jomah J, Bahi AW, Mousa KP, et al. Treatment of vaginal relaxation syndrome with an erbium:YAG laser 360° scanning scope via automatic dual mode technique. *Eur J Plast Surg* 2019;42(2):169–176.

54. Lordêlo P, Dantas Leal MR, Brasil CA, et al. Radiofrequency in female external genital cosmetics and sexual function: A randomized clinical trial. *Int Urogynecol J* 2016;27(11):1681–1687.

55. Fistonic I, Sorta Bilajac Turina I, Fistonic N, et al. Short time efficacy and safety of focused monopolar radiofrequency device for labial laxity improvement—Noninvasive labia tissue tightening. A prospective cohort study. *Lasers Surg Med* 2016;48(3):254–259.

56. U.S. Food and Drug Administration. FDA warns against use of energy-based devices to perform vaginal "rejuvenation" or vaginal cosmetic procedures: FDA safety communication. Accessed December 29, 2019. https://www.fda.gov/medical-devices/safety-communications/fda-warns-against-use-energy-based-devices-perform-vaginal-rejuvenation-or-vaginal-cosmetic

57. Ahluwalia J, Avram MM, Ortiz AE. Lasers and energy-based devices marketed for vaginal rejuvenation: A cross-sectional analysis of the MAUDE database. *Lasers Surg Med* 2019; 51(8):671–677.

58. Park HJ, Jung KH, Kim SY, et al. Hyaluronic acid pulmonary embolism: A critical consequence of an illegal cosmetic vaginal procedure. *Thorax* 2010;65(4):360–361.

59. Goodman MP, Placik OJ, Benson RH III, et al. A large multicenter outcome study of female genital plastic surgery. *J Sex Med* 2010;7(4 Pt 1):1565–1577.

CHAPTER 61

VAGINAL ATROPHY AND COMMON SKIN DISORDERS OF THE VULVA AND VAGINA

Anita H. Chen

VAGINAL ATROPHY

Introduction

Menopause is characterized by loss of ovarian function and as life expectancy has risen, women can spend 30 or more years living with changes that affect them physically, emotionally, functionally, and histologically.[1] Menopause symptoms include vasomotor symptoms, sleep disturbances, changes to sexual function, urinary tract symptoms, and vulvovaginal symptoms. Hypoestrogenic changes can occur to the labia majora, labia minora, clitoris, introitus, vagina, urethra, and bladder; these physical changes have been referred to as vulvovaginal atrophy (VVA), vaginal atrophy, and atrophic vaginitis. Resulting symptoms include vaginal dryness, burning, and irritation; sexual symptoms of dyspareunia and impaired function; urinary symptoms of urgency, dysuria, and recurrent urinary tract infection.[2] In 2014, the North American Menopause Society and the International Society for the Study of Women's Sexual Health proposed the term genitourinary syndrome of menopause (GSM). GSM acknowledges the changes that occur to the lower urinary tract as well as the vulvar and vaginal tissues from postmenopausal estrogen deficiency and specifically avoids the negative connotations associated with the term atrophy.[2,3] As many as 84% of postmenopausal women will experience GSM symptoms from decreased estrogen levels.[4] GSM is a clinical diagnosis and is made with a combination of characteristic examination findings and bothersome symptoms which are known to be chronic and progressive.[3,4] VVA is a subset of GSM. Vaginal physiology and resulting symptomatology is an indicator of the levels of circulating estrogen.[5] The prevalence of GSM is not well established; however, a longitudinal study evaluating presence of vaginal dryness symptoms by age group found that 3% of women of reproductive age, 4% of women in early menopause transition, 21% of women in later years of menopause transition, 40% of women 3 years after menopause, and 83% of women 6 years after menopause

reported symptoms.[6] The incidence of GSM symptoms in women visiting a gynecology or menopause clinic is over 90%.[7]

Anatomy and Physiology

The female genital and lower urinary tract both arise from the primitive urogenital sinus and share common estrogen receptor function.[8] The vaginal wall consists of nonkeratinized stratified squamous vaginal epithelium; lamina propria with dense connective tissue rich in blood and lymphatic vessels; muscular layer of smooth muscle; and tunica adventitia with loose connective tissue, collagen, and elastic fiber.[9] Although sometimes referred to as mucosa, glands are not present. Vaginal epithelium is composed of deep immature parabasal cells, intermediate cells, and mature superficial cells which store glycogen in the presence of estrogen.[8] The ratio of these cell types change over a woman's lifetime and is based on estrogen stimulation. Before menarche, the vaginal cytology is composed primarily of parabasal cells, whereas superficial cells are most prominent during the reproductive years. Declining estrogen levels in menopause result in a return of parabasal cell predominance with fewer intermediate and superficial cells.[10]

Estrogen, progesterone, and androgen have important effects on the genitourinary system.[11] Androgen receptors have been detected in the genitourinary system and contribute to the maintenance of tissue structure and function.[11] Androgen receptors are most dense in the external genitalia, whereas progesterone receptors are found in the vagina and vulvovaginal transitional epithelium.[4] Vaginal physiology is dominated by estrogen. Estrogen receptors are most dense in the vagina and are also located in the vulva, urethra, and trigone of the bladder.[4] Two estrogen receptors have been identified, designated as estrogen receptor alpha (ER-α) and estrogen receptor beta (ER-β) with relative expression and actions of the two receptors varying among tissues.[12] In premenopause, the vagina, vulva, pelvic floor skeletal muscles, urethra, and bladder trigone display a significant number of both α and β estrogen receptors. In the vagina, estrogen receptors are expressed in the epithelium, stroma, and muscle cells[13] and expression of ER-α decreases after menopause. Estrogen therapy increases ER-α receptor content, although not to premenopausal levels; ER-β, however, exhibits a dramatic decline after menopause, regardless of exogenous estrogen supplementation.[12] These findings indicate that the beneficial response to exogenous estrogen after menopause is modulated by ER-α receptors.[12] Estrogen affects thickness and elasticity of the vagina by maintaining collagen content of the epithelium, keeps the epithelial surface moist by maintaining intercellular acid mucopolysaccharides and hyaluronic acid, and maintains optimal genital blood flow.[13,14]

Estradiol levels from premenopausal to postmenopausal state can decrease approximately 95%. This marked decrease in serum estrogen along with the normal aging process results in many of the changes that comprise vaginal atrophy. With decreasing estrogen, the vaginal epithelium and lamina propria thins, smooth muscle atrophies, blood flow decreases, and tissue elasticity decreases from fusion and hyalinization of collagen fibers and fragmentation of elastin; loss of vaginal rugal folds results in a shortened and narrow vagina with loss of distensibility and thinning of the epithelium become apparent.[5,8,13] Reduction of blood supply leads to a decrease in volume of transudate and other glandular secretions.[5,13] Thinning of the vaginal epithelium leads to susceptibility for inflammation and infection. As the epithelium thins, glycogen which is stored in mature cells decreases; this results in a reduction of lactic acid production by lactobacilli, causing an increase in vaginal pH.[10,15] This change in vaginal microbiota can result in colonization by pathogenic organisms resulting in vaginal and urinary tract infections.[16,17] Hypoestrogenic changes to the urethral epithelium and suburethral plexus along with loss of protective urogenital lactobacilli increase risk of recurrent urinary tract infections after menopause.[18]

Impact on Quality of Life

Vasomotor symptoms of hot flashes or night sweats can affect up to 80% of women across the menopause transition and is a motivator for seeking medical care.[19] Of the women who suffer from menopausal symptoms, approximately 50% will have GSM symptoms.[20] Studies indicate that vasomotor symptoms can improve over time; however, symptoms of GSM can be progressive and may not resolve without treatment.[3,4,21] GSM has significant negative impact on a woman's quality of life and sexual health. Quality of life surveys conducted in multiple countries including the United States have reported negative effects on women's lives (75% to 80%), adverse effects on intimacy (75% to 85%), and impact on personal relationships (33% to 47%).[22–25]

Despite these findings, large-scale surveys of menopausal women and their physicians demonstrate that GSM is often ignored by women and overlooked by clinicians and up to one-third of the women surveyed wanted their physician to start the conversation.[26,27] Vaginal dryness is the most prevalent and also the most bothersome symptom of GSM.[7,28]

Investigators have analyzed the relationship of vaginal atrophy with subjective symptoms of vaginal dryness and the Female Sexual Function Index (FSFI) score, a questionnaire of 19 questions around the domains of desire, arousal, orgasm, dyspareunia, lubrication, and sexual satisfaction.[29] They found that vaginal dryness was the one symptom which most closely related to all domains of female sexuality, thereby identifying a treatable factor that could improve female sexual function during the menopause transition.[30] Women whose symptoms of GSM are confirmed by physical examination have even lower quality of life and sexual function scores.[7,31,32]

Surveys evaluating menopausal women's understanding of VVA found that almost 75% have not discussed concerns with their clinician.[20,25,27,33,34] In addition, a survey querying physicians who self-identified as providing care to menopausal women with GSM found that up to 15% of women with symptomatic VVA were not offered any form of treatment.[21] Likely, this percentage would be even higher for providers who infrequently treated women with GSM concerns.[21,35] Potential explanations for these findings include the assumption that women and health care providers may feel symptoms are a natural part of aging, may be embarrassed to discuss symptoms, may not have sufficient knowledge about disease progression or long-term treatment strategies, or may not have adequate time during the visit.[6,22,32–34]

Clinical Manifestations

As mentioned earlier, common presenting symptoms of GSM include vaginal dryness (75%), dyspareunia (38%), vaginal itching, discharge, and pain (15%).[5,8] Urinary symptoms include urinary frequency, dysuria, and increased risk for urinary tract infection.[6,17] Symptoms may progress to the point of precluding penetrative sexual activity.[4] Some women report discomfort even with activity such as sitting or wiping.[4] Of the different symptoms, vaginal dryness is the only symptom to increase with years since menopause.[28] Dyspareunia symptoms decreased after the first 6 years since menopause, likely a reflection of less frequency of sexual activity over time from sexual discomfort or aging.[28]

Evaluation

Evaluation of GSM includes a medical history and pelvic examination. Women who are peri- or postmenopausal should be asked about symptoms of urogenital atrophy during their visit as many women are hesitant to bring up symptoms.[26] It is important to detail the obstetric and gynecologic history including menstrual history. Other contributors to low estrogen status such as use of selective estrogen receptor modulators (SERMs) and aromatase inhibitors (AIs) should be assessed.[5] Responses to previous intervention should be reviewed and a pertinent sexual history should be taken to ascertain whether symptoms impact sexual activity and cause distress. A thorough review of systems focusing on history of pelvic radiation, exposures to irritants or allergens, and infectious or inflammatory conditions can aid in differential diagnosis. Quality-of-life issues should be assessed, and impact of symptoms on daily activities, sexual activity, and partner relationships should be reviewed. The clinician should have a discussion about the woman's therapeutic goals.

Office pelvic exam begins after a review of the exam process and informed consent is obtained. Providing the patient with a mirror during the pelvic exam may be helpful to mutually evaluate areas of concern. The appropriate size speculum with adequate lubrication should be used as even gentle contact with atrophic changes can result in pain and bleeding. Common changes on physical examination include a decrease in pubic hair, loss of labial adipose, thinning and resorption of the labia minora, narrowing of the introitus, and increased vaginal pH.[2] The urethral meatus may appear more prominent and erythematous as the mons pubis, labia majora, and minora lose bulk (Fig. 61.1). Speculum examination findings include reduced vaginal caliber, smooth, shiny, pale mucosa with loss of folds, loss of cervical length with cervix flush with the vaginal apex, and obliteration of the vaginal fornices.[4] The vagina may appear erythematous, develop petechiae, and become more friable with inflammation.[4] The prevalence of objective signs increase with time since menopause, reaching 90% with findings of mucosal pallor and rugae thinning, 80% mucosal fragility, and 51% presence of petechiae.[17] Pelvic examination also evaluates for other vulvar and vaginal conditions including contact dermatitis, inflammatory vaginitis, vulvar dermatoses, and neoplasm.[4] Visual assessments of the vagina appear to be a useful measurement to diagnose VVA; however, there is no consensus on best visual assessment tool.[36]

Laboratory tests are not usually necessary for diagnosis and evaluation of GSM; however, these exclude other etiology such as infectious vaginitis or urinary tract infection. pH testing, performed by placing a piece of litmus paper on the lateral vaginal wall at the time of speculum exam, will typically show a pH >5.0.[37] Vaginal maturation index (VMI) is a quantification of the estrogenic effect on vaginal cytology and describes the relative proportions of parabasal, intermediate, and superficial cells.[14] A vaginal smear is collected from the lateral wall of the upper third of the vagina. VMI is reported as the

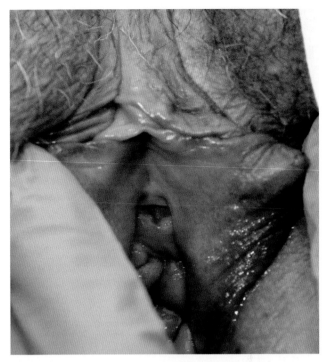

FIGURE 61.1 VVA. Urethral caruncle presenting as a bright, red, fleshy protuberance from the distal urethral as a result of shrinkage of the surrounding vaginal epithelium from decreased estrogen. (Courtesy of Dr. Anita Chen.)

percentage of superficial, intermediate, and parabasal cells and indicates the degree of tissue maturation.[38] With menopause, superficial cells are either diminished or disappear, and intermediate and parabasal cells increase.[37] Measurement of pH and VMI have limited utility in the clinical setting as these measures are not typically obtained.[36]

Management of Genitourinary Syndrome of Menopause

Despite the prevalence of symptoms, treatment for GSM remains low. More than half of women who are symptomatic have never used therapy.[4] In addition, lifestyle modifications which have been shown to reduce symptoms of GSM such smoking cessation, increased coital activity, and pelvic floor physiotherapy are not routinely discussed.[8,38] Management strategies will vary according to symptom severity, and life-long management is essential.

Lubricants and moisturizers

Lubricant and moisturizers are useful for women with mild to moderate vaginal dryness and are recommended as first-line therapy (Table 61.1).[4] Vaginal moisturizers are commercially available insoluble hydrophilic cross-linked polymer bioadhesives that adhere to the vaginal

TABLE 61.1

Topical Nonhormonal Treatments for Genitourinary Syndrome of Menopause

LUBRICANTS	MOISTURIZERS
Water based	Replens
Astroglide Liquid	Me Again
Astroglide Gel Liquid	Feminease
Astroglide	K-Y SILK-E
Good Clean Love	Luvena
Just Like Me	Revaree
K-Y Jelly	Silken Secret
Pre-Seed	Hyalo-gyn
Slippery Stuff	
Liquid Silk	
YES WB	
SYLK	
Sliquid	
Silicone based	
Astroglide X	
ID Millennium	
K-Y Intrigue	
Pink	
Pjur Eros	
Uberlube	
Sliquid	
Oil based	
Elégance Women's Lubricants	
Olive oil	
YES OB	

From The 2020 genitourinary syndrome of menopause position statement of the North American Menopause Society. *Menopause* 2020;27(9):976–992.

wall by retaining water.[38] These products trap moisture, improve vaginal pH balance, and reduce itching and are meant to be used on a regular basis as they tend to have a longer lasting effect.[38–40] Some vaginal moisturizers contain hyaluronic acid, a polymer that has a high capacity to bind water.[38] Data, however, have not shown that products containing hyaluronic acid have a greater benefit than those that do not.[4]

Lubricants are used for short-term relief of vaginal dryness during intercourse to reduce dyspareunia.[38] Lubricants are also commercially available and may be water, silicone, or oil based. These products decrease friction during intercourse to relieve discomfort related to vaginal dryness.[39] Water-based lubricants are non-staining and are associated with fewer genital symptoms than silicone-based lubricants.[40] Oil-based lubricants can cause breakdown of latex condoms, but most water- and silicone-based lubricants are latex safe. Even though clinicians commonly recommend use of over-the-counter lubricants and moisturizers, there is limited data on safety and effectiveness. A study evaluating the

safety of lubricants found that iso-osmolar (pH 4.0) water-based gels and silicone-based gels were the safest in regard to cellular toxicity and epithelial damage.[41] Mild to moderate symptoms of vaginal dryness can be managed by routine, two to three times per week use of vaginal moisturizing agents with vaginal lubricants added during sexual intercourse.[42] Although these products may improve discomfort during intercourse and also increase vaginal moisture, they do not reverse atrophic vaginal changes.

Low-dose vaginal estrogen

Vaginal estrogen therapy is a common second-line treatment for GSM not responding to first-line therapy; it is administered via cream, ring, insert, or tablet (Table 61.2). There are two vaginal creams commercially available: a 17β-estradiol vaginal cream and a conjugated estrogen cream. Vaginal creams can be applied digitally or with the supplied plastic applicator. The only vaginal tablet product currently available in the United States contains 10 μg of estradiol hemihydrate. The tablet is placed vaginal with a single-use plastic applicator. There are two estrogen vaginal rings available, only the 17β-estradiol silastic vaginal ring delivers low-dose hormone to the vaginal tissues without systemic levels of hormone. The estradiol acetate ring provides systemic levels of hormone.[43] Vaginal rings are placed in the vagina and switched out every 3 months. For women who prefer not to use an applicator, vaginal estrogen inserts are available in 4- and 10-μg doses; these are digitally placed in the vagina. Different vaginal estrogen therapy have variable rates of systemic absorption; however, overall vaginal preparations have minimal systemic absorption, are generally safe, do not require concomitant progesterone therapy for endometrial protection, and have similar efficacy.[4,44–46] These local preparations may be more effective than the systemic estrogen therapy for treatment of GSM as some woman receiving systemic estrogen therapy for menopausal symptoms often have persistent GSM symptoms.[3] Endometrial evaluation should be performed if a woman reports abnormal uterine bleeding; otherwise, routine endometrial surveillance is not recommended.[4,42]

For postmenopausal women, topical vaginal estrogen use can decrease recurrent urinary tract infections and improve overactive bladder symptoms with reduction in urinary urgency and frequency.[18,47,48] Trials have shown an increased incidence of stress incontinence in users of systemic estrogen; however, users of vaginal estrogen have demonstrated a decreased incidence of incontinence in addition to reduced urinary urgency.[47]

The American College of Obstetricians and Gynecologists and the North American Menopause Society advise that low-dose vaginal estrogen therapy may be used as long as needed.[4,42,49] In fact, if hormone

TABLE 61.2

Topical Vaginal Therapies

PREPARATION	FORMULATION	BRAND	SUGGESTED CLINICAL DOSING	GENERIC AVAILABILITY
Vaginal cream	Conjugated estrogen	Premarin	0.625 mg per 1 g cream. Use 0.5–1 g nightly for 2 wk and then three times per week.	No
	17 β-Estradiol	Estrace	0.1 mg per 1 g cream. Use 0.5–1 g nightly for 2 wk and then three times per week.	Yes
Vaginal tablet	Estradiol	Vagifem	10-μg tablet daily for 2 wk and then twice weekly	Yes
Vaginal insert	Estradiol	Imvexxy	4- or 10-μg insert daily for 2 wk and then twice weekly	No
	Prasterone (DHEA)	Intrarosa	6.5-mg insert daily	No
Vaginal ring	17 β-Estradiol	Estring	2 mg delivers 7.5 μg daily; change every 90 d.	No

therapy is discontinued, GSM will recur.[4] Data from the Women's Health Initiative and the Nurses' Health Study have shown no increase in risk of invasive breast cancer, stroke, colorectal cancer, endometrial cancer, pulmonary embolism or deep vein thrombosis, coronary heart disease, or death with vaginal estrogen.[50] Despite this data, the current U.S. Food and Drug Administration (FDA) package labeling for low-dose vaginal estrogen has not changed and remains the same as that for systemic formulations with a black-box warning of risk of endometrial cancer, myocardial infarction, stroke, invasive breast cancer, pulmonary embolism, and dementia.[51] GSM symptoms can be successfully managed with local estrogen therapy; however, surveys aimed at evaluating the attitudes of menopausal women regarding use of vaginal hormone therapy have shown that women avoid or discontinue vaginal estrogen therapy because of concerns of risk, side effects, and cost.[25,27]

Selective estrogen receptor modulators

SERMs are synthetic nonsteroidal agents that exert estrogen agonist or antagonist effects based on target tissue. Ospemifene and lasofoxifene show the most targeted beneficial effects for treatment of GSM.[52] Ospemifene is the only SERM currently FDA approved for the treatment of moderate to severe dyspareunia caused by VVA in menopausal women with or without a uterus.[4,38,53] Histologically, ospemifene has been found to increases cell maturation and ER-α expression of the vaginal epithelium.[54] Additional effects to the vagina and vulva vestibule include increased epithelial thickness, glycogen content, collagen content, and proliferation index.[55] An oral dose of 60 mg per day exerts estrogenic defects on the vulva vaginal tissue resulting reduction of severity of vaginal dryness and

dyspareunia with improvements of VMI, vaginal pH, and FSFI scores.[56,57] Safety data for ospemifene show no detrimental impact on breast, bone, and cardiovascular health and no endometrial hyperplasia or carcinoma were observed.[58-60] There is not enough data, however, to demonstrate safety in patients with personal history or high risk of breast cancer or for women with increased risk of thromboembolic events.[4] Treatment adverse events include hot flushes (6.3%) and vaginal bleeding (1.3%).[58]

Other SERMs under investigation for improvement of GSM symptoms include lasofoxifene and bazedoxifene used in combination with conjugated equine estrogen. It should be noted that bazedoxifene alone and raloxifene do not exert a positive effect on the vagina. Tamoxifen exerts a mixed effect on the vagina and has been reported to cause dyspareunia, increased vaginal discharge, and vaginal dryness.[52]

Vaginal dehydroepiandrosterone

Clinical trials with daily use of vaginal dehydroepiandrosterone (DHEA) (prasterone) have found improvement in GSM symptoms, specifically dyspareunia, vaginal pH, and VMI.[3,61] Prasterone is a precursor of intracellular sex steroid androgens and estrogens. The intracellular transformation of DHEA into estrogen results in maturation of the parabasal cells into intermediate and then superficial cells with increase in density of collagen.[61] Prasterone tablets are administered intravaginally with a single-use plastic applicator on a nightly basis. Research has shown that serum estrogens and androgens and their metabolites remain in the normal postmenopausal range; however, safety in women with breast cancer or taking AIs is unknown as this group was excluded from the study.[61-63]

Therapy under investigation

Energy-based devices have been used to treat GSM. The most commonly used are the fractional microablative carbon dioxide (CO_2) laser, nonablative photothermal erbium-doped:yttrium aluminum garnet (Er:YAG) laser, and radio frequency (RF) laser. The CO_2 fractional microablative laser burns a grid of tiny holes on the surface tissue; this microtrauma induces a healing response to increase production of collagen, elastin, and glycogenated cells.[8,38,64] The nonablative Er:YAG laser produces a photothermal effect by heating underlying tissue resulting in an increase in heat shock proteins and collagen production without harming the surface.[64] GSM treatment of the vaginal wall with CO_2 or Er:YAG laser has been reported in small studies with short-term follow-up and the number of publications continue to grow.[65–68] Nonablative RF devices which emit focused electromagnetic waves that heat the superficial layers of tissue are used to remodel the vaginal and vulvar tissue. Small case series have found benefit on vaginal, sexual, and urinary symptoms.[69] Randomized controlled trials comparing microablative laser therapy to vaginal estrogen have demonstrated similar effects, and investigation of laser therapy as a treatment option for breast cancer survivors have been conducted.[70–73] Typically, laser treatment is performed as a series of three sessions, 4 to 6 weeks apart with one session per year as maintenance therapy. A recent review of published literature found that these short-term, small longitudinal studies appear to demonstrate reductions in GSM symptoms. In the absence of clinical practice guidelines supported by high-level evidence, clinical consensus statements are created based on rigorous criteria and expert opinion after review of the available literature. A clinical consensus statement from a global group of experts summarized that energy-based therapy to the vagina results in thickening of glycogen-enriched epithelium, neovascularization, collagen growth in the lamina propria, increased lactobacilli, reduced pH, vaginal wall tightening, and improved urinary control with favorable safety profile.[74] The American Urogynecologic Society published a consensus statement on vaginal energy-based devices in 2020 to provide guidance.[75] Consensus in efficacy outcomes were reached for the statements that energy-based therapy demonstrated up to 1 year efficacy in conditions of VVA, vaginal dryness, and dyspareunia with positive short-term effect on sexual function.[75] The preferred energy device, optimal number of treatments, timing of maintenance therapy, and add-on treatments such as estrogen need to be further studied.[74,75] As of this writing, the FDA has not approved laser therapy and both the FDA and several professional organizations have recommended against widespread use without long-term and well-controlled studies to evaluate safety and efficacy of the various lasers.[76–79]

Regenerative medication applications have expanded into the field of gynecology.[80] When tissue injury occurs, the body responds by increasing delivery of platelets to the injured area. Platelets contain high concentrations of cytokines, growth factors, and other substances that initiate wound healing. Release of growth factors and cytokines upon platelet activation promote wound healing via a response cascade that includes cell proliferation and migration, extracellular matrix synthesis, remodeling, angiogenesis, and epithelialization.[81,82] For this procedure, an individual's whole blood is drawn and centrifuged to remove red blood cells, resulting in platelet-rich plasma (PRP) which has a platelet concentration of 4 to 7 times baseline. Autologous PRP is then injected into the area of concern. Pilot studies, case series, and case reports of PRP for treatment of VVA and lichen sclerosus have shown promising, preliminary short-term results.[83–86] More research is required to confirm the efficacy and safety of use of PRP to treat symptoms of GSM.

Oxytocin is a neuropeptide released by the posterior pituitary gland. Local vaginal oxytocin treatment is thought to increase cell proliferation and when placed topically in the vagina can increase vaginal thickness.[87] Small randomized controlled trials evaluating the effect of topical oxytocin on vaginal atrophy have been reported. A trial of oxytocin intravaginal gel 100 or 400 IU for 7 weeks resulted in improved maturation values and decreased pH.[88] A multicenter, prospective, randomized controlled trial of 140 women with symptoms of VVA were treated with 400 IU of topical oxytocin gel or placebo for 30 days.[89] Serum estradiol level, visual and colposcopic evaluation, and vaginal biopsy for histology was obtained pre- and posttreatment. The authors concluded that topical oxytocin gel was useful in the restoration of vaginal epithelium with no side effects.[89] In other trials, oxytocin gel 400 IU for 8 weeks compared to placebo demonstrated improved VMI, decrease in vaginal pH, and subjective improvement of symptoms including sexual dysfunction.[90,91] Further studies need to be conducted to determine long-term effects.

Special Considerations

Aging and the menopause transition can result in symptoms of GSM for women; however, cancer patients and survivors often undergo treatments that can trigger, worsen, or induce earlier vulva vaginal issues.[92,93] Breast cancer is the most common cancer among women worldwide, and hormone receptor–positive breast cancer accounts for 75% of breast cancers.[94–96] A survey found that 71% of breast oncologists treat GSM with nonhormonal therapy.[97] The FDA has not approved low-dose vaginal estrogen in women with breast cancer; however, off-label use of estradiol tablet and insert have not been shown to increase serum estradiol levels above the postmenopausal range.[98,99] The American College of Obstetricians and Gynecologists, the North American Menopause Society, and the Endocrine Society recommend a shared decision-making process, in coordination with a breast oncologist, to determine low and ultra–low-dose vaginal estrogen use in women with GSM and breast cancer when nonhormonal therapies are ineffective.[4,43,100] Despite these endorsements, the WISDOM survey found that most physicians were comfortable prescribing low-dose vaginal estrogen for symptoms of GSM; however, comfort level decreased when the patient had an elevated risk or a personal history of breast cancer.[21,101] Data among women with a personal history of breast cancer including those women currently undergoing treatment, who use a vaginal estrogen for treatment of GSM, do not show an increased risk of breast cancer recurrence or mortality.[39]

For the last 50 years, the mainstay of treatment of hormone receptor–positive breast cancer has been estrogen receptor–targeted therapy.[99] Tamoxifen and AIs have antiestrogen activity within the breast but different effects on urogenital tissue. Tamoxifen is a nonsteroidal triphenylethylene derivative that binds to estrogen receptors and has both antagonistic and agonistic effects, resulting in less severe symptoms of GSM.[99] For those who have symptoms refractive to first-line therapy, vaginal estrogen may be used as tamoxifen would exert a competitive effect with the estrogen receptor in the presence of a mild or temporary serum estradiol elevation.[43,99] AIs act to block conversion of androgens to estrogens, resulting in an estrogen deficient state. AIs are recommended for postmenopausal and premenopausal women in combination with ovarian suppression who have hormone-positive breast cancer. Current duration of treatment with adjuvant endocrine therapy is 10 years.[102] Breast cancer patients who take AIs have a 50% incidence of GSM symptoms, and symptoms may be more severe.[4] A meta-analysis to determine the safety of local hormonal treatment of VVA in women with breast cancer on AI found the absence of clinically relevant circulating estradiol levels with use of low or ultralow intravaginal estrogen administration, thus providing indirect evidence for safety of use.[93] Some studies have shown an initial small elevation in serum estradiol levels with the vaginal ring, potentially reversing effects of AIs; however, this rise was not sustained over time.[43,99] Of note, however, is that the threshold for systemic estrogen levels associated with breast cancer recurrence risk has not been determined, and the main reason that breast oncologists hesitate to prescribe vaginal estrogen therapy is the fear of increased cancer recurrence and possible interference with endocrine therapy.[97] Large prospective randomized clinical control trials are needed to establish long-term safety in this population.[43,93]

Endometrial cancer is the sixth most common cancer in women worldwide, and women who are menopausal are at greater risk. Endometrial cancer survivors may have preexisting menopausal symptoms, symptoms that occur after oophorectomy, or that develop after menopause inducing treatment. The available evidence does not suggest harm if hormone replacement therapy is used after surgical treatment of early-stage I endometrial cancer, but more research is needed.[103]

COMMON SKIN DISORDERS OF THE VULVA AND VAGINA

Introduction

The vulva structures include the mons pubis, labia majora, labia minora, clitoris, clitoral bulb, vestibule, and hymen.[9,104] The mons pubis is composed of adipose tissue overlying fascia and covered with hair-bearing skin. The labia majora are prominent paired cutaneous lateral folds of hair-bearing skin and adipose tissue that extend from the mons pubis and extend inferiorly to form the posterior fourchette. The lateral surface of the labia majora is keratinized, whereas the medial side is modified mucous membrane composed of partially keratinized epithelium, subtle hair follicles, apocrine sweat glands, and sebaceous glands.[104,105] The labia minor are hairless folds of skin located medial to the labia majora. Anteriorly, the labia minor separates into two folds; the superior fold runs over the glans of the clitoris and forms the clitoral hood. The inferior fold inserts into the inferior portion of the clitoris to form the frenulum. The posterior portions of both labia minora merge with the labia majora at the posterior fourchette. The labia minora, clitoral hood, and posterior fourchette are also composed of partially keratinized, modified mucous membrane.[105] Hart's line delineates the change from the modified mucous membrane of the labia minora to the mucous membrane of the vestibule.[106] A wide spectrum of benign, premalignant, and malignant lesions may occur on the vulva, and patients with these conditions may present to a variety of clinicians including gynecologist, primary care providers, and dermatologist. Clinicians need to differentiate between normal variance, benign conditions, and more worrisome pathology. The following text reviews common benign skin disorders of the vulva and vagina.

History

In addition to the standard medical history which include review of systemic illnesses, medications, and known allergies, answers to more directed questions can aid in formulating a differential diagnosis of skin disorders of the vulva and vagina. Common questions include onset; duration with associated changes; location; exacerbating and relieving factors; associations with vaginal complaints; and accompanying symptoms including presence of pain, burning, bleeding, and discharge. Additional questions of whether other family members have similar conditions, presence lesions in other areas such as of the mouth or anus, and presence of urinary or fecal incontinence can assist in making a diagnosis. Previous evaluation, laboratory studies, biopsy results, and treatments should be documented and attempts made to obtain results. The clinician should also assess impact on quality of life and sexual activity.

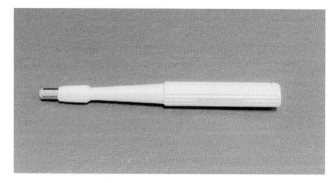

FIGURE 61.2 Keyes punch.

Examination

Informed consent is obtained prior to examination and the clinician should have a detailed discussion with the patient in regard to the planned examination. A chaperone should be present and the patient should be offered a mirror to participate in the examination and assist in identifying areas of concern. Positioning should be in low lithotomy with stirrups so that the entire vulva and external genitalia can be examined and adequate lighting is essential. Documentation of the lesion with photography and/or diagrams is helpful to objectively document the location, size, and features of the lesions. Measurements and mention of adjacent anatomic landmarks help to facilitate accurate lesion localization and future clinical comparison.

Biopsy

Vulvar and vaginal biopsies are usually performed in the office. Biopsies are performed for histologic confirmation or to aid in diagnosis of an infectious etiology. In some cases, the pathologist may report the histologic findings without a specific diagnosis. Biopsy results can be affected by sampling and interpretation error or the histologic findings may be nonspecific. Clinical–pathologic correlation, however, should aid in diagnosis.[107] Indications for biopsy include lesions that are suspicious for malignancy, uncertain diagnoses after visual inspection, lesions which do not resolve after standard therapy, to address patient concerns, and patients with chronic conditions such as lichen sclerosis who developed new or concerning changes.

When performing a biopsy, the indications and procedure should be reviewed with the patient. This discussion should include review of risks which include bleeding, infection, scarring, allergic reaction, and the possibility of nondiagnostic biopsy. After obtaining informed consent, the clinician and chaperone should ensure that all needed equipment is available. Once the patient has positioned herself on the examination table, the selected biopsy site is

prepped with a cleansing solution. Ulcerative and erosive lesions are sampled at the edges to include half of the erosion and half normal skin.[108] Indurated areas are biopsied in their thickest region. Conditions with multiple morphologies may need more than one biopsy for diagnosis.

A topical anesthetic such as lidocaine and prilocaine cream can be applied to desensitize the skin prior to injection of an anesthetic. The topical anesthetic should be applied sparingly and left on for approximately 15 minutes on modified mucous membranes and slightly longer on keratinized skin. Effectiveness is enhanced when applied under occlusion. After the appropriate time, the site is infiltrated with 1% to 2% lidocaine with or without epinephrine. Once adequate anesthesia has been attained, the biopsy can be easily performed with a Keyes skin punch. Keyes punches are available in various diameters, ranging from 2 to 6 mm (Fig. 61.2). Size selection is based on lesion dimension and goals of sampling versus excision. A punch biopsy samples the squamous epithelium of the epidermis, submucosal dermis, and subcutaneous tissue.[109] The skin is held taut for stabilization and gentle downward pressure is exerted as the punch is rotated. Rotational pressure should stop once the hub is reached. Care should be taken to not perform too deep of a biopsy as this will leave a depressed scar. The tissue disc core is then freed at its base with fine scissors. The advantage of a punch biopsy is the ability to sample deeper tissue with good cosmesis. For routine histologic examination, the sample should be fixed in formalin. Following biopsy, direct pressure is placed. Silver nitrate stick or Monsel paste may be used to control bleeding.[109] Punch biopsies that are 4 to 6 mm may require closure with a simple interrupted suture of a fine, rapidly absorbable suture to obtain hemostasis and edge approximation. The patient is instructed on perineal care and nonnarcotic oral analgesics may be used as needed. The International Society for the Study of Vulvovaginal Disease has classified vulvar dermatologic disorders into pathologic subsets and their clinical correlates to aid clinicians in formulation of a diagnosis.[107]

Dermatitis

Vulvar dermatitis, formally referred to as eczema, has traditionally been divided into endogenous dermatitis (seborrheic dermatitis, atopic dermatitis, lichen simplex chronicus) and exogenous dermatitis (allergic or irritant contact dermatitis). Clinically, however, it is often difficult to distinguish between the subtypes and patients often present with a mixed picture. The main symptom is pruritis; additional symptoms include pain and superficial dyspareunia.[110] Many patients with vulvar dermatitis have a history of asthma, allergic rhinitis, sinusitis, or atopic dermatitis on other parts of the body; therefore, a history of allergy elsewhere on the body and examination of other sites are diagnostically helpful.

Contact dermatitis, both irritant and allergic, should be considered in evaluation of women with vulvar complaints and compatible clinical findings as the vulva is susceptible to irritants and allergens. Vulvar contact dermatitis is more often caused by irritants than allergens.[111] Clinical features vary and range from mild poorly demarcated erythema to severe skin thickening or lichenification. Edematous papules and vesicles which can erode and ulcerate may be present.[111] Flaking skin is a telltale sign as allergic stimulation leads to epithelial proliferation. Bacterial and fungal cultures may be required to exclude superimposed infection as vulvar skin affected by allergic dermatitis is more susceptible to bacteria and yeast colonization. Patch testing is not always helpful as the tougher skin of the back may not disclose vulvar sensitivities; however, it should be considered in patients not responding to standard therapy or those with preexisting dermatoses.[106]

Allergic contact dermatitis is a delayed hypersensitivity reaction, presenting 2 to 7 days after antigen exposure.[106] This can occur as a primary process and also as a secondary complication in preexisting vulvar dermatoses. A variety of agents have been implicated as causes, and these include fragrances, preservatives, and medications that patients may use to manage vulvar pruritis (Table 61.3). Management of allergic contact dermatitis includes identification of allergens, specifically topical products applied to the skin.[112] The vulva should be cleansed no more than once daily using only lukewarm water without soap, fragrance, or detergent.[106] Sitz baths or handheld shower sprays to the vulva may be helpful for cleansing and for pain relief or itching. Use of washcloths, loofas, and sponges should be avoided and patients should be instructed on patting the vulva dry with avoidance of rubbing which can cause additional friction. Additional recommendations include liberal application of a gentle nonallergic emollient and use of loose-fitting cotton clothing until the dermatitis has resolved.[106]

Topical corticosteroids are the foundation for treatment of vulvar dermatoses (Table 61.4). For vulvar application, ointment formulations are the preferred vehicle as they exhibit better penetration and cause less irritation.[106,112–114] A low- to medium-potency ointment such as 0.1% hydrocortisone applied twice daily for 4 to 6 weeks may be required for resolution.[106] Occasionally, a super-high-potency topical steroid such as clobetasol 0.05% ointment may be necessary for 3 to 4 weeks and then tapered.[112] It is important to ensure that the prescribed topical corticosteroid is not precipitating vulvar allergic dermatitis. Systemic steroids may be required in severe or refractive cases.[106]

Irritant contact dermatitis results from exposure to agents that cause direct injury to keratinocytes and the lipid barrier and is characterized by a burning sensation.[106] Irritant contact dermatitis can be acute, occurring within minutes to hours; or chronic, resulting from repeated exposures that can cause damage to the skin barrier.[115] Recognizing and eliminating potential irritants is the first step toward treatment. Common vulvar irritants include oxalate in urine, propylene glycol containing creams and lotions, and abrasive toilet paper. Exacerbating factors include stress, heat, premoistened personal hygiene wipes, and candidiasis. Irritant contact dermatitis may be seen in older patients from overzealous cleaning, urinary or fecal incontinence, or chronic diarrhea. A burning reaction after application of a topical cream suggests compromise of the skin barrier that would have otherwise prevented entry of the irritant. Regular use of bland emollients and discontinuation of soap is recommended. Patients may benefit from using a squirt bottle to rinse the vulva after urination. Using liquid rather than powder detergent may also be helpful. Twice daily or more frequent application of a skin moisturizer also helps to heal the skin and continued use may prevent recurrence of symptoms.

Lichen Simplex Chronicus

Lichen simplex chronicus originates from an itch–scratch cycle that leads to chronic trauma from rubbing and scratching. It is commonly associated with a personal or family history of atopy.[110] Women complain of an itch that generates an overwhelming need to scratch in order to obtain relief.[115,116] Symptoms can cause distress to activities of daily living, exercise, sexual activity, and psychological well-being.[115] The keratinized vulva become thickened with accentuated skin marking (lichenified) and may appear erythematous and exhibit hyperpigmentation with scales.[116] Excoriations and irregular erosion are signs of scratching.[115] Skin changes most commonly involve the labia majora but can also involve the labia minora, perineum, vestibule, and perianal skin.[115] Changes may be more prominent on one side secondary to scratching with the dominant hand.[111] Patients who scratch extensively will demonstrate hypopigmented or white and atrophic scars; postinflammatory hyperpigmentation can also occur.[115,116] Biopsy is typically not

TABLE 61.3			
Common Vulvar Allergens and Irritants			
COMMON VULVAR ALLERGENS		**COMMON VULVAR IRRITANTS**	
Anesthetics	Benzocaine Procaine Tetracaine	**Body fluids**	Feces Semen Sweat Urine Vaginal discharge
Antibiotics	Bacitracin Neomycin Polymyxin Sulfonamides	**Overzealous washing and hygiene**	
Antifungals	Imidazoles Nystatin	**Feminine hygiene products**	Douches: acid or alkaline Lubricants Pads due to friction
Corticosteroids	Steroid component Vehicle component	**Heat**	
Emollients	Glycerin Lanolin Propylene glycol	**Medications**	Topicals containing: Alcohol Propylene glycol Phenols Bichloracetic acid Trichloroacetic acid Chemodestructive agents Fluorouracil Imiquimod Podophyllin
Fragrance	Balsam of Peru Fragrance mix I and II	**Soaps and detergents**	
Pads	Acetyl acetone Formaldehyde Fragrance Methacrylates		
Preservatives	Benzalkonium chloride Maleic acid Paraben mix Quaternium-15		
Rubber and latex			
Spermicides			

Adapted from Schlosser BJ. Contact dermatitis of the vulva. *Dermatol Clin* 2010;28(4):697–706; and Woodruff CM, Trivedi MK, Botto N, et al. Allergic contact dermatitis of the vulva. *Dermatitis* 2018;29(5):233–243.

needed for diagnosis or treatment but may be indicated if there are concerns for inflammatory conditions or suspicion of malignancy.[115]

Combination therapy is often needed and include topical corticosteroids, nighttime sedation, antipruritic treatment, treatment of secondary infections, avoidance of triggers, and identification and treatment of underlying conditions.[115] Topical lidocaine jelly 2% may be applied as needed for symptomatic relief until topical corticosteroids take effect.[115] A pea-sized amount of a medium- or high-potency steroid can be used daily to twice daily for a few weeks to a few months (see Table 61.4). Once symptoms improve, use should be tapered to only a few times a week as needed for recurrent symptoms. Bacterial superinfection can be treated with cephalexin 500 mg twice weekly for a week. Fungal prophylaxis with fluconazole 150 or 200 mg weekly can be used for secondary yeast infections.[115]

TABLE 61.4

Topical Corticosteroid Ointments According to the United States Classification System

CLASSIFICATION	GENERIC
Super high potency Group 1	Betamethasone dipropionate, augmented 0.05% Clobetasol propionate 0.05% Halobetasol propionate 0.05%
High potency Group 2	Amcinonide 0.1% Betamethasone dipropionate 0.05% Desoximetasone 0.25% Diflorasone diacetate 0.05% Fluocinonide 0.05% Halcinonide 0.1%
High potency Group 3	Betamethasone valerate 0.1% Fluticasone propionate 0.005% Mometasone furoate 0.1% Triamcinolone acetonide 0.5%
Medium potency Group 4	Fluocinolone acetonide 0.025% Flurandrenolide 0.05% Hydrocortisone valerate 0.2% Triamcinolone acetonide 0.05%, or 0.1%
Lower mid potency Group 5	Desonide 0.05% Hydrocortisone butyrate 0.1% Triamcinolone acetonide 0.025%
Low potency Group 6	Alclometasone dipropionate 0.05%
Least potency Group 7	Hydrocortisone 0.5%, 1% or 2.5%

NOTE: Ointment is the preferred vehicle when treating the vulva because it serves as an emollient, does not burn when applied, and causes less allergic contact dermatitis.

Nonsedating (cetirizine, fexofenadine) and sedating (diphenhydramine, hydroxyzine) antihistamines may be used to reduce pruritis and improve sleep by stopping nighttime scratching.[110,114,116] Neuromodulators such as amitriptyline and gabapentin have been used for neuropathic itch.[116] Similar to contact dermatitis, patients should be instructed to wash with water only, avoid use of soap, irritants, allergens, and rubbing of the skin. Vulvar skin can be hydrated by soaking in a tub of warm water followed by application of a bland emollient.[110,115] Short fingernails and wearing gloves during sleep may be helpful as a significant amount of rubbing or scratching tends to occur at night.[115,116] Although lichen simplex chronicus is a chronic disease, multimodal treatment can result in remission, and

unlike inflammatory vulvar dermatoses, this condition does not usually lead to scarring or cancer.[110,116]

Psoriasis

Psoriasis is a common, chronic skin disorder thought to be immune mediated with genetic predisposition.[110] Skin cells multiply faster than normal, resulting in clearly delineated red and scaly plaques of thickened skin. Erythematous, smooth, clearly demarcated plaques can affect the labia majora and extend to the mons pubis and is seen in 29% to 46% of women with psoriasis (Fig. 61.3)[110,111] The labia minora are unaffected as psoriasis is usually confined to hair-bearing areas. Diagnosis can be straightforward and made from a combination of the clinical appearance in the genital region with typical lesions elsewhere on the body, although the characteristic scale may be absent in the genital area (Fig. 61.4).[110,115] Topical agents used for other areas of the body may not be suitable for the genital region. Moderately potent topical corticosteroid combined with antibiotic and antifungal preparations remain most useful for treatment of genital psoriasis (see Table 61.4).[110,117] There are no universal treatment regimens for genital psoriasis.[117]

Lichen Sclerosus

Lichen sclerosus is a chronic inflammatory disease of the skin and can present anywhere from childhood to old age. Females have a bimodal peak at prepuberty and postmenopausal.[112] The cause of lichen sclerosus is unknown, although there may be a genetic predisposition (10% with a positive family history), as well as associations with human leukocyte antigen, excess of the enzyme elastase, and autoimmune disorders such as thyroid disease, vitiligo, alopecia areata, and pernicious anemia.[110,118] Lichen sclerosus preferentially affects the

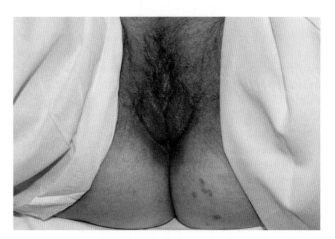

FIGURE 61.3 Psoriasis of the vulva. (Courtesy of Dr. Anita Chen.)

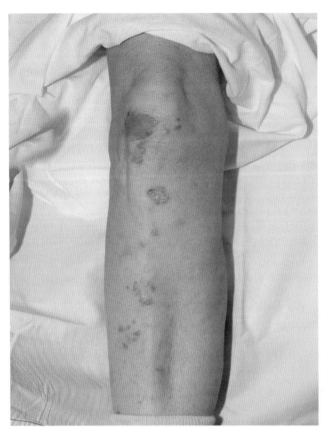

FIGURE 61.4 Psoriasis of the lower extremity exhibiting red, raised, erythematous plaques with scale. (Courtesy of Dr. Anita Chen.)

disease severity.[118] Biopsy for histologic examination is performed if the disease is refractive to appropriate treatment or if there is concern for malignancy. Suspicious findings include nonhealing erosion/ulcers, areas of persistent erythema, hyperkeratotic papules, friable nodules, and areas of irregular pigmentation.[118] A nonspecific biopsy does not rule out lichen sclerosis, although classic histologic findings will confirm the diagnosis.[119] Repeat biopsies over time are sometimes required to establish the diagnosis especially in those who have been previously treated with potent topical corticosteroids. Women should be asked to avoid use of topical corticosteroids for 2 to 3 weeks prior to biopsy.[120]

Genital lichen sclerosus is generally a steroid responsive condition, and therefore, the treatment of choice is a class I super-high-potency topical corticosteroid (see Table 61.4).[119,121] There is no standard on regimen of super-high-potency topical steroid ointment treatment.[121,122] Treatment can be started with twice daily application to the affected area for 1 month, daily for 2 months, and then tapered over 2 weeks to once- or twice-a-week applications or to a lower strength corticosteroid.[114] Intermittent maintenance therapy may be required to control symptoms, and symptom improvement usually exceeds objective improvement. The initial follow-up should occur at 3 months following initiation of super-high-potency steroids and then again

anogenital area (80%); however, it can also occur anywhere in the body (20% of cases) (Fig. 61.5).[111,112] The characteristic appearance of lichen sclerosus is vulvar hypopigmentation with thin crinkled atrophic skin in a classic figure-of-eight distribution around the vulva, perineal body, and perianal skin.[115] Normal architecture may be obliterated with loss of labia minora, clitoral hood, and urethral meatus. Petechiae, fissuring, and erosion are indicators of active disease.[112] Normal architecture of the clitoral hood, labia minora, posterior fourchette, and vaginal introitus may be obliterated with scarring.[118] In severe cases, the introitus may be almost completely agglutinated, leading to voiding dysfunction.[118] Ivory, white, atrophic, or thickened skin with ecchymosis and hemorrhage from repeated scratching of the thinned labia minor may be seen.[119] Vaginal and cervical tissues are not usually involved by lichen sclerosus.

Up to 40% of patients with lichen sclerosus are asymptomatic; however, those that present to specialist are very symptomatic with severe itching, often worse at night, and pruritis can progress to pain.[115,118] Associated symptoms include dysuria, urethral and vaginal discharge, dyspareunia, and burning pain. Symptom severity does not necessarily correlate with

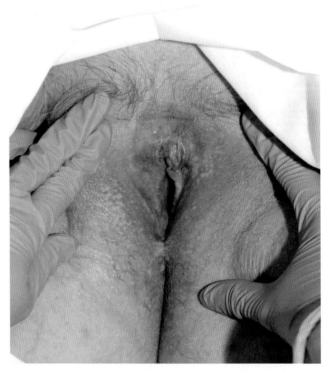

FIGURE 61.5 Lichen sclerosus with white papules of the labia majora and white plaque over the perineum. Involution of the right labia minora is present. (Courtesy of Dr. Anita Chen.)

in 6 months.[119] For patients who do not have symptom improvement with super-high-potency corticosteroids, topical tacrolimus 0.1% and 0.03% ointments and pimecrolimus 1% cream can be considered.[113,114] Tacrolimus and pimecrolimus are calcineurin inhibitors with immunomodulating and anti-inflammatory effects; long-term safety data for these second-line topical agents has not been established.[113]

Patients with Lichen sclerosus need long-term follow up due to risk of scarring and development of cancer. Lichen sclerosus is associated with an increased risk for vulvar squamous cell carcinoma with lifetime risk up to 5%.[112,118] Hypertrophic vulvar lesions and age older than 60 years are risk factors for development of squamous cell carcinoma in women with lichen sclerosis; therefore, persistent hyperkeratotic lesions should be biopsied.[119]

Lichen Planus

Lichen planus is thought to be a T-cell–mediated inflammatory disease of the skin and mucous membranes resulting from an autoimmune response to altered self or exogenous antigens.[118] The classic lesion is a violaceous to pink flat-topped papule.[123] Lichen planus frequently affects the flexor surfaces of the forearms, dorsal aspect of the hands, anterior lower legs, neck, and presacral area (Fig. 61.6).[123] Up to 50% of patients with lichen planus have oral involvement of the buccal mucosa, tongue, and gingiva (Fig. 61.7).[123,124] Lichen planus also affects the vulva and vagina (Fig. 61.8). Risk of squamous cell carcinoma in lichen planus depends on location. There is no cancer risk on extragenital skin; however, oral, esophageal, and vulvar lichen planus should be monitored for development of squamous cell carcinoma.[108]

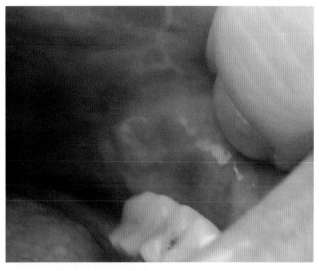

FIGURE 61.7 Oral lichen planus. Patient with vulvovaginal gingival lichen planus. (Courtesy of Dr. Anita Chen.)

Half of women with oral lichen planus also have vulvovaginal lichen planus.[123] Vulvar lichen planus is categorized into three main groups according to their clinical presentation.[110] The classic type presents with flat-topped polygonal papules on the labia majora with pruritis as the presenting symptom, although some

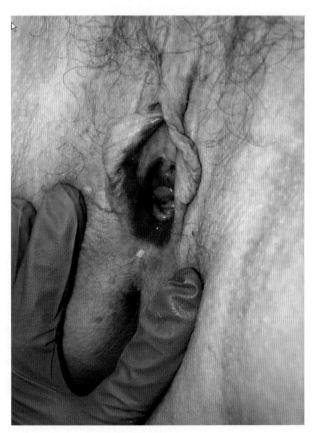

FIGURE 61.8 Vulvar lichen planus. (Courtesy of Dr. Anita Chen.)

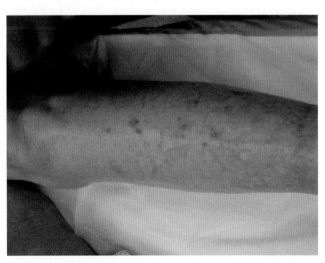

FIGURE 61.6 Cutaneous lichen planus of the lower extremity. (Courtesy of Dr. Anita Chen.)

are asymptomatic.[110,123] The least common form of vulvar lichen planus is the hypertrophic type. This type typically involves the perineum and perianal skin and spares the vagina. Patients present with extensive white, thickened, and hyperkeratotic papules and plaques of the mucous membranes.[110,123,124] The third type, erosive vulvovaginal lichen planus, is found in postmenopausal women and is usually accompanied by oral disease.[110,112] Patients tend to seek care as they can develop symptoms of severe pain, soreness, and dyspareunia. Chronic erosive lichen planus can lead to significant scarring and distortion of anatomy with resorption of labia minora and clitoral hood resulting in clitoral burying (68%) and narrowing of the introitus (59%) (Fig. 61.9).[118] Unlike lichen sclerosus, vaginal involvement is common and can produce discharge (25%) and adhesions.[112] Urethral stenosis leading to voiding dysfunction can also occur.[118]

On vulvar examination, erosions can have a lacey white periphery, and this is a good area to biopsy for confirmation of the diagnosis.[111] Vaginal findings include erythematous patches or erosions.[112] Vulvovaginal gingival lichen planus is a term used when genital and oral involvement are present, it is a severe variant of erosive lichen planus with a predilection for scarring and

TABLE 61.5	
Clinicopathologic Diagnostic Criteria for Vulvar Lichen Planus	
Signs	Color: glazed red
	Contour: macule or patch
	Demarcation: well demarcated
Sites	Labia minora
	Vestibule
	Vagina
Histology	Lymphocytic infiltrate
	Basal cell layer damage: regenerative or degenerative
	Absence of subepithelial sclerosis

Adapted from Day T. Clinicopathologic diagnostic criteria for vulvar lichen planus. *J Low Genit Tract Dis* 2020;24(3):317–329.

stricture formation.[118] The International Society for the Study of Vulvovaginal Disease developed consensus criteria for the clinicopathologic diagnosis of erosive lichen planus incorporating five criteria based on clinical appearance, site, and three histopathologic features (Table 61.5).[125]

Treatment begins with local and supportive care, and patients should be counseled that symptom control may be challenging if multiple sites of erosive lichen planus are involved.[112,113] Treatment regimens are based on limited evidence and expert opinion; typically, treatment is initiated with a super-high-potency topical steroid ointment such as clobetasol 0.05% or betamethasone dipropionate, augmented 0.05%, and a pea-sized amount applied twice daily for 1 month and then reevaluated (see Table 61.4).[112–114] Many patients will experience symptom improvement, but some may need daily or every other day application for up to 3 months.[108,118] Once symptoms improve, therapy should be tapered by lowering the steroid potency or decreasing frequency of application.[108] For erosive lichen planus that is refractive to topical corticosteroid therapy, topical tacrolimus 0.1% ointment or intralesion injection with triamcinolone acetonide can be considered.[112,113] As with all inflammatory vulvar dermatoses, secondary infections and contact dermatitis should be identified and treated.

Erosive lichen planus of the vagina can be treated with 25-mg hydrocortisone acetate suppositories twice daily and then tapered to a symptom-free maintenance dose of once or twice weekly.[113,118] If the 25-mg dose is of insufficient potency for benefit, compounded vaginal suppositories of 200 or 300 mg can be used at bedtime with tapering of use frequency once symptoms improve.[112] Regular use of vaginal dilators should be considered to avoid and treat vaginal agglutination and stenosis.[118] Vaginal synechiae may require surgical lysis under anesthesia with addition of intraoperative and

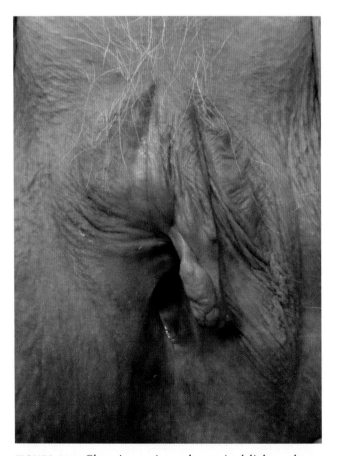

FIGURE 61.9 Chronic erosive vulvovaginal lichen planus demonstrating loss of architecture and agglutination over the clitoral hood with resorption of labia minor and introital narrowing. (Courtesy of Dr. Anita Chen.)

postoperative vaginal dilators and topical estrogen therapy as needed.[118]

Systemic therapies for treatment of erosive lichen planus are available and can be combined with topical therapy. Systemic agents include prednisone, methotrexate, mycophenolate mofetil, hydroxychloroquine, azathioprine, cyclosporine, cyclophosphamide, tacrolimus, and tumor necrosis factor α blockers; only systemic corticosteroids have shown a consistent predictable benefit.[112,114]

After symptom control has been maintained, follow-up every 6 to 12 months should continue for monitoring of disease activity and potential complications. Long-term multidisciplinary collaboration is crucial to maximize response. Development of premalignant intraepithelial neoplasia and squamous cell carcinoma of the vulva have been reported.[118]

Aphthous Ulcers

Genital aphthae can present on the medial labia minora and vestibule and, less commonly, on the labia majora, vagina, and cervix.[112] Aphthous ulcers result from a reactive, immunologic reaction and may be associated with acute viral infection such as Epstein-Barr virus, neoplasms, and nutritional deficiencies.[111,112] Noninfectious genital ulcers are more common than ulcers arising from infections. Prevalence is unknown and approximately 90% of cases are idiopathic.[111] On examination, multiple ulcers are present, appearing deep with a white fibrin base, sometimes described as "craterlike."[111,112] Genital lesions may also arise from conditions such as inflammatory bowel disease, myeloproliferative disease syndromes, and Behçet disease.[111] Sexually acquired infections should also be included in the differential.

Treatment is directed at symptom reduction with topical anesthetics, sitz baths, and analgesics. Super-high-potency topical corticosteroid ointments may be of benefit; however, oral prednisone 40 to 60 mg per day may be required.[112] Oral doxycycline 100 mg daily may be used to prevent recurrences.[112]

CONCLUSION

With our aging population, health care providers will be challenged by a higher incidence of patients presenting with postmenopausal symptoms. GSM and skin conditions of the vulva and vagina can significantly impact a woman's quality of life and sexual activity. Perimenopausal and postmenopausal women who present for annual examination should be queried about symptoms related to the vagina and vulva so that conditions such as GSM, vulvar dermatoses, vulvovaginal infections, and pelvic floor disorders can be evaluated. VVA when left untreated leads to progressive symptoms, urogynecologic dysfunction, decreased quality of life, and impaired sexual function. Treatment options are varied,

and the primary goal is to alleviate symptoms with management tailored to the individual patient. For women with GSM that use low-dose vaginal estrogen therapy, a discussion in regard to pros and cons of method of application is helpful to guide in preference decision-making as efficacy is similar among the topical formulations.

Symptoms similar to GSM may occur with other skin conditions of the vulva and vagina as menopause is associated with a decline in skin barrier function and immunity.[111] Women with allergic or inflammatory conditions who do not respond to usual therapy may warrant biopsy and consideration of referral to a specialist. A multidisciplinary approach is beneficial to optimize patient outcomes.

References

1. Arias E. United States life tables, 2017. *Natl Vital Stat Rep* 2019;68(7):1–66.
2. Portman DJ, Gass ML. Genitourinary syndrome of menopause: New terminology for vulvovaginal atrophy from the International Society for the Study of Women's Sexual Health and the North American Menopause Society. *Menopause* 2014;21(10):1063–1068.
3. Faubion SS, Sood R, Kapoor E. Genitourinary syndrome of menopause: Management strategies for the clinician. *Mayo Clin Proc* 2017;92(12):1842–1849.
4. The 2020 genitourinary syndrome of menopause position statement of the North American Menopause Society. *Menopause* 2020;27(9):976–992.
5. Sturdee DW, Panay N. Recommendations for the management of postmenopausal vaginal atrophy. *Climacteric* 2010;13(6):509–522.
6. Palma F, Volpe A, Villa P, et al. Vaginal atrophy of women in postmenopause. Results from a multicentric observational study: The AGATA study. *Maturitas* 2016;83:40–44.
7. Palacios S, Nappi RE, Bruyniks N, et al. The European Vulvovaginal Epidemiological Survey (EVES): Prevalence, symptoms and impact of vulvovaginal atrophy of menopause. *Climacteric* 2018;21(3):286–291.
8. Gandhi J, Chen A, Dagur G, et al. Genitourinary syndrome of menopause: An overview of clinical manifestations, pathophysiology, etiology, evaluation, and management. *Am J Obstet Gynecol* 2016;215(6):704–711.
9. Mitchell CM, Waetjen LE. Genitourinary changes with aging. *Obstet Gynecol Clin North Am* 2018;45(4):737–750.
10. Anderson DJ, Marathe J, Pudney J. The structure of the human vaginal stratum corneum and its role in immune defense. *Am J Reprod Immunol* 2014;71(6):618–623.
11. Traish AM, Vignozzi L, Simon JA, et al. Role of androgens in female genitourinary tissue structure and function: Implications in the genitourinary syndrome of menopause. *Sex Med Rev* 2018;6(4):558–571.
12. Gebhart JB, Rickard DJ, Barrett TJ, et al. Expression of estrogen receptor isoforms alpha and beta messenger RNA in vaginal tissue of premenopausal and postmenopausal women. *Am J Obstet Gynecol* 2001;185(6):1325–1331.
13. Nappi RE, Martini E, Cucinella L, et al. Addressing vulvovaginal atrophy (VVA)/genitourinary syndrome of menopause (GSM) for healthy aging in women. *Front Endocrinol (Lausanne)* 2019;10:561.

14. Nappi RE, Palacios S. Impact of vulvovaginal atrophy on sexual health and quality of life at postmenopause. *Climacteric* 2014;17(1):3–9.

15. Miller EA, Beasley DE, Dunn RR, et al. Lactobacilli dominance and vaginal pH: Why is the human vaginal microbiome unique? *Front Microbiol* 2016;7:1936.

16. Brotman RM, Shardell MD, Gajer P, et al. Association between the vaginal microbiota, menopause status, and signs of vulvovaginal atrophy. *Menopause* 2018;25(11):1321–1330.

17. Cagnacci A, Carbone MM, Palma F. Prevalence and association between objective signs and subjective symptoms of vaginal atrophy: The AGATA study. *Menopause* 2016;23(10):1139–1145.

18. Dueñas-Garcia OF, Sullivan G, Hall CD, et al. Pharmacological agents to decrease new episodes of recurrent lower urinary tract infections in postmenopausal women. A systematic review. *Female Pelvic Med Reconstr Surg* 2016;22(2):63–69.

19. Avis NE, Crawford SL, Green R. Vasomotor symptoms across the menopause transition: Differences among women. *Obstet Gynecol Clin North Am* 2018;45(4):629–640.

20. Parish SJ, Nappi RE, Krychman ML, et al. Impact of vulvovaginal health on postmenopausal women: A review of surveys on symptoms of vulvovaginal atrophy. *Int J Womens Health* 2013;5:437–447.

21. Kingsberg SA, Larkin L, Krychman M, et al. WISDOM survey: Attitudes and behaviors of physicians toward vulvar and vaginal atrophy (VVA) treatment in women including those with breast cancer history. *Menopause* 2019;26(2):124–131.

22. Simon JA, Kokot-Kierepa M, Goldstein J, et al. Vaginal health in the United States: Results from the Vaginal Health: Insights, Views & Attitudes survey. *Menopause* 2013;20(10):1043–1048.

23. Nappi RE, Palacios S, Bruyniks N, et al. The burden of vulvovaginal atrophy on women's daily living: Implications on quality of life from a face-to-face real-life survey. *Menopause* 2019;26(5):485–491.

24. Nappi RE, Kokot-Kierepa M. Vaginal health: Insights, views & attitudes (VIVA)—Results from an international survey. *Climacteric* 2012;15(1):36–44.

25. Krychman M, Graham S, Bernick B, et al. The Women's EMPOWER Survey: Women's knowledge and awareness of treatment options for vulvar and vaginal atrophy remains inadequate. *J Sex Med* 2017;14(3):425–433.

26. Nappi RE, Kokot-Kierepa M. Women's voices in the menopause: Results from an international survey on vaginal atrophy. *Maturitas* 2010;67(3):233–238.

27. Kingsberg SA, Krychman M, Graham S, et al. The Women's EMPOWER Survey: Identifying women's perceptions on vulvar and vaginal atrophy and its treatment. *J Sex Med* 2017;14(3):413–424.

28. Palma F, Xholli A, Cagnacci A. The most bothersome symptom of vaginal atrophy: Evidence from the observational AGATA study. *Maturitas* 2018;108:18–23.

29. Meston CM, Freihart BK, Handy AB, et al. Scoring and interpretation of the FSFI: What can be learned from 20 years of use? *J Sex Med* 2020;17(1):17–25.

30. Cagnacci A, Venier M, Xholli A, et al. Female sexuality and vaginal health across the menopausal age. *Menopause* 2020;27(1):14–19.

31. Particco M, Djumaeva S, Nappi RE, et al. The European Vulvovaginal Epidemiological Survey (EVES): Impact on sexual function of vulvovaginal atrophy of menopause. *Menopause* 2020;27(4):423–429.

32. Palma F, Della Vecchia E, Cagnacci A. Medical and patient attitude towards vaginal atrophy: The AGATA study. *Climacteric* 2016;19(6):553–557.

33. Kingsberg SA, Wysocki S, Magnus L, et al. Vulvar and vaginal atrophy in postmenopausal women: Findings from the REVIVE (REal Women's VIews of Treatment Options for Menopausal Vaginal ChangEs) survey. *J Sex Med* 2013;10(7):1790–1799.

34. Nappi RE, Kingsberg S, Maamari R, et al. The CLOSER (CLarifying Vaginal Atrophy's Impact On SEx and Relationships) survey: Implications of vaginal discomfort in postmenopausal women and in male partners. *J Sex Med* 2013;10(9):2232–2241.

35. Shifren JL. The WISDOM survey: Toward wiser care of women with vulvovaginal atrophy. *Menopause* 2019;26(2):115–117.

36. Simon JA, Archer DF, Kagan R, et al. Visual improvements in vaginal mucosa correlate with symptoms of VVA: Data from a double-blind, placebo-controlled trial. *Menopause* 2017;24(9):1003–1010.

37. Lev-Sagie A. Vulvar and vaginal atrophy: Physiology, clinical presentation, and treatment considerations. *Clin Obstet Gynecol* 2015;58(3):476–491.

38. Alvisi S, Gava G, Orsili I, et al. Vaginal health in menopausal eomen. *Medicina (Kaunas)* 2019;55(10):615.

39. Crean-Tate KK, Faubion SS, Pederson HJ, et al. Management of genitourinary syndrome of menopause in female cancer patients: A focus on vaginal hormonal therapy. *Am J Obstet Gynecol* 2020;222(2):103–113.

40. Edwards D, Panay N. Treating vulvovaginal atrophy/genitourinary syndrome of menopause: How important is vaginal lubricant and moisturizer composition? *Climacteric* 2016;19(2):151–161.

41. Dezzutti CS, Brown ER, Moncla B, et al. Is wetter better? An evaluation of over-the-counter personal lubricants for safety and anti-HIV-1 activity. *PLoS One* 2012;7(11):e48328.

42. ACOG Practice Bulletin No. 141: Management of menopausal symptoms. *Obstet Gynecol* 2014;123(1):202–216.

43. Farrell R. ACOG Committee Opinion No. 659: The use of vaginal estrogen in women with a history of estrogen-dependent breast cancer. *Obstet Gynecol* 2016;127(3):e93–e96.

44. Santen RJ. Vaginal administration of estradiol: Effects of dose, preparation and timing on plasma estradiol levels. *Climacteric* 2015;18(2):121–134.

45. Lethaby A, Ayeleke RO, Roberts H. Local oestrogen for vaginal atrophy in postmenopausal women. *Cochrane Database Syst Rev* 2016;2016(8):CD001500.

46. The 2017 hormone therapy position statement of the North American Menopause Society. *Menopause* 2018;25(11): 1362–1387.

47. Rahn DD, Ward RM, Sanses TV, et al. Vaginal estrogen use in postmenopausal women with pelvic floor disorders: Systematic review and practice guidelines. *Int Urogynecol J* 2015;26(1):3–13.

48. Baber RJ, Panay N, Fenton A. 2016 IMS recommendations on women's midlife health and menopause hormone therapy. *Climacteric* 2016;19(2):109–150.

49. Pinkerton JV, Kaunitz AM, Manson JE. Vaginal estrogen in the treatment of genitourinary syndrome of menopause and risk of endometrial cancer: An assessment of recent studies provides reassurance. *Menopause* 2017;24(12):1329–1332.

50. Crandall CJ, Hovey KM, Andrews CA, et al. Breast cancer, endometrial cancer, and cardiovascular events in participants who used vaginal estrogen in the Women's Health Initiative Observational Study. *Menopause* 2018;25(1):11–20.

51. Manson JE, Goldstein SR, Kagan R, et al. Why the product labeling for low-dose vaginal estrogen should be changed. *Menopause* 2014;21(9):911–916.

52. Pinkerton JV, Stanczyk FZ. Clinical effects of selective estrogen receptor modulators on vulvar and vaginal atrophy. *Menopause* 2014;21(3):309–319.

53. DeGregorio MW, Zerbe RL, Wurz GT. Ospemifene: A first-in-class, non-hormonal selective estrogen receptor modulator approved for the treatment of dyspareunia associated with vulvar and vaginal atrophy. *Steroids* 2014;90:82–93.

54. Alvisi S, Baldassarre M, Martelli V, et al. Effects of ospemifene on vaginal epithelium of post-menopausal women. *Gynecol Endocrinol* 2017;33(12):946–950.

55. Alvisi S, Baldassarre M, Gava G, et al. Structure of epithelial and stromal compartments of vulvar and vaginal tissue from women with vulvo-vaginal atrophy taking ospemifene. *J Sex Med* 2018;15(12):1776–1784.

56. Portman DJ, Bachmann GA, Simon JA. Ospemifene, a novel selective estrogen receptor modulator for treating dyspareunia associated with postmenopausal vulvar and vaginal atrophy. *Menopause* 2013;20(6):623–630.

57. Reid RL, Black D, Derzko C, et al. Ospemifene: A novel oral therapy for vulvovaginal atrophy of menopause. *J Obstet Gynaecol Can* 2020;42(3):301–303.

58. Archer DF, Goldstein SR, Simon JA, et al. Efficacy and safety of ospemifene in postmenopausal women with moderate-to-severe vaginal dryness: A phase 3, randomized, double-blind, placebo-controlled, multicenter trial. *Menopause* 2019;26(6): 611–621.

59. Archer DF, Simon JA, Portman DJ, et al. Ospemifene for the treatment of menopausal vaginal dryness, a symptom of the genitourinary syndrome of menopause. *Expert Rev Endocrinol Metab* 2019;14(5):301–314.

60. Simon JA, Altomare C, Cort S, et al. Overall safety of ospemifene in postmenopausal women from placebo-controlled phase 2 and 3 trials. *J Womens Health (Larchmt)* 2018;27(1):14–23.

61. Labrie F, Archer DF, Koltun W, et al. Efficacy of intravaginal dehydroepiandrosterone (DHEA) on moderate to severe dyspareunia and vaginal dryness, symptoms of vulvovaginal atrophy, and of the genitourinary syndrome of menopause. *Menopause* 2018;25(11):1339–1353.

62. Archer DF, Labrie F, Montesino M, et al. Comparison of intravaginal 6.5 mg (0.50%) prasterone, 0.3 mg conjugated estrogens and 10 μg estradiol on symptoms of vulvovaginal atrophy. *J Steroid Biochem Mol Biol* 2017;174:1–8.

63. Labrie F, Archer DF, Martel C, et al. Combined data of intravaginal prasterone against vulvovaginal atrophy of menopause. *Menopause* 2017;24(11):1246–1256.

64. Mounir DM, Hernandez N, Gonzalez RR. Update: The clinical role of vaginal lasers for the treatment of the genitourinary syndrome of menopause. *Urology* 2021;151:2–7.

65. Athanasiou S, Pitsouni E, Grigoriadis T, et al. Microablative fractional CO_2 laser for the genitourinary syndrome of menopause: Up to 12-month results. *Menopause* 2019;26(3):248–255.

66. Filippini M, Luvero D, Salvatore S, et al. Efficacy of fractional CO_2 laser treatment in postmenopausal women with genitourinary syndrome: A multicenter study. *Menopause* 2020;27(1):43–49.

67. Sokol ER, Karram MM. An assessment of the safety and efficacy of a fractional CO_2 laser system for the treatment of vulvovaginal atrophy. *Menopause* 2016;23(10):1102–1107.

68. Zerbinati N, Serati M, Origoni M, et al. Microscopic and ultrastructural modifications of postmenopausal atrophic vaginal mucosa after fractional carbon dioxide laser treatment. *Lasers Med Sci* 2015;30(1):429–436.

69. Photiou L, Lin MJ, Dubin DP, et al. Review of non-invasive vulvovaginal rejuvenation. *J Eur Acad Dermatol Venereol* 2020;34(4):716–726.

70. Quick AM, Zvinovski F, Hudson C, et al. Fractional CO_2 laser therapy for genitourinary syndrome of menopause for breast cancer survivors. *Support Care Cancer* 2020;28(8):3669–3677.

71. Arêas F, Valadares ALR, Conde DM, et al. The effect of vaginal erbium laser treatment on sexual function and vaginal health in women with a history of breast cancer and symptoms of the genitourinary syndrome of menopause: A prospective study. *Menopause* 2019;26(9):1052–1058.

72. Cruz VL, Steiner ML, Pompei LM, et al. Randomized, double-blind, placebo-controlled clinical trial for evaluating the efficacy of fractional CO_2 laser compared with topical estriol in the treatment of vaginal atrophy in postmenopausal women. *Menopause* 2018;25(1):21–28.

73. Paraiso MFR, Ferrando CA, Sokol ER, et al. A randomized clinical trial comparing vaginal laser therapy to vaginal estrogen therapy in women with genitourinary syndrome of menopause: The VeLVET Trial. *Menopause* 2020;27(1):50–56.

74. Tadir Y, Gaspar A, Lev-Sagie A, et al. Light and energy based therapeutics for genitourinary syndrome of menopause: Consensus and controversies. *Lasers Surg Med* 2017;49(2):137–159.

75. Alshiek J, Garcia B, Minassian V, et al. Vaginal energy-based devices. *Female Pelvic Med Reconstr Surg* 2020;26(5):287–298.

76. Preti M, Vieira-Baptista P, Digesu GA, et al. The clinical role of LASER for vulvar and vaginal treatments in gynecology and female urology: An ICS/ISSVD best practice consensus document. *Neurourol Urodyn* 2019;38(3):1009–1023.

77. Shobeiri SA, Kerkhof MH, Minassian VA, et al. IUGA committee opinion: Laser-based vaginal devices for treatment of stress urinary incontinence, genitourinary syndrome of menopause, and vaginal laxity. *Int Urogynecol J* 2019;30(3):371–376.

78. American College of Obstetricians and Gynecologists. Fractional laser treatment of vulvovaginal atrophy and U.S. Food and Drug Administration clearance (Position statement). Accessed October 1, 2020. https://www.acog.org/clinical-information/policy-and-position-statements/position-statements/2018/fractional-laser-treatment-of-vulvovaginal-atrophy-and-us-food-and-drug-administration-clearance

79. U.S. Food and Drug Administration. FDA warns against use of energy-based devices to perform vaginal 'rejuvenation' or vaginal cosmetic procedures: FDA safety communication. Accessed October 1, 2020. https://www.fda.gov/medical-devices/safety-communications/fda-warns-against-use-energy-based-devices-perform-vaginal-rejuvenation-or-vaginal-cosmetic

80. Dawood AS, Salem HA. Current clinical applications of platelet-rich plasma in various gynecological disorders: An appraisal of theory and practice. *Clin Exp Reprod Med* 2018;45(2):67–74.

81. Sundman EA, Cole BJ, Karas V, et al. The anti-inflammatory and matrix restorative mechanisms of platelet-rich plasma in osteoarthritis. *Am J Sports Med* 2014;42(1):35–41.

82. Pietrzak WS, Eppley BL. Platelet rich plasma: Biology and new technology. *J Craniofac Surg* 2005;16(6):1043–1054.

83. Kim SH, Park ES, Kim TH. Rejuvenation using platelet-rich plasma and lipofilling for vaginal atrophy and lichen sclerosus. *J Menopausal Med* 2017;23(1):63–68.

84. Hersant B, SidAhmed-Mezi M, Belkacemi Y, et al. Efficacy of injecting platelet concentrate combined with hyaluronic acid for the treatment of vulvovaginal atrophy in postmenopausal women with history of breast cancer: A phase 2 pilot study. *Menopause* 2018;25(10):1124–1130.

85. Casabona F, Priano V, Vallerino V, et al. New surgical approach to lichen sclerosus of the vulva: The role of adipose-derived mesenchymal cells and platelet-rich plasma in tissue regeneration. *Plast Reconstr Surg* 2010;126(4):210e–211e.

86. Behnia-Willison F, Pour NR, Mohamadi B, et al. Use of platelet-rich plasma for vulvovaginal autoimmune conditions like lichen sclerosus. *Plast Reconstr Surg Glob Open* 2016;4(11):e1124.

87. Kallak TK, Uvnäs-Moberg K. Oxytocin stimulates cell proliferation in vaginal cell line Vk2E6E7. *Post Reprod Health* 2017;23(1):6–12.

88. Al-Saqi SH, Uvnäs-Moberg K, Jonasson AF. Intravaginally applied oxytocin improves post-menopausal vaginal atrophy. *Post Reprod Health* 2015;21(3):88–97.

89. Torky HA, Taha A, Marie H, et al. Role of topical oxytocin in improving vaginal atrophy in postmenopausal women: A randomized, controlled trial. *Climacteric* 2018;21(2):174–178.

90. Zohrabi I, Abedi P, Ansari S, et al. The effect of oxytocin vaginal gel on vaginal atrophy in postmenopausal women: A randomized controlled trial. *BMC Womens Health* 2020;20(1):108.

91. Abedi P, Zohrabi I, Ansari S, et al. The impact of oxytocin vaginal gel on sexual function in postmenopausal women: A randomized controlled trial. *J Sex Marital Ther* 2020;46(4): 377–384.

92. Carter J, Stabile C, Seidel B, et al. Vaginal and sexual health treatment strategies within a female sexual medicine program for cancer patients and survivors. *J Cancer Surviv* 2017;11(2):274–283.

93. Pavlović RT, Janković SM, Milovanović JR, et al. The safety of local hormonal treatment for vulvovaginal atrophy in women with estrogen receptor-positive breast cancer who are on adjuvant aromatase inhibitor therapy: Meta-analysis. *Clin Breast Cancer* 2019;19(6):e731–e740.

94. DeSantis CE, Ma J, Gaudet MM, et al. Breast cancer statistics, 2019. *CA Cancer J Clin* 2019;69(6):438–451.

95. Bray F, Ferlay J, Soerjomataram I, et al. Global cancer statistics 2018: GLOBOCAN estimates of incidence and mortality worldwide for 36 cancers in 185 countries. *CA Cancer J Clin* 2018;68(6):394–424.

96. Chumsri S, Howes T, Bao T, et al. Aromatase, aromatase inhibitors, and breast cancer. *J Steroid Biochem Mol Biol* 2011;125(1–2):13–22.

97. Biglia N, Bounous VE, D'Alonzo M, et al. Vaginal atrophy in breast cancer survivors: Attitude and approaches among oncologists. *Clin Breast Cancer* 2017;17(8):611–617.

98. Santen RJ, Mirkin S, Bernick B, et al. Systemic estradiol levels with low-dose vaginal estrogens. *Menopause* 2020;27(3):361–370.

99. Sussman TA, Kruse ML, Thacker HL, et al. Managing genitourinary syndrome of menopause in breast cancer survivors receiving endocrine therapy. *J Oncol Pract* 2019;15(7):363–370.

100. Stuenkel CA, Davis SR, Gompel A, et al. Treatment of symptoms of the menopause: An Endocrine Society clinical practice guideline. *J Clin Endocrinol Metab* 2015;100(11): 3975–4011.

101. de Villiers TJ, Hall JE, Pinkerton JV, et al. Revised global consensus statement on menopausal hormone therapy. *Climacteric* 2016;19(4):313–315.

102. Burstein HJ, Lacchetti C, Anderson H, et al. Adjuvant endocrine therapy for women with hormone receptor-positive breast cancer: ASCO clinical practice guideline focused update. *J Clin Oncol* 2019;37(5):423–438.

103. Edey KA, Rundle S, Hickey M. Hormone replacement therapy for women previously treated for endometrial cancer. *Cochrane Database Syst Rev* 2018;(5):CD008830.

104. Yeung J, Pauls RN. Anatomy of the vulva and the female sexual response. *Obstet Gynecol Clin North Am* 2016;43(1):27–44.

105. Mauskar MM, Marathe K, Venkatesan A, et al. Vulvar diseases: Approach to the patient. *J Am Acad Dermatol* 2020;82(6): 1277–1284.

106. Woodruff CM, Trivedi MK, Botto N, et al. Allergic contact dermatitis of the vulva. *Dermatitis* 2018;29(5):233–243.

107. Lynch PJ, Moyal-Barracco M, Scurry J, et al. 2011 ISSVD terminology and classification of vulvar dermatological disorders: An approach to clinical diagnosis. *J Low Genit Tract Dis* 2012;16(4):339–344.

108. Mauskar M. Erosive lichen planus. *Obstet Gynecol Clin North Am* 2017;44(3):407–420.

109. Selim MA, Hoang MP. A histologic review of vulvar inflammatory dermatoses and intraepithelial neoplasm. *Dermatol Clin* 2010;28(4):649–667.

110. van der Meijden WI, Boffa MJ, Ter Harmsel WA, et al. 2016 European guideline for the management of vulval conditions. *J Eur Acad Dermatol Venereol* 2017;31(6):925–941.

111. Matthews N, Wong V, Brooks J, et al. Genital diseases in the mature woman. *Clin Dermatol* 2018;36(2):208–221.

112. Mauskar MM, Marathe K, Venkatesan A, et al. Vulvar diseases: Conditions in adults and children. *J Am Acad Dermatol* 2020;82(6):1287–1298.

113. Diagnosis and management of vulvar skin disorders: ACOG Practice Bulletin summary, Number 224. *Obstet Gynecol* 2020;136(1):222–225.

114. Stockdale CK, Boardman L. Diagnosis and treatment of vulvar dermatoses. *Obstet Gynecol* 2018;131(2):371–386.

115. Stewart KM. Clinical care of vulvar pruritus, with emphasis on one common cause, lichen simplex chronicus. *Dermatol Clin* 2010;28(4):669–680.

116. Chibnall R. Vulvar pruritus and lichen simplex chronicus. *Obstet Gynecol Clin North Am* 2017;44(3):379–388.

117. Czuczwar P, Stępniak A, Goren A, et al. Genital psoriasis: A hidden multidisciplinary problem—A review of literature. *Ginekol Pol* 2016;87(10):717–721.

118. Schlosser BJ, Mirowski GW. Lichen sclerosus and lichen planus in women and girls. *Clin Obstet Gynecol* 2015;58(1):125–142.

119. Murphy R. Lichen sclerosus. *Dermatol Clin* 2010;28(4): 707–715.

120. Thorstensen KA, Birenbaum DL. Recognition and management of vulvar dermatologic conditions: Lichen sclerosus, lichen planus, and lichen simplex chronicus. *J Midwifery Womens Health* 2012;57(3):260–275.

121. Kirtschig G, Becker K, Günthert A, et al. Evidence-based (S3) guideline on (anogenital) lichen sclerosus. *J Eur Acad Dermatol Venereol* 2015;29(10):e1–e43.

122. Chi CC, Kirtschig G, Baldo M, et al. Topical interventions for genital lichen sclerosus. *Cochrane Database Syst Rev* 2011;2011(12):CD008240.

123. Lewin MR, Hick RW, Selim MA. Lichenoid dermatitis of the vulva: Diagnosis and differential diagnosis for the gynecologic pathologist. *Adv Anat Pathol* 2017;24(5):278–293.

124. Mirowski GW, Goddard A. Treatment of vulvovaginal lichen planus. *Dermatol Clin* 2010;28(4):717–725.

125. Day T, Wilkinson E, Rowan D, et al. Clinicopathologic diagnostic criteria for vulvar lichen planus. *J Low Genit Tract Dis* 2020;24(3):317–329.